ALLERGY

Commissioning Editor: Karen Bowler
Development Editor: Cecilia Murphy
Project Manager: Gemma Lawson
Design Manager: Jayne Jones
Illustration Buyer: Gillian Murray
Illustrator: Martin Woodward
Marketing Manager(s) (UK/USA): Clara Toombs and Lisa Damico

ALLERGY

THIRD EDITION

Stephen T. Holgate, MD, DSc, FRCP, FRCPath, FF Biol, F Med Sci
MRC Clinical Professor of Immunopharmacology, University of Southampton, Southampton General Hospital, Southampton, UK

Martin K. Church, MPharm, PhD, DSc
Professor of Experimental Immunopharmacology, Division of Infection, Inflammation and Repair, University of Southampton, Southampton General Hospital, Southampton, UK

Lawrence M. Lichtenstein, MD, PhD
Professor of Clinical Immunology, Johns Hopkins University, School of Medicine, Baltimore, MD, USA

MOSBY

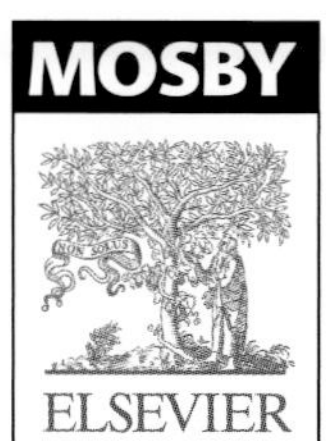

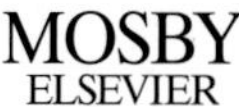

An imprint of Elsevier Ltd

First published 2006
First edition 1993
Second edition 2001
Reprint 2007

Cover image: SEM of a dust mite
Credit: Photo Insolite Realite & v. Gremet/Science Photo Library

ISBN-13: 978-0-323-03227-8
ISBN-10: 0-323-03227-3

British Library Cataloguing in Publication Data
A catalogue record for this book is available from the British Library

Library of Congress Cataloging in Publication Data
A catalog record for this book is available from the Library of Congress

---

Notice

Medical knowledge is constantly changing. Standard safety precautions must be followed, but as new research and clinical experience broaden our knowledge, changes in treatment and drug therapy may become necessary or appropriate. Readers are advised to check the most current product information provided by the manufacturer of each drug to be administered to verify the recommended dose, the method and duration of administration, and contraindications. It is the responsibility of the practitioner, relying on experience and knowledge of the patient, to determine dosages and the best treatment for each individual patient. Neither the publisher nor the author assume any liability for any injury and/or damage to persons or property arising from this publication.

The Publisher

Printed in China
Last digit is the print number: 9 8 7 6 5 4 3 2

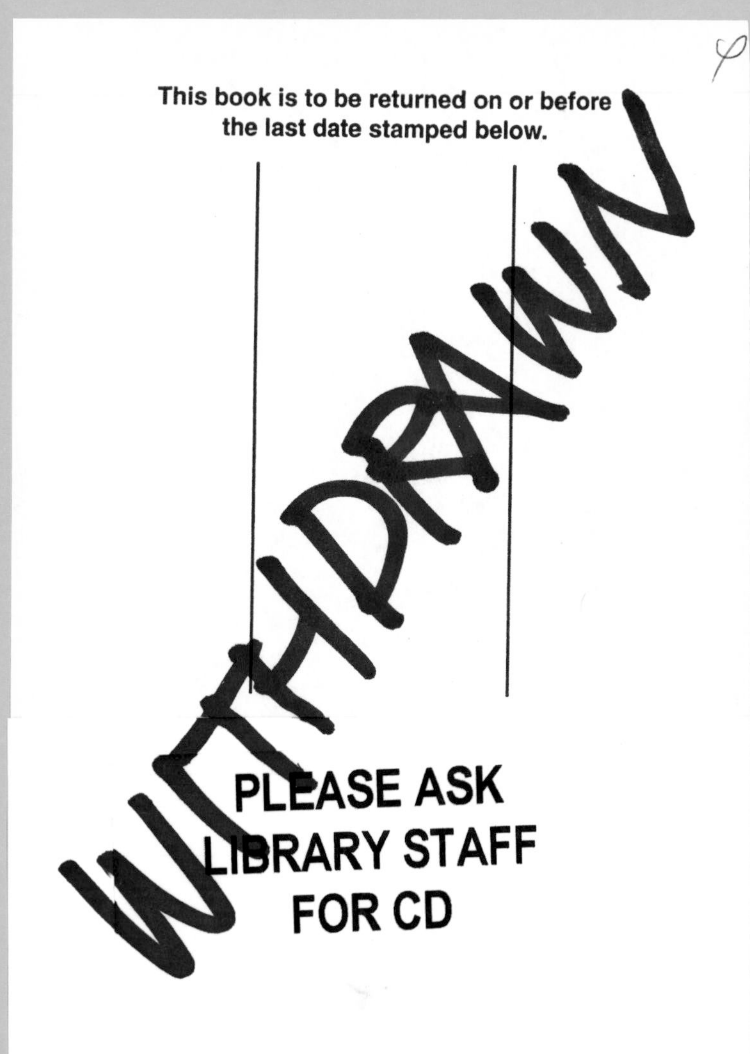

Contents

List of Contributors

Mitsuru Adachi, MD
First Department of Internal Medicine
Showa University School of Medicine
Shingawa-ku, Tokyo
Japan

N Franklin Adkinson Jr., MD
Professor of Medicine
Clinical Immunology Unit
Johns Hopkins Asthma & Allergy Center
Baltimore, MD
USA

Neil Alexis, MD
Assistant Professor
Department of Pediatrics
Division of Immunology and Infectious Disease
US EPA Human Studies Facility
University of North Carolina at Chapel Hill
Chapel Hill, NC
USA

Andrew J Beavil, BsC, PhD
Senior Lecturer in Asthma
King's College London
MRC & Asthma UK Centre in Allergic Mechanisms of Asthma
New Hunt's House
Guy's Hospital
London, UK

Rebecca L Beavil, BSc, PhD
Research Fellow
King's College London
The Randall Division of Cell and Molecular Biophysics
New Hunt's House
Guy's Hospital
London, UK

Thomas Bieber, MD, PhD
Professor and Chairman
Director of the Department of Dermatology
University of Bonn
Bonn, Germany

Stephan C Bischoff, MD
Professor of Medicine
Department of Clinical Nutrition and Prevention
University of Hohenheim
Stuttgart, Germany

David H Broide, MB, ChB
Professor of Medicine
Division of Allergy and Immunology
University of California - San Diego
La Jolla, CA
USA

Roger J Buckley, MA, FRCS, FRCOphth, HonFCOptom
Bausch & Lomb Professor of Ocular Medicine
Department of Optometry and Ophthalmic Dispensing
School of Applied Sciences
Anglia Ruskin University
Cambridge, UK;
Honorary Consultant Ophthalmologist
Moorfields Eye Hospital
London, UK

William W Busse, MD
Professor of Medicine
Allergy and Immunology, Department of Medicine
University of Wisconsin - Madison Medical School
Madison, WI
USA

Virginia L Calder, BsC, PhD
Lecturer in Immunology
Division of Clinical Ophthalmology
Institute of Ophthalmology
University College London
London, UK

Thomas B Casale, MD
Professor of Medicine
Chief, Division of Allergy/Immunology
Creighton University
Omaha, NE
USA

Mariana Castells, MD, PhD
Assistant Professor of Medicine, Harvard Medical School
Brigham & Women's Hospital
Boston, MA
USA

Ernest N Charlesworth, MD
Associate Professor of Medicine
Department of Allergy & Immunology
University of Texas Medical Branch at Galveston
Galveston, TX
USA

Martin K Church, MPharm, PhD, DSc
Professor of Experimental Immunopharmacology
Division of Infection, Inflammation and Repair
University of Southampton
Southampton General Hospital
Southampton, UK

Julian Crane, MBBS, FRCP, FRACP
Professor of Clinical Epidemiology
Department of Medicine
Wellington School of Medicine and Health Sciences
Wellington, New Zealand

Adnan Custovic, MSc, DM, MD, PhD
Professor of Allergy
North West Lung Centre
Wythenshawe Hospital
Manchester, UK

Graham Devereux MA, MD, PhD, FRCP(Ed)
Senior Clinical Lecturer
Department of Environmental and Occupational Medicine
University of Aberdeen
Aberdeen, UK

Stephen R Durham, MA, MD, FRCP
Professor of Allergy and Respiratory Medicine
Head, Allergy and Clinical Immunology
National Heart and Lung Institute
Imperial College School of Medicine and Royal Brompton Hospital
London, UK

Leonardo M Fabbri, MD
Professor of Respiratory Medicine
Department of Respiratory Diseases
University of Modena and Reggio Emilia
Modena, Italy

Anna Feldweg, MD
Instructor of Medicine
Harvard Medical School
Brigham and Women's Hospital
Boston, MA
USA

Anthony J Frew, MA, MD, FRCP
Professor of Allergy and Respiratory Medicine
Department of Respiratory Medicine
Brighton General Hospital
Brighton, UK

Peter S Friedmann, MD, FRCP, FMedSci
Professor of Dermatology
University of Southampton
Dermatopharmacology Unit
Southampton General Hospital
Southampton, UK

David BK Golden, MD
Associate Professor of Medicine
Johns Hopkins University
Baltimore, MD
USA

Clive E Grattan, MA, MD, FRCP
Consultant Dermatologist
Dermatology Centre
Norfolk and Norwich University Hospital
Norwich, UK

Catherine M Hawrylowicz, PhD, BSc
Senior Lecturer
Department of Asthma Allergy and Respiratory Medicine
Division of Asthma Allergy & Lung Biology
Guy's, King's and St Thomas' School of Medicine
London, UK

David J Hendrick, MSc, MD, FRCP
Professor of Occupational Respiratory Medicine, Newcastle University
Consultant Physician
Department of Respiratory Medicine
Royal Victoria Infirmary
Newcastle upon Tyne, UK

Melanie Hingorani, MA, MBBS, MD, FRCOphth
Consultant Ophthalmic Surgeon
Eye Department
Hinchingbrooke Hospital
Huntingdon, UK

Stephen T Holgate, MD, DSc, FRCP, FRCPa, F Med Sci
MRC Clinical Professor of Immunopharmacology
University of Southampton
Southampton General Hospital
Southampton, UK

Patrick G Holt, DSc, FRCPath, FAA
Deputy Director
Division of Cell Biology
Telethon Institute for Child Health Research
Perth, Western Australia

Alexander Kapp, MD, PhD
Professor of Medicine
Department of Dermatology and Allergology
Hannover Medical School
Hannover, Germany

M Thirumal Krishna PhD, MRCP(UK), MRCPath, DNB
Consultant Immunologist and Honorary Senior Clinical Lecturer
Department of Immunology
Birmingham Heartlands Hospital
Birmingham, UK

Lawrence M Lichtenstein, MD, PhD
Professor of Clinical Immunology
Johns Hopkins University
School of Medicine
Baltimore, MD
USA

Susan Lightman, PhD, FRCP, FRCOphth, FMedSci
Professor of Clinical Ophthalmology
Department of Clinical Opthalmology
Moorfields Eye Hospital
London, UK

Donald W MacGlashan Jr, MD, PhD
Professor of Medicine
Johns Hopkins Asthma and Allergy Center
Division of Clinical Allergy and Immunology
Baltimore, MD
USA

Piero Maestrelli, MD
Professor of Occupational Medicine
Department of Environmental and Public Health
University of Padova
Padova, Italy

Sohei Makino, MD, PhD
Professor of Medicine
Department of Medicine
Dokkyo University School of Medicine
Mibu, Tochigi
Japan

Jean-Luc Malo, MD
Professor
Université de Montréal School of Medicine
Montréal, Quebec
Canada

Charles McSharry, MD, PhD, MRCPath
Principal Clinical Immunologist
Department of Immunology
Glasgow Biomedical Research Centre
University of Glasgow
Glasgow, Scotland

Natalija Novak, MD
Head of Allergy Unit
Department of Dermatology
University of Bonn
Bonn, Germany

Paul M O'Byrne, MB, FRCPI, FRP(C)
EJ Moran Campbell Professor of Medicine
McMaster University
Hamilton, Ontario, Canada

Hans Oettgen, MD, PhD
Clinical Director
Division of Immunology
Children's Hospital
Associate Professor of Pediatrics
Harvard Medical School
Boston, MA
USA

Romain A Pauwels, MD, PhD
Formerly Professor of Medicine
Department of Respiratory Medicine
University Hospital
Ghent, Belgium

David Peden, MD
Center for Environmental Medicine and Lung Biology
University of North Carolina at Chapel Hill
Chapel Hill, NC
USA

Carl G A Persson, PhD
Professor
Department of Clinical Pharmacology
Lund University Hospital
Lund, Sweden

Thomas A E Platts-Mills, MD, PhD
Department of Medicine, Division of Allergy and Immunology
University of Virginia
Charlottesville, VA
USA

Jacqueline A Pongracic, MD
Assistant Professor of Pediatrics and Medicine
Northwestern University Feinberg School of Medicine
Chigaco, IL
USA

Jay J Prochnau, MD
Staff Allergist
Department of Allergy and Asthma
Arnett Clinic
Lafayette, IN
USA

Ilona G Reischl, PhD
Head of National Affairs
Science and Information Division
Austrian Medicines and Medical Devices Agency
Vienna, Austria

Hirohisa Saito, MD, PhD
Professor of Pediatrics
Department of Allergy Immunology
National Research Institute for Child Health & Development
Setagaya-ku, Tokyo
Japan

Glenis K Scadding, MA, MD, FRCP
Consultant Allergist and Rhinologist
Royal National Throat, Nose and Ear Hospital
London, UK

Albert L Sheffer, MD
Clinical Professor of Medicine
Harvard Medical School
Brigham & Women's Hospital
Boston, MA
USA

Hans-Uwe Simon, MD
Professor of Pharmacology and Chairman
Department of Pharmacology
University of Bern
Bern, Switzerland

Estelle Simons, MD, FRCPC
Professor
Department of Pediatrics & Child Health
Professor
Department of Immunology
University of Manitoba
Winnipeg, MB
Canada

Peter DL Sly, MBBS, MD, DSc, FRACP
Head of Division
Division of Clinical Sciences
Telethon Institute for Child Health Research
Perth, Western Australia

Geoffrey A Stewart, PhD
School of Biomedical, Biomolecular and Chemical Sciences
The University of Western Australia
Perth, Western Australia

Philip J Thompson, MBBS, FRACP, MRACMA, FCCP
Director, Asthma and Allergy Research Institute Inc SCGH
Director, Centre for Asthma, Allergy and Respiratory Research
Associate Professor of Respiratory Medicine
Department of Medicine
University of Western Australia
Editor in Chief, Respirology
Director, Chimes Estate
Clinical Professor
Curin University
Perth, Western Australia

Erika von Mutius, MD, MSc
Head
Asthma and Allergy Department
Munich University Children's Hospital
Munich, Germany

Ulrich Wahn, MD
Professor of Pediatrics, Director
Department for Pediatric Pneumology and Immunology
Charité
Berlin, Germany

Andrew J Wardlaw, FRCP, PhD
Professor of Respiratory Medicine
Department of Infection, Immunity & Inflammation
University of Leicester Medical School
Glenfield Hospital
Leicester, UK

Thomas Werfel, MD
Professor of Medicine
Department of Dermatology and Allergology
Hannover Medical School
Hannover, Germany

Burton Zweiman, MD
Professor of Medicine and Neurology
Allergy and Immunology Section
Pulmonary, Allergy and Critical Care Division
Department of Medicine
University of Pennsylvania School of Medicine
Philadelphia, PA
USA

Preface to the Third Edition

Allergic diseases, including asthma, rhinitis, conjunctivitis, dermatitis and food allergies are major contributors to morbidity and sometimes cause mortality in the civilized world. Also, their incidence and severity are still rising. Over the past decades, genetics together with both basic and clinical immunology have made great strides in understanding the disease processes in allergy.

In 1992, we published the first edition of an entirely new text on allergic diseases and their mechanisms based on specifically designed, clear and informative diagrams. This allowed us to produce a text which found a unique niche between the more heavily referenced books and the more superficial guides. In this edition, the reader was introduced to the individual cells that participate in the allergic response and this information was then built on to describe the histopathological features, diagnoses and treatment of allergic responses occurring in all major organs.

When preparing the second edition, we took note of the feedback of many clinicians who asked us if we could put primary emphasis on the clinical manifestations of allergy and augment this with a solid scientific background. This we attempted to do starting with an entirely new chapter on the principles of allergy diagnosis, a skill which is crucial to all practicing physicians. This was followed by a series of chapters focusing on the histopathology, diagnosis and management of allergic disease in individual organs. The Basic Mechanisms of Allergy section was been substantially revised and updated. In our preparation of this section, we attempted to bring together various aspects of the biology of allergic disease and combine them in integrated chapters.

In the third edition, we have followed the same format as for the second edition. In addition, we have recognised the importance of allergic disease in children and have included a chapter devoted to its diagnosis and treatment. Also, it is now becoming obvious that allergy develop very early in life, the 'allergic march' often starting before birth. Consequently, we have added a chapter on the early life origins of allergy and asthma. Finally, the great advances in our knowledge about the scientific basis of allergic diseases, particularly the relationship between genes and the environment, has necessitated the updating of most chapters, particularly those dealing with the scientific basis of allergy.

Again, to make sure that each chapter had international authority, we often invited two or more authors from different countries to work together to produce their text. While this approach is not without its logistical problems, we believe it to have produced a more authoritative text and we thank all the authors for their forbearance.

As readers, we hope that you will appreciate the novelty of our approach to allergy and that you find the text enjoyable and educative to read. As we requested in the first and second editions, please give us your feedback on the book so that we can refine it even further in the future.

STH, MKC, LML, 2006

SECTION ONE

CLINICAL

Chapter 1

Definition:

Successful management of allergic disease is dependent on the accurate diagnosis of the problem and its likely causes. This chapter describes allergy diagnosis from taking a history to specific allergy tests.

Principles of Allergy Diagnosis

Stephen R Durham and Martin K Church

INTRODUCTION

This chapter focuses on the diagnosis of IgE-mediated allergy. It is important to define terms and the following are recommendations:

- 'Atopy' refers to IgE hyperresponsiveness and represents a predisposition to allergic diseases.
- 'Allergy', by contrast, refers to the clinical expression of atopic IgE-mediated disease (Table 1.1).

Thus atopic individuals may or may not have clinical symptoms (Fig. 1.1). Some 30–40% of individuals in developed countries are atopic whereas only a proportion has allergic diseases, which include asthma (5–10%), rhinitis (10–20%), and food allergy (1–3%). In population studies allergic diseases peak at different ages. Food allergy and atopic eczema are predominant in early childhood whereas asthma shows a biphasic peak, and rhinitis peaks in the second or third decade (Fig. 1.2).

Allergic diseases are manifest as hyperresponsiveness in the target organ, whether skin, nose, lung, or gastrointestinal (GI) tract. This hyperresponsiveness may have both IgE-mediated and non-IgE-mediated components (Fig. 1.3). The situation is further complicated because allergen exposure in allergic subjects may increase target organ hyperresponsiveness, which results in exaggerated symptoms on exposure to non-specific irritants (tobacco smoke, changes in temperature, etc.) in allergic subjects. Only a proportion of atopic subjects develop disease and atopic individuals may have causal factors in their disease independent of their atopic status (see Fig. 1.3). Furthermore, increased non-specific responsiveness lowers the threshold for symptoms on subsequent allergen exposure (Fig. 1.4).

Diagnosis of IgE-mediated allergy depends on the history and results of skin tests or radioallergosorbent tests (RAST), which are occasionally supplemented by a

Table 1.1 Definitions of IgE-mediated disease. Note that allergy may involve immunologic mechanisms other than IgE, e.g. extrinsic allergic alveolitis or contact eczema

IgE-mediated Disease – Definitions	
Atopy	A tendency for exaggerated IgE responses, defined clinically by the presence of one or more positive skin prick tests (or caused serum allergens) i.e. a *predisposition* to develop allergy
Allergy	The clinical *expression* of atopic disease, including asthma, rhinitis, eczema, and food allergy

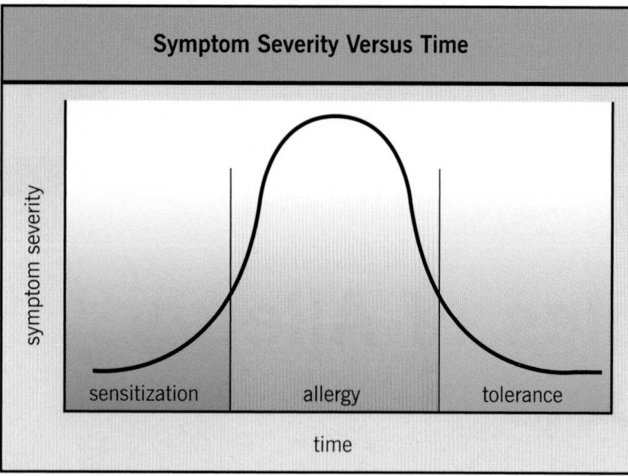

Fig. 1.1 Positive skin tests may not be associated with clinical symptoms (allergy).

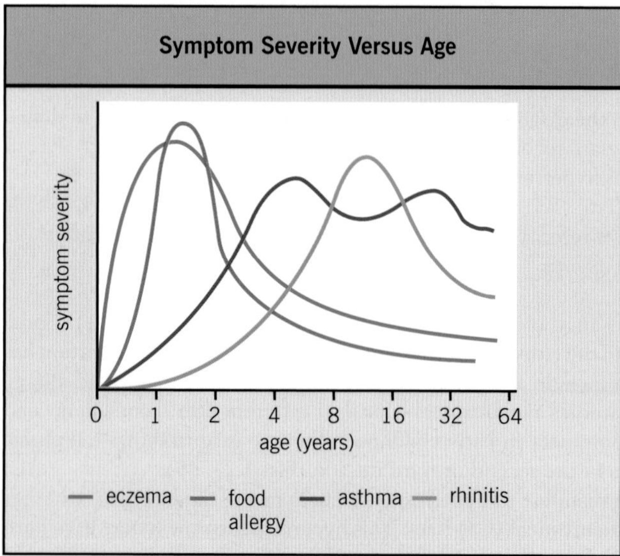

Fig. 1.2 Manifestations of allergy differ with age.

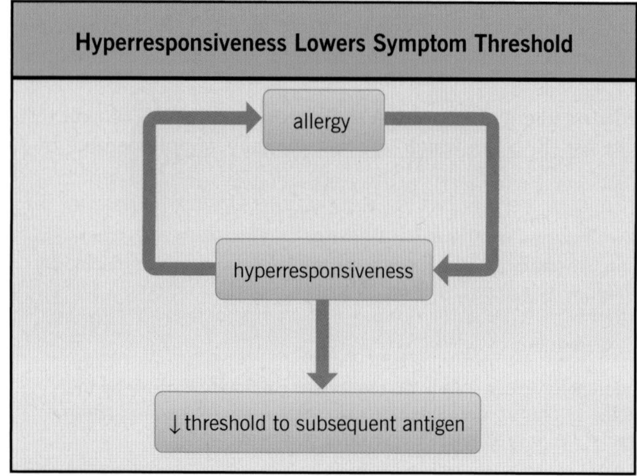

Fig. 1.3 Allergy increases target organ hyperresponsiveness, which lowers the threshold to subsequent allergen exposure.

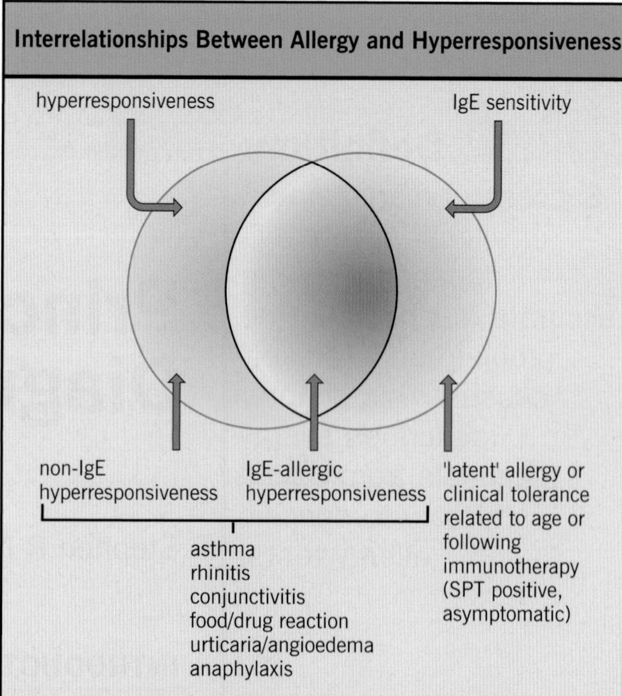

Fig. 1.4 Interrelationships between allergy and hyperresponsiveness, which may have both IgE-mediated and non-IgE-mediated components. SPT, skin prick test.

therapeutic trial of avoidance of the suspected allergen or provocation testing in the target organ. These parameters are discussed and a diagnostic approach is recommended.

ALLERGY HISTORY

Before taking an allergy history, a professional but friendly manner, the early establishment of eye contact, and the avoidance of extraneous distractions should put patients at their ease. The history need not be time consuming although patients should be allowed to give their own accounts of symptoms followed by structured prompts or questions to cover points listed in Table 1.2. A recent study showed that standardized questions put to the parents of children (aged 1–17 years) by a trained interviewer were highly predictive of answers obtained by an experienced pediatric allergist (Table 1.3).

Patient's account

The frequency and severity of symptoms, as well as the dominant symptom, should be established. For example, if nasal watery discharge is accompanied by nasal and palatal itching and associated eye symptoms, this is highly suggestive of allergy and a history of potential allergic triggers, e.g. pets, pollen, and house dust mites. Any occupational causes should be recorded.

Trigger factors

Patients with mite sensitivity may complain of immediate symptoms during activities such as bed making, dusting, and vacuum cleaning. The symptoms are frequently worse on

Table 1.2 Elucidating the history of a patient's allergy. The history need not be time consuming although the patient should be allowed to give his or her own account of symptoms followed by structured prompts or questions to cover the given points

Allergy History
Put the patient at his or her ease
Listen to the patient's account of the symptoms
What is the frequency or severity of the symptoms?
Are the symptoms seasonal or perennial?
Are there any trigger factors (allergic or non-allergic)?
Ask about any impact on lifestyle, i.e. work or school, leisure time and sleep
Ask about occupation and hobbies
Ask about possible allergens in the home
Ask about food allergies and any adverse reactions to drugs
Is there a personal or family history of asthma, rhinitis, and eczema?
Ask about the influence of prior treatment, i.e. efficacy, side-effects, compliance and the patient's concerns about treatment
Ask the patient what his or her main problem is

entering damp, older buildings, and better when the subject is outside, particularly in dry areas.

Are symptoms worse on exposure to pets? First, confusion may arise when there are several pets. Also the absence of known contact with pets does not exclude sensitization to animals or symptoms on exposure. A recent study from Sweden confirmed high levels of the major allergens of cat (Fel d 1) and dog (Can f 1) on the chairs and desks in schools but not on the floors. This suggested contamination from the clothes of children who owned pets. Horse dander is an exquisite allergen and even contact with the clothing or livery of owners and riders may frequently provoke symptoms in horse-allergic subjects.

Seasonal pollenosis is usually evident from the clinical history although it will vary according to geographic areas (Fig. 1.5). Within the UK, tree pollen is predominant in March and April, and grass pollen peaks in June and July; weed pollens are most prevalent in late summer, and molds during the late summer and fall months. The dominant pollens and their timing vary across Europe. Tree pollen occurring in April and May is the dominant problem in Scandinavia; in the UK it is grass pollen and, following an early grass pollen season (April and May) in southern Europe, the dominant pollens are *Parietaria* and olive during the summer months.

Allergic versus non-allergic triggers

Patients with inhalant allergies from whatever cause develop hyperresponsiveness in the target organ. Certain features in the history may point to either allergic or non-allergic triggers as

Table 1.3 Accuracy of standardized questions put to the parents of children (aged 1–17 years) by a trained interviewer, used for predicting answers obtained by an experienced pediatric allergist

Accuracy of Standardized Questions

Questions	Accuracy (%)
Months when symptoms are worse	94
Worse in bed at night	95
Worse in morning when awakening	96
Better when outside	95
Better when in dry area of the country	96
Worse when with dogs	97
Worse when with cats	97
Worse when vacuuming or dusting	93
Worse when blankets are shaken	96
Worse when among trees in March and April	85
Worse when in grass	97
Number of patients interviewed: 151	
Accuracy (%) $\frac{\text{(True positive + True negative) x 100}}{\text{(True positive + True negative + False positive + False negative}}$	

Data modified from Murray AB, Milner RA. The accuracy of features in the clinical history for predicting atopic sensitization to airborne allergens in children. J Allergy Clin Immunol 1995; 96:588–596.

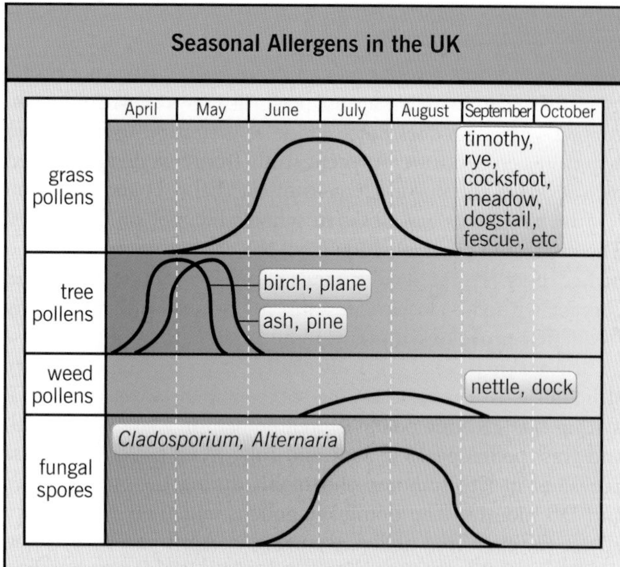

Fig. 1.5 Seasonal allergens may be present for most of the year. Pollenosis is usually evident from the clinical history although the timing will vary according to geographic areas.

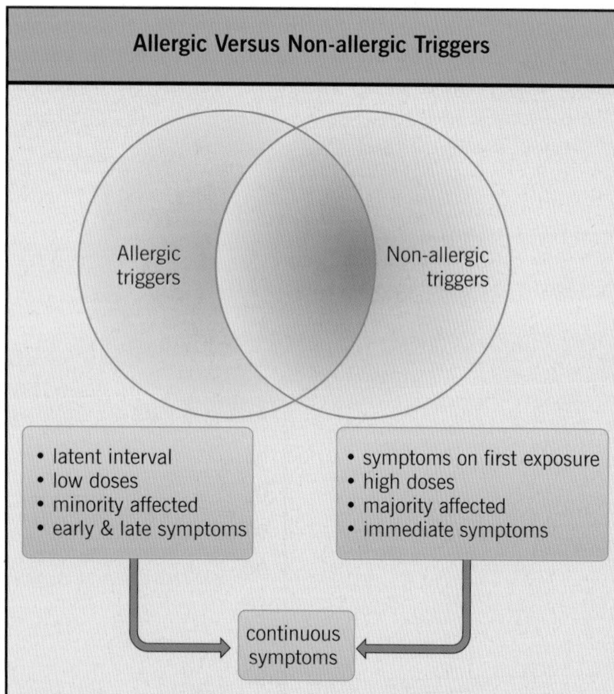

Fig. 1.6 Features suggesting an allergic or non-allergic trigger as the cause of symptoms.

the dominant causes of symptoms (Fig. 1.6). In general, allergen-induced symptoms require a period of sensitization (the latent interval). They may occur at very low allergen concentrations and affect only a proportion of exposed and sensitized individuals; symptoms may be 'early' (i.e. from minutes to 1–2 hours) or 'late' (3–24 hours). Continual low allergen exposures, however, have been shown to provoke only late symptoms, in the absence of an immediate response following either natural or experimental allergen exposure. Such isolated late symptoms may not necessarily be attributed to allergen exposure several hours earlier. In contrast, irritant triggers tend to provoke symptoms on first exposure, require high exposure concentrations and affect the majority of exposed subjects to a lesser or greater extent.

Irritant-induced symptoms tend only to be immediate, with resolution within minutes or hours. A good example is the patient with non-allergic, non-infective rhinitis who typically complains of symptoms on exposure to changes in temperature, tobacco smoke, pollutants, perfumes, domestic sprays, bleach, and stressful circumstances. However, these distinctions should be regarded as only a guide since there is considerable overlap. There is no doubt that perennial allergens – resulting in repeated early and late symptoms – result in increased target organ hyperresponsiveness with heightened sensitivity to non-specific triggers. In these circumstances symptoms may become continuous and a causal relationship between allergen exposure and symptoms may not be evident to either the patient or the clinician (see Fig. 1.6).

Quality of life

It is important to assess the impact of allergic symptoms on the patient's lifestyle, e.g. impairment of work, time off work (or school), interference with leisure activities (including sports and hobbies), and sleep disturbance.

Family history

A personal and family history of asthma, rhinitis, eczema, or food allergy, or adverse reactions to drugs should be established in all cases. A history of allergens in the home should be obtained, including such details as pet ownership, presence of carpets, central heating, double glazing, and nature of soft furnishings in the bedroom and living areas. Old, damp accommodation will favor the growth of house dust mites and molds.

Influence of treatment

The effect of previous attempts at avoidance should be ascertained, bearing in mind that several months of vigorous environmental control or avoidance, or respiratory protection, may be required before any improvement may become apparent. Similarly, the response to pharmacologic treatment including benefit and possible associated side-effects should be noted. Compliance with medication should be carefully assessed in every case, particularly where there has been an apparent poor response to treatment. Patients' knowledge and potential fears about their conditions and the treatments should be explored.

Useful leading questions include:

- 'Are you concerned about any side-effects of your steroid inhaler/nasal spray/creams?'
- 'Do you find it difficult to always remember to use your inhaler?'
- 'How often do you collect repeat prescriptions for your medicines?'

What is your main problem?

It is often helpful to ask patients at the end of the interview to recap their main problem.

Table 1.4 Common examples of causes of occupational asthma

Occupational Allergy	
Agent	**At-risk employment**
Laboratory animals	Scientific, animal-house work, etc.
Flour	Baking
Biological enzymes	Soap powder industry work
Wood dusts	Saw milling, furniture manufacture
Latex rubber gloves	Health workers
Bleaching agents, hair dyes	Hairdressing
Isocyanates	Paint spraying, printing industry
Colophony (solder fumes)	Electronics industry

ALLERGY HISTORY – SPECIAL CASES

Occupational history

An occupational history should be obtained in all patients with asthma, rhinitis, and eczema. In contrast to occupational asthma (OA) (Table 1.4), occupational rhinitis is less well documented although likely to be very common, with or without associated asthma. Knowledge of potential occupational causes is important. Symptoms tend to occur within the workplace or during the evening following work; they may improve at weekends and during holiday periods. OA, at least within the UK, is a registered and compensatable industrial disease – 5% of adult onset asthma may be attributed to an occupational cause. The associated loss of self-esteem, together with financial and social difficulties, may provoke symptoms of depressive illness and even suicidal tendencies. Moreover, symptoms may persist in up to 50% of cases for months or even years following termination of the occupational exposure. For these reasons an occupational cause should be established early and certainly not missed. A history of all occupations since leaving school should be obtained if a critical timing of exposure to a potential occupational sensitizer and onset of symptoms is not to be missed. Allergic contact eczema (Table 1.5) may also result from common sensitizers in the home and workplace.

Table 1.5 Examples of allergic contact eczema

Allergic Contact Eczema	
Agent	**Source**
Nickel	Coins, watches, jewellery
Cobalt	Metal-plated objects, wet cement
Fragrances	Cosmetics
Lanolin	Cosmetics, moisturizing creams
p-Phenylenediamine	Hair dye, fur dye
Epoxy resins	Adhesives

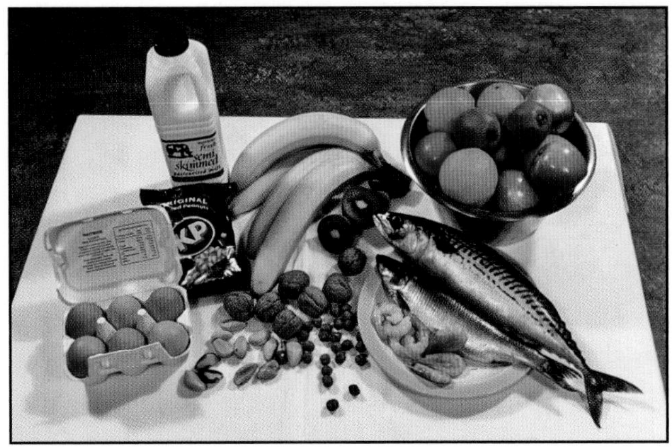

Fig. 1.7 Common allergenic foods.

Food allergy and intolerance

The accurate diagnosis of food allergy is critically dependent on a good history. Up to 20% of the population may perceive food as a cause of their symptoms, whereas the prevalence of true food allergy is around 1%; food allergy tends to occur in highly atopic subjects with a strong personal and family history of allergies. A clear association between ingestion (or contact) with the food and symptoms may be elicited. Only a limited number of foods commonly provoke symptoms: in children the culprits are eggs, milk, and peanuts; in adults they are fish, shellfish, fruit, peanuts, tree nuts, etc. (Fig. 1.7). Frequently, more than one organ system is involved; i.e. true food allergy is a rare cause of isolated asthma in adults, although severe food-induced allergy may provoke asthma associated with other typical organ involvement, e.g. lip tingling, angioedema, nettle rash, nausea, and vomiting.

This is in contrast to the typical patient presenting with non-IgE-mediated food intolerance; the symptoms tend to be non-specific or confined to one organ. There is often no clear history of provoking foods. Alternatively, atypical foods, such as yeast and wheat, are perceived to be involved, with no clear association between ingestion and exposure or delayed symptoms following ingestion. Such patients are either non-atopic or the symptoms occur independently of their atopic status; the latter patients, unlike those with typical food allergy, are unlikely to be highly atopic on the basis of their personal or family history, or via the detection of allergen-specific IgE on skin prick testing or RAST testing.

Non-IgE-mediated food-induced reactions may occur following the ingestion of preservatives such as salicylates, benzoates, and tartrazine. Common products containing preservatives include meat pies, sausages, cooked ham and salami, colored fruit drinks, confectionery, and wine (Fig. 1.8). No diagnostic tests are available and diagnosis depends upon the history and observation of the effect of exclusion diets and, where necessary, blinded food challenges.

Several clinically relevant cross-reactions may occur between certain inhalant allergens and foods (Table 1.6). A common example is oral allergy syndrome in patients with springtime hayfever (i.e. sensitivity to birch pollen) and oral itching and lip swelling on eating apples (particularly green apples), hazelnuts, and stone fruits (peaches, plums, etc.). Such reactions tend not

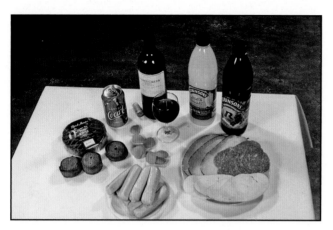

Fig. 1.8 Common products containing preservatives.

Table 1.6 Some clinically relevant cross-reactions between inhalant allergens and foods

Cross-reactions Between Inhalant Allergens and Foods	
Inhalant allergen	**Food**
Birch pollen	Hazelnut, apple, pear, stone fruits (e.g. peaches, plums, and cherries)
Ragweed pollen	Melon, bananas
House dust mite	Snails
Latex	Banana, chestnut, avocado, kiwi fruit (a.k.a. Chinese gooseberry)

to be severe and cooked fruits are well tolerated, indicating the labile nature of the allergens responsible.

Anaphylaxis

Anaphylaxis by definition (Table 1.7) may be life threatening. The differential diagnosis depends upon the history of provoking factors and, where possible, an eyewitness account should always be obtained. The differential diagnosis includes anaphylactoid reactions, syncope, and psychogenic reactions, as well as other medical conditions such as myocardial infarction, epilepsy, and metabolic or other causes of loss of consciousness. Also, airway obstruction due to a foreign body could be the cause.

EXAMINATION

Physical examination is required for all patients, although the extent will be guided by the history (Table 1.8).

Skin

When rash is the presenting symptom, the entire skin, including hair and nails, should be examined. Individual lesions of urticaria may coalesce, are intensely itchy and, characteristically, last several hours (generally less than 24 hours).

Table 1.7 Anaphylaxis. The presence of one major and two minor features (arbitrarily) may be regarded as diagnostic. If in doubt, give epinephrine!

Features of Anaphylaxis
Major
Respiratory difficulty (either severe asthma or stridor due to laryngeal edema) Hypotension (fainting, collapse, loss of consciousness)
Minor
Itching (particularly the hands, feet, groin, and scalp) Erythema Urticaria Angioedema Asthma (mild or moderate) Rhinoconjunctivitis Nausea, vomiting, abdominal pain Palpitations Sense of impending doom

Urticarial lesions that remain fixed, persist for longer than 24 to 48 hours, or leave a residual bruise, should raise the possibility of an underlying vasculitic cause. Dermographism is a common accompaniment of urticaria or it may be the only manifestation, and may confound the interpretation of skin prick tests. Urticaria is evident as raised irregular wheals usually on a red base; there may be associated subcutaneous swellings (angioedema). In view of the episodic nature of urticaria, examination results may be entirely normal.

The distribution of eczema varies with age. Eczema during infancy is prominent on the face and trunk, whereas later in childhood the typical flexural distribution develops. This is frequently associated with artifactual excoriation, sometimes with associated bleeding, and there may be evidence of secondary infection. The skin is dry and in chronic cases may be thickened due to hyperkeratinization.

Nose

External examination of the nose may reveal a transverse skin crease, which is rare. Internal inspection of the nasal mucosa may reveal the typical appearance of a pale, watery swollen bluish mucosa in allergic patients but only if symptomatic at the time of examination. Structural causes of obstruction should be excluded. Oropharyngeal candidiasis may occasionally be evident in patients on inhaled corticosteroids. The larynx should be examined in cases where there is associated hoarseness although this will usually be due to concomitant inhaled corticosteroid therapy for asthma when the larynx appears normal, although occasionally a 'midline chink' on adduction of the cords may be evident.

Chest

In patients with asthma the shape of the chest (pigeon chest deformity) may indicate chronic, poorly controlled asthma.

Table 1.8 Examination of the allergic patient. Physical examination is required for all patients although the extent will be guided by the history

Examination of the Allergic Patient

Organ	Technique	Comments
General	Appearance	Does patient look well or ill, mood, attitude to interview?
	Height, weight	Failure to thrive?
	Inspection of skin including scalp, hair, nails, and buccal mucosa	Dry skin, excoriations? Flexural eczema? Infection? Urticaria or angioedema? Drug rash?
	Look for evidence of corticosteroid side-effects?	Striae, truncal obesity, bruising, proximal myopathy, hypertension, cataracts?
Eyes	Inspection of eyes and/or eversion of upper lid	Presence of allergic 'shiners' Conjunctiva in allergic conjunctivitis often appears normal
Nose	External inspection of nose and use of auroscope attachment with ophthalmoscope Ideally, use of head mirror or flexible or rigid endoscopy	Deformity? Transverse skin creases? Nasal mucosa may appear normal or pale bluish, swollen with watery secretions but *only if* patient is symptomatic Exclude structural problems (polyps, deflected nasal septum)
Chest	Inspection	Hyperinflation? Pigeon chest deformity?
	Auscultation	Presence of stridor? Wheeze?

There may be a barrel chest with hyperresonance on percussion, diminished breath sounds and an audible wheeze. Peak flow monitoring and spirometry, together with an assessment of reversibility (either before or after a bronchodilator), or repeated peak flow measurements at home in order to detect diurnal variation will confirm or exclude the reversibility of airflow obstruction (i.e. asthma) in the majority of cases. Measurements of airway hyperresponsiveness by means of histamine or methacholine inhalation testing may be helpful, particularly in mild cases where lung function may be normal and response to a bronchodilator is absent. In these circumstances, a low-histamine PC_{20} [i.e. a provocation concentration which causes a 20% reduction in FEV_1 (forced expiratory volume in 1 second)] within the asthmatic range (less than 8 mg/mL) would confirm the need for a trial of bronchodilator therapy and further peak flow monitoring.

Rarely, rhinitis and asthma or urticaria may be a presenting feature of underlying systemic vasculitic illness such as Churg–Strauss syndrome when purpura, other vasculitic rash, cardiomegaly, pericardial rub, peripheral neuropathy, proteinuria or hematuria, and the presence of casts on routine urine testing, may be evident. Generally these patients are ill, have weight loss and recurrent fevers, and there is leukocytosis, a raised eosinophil count, and considerable elevation of the erythrocyte sedimentation rate.

SKIN PRICK TESTS

Techniques

Skin prick tests (SPTs) provide important objective information, although they must always be interpreted in the light of the clinical history. SPTs (or RAST tests) using a limited number of common allergens (for example, in the UK, cat, dog, house dust mite, and grass pollen) may confirm or exclude atopy (Fig. 1.9). They identify sensitization to a particular allergen, although they cannot predict their clinical relevance independent of the history. However, a recent study suggests that for house dust mite and grass pollen allergens an immediate skin wheal of 30 mm^2 (approximate diameter 6 mm) provides a useful cut-off point for separating patients with clinical symptoms on exposure to the relevant allergen rather than subclinical sensitization alone (Phazet, Pharmacia). Similarly, in the same study, a serum allergen-specific IgE test (Pharmacia CAP system) of approximately 10 kU/L segregated those with symptoms compared to those without symptoms on exposure to the relevant allergen. However, it is not clear how applicable these results are to individual subjects, as opposed to large groups, and so further studies are required.

SPTs, in general, tend to be more sensitive, whereas allergen-specific IgE measurements may be more specific.

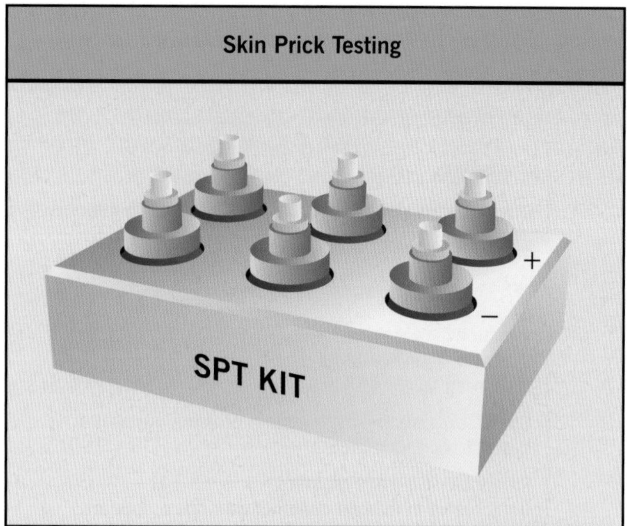

Fig. 1.9 A few common allergens used for skin prick testing will confirm or exclude the presence of atopy in the vast majority of patients. For the UK these are house dust mite, cat, dog, grass pollen, and positive (histamine 10 mg/mL) and negative (allergen diluent) controls.

Table 1.10 Practice points for skin prick tests

Skin Prick Tests – Practice Points
Skin prick testing requires training, both for performance and interpretation of results
Check that patient is not taking antihistamines
Oral corticosteroids do not (significantly) inhibit skin prick tests
Include positive (histamine) and negative (allergen diluent) controls
Skin prick tests may be performed on the flexor aspect of the forearm (or back) using sterile lancets (see Fig 1.10)
The procedure should be painless and not draw blood
A positive test (arbitrarily) is 2 mm or more greater than negative control. A positive skin prick test is usually at least 6 mm when concordant with clinical history of sensitivity
Demographism may confound results (although it is evident as a positive response with the negative control solution)
Skin tests should not be performed in the presence of severe eczema

Table 1.9 Uses of skin prick tests – a particular advantage is their educational value for patients

Skin Prick Tests – Uses
Allow diagnosis (or exclusion) of atopy
Provide supportive evidence (with clinical history) for diagnosis (or exclusion) of allergy
Educational value, providing a clear illustration for patients that may reinforce verbal advice
Essential when expensive or time-consuming allergen avoidance measures, removal of a family pet, or immunotherapy, are being considered
Serum allergen-specific IgE concentrations generally provide the same information if skin tests are unavailable

Lancet for Skin Prick Testing

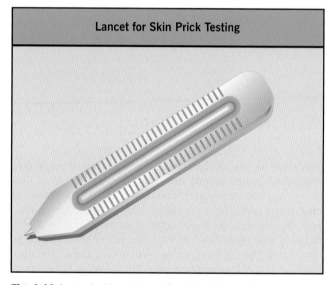

Fig. 1.10 A standard lancet used for skin prick testing.

The reliability of skin test extracts will depend on their containing adequate concentrations of all major allergenic determinants. Extracts should be biologically standardized in order to avoid batch-to-batch variation, and manufacturers' advice on shelf life and storage (generally at +4°C) should be observed. Uses of skin tests are summarized in Table 1.9. A particular advantage is their educational value for patients. Their peak performance and the interpretation of SPTs require training. Practice points are summarized in Table 1.10, and a standard lancet for SPTs is shown in Figure 1.10.

For routine clinical use the skin wheal is recorded as the mean of the longest diameter and the orthogonal diameter, i.e. the diameter at 90° to the midpoint of the longest diameter, excluding pseudopodia. Results are compared with the negative control (allergen diluent), as in Figure 1.11. A positive test is 2 mm or more greater than the negative control. However, as mentioned above, a skin wheal 6 mm or more across is more likely to be clinically relevant, although this may not always be the case. For the purposes of research, particularly when changes in immediate cutaneous allergen sensitivity may be important, more precision is required. In these circumstances a dose response curve using half log or log allergen concentrations may be constructed and the result expressed as the provocation concentration of allergen to cause a skin wheal of a given size, generally 4–6 mm, since this represents the linear portion of the dose response curve for many subjects. An example is given in Figure 1.12.

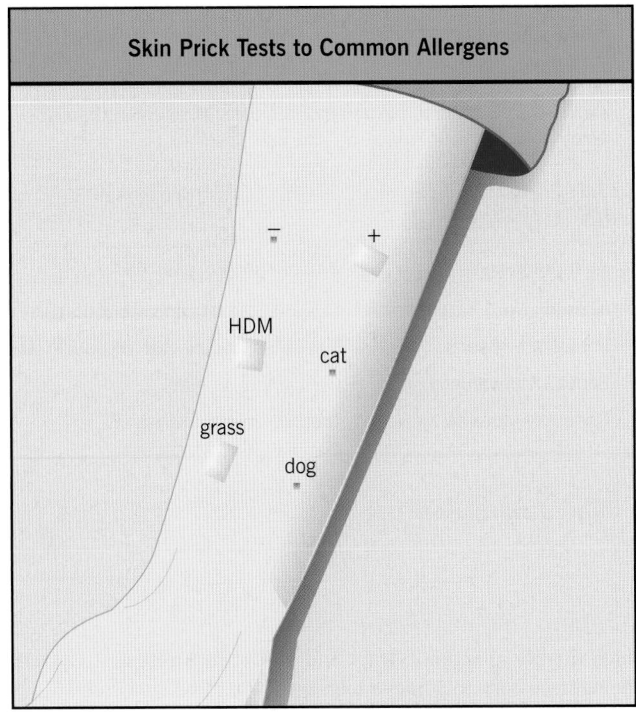

Fig. 1.11 Skin prick tests to common allergens on the forearm. Compared to the negative control, results indicate the presence of allergen-specific IgE to house dust mite (HDM) and grass pollen (grass).

Allergen PC_6 (provocation concentration to cause 6 mm skin wheal)

skin wheal diameter (mm)
provocation concentration of allergen (Bu/mL)
560 Bu/mL
14 000 Bu/mL

Fig. 1.12 Log dose response curve illustrating allergen PC_6, i.e. the provocation concentration of allergen causing a 6 mm skin wheal. The choice of wheal sizes is arbitrary and, ideally, should lie on the linear part of the curve. The results are from two patients following skin prick tests with grass pollen extract.

General practice

Whether or not skin prick testing should be performed routinely in general practice remains a matter of debate. A pilot study evaluated skin prick testing in children and adults in 320 patients in 16 general practices in the UK. The study involved 2 days' training in allergy, combined with instruction in skin prick testing with four common allergens (and positive and negative controls) followed by reinforcement on a further training day, including the interpretation of results. Participating nurses found that the technique was simple, relatively easy to incorporate into their routine assessment of new referrals to the asthma clinic, and acceptable to both adults and children. The procedure undoubtedly increased the nurses' awareness of the role of allergy in patients' asthma, although the study was not linked to specific outcomes. An important finding was the value of negative results of SPTs, which excluded atopy in these patients and enabled the investigators to advise patients against inappropriate allergen avoidance measures. The nurses also found the visual illustration provided by positive results helpful to reinforce advice. Further studies linked to specific outcome measures are still required.

Hospital practice

In hospital practice a routine panel of SPTs might include house dust mite, cat or dog hair, horse dander, molds (*Aspergillus fumigatus*, *Cladosporium* and *Alternaria*), and pollens (birch, mixed trees, timothy, or mixed grasses and weed), as well as positive and negative controls. Skin prick testing with foods should be confined to hospital practice, in view of the slight increase in risk of systemic reactions. However, skin prick testing with inhaled allergens is extremely safe and may be performed by a nurse without medical supervision, although epinephrine should be immediately available as a precaution.

Skin testing with fresh food (see Fig. 1.12) has been shown to be both more sensitive and specific than the use of allergen extracts for eggs (yolk and egg white) and fresh fruit.

Skin testing is useful for penicillin (major determinants, penicilloyl–polylysine) and the minor determinant mixture (benzylpenicillin, penilloate). A negative test excludes IgE–penicillin sensitivity in the vast majority of patients, whereas a positive test is less effective in predicting the result of provocation tests; skin tests are not helpful for other manifestations of penicillin allergy. SPTs with other antibiotics (such as cephalosporins and amoxicillin) may be performed although these have higher false-negative and false-positive rates.

Similarly, skin prick testing with latex, neuromuscular blocking drugs, and certain anesthetic agents may provide useful information but with limitations (see Chs 9 and 10).

IN VITRO TESTS

Total IgE

The concentration of total serum IgE is approximately 10 000 times less than that of serum IgG and therefore requires sensitive tests for its determination. IgE concentration is approximately 1 ng/mL in cord blood and increases throughout life to concentrations of up to 200 ng/mL in non-allergic adults and 3–600 ng/mL, or even higher, in allergic adults. It is still questionable whether an increased IgE concentration in cord

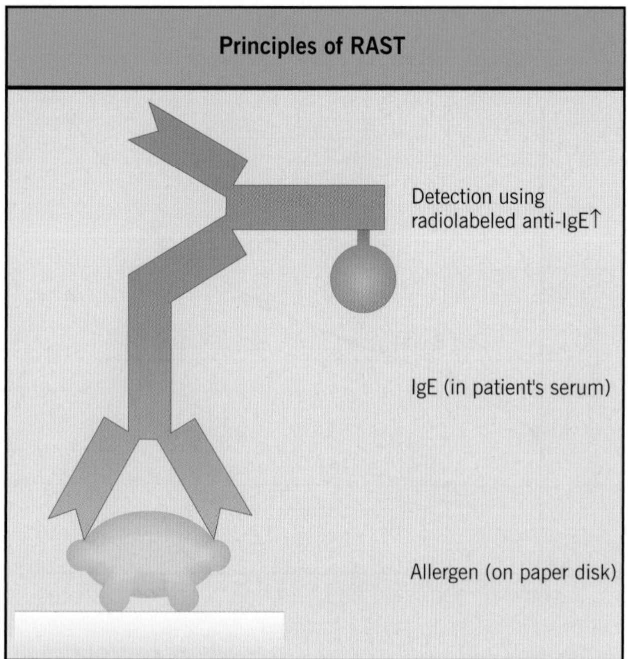

Fig. 1.13 Principles of RAST for measuring allergen-specific IgE in serum. ELISA tests involve the detection of the patient's IgE bound to allergen in the liquid phase using enzyme-linked anti-IgE. ELISA, enzyme-linked immunosorbent assay; RAST, radioallergosorbent test.

blood is of any prognostic value as several conditions, including parasite infestation, are associated with elevated levels. About half of IgE allergic patients will have a total IgE within the normal range, and therefore the predictive value of the test is rather limited. However, as higher serum IgE levels are often seen in hyperreactivity diseases in which large parts of skin and mucosa are involved, an elevated total IgE should stimulate further investigations of allergen-specific IgE.

Allergen-specific IgE

Immunoassays

Determination of allergen-specific IgE in serum is made by radioimmunoassays (RIA), enzyme-linked immunosorbent assays (ELISA), or chemiluminescence methods, usually by specialized immunology or clinical chemistry laboratories. The best known test for allergen-specific IgE is RAST (Fig. 1.13). In this test, individual allergen extracts are chemically bound to plastic tubes or wells in a multiwell plate. Any number or variety of allergens can be requested. A small aliquot of the patient's serum is added and any IgE specific for that particular allergen binds to the tube or plate. After thorough washing, radiolabeled anti-IgE is added and, after a predetermined period of incubation, further washed and the radioactivity counted. In an ELISA, the anti-IgE is labeled with an enzyme capable of causing a quantitative colorimetric reaction with an added substrate. In chemiluminescence assays, the anti-IgE is labeled with a substance, such as luciferase, capable of emitting photons. The result is semiquantitative and expressed on an arbitrary scale with reference to a standard. The sensitivity of these techniques varies with the different extract systems, a high quality allergen extract and an optimal detection system being necessary to achieve high sensitivity and specificity.

Also, there are more sophisticated tests for the standardization of allergens by use of a serum of known specificity. These tests include crossed radioimmunoelectrophoresis (CRIE) (see Fig. 17.8). SDS-PAGE followed by immunoblot, and RAST inhibition. CRIE, in particular, is essential for the standardization of allergen extracts for use in the above tests for allergen-specific IgE. Furthermore, CRIE and RIA may be used to assay allergen-specific IgG subclasses for monitoring allergen-specific immunotherapy, although their value in determining the clinical outcome is limited.

For inhalant allergies, the sensitivity of the RAST system is 60–80% and the specificity is higher than that of the SPTs, often as high as 90%. The technique is not, therefore, the best means of selecting the total number of allergen-sensitive patients, but if the RAST is positive most patients will be allergen sensitive, indicating high specificity. The advantages of RAST compared to SPTs are compared in Table 1.11.

Table 1.11 Advantages of skin prick tests compared with serum allergen-specific IgE RAST. Both have a high sensitivity but low specificity, i.e. a negative test is more effective for excluding the clinical relevance of a particular allergen than a positive test for confirming clinical relevance

Skin Prick Tests Compared with Serum Allergen-Specific IgE Test

Skin prick test	Serum-specific IgE RAST
Inexpensive	Not affected by concurrent drugs
Immediate results	Not influenced by skin disease
Educational value	Completely safe
Generally more sensitive	Testing for wider range of possible allergens

RAST, radioallergosorbent test.

Basophil histamine release

Allergy screening may also be performed by assessing histamine released from blood basophils after the addition of allergen extract. In this test, blood samples, which may be as small as 20 μL for each allergen, are pipetted into the wells of an ELISA plate precoated with the suspected allergens. The plate is then incubated at 37°C for up to 1 hour and the resultant histamine release estimated by fluorescence or RIA. Basophil histamine release, which is usually performed by specialist laboratories, takes only a few hours to perform. This test, which has a sensitivity and specificity similar to that of RAST, is semi-quantified on the basis of the concentration of the allergen extract which gives rise to a certain amount of histamine released. As the basophils of about 5% of the population do not release histamine in vitro, a positive response to anti-IgE, used as a positive control, is absolutely necessary to validate a negative result. Furthermore, as the majority of the population has some circulating IgE, a positive result to anti-IgE is not indicative of the presence of allergy.

Table 1.12 Measurement of environmental allergens

Measurement of Environmental Allergens		
Measurement	**Allergens**	**Detection**
Pollen, spore counts in relation to diary symptom/medications	Grass, trees, weeds, molds	Burkard spore trap (or other device) followed by microscopy; counts expressed as particles per cubic meter
Dust sampling and allergen detection	House dust mite, laboratory animals, domestic pets, cockroaches	Vacuum cleaning or collection of settled dust, followed by allergen extraction and detection using RAST inhibition or specific immunoassay
Air sampling and allergen detection	House dust mites, laboratory animals, domestic pets	Personal air sampler, followed by allergen extraction from air filter and detection using RAST inhibition or specific immunoassay
Culture for mold identification	Molds such as *Aspergillus Cladosporium* and *Alternaria*	Specialized microbiological culture techniques
Occupational agents	Isocyanates	Isocyanate meter

RAST, radioallergosorbent test.

Measurement of environmental allergens

A number of naturally occurring protein antigens in the patient's environment may give rise to sensitization and stimulation of IgE production. Many of these allergens are well known or visible; others are hidden and have to be determined by a thorough medical history and analysis of the environment.

Different biological and immunochemical methods are presently available for the demonstration of allergens in air and in dust sampling (Table 1.12). Determining the relationship between symptoms and allergens and the decrease in symptoms during allergen reduction makes up a part of the testing for allergy.

A simple technique for sampling dust is to use a vacuum cleaner with a special filter which retains small particles found in the dust. The dust is extracted 1:3 (w/v) in saline for an hour; the presence of a detergent in the buffer may be required for optimal extraction and the allergen content is identified and quantified by immunochemical techniques. For some purified allergens, monoclonal antibodies have been produced, thereby enabling quantification (in nanograms of major allergen per gram of dust). Other devices for collecting airborne allergens are available, e.g. stationary high volume air samplers and portable air samplers. Mold spores can be identified and quantified in the home, the working place of the patient, or the outdoor air.

PROVOCATION TESTS

Provocation tests are only occasionally required for routine allergy diagnosis. They are reserved for cases of diagnostic difficulty and when there is discordance between the clinical history and the results of objective tests. For example, occasionally patients will give a clear history of summer hay-fever in the absence of a positive SPT or RAST to grass pollen or other prevalent seasonal allergens; one careful study found 11% of the total number of cases to be due to this circumstance.

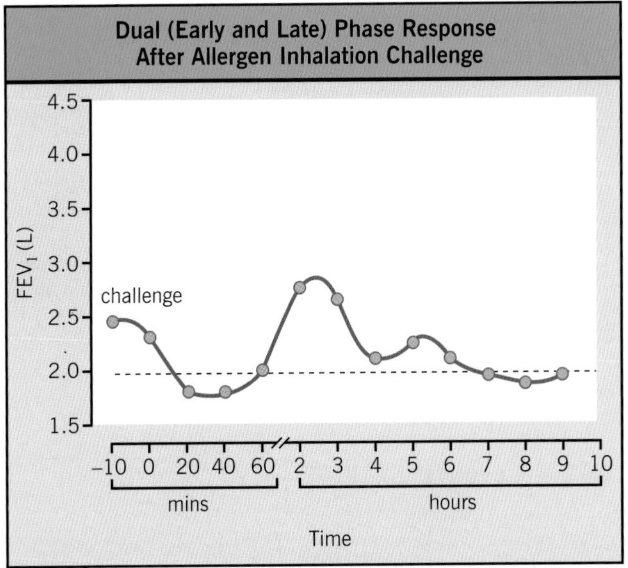

Fig. 1.14 Allergen provocation with house dust mite resulting in the development of early and late asthmatic responses. FEV, forced expiratory volume.

This raises the possibility of IgE sensitivity in the target organ in the absence of positive SPT or RAST. Specific provocation tests may be of value in these circumstances.

A recently described alternative involves immunostaining of nasal biopsies using biotinylated allergens in order to detect allergen-specific IgE-bearing cells directly within the nasal mucosa. This approach is invasive and not available for routine use. Similarly, allergen bronchial provocation is rarely indicated for routine diagnosis although this is of value for research and in the evaluation of new potential therapeutic agents (Fig.1.14). The methods, uses, and limitations of allergen provocation to the nose, conjunctiva, lung, and GI tract are covered elsewhere.

The evaluation of target organ hyperresponsiveness is of value in epidemiology, basic research, and the evaluation of new therapeutic agents. These tests, in contrast to allergen provocation, may have more value in the routine clinical assessment of individual patients. Examples include the elicitation of physical causes of urticaria using locally applied ice, heat, pressure, or UV light. Histamine or methacholine inhalation testing defines non-specific airway hyperreactivity and may be helpful in identifying patients with bronchial asthma when baseline lung function is normal and there is no immediate response to a bronchodilator. In such cases, increased airway responsiveness indicates the need for a therapeutic trial and further lung function monitoring.

DIAGNOSTIC TESTS THAT ARE NOT RECOMMENDED

There are many unproven 'diagnostic' tests performed by ecologists and alternative practitioners. These tests are of unproven value, are often time consuming and expensive and are therefore not to be recommended (Table 1.13).

Table 1.13 'Diagnostic' tests that are of unproven value and are therefore not recommended

'Diagnostic' Tests of Unproven Value
Neutralization provocation (Miller) tests (based on multiple skin tests; environmental allergens include smoke, petrol, tobacco, etc.)
Leukocytotoxic tests
Hair analysis
Vega testing (a 'black box' electrical test). The test is based on the addition of food extracts to a chamber contained within an electrical circuit completed by the patient
Applied kinesiology (based on muscle weakness)
Auricular cardiac reflex testing (based on pulse rate)

DIAGNOSTIC APPROACH

Allergy diagnosis depends primarily on the clinical history. This history, aided by a physical examination and objective tests of IgE sensitivity (either skin tests or serum IgE measurements), is used to focus on the following questions:

- Is the patient atopic?
- Does allergy contribute to the patient's symptoms?
- What are the clinically relevant allergens?

Several investigators have evaluated various diagnostic tests in terms of their sensitivity, specificity, and negative and positive predictive value (Table 1.14). In general, no tests, even when combined with a careful history, will confirm or exclude relevant allergy in every individual case. Dreborg emphasized the relative lack of prospective studies examining the efficiency of these various tests and pointed out the importance of studying defined populations. For example, skin tests are likely to be more predictive of clinically relevant allergy (lower false-positive rate) in patients studied from a specialist allergy clinic, compared to those from a general practice, where the proportion of 'allergic' patients is likely to be lower. In contrast (as Eriksson found) a negative skin test is likely to have more negative predictive value in a general practice population compared to a specialist allergy clinic.

A simple diagnostic approach is presented in Figure 1.15. There should be a high index of suspicion for allergy in patients presenting with symptoms of asthma, rhinitis, or eczema, particularly if there is an associated personal or family history of other atopic disease. Whether or not allergy is suspected on the basis of the initial history, it is the authors' view that a limited number of SPTs, and possibly RAST, to several common aeroallergens (generally four) should be performed in the majority of patients to confirm or exclude atopy; a physical examination should also be included. When both the clinical history and results of SPTs or RAST are negative, one can exclude allergy with a high degree of confidence and no specific treatment for allergy is indicated. Similarly, when the history and tests are both positive, then allergen avoidance measures, and in selected cases immunotherapy, should be carefully con-

Table 1.14 Definition of test characteristics

Allergy Test Characteristics			
Patient group	**Diagnostic test (positive)**	**Diagnostic test (negative)**	**Total**
Allergics	True positive (TP)	False negative (FN)	TP + FN
Non-allergics	False positive (FP)	True negative (TN)	FP + TN
Total	TP + FP	FN + TN	
Sensitivity: TP/(TP + FN)			
Specificity: TN/(FP + TN)			
Predictive value of negative test (PV_{neg}): TN(FN + TN)			
Predictive value of positive test (PV_{pos}): TP(TP + FP)			

From Murray AB, Milner RA. The accuracy of features in the clinical history for predicting atopic sensitization to airborne allergens in children. J Allergy Clin Immunol 1995; 96:588–596.

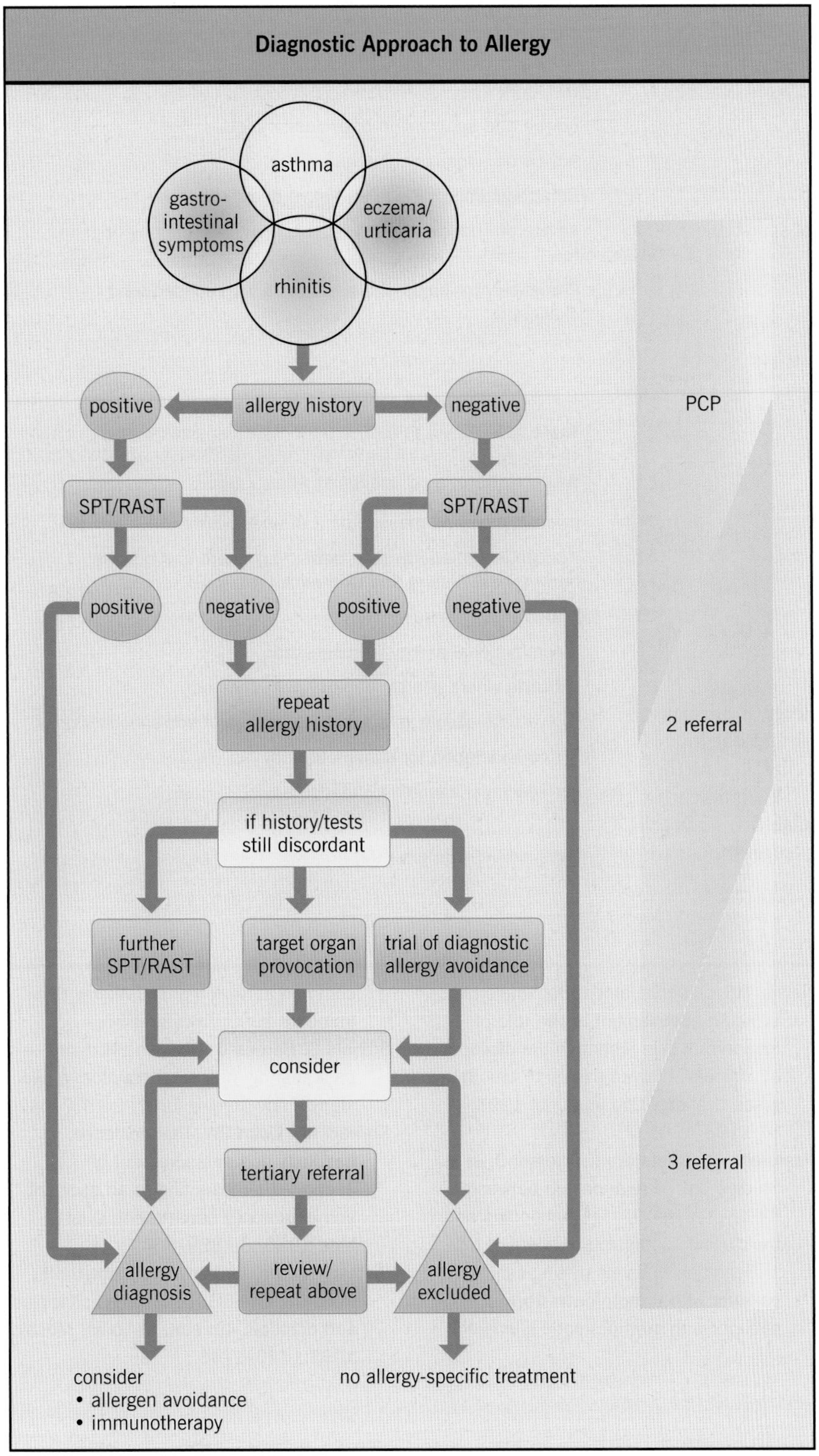

Diagnostic Approach to Allergy

asthma
gastro-intestinal symptoms
eczema/urticaria
rhinitis
allergy history
positive
negative
SPT/RAST
SPT/RAST
positive
negative
positive
negative
repeat allergy history
if history/tests still discordant
further SPT/RAST
target organ provocation
trial of diagnostic allergy avoidance
consider
tertiary referral
allergy diagnosis
review/ repeat above
allergy excluded
consider
• allergen avoidance
• immunotherapy
no allergy-specific treatment
PCP
2 referral
3 referral

Fig. 1.15 Diagnostic approach to allergy. PCP, primary care physician; RAST, radioallergosorbent test; SPT, skin prick test.

sidered for each individual patient. Where there is discordance, above all, the history should be reassessed.

Specialist referral and, occasionally, more sophisticated tests or specific provocation testing may be required. When the specific allergy diagnosis remains uncertain, the threshold for when to intervene with a therapeutic trial of potentially time consuming and expensive avoidance measures (or the removal of a family pet) will depend on factors such as the disease severity, the requirement for pharmacotherapy, and the likelihood of successful intervention with either allergen-specific avoidance or immunotherapy. The importance of the role of the specialist nurse in the allergy clinic cannot be overemphasized

Table 1.15 The role of the specialist nurse in the allergy clinic

The Specialist Nurse in the Allergy Clinic
Skin prick testing
Asthma education, self-management plans
Spirometry and peak expiratory flow recording
Checking inhaler technique; correct use of nasal sprays and drops
Advice on avoidance of allergens
Instruction on self-administration of epinephrine
Liaison with parents, school nurses, pharmacists, etc.
Involvement in allergen injection immunotherapy

Table 1.16 The role of the dietitian in the allergy clinic

The Dietitian in the Allergy Clinic
Advice and supervision of exclusion diets
Advice on adequacy of diets
Reintroduction of foods that have been withdrawn
Advice on reducing additives, preservatives and colorings in food
Preparation of foods and assistance with blinded food challenges

(Table 1.15). Also, in patients with food allergy, a specialist dietitian (Table 1.16) is indispensable. An important question is when to refer a patient to a specialist allergy clinic for further diagnostic procedures and advice on therapy. This is likely to vary, depending on the level of expertise available in primary care and the availability of allergy clinics; suggestions are included in Table 1.17.

Table 1.17 When to refer a patient to a specialist allergy clinic

When to Refer to a Specialist Allergy Clinic
Investigation and management of anaphylaxis
If diagnosis of allergy is in doubt, e.g. there is a discord between the history and skin prick test/RAST results
If food allergy is suspected
If occupational allergy is suspected
Urticaria where allergic etiology is suspected
To evaluate allergy as a suspected cause of non-specific illness
For consideration for immunotherapy
For specialist allergen-avoidance advice

RAST, radioallergosorbent test

FURTHER READING

Dreborg S. Allergy diagnosis. In: Mygind N, Naclerio RM, eds. Allergic and non-allergic rhinitis: clinical aspects. Copenhagen: Munksgaard; 1993:82–94.

Durham SR, ed. ABC of allergies. London: British Medical Journal Books; 1998.

Eriksson NE. Diagnosis of IgE mediated allergy in clinical practice. Allergol Immunopathol 1994; 22:139–151.

Murray AB, Milner RA. The accuracy of features in the clinical history for predicting atopic sensitisation to airborne allergens in children. J Allergy Clin Immunol 1995; 96:588–596.

Nelson HS, Oppenheimer J, Buchmeier A, et al. An assessment of the role of intradermal skin testing in the diagnosis of clinically relevant allergy to timothy grass. J Allergy Clin Immunol 1996; 97:1193–1201.

Pastorello EA, Cristoforo I, Ortolani C, et al. Studies on the relationship between the level of specific IgE antibodies and the clinical expression of allergy: 1. Definition of levels distinguishing patients with symptomatic from patients with asymptomatic allergy to common aeroallergens. J Allergy Clin Immunol 1995; 96:580–587.

Sibbald B, Barnes G, Durham SR. Skin prick testing in general practice: a pilot study. J Adv Nursing 1997; 26:537–542.

Stewart AG, Ewan PW. The incidence, aetiology and measurement of anaphylaxis presenting to an accident and emergency department. Quart J Med 1996; 89:859–864.

Sullivan TG. Drug allergy. In: Middleton E, Reed CE, Ellis EF, et al. Allergy: principles and practice. 4th edn. St Louis: Mosby; 1993:1726–1746.

Chapter 2

Definition:
Asthma is a chronic inflammatory disorder in which the airway smooth muscle undergoes exaggerated contraction and is abnormally responsive to external stimuli.

Asthma

Thomas AE Platts-Mills, Mitsuru Adachi, Romain A Pauwels, and Stephen T Holgate

INTRODUCTION

The symptoms of asthma occur together with variations in the diameter of medium-size airways such that it is increasingly difficult to exhale. Narrowing of the airways can occur because of smooth muscle contraction, edema or swelling of the wall, or increased mucus in the airways. However, it is increasingly clear that the pathologic event underlying most cases of asthma is chronic inflammation of the airway walls. The elements of this inflammation will be discussed in Chapters 21, 22, and 23. The best-defined and most commonly identified cause of this inflammation is inhalation of allergens. Sometimes, the relationship of these foreign proteins to the symptoms of asthma may be obvious to the patient (e.g. when wheezing or coughing starts within 10 minutes of entering a house that has a cat in it). On the other hand, many patients who are allergic to dust mites are not aware of the association between exposure and their symptoms. By contrast, most patients with asthma are well aware that their lungs vary in tightness and that many non-specific stimuli such as exercise, cold air, or passive smoking can trigger attacks. The fact that the lungs of patients with asthma can react to otherwise 'trivial' stimuli such as cold air is referred to as bronchial hyperresponsiveness. This hyperresponsiveness can be demonstrated in the clinic by using histamine or methacholine, which narrow the airways directly, or by cold air or exercise challenge, which are indirect stimuli that narrow the airways following the release of secondary mediators.

The relationship between inflammation in the airways of a patient and either the symptoms of asthma or bronchial hyperresponsiveness is not simple. Thus, it is not possible to define the severity of asthma on the basis of a measurement of inflammation in the lungs. Nonetheless, the production of mediators by eosinophils, T cells, and mast cells is of central importance in understanding the pathophysiology of asthma as well as being a target for treatment. Estimating the prevalence of asthma is dependent on the method used to define the disease, and in addition the prevalence varies markedly between countries and between different communities within a country.

The main problem in defining the disease is that the disease varies from occasional episodes of chest tightness or wheezing that can easily be reversed to a life-threatening disease with continuous airway obstruction that requires high-dose inhaled corticosteroid or oral corticosteroid treatment. Because of this variability, any discussion of etiology, pathogenesis, or treatment is dependent on a system for classifying the disease.

THE CLASSIFICATION OF ASTHMA

Classification of bronchial asthma can be based on age, etiology, associated characteristics, or severity. Classifications based on severity have been primarily designed as an approach to treatment. Thus, management of mild intermittent disease may require only bronchodilator treatment, but frequent attacks with or without persistent mild

Table 2.1 Classification of asthma and chronic airway obstruction, based on age of onset and etiology

Classification of Asthma and Chronic Airway Obstruction		
Age of onset	**Disease**	**Contributing factors and special features**
Infants ≤ 2 years old	Bronchiolitis/wheezing, single or multiple episodes Bronchopulmonary dysplasia	Respiratory syncytial virus, maternal smoking, and small lungs at birth Prematurity
Children	Allergic asthma	Family history, sensitization to common allergens and intercurrent rhinovirus infection
Adults 20–60 years old	Allergic asthma Allergic bronchopulmonary aspergillosis Late onset /intrinsic asthma Other forms of airway obstruction	Sensitization to indoor allergens and rhinovirus infection High IgE, transient infiltrates, eosinophilia Sinusitis, polyps, aspirin sensitivity Hyperventilation, vocal cord syndrome
> 45 years old	Intermittent wheezing complicating chronic obstructive lung disease	Fixed obstruction, FEV_1 ≤ 35% predicted following prolonged smoking

FEV_1, forced expiratory volume in 1 second.

symptoms require a comprehensive approach to controlling inflammation as well as bronchodilator treatment. Severe asthma can become a major clinical problem that requires specialist care and many different approaches to treatment.

The pattern of disease presenting at different ages is distinct (Table 2.1). In the first 2 years of life, wheezing and bronchiolitis are not distinguishable, and the commonest cause of these episodes is infection with the respiratory syncytial virus (RSV). Infection with RSV is almost universal in the first 2 years of life and in most cases does not result in more than a mild upper respiratory infection. An important risk factor for the severity of bronchiolitis or asthma during RSV infection is the size of the lungs at birth. The two major factors that influence the size of the lungs at birth are prematurity and maternal smoking.

In older children and young adults, by far the most commonly identified cause of asthma is sensitization to one of the common inhalant allergens, particularly those encountered indoors. Other important risk factors include a family history of asthma, infection with common cold viruses, especially rhinoviruses, and housing conditions.

Allergen provocation of the lungs of asthmatic patients can induce bronchoconstriction, inflammation in the bronchi, and prolonged increases in bronchial reactivity. In keeping with this, allergen-activated inflammation has become a major target for treatment. This includes reducing exposure to allergens and pharmacologic approaches to counteract the inflammatory mediators (e.g. cromolin sodium, topical corticosteroids, and leukotriene-modifying drugs).

People with allergic asthma represent the largest group of asthma patients requiring treatment, and in addition they are also the group on whom most epidemiology studies have been focused. Thus, most of the population-based evidence for the increased prevalence of asthma has concerned school children or young adults.

Asthma that presents after the age of 20 years provides a complex problem both in management and in investigation. For this age group there is a wider differential diagnosis, and all cases with persistent symptoms require investigation. Major causes include simple allergic asthma in adults, intrinsic asthma associated with chronic hyperplastic sinusitis, allergic bronchopulmonary aspergillosis, wheezing associated with chronic obstructive lung disease, and the many different causes of airway obstruction that are not related to generalized airway reactivity.

Allergic asthma in children

The two strongest risk factors for asthma in childhood are a family history and immediate hypersensitivity to common allergens. This immune response includes both IgE antibodies and helper T cells type 2 (Th2), both of which are thought to contribute to the inflammation in the respiratory tract (see Ch. 21). Children who mount an immune response to inhalant allergens have an increased risk of developing asthma because of this combination of genetics and exposure. However, it is sensitization to indoor allergens (e.g. dust mites, cats, dogs, and cockroaches) that is strongly associated with asthma (Fig. 2.1). By contrast, in some recent studies, immediate hypersensitivity to grass or other pollens has not been found to be significantly associated with asthma. The implication is that a large part of the allergen exposure that contributes to the inflammation in the lungs of patients with perennial asthma occurs inside houses.

The evidence for a causal relationship between exposure to dust mite allergens and asthma has come from many different experiments (Table 2.2). The important features are that:

- there is a very strong association between sensitization to indoor allergens and asthma;
- bronchial challenges with the relevant allergens can replicate many features of the disease – acute and delayed airway narrowing, inflammation (which includes an influx of eosinophils), and prolonged increases in non-specific bronchial hyperresponsiveness; and
- reducing exposure to allergens, whether in the house, hospital room, or sanatorium, can decrease symptoms of asthma.

Thus, the classification of allergic or 'extrinsic' asthma implies not only that the patient has a positive skin test to an allergen but also that exposure to this allergen is contributing to the

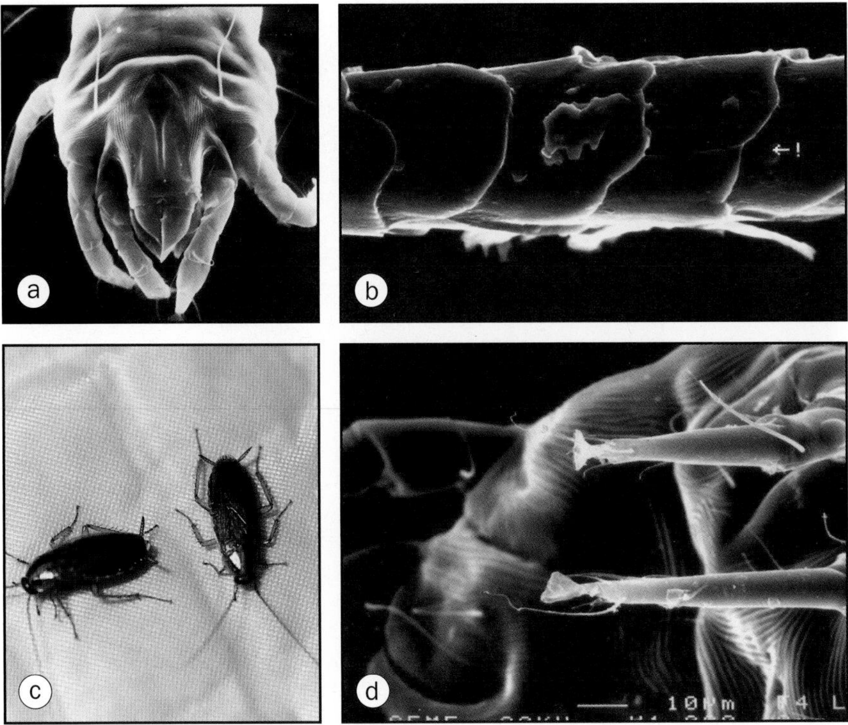

Fig. 2.1 Allergens. (a) Dust mite. (b) Cat hair. (c) Cockroach. (d) Mite legs.

Table 2.2 Evidence that exposure to indoor allergens is causally related to asthma

Evidence for Indoor Allergens as Cause of Asthma
There is a very strong association between sensitization to indoor allergens and asthma
The observations about allergens in houses, sensitization of asthmatics and the association with asthma have been made in many different countries
The association is only with asthma, not with any other lung disease
Bronchial challenge with allergens can reproduce many of the findings of asthma including eosinophil infiltrates and persistent increases in bronchial reactivity
Reducing exposure to dust mites in a sanatorium or in the home is an effective treatment for asthma
The mechanism by which allergen exposure causes sensitization and subsequent diseases is biologically plausible

disease. The main allergens that are associated with asthma have been purified, cloned, and sequenced (Table 2.3). The immune response to these proteins is very well defined and includes IgE antibodies, IgG4 antibodies, and Th2 lymphocytes. Although this immune response to indoor allergens is well defined as a 'risk factor' for asthma, it is not clear why some allergic people have bronchial hyperreactivity and asthma while other apparently equally allergic people do not. In part, this may relate to the many factors that can increase the inflammatory response in allergic people and the many triggers that can induce wheezing. These factors include viral infections, ozone, and passive smoking, all of which are stimuli that induce an epithelial stress response (Fig. 2.2). It is plausible that a fundamental abnormality in asthma is an impaired ability to restitute the epithelium in response to environmental stress (Fig. 2.3).

Asthma in adults

Allergic asthma

Asthma in adults is more difficult to classify than asthma in children because there are several overlapping entities and, in addition, a larger number of alternative causes for symptoms of this kind. Among adults with asthma, 30–70% are allergic, depending on the population studied and the severity of the disease. The allergic patients include childhood onset cases, patients who present for the first time, and those allergic patients whose disease goes into remission in their teens but subsequently relapses. The evidence for a direct role of allergens in adults is less complete than it is in children. However, bronchial provocation with allergens can mimic many aspects of the disease, allergen avoidance can reduce both the symptoms and the requirement for medicines, and the epidemiologic association between allergen sensitization and asthma in adults has also been found in many countries. In addition, the pattern of sensitization among adults who present to an emergency room with asthma reflects the allergens found in their houses. Patients in this group have positive prick tests to allergens, intermittent wheezing, and significant bronchial hyperreactivity. In addition, their total serum IgE ranges from high normal to high (100 IU/mL up to about 1000 IU/mL), and in general they have moderate eosinophilia (200–500 eosinophils per mL). In most cases of allergic asthma in adults, chest X-ray is clear and computed tomography (CT) of the sinuses is either normal or shows only mild changes (Fig. 2.4).

Table 2.3 Allergens associated with asthma

Allergens Associated with Asthma				
	Species	**Allergen**	**Assays**	**Size of airborne particles**
INDOOR				
Arthropods:				
Dust mites	*Dermatophagoides pteronyssinus*	Der p 1	mAb ELISA	1–30 µm
	D. farina	Der f 1	mAb ELISA	1–30 µm
Cockroach	*Blattella germanica*	Bla g 2	mAb ELISA	> 10 µm
Domestic animals:				
Cat	*Felix domesticus*	Fel d 1	mAb ELISA	2–10 µm
Dog	*Canis familiaris*	Can f 1	mAb ELISA	2–10 µm
Rodents:				
Mouse	*Mus muscularis*	Mus m 1	Polyclonal RIA	2–10 µm
Rat	*Rattus norweigicus*	Rat n 1	mAb	2–10 µm
OUTDOORS/INDOOR				
Molds:	*Alternaria alternata*	Alt a 1	mAb/Polyclonal	10–14 µm
	Aspergillus fumigatus	Asp f 1	mAb	2 µm
Pollens:				
Rye Grass	*Lolium perenne*	Lol p 1	Microscopic pollen count	15–30 µm
Ragweed	*Ambrosia elatior*	Amb a 1		
Oak	*Quercus*			

ELISA, enzyme-linked immunosorbent assay; mAb, monoclonal antibody; RIA, radioimmunoassay.

Allergic bronchopulmonary aspergillosis

When patients with asthma develop a more severe course (i.e. they require corticosteroids), have persistent symptoms, or start producing sputum, the diagnosis of allergic bronchopulmonary aspergillosis (ABPA) should be considered. In most cases, ABPA is a complication of pre-existing allergic asthma. The diagnostic features are:

- total IgE > 400 IU/mL (however total IgE can be suppressed by chronic oral corticosteroid treatment);
- persistent eosinophilia (500/mL^3);
- productive sputum, which may be brown, orange, or gray in color and which may grow *Aspergillus fumigatus* or other fungi;
- transient infiltrates on chest X-ray;
- central bronchiectasis on fine section CT scan of chest;
- immediate hypersensitivity to *A. fumigatus* as judged by skin tests or serum IgE antibodies; and
- precipitins against the fungus or high-titer specific IgG antibodies.

Colonization of the lungs with *Aspergillus* is very common among patients with cystic fibrosis, and these children often have high total serum IgE and IgE antibodies to the fungus. Almost all these children have lung damage, including bronchiectasis, but in general they do not have significant eosinophilia. Other fungi can occasionally cause a very similar syndrome (e.g. allergic bronchopulmonary curvulariosis or allergic bronchopulmonary candidiasis).

Intrinsic asthma

Intrinsic asthma was defined in 1947 by Rackemann, who drew attention to patients presenting in adult life who showed:

- negative skin tests to common allergens;
- no family history of atopic disease;
- persistent eosinophilia;
- a severe course (often requiring oral corticosteroids and therefore over-represented in tertiary care clinics and among hospitalized patients); and
- no improvement when admitted to hospital.

In 1956, Samter added the observation that some of these patients had nasal polyps, sinusitis, and aspirin sensitivity. In this form of asthma there is greatly enhanced production of cysteinyl leukotrienes by mast cells and eosinophils with a selective upregulation of leukotriene C_4 synthase, the terminal enzyme in the generation of these mediators. Although sinusitis is not present in all cases of intrinsic asthma, it is common.

Among adults aged over 40 years who develop severe asthma for the first time, almost 50% may have intrinsic asthma, although these patients do not represent more than 10% of the total population with asthma. In a random sample of adults presenting with asthma to an emergency room, almost 30% have extensive sinusitis on CT. However, this figure includes both those with polypoid sinusitis typical of intrinsic asthma and those with acute sinusitis related to intercurrent viral infection (Fig. 2.4).

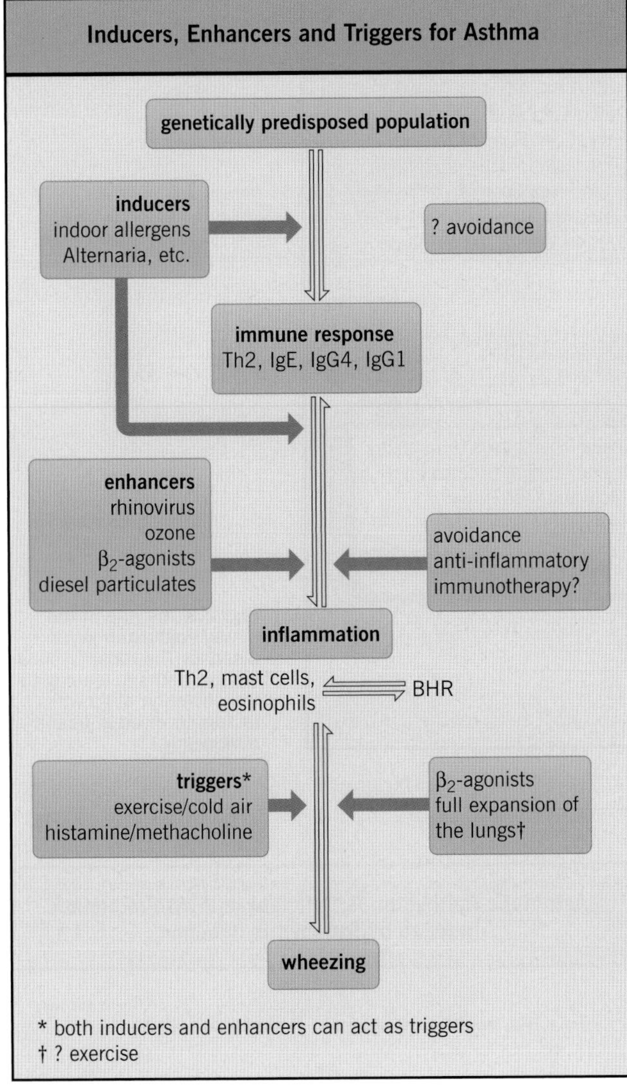

Fig. 2.2 Causes of asthma.

Late-onset asthma, which is frequently not associated with atopy, may be linked to the workplace. Occupational exposure to sensitizing chemicals (e.g. isocyanates) is an important cause of asthma as the timely removal from exposure can cure the disease or at least prevent progression. In atopic people, exposure to complex molecules (e.g. proteins in rodent urine), may also lead to occupational asthma. The diagnosis is best established by a careful history, monitoring the peak expiratory flow rate both in and out of work, and occasionally by controlled provocation with the suspected agent or agents.

Virally-induced asthma

Viruses are the most common trigger, up to 85%, of acute asthma exacerbations.

Also, virus infection is associated with particularly severe acute symptoms, with more severe airflow obstruction, and a longer length of stay in hospital. Furthermore, in this condition corticosteroids offer only limited amelioration. The most common pathogens associated with asthma exacerbations are rhinoviruses to which asthmatics are particularly susceptible because of the higher levels of intercellular adhesion molecule-1 (ICAM-1) on the surface of the epithelial cells lining the bronchial tree. Infection leads to increased bronchial inflammation, which, unlike allergic asthma, is neutrophil rather than eosinophil dominated, and increased bronchial responsiveness.

But why should the airways of asthmatics respond so dramatically to virus infection when those of non-asthmatics do not? The answer appears to lie in the ability of the bronchial epithelial cells (BEC) to synthesize interferon β (IFNβ) (Fig. 2.5). Infection of normal BEC with rhinovirus stimulates a large increase in the synthesis of IFNβ which in turn induces apoptosis and termination of the infection. In bronchial cells from asthmatic subjects, however, the synthesis of IFNβ, the stimulus for apoptosis, is greatly reduced. As a result, the cells survive and the virus replicates until death by necrosis occurs and causes inflammation and asthma exacerbation. In addition, the virions released by the necrotic cell are free to infect further bronchial epithelial cells. Addition of IFNβ before or during rhinovirus infection of asthmatic epithelial cells restores their ability to eliminate the virus.

Chronic obstructive lung disease

Chronic bronchitis with emphysema, which is also known as chronic obstructive pulmonary disease (COPD), is in most cases a sequel to many years of active smoking. The damage caused by smoking is slow:

- after 5–10 years of smoking, the effect on spirometry may not be detectable;
- after 20 years of smoking, the forced expiratory volume in 1 second (FEV_1) and the forced vital capacity (FVC) are usually decreased; and
- after 30–50 years of smoking, the disease becomes a major clinical problem.

This means that it is unusual for patients to present before the age of 50 years with severe fixed obstruction.

The dominant symptoms of COPD are coughing and shortage of breath on activity, but some patients present with acute breathlessness and wheezing, which is difficult to distinguish from asthma. The treatment of acute episodes in patients with COPD is similar to that of asthma, including bronchodilators, corticosteroids, and theophylline. In addition, many of these patients show significant reversibility and moderate, non-specific bronchial hyperreactivity to methacholine. The basis for the inflammation in these patients is not clear, but it is usually not related to allergy. In a few patients, colonization of the lungs with fungi may exacerbate the disease; however, even in these cases the patients are usually not 'allergic' to the fungi as judged by skin tests or IgE antibodies.

Establishing that a patient has fixed obstruction is best achieved by spirometry when the patient has been optimally treated. Thus, 2 weeks of full treatment with high-dose inhaled corticosteroids or oral prednisone (about 40 mg/day) is usually sufficient to establish the optimal lung function for that patient. Reversibility of airway obstruction is usually defined in terms of percentage change; however, if obstruction is severe, even a 15% change may represent very little improvement (e.g. a 15% improvement in an FEV_1 of 0.8 L gives an FEV_1 of 0.9 L). Thus, it is necessary to know both the response to bronchodilator and the best FEV_1 and FVC achieved after treatment.

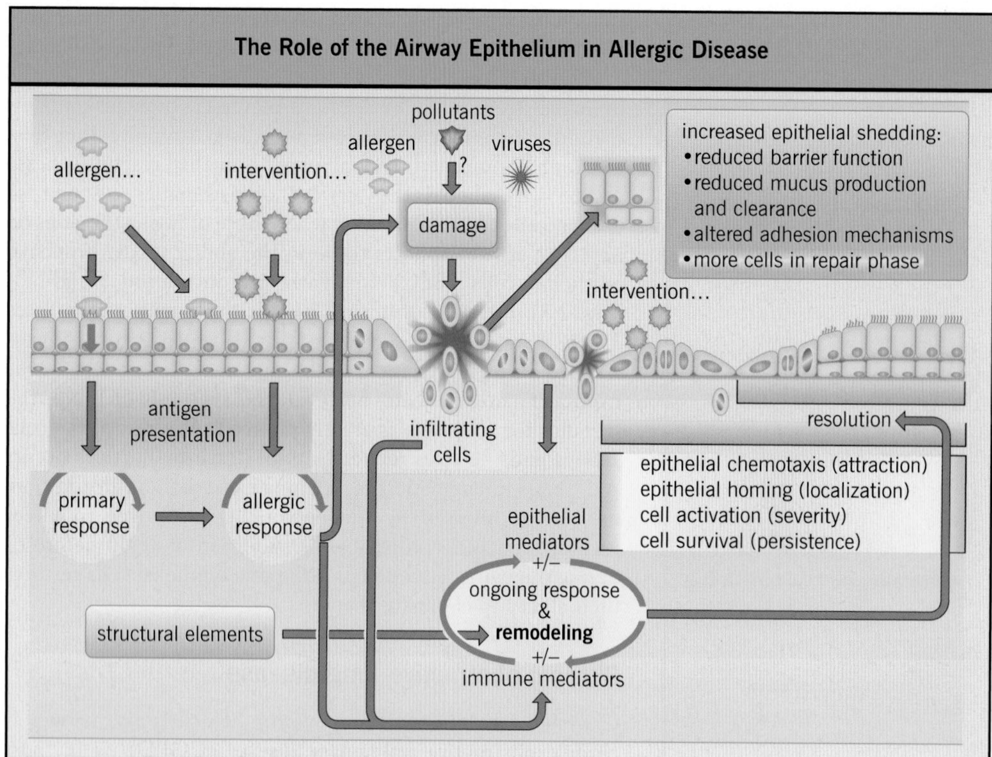

Fig. 2.3 The role of the airway epithelium in disease. The repair cycle in chronic asthma, leading to the secretion of growth factors involved in tissue remodeling.

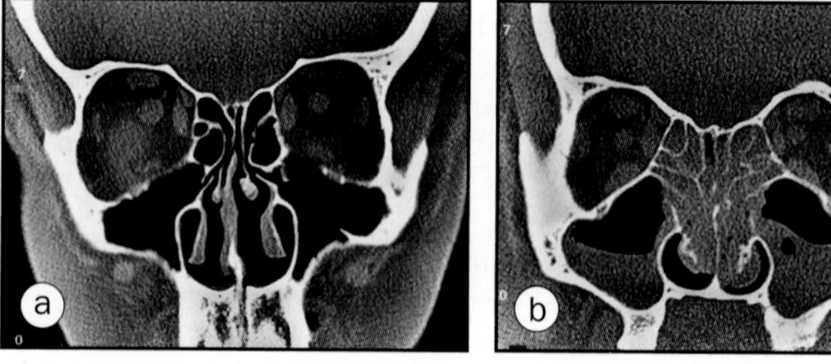

Fig. 2.4 Computed tomography (CT) scan of the sinus. (a) Normal scan. (b) Scan from a patient with severe polypoid changes.

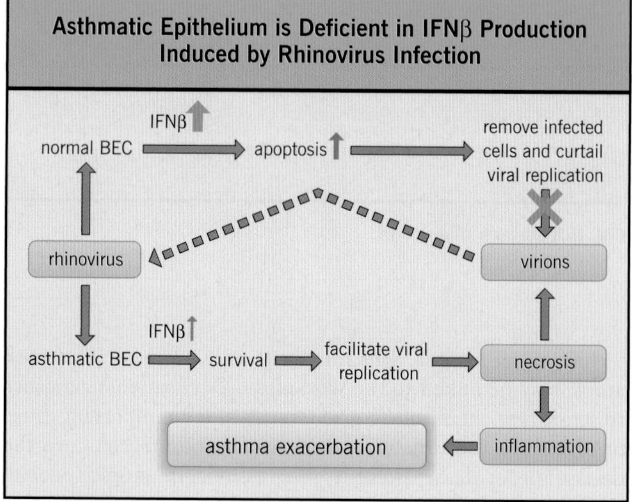

Fig. 2.5 Model of the mechanism of viral asthma. Please see text for explanation. BEC, bronchial epithelial cells; IFNβ, interferon β. (Drawn from Wark PA, Johnston SL, Bucchieri F, et al. Asthmatic bronchial epithelial cells have a deficient innate immune response to infection with rhinovirus. J Exp Med 2005; 201:937–947.)

ANATOMY AND PHYSIOLOGY OF THE BRONCHI

The pathophysiology of asthma involves the nasal passages, the paranasal sinuses, the mouth, the larynx, trachea, and the bronchial tree. Each of these may be inflamed and to some degree obstructed, and each can play an important role in symptoms. The anatomy and physiology of the nasal passages and sinuses are considered in Chapter 4. The major focus of asthma is large, medium and small bronchi, all of which can become inflamed, swollen, and hyperresponsive. The bronchial tree has approximately 16 divisions, or generations, before reaching the terminal, or respiratory, bronchioles. In uncomplicated asthma, the remaining five to seven divisions of the bronchioles and alveolae are normal. The bronchi have cartilage in their walls, which forms complete rings in the trachea; it is present as plates as the bronchi divide but it is absent from the smallest bronchi. All bronchi have smooth muscle in their walls (Fig. 2.6).

The blood supply to the lungs comes from two sources. The pulmonary circulation coming from the pulmonary arteries provides venous (i.e. unoxygenated) blood to the alveoli for gas exchange. The bronchial circulation comes from the aorta and provides blood supply to the bronchial walls. The branches of

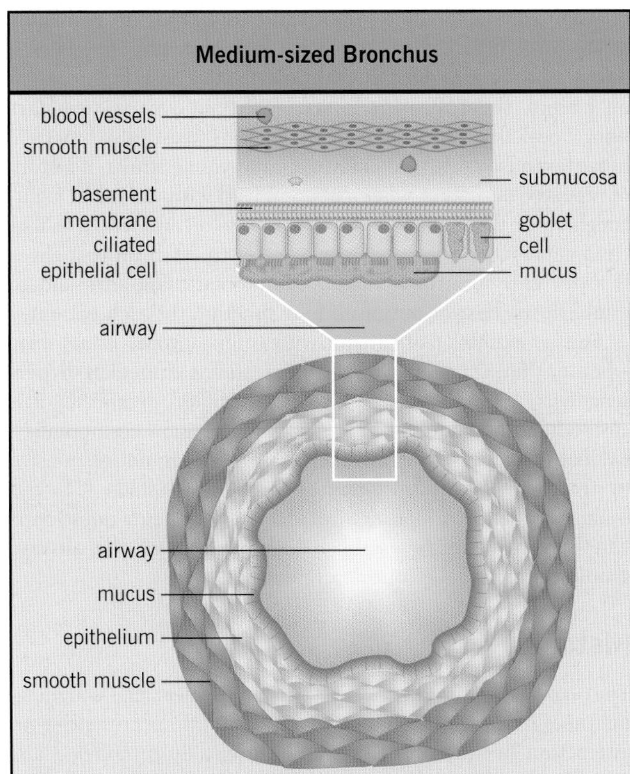

Fig. 2.6 The anatomy of a medium-sized bronchus. The changes in the bronchi that occur in asthma are: (1) increased mucus production; (2) subbasement membrane thickening; (3) epithelial desquamation; (4) submucosal edema; (5) hypertrophy of smooth muscle; (6) infiltration of submucosa and epithelium with mast cells, eosinophils, T cells and basophils.

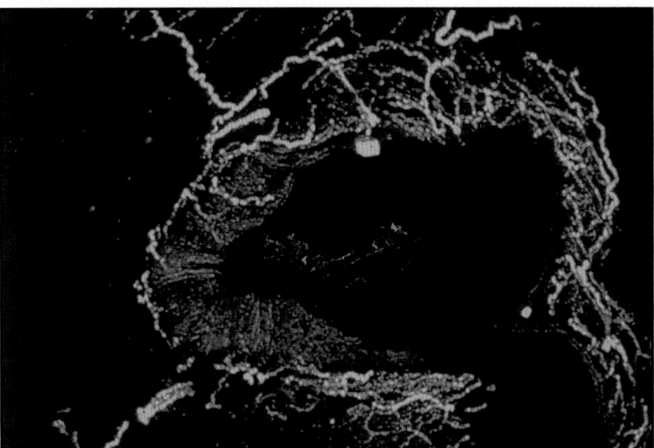

Fig. 2.7 Three-dimensional confocal microscopic reconstruction of sensory nerves surrounding a small asthmatic airway. (Courtesy of J. Polak, RPMS, London.)

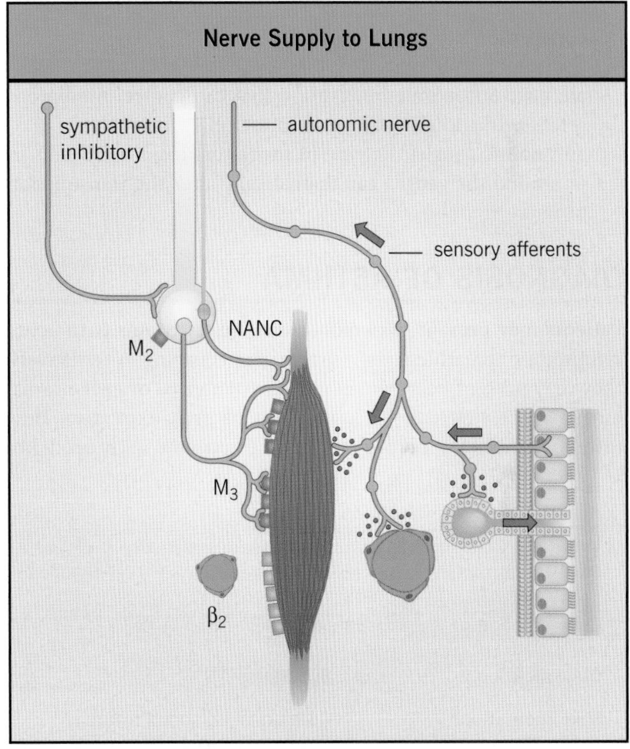

Fig. 2.8 The nerve supply to the airways. The efferent innervation of smooth muscle is cholinergic through M_3 receptors, and sympathetic inhibitory fibers act on adrenergic receptors of the parasympathetic ganglia. Inhibition of smooth muscle is through circulating epinephrine from the adrenal medulla. Activation of sensory non-myelinated fibers with axon reflexes can release neuropeptides [e.g. neurokinin A, substance P, and calcitonin gene-related peptides (CGRP)]. NANC fibers, non-adrenergic non-cholinergic fibers.

the bronchial arteries and veins provide a plexus in the submucosa and around the smooth muscles. Changes in the walls of the vessels allow edema formation and influx of inflammatory cells; in addition, simple changes in the blood vessels may contribute to the thickness of the wall.

The bronchi are lined with a mixture of ciliated and serous cells. For most of the bronchial tree, 60% of the cells are ciliated; however, in the trachea and main bronchi the epithelium is pseudostratified. The proportion of ciliated cells increases as the bronchi divide. The serous cells play a major role in controlling airway lung fluid; in addition, there are goblet cells in the epithelium and mucous glands in the bronchial wall and these goblet cells provide the mucous blanket. The best-recognized part of inflammation in asthma is an influx of eosinophils with associated damage, which includes desquamation of the epithelial cell layer (see Fig. 2.3). The response to allergens or other antigens can also include a marked increase in goblet cells and mucus production. The products of this inflammation may be demonstrable in the sputum as mucus, Charcot–Leyden crystals, eosinophil cationic protein, and whorls of desquamated epithelium (Creola bodies) which are indicative of an interaction between infiltrating eosinophils and the epithelium.

Innervation of the bronchi

The bronchi receive nerves from the parasympathetic nervous system, including efferent cholinergic fibers and non-myelinated sensory nerves (C fibers) and from the sympathetic nervous system, primarily from postganglionic adrenergic fibers to the parasympathetic ganglia; the bronchi also receive non-cholinergic, non-adrenergic (NANC) inhibitory fibers, which travel with the cholinergic fibers and provide the only direct neuronal bronchodilator pathway (Fig. 2.7). These nerves provide innervation to smooth muscle, blood vessels, mucous glands, the epithelium, and mast cells. Cholinergic fibers from local ganglia stimulate contraction of the smooth muscles and the muscarinic receptor via an M_3 receptor (Fig. 2.8). Adrenergic inhibitory control of the smooth muscle comes from two routes – noradrenaline released from postganglionic inhibitory fibers to the vagal ganglia, and epinephrine released into the circulation from the adrenal medulla. There is no direct sympathetic innervation to the smooth muscle. In addition, fibers of the NANC system run with the vagus nerve, and their postganglionic fibers innervate smooth muscle. The mediator for the NANC fibers that relaxes smooth muscle is thought to be nitric oxide.

There are two additional elements to the innervation of the bronchi, which may be relevant to the pathophysiology of asthma:

- Sensory fibers that supply the epithelium, blood vessels, and mucous glands contain several mediators, including substance P, neurokinin A, and calcitonin gene-related peptide. Release of these mediators can be triggered by axon reflexes from other sensory endings. The nerve endings can be stimulated by many inflammatory mediators, including bradykinin, mast cell tryptase and leukotrienes. Damage to the bronchial epithelium exposes sensory nerve endings and can potentially increase reflex stimulation of mucus production, vascular leakage, and smooth muscle contraction.
- Sectioning of mast cells in tissues reveals that most, if not all, have autonomic innervation that can control mediator release. In addition, there are mast cells within the autonomic ganglia. Release of mediators from mast cells in or around the ganglia can dramatically alter the transmission of nerve impulses.

DIAGNOSIS OF ASTHMA

Patients may present to clinics or emergency rooms with acute symptoms of breathlessness, wheezing, or coughing. Alternatively, they may present between episodes with normal or near-normal lungs. In the first case, measurement of peak expiratory flow rate or spirometry before and after treatment with bronchodilators will generally establish the diagnosis of reversible airway obstruction. In patients who present without physical signs in the chest or decreased airflow, the diagnosis is dependent on history, serial measurements of airflow over several days using a peak flow meter, or provocation tests to establish bronchial hyperresponsiveness. In children and in young adults, a history of repeated attacks of wheezing combined with waking at night, coughing, or wheezing may be sufficient to recommend a trial of treatment. However, it is always better to establish that there is a decrease in airflow during symptomatic episodes and to establish the best or optimum lung function for each patient.

Further evaluation of patients with asthma involves establishing whether they are allergic (with skin tests for immediate hypersensitivity, measurements of total serum IgE or specific IgE antibodies, and routine blood count focusing on eosinophilia). Evaluation of persistent or severe cases that are not responsive to treatment may also require chest X-ray, sinus CT, and evaluation of the upper airway. The more difficult question is whether any tests to establish inflammation of the airways should be part of the routine evaluation.

History

The cardinal symptoms of asthma are wheezing, coughing, tightness in the chest, and shortage of breath, representing an interaction between inflamed and chronically remodeled airways. In all patients the symptoms fluctuate in intensity, and in the majority of patients the symptoms are intermittent. Thus, most patients have normal or near-normal lung function and no symptoms between episodes. Attacks may occur spontaneously (often at night or first thing in the morning), after exercise, or shortly after exposure to a known trigger factor. In order to define the history, the patient must be questioned about the age at onset of symptoms and about the details of the attacks (Table 2.4). The history should also include details of the

Table 2.4 Classification of asthma based on severity of disease. Occasional patients have rare severe attacks (or even only one severe attack) that requires emergency treatment but have no significant symptoms otherwise

Classification of Asthma Based on Severity			
Classification	**Symptoms**	**Best FEV_1**	**Investigation**
Mild intermittent	Occasional episodes reverse spontaneously or with one dose of bronchodilator	90–100%	History only
Moderate intermittent	Occasional episodes but may require more treatment Attacks after exercise	90–100%	Peak flow meter
Mild persistent	Symptoms several times per week Attacks after exercise Requires regular treatment	> 90%	Spirometry, evaluate etiology, peak flow monitoring, CXR
Moderate persistent	Frequent symptoms, some difficult attacks Difficulty with exercise Requires regular treatment	85–95%	Evaluate causes of increasing severity
Severe persistent	Persistent symptoms requiring continuous treatment, emergency visits and/or hospitalization	60–80%	Spirometry, DLCO, Sinus CT. Re-evaluate causes including sinusitis, aspirin sensitivity, fungal infection, etc.

CT, computed tomography; CXR, chest X-ray; DLCO, diffusion capacity of the lung for carbon monoxide; FEV_1, forced expiratory volume in 1 second.

response of attacks to treatment. Evidence of severity is based on the occurrence and frequency of acute episodes, emergency room visits, or hospitalizations as well as on treatment requirements, especially the use of bronchodilators and inhaled or oral corticosteroids.

Careful questioning about factors that influence symptoms should distinguish between non-specific triggers (e.g. cold air, passive smoking, emotional events, or strong perfumes) and specific reactions that suggest that the patient is allergic (e.g. seasonal hayfever or nasal, eye, or lung symptoms following exposure to known sources of allergens such as domestic animals). Questions about seasonal variations in symptoms are important; however, some patients who are allergic to common indoor allergens do not describe seasonal variation and, conversely, some patients whose attacks are triggered by viral infection report seasonal exacerbations in the autumn. Therefore, the presence or absence of seasonality is not a basis for distinguishing between allergic and non-allergic cases. It is also helpful to ask directed questions about the environment in terms of dampness, mold, domestic animals, pests, and house furnishings. In addition, patients may be aware of reacting specifically to exposures in other houses. Similarly, it is important to know where a child spends time (e.g. other bedrooms, houses of friends or family members, day care centers).

Attacks of asthma vary from transient wheezing that recovers rapidly either spontaneously or after treatment with a bronchodilator, to episodes that develop over minutes, hours, or days into severe symptoms that are not responsive to any inhaled medicine. It is essential to know both the severity and the frequency of attacks. In many cases, chest symptoms develop without preceding evidence of an attack; however, in other cases, the attack is preceded by or associated with nasal or sinus symptoms or productive cough.

Nasal or sinus symptoms

At least half the patients who are being treated for asthma also have nasal or sinus symptoms of some kind. In many cases, the symptoms are allergic and are consistent with exposure to allergens and the pattern of positive skin tests. However, many patients report episodes of nasal pressure or pain associated with mucopurulent discharge. Patients may give a history that these symptoms respond to antibiotics. However, the history is a very poor indication of the extent of changes found on sinus CT, and some of these patients will respond to treatment for known allergic disease (i.e. allergen avoidance and local anti-inflammatory treatment).

Sinus CT should be reserved for patients who have recurrent episodes that are not responsive to treatment. However, there are many different patterns of sinus disease, and the treatment is not well defined. Extensive sinusitis on CT scan (see Fig. 2.4) is a common feature of intrinsic asthma. In such cases, nasal polyps, eosinophilia, and aspirin sensitivity are also common. Moderate degrees of sinus abnormality are common and may be associated with recurrent episodes of bacterial infection; however, it is not clear to what degree these abnormalities are associated with asthma. Furthermore, very few of these 'infections' are diagnosed bacteriologically. Sinusitis with nasal polyps is very common in cystic fibrosis and the presence of polyps should trigger a sweat test in all patients who are aged less than 25 years. Finally, sinusitis with extensive changes on CT can occur during acute rhinovirus infection. Some adults presenting with acute asthma have extensive sinus abnormalities that resolve over the following few weeks, strongly suggesting that an acute viral infection triggered the asthma attacks (Fig. 2.9).

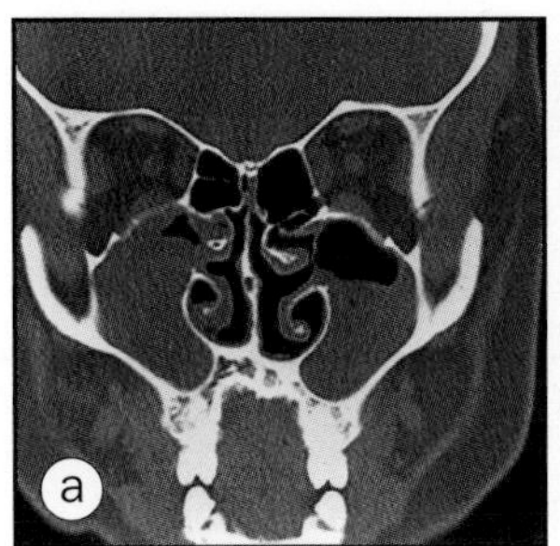

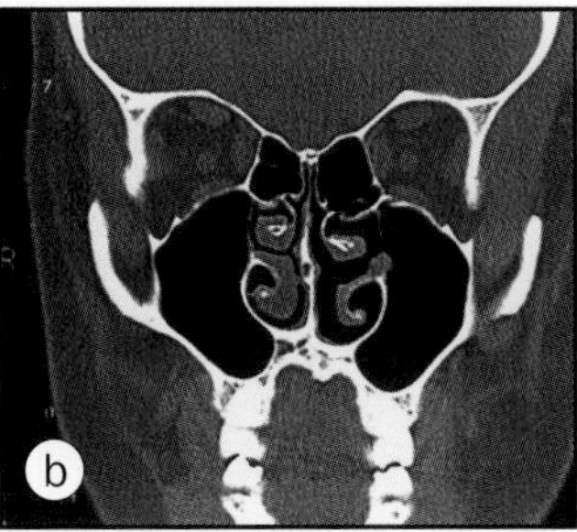

Fig. 2.9 Computed tomography (CT) scans of the sinus. (a) Scan at the time of an acute attack of asthma. (b) Scan 4 months later.

Evaluation of lung function

Clinical examination of the chest may identify wheezing, prolonged expiration, and poor air entry, but it is an unreliable method of estimating the extent of airway obstruction. The simplest technique for monitoring obstruction is the use of the peak flow meter, which measures the maximum rate of expiratory flow in liters per minute (Fig. 2.10). Peak flow meters are ideal for home monitoring because they are simple to use, inexpensive, and portable. A chart showing repeated measurements over 2 weeks may establish diurnal variation, major changes from day to day, or consistently normal values. However, the results are dependent on effort, require consistent recording by the patient or parents, and do not provide information about the pattern of flow. Spirometry provides a record of the FEV over time; this is most commonly expressed as:

- the FEV for the first second (FEV_1);
- the midflow FEV (FEV 25–75%); and
- the FVC, which is the forced volume over 6 seconds (FVC_6).

In addition, spirometry can provide visual comparison of repeated curves before and after treatment, which can yield clear evidence of reversible airway obstruction. In children or young adults with mild or moderate disease, this is sufficient to establish the diagnosis. In patients with severe disease, spirometry may demonstrate minimal reversibility following bronchodilator therapy (i.e. < 15% increase) or may demonstrate reversibility (i.e. > 15% increase) but still show marked obstruction. In such cases, further lung function studies (e.g. diffusion capacity for carbon monoxide and measurements of lung volume, both of which are normal in uncomplicated asthma) may be required to rule out other diagnoses. However, the most useful investigation is to repeat spirometry after 3 weeks' treatment with high-dose inhaled or oral corticosteroids plus bronchodilators. The diagnosis of fixed or irreversible obstruction should be considered only in patients who have obstruction after 2 or 3 weeks of such treatment.

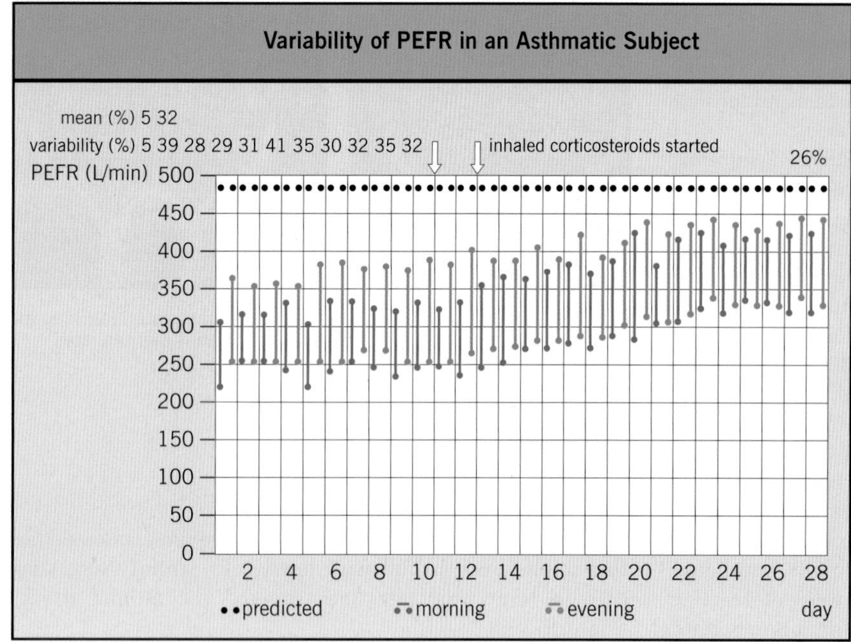

Fig. 2.10 Peak flow data. Daily peak flow records taken before and after bronchodilator in the mornings and evenings for 1 month. PEFR, peak expiratory flow rate.

Tests for bronchial hyperreactivity

In patients who have normal lung function (i.e. $FEV_1 > 90\%$ predicted), hyperreactivity or hyperresponsiveness can be demonstrated by several different provocation tests (Table 2.5). Bronchial provocation using specific allergen extract in fine droplets from a nebulizer will produce acute airway obstruction in sensitive patients. However, a similar response, generally requiring a higher dose, occurs in allergic patients who do not have asthma. Furthermore, allergens to which people are exposed naturally are in the form of particles that vary in diameter from 2 μm to 20 μm, not in the form of nebulized droplets (Fig. 2.11). Thus, bronchial challenge with allergen is not a test for asthma and provides little clinical information that cannot be obtained from skin tests. Non-specific challenge tests to identify bronchial hyperresponsiveness include exercise, inhalation of dry or cold air, histamine, and methacholine.

Exercise challenge

Four minutes of exercise that is sufficiently vigorous to increase the heart rate to 80% of maximum, or random running, will generally be enough to provoke a fall in FEV_1 or peak flow in patients with bronchial hyperreactivity. This test of bronchial hyperresponsiveness is dependent on evaporation from the respiratory tract, and humidification of the inspiratory air will prevent the response. In turn this means that results are very strongly influenced by ambient humidity.

Cold air challenge

Using cold air (which is by definition dry) for the challenge achieves a very similar effect by inducing evaporation from the lungs, and it is easier to control the conditions of the challenge. Whether exercise or cold air challenge induces mediator release is not entirely clear, because it has proved difficult to measure mediators in the lung after challenge. On the other hand, these responses can be inhibited by cromolin, nedocromil, corticosteroids, or leukotriene antagonists, which strongly suggests that mediator release is involved.

Histamine challenge

Histamine challenge to demonstrate bronchial hyperreactivity was first introduced by Samter in 1935 and adapted by Tifeneau in 1949. There are many different techniques, including tidal breathing over 2 minutes, sequential puffs from a hand-held inhaler, and the use of a dosimeter. The techniques are different in that the response of the lungs to challenge is altered by full inspiratory maneuvers. The advantage of histamine is that it is a natural substance and has a very short half-life in vivo. The disadvantage is that it can cause unpleasant flushing. As with all challenges, histamine challenge can cause rapid increases in lung resistance; it should therefore be started at a low dose, and it requires medical supervision.

Methacholine challenge

Methacholine is an analog of the cholinergic mediator for smooth muscle contraction in the lung. The assumption is that methacholine challenge works by acting on smooth muscle, although there are other possible pathways and in vitro experiments do not demonstrate very marked hyperresponsiveness of smooth muscle from patients with asthma. A concept that goes some way towards explaining bronchial hyperresponsiveness is thickening of the airway wall. In the submucosa, this thickening will lead to a disproportionate reduction in airway caliber for a given degree of airway smooth muscle shortening; in the adventitia outside the smooth muscle, it will distribute elastic contractile forces over a greater surface area and therefore reduce protection from airway closure. Nonetheless, methacholine provides consistent bronchial challenge results and is very

Table 2.5 Provocation tests for specific and non-specific bronchial reactivity

Tests for Bronchial Reactivity	Response Immediate–15 min	Response Late 2–8 hours	Depends on BHR	Blocked by	Mechanism
Specific:					
Relevant allergen	++	++	No	Cromolyn, etc.	Triggering of mast cells through specific IgE
Non-specific:					
Exercise or cold air	++	±	Yes	Cromolyn, etc. Antileukotrienes short- and long-acting β_2-agonist	Evaporation of water → hyperosmolar triggering
Histamine*	++	No	Yes	Antihistamine	Direct action on blood vessels, muscles, etc.
Methacholine*	++	No	Yes	Anticholinergics	Direct action on smooth muscles
Others:*					
Water	++	No	Yes	Cromolyn, etc.	
Hypertonic saline	++	No	Yes	Cromolyn, etc.	
Adenosine	++	No	Yes	Theophylline, cromolin nedocromil	
SO_2	++	No	±	Nedocromil, cromolin	

*Given as nebulized drops approximately 2 µm in diameter.

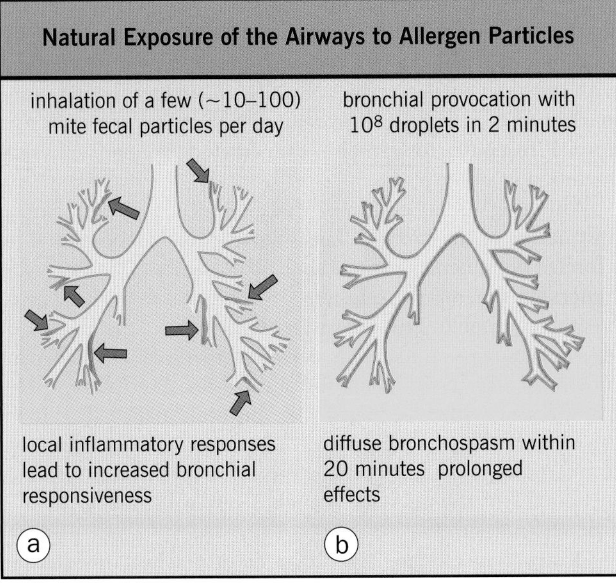
Natural Exposure of the Airways to Allergen Particles
inhalation of a few (~10–100) mite fecal particles per day
bronchial provocation with 10^8 droplets in 2 minutes
local inflammatory responses lead to increased bronchial responsiveness
diffuse bronchospasm within 20 minutes prolonged effects
a
b

Fig. 2.11 Lung exposure. (a) The natural exposure of the airways to allergen particles – inhalation of a few (10–100) mite fecal particles per day. Local inflammatory responses lead to increased bronchial responsiveness. (b) Exposure to nebulized extract or histamine – bronchial provocation with $\geq 10^8$ droplets in 2 minutes. There is diffuse bronchospasm within 20 minutes, with or without prolonged effects.

widely used for routine clinical testing (Fig. 2.12). The standard technique uses a dosimeter, but it can also be given by tidal breathing. Methacholine challenge is well tolerated and recovery after challenge is rapid.

With all testing of non-specific bronchial hyperresponsiveness, it is assumed that the test does not itself increase bronchial hyperresponsiveness. This is in contrast to allergen challenge, which can produce a late reaction (after 6 hours) and is often followed by prolonged increases in bronchial hyperresponsiveness. With histamine challenge there have been no reports of late reactions or persistent effects on the lung. Most exercise challenges are not followed by late reactions. However, the response to exercise is thought to involve mediator release, and there have been occasional reports of late reactions. Thus it is legitimate to ask whether repeated exercise challenge that results in bronchoconstriction will increase non-specific bronchial hyperresponsiveness. The evidence about methacholine challenge is less clear than that about histamine, because there have been occasional reports of prolonged effects following repeated challenges.

Other causes of intermittent symptoms that suggest asthma

Asthma is characterized by widespread inflammation of the bronchi, with hyperreactivity that is present in all lobes of the

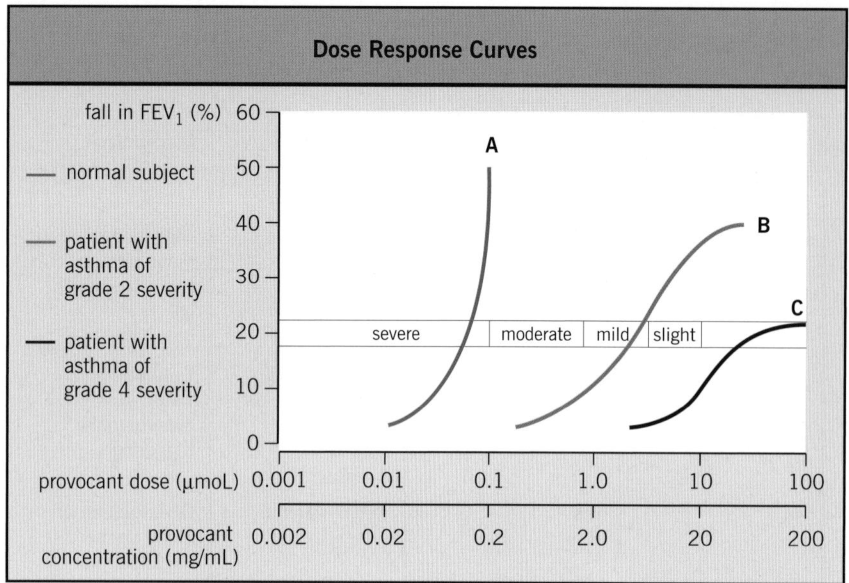

Fig. 2.12 The response of the airways to methacholine challenge. Fall in FEV_1 plotted against amount of provocant (methacholine) that causes that fall.

lung. In keeping with this, most diseases that involve localized obstruction, cardiac or other medical causes of shortage of breath, and simple hyperventilation do not present with the typical history of asthma or with typical reversible spirometry. Nonetheless, many patients present in a sufficiently unusual way that they are diagnosed as having asthma and may be erroneously treated for asthma. These alternative diagnoses can be classified as:

- medical conditions involving the lungs that present with symptoms suggestive of asthma;
- syndromes characterized by abnormal breathing in which the lungs are structurally normal; and
- cases of local airway obstruction that present with wheezing that is audible to the patient or on examination.

On occasion, asthma may present solely as cough without evidence of airway obstruction or bronchial hyperreactivity. In this 'cough variant' form, sputum eosinophilia is invariably present.

Many different medical conditions present with cough or shortage of breath (with or without wheezing) and can easily be confused with asthma. These include:

- cardiac failure with acute pulmonary edema;
- cardiac failure secondary to myocardial infarction;
- pulmonary embolism;
- pneumonia; and
- tracheobronchitis.

Chest pain may confuse the situation because anterior chest pain is fairly common in severe cases of asthma. This pain in adults routinely induces work-up for myocardial infarction. The distinction from pulmonary edema is important because narcotics are contraindicated in asthma. Similarly, the recognition of pulmonary embolism as a cause of wheezing and shortage of breath is very important because heparin is life saving in pulmonary embolus. Bronchitis secondary to bacterial or viral infection can produce symptoms that are very similar to the symptoms of that minority of patients with asthma who present primarily with a cough or who have a productive cough.

There are several conditions that present as shortage of breath in which the lungs are not abnormal. The commonest of these is hyperventilation syndrome. If the patient makes severe expiratory noises, these noises are often interpreted as wheezing. However, such patients will have normal spirometry if they can be persuaded to comply. In addition, they have blood gases that are typical of hyperventilation (i.e. normal pO_2 and very low pCO_2). Paradoxical closure of the vocal cords on expiration, the so-called vocal cord syndrome, may present with typical symptoms, but in many cases it is difficult to diagnose. Improvement in symptoms while talking, inconsistent pulmonary function tests, and an absence of markers of atopy or inflammation (i.e. eosinophil count $< 0.01 \times 10^9$/L, or exhaled nitric oxide parts per billion) are all suggestive. The diagnosis should also be considered in patients who rapidly recover fully normal lung function and do not respond consistently to treatment with systemic corticosteroids. Finally, an apparently increasing number of normal people present with shortage of breath as a normal response to exercise exacerbated by poor physical condition or obesity.

Wheezing is a common feature of localized partial obstruction of the bronchi. Local obstruction can be caused by a foreign body, benign tumors such as an adenoma, or malignant tumors. In general, these lesions do not give rise to shortage of breath or variable airway resistance. However, the degree of obstruction may vary with associated inflammation. Malignant tumors are usually visible on the chest X-ray; alternatively, they may present with bleeding. However, even malignant tumors can occasionally present as airway obstruction that is responsive to treatment, including corticosteroids. In doubtful cases, fine-section CT of the chest or bronchoscopy will usually reveal a local obstruction.

Obstruction of the large bronchi or trachea can also be caused by the rare syndrome of bronchomalacia or tracheomalacia, and in some cases the obstruction is intermittent. This diagnosis should also be clear on chest CT. Obstruction of the trachea (e.g. by a tumor) outside the chest can present with symptoms of shortage of breath, but the primary finding is usually inspiratory stridor.

MANAGEMENT OF ASTHMA

The fluctuating nature of airway obstruction in asthma means that patients have to play a major role in controlling the symptoms themselves and therefore have to make appropriate decisions. Effective education early in the course of the disease can create a well-informed, confident patient (or parent) who will manage the disease (Table 2.6). This allows less interruption of normal life, better long-term outcome, and dramatically reduces use of emergency services. The essence of a management plan is that:

- it is simple and effective at controlling symptoms;
- it has minimum risk of severe side-effects; and
- it will achieve the best long-term outcome in terms of lung function.

Table 2.6 Role of education in asthma management

Asthma Management

1. Education about the nature of the disease and the distinction between causes of inflammation and triggers of acute shortage of breath
2. Techniques for using inhaler, spacers and nebulizers, distinction between those inhalers that help to control the disease and bronchodilators suitable for short-term use
3. Home monitoring:
   - Use of peak flow meter
   - Establish normal variability and personal best
   - Regular monitoring in a minority of cases only
   - Use of meter to help assess attacks and to design response to attacks
4. Side-effects of asthma medications:
   - Excess bronchodilator use
   - Inhaled steroids
   - Oral steroids
   - Theophylline
5. Action plan for treating exacerbations
6. Measures to decrease exposure
   - Education on relevant avoidance measures: dust mites, domestic animals, cockroach, fungi, pollens, etc.

This requires an evaluation of severity (see the history and diagnosis sections above) based on frequency of attacks, severity of attacks, and previous response to treatment. One of the greatest difficulties is encouraging patients to comply with preventative measures when their symptoms are relatively well controlled. A clear understanding of the nature of asthma and the objectives of treatment is therefore of great value. Effective management of asthma requires a partnership between the patient and the health professional.

Drug treatment

The primary classification of drugs used in asthma (Table 2.7) recognizes:

- bronchodilators, which can relieve symptoms rapidly (relievers); and
- antiinflammatory drugs, which decrease the underlying inflammation in the lungs, and therefore can control symptoms over a longer period of time (controllers).

None of the currently available drugs can be said to offer a cure for the disease. There are several drugs that defy classification but play an important role in some cases. In particular these include:

- theophylline, which may act as an A2b-adenosine antagonist and as a phosphodiesterase inhibitor;

Table 2.7 Properties of the commonly used asthma drugs

Commonly-Used Asthma Drugs

	Action			Protects against			
				Exercise	Allergen		
Steroids	**Route**	**Controls**	**Bronchodilators**		**Early**	**Late**	**Frequency/ dosage**
Steroids	Inhaled	+ + +	–	+	–	+ +	Daily/b.i.d
	Oral	+ + +	–	–	–	+ +	Daily
Cromolin	Inhaled	+	–	+ +	+ +	+	q.i.d.
Nedocromil sodium						+ +	
β_2 – Adrenergic agonist	Inhaled	–	+ + +	+ + +	+ +		As needed
	Oral	–	+ +	nr	nr	–	t.i.d.
	Injected					nr	
Long-acting β_2-adrenergic agonist (LABA)	Inhaled	+ +	+ +	+ + +	+ +	+ +	b.i.d., nocturnal, or before exercise
Theophylline	Oral	+ +	+	+	+	–	b.i.d., or as needed
Ipratropium bromide	Inhaled	–	+	+ +	–	–	t.i.d.
Leukotriene antagonists	Oral	+ + or ±	±	+ +	–	–	Daily or b.i.d.

nr, Not relevant.

- salmeterol and formoterol, which are long-acting β_2-agonists; and
- the recently introduced leukotriene-modifying drugs, including both receptor antagonists (montelukast, zafirlukast) and 5-lipoxygenase inhibitors (zileuton), which may have both bronchodilator and controlling effects.

β_2-Adrenergic agonists

β_2-Adrenergic agonists are the primary treatment for bronchospasm both in daily life and in the emergency situation. The inhaled, short-acting β_2-selective agonists generally act within 10 minutes and are very effective at relieving symptoms. Almost all patients with asthma should be taught how to use an inhaler and provided with one. However, these agonists have no controlling effects, and there is some evidence that excessive use of adrenergic agonists without an anti-inflammatory drug can increase bronchial hyperreactivity. In most cases β_2-adrenergic agonists should be prescribed for use in response to increased symptoms or decreased peak flow. In addition, patients should be told that they may need alternative or additional treatment if they require more than two or three doses of bronchodilator per week. Long acting β_2-agonists (LABAs) are used as a supplement to inhaled corticosteroids in patients who remain symptomatic despite moderate to high doses of corticosteroids. They may be administered separately twice daily or as combination therapy with an inhaled corticosteroid in a single inhaler device. LABAs should never be given in the absence of inhaled corticosteroid.

Inhaled cromolin sodium

In 1970, cromolin sodium was shown to control the increase in bronchial hyperreactivity that can occur in allergic patients during the pollen season. In addition, cromolin sodium can protect against the effects of exercise challenge and against both the immediate and delayed effects of allergen bronchial challenge. Although the antiinflammatory or controlling effects of this drug are considered to take 2 weeks for full effect, the protective effect against a challenge is present in 20 minutes. Regular inhaled cromolin sodium provides effective long-term control of asthma in many children, but it needs to be given frequently (four times per day) for optimum effects.

Inhaled corticosteroids

Corticosteroid inhalers (dry powder or metered dose inhalers) have become the primary antiinflammatory treatment for adults and are very widely used in children. Systemically active corticosteroids (e.g. prednisone or dexamethasone) can be inhaled, but the corticosteroids currently used have been developed specifically for local use in the nose or lungs. These modifications are designed to increase local bioavailability and decrease systemic side-effects. The details of local action, absorption, and systemic half-life are different for each preparation.

Local steroids should be used on a regular basis once or twice daily but can also be used as part of an action plan. Regular dosage in children should be kept below 800 μg per day to minimize systemic side-effects. In mild exacerbations the dose can be doubled, and in significant attacks the dose should be increased up to 2 mg per day (i.e. 800 μg of budesonide, or equivalent dose of flunisolide or fluticasone three times per day). In the case of metered dose inhalers, large volume spacers are advised to reduce oropharyngeal deposition (and therefore the swallowed dose) and to increase the efficiency of intrapulmonary deposition.

New treatment with antiimmunoglobulin E antibody in allergic asthma

Treatment of adult and pediatric allergic moderate-to-severe asthma with humanized monoclonal anti-IgE antibody (omalizumab) results in the decrease in asthma exacerbation rates and usage of inhaled and oral corticosteroids. In addition, improvements of lung function, asthma symptoms, and asthma-related quality of life were observed. Treatment with omalizumab leads to decreased IgE levels and partial inhibition of early and late asthmatic responses after allergen bronchoprovocation in allergic asthma. In a range of studies omalizumab also shows reductions in multiple markers of airway inflammation, including eosinophils and high-affinity receptors for IgE. Although omalizumab is more expensive than other controller medications for asthma, it has been demonstrated to save overall treatment costs when used for a restricted group of patients with severe asthma.

Specific immunotherapy (SIT) is effective in patients with allergic rhinitis and allergic asthma if adequate doses of allergens are administered. However, the risks of systemic anaphylactic reactions must be considered. Therefore, treatment with both SIT and omalizumab would provide better clinical efficacy with less adverse events than either treatment given alone. Indeed, a recent clinical study of combined treatment with omalizumab and SIT in polysensitized children and adolescents with seasonal allergic rhinitis showed that combined treatment was more effective than SIT alone by decreasing symptom loads during the pollen season. Therefore, anti-IgE antibody represents a novel therapeutic approach for severe allergic asthma.

Management plans

There is no shortage of guidelines for asthma treatment and all of the national and international guidelines include progressive increases in therapy based on severity. However, many other factors influence the design of treatment plans, including past experience with different drugs, the patient's enthusiasm for, compliance with, and prejudice against corticosteroid inhalers, economics, and the patient's level of anxiety about the symptoms. Effective management of patients with moderate or severe persistent disease includes the use of many different drugs. In addition, it may be necessary to tolerate rather poor control if the patient is emotionally or intellectually opposed to some forms of treatment or close monitoring.

The introduction of guidelines for the management of asthma has moved the control of airway inflammation with a combination of environmental measures and controller drugs to the center of management. In order to target therapy effectively, it is important to assess the severity of the asthma. Classifying symptoms as intermittent or persistent and then recognizing attacks as mild, moderate, or severe gives rise to five major groups (Table 2.8). Needless to say, there are many cases that do not fit these groups. However, the key steps involved in management are:

- Does the patient have asthma? If so, establish best lung function, and educate on home monitoring.
- Provide a method of relief of symptoms, plus education about the use of inhalers and how to respond to attacks.

Table 2.8 Severity-based asthma treatment. Skin tests, or in vitro assays plus specific advice; immunotherapy in seasonal cases related to pollen and other highly allergic cases

Severity-Based Asthma Treatment

	Treatment plan			
Symptoms	**β_2-Agonist short acting**	**Regular**	**Action plan**	**Education steps from Table 2.6**
Intermittent: Occasional symptoms or only after exercise	p.r.n.	Not necessary	No	1 and 2
Symptoms 2–3 times per week	p.r.n.	In some cases	+ or –	1,2,3, (6)
Persistent: Mild to moderate	p.r.n.	Cromolin inhaled steroid/ theophylline	Yes	2,3,4, (5), 6
Moderate with attacks	p.r.n.	Inhaled steroids and others	Yes	1,2,3,4,5,6
Severe	p.r.n.	High-dose inhaled steroids and others	Yes	1,2,3,4,5,6

p.r.n., as required.

Table 2.9 Examples of an action plan

Action Plans

Case A. Intermittent symptoms with occasional episodes of prolonged wheezing

1. Take bronchodilator, two puffs, repeated every hour until symptoms improve. [Use peak flow meter if available.]
2. If deteriorating or no improvement after 4 hours, consult physician or call emergency number. [Take action if peak flow is < 80% of best]

Case B. Persistent symptoms with mild to moderate attacks several times per year

1. Increase bronchodilator either from an inhaler or nebulizer. Measure peak flow.
2. If no response [i.e. peak flow ≤ 80% of best] increase treatment:
 – maintain increased dose of bronchodilator;
 – increase or add high dose inhaled steroids, up to 3000 μg/day BDP or equivalent;
 – add delayed release oral theophylline, 300 mg in the evening or 200–300 mg t.i.d.
3. If no response within 2 days or deterioration, consult physician or call emergency number

Case C. Persistent symptoms with severe attacks requiring emergency treatment or oral steroids

1. Increased inhaled steroids promptly if symptoms not responsive to bronchodilator; dose increased up to at least 3000 μg/day BDP or equivalent
2. Add oral theophylline to maximum tolerated dose to give blood level 10–15 μg/mL
3. If deteriorating or no response within 24 hours and peak flow persistently < 70% of best, start or increase oral steroids. Using standard dosage, i.e. 50 mg/day for 6 days, or 60 mg tailing to 10 mg over 12 days. Consult physician if starting oral steroids. Seek advice if not responding within 24 hours on steroids

Emergency telephone numbers will depend on the system but all patients with asthma should know how to obtain emergency advice or treatment. Some patients start attacks with increased sinus symptoms and may require antibiotics. However, antibiotics are not part of the normal management of acute attacks of asthma. All patients who receive courses of corticosteroids should be fully educated about the acute and chronic side-effects of these drugs. BDP = beclomethasone dipropionate.

- Does the patient need regular treatment?
  - inhaled, or oral, controlling drugs on a daily basis;
  - skin testing combined with education about the role of allergens and methods for avoidance.
- Assess the requirement for additional treatment:
  - management of exercise-induced exacerbations;
  - increased treatment in patients with persistent symptoms;
  - specific action plans.

Action plans

Patients who have persistent symptoms, with or without exacerbations, should be given an action plan to guide their self-management. In most cases, the plan should be written down (Table 2.9). However, the plans vary a great deal depending on the severity of disease and the level of understanding of the patients. The simplest action plan is for the patient to take extra puffs of bronchodilator if they feel 'tight' and to call their doctor if symptoms do not resolve within 3–4 hours. By contrast, for patients who are prone to severe attacks, the action plan will include indications for:

- increasing bronchodilators;
- increasing routine treatment (usually in terms of changes in peak expiratory flow rate);
- adding other medications, such as long-acting β_2-agonists, theophylline, or nebulized bronchodilator; and
- increasing inhaled corticosteroids and starting oral corticosteroids.

Although many clinics have printed action plans, these cannot replace education, including discussion of each step with the patient. Writing the plan down with the patient is more effective than using preprinted forms since a clear understanding of the steps required to control asthma in its different phases is essential for good management. Time spent explaining an asthma plan is time well spent.

Allergen avoidance

The majority of children and young adults with asthma are allergic to one or more of the common inhaled allergens. Evidence that inhalation of these allergens contributes to the disease has come both from the demonstration that allergen challenge can produce the inflammation that is typical of asthma, and studies on allergen avoidance. The avoidance studies in sanatoria, hospital rooms, and patients' houses have shown that decreased exposure to dust mites can improve symptoms and non-specific bronchial hyperreactivity (Table 2.10). In addition, it has been shown that reductions in bronchial hyperresponsiveness are paralleled by decreased numbers of eosinophils in induced sputum. The logical conclusion is that allergen avoidance is the primary form of antiinflammatory treatment for asthma. Certainly it should be included in the management of all allergic patients with persistent symptoms.

Although many different allergens can contribute to asthma (see Table 2.3), the dominant allergens in most studies have been those that are found indoors. Furthermore, the measures that can decrease exposure to outdoor pollens and molds are not well established. The measures for decreasing exposure in houses are allergen specific. The techniques for reducing exposure to dust mites are almost completely different from those that are useful in controlling exposure to domestic animals or the allergens derived from the German cockroach. The conclusion is that advice about avoidance is dependent on identifying the specific sensitivity of the patient. Since histories are not a reliable method of defining immediate hypersensitivity, advice on avoidance should reflect the results of skin testing or serum assays for IgE antibodies. Skin testing using prick or lancet techniques is simple, safe, and highly informative for most of the major allergen sources (see Ch. 1). Serum assays using the radioallergosorbent technique or modifications of this test are generally less sensitive. However, in vitro assays provide a reliable test with less discomfort for the patient, can be standardized, and – for some allergens such as molds – may be more sensitive.

The primary problem in allergen avoidance is encouraging the patient to carry out the recommended steps, which by the very nature of the intervention will only be beneficial over the long term. In the case of occupational asthma, when there is clear identification of a sensitizing chemical, removal of the patient from areas of exposure is relatively straightforward. However, with asthma that is activated by major allergens, avoidance becomes more difficult. Without detailed education about both the objectives and the practical steps, patients are unlikely to carry out measures that require effort and expense. Thus, as with so many aspects of asthma management, the success is dependent on adequate education and full involvement by the patient and the patient's family.

Table 2.10 Measures recommended for allergen avoidance. These recommendations are only for patients who have been demonstrated to be allergic on the basis of skin tests or in vitro assays for IgE antibodies

Measures Recommended for Allergen Avoidance
Dust mites
Bedrooms:
Impermeable covers for mattress and pillows
Wash all bedding regularly at 130°F/60°C
Vacuum clean weekly (wearing a mask)
Remove carpets, stuffed animals and clutter
Rest of house:
Minimize carpets and upholstered furniture
Reduce humidity
Treat carpets with benzyl benzoate or tannic acid
Cats and dogs
Keep animals outside, or remove
Reduce reservoirs and clean weekly
Room air filters with HEPA quality
Wash animal weekly to reduce allergen going in reservoirs or airborne
Cockroaches
Obsessional cleaning to remove accumulated allergen and control all food sources
Bait stations, bait paste and/or boric acid
Close up cracks, etc. to reduce sites for breeding

HEPA, high-efficiency particulate air filter.

Exercise

The ability of patients to be able to participate in normal exercise is a special concern in management (and sometimes the primary concern). It is one of the best markers of good control and also a primary aspect of the long-term health of the patient. Physical exercise is good for human beings including those who have asthma. In addition, many patients and physicians agree that exercise is specifically good for asthma.

A regimen for controlling exercise-induced bronchospasm is part of the management plan for all patients. Examples of such regimens might be:

- two puffs of a short-acting β_2-agonist 10 minutes before exercise;
- two puffs of cromolin sodium or nedocromil sodium 20 minutes before exercise plus two puffs of a β_2-agonist immediately before exercise; or
- a long-acting β_2-agonist 1 hour before exercise – both salmeterol and formoterol are long-acting β_2-agonists and are of special value in patients with exercise-induced asthma but should not be taken in the absence of an inhaled corticosteroid.

Recent studies indicate that the leukotriene receptor antagonists (e.g. montelukast, pranlukast) are effective in controlling exercise-induced asthma. However, it is important to recognize that the response to exercise is a reflection of non-specific bronchial hyperresponsiveness; in cases that are not easily controlled, treatment should be directed at the underlying inflammation of the lungs. This can include specific allergen avoidance, regular treatment with leukotriene antagonists, and inhaled cromolin sodium, theophylline, or inhaled corticosteroids (each of which have been shown to help control the response to exercise).

In addition, all patients should be encouraged to establish a plan for normal exercise. The important principle in exercise is that slow warming up, walking or jogging, decreases subsequent responses to more vigorous exercise. Thus, all patients should design a regimen, including pretreatment if necessary, for prolonged (i.e. more than 30 minutes), regular exercise that they can do without developing bronchospasm.

OUTCOMES OF ASTHMA – NATURAL COURSE AND THE IMPACT OF MANAGEMENT

In most patients, the long-term outcome of asthma is good. Only a small minority of patients who experience wheezing and require treatment will develop severe disease. In childhood, remission is common, although some of this may relate to misdiagnosis of virus-induced wheezing or asthma. Although up to 70% of patients have a complete remission, many of these patients will still have bronchial hyperresponsiveness and some will relapse. The factors that influence remission and relapse are poorly understood. However, highly allergic children (especially those with ongoing eczema) and those who experience symptoms before the age of 3 years are less likely to have a remission. In a birth cohort in Dunedin, New Zealand, the risk factors for persistence of asthma from childhood to adulthood or for relapse after remission during adolescence were sensitization to house dust mites, airway hyperresponiveness to methacholine, female sex, smoking, and early age at onset. When asthma starts in adult life, it is more likely to become severe and less likely to remit.

Although most physicians believe that good management influences the long-term outcome of asthma, this has not yet been proven. Until recently there was very little evidence that medical management had decreased rates of hospitalization or mortality. It is now clear that the introduction of inhaled corticosteroids has played an important role in decreasing hospitalization for asthma in Scandinavia. By contrast, in many areas of the world (e.g. the UK, Australia, Japan, and major cities of the USA) asthma remains severe, and it is not clear that management has yet made a major impact. It is commonly implied that the severity of the disease is primarily due to poor medical care and that the full application of the guidelines for the management of asthma would reverse the present situation. The equally plausible view is that the disease has become both more common and more severe.

Another important factor is the influence of the Th2-mediated inflammation on the formed airway elements, leading to remodeling. This would explain why drugs such as the long-acting β_2-agonists and leukotriene receptor antagonists, when added to a regimen of inhaled corticosteroids in moderate to severe asthma, are more efficacious than simply doubling the dose of inhaled corticosteroid (Fig. 2.13).

Most patients with intermittent asthma have normal or near-normal lung function between attacks. By contrast, patients with moderate or severe persistent disease often have an FEV_1 of < 80% of the predicted value. Follow-up of adults with persistent symptoms of asthma has found accelerated decline in lung function comparable to that of smokers. The nature of

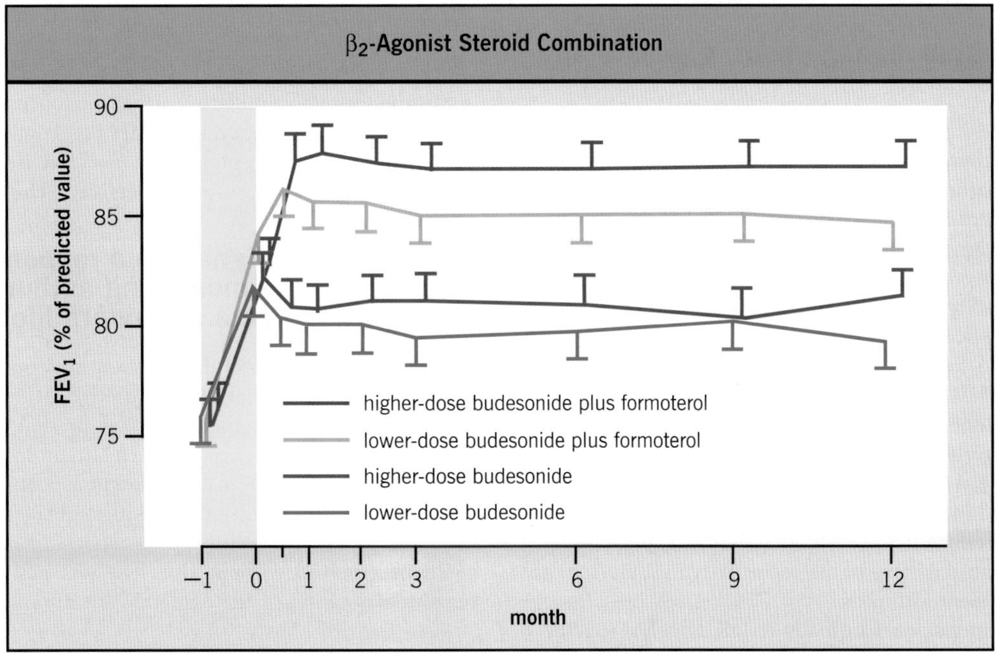

Fig. 2.13 The effect of adding the long-acting inhaled β_2-adrenoceptor agonist formoterol on to high- and low-dose inhaled budesonide on FEV_1, as an index of airway caliber in a 12-month randomized controlled trial in symptomatic asthma (the FACET study). [Modified from Pauwels RA, Lofdahl CG, Postma DS, et al. Effect of inhaled formoterol and budesonide on exacerbations of asthma. Formoterol and Corticosteroids Establishing Therapy (FACET) International Study Group. N Engl J Med 1997; 337(20):405–411.]

the long-term damage is not clear. There are changes in the lungs of children and adults with asthma that are more marked in those who have had disease for many years. These include the deposition of repair collagens (types I, III, and V) beneath the basement membrane of the bronchi. These changes, which are sometimes described as 'remodeling', are thought to occur secondary to the release of cytokines, growth factors and other mediators from mast cells, T cells, eosinophils and epithelial cells. This has led to the view that aggressive early anti-inflammatory treatment should improve long-term outcome. However, it has not been established that the changes seen in the lung structure are the cause of the decreased lung function, or that early use of inhaled antiinflammatory drugs will prevent these changes. There is, however, good evidence for proliferative responses of epithelial cells, fibroblasts, smooth muscle cells, and blood vessels. The challenge that now faces us is to determine the mechanisms and significance of this.

Chronic airway inflammation is a major cause of symptoms and abnormal airway physiology in asthma, even in mild disease. Since this inflammation might lead to changes in airway structure (remodeling), causing irreversible airflow limitation and persistent symptoms, the long-term effect of early intervention with inhaled corticosteroids in patients with mild persistent asthma of recent onset was investigated in the START study (inhaled steroid treatment as regular therapy in early asthma study). Long-term, once-daily treatment with low-dose inhaled corticosteroids decreased the risk of severe exacerbations and improved asthma control in these patients with mild persistent asthma. Although the benefit of inhaled corticosteroids was also noted in lung function measurements, the accelerated decline in lung function over time was only partially prevented by this treatment. It is thus tempting to speculate that, besides chronic airway inflammation, other pathways could be involved in the pathogenesis of airway remodeling.

NEW APPROACHES TO THERAPY

Pharmaceutical management: agonists and antagonists

Given the evidence that asthma is an inflammatory disease, it is logical to try to manage the disease by blocking the mediators of the inflammatory response. Examples of this approach are the development of cromolin sodium, delayed-release theophylline, leukotriene antagonists, leukotriene synthesis inhibitors, and the locally active corticosteroids. Many different approaches are being developed that range from traditional antagonists to antisense DNA. These approaches include the development of:

- highly active, low-molecular-weight vascular cell adhesion molecule-1 (VCAM-1) antagonists that can prevent eosinophil adhesion;
- a soluble interleukin-4 (IL-4) receptor that can block the activity of IL-4 in vivo, which is in clinical trials;
- a humanized monoclonal antibody to IL-5 that can effectively reduce blood eosinophil numbers, but fails to improve clinical indices of disease activity in subjects with severe persistent asthma;
- humanized monoclonal antibody to IgE, which is specific for the site on human IgE that binds to the high-affinity IgE receptor on mast cells – this molecule has already shown promise in clinical trials; and is currently licensed for use in severe allergic asthma in the USA and Europe. Omalizumab is administered subcutaneously as an injection once every month or two weeks depending upon the total serum IgE level and body weight. Omalizumab is the first therapy that specifically targets the IgE molecule.
- antisense DNA, which is designed to block the production of target mediators or their receptors – short sections of DNA that are antisense will block DNA transcription, and, in theory, antisense DNA can be delivered as a pharmaceutical agent directly to the lung and would be active for a period of days.
- anti-TNF therapy for severe disease.

Altering the immune response – immune deviation versus immunotherapy

The best defined target for traditional immunotherapy is the allergen-specific CD4+ T cell. Many different approaches have been proposed to act on these T cells or to deviate the response before initial exposure to allergen (Fig. 2.14).

Recombinant allergens can be modified by random or site-directed mutagenesis in such a way that they have greatly reduced reactivity with specific IgE antibodies but maintain T-cell responses. These molecules would presumably provide a safer version of traditional immunotherapy.

In animal models, DNA plasmids have shown promise both as a method of replacing deficient genes and also as a method of providing transient expression of foreign proteins. Furthermore, the DNA in plasmids includes immunostimulatory signals that can influence the immune response in the direction of either a helper T cells type 1 (Th1) or a Th2 response. Thus DNA plasmids, including the gene for an allergen, can be designed to alter an existing immune response.

Modifying the immune response could be achieved either by immunizing children before they make a natural response or by altering an existing response. Typical approaches are:

- to give nasal or oral immunization to at-risk children, using native protein, in order to try to induce tolerance;
- to immunize with antigen linked to IL-12, which will create a Th1 bias; or
- to use immunostimulatory signal sequences of DNA, such as synthetic oligodeoxynucleotides that contain CpG motifs, linked directly to proteins; the objective is to create a Th1 response that will prevent or replace a Th2 response.

Approaches designed as a response to the epidemiology of increasing asthma – how to reverse the effects of modern life

The increase in the prevalence of asthma and its morbidity during the second half of the twentieth century is such that at least three-quarters of the cases that present to clinics or to hospitals would not have required treatment in the 1950s. This increase correlates with many different aspects of modern life. We do not want to reverse the conquest of the major infectious diseases; however, there are some aspects of modern life that could be reversed without risk. The changes that have been suggested as causes of the epidemic are summarized below.

Changes in housing

Changes in housing that were designed to make houses more comfortable but that have increased exposure to indoor

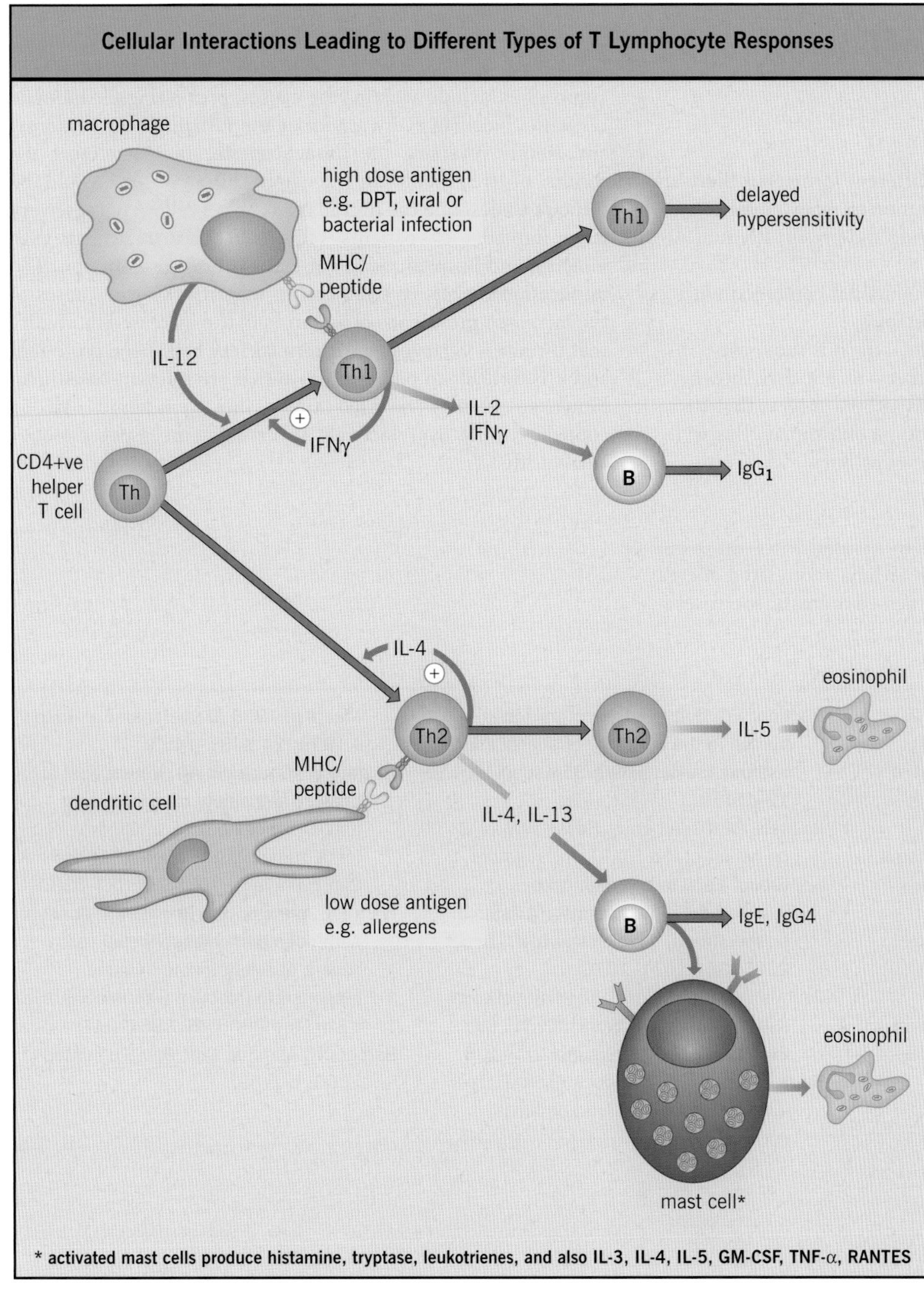

Fig. 2.14 Cellular interactions leading to different types of T lymphocyte responses. DPT, diptherial-pertussis-tetanus.

allergens may have contributed to increasing sensitization and could easily be changed (see Table 2.10).

Decreased rates of infections in early childhood

The incidence of infections in early childhood has decreased as a result of vaccination, decreased family size, and the introduction of antibiotics. The evidence that viral infections have decreased is not clear, neither is it obvious how this would have contributed to increasing asthma. By contrast, there is no doubt that bacterial infections in childhood have decreased. Bacterial infections are thought to create a bias towards Th1 responses by stimulating IL-12 production.

Decreased physical exercise

In many Western countries there has been a dramatic decrease in physical exercise such that children typically do several hours of exercise per week rather than the several hours per day that was normal in 1950. The mechanism by which exercise may protect the lungs is not clear, but full inspiration decreases lung resistance and gentle exercise can protect against exercise-induced asthma.

Changes in diet

Changes in diet have taken many different forms, but there are several aspects that have been common to many countries:

- the pervasive presence of coloring and preservatives in modern diet;
- the increased consumption of animal fat combined with decreased consumption of vegetables;
- excess protein and caloric intake, which is the most consistent feature of Western diet – recent data showing a correlation between obesity and asthma suggest that there has been a change in the phenotype of asthmatics as well as an increase in the prevalence of asthma.

CONCLUSION

In parallel with the rising trends in asthma and related allergic diseases, the past 40 years have witnessed dramatic increases in the understanding of both the immunology and the mechanisms of inflammation that are related to asthma. This understanding has led to some major new approaches to treatment. These approaches include avoiding the causes, preventing the immune response, blocking every aspect of the inflammatory response, and simply reversing the bronchospasm. In many cases the results of treatment are excellent. However, it would be difficult to describe the overall results as excellent because very large numbers of patients require regular treatment with inhalers, and hospitalization for asthma remains common. The implication is that we still need to identify the true causes of the increased prevalence of asthma and the increased morbidity that it causes. Changes in Western society have been profound, and it is difficult to pinpoint those that are relevant to asthma. However, it may be that the asthma epidemic will be controlled only by selectively reversing some aspects of our current life.

FURTHER READING

Allergy and Asthma. Nature 1999; 402 (6760):B1–B39.

Barnes PJ, Alving K, Kharatonov SA, et al. Exhaled markers in airway disease. Eur Respir Rev 1999; 9:207–253.

Chung KF, Barnes PJ. Cytokines in asthma. Thorax 1999; 54:825–857.

Chung KF, Godard P. Difficult therapy-resistant asthma. ERS Task Force Report. Eur Respir Rev 2000; 10:1–101.

Klinman DM. Immunotherapeutic uses of CpG oligodeoxynucleotides. Nat Rev Immunol 2004; 4:249–258.

Martinez FD, Holt PG. Role of microbial burden in the aetiology of allergy and asthma. Lancet 1999; 354(suppl II): 12–15.

Pauwels RA, Pedersen S, Busse WW, et al on behalf of the START Investigators Group. Early intervention with budesonide in mild persistent asthma: a randomized, double-blind trial. Lancet 2003; 361:1071–1076.

Postma DS, Gerritesen J. The link between asthma and COPD:bronchitis VL. Clin Exp Allergy 1999; 29(suppl 2):2–128.

Sterk PJ, Buist SA, Woolcock AT, et al. The message from the World Asthma Meeting, 1998 (Barcelona). Eur Respir J 1999; 14:1435–1453.

Holgate ST, Chuchalin AG, Hebert J, et al. Efficacy and safety of recombinant anti-immunoglobulin E antibody (omalizumab) in severe allergic asthma. Clin Exp Allergy 2004; 34:632–638.

Wark PA, Johnston SL, Bucchieri F, et al. Asthmatic bronchial epithelial cells have a deficient innate immune response to infection with rhinovirus. J Exp Med 2005; 201:937–947.

Barbers R. Asthma. Curr Opin Pulm Med 2000; 6:1–89.

Chapter 3

Extrinsic Allergic Alveolitis

David J Hendrick and Charles McSharry

Definition:
Extrinsic allergic alveolitis (synonym: hypersensitivity pneumonitis) describes an interstitial and bronchioloalveolar disease of the lungs caused by an immune-mediated hypersensitivity response. It is associated with repeated exposure to a variety of inhaled organic dusts and reactive chemicals, but only a proportion of exposed subjects become affected. Notable examples are farmers' lung (due to actinomycetes contaminating farm produce) and bird fanciers' lung (due to secreted avian antigens). The disease has considerable potential as a model of allergic lung disease, since the populations at risk can often be identified precisely, the relevant antigens can be purified, and the clinical and immunologic consequences of antigen exposure can be examined.

INTRODUCTION

Extrinsic allergic alveolitis (EAA) is found in many occupational and environmental settings and has a worldwide distribution. It is most commonly a consequence of the release of antigenic products from the microbial contamination of farm produce, but microbial proliferation may occur in other settings, and occasionally antigenic respirable dusts from other sources are responsible (particularly birds). The underlying inflammatory response primarily affects the lung parenchyma, and in a diffuse manner. It is not confined to the alveoli, and for this reason the term hypersensitivity pneumonitis may be preferable.

The parenchymal nature of the disorder was not clearly distinguished from asthma until 1932, when Campbell published a report describing three English farm workers; the term farmers' lung was introduced later in 1944. Nonetheless, EAA was recognized in Iceland in the nineteenth century, and probably contributed to the occupational ailments of grain workers graphically described by Ramazzini in the eighteenth century. It was not until 1961, when Pepys and colleagues demonstrated the presence of precipitins to antigens of moldy hay in patients suffering from farmers' lung, that the idea of an allergic etiology gained general acceptance. These and other investigators showed that the main sources of antigen were contaminating thermophilic actinomycetes, *Micropolyspora faeni* [syn: *Saccharopolyspora* (or *Faeni*) *rectivirgula*] and *Thermoactinomyetes* sp., and other organisms including *Aspergillus umbrosus* (in Scandinavia) and *Trichosporon* sp. The latter typically appears in the summer months in humid environments and subsides spontaneously in mid-fall. It is most prevalent in Japan (Japanese summer-type hypersensitivity pneumonitis). Similar pulmonary effects sometimes follow the therapeutic use of a number of drugs, but toxic as well as hypersensitivity mechanisms are often involved, and the drugs are not administered by inhalation. They will not be considered further in this chapter.

For penetration and deposition of dust to occur predominantly in the gas exchanging tissues, particle size should be largely confined to 0.5–5 μm. This encompasses the diameters of many bacterial and fungal spores, and a large number of microbial species are now recognized to cause EAA. In addition, the disease has been noted to follow exposure to a variety of antigens derived from animal, vegetable, and chemical sources in both the workplace and the home. Table 3.1 lists some of the various causal agents and the common names of the associated disease. The clinical presentation among the different examples is similar, and the underlying hypersensitivity reactions are largely common to all. Although a particular antigen may be specific to a given example of EAA, there is no 'EAA-specific' antigen as such; rather, it is the amount of antigen contact and the level of individual susceptibility that determines disease outcome.

Farmers' lung patients, and some exposed symptom-free individuals, develop precipitating antibodies in serum (precipitins) against epitopes expressed on

Table 3.1 Agents reported to cause extrinsic allergic alveolitis (EAA)

Some Agents Reported to Cause Extrinsic Allergic Alveolitis

Agent	Source	Common name
Microorganisms		
Alternaria	Paper mill wood pulp	Wood pulp workers' lung
Aspergillus clavatus	Whiskey malting	Malt workers' lung
Aspergillus fumigatus/umbrosus	Vegetable compost	Farmers' lung
Aspergillus versicolor	Dog bedding (straw)	Dog house disease
Aureobasidium pullulans	Redwood	
Bacillus subtilis	Domestic wood	
Cephalosporium	Sewage	Sewage workers' lung
Cryptostroma corticale	Maple	Maple bark strippers' lung
Graphium	Redwood	Sequoiosis
Lycoperdon	Puffballs	Lycoperdonosis
Merulius lacrymans	Domestic wood	
Mucor stolonifer	Paprika	Paprika splitters' lung
Penicillium casei	Cheese	Cheese washers' lung
Penicillium chrysogenum	Domestic wood	
Penicillium cyclopium		
Penicillium frequentens	Cork	Suberosis
Saccharomonospora viridis	Logging plant	
Sporobolomyces	Horse barn straw	
Streptomyces albus	Soil, peat	
Thermophilic actinomycetes *(Faeni rectivirgula, Thermoactinomyces sacchari, T. vulgaris)*	Hay, straw, grain, mushroom compost, bagasse	Farmers' lung, mushroom workers' lung, bagassosis
Trichosporon cutaneum		Japanese Summer-type hypersensitivity pneumonitis
Various bacteria, fungi, amoebae, and nematode debris	Air conditioners, humidifiers,and rotting vegetation	Humidifier lung, ventilation pneumonitis, sauna takers' lung
Animals		
Arthropods (*Sitophilus granarius*)	Grain dust	Weevil disease
Birds	Bloom, excreta	Bird fanciers' lung
Fish	Fish meal	Meal workers' lung
Mammals		
Pituitary (cattle, pig)	Pituitary extracts	Pituitary snuff takers' lung
Hair	Fur	Furriers' lung
Mollusc shell	Nacre-button manufacture	
Urine (rodents)	Urinary protein	Rodent handlers' lung
Vegetation		
Coffee	Coffee bean dust	Coffee workers' lung
Wood (*Gonystylus bacanus*)	Wood dust	Wood workers' lung
Chemicals		
Acid anhydrides	Epoxypolyester paint	
Bordeaux mixture (fungicide)	Vineyards	Vineyard sprayers' lung
Cobalt dissolved in solvents	Tungsten carbide grinding	
Diphenylmethane diisocyanate	Plastics industry	
Hexamethylene diisocyanate		
Pauli's reagent	Laboratory	
Pyrethrum	Insecticide spray	
Toluene diisocyanate	Plastics industry	
Trimellitic anhydride		

(glyco)protein antigens in the inhaled organic dust. Thermophilic actinomycetes are ubiquitous, and approximately 10 per 100 000 in the general population have precipitins against extracts of these organisms. Surveys of farmers have shown that a minority (approximately 10%) have precipitins. A proportion of these (about 50%) are asymptomatic, but some have abnormal pulmonary function tests or radiographs, which suggests subclinical disease. Studies of EAA among farmers suggest an incidence of around 0.5% per year, and a prevalence of up to 10%, depending on region, climate, and farming practice. Among people exposed to birds, the prevalence is estimated at between 20 and 20 000 per 100 000 persons, depending on intensity of

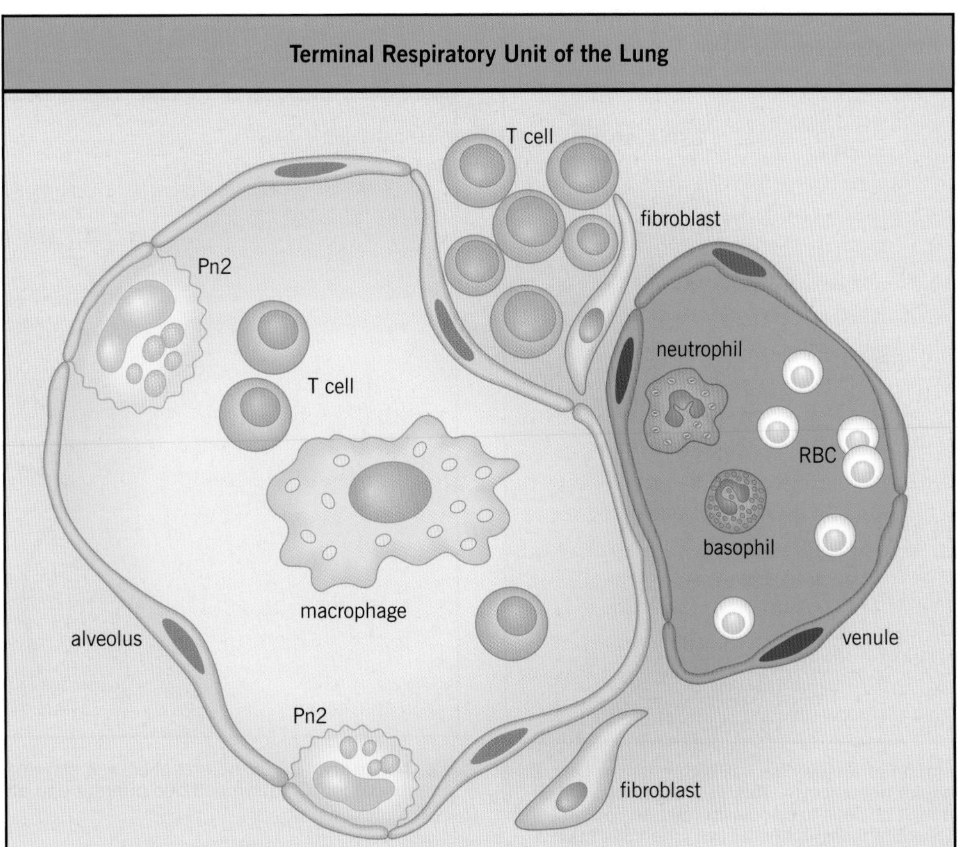

Fig. 3.1 A representation of the terminal respiratory unit of the lung. This illustrates an alveolar sac and an adjacent capillary. Gas exchange is facilitated by their close approximation, and normally the combined thickness of capillary endothelium plus simple squamous alveolar epithelium separating blood from air is extremely thin. The septa between the alveolar spaces contain the capillary lumens. Very fine collagen and elastic fibers also accompany the capillaries to provide mechanical support and elastic recoil. In extrinsic allergic alveolitis (EAA) this interstitium is infiltrated by inflammatory cells, predominantly lymphocytes and macrophages, which may restrict gas exchange. There is hyperplasia of the type 2 pneumocytes (Pn 2) and a marked increase in the number of alveolar lymphocytes. A higher power view of an alveolar space in EAA demonstrates numerous small mainly lymphocytic mononuclear cells, and large foamy macrophages with abundant, light pink cytoplasm (stained with hematoxylin and eosin), and central, vesicular nuclei. The macrophages are activated and have a characteristic lipid laden 'foamy' appearance. In chronic disease there is increased collagen deposition by activated fibroblasts.

exposure. The incidence and prevalence of EAA worldwide remain unknown, but vary considerably from country to country, and region to region, depending on climate, local industry, and working practices.

The usual low prevalence of EAA in at-risk populations implies that individual susceptibility is necessary for the development of disease, as well as environmental factors. The primary consideration relating to susceptibility is individual immune responsiveness to the inhaled antigens. Many individuals with antibody do not have symptoms, but disease without antibody is conspicuous by its rarity. Antibody seems necessary but not sufficient for disease. There is a caveat in that smoking suppresses precipitin responses, and it is unclear whether it fully suppresses EAA in parallel. A direct causal role for antibody in EAA is still controversial but its association with EAA may be clarified by replacing the precipitin method with more sensitive techniques which can quantify antibody concentration. Commercial enzyme-immunoassay methods have recently been established as a laboratory adjunct in the clinical assessment of EAA among bird breeders and farmers. These can quantify antibody within the dynamic range associated with disease. This could allow international standardization and quality control, and facilitate comparison of results between centers. In addition to improved diagnosis, this may improve the understanding of the immunopathogenic mechanisms of EAA.

ANATOMY AND PHYSIOLOGY OF THE ALVEOLI

The alveoli represent the terminal respiratory units of the lung. The term alveolar tissue applies to that anatomic part of the lung which contains the alveoli and is capable of gas exchange – it includes both the alveolar ducts and sacs (Fig. 3.1). The respiratory bronchioles are also, in part, composed of alveolar tissue. The term pulmonary parenchyma is commonly used to describe the overall gas-exchanging portion of the lung and it is essentially equivalent to the term alveolar tissue. Much of the lung is composed of supporting mesenchymal tissue, with a single layer of epithelium lining the alveolar spaces. Approximately 95% of the alveolar surface is covered with a simple squamous epithelium, the cells of which are referred to as type 1 alveolar cells (or type 1 pneumocytes). They are vulnerable to injury, and denudation of the epithelium is seen in many alveolar diseases. Type 2 alveolar cells, or granular pneumocytes, make

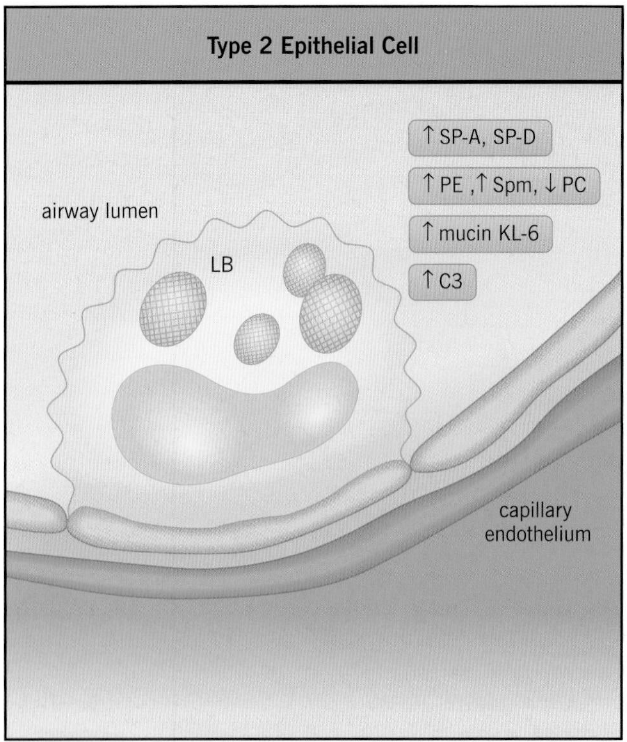

Fig. 3.2 A representation of an alveolar wall highlighting a type 2 epithelial cell or granular pneumocyte. This is a large, rounded or cuboidal cell, with a high nucleus-to-cytoplasm ratio, in contrast to the very flat type 1 alveolar lining epithelial cell. The cells have a deeply blue-stained, vacuolated cytoplasm after May–Grunwald–Giemsa-staining. The large vesicles in the cytoplasm are lamellar bodies (LB) containing the precursor of alveolar surfactant lipids and proteins. In extrinsic allergic alveolitis (EAA) there is increased production of surfactant protein-A (SP-A) and SP-D, and increased phospholipid synthesis, mainly immunostimulatory phosphatidylethanolamine (PE) and sphingomyelin (Spm), with a reduced production of immunosuppressive phosphatidylcholine (PC). The levels of these correlate with the alveolar accumulations of lymphocytes, mast cells and 'foamy' macrophages. The presence of reactive type 2 cells in bronchoalveolar lavage fluid is characteristic of patients with EAA and is not observed in sarcoidosis. KL-6, Krebs von den Lungen-6;

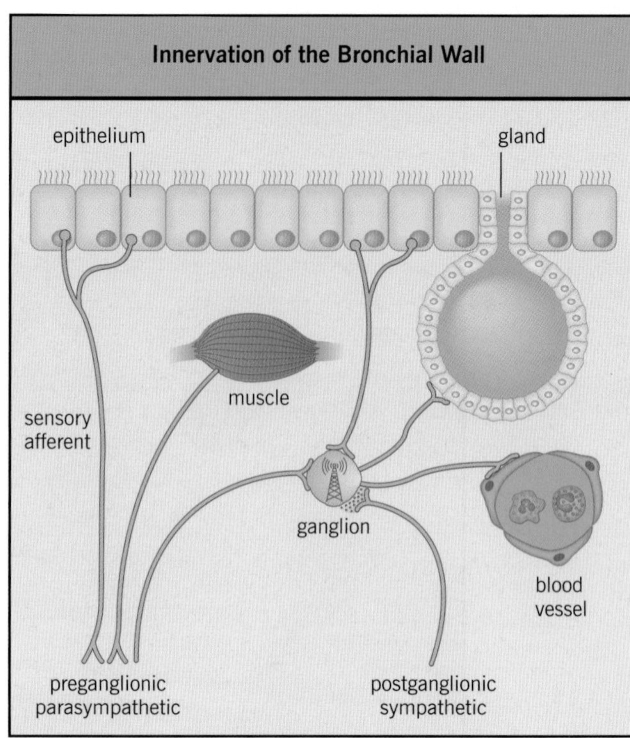

Fig. 3.3 Innervation of the bronchial wall showing the parasympathetic and sympathetic efferent and afferent pathways.

up the remaining 5% of the alveolar surface (Fig. 3.2). These are angular cells, which contain more organelles in their cytoplasm and microvilli and produce the surfactant that lines the alveolar surface. Repair of injured alveolar epithelium comes from proliferation of type 2 granular pneumocytes, which can divide and differentiate into either type 1 or 2 cells.

The alveolar epithelial cells rest on a basement membrane that is generally adjacent to, but discrete from, the endothelial cells of the capillaries. The potential space between them constitutes the interstitium, and incorporates fibrous tissue, nerves, and lymphatics. The capillaries within the alveolar wall form a dense reticular network of interconnecting channels. Other cell types include interstitial fibroblasts, which play a maintenance role in the fibrous skeleton of alveolar tissue, and pulmonary macrophages, which are found in the alveolar spaces and, at times, in the interstitium. These macrophages are derived from bone marrow, and are capable of limited local division.

Two autonomic nervous systems – the cholinergic, or parasympathetic, and the adrenergic, or sympathetic – as well as a third non-adrenergic non-cholinergic nervous system have been described in the lung (Fig. 3.3). The afferent parasympathetic preganglionic fibers travel in the vagus nerves, and convey impulses centrally from irritant or cough receptors located next to epithelial cells lining the airways. Stimulation of these may be important in EAA because one of the signal symptoms is unexplained chronic non-productive cough. The non-adrenergic non-cholinergic nervous system has both inhibitory and excitatory limbs. Certain neurotransmitter peptides are active in the inhibitor limb (e.g. vasoactive intestinal peptide) and others are active in the excitatory limb (e.g. substance P). There is a recent description of increased nerve growth factor (NGF) associated with pigeon fanciers' lung suggesting a possible neuropeptide link between the cells which produce and respond to NGF, including mast cells and lymphocytes (both of which are markedly increased in number in EAA), and sensory nerve cells.

PATHOGENESIS OF EXTRINSIC ALLERGIC ALVEOLITIS

Many of the histologic changes associated with EAA occur also in other interstitial lung diseases. Because the natural history of many interstitial diseases of unknown origin involves progressive evolution through these same histologic phases, knowledge about immune pathogenesis gained from studies of EAA may provide a way to understand the causes and development of these also. There is a rich tapestry of histologic features to explore, and hypotheses on pathogenic mechanisms can be proposed to account for them.

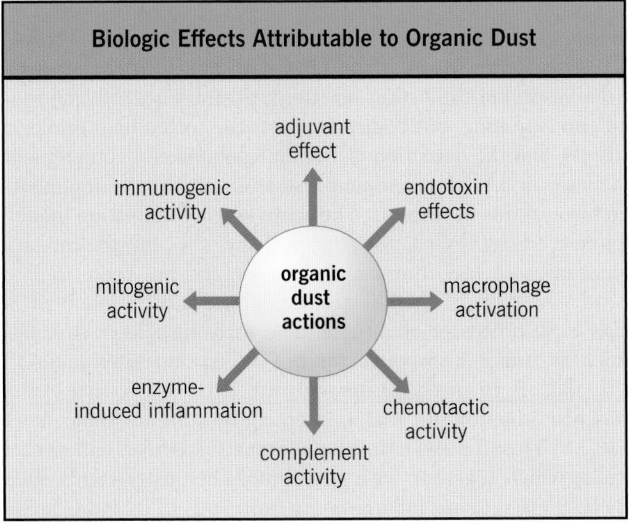

Fig. 3.4 Some biological effects attributable to organic dusts.

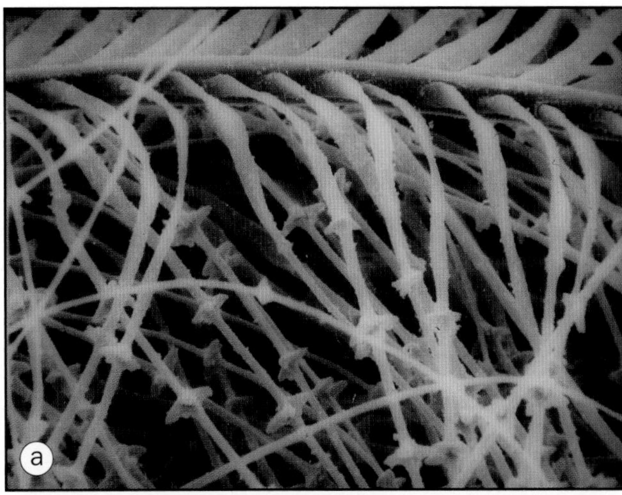

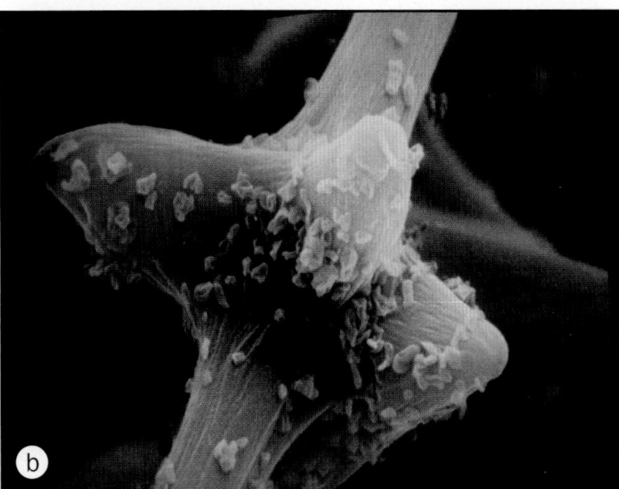

Fig. 3.5 A scanning electron micrograph of a pigeon feather (a) showing the particles of powder-down or 'bloom' on the feather barbs (b). This waxy bloom coats the feathers and confers waterproofing. Bloom dust looks like talcum powder; it is abundant in pigeon lofts and is readily airborne. The bloom particles, approximately 1 μm in diameter, are composed largely of keratin, and have a favorable aerodynamic size to penetrate and sediment in the peripheral airways. The bloom particles are coated with pigeon serum proteins. These soluble antigens are transported into the lung and their immunogenicity is enhanced by the insoluble irritant/adjuvant nature of the bloom particles. (Photograph courtesy of Dr Gavin Boyd.)

Pathophysiology

The typical histologic features of lung biopsy in EAA are similar regardless of causative antigen, and depend on stage of disease. Biopsies are generally taken from patients with long-standing lung disease, and show a lymphocytic infiltrate, with minimal evidence for immune complexes or complement deposition. However, in experimental models of early disease, shortly after antigen contact, there is edema, vasculitis and a neutrophil influx. Over the following days or weeks, there develops a diffuse interstitial infiltrate at the terminal bronchioles extending into the parenchyma. It represents a bronchiolocentric inflammation with preferential involvement of the centrilobular regions. The interstitial pneumonitis is composed predominantly of lymphocytes, plasma cells, and foamy macrophages. Small and loosely formed granulomata are observed. The lymphocyte infiltrate is predominantly CD8+ but over time this normalizes to a predominance of CD4+ cells in chronic disease. There is proliferation of type 2 pneumocytes and fibroblasts, and fibrosis secondary to the pneumonitis may include emphysematous changes. In severe cases, irreversible alterations in the lung architecture (referred to as 'honeycombing') may follow. The severity of the fibrosis, along with radiographic evidence of honeycombing, is the best predictor of mortality.

In EAA, the total number of cells recovered by bronchoalveolar lavage (BAL) fluid may be increased up to fourfold compared to normal, and of these the proportion of lymphocytes may be up to 70%. The composition of lymphocyte types in the BAL fluid and respiratory tract is also altered. The ratios of CD4+ T-helper to CD8+ T-cytotoxic lymphocytes locally in the respiratory tract and BAL are normally consistent with those in blood, but in acute EAA there is a significant increase in the number of cytotoxic T cells, B cells and plasma cells.

These changes may be caused directly by the inhaled dusts or by the response to them. The intrinsic, immunologically non-specific nature of the causative organic dusts may explain some aspects of the pathology of EAA. They produce a variety of similar biological effects (Fig. 3.4). In particular they can serve as potent immunologic adjuvants, by stimulating alveolar macrophages and directly activating the alternative and lectin-binding pathways of complement. This provides the necessary mediator stimuli for increasing vascular permeability and promoting chemotactic migration of neutrophils and other cells into the lung. Organic dusts commonly contain toxic substances, many of which have enzymatic activities, while other agents produce scavenger receptor-mediated macrophage enzyme release and non-specific lymphocyte blastogenesis. The inflammatory consequences of these direct effects, and of those modulated by complement and macrophages, are important factors in the pathogenesis of EAA. Examples of the dusts associated with pigeon fanciers' lung and farmers' lung are shown in Figures 3.5 and 3.6 respectively.

Dust exposures can be similar in symptomatic and symptom-free subjects; therefore the main determinant of disease outcome is likely to be individual susceptibility. This may involve a genetic predisposition associated with a particular HLA haplotype responsive to antigen, or a polymorphism regulating the production of an important mediator or mediator receptor. Susceptibility appears to be associated with specific immune responsiveness to the inhaled dust antigen. The detail of some of the specific questions can be addressed by studying experimental models of EAA.

Experimental models

There are numerous animal models with which to study the immunopathogenic mechanisms of EAA. A common protocol for the induction and monitoring of the disease in rabbits is illustrated in Figure 3.7. The most natural model of EAA is that occurring in cattle (bovine farmers' lung) exposed to the same moldy hay as farmers, but mice (*Mus musculus*) are the tools of choice for immunologists, and with inbred strains, and gene-insertion or deletion techniques, there have been major advances in our understanding of EAA.

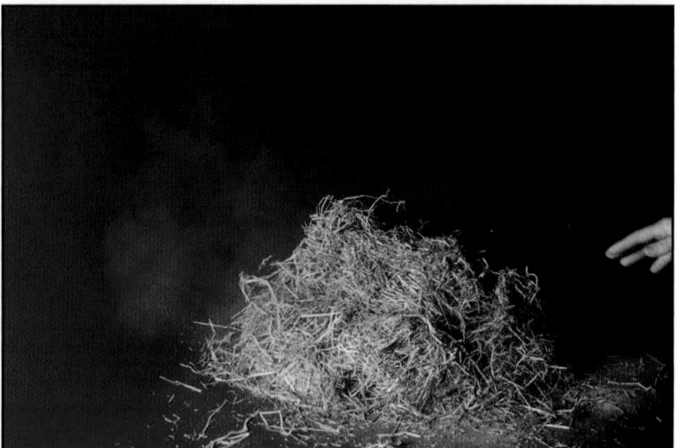

Fig. 3.6 An open bale of moldy hay contains an abundance of *Faeni rectivirgula* spores. These spores are approximately 1 μm in diameter and are readily aerosolized when the hay is disturbed. (Photograph courtesy of Dr Gavin Boyd.)

Immune-complex-induced tissue injury, as originally postulated by Pepys, is thought to play a role in the pathogenesis of EAA. The development of symptoms 4–8 hours after exposure (reminiscent of the Arthus reaction), the presence of high levels of precipitating antibodies against the offending etiologic agents, and the detection of immunoglobulin and complement deposits in BAL fluid and lung lesions are among the arguments in favor of this hypothesis. The acute lung inflammation model, pioneered by Ward, is triggered by the intrapulmonary deposition of IgG immune complexes, and has been used to study the roles of chemokines, cytokines, and complement in the early processes of disease. The early response cytokines, such as tumor necrosis factor α (TNFα) and interleukin-1β (IL-1β), are required for upregulation of the expression of the vascular adhesion molecules, intercellular adhesion molecule-1 (ICAM-1) and E-selectin on pulmonary vascular endothelial cells, which together with neutrophil chemoattractants such as IL-8 macrophage inflammatory protein-2, LTB_4 and C5a are required for the recruitment of neutrophils into the alveolar compartment. This is associated with rapid (within 30 minutes) activation of the signal transducer and activator of transcription-3 (STAT-3) protein in macrophages. This may be of importance because there are several isotypes of STAT and the relative expression of STAT-3 compared with STAT-1 is an indicator of chronicity in experimental arthritis. The more chronic inflammation associated with asthma involves the expression of the adhesion molecule, vascular cell adhesion molecule-1 (VCAM-1) on vascular epithelium. Its ligand very late antigen-4 (VLA-4) (the integrin $\alpha_4\beta_1$) is expressed along with ICAM-3 on lung lymphocytes in EAA, and in asthma (Fig. 3.8).

Although antibodies are related to antigen exposure and are not diagnostic of disease per se, it is likely that immune complexes of a certain antigen-antibody combining ratio, rather than the antibody itself, can release proinflammatory cytokines and cause granuloma formation. Also, disease outcome may depend on the relative expression of stimulatory Fcγ receptors CD16 and CD64, or the FcγR11β isoform of CD32 which is an inhibitory regulator of immune-complex cell activation.

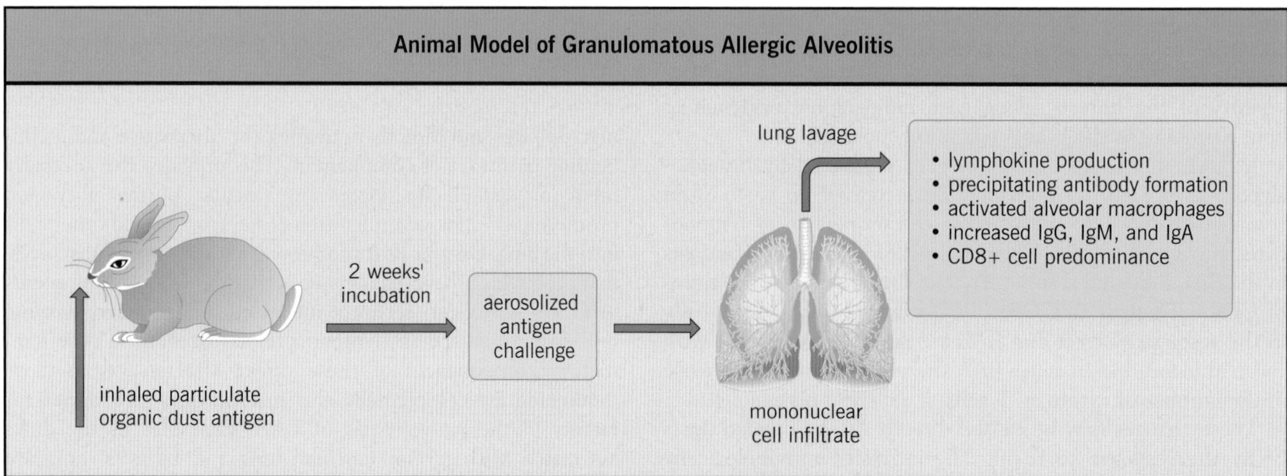

Fig. 3.7 Rabbit model of extrinsic allergic alveolitis (EAA). Aerosol challenge with particulate organic dust, or related antigens after systemic immunization, results in an early neutrophilic infiltrate followed by granulomatous lesions compatible with those in cell-mediated allergic tissue injury. The presence of lung lesions seen on histology is associated with local inflammatory cytokine production, antibody formation, and the presence of activated alveolar macrophages plus a predominance of CD8+ T lymphocytes.

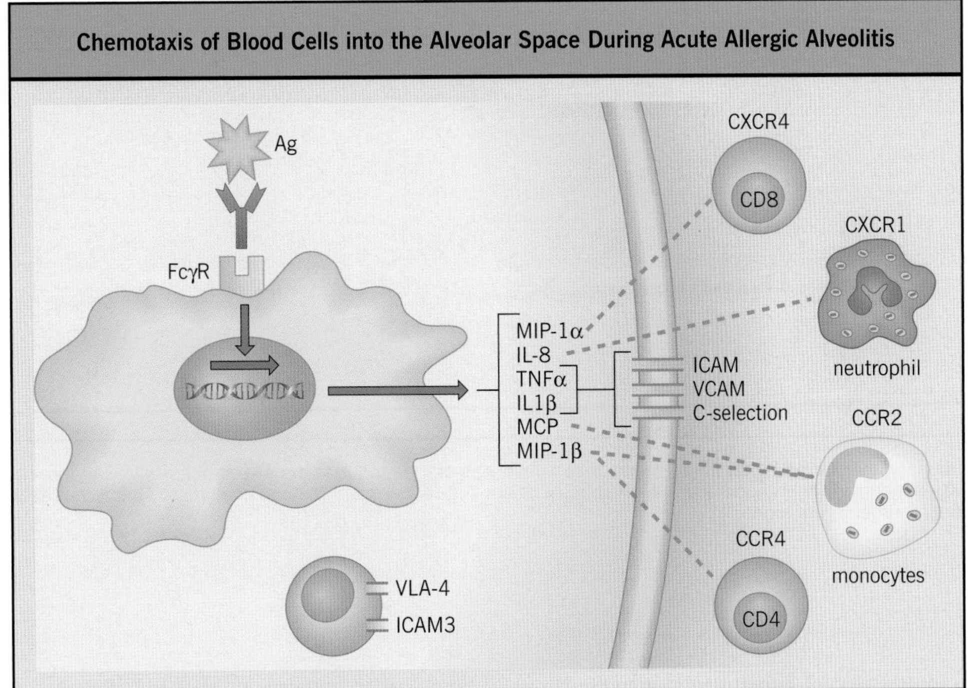

Fig. 3.8 Cellular recruitment into the alveoli in EAA. Antigen reaching the alveolar spaces is bound by IgG antibody, and this antigen-antibody complex is bound by IgG receptors on alveolar macrophages. This triggers synthesis of cytokines which up-regulate the expression of adhesion molecules, and cytokines which have chemotactic activity (chemokines), and these together regulate the influx of inflammatory cells accounting for the different phases of alveolitis. Acute inflammatory cytokines, such as tumor necrosis factor-α (TNFα) and interleukin (IL)-1β induce the expression of intercellular adhesion molecule-1 (ICAM-1) and E-selectin which along with chemokines such as IL-8 binding its specific chemokine receptor CXCR1 rapidly recruit neutrophils. This may partly explain the transient airway neutrophilia seen after acute antigen exposure. More chronic antigen exposure is associated with expression of vascular cell adhesion molecule-1 (VCAM-1), and the typical alveolar profile in EAA is of increased lymphocytes expressing its ligand the integrin very late antigen-4 (VLA-4) and ICAM-3. CD8 T-lymphocytes responding to the cytokine macrophage inflammatory protein (MIP)-1α binding its specific chemokine receptor CXCR4 are recruited and predominate for some weeks after antigen exposure. CD4 T-lymphocytes responding to the cytokine MIP-1β binding its specific chemokine receptor CCR4 are recruited and predominate thereafter. Throughout this time the macrophage count is markedly increased supported by the recruitment of monocytes by the chemokine monocyte chemoattractant peptide (MCP) binding its specific chemokine receptor CCR2.

Immune complex activation of alveolar macrophages may be a prerequisite to cell-mediated lung injury. Proinflammatory cytokines stimulated by immune complexes are involved in the formation of granulomata of the type seen in EAA. In addition to immune complex tissue injury there has been mounting evidence for the participation of lymphocyte-mediated tissue injury in the pathogenesis of EAA. For example, agents and procedures that inhibit cell-mediated hypersensitivity (e.g. corticosteroids, ciclosporin, antiserum against certain pro-inflammatory cytokines, and neonatal thymectomy) have either markedly diminished or prevented the development of forms of granulomatous pneumonitis in animal experiments. EAA has also been transferred passively by sensitized lymphocytes followed by respiratory tract challenge, whereas such transfer is generally unsuccessful with hyperimmune serum.

In animal models, aerosol challenge with simple soluble antigen generally results in immune tolerance; clinical disease seems to require prior systemic sensitization with adjuvant. In models of pigeon breeders' EAA, long-term aerosol exposure to soluble antigens from pigeon serum resulted in antibody formation without detectable pulmonary inflammation. However, when the lung was primed with the adjuvant Bacille Calmette-Guérin (BCG) and then exposed to the same antigens by aerosol, granulomatous lesions resembling those of EAA occurred in association with T-cell-dependent hypersensitivity to the inhaled antigens. This model might have relevance for humans, since many people are exposed to relevant etiological agents for long periods with the consequent development of precipitating antibodies, but with little evidence of inflammatory changes in the lung. Particulate organic dusts e.g. *M. faeni* spores, on the other hand, seem to have endogenous adjuvant activity. When inhaled, these spores cause an early (6 hours) neutrophilic infiltrate followed by granulomatous lesions compatible with cell-mediated immune tissue injury. The importance of lymphocytes to this process is shown by passive transfer of sensitivity with specifically sensitized lymph node and spleen cells (Fig. 3.9). When followed by aerosol antigen challenge, this results in the production of granulomatous lesions closely resembling those observed in human EAA.

Cytokines

The pathogenesis of EAA is likely to be regulated by cytokines. The influenza-like symptoms associated with acute disease are reminiscent of the adverse symptoms termed 'cytokine-fever' associated with cytokine therapy. The immune response associated with antigen exposure is cytokine mediated and granuloma formation generally requires the contribution of TNFα and IFNγ, implying a Th1 polarized lymphocyte response. Some Th1 lymphocyte-derived cytokines have been shown to

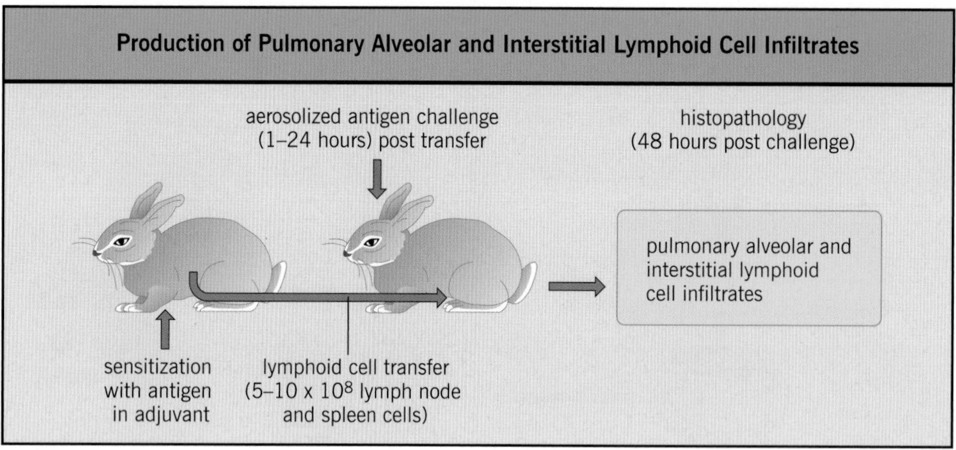

Fig. 3.9 Typical pulmonary alveolar and interstitial lymphoid cell infiltrates can be induced in naive rabbits following the intraperitoneal transfer of specifically sensitized lymph node and spleen cells, with subsequent aerosol antigen challenge. This is not achieved by challenge after transfer of hyperimmune serum alone.

be involved in the production of experimental granulomatous reactions. Administration of neutralizing antibody against several of these, particularly TNFα, but also IL-2, IL-12 and INFγ, can markedly decrease pulmonary granulomatous responses.

Other cytokines appear to play an important inhibitory role; for example, administration of recombinant (r)IL-6 in the mouse model of actinomycete-induced EAA markedly diminishes the recruitment of inflammatory cells into the lungs, as well as reducing the ensuing fibrotic response. On the other hand, mice challenged with actinomycete antigen via the respiratory tract and given anti-IL-6 antibody develop a sustained neutrophilic response followed by a more significant fibrosis than that seen in control mice. Administration of rIL-10 reduces the pulmonary granuloma formation induced by schistosome egg antigens. The lymphoid cells from these rIL-10-treated mice produce low levels of IL-2 and IFNγ, suggesting that IL-10 functions by downregulating Th1 responses. A counterpoint to this was the observation of an increased susceptibility to EAA in C57BL/6 mice rendered genetically deficient in IL-10 production (IL-10-/-). These IL-10-/- mice had strikingly higher cell counts in BAL fluid and a marked increase in granuloma formation when compared to their wild-type littermates.

The research groups of Schuyler and Hunninghake studied this association between Th1- or Th2-bias and EAA susceptibility in a murine model. It was shown that Th1-biased C57BL/6 mice are susceptible to EAA, whereas Th2-biased DBA/2 mice are resistant. DBA/2 mice can become sensitized if they are given exogenous IL-12, a potent Th1 signal cytokine, at the time of antigen exposure. The basis of this susceptibility is thought to lie with the regulation of IL-12 by IL-4. Splenocytes from Th-1 biased, disease-susceptible C57BL/6 mice exhibited decreased stability of IL-4 mRNA relative to splenocytes from DBA/2 mice. This suggests that mRNA stability may serve as an important mechanism underlying susceptibility to EAA, and perhaps also to Th1/Th2 immune polarization in general. The induction of EAA in Th2-biased BALB/c mice seemed to require activated/memory Th1 cells (characterized by the adoptive transfer of cells with the phenotype CD45Rb-, CD44+, CD25 low and α_4 integrin CD49d+). The requirement for T-cell activation for experimental EAA was confirmed by the administration of the synthetic molecule CTLA-4-Ig which prevented disease development in experimental EAA. This molecule is an antagonist of the CD28/B7 interactions that were essential for T-cell activation and differentiation.

Experimental EAA induced by *S. rectivirgula* in mice with either a Th1 or a Th2 bias is not altered by treatment with neutralizing antibody to IFNγ or IL-4. However disease susceptibility can be passively transferred with *S. rectivirgula*-specific CD4+ cells taken from either sensitized C3H/HeJ (Th1 bias) or BALB/c mice (Th2 bias). This suggests that other aspects, in addition to genetic background and cytokine environment at the site of initial sensitization, determine the development of EAA. A more detailed study of this strain-dependency by microarray technology may determine the relevant cytokine (and other) gene expression involved in pathogenesis.

A strong candidate for further investigation is the chemokine family of molecules which coordinate the recruitment of cells into an inflammatory site. For example the neutrophil chemotactic cytokine IL-8 induces and activates neutrophil accumulation in vivo in the lungs, whereas administration of anti-IL-8 blocks the recruitment of neutrophils and protects against lung injury in experimental rat models of EAA. In vitro *S. rectivirgula* can directly induce the secretion of the C-C chemokines macrophage inflammatory protein-1α (MIP-1α) and monocyte chemoattractant protein-1 (MCP-1) from murine macrophage cell lines. Similarly, after single intratracheal administration of *S. rectivirgula* in C57BL/6 and BALB/c mice there is a marked appearance of MIP-1α and MCP-1 in BAL fluid, followed by neutrophilia (24–48 hours), then lymphocytosis (48–72 hours). More recent work however suggests that MCP-1 and CCR-2 expression are not necessary for this alveolitis.

This influx of lymphocytes and the development of granulomata can be blocked with analogs of sialyl Lewis X which bind E- and P-selectins, thus preventing the initial stages of leukocyte influx at which circulating cells adhere to endothelium. The subsequent movement of T lymphocytes into the interstitium has been shown to be dependent on their expression of CXCR3. The chemoattractants associated with this include the IFNγ-inducible CXC chemokine ligand 9 (CXCL9) and CXCL11. Levels of these chemokines are greatly reduced in IFNγ(-/-) mice which do not form granuloma in this model. Some of these interactions are illustrated on Figures 3.8 and 3.10.

In conclusion

Animal models allow the investigation of specific research questions relating to EAA – primarily to generate hypotheses to be tested in human disease. *Mus musculus* and *Homo sapiens* have 65 million years of evolutionary diversification, and their respirable microenvironments are different. There is increasing recognition of interspecies discrepancies in immune mechanisms which should be taken into account when using mice as preclinical models of human disease. Thus the immunopathologic findings in animal models require confirmation in human studies of EAA.

DIAGNOSIS OF EXTRINSIC ALLERGIC ALVEOLITIS

An algorithm for the diagnosis of EAA is shown in Figure 3.11 and discussed, in detail, below.

Symptom presentation

The disease may present in an acute, intermediate, or chronic form. Major symptoms are cough, dyspnea, and weight loss.

Acute form

The acute form of EAA is the most easily recognized because symptoms are often quickly distressing and incapacitating, and have a high degree of specificity. Following the sensitizing period of exposure, which may vary from weeks to years, affected patients experience repeated episodes of an influenza-like illness accompanied by coughing and undue breathlessness some hours (usually 4–8 hours) after commencing exposure to the relevant organic dust. The systemic influenza-like symptoms generally dominate those that are essentially respiratory in nature, and patients complain mostly of malaise, fever, chills, widespread aches and pains (particularly headache), anorexia, and tiredness. They are unlikely to exercise, may well go to bed, and may therefore be unaware of shortness of breath. They are, however, likely to develop a dry cough without wheeze and some difficulty in taking deep satisfying breaths. Occasionally, there is an asthmatic or bronchitic response in addition to that in the gas-exchanging tissues, and wheezing or productive cough becomes a further feature.

Affected patients soon learn to associate symptoms with a causative environment despite the delay in onset after exposure begins. Recognition is particularly easy for groups such as farmers and pigeon fanciers as the risks are likely to be well known. However, in some cases there may be a tendency to deny such a relationship for fear of compromising the ability to pursue a livelihood or hobby, and the clinical history may appear much less convincing than it should.

The severity and duration of symptoms depend on the exposure dose as well as individual susceptibility. With a relatively low level of acute exposure, symptoms are mild and persist for a few hours only. When occupation is responsible, the affected worker may feel unwell at home during the following evening or night and be fully recovered by the next morning. Consequently, the relevance of the workplace may be obscured. When severe responses follow particularly heavy exposures, the relation of the one to the other will be more

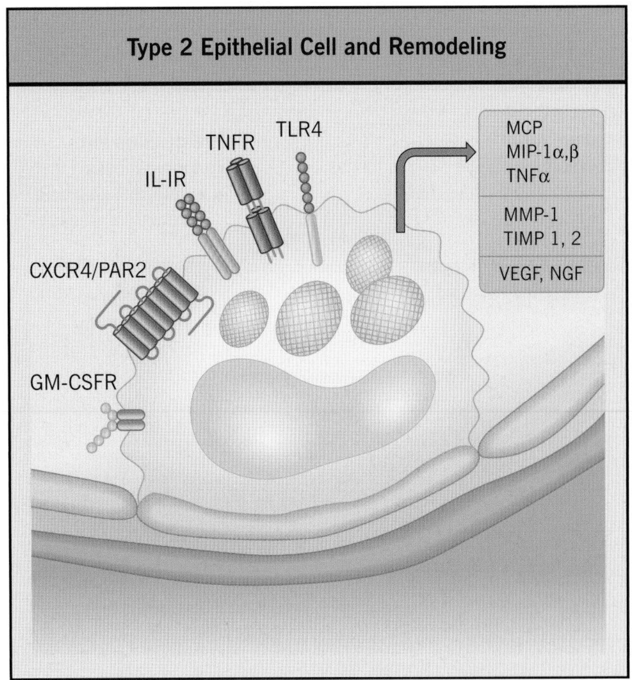

Fig. 3.10 The type 2 epithelial cell has receptors (R) for, and responds to, cytokines including interleukin-1β (IL-1β), tumor necrosis factor α (TNFα), IL-13 and granulocyte–macrophage colony-stimulating factor (GM-CSF). The latter induces hyperplasia of the type 2 cell and foamy macrophages; both characteristic of extrinsic allergic alveolitis (EAA). Other receptors include chemokine receptors, predominantly CXCR4 (its ligand is stromal derived factor-1α), and protease activated receptors (PAR2). The cells respond to lipopolysaccharide (LPS) [suggesting also Toll-like receptor 4 (TLR4)] and TNFα by increasing intracellular cyclic guanosine monophosphate (cGMP), and release a range of proinflammatory cytokines and chemokines including monocyte chemoattractant protein (MCP), macrophage inflammatory protein-1α (MIP-1α), and MIP-2α. These are chemotactic for lymphocytes and, along with TNFα, contribute to the development of local ectopic lymphoid granuloma and germinal center formation.
The type 2 epithelial cell has a major role in tissue repair. It contributes to the regeneration of all epithelial cells after damage, most notably following hypoxia, radiation, and the inhalation of silica and the antigens responsible for extrinsic allergic alveolitis (EAA). The type 2 cells also provide mediators for remodeling of extracellular matrix including increased production of transforming growth factor β (TGFβ), tissue inhibitor of metalloproteinase-1 (TIMP-1) and TIMP-2 but constitutive production of matrix metalloprotease-1 (MMP-1). Type 2 epithelial cells synthesize a high molecular weight sialoglycoprotein KL-6 (Krebs von den Lungen-6) belonging to cluster 9 of the mucin MUC1 classification. In diseases where these cells rapidly proliferate, such as EAA, KL-6 levels are extremely high in bronchoalveolar lavage (BAL) fluid and serum. Monitoring serum KL-6 levels reflects the severity of, and is a useful indicator for the effectiveness of corticosteroid therapy in, interstitial lung disease including EAA. In addition to structural proteins, the type 2 cells produce vascular endothelial growth factor (VEGF) and nerve growth factor (NGF), promoting angiogenesis and new nerve growth and survival. These last mediators have receptors on lymphocytes and newly ascribed immunomodulatory functions, and they may prove to have important roles in immune hypersensitivity diseases such as EAA.

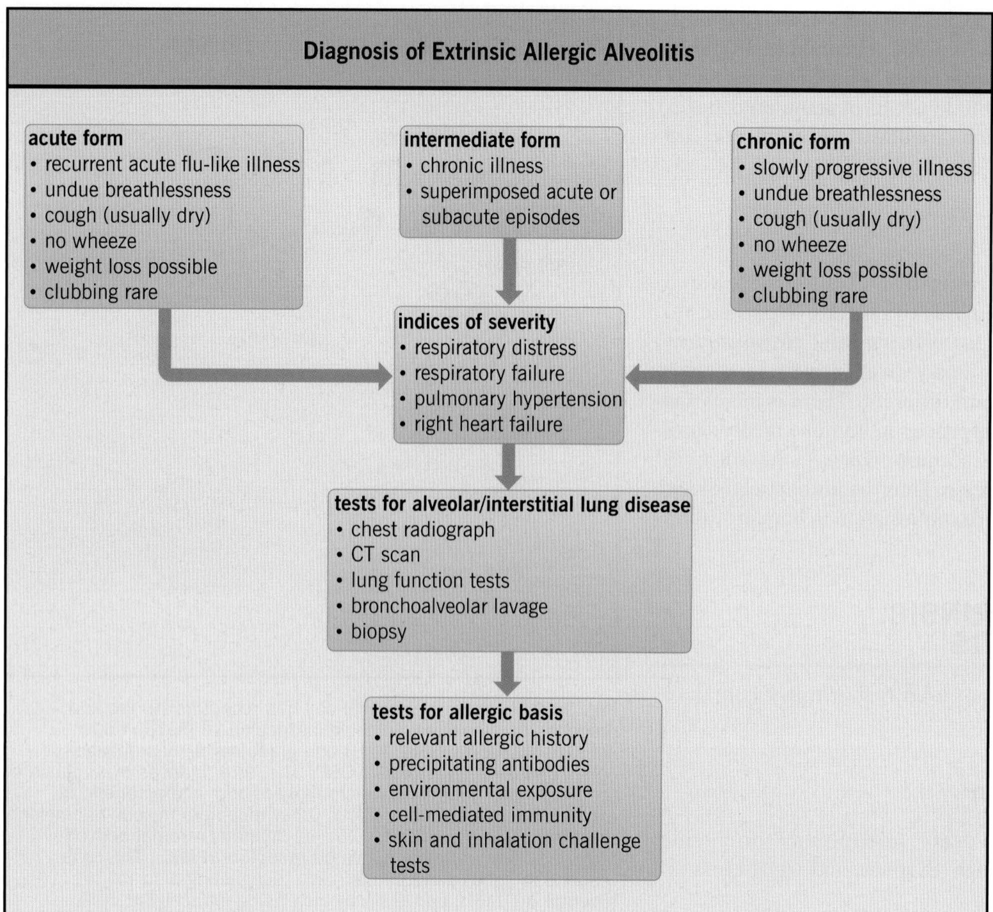

Fig. 3.11 Diagnostic flow chart for extrinsic allergic alveolitis. CT, computed tomography.

obvious and complete remission may require several days or even weeks. Such responses are occasionally life threatening.

Chronic form

In some subjects EAA expresses itself much less dramatically though there is greater potential for serious disablement. There is a slowly increasing loss of exercise tolerance owing to shortness of breath with no systemic upset apart from an occasional prominent loss of weight. This is the result of diffuse pulmonary fibrosis which has often been progressing for years before the affected person seeks advice. The slower the progression and the longer the delay, the greater is the likelihood of permanent fibrotic damage. Eventually hypoxia and pulmonary hypertension may supervene and the right heart fails. There are no acute exacerbations and each day and each month are much like any other.

The chronic form of EAA is typically seen in patients who keep a single budgerigar/parakeet in the home. The level of antigenic exposure to avian dust is comparatively trivial – compared with the farm worker forking bales of heavily contaminated hay in a poorly ventilated barn – but it is encountered almost continuously, particularly if the affected person is a housewife or an elderly pensioner largely confined to the home. These different exposure patterns are generally responsible for the distinct clinical forms of EAA, although differences in host responsiveness exert an important additional influence. Consequently, there may be considerable variability in the symptomatic features among individuals affected by the same source of antigenic exposure. Over recent years it has also been recognized that farmers affected by EAA may develop severe and disabling emphysema, despite never having smoked, and so it appears that lung destruction as well as fibrosis may characterize the chronic form of EAA.

Intermediate form

The acute form of EAA can be produced by inhalation-provocation testing in patients with the chronic form of the disease. This emphasizes the major role that dose exerts in determining the clinical nature of the response that occurs. Depending on the exposure dose and host responsiveness, a variety of intermediate forms of EAA can be recognized and some patients will experience different patterns of response at different times. In subjects predominantly manifesting the chronic form of the disease, for example, it is possible for a limited degree of recovery to follow cessation of exposure and for an acute exacerbation to occur. In general, however, the individual affected by the chronic form of EAA should be satisfied if no further progression occurs following cessation of exposure because, in some cases, fibrotic damage continues regardless.

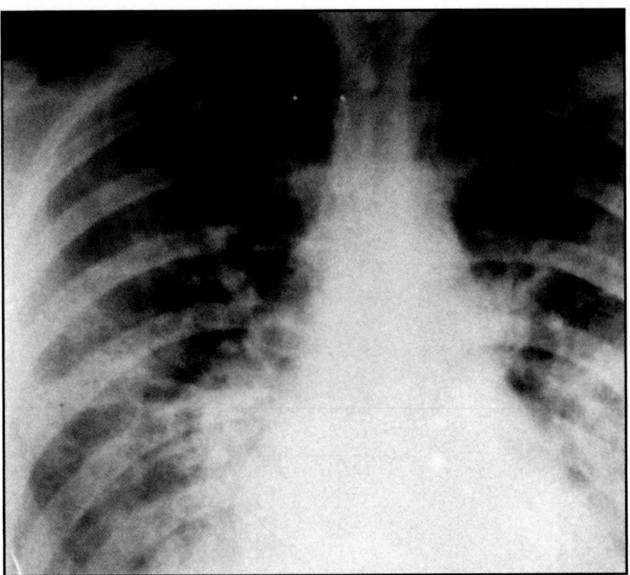

Fig. 3.12 Patchy bilateral infiltrates in a patient with humidifier lung. The lesions cleared after removal of duct work, and cleaning and replacement of the humidifier and the residual water pan, which contained a heavy growth of actinomycetes and other microorganisms.

Physical examination

In exceptionally severe cases of the acute form of EAA, life-threatening respiratory failure may develop and emergency admission to a hospital becomes necessary – death is very uncommon but not unknown. Respiratory distress at rest with fever and gravity-dependent crackles comprise the major physical signs, with breathing being fast but shallow. Clubbing is very rarely seen. Hypoxia is typically accompanied by hypocapnia and a chest radiograph shows a diffuse alveolar filling pattern (Fig. 3.12). Spontaneous recovery can be expected to begin within 12–24 hours and can be accelerated with corticosteroid therapy.

In the chronic form of the disease the major physical signs are similar to those of other varieties of pulmonary fibrosis, although clubbing is rare and crepitations may not be readily evident, and it may be extremely difficult to distinguish this form of EAA from cryptogenic fibrosing alveolitis, sarcoidosis, or other slowly progressive forms of pulmonary fibrosis.

Investigation

Establishing a diagnosis of EAA involves several areas of investigation apart from the clinical history: an assessment of the nature and severity of the pulmonary disorder, an environmental evaluation, and tests to establish hypersensitivity. The diagnosis should be considered in all patients presenting with relevant acute or chronic symptoms who have regular exposure to organic dusts or animal proteins in domestic, occupational, or avocational settings. In all but the chronic form, a careful history should reveal symptom remission after extended removal from the source of antigen.

Pulmonary assessment

In many cases EAA is first suspected after the presence of diffuse alveolitis or progressive pulmonary fibrosis is established.

Radiographs

In the acute form of the disease a chest radiograph will commonly show no abnormality unless symptoms are moderately severe. Normal radiographic appearances are particularly common with humidifier lung, possibly because the antigen is largely present in soluble rather than particulate form. When the radiograph is abnormal there is a widespread alveolar filling pattern, particularly in the lower and middle zones. This may resolve within a mere 24–48 hours once exposure has ceased. In more subacute forms, irregular small 'reticular' opacities simulating asbestosis are seen within the same distribution. Occasionally a more nodular pattern occurs. The opacities may persist for several weeks despite cessation of exposure, and if exposure continues, honeycombing may develop. In contrast, the upper zones are predominantly affected by the irreversible fibrotic process that characterizes the chronic form of EAA. This may simulate sarcoidosis or even tuberculosis and may lead to considerable shrinkage and distortion. In practice, the radiographic appearances vary considerably from patient to patient and correlate poorly with the clinical severity of the disease.

Computed tomography (CT) scans

CT scans provide a much clearer picture of the type and extent of radiographic abnormality, particularly when thin-section, high-resolution techniques are used, but they have shown that no single feature or pattern is pathognomonic. Investigation within hours of exposure has been limited and experience is largely confined to patients with subacute and chronic disease. Increased density of the lung parenchyma, demonstrated by 'ground-glass' attenuation in the lower and mid zones, has been the most prominent finding in the subacute form of EAA followed, almost equally, by reticular or nodular infiltration. Expiratory images may show a mosaic pattern due to patchy air trapping, which indicates bronchiolar involvement. Unaffected bronchioles allow the distal lobule to deflate normally (the parenchyma becomes denser), but those that are sufficiently involved become obstructed during expiration and so prevent deflation (the parenchyma remains lucent). Neither lymph node enlargement nor pleural involvement is characteristic. The CT scan is appreciably more sensitive than the plain chest radiograph and shows a more uniform involvement of the lung fields in subacute disease than does the plain chest radiograph. With chronic disease, the CT scan shows a similar pattern of fibrosis and disruption to the plain radiograph, but again is considerably more sensitive.

The abnormal features in the acute and subacute forms may be simulated by pulmonary congestion from cardiac disease, but the latter is markedly gravity dependent, and so changes when the subject moves from a supine to prone position. By contrast, the abnormalities signifying inflammatory or fibrotic diseases of the lung do not vary with posture. CT scanning for the investigation of EAA should consequently include both supine and prone views.

Pulmonary function studies

The pattern of results from tests of lung function varies according to severity and recent activity and, as with asthma,

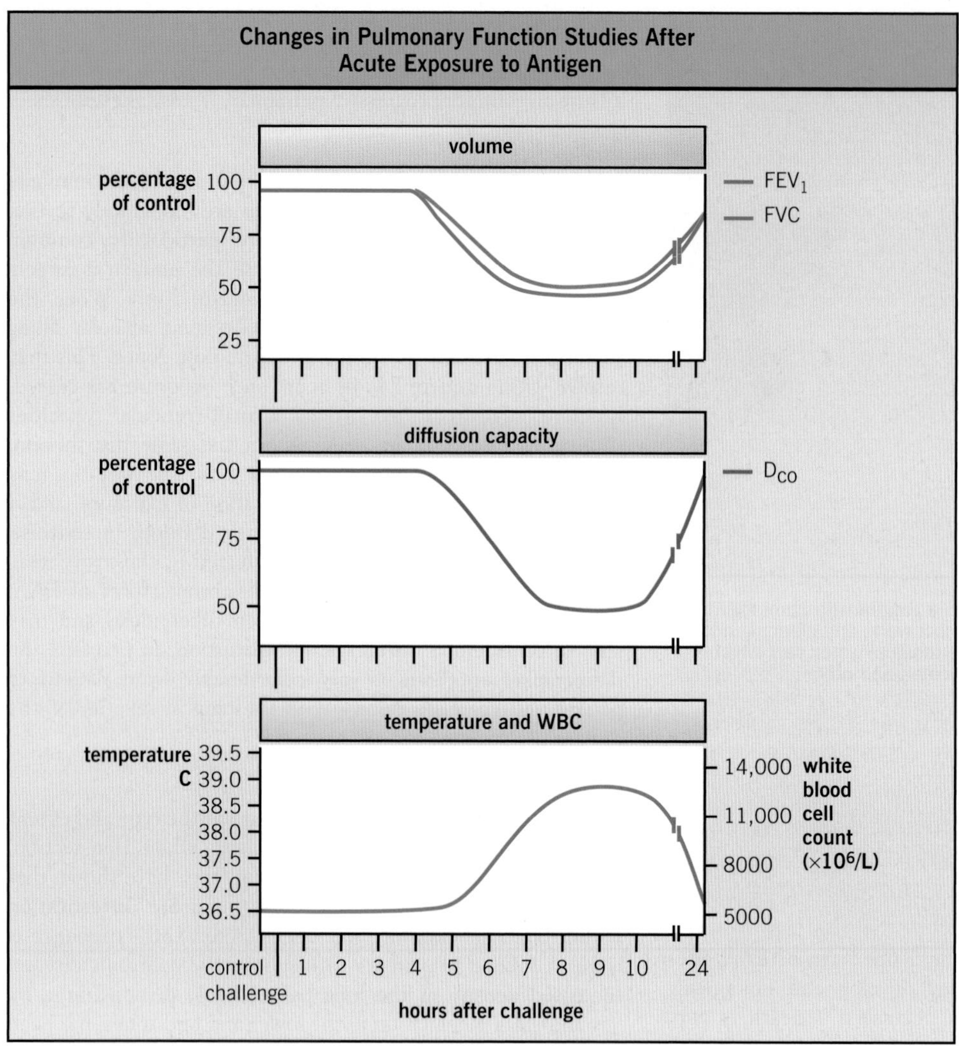

Fig. 3.13 Illustrative changes in pulmonary function studies and peripheral blood cell analysis following acute exposure to antigen (from a patient with pigeon breeder's disease). Note similar decrease in forced expiratory volume in 1 second (FEV_1) and forced vital capacity (FVC), indicating ventilatory restriction not obstruction, plus diminished carbon monoxide diffusing capacity (DLCO), commencing 5 hours after exposure. Typical rises in temperature and total white cell count were also noted at this time.

may reveal little of note in the acute form of the disease when there has been little recent exposure. When lung function is impaired the pattern suggests parenchymal or interstitial disease but is otherwise non-specific. There is impaired carbon monoxide gas transfer [diminished carbon monoxide diffusing capacity (DLCO) and carbon monoxide transfer coefficient (KCO)] with restricted ventilation [diminished FVC with normal or increased FEV_1:FVC ratio (FVC, forced vital capacity; FEV_1 the forced expiratory volume in 1 second)], decreased compliance and, in the more severe examples, hypoxemia with hypocapnia – particularly on exercise. Although total lung capacity is reduced, residual volume is often increased suggesting air trapping as a result of bronchiolar involvement. Occasionally there is also obstruction of the large airways but this implies a coincidental asthmatic or bronchitic effect. The changes following an acute exposure in an affected pigeon fancier are shown in Figure 3.13.

Lung biopsy

A transbronchial, video-assisted thoracoscopic, or open lung biopsy may be required when other diagnostic procedures are not sufficiently definitive in distinguishing EAA from cryptogenic fibrosing alveolitis, or other diffuse infiltrative or fibrotic disorders of the lung, but it is not commonly needed. The recent popularity of video-assisted thoracoscopic techniques has made adequate-volume biopsy more readily available. It may be particularly useful in the subacute or chronic forms of the disease when hypersensitivity is less obvious or when, acutely, there has been an unduly heavy exposure to microbial spores and there is a suspicion of microbial invasion. BAL, although more readily performed and less hazardous, has not proved to be as definitive as biopsy and remains a complementary rather than an alternative investigatory procedure.

Environmental evaluation

If a causal agent has to be identified from an unexpected or previously unrecognized source, direct air sampling of the suspected environment may be required using industrial hygiene techniques, coupled (if appropriate) with microbiologic investigations. A recent domestic example in North America showed that fungal contamination centered on damp fiberglass insulation in a basement with *Aureobasidium pullulans* (the microorganism associated with sequoiosis), *Saccharopolyspora rectivirgula* (a microorganism associated with farmers' lung), and a species of *Humicola* was the probable cause of a housewife's EAA. This illustrates importantly that such a cause is not confined to Japan or to summer, or to species of *Trichosporon*, or to redwood

Table 3.2 Diagnostic features of positive inhalation-challenge tests

Diagnostic Features of Positive Inhalation-Challenge Tests	
Diagnostic changes within 3–6 hours of challenge exposure	**Sensitivity (%)**
Increase in body temperature to > 37.2°C	78
Increase in circulating neutrophils by ≥ 2.5 × 10^9/L	68
Decrease in circulating lymphocytes by ≥ 0.5 × 10^9/L to lymphopenia (i.e. 1.5 × 10^9/L)	52
Decrease in forced vital capacity by ≥ 15%	48
Increase in exercise minute volume by ≥ 15%	85
Increase in exercise respiratory frequency by ≥ 25%	64

The diagnostic cut-offs were chosen to produce specificities of 95%

(sequoia) workers or farm workers. Although the fiberglass was removed, fungal growth could not be completely eliminated and her degree of susceptibility was such that only an eventual house move brought satisfactory control.

Immunologic assessment

Respirable antigenic dusts stimulate immune responses in most (perhaps all) exposed subjects, yet disease such as EAA becomes evident in only a minority. This creates difficulty in assessing which immunologic tests, among the many with diagnostic potential, are best able to separate subjects with disease from those who are exposed but unaffected. The matter is complicated because symptom perception varies enormously from subject to subject, and so some with symptoms have no demonstrable disease, while others without symptoms show unequivocal physiologic or radiographic abnormalities. In general, immunologic tests identify subjects with exposure more readily than they identify disease among the subjects who are exposed. A positive immunologic test does, however, indicate that the exposed subject has mounted an immune response, and so usefully separates an exposed subject in whom EAA is plausible from one in whom it is improbable. Furthermore, the greater the strength of an immune response, the greater is the probability of disease. This implies potential diagnostic benefit from tests which display results quantitatively over a range compared with those which give positive or negative results only. Nevertheless, in practice a negative test goes a long way to excluding EAA.

A caveat needs to be applied to smokers, since smoking diminishes many immune responses. When immunologic tests do not favor EAA, the diagnosis is rarely made, but it may not be adequately excluded. There is consequently some doubt as to whether smoking diminishes the risk of EAA in proportion to the degree that it diminishes immune responsiveness. Thus, a negative immunologic test in a current smoker does not exclude EAA with the same degree of confidence that it does in a current non-smoker.

Inhalation challenge testing

Inhalation challenge tests provide the gold standard for the diagnosis of EAA, whether in the natural setting or in the laboratory. A return to the suspected environment after a week or so without exposure offers the simplest method of producing the 'challenge', but may not be sufficient to generate an unequivocally positive response in subjects with the chronic form of the disease. It may, however, be the only practical method if the suspected environment harbors no obvious source of allergen, or if there are many potential candidates. A positive response will confirm that the subject is affected, but will not identify the causal agent. When a definitive diagnosis is particularly important, laboratory-based inhalation-challenge testing can be used. These tests employ a variety of techniques from nebulizing soluble extracts to recreating environmental exposures in an exposure chamber. Ideally the 'challenge' is conducted in a double-blind fashion, neither the test subject nor the immediately supervising physician knowing whether the test allergen is being used or a dummy control.

The influenza-like component of positive reactions is often uncomfortable and, if excessive doses are administered, these tests can be hazardous. Moreover, objective evidence for positive reactions may be difficult to obtain from conventional lung function testing. Consequently, tests of this nature should be restricted to centers with special expertise. Personal experience from 144 inhalation-challenge tests of evaluating objective changes in body temperature, circulating neutrophil and lymphocyte numbers, FVC, and exercise tests is summarized in Table 3.2. Together, these monitoring tests provide high specificity and high sensitivity. Auscultation, chest radiography, measurement of gas transfer, and arterial blood gas analysis are often too insensitive to provide useful diagnostic information.

Serum antibody

High levels of a precipitating antibody, which reacts with the offending antigen, are characteristically detectable by simple double gel diffusion in the serum of individuals with EAA, particularly those with the acute form of the disease. More sensitive techniques than precipitin formation [e.g. counter-current electrophoresis or quantitative enzyme-linked immuno-sorbent assay (ELISA)] are sufficiently sensitive to detect antibodies against organic dust antigen in virtually all patients. The predominant antibody class is IgG and healthy control subjects with no apparent exposure to a particular aero-antigen will have very low antibody levels. Exposed individuals will have a range of levels of antibody and it is important to consider testing asymptomatic as well as symptomatic subjects. In general, antibodies can be detected in large numbers of asymptomatic subjects with exposure but higher antibody titers are associated more strongly with acute disease, and sero-negative EAA is rare. Thus, antibodies do not usefully identify EAA (this depends on symptoms, physical signs, lung function tests, radiologic imaging, and BAL), but once EAA becomes a plausible/probable diagnosis, IgG antibodies are indispensable in identifying the probable antigenic agent.

For diagnostic purposes, the identification of serum antibody is useful to confirm 'meaningful' exposure. It is reasonable for screening purposes to check any suspected organic dust for antigenic activity by simple agar double gel diffusion. Quantifying antibody by ELISA is an additional laboratory adjunct in the assessment of disease. It is extremely useful for monitoring decreasing IgG antibody titers, since this confirms compliance with advice to avoid antigen contact.

Assays for cell-mediated immunity

A distinctive characteristic of acute EAA is the marked increase in lymphocyte numbers in the interstitium and air spaces. This reflects the involvement of cell-mediated immune (CMI) responses, but in vitro tests for CMI responses (e.g. antigen-induced lymphocyte proliferation and cytokine production) do not yet have any practical clinical application. There are no standard conditions for doing these tests and, as with serum precipitins, they have been shown to be positive in many exposed, asymptomatic individuals. At present, these tests have more value in research than diagnosis.

Skin tests

Skin tests, as diagnostic aids, can be performed with certain antigens associated with EAA, such as serum proteins or purified fungal extracts, though, in most cases, non-irritant antigenic extracts are not commercially available for testing in humans. Furthermore, administration by intracutaneous injection rather than 'pricking' may be necessary to achieve adequate dosage. This carries a potential hazard if there is IgE hypersensitivity in the recipient or an unrecognized infective agent in the extract. When positive, the skin test often reveals an immediate wheal and flare reaction followed by a late-phase response at 4–6 hours and, occasionally, delayed reactivity at 24–72 hours. Delayed skin reactivity is more difficult to demonstrate in humans, possibly because of the removal of antigen during the associated immediate skin reaction. As in the case of serum precipitins, positive skin reactivity can often be demonstrated in exposed but asymptomatic individuals. The main limitation to diagnostic skin testing is the lack of standard antigen preparations and the fact that most antigen extracts associated with EAA are likely to contain irritant or toxic components, perhaps from sterilizing components, which make the interpretation of any responses difficult. Prick testing with common allergens is unhelpful other than to identify an atopic predisposition, which is uncommon in patients with EAA. Occasionally, respiratory symptoms among subjects exposed to birds may be due to asthma and to immediate hypersensitivity to either avian serum proteins or bird mites. This can be confirmed by immediate responses to prick tests.

Bronchoalveolar lavage

Analyses of cell phenotype and humoral factors in BAL fluid may provide very useful supportive information for the diagnosis of EAA. Once established EAA is, like sarcoidosis, associated with a T-lymphocyte and macrophage response in BAL fluid. Lymphocytes usually represent 10–20% of recovered cells but in EAA the percentage may reach a level of about 70% (rather more than in sarcoidosis), with large numbers of cytotoxic CD8+ T lymphocytes rather than helper CD4+ T lymphocytes, as well as increased plasma and natural killer (NK) cell numbers. Lymphocytosis, however, is often seen in asymptomatic although similarly exposed subjects (Fig. 3.14). Even though there is usually a predominance of cytotoxic CD8+ lymphocytes, the CD4+ helper lymphocytes are also increased in numbers following exposure. A CD4:CD8 ratio of less than 1 is compatible with acute disease, but this approaches a more normal 2:1 ratio as disease becomes more chronic. During the hours immediately following exposure a polymorphonuclear leukocytosis may dominate, simulating cryptogenic fibrosing alveolitis.

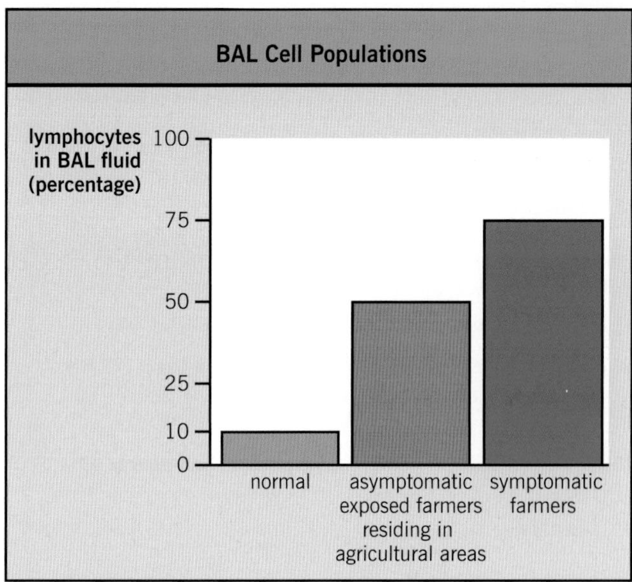

Fig. 3.14 A comparison between the lymphocyte proportion in bronchoalveolar lavage (BAL) fluid from asymptomatic and symptomatic farmers with the proportion in healthy control subjects.

These local T cells bear class II histocompatibility antigen (HLA-DR), and the markers CD25 and CD69 indicating activation. These activation markers are not necessarily related to a regulatory function and can be detected on activated lymphocytes of both helper and cytotoxic subsets. The presence of these cells probably reflects ongoing local, T-cell-dependent immune processes and not necessarily disease, because they are present, albeit in lesser numbers, in subjects who are exposed but remain asymptomatic.

Various humoral factors have been measured in the airway fluid retrieved by BAL. There is antibody activity which seems to be proportional to the peripheral blood level. Elevated levels of total IgG, IgA, and IgM have also been demonstrated in BAL fluids, as have high levels of certain proinflammatory cytokines, as discussed in the Pathogenesis section. Other BAL findings in asymptomatic healthy farmers who were non-smokers revealed elevated levels of albumin, fibronectin, and angiotensin-converting enzyme, which suggests that healthy farmers exposed to appropriate mold-laden composts may exhibit subclinical alveolitis including accumulation of inflammatory cells in the airways. These data suggest that there is ongoing lung inflammation in subjects exposed to antigens of EAA, but only a proportion of these go on to develop symptoms.

In summary, BAL may be of practical diagnostic value if used to investigate diffuse interstitial lung disease, since a high lymphocyte count with CD4:CD8 ratio < 1 will alert the clinician to the possibility of EAA; and serological tests for IgG antibody are indispensable in showing that an immunologic response has been generated to a recognized cause of EAA. For practical purposes, failure to demonstrate a relevant IgG antibody makes a diagnosis of EAA improbable, though the confidence with which this applies to current smokers is yet to be clarified.

DIFFERENTIAL DIAGNOSIS

Acute EAA is not the only disorder characterized by systemic influenza-like symptoms and respiratory distress, following an unusually heavy exposure to microbially contaminated vegetable produce. In 1986, an international symposium considered a further disorder which occurs within hours of heavy respiratory exposure to dust containing fungal toxins, particularly those released on decapping silos. This is the result of direct toxicity rather than hypersensitivity. Although illness from fungal toxin ingestion (mycotoxicosis) has been recognized for some time, respiratory exposure was not considered hazardous until recently. Rather than pulmonary mycotoxicosis, the term organic dust toxic syndrome (ODTS) was the recommended description. Its effects are usually mild and self-limiting but severe respiratory embarrassment may occur and there is a small risk of ongoing and potentially fatal fungal invasion of the lungs. This risk could be enhanced if corticosteroid treatment is given, and death has occurred because of this despite normal immunocompetence. Not only does ODTS occur in circumstances which favor the occurrence of EAA, but its clinical features have much in common with EAA and, to a lesser extent, with nitrogen dioxide toxicity which also affects silo workers. Indeed, there is so much overlap that it may be very difficult to distinguish one disorder from the other in the individual (Table 3.3).

The acute form of EAA can only be the result of an acute and recent exposure to the relevant causal antigen (a matter of hours). With the exceptions of ODTS and nitrogen dioxide toxicity, this limits the opportunity for diagnostic error although the circumstances of an unusually heavy exposure may be subtle. For example, a pigeon fancier might spend rather less time than usual with his birds, but much more time than usual in the confined environment of his hazardous car – hazardous because of pigeon dust accumulated from the regular transport of his racing birds for training exercises.

Just as acute and heavy exposures to organic dust may, on the one hand, cause disorders other than EAA, they may, on the other hand, be quite irrelevant and purely coincidental to the acute respiratory disorder with which a patient presents. Consequently, the differential diagnosis should include some consideration of other acute disorders of the lung parenchyma and interstitium such as infections, other immunologic disorders, drug reactions, and even paraquat poisoning, which sometimes occurs accidentally in farm workers. In bird keepers the diagnosis of viral, mycoplasma, and chlamydial infection may itself be confounded by false-positive microbial antibody tests. This is the result of cross-reactions between pre-existing avian antibodies and egg protein in the microbial culture material used to provide the test agents.

When subacute or chronic forms of EAA are encountered, the differential diagnosis lies with other diffuse infiltrative and fibrotic disorders of the lung. Those most frequently resembling EAA include diffuse idiopathic pulmonary fibrosis (cryptogenic fibrosing alveolitis), sarcoidosis, pneumoconiosis, tuberculosis, and metastatic cancer although a huge variety of less common disorders may also need to be considered.

NATURAL HISTORY AND PROGNOSIS

Little is known about the natural history and prognosis of EAA after chronic long-term exposure, and there is a degree of inconsistency among the reports that have been published. One study of patients with farmers' lung revealed a 5-year morbidity rate of 30% and another of Mexican patients with pigeon fanciers' lung suggested a 5-year mortality as high as 25%. Respiratory disability in these cases was caused mainly by pulmonary fibrosis. In general, when individuals continue to work after experiencing one or more acute attacks they may be subject to recurrent acute attacks and to progressive and permanent fibrotic damage (i.e. the chronic form of the disease). Fortunately, such a course is usually followed in only a minority of affected subjects. The reasons why some individuals develop fibrosis are extremely important but unresolved. The matter was addressed in a recent study describing tissue inhibitors of metalloproteinase (TIMP), the protein with regulates collagenase function. A haplotype variant of the TIMP-3 promoter was found to protect against susceptibility in pigeon breeders' EAA (Fig. 3.10).

A survey of 1992 farm workers, presenting with the acute form of farmers' lung and followed over 2–40 years, showed that, while the majority continued to live on farms, only a minority developed radiographic evidence of pulmonary fibrosis (39%) or impairment of carbon monoxide gas transfer (30%). As many as 28% gave histories of chronic productive cough and 25% had airway obstruction. This illustrates: first, that farm (and other occupational) dusts may cause chronic bronchitis and asthma as well as EAA; and second, that chronic forms of farmers' lung may involve emphysema as well as fibrosis. A similar 10-year outcome has been reported in 24 pigeon fanciers with the acute form of EAA. Again, the majority elected to continue the antigenic exposure despite medical advice to the contrary. Fanciers had attempted to regulate their exposure to the birds by use of masks and by spending less time in their lofts, but this is an unlikely explanation for the benign course of their disease, as levels of antibody to pigeon antigen remained high, suggesting that appreciable antigen exposure was still occurring.

It seems that in some cases, perhaps in the majority, important protective mechanisms emerge which lead to tolerance from the effects of further acute exposures or at least prevent the development of damaging fibrosis. Such tolerance, perhaps associated with the production of antiinflammatory cytokines and related suppressor factors, has been the rule rather than the exception in most animal models of EAA. Rodents exposed to aerosols of soluble antigen develop immunologic tolerance which can only be circumvented by co-administration of immunologic adjuvant, which then induces EAA. Similarly in humans, the majority of subjects newly exposed to aerosolized antigens do not develop symptoms and disease. The nature of this inherent non-responsiveness is unknown, but understanding it could be very important in understanding many chronic disorders. There are likely to be several mechanisms, and in

Table 3.3 Features of nitrogen dioxide pneumonitis, organic dust toxic syndrome (ODTS) and acute farmers' lung

Features of Nitrogen Dioxide Pneumonitis, ODTS and Acute Farmers' Lung			
Features	**Nitrogen dioxide pneumonitis**	**Organic dust toxic syndrome**	**Acute farmers' lung**
Susceptibility in smokers	Unknown	Unknown	Decreased
Relation to time of harvest	Days	Months–years	Months–years
Microbial decomposition of harvest product	Little	Marked	Variable
Confined exposure space	+ + +	+	+
Previous episodes	–	+	+ +
Symptoms			
Dry cough	+ +	+ +	+ +
Breathlessness	+ +	+ +	+ +
Wheeze	–	–	–
Systemic upset	+	+	+
Signs			
Basal cracks	+	+	+
Fever	+	+	+
Time of onset after beginning exposure	1–10 hours	1–10 hours	1–10 hours
Duration	Hours–days	Hours–days	Hours–days
Investigations			
Leukocytosis	+	+	+
Radiograph (small irregular opacities, alveolar shadows)	+	+	+
Restricted ventilation	+	+	+
Reduced gas transfer	+	+	+
Hypoxia	+	+	+
Fungi from secretions/biopsy	–	+ + +	+
Methemoglobinemia	+	–	–
Serum precipitins	–	–	+ (– in smokers)
Response to steroids	+	–	+ +
Life threatening	Not uncommon	Occasionally	Rarely

some cases cigarette smoking may be relevant. Among pigeon fanciers, the smokers do not generally make IgG responses to avian antigens and appear not to develop EAA. This may be a consequence of the lower inducible macrophage cytokine production, which is thought to explain the association between smoking or nicotine therapy with the prevention or resolution of another mucosal disease, ulcerative colitis. A further but unexplored possibility is that a diagnosis of EAA has been excluded inappropriately in smokers simply because antibody tests are negative. Such bias could have distorted the epidemiologic evidence.

Another example of tolerance is reflected in the periodicity of the clinical response shown by some subjects with EAA – particularly those sensitized to humidifier contaminants at work. Although they show a typical acute EAA response on the first day at work after a weekend break, symptoms over the following days lessen or even cease. The mechanisms for this are unknown, but suggest either an exposure-dependent depletion of active mediators which can reaccumulate during periods away from antigen exposure, or the downstream induction of antiinflammatory mediators. There is some evidence for this latter suggestion among pigeon fanciers. They have a typical serum pattern of marginally higher than normal C-reactive protein and proinflammatory TNFα and IL-6 levels, but very markedly raised IL-1 receptor antagonist (IL-1Ra) levels. IL-1Ra is an antiinflammatory cytokine which binds and blocks the function of the IL-1 receptor. The IL-1Ra levels correlate with the IgG antibody titers suggesting a steady-state of antigen exposure and control of inflammation which may prevent symptoms. This response may be biologically useful in order to minimize tissue damage to intermittent antigen exposure. However, this damping of acute symptoms may disguise the insidious progression of fibrotic disease.

Individuals in a particular aero-environment who have no immunologic or clinical reactivity to antigen may exhibit one further example of tolerance. They may have a counterpart to functional regulatory CD4+/CD25+ T cells, which prevent hypersensitivity to common allergens among non-atopic individuals. In asthma patients these cells are functionally deficient, and this may also be the case in subjects who develop EAA. There is indirect evidence for this, since the function of these regulatory cells is enhanced by steroid treatment and steroid therapy provides the mainstay in the pharmaceutical management of EAA. Some of these aspects are illustrated on Fig. 3.15.

MANAGEMENT OF EXTRINSIC ALLERGIC ALVEOLITIS

General principles

Disease management centers on reducing any further exposure to a minimum: there is no place for desensitization. Ideally the causal environment is avoided completely, or changed so that the causal agent is eliminated completely. This may mean a profound loss in income or great expense, and is often unrealistic; nor is it fully justified on purely medical grounds since continued exposure does not inevitably lead to progressive disease. Affected individuals who continue to work in the occupation responsible for their disease can often reduce exposure substantially by changing the pattern of their particular duties. An alternative is the use of industrial respirators which filter out 98–99% of respirable dust from the ambient air. They are particularly valuable when exposures are intermittent and short, but may be uncomfortably hot when worn for long periods or during heavy work. There is, of course, an obligation for the employer to provide a safe working environment, and improved industrial hygiene procedures may be required.

Whatever course is followed continued exposure should be accompanied by regular medical surveillance. If there is no progression, it is reasonable for some exposure to continue. When there is progressive disease, exposure should cease. This may involve a loss of earnings and may entitle an affected worker to compensation. Some individuals with progressive disease refuse to change their occupation or hobby (or are unable to change their domestic environment), and the physician must weigh the possible advantages of long-term corticosteroid therapy against the well-known risks.

Reduction of antigenic contamination

Sometimes the antigen can be removed entirely from the affected subject's environment, or its accumulation can be prevented. This will not only help control his/her disease, but will prevent sensitization in other exposed individuals. For example, simply altering the moisture content or pH of moldy bagasse has resulted in the diminution and even disappearance of bagassosis in those areas of the world where it was originally described. Certain other organic materials (e.g. mushroom compost) can be rendered sterile by exposure to high temperatures, and drying hay and cereal crops before storage can greatly diminish the potential for microbial contamination.

In cases where ventilation and humidification systems are responsible for EAA, major mechanical alterations may be necessary and the methods of humidification and temperature control may need to be changed. It is crucial to reduce the ease with which normal airborne microbial contaminants are able to proliferate in the stagnant collections of water which inevitably occur in these systems. There may be a role for certain biocidal sterilizing agents but these are likely to become airborne and respirable and so must have low intrinsic toxicity and sensitizing potency. The manufacture (but not necessarily the use) of isothiazolinones, for example, carries a small risk of sensitization and hence of skin rashes, rhinitis, or asthma. In large manufacturing plants, the use of recirculated filtered air is most economical but effective filters are expensive and can become contaminated themselves, increasing rather than decreasing the load of respirable microbial antigen in the working environment. The use of heat exchangers minimizes the cost of temperature control if contaminated exhaust air is not recirculated, but it does not conserve water and so may be inordinately expensive for plants that need to maintain high levels of humidity.

Drug treatment

Many mild acute febrile episodes will abate spontaneously when the patient is removed from the offending environment. Severe attacks require treatment with corticosteroids although there is still some debate over their usage for attacks of only moderate severity. One recent investigation failed to demonstrate any long-term functional differences between groups treated randomly with corticosteroids or placebo for the initial acute episode of farmers' lung. The corticosteroid group did, however, recover more quickly. Supplemental oxygen and bronchodilators may also be required if there is hypoxemia and airway obstruction and, in life-threatening cases, there may be a need for a period of mechanical ventilation.

Novel therapeutic approaches will follow from improved understanding of the disease mechanisms, and a number of new approaches are under investigation. There are case reports showing improvement in farmers' lung when subjects were treated empirically with erythromycin because their symptoms were thought to be due to atypical pneumonia. In experimental EAA, erythromycin has been shown to be therapeutic. It had no effect on cytokines, but reduced ICAM-1 and neutrophils in BAL fluid and myeloperoxidase in the lung, suggesting a block on the early inflammatory events. Pentoxifylline has anti-inflammatory effects on cytokine regulation using ex vivo alveolar macrophages from EAA patients, suggesting a basis for clinical trials. More specifically, there is increasing evidence supporting a pivotal role for TNFα in granuloma formation and in causing the acute symptoms of EAA. Recent observations associating EAA with a particular polymorphism for increased production of TNFα suggest a possible therapeutic role for anti-TNFα therapy using humanized anti-TNFα (infliximab) or recombinant soluble TNFα receptor (etanercept). The value of these interventions will require appropriate clinical trials.

CONCLUSIONS

EAA develops as a result of a complex series of events involving initial non-specific inflammation, followed by immunologically specific sensitization and a genetically controlled granulomatous inflammatory response. An overview of these mechanisms, as currently understood, is shown in Figures 3.8 and 3.10, with some regulatory processes in Figure 3.15.

If left unrecognized and untreated, EAA in the individual may progress to an irreversible phase characterized by the progression of pulmonary fibrosis. A failure of recognition may additionally allow other exposed individuals to become affected. In consequence, considerable importance attaches to an early diagnosis and the prompt identification and control of the causal antigen.

ACKNOWLEDGEMENT

We have retained some of the text and format prepared for this chapter by the late JE Salvaggio in Allergy I and Allergy II.

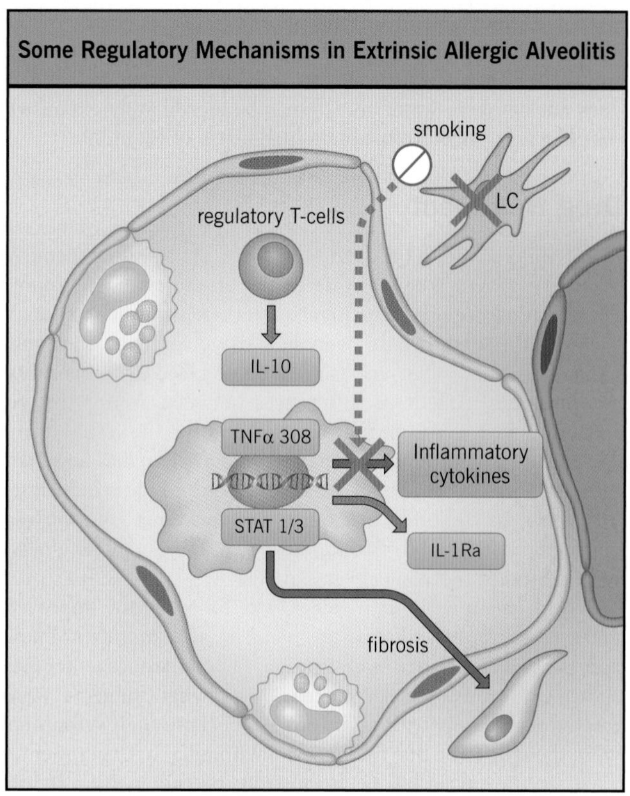

Fig. 3.15 A simplistic scenario for several proposed regulatory mechanisms in EAA. Most subjects exposed to antigenic aerosols associated with EAA do not develop progressive disease, therefore the default position may be anti-inflammatory. Despite evidence of antibody and lymphocyte responses in most exposed subjects there is evidence of anti-inflammatory cytokines including high concentrations of interleukin-1 receptor antagonist (IL-1Ra), which can regulate the inflammatory response, and IL-10 produced by regulatory T cells, which can modulate local T cell proliferation. Cigarette smoking inhibits the immune response to inhaled antigens partly by abrogating local antigen presenting cells and by deactivating alveolar macrophages. On the other hand, disease susceptibility and progression may be related to cytokine polymorphisms, for example an increase in the allele frequency of the promoter region of the tumor necrosis factor gene ($TNF\alpha^{308}$) has been associated with disease, and the relative expression of the regulatory molecules signal transducer and activator of transcription (STAT)-1 and -3 determines the extent of the fibrotic response.

FURTHER READING

American Thoracic Society/European Thoracic Society. International Multidisciplinary Consensus Classification of the Idiopathic Interstitial Pneumonias. Am J Respir Crit Care Med 2002; 165:227–304.

Ando M, Konishi K, Yoneda R, et al. Difference in the phenotypes of broncho-alveolar lavage lymphocytes in patients with summer-type hypersensitivity pneumonitis, farmer's lung, ventilation pneumonitis, and bird fancier's lung: report of a nationwide epidemiologic study in Japan. J Allergy Clin Immunol 1991; 87:1002–1009.

Dangeman KH, Cole SR, Hodgson MJ, et al. The hypersensitivity pneumonitis diagnostic index: use of non-invasive testing to diagnose hypersensitivity pneumonitis in metalworkers. Am J Indust Med 2002; 42:150–162.

Facco M, Trentin L, Nicolardi L, et al. T cells in the lung of patients with hypersensitivity pneumonitis accumulate in a clonal manner. J Leukoc Biol 2004; 75:798–804.

Gudmundsson G, Hunninghake GW. Mice deficient in interleukin-10 production develop more severe hypersensitivity pneumonitis. J Invest Med 1997, 244A.

Johnston I. (Chairman), British Thoracic Society, Standards of Care Committee. The diagnosis, assessment and treatment of diffuse parenchymal lung disease in adults. Thorax 1999; 54(suppl 1):S1–S28.

Kupeli E, Karnak D, Kayacan O, et al. Clues for the differential diagnosis of hypersensitivity pneumonitis as an expectant variant of diffuse parenchymal lung disease. Postgrad Med J 2004; 80:339–345.

Lacasse Y, Selman M, Costabel U, et al. EAA Study Group. Clinical diagnosis of hypersensitivity pneumonitis. Am J Respir Crit Care Med 2003; 168:952–958.

McSharry C, Anderson K, Bourke SJ, et al. Takes your breath away – the immunology of allergic alveolitis. Clin Exp Immunol 2002; 128:3–129.

Patel AM, Ryu JH, Reed CE. Hypersensitivity pneumonitis: current concepts and future questions. J Allergy Clin Immunol 2001; 108:661–670.

Pérez-Padilla R, Salas J, Chapela R, et al. Mortality in Mexican patients with chronic pigeon breeder's lung compared to those with usual interstitial pneumonitis. Am Rev Respir Dis 1993; 148:49–53.

Schenker MB. Respiratory health hazards in agriculture. Am J Respir Crit Care Med 1998; 158:S1–S76.

Chapter 4

Definition:

Rhinitis can be defined as symptoms of nasal irritation, sneezing, rhinorrhea, and nasal blockage lasting for at least 1 hour a day on most days.

Rhinitis

Glenis K Scadding and Martin K Church

INTRODUCTION

Most people will experience nasal symptoms at times as a normal defense mechanism, and the threshold at which such symptoms are perceived as a problem varies. The diagnosis of rhinitis is based on the subjective reporting of nasal complaints in the absence of upper respiratory tract infection, other diseases, or structural abnormalities. To date, investigations for rhinitis have low sensitivity and specificity and the diagnosis, therefore, must be made predominantly on the basis of the clinical history – the above definition may exclude a proportion of cases with mild disease. Diary recording of symptoms and their circumstances over a 2-week period may be helpful in borderline cases.

Readers should note that according to current guidelines rhinitis is now referred to as intermittent or persistent rather than seasonal or perennial as was the case previously.

CLASSIFICATION OF RHINITIS

Rhinitis occurs mostly in patients aged 15–25 years, and is less common in older patients. As with other allergic diseases, the prevalence of rhinitis is steadily increasing (Fig. 4.1).

Patients present with nasal irritation, sneezing, rhinorrhea, and nasal blockage, symptoms which may be intermittent or persistent. In allergic rhinitis there is usually a clear relationship with exposure to known allergens, most frequently pollens in intermittent rhinitis, and house dust mite or household pets in persistent rhinitis. The identification of an allergic trigger in the latter group is often difficult. In some patients there is no evidence of allergy. Some of these have autonomic rhinitis, the major symptom of which is rhinorrhea, and, in the remainder, no allergen can be detected even though their symptoms are similar to those of allergic rhinitis (Fig. 4.2). Mixed forms of rhinitis with allergic and autonomic features also exist.

Certain systemic disorders such as Wegener's granulomatosis and sarcoidosis can present with rhinitis.

Allergic rhinitis

Atopy, defined as the ability to produce high levels of IgE directed against common allergens, is very prevalent among young adults, with approximately 50% of individuals aged 18–45 years having at least one positive skin prick test (SPT) to common inhalant allergens. The prevalence of allergic rhinitis is over 10% in the 15–25 year age group, approximately half of whom seek medical advice (see Fig. 4.1).

The important allergens in allergic rhinitis vary in different parts of the world: in the UK grass pollinosis is commonest, in some parts of North America ragweed predominates, in Scandinavia birch pollen is common, while in Mediterranean areas

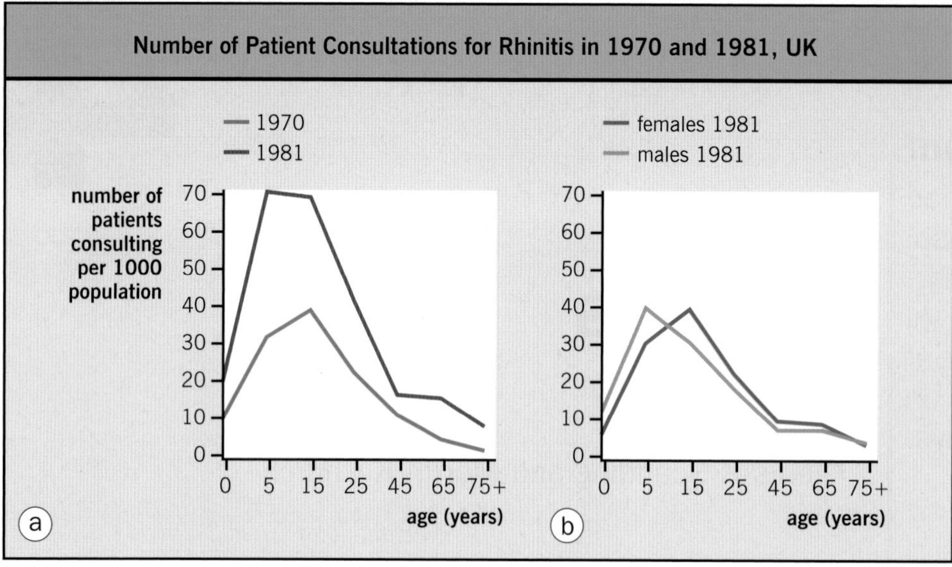

Fig. 4.1 (a) Number of patients consulting their family doctor for treatment of seasonal rhinitis in the UK in 1970 and 1981. (b) Number of men and women consulting their family doctor for treatment of seasonal rhinitis in the UK 1981. [Adapted with permission from Fleming DM, Crombie DL. Prevalence of asthma and hay fever in England and Wales. Br Med J (Clin Res Ed). 1987; 294:279–283.]

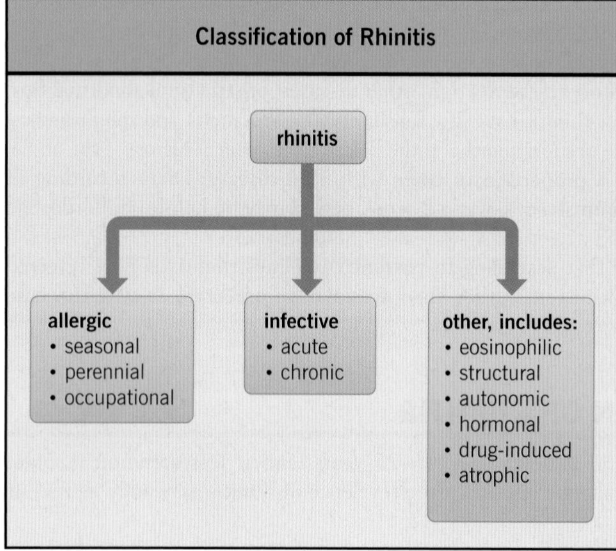

Fig. 4.2 Classification of rhinitis.

Table 4.1 Major allergens worldwide

Major Allergens Worldwide	
Type of allergen	**Examples**
Major pollen allergens	**Grasses and weeds** Ragweed (USA) Bermuda grass (USA) Timothy grass (UK) Cocksfoot (orchard) grass (UK) **Trees** Silver birch (Sweden) Japanese cedar (sugi tree) (Japan) Oak (USA and UK) Mesquite tree (South Africa, South America, and Asia)
Domestic and occupational allergens	Mite Domestic pets Flour (bakers) Solder (solderers) Latex (health workers)

Parietaria species (a nettle-like weed) and olive tree pollen are common allergens (Table 4.1). In tropical climates, allergenic pollens may be present all year round; consequently the symptoms of pollen allergy may be persistent. Conversely, classically persistent allergens, such as the house dust mite, provoke intermittent symptoms in temperate climates where there are increased levels of mite allergens during the autumn (see Table 4.1). Molds are uncommon causes of allergic rhinitis, owing to their small size, as they are more likely to be deposited in the lower airway by gravity-dependent sedimentation or inertial impaction than in the upper airway by turbulent airflow. However, occasionally small quantities of mold trapped in the sinuses result in a marked eosinophilic inflammatory response with the formation of nasal polyposis. This is termed allergic fungal sinusitis.

Occupational agents also cause allergic rhinitis (see Table 4.1). In fact, rhinitis is a more common manifestation of sensitization than asthma, the nasal mucosa being more accessible to deposition of dusts and vapors (e.g. baker's flour, isocyanates, wood dusts, and animal allergens), all of which can be associated with an IgE-mediated allergic response. Occupational rhinitis always precedes or accompanies the development of occupational asthma, never the other way round. Food allergens are also sometimes a source of symptoms, particularly in children, but rhinitis is very uncommon as an isolated feature of food allergy. Some food additives, such as metabisulphite, can also provoke generalized allergic symptoms, including rhinitis.

It is likely that much allergic sensitization occurs in very early life when the immune system is immature (Table 4.2). The inheritance of atopy is likely to be polygenic. Gene linkage studies have suggested an autosomal-recessive inheritance for elevated total IgE levels, but there are several levels of genetic control for specific and total IgE, skin test positivity, and disease specificity. There is also a higher prevalence of rhinitis

Table 4.2 Factors contributing to the development of rhinitis

Factors Contributing to the Development of Rhinitis	
Increased by	**Decreased by**
Atopy	Early infection with hepatitis A
Month of birth (May and June)	BCG vaccinations
Male gender	
First born	
Smoking	
Early allergen exposure	
Viral infection	
Environmental pollution	

in boys than in girls. This may be genetically determined, as IgE levels are higher in boys from birth.

Environmental influences in the first year of life are important in the onset of allergic disease. Rhinitis is more common in individuals born in spring and summer. This was initially thought to indicate the influence of tree or grass pollen exposure in the first weeks of life. However, non-atopic rhinitis is also more common in those born in spring and summer, indicating that factors other than environmental pollens are responsible for this seasonality. There is evidence that early respiratory infections have a role in initiating IgE dysregulation, a fundamental feature of allergic disease. As the onset of allergic disease in children born to atopic parents is temporally related to early respiratory infections, it has been proposed that exposure of infants born in spring or summer to winter viral respiratory infections occurs at a vulnerable time, (i.e. after protective maternal immunoglobulins have fallen to a low level but before the infant's own immune system has developed fully). This theory is supported by detailed studies of infants with respiratory syncytial virus bronchiolitis showing the presence of virus-specific IgE and raised total circulating IgE, suggesting a direct association of viral infection with IgE.

Socioeconomic factors are also important. A strong inverse relationship between hayfever and family size has been noted, with first-born children being at greatest risk. This relationship is independent of the social class of the father. Children with antibodies to hepatitis A and those with positive skin tests to *Mycobacterium tuberculosis* (i.e. those from less clean environments), are less likely to have allergic rhinitis. This suggests that early infection with hepatitis A and *Mycobacterium tuberculosis* may protect against the development of atopy, possibly because of increased production of interferon γ (IFNγ). IgE production is enhanced by cigarette smoking and, in infants and young children, parental smoking contributes to allergic sensitization and is associated with wheezing and the risk of rhinitis. The relative risk of rhinitis is doubled for children who live in damp houses and have parents who smoke. Modern energy-efficient 'tight' buildings encourage the growth of house dust mites and molds, because of higher humidity and warmth, and so increase exposure to potential allergens.

Environmental pollution may also contribute to allergic sensitization. Epidemiologic studies in Japan have shown that the prevalence of Japanese cedar pollen rhinitis is higher in urban than in rural environments. Studies in mice have also shown that diesel exhaust particles have an adjuvant effect on sensitization to ovalbumin when both are inoculated intranasally.

Non-allergic rhinitis

Non-allergic rhinitis is defined by the absence of positive SPTs or radioallergosorbent test (RAST) to common allergens. Ideally, it should include a negative response to likely nasal allergen challenge since local nasal IgE synthesis has been demonstrated. In practice, the diagnosis is usually dependent on there being no offending allergen apparent from the clinical history. As advancing age is associated with reduced IgE levels and a reduced prevalence of positive SPTs, this may be a confounding factor when assigning rhinitics into atopic and non-atopic subgroups. Such age-related changes contribute to the fall in the apparent prevalence of allergy among persistent rhinitics from around 80% in childhood to below 20% in elderly people. Epidemiologic studies of a population of nearly 3000 patients in Tucson, Arizona, have shown that the prevalence of symptoms of rhinitis is as high as 30% even in those with very low age-adjusted serum IgE scores. This emphasizes that there is a non-allergic subgroup to rhinitis.

The contribution of environmental pollutants and occupational agents to non-allergic rhinitis is uncertain. Well recognized occupational sensitizers do not necessarily involve an IgE-mediated mechanism. Fewer than 20% of patients with symptoms caused by isocyanates have a raised specific IgE level. Furthermore, it is likely that there are many unrecognized agents which may contribute to the development of rhinitis.

Non-allergic rhinitis may be subdivided into eosinophilic and non-eosinophilic subgroups. The latter includes individuals with autonomic rhinitis where parasympathetic overdrive occurs, replacing the normal alternating sympathetic tone which leads to the nasal cycle and maintains patency. Patients with a history of predominantly watery rhinorrhea without eosinophilic secretions may be included in the autonomic subgroup, although ideally this group should be defined by a therapeutic response to parasympathetic blockage. The term vasomotor rhinitis should be abandoned because it is misused for patients who demonstrate mucosal hyperreactivity secondary to allergic rhinitis. Predominantly unilateral rhinorrhea may represent a leak of cerebrospinal fluid. The presence of eosinophils in nasal secretions may be demonstrated by light microscopy. The eosinophilic subgroup is very similar to the allergic rhinitis group, except for the absence of an identifiable allergen.

Nasal polyps

Nasal polyps occur most commonly in males aged between 30 and 40 years. In childhood, polyps are predominantly associated with cystic fibrosis and differ from those in adulthood in that the accompanying nasal secretions are purulent with a high neutrophil content, and that they usually respond poorly to corticosteroids. The more commonly found nasal polyps may occur in association with both asthma (7% of cases) and rhinitis (2%), but they do not have a clearly allergic etiology despite predominant nasal secretion eosinophilia. In fact, polyps are more common in non-atopic asthmatics than in atopic asthmatics. There is an association of nasal polyposis with asthma and aspirin sensitivity, the mechanism probably involves increased leukotriene synthesis plus decreased prostaglandin

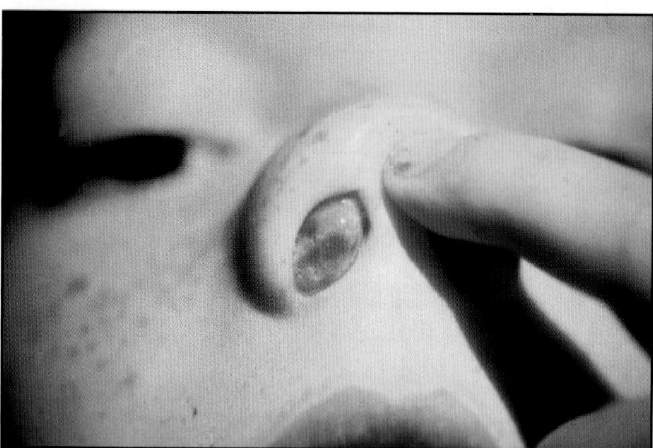

Fig. 4.3 Nasal polyps. (Courtesy of Mr D Gatland, St Bartholomew's Hospital, London.)

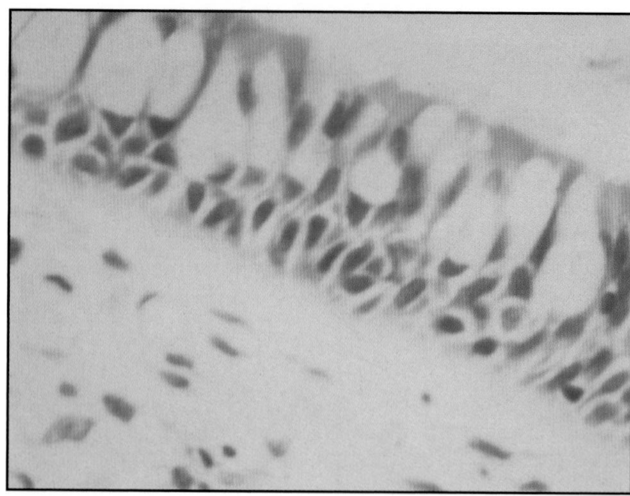

Fig. 4.5 Pseudostratified ciliated columnar epithelium of the nasal mucosa. (Courtesy of Dr M Calderon-Zapata, St Bartholomew's Hospital, London.)

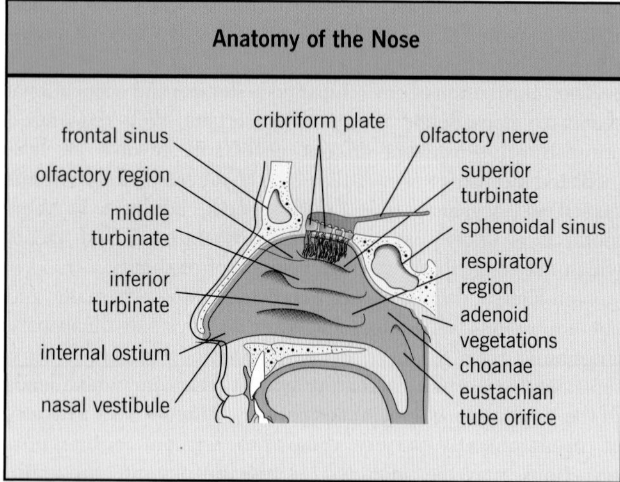

Fig. 4.4 Gross nasal anatomy in sagittal section.

E2 secondary to COX1 inhibition. Upregulation of the leukotriene receptors also appears relevant. The predominant symptoms of polyposis are nasal blockage and anosmia, sometimes with watery discharge. Symptoms are rarely unilateral, although this may occur in teenagers with choanal polyps, which arise from the maxillary sinuses. More usually, nasal polyps arise from the ethmoid sinuses as well as from the mucosa overlying the turbinates. Polyps can be seen at rhinoscopy as pale gray–yellow rounded masses (Fig. 4.3). Clinically, they can cause purulent sinusitis due to obstruction of the ostia of the paranasal sinuses.

ANATOMY AND PHYSIOLOGY OF THE NOSE

The nasal cavity commences at the internal ostium, a narrow slit-like orifice about 1.5 cm from the nostrils (Fig. 4.4). The internal ostium is the narrowest part of the respiratory tract with a cross-sectional area of approximately $0.3\ cm^2$. The inferior, middle, and superior turbinates form the lateral wall, and the nasal septum forms the medial wall, of the nasal cavity. The turbinates contribute to the irregular outline of the nasal cavity, which is important to its air-conditioning and air-filtering functions. The nasolacrimal duct opens into the inferior meatus, the portion of the nasal cavity lateral to the inferior turbinate. The orifices of the frontal, maxillary, and anterior ethmoidal sinuses open into the middle meatus, lateral to the middle turbinate.

The epithelium changes from stratified squamous in the nasal vestibule to a squamous and transitional epithelium lining the anterior one-third of the cavity. The remaining portion is lined by ciliated pseudostratified columnar epithelium typical of the respiratory tract (Fig. 4.5), except in the upper part of the cavity where olfactory epithelium is present. The number of goblet cells is highest in the posterior nasal cavity, similar to that in the trachea and main bronchi.

The epithelium rests on the basement membrane (lamina lucida, lamina densa, and lamina reticularis), a layer of connective tissue composed of collagen types III, IV, and V, laminin, and fibronectin. The underlying lamina propria is characterized by high vascularity (Fig. 4.6). The arterioles have no internal elastic lamina and a porous basement membrane, which increases permeability and allows greater access for pharmacologic agents. There is an extensive capillary network, and the capillaries are fenestrated, allowing rapid transit of fluid across the capillary wall. Large cavernous vascular sinusoids are present in the lamina propria on the turbinates. These contribute to heating and humidification of inspired air. Beneath the lamina propria are periosteum and bone.

Innervation

Sensory innervation

The trigeminal nerve supplies afferent (sensory) fibers to the nasal mucous membrane. Activation of these fibers produces the sensations of irritation or pain, which often results in sneezing (Fig. 4.7). Olfaction is affected by fibers from the first cranial nerve which enter the roof of the nose via the cribriform plate (see Fig. 4.4).

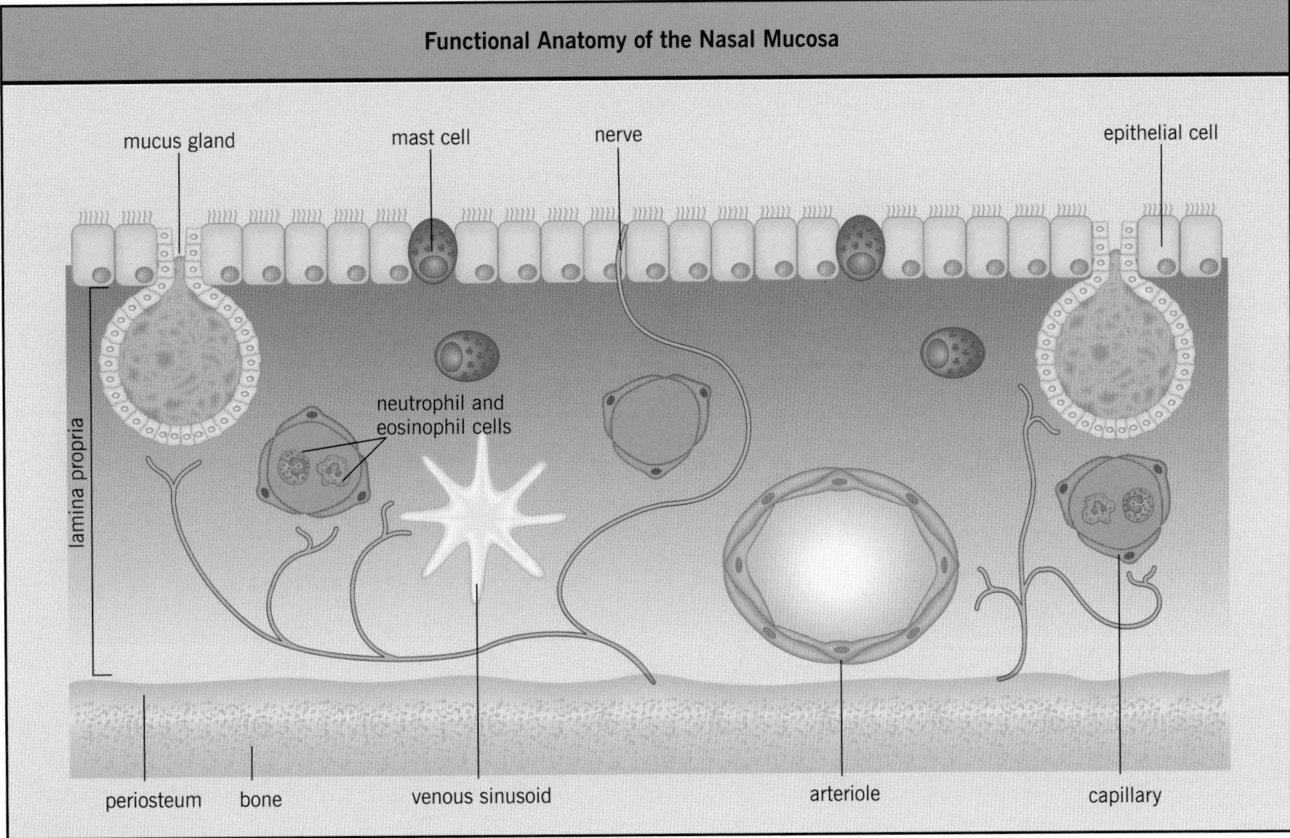

Fig. 4.6 Functional anatomy of the nasal mucosa.

Vascular innervation

Sympathetic fibers, which mainly follow the blood vessels, predominate. Release of their co-transmitters – noradrenaline and neuropeptide Y – causes vasoconstriction and maintains the sympathetic tone of the sinusoids. Sympathetic tone fluctuates throughout the day with an increase in patency in alternate nostrils every 2–4 hours (the nasal cycle).

Parasympathetic fibers, arising in the sphenopalatine ganglion to form the vidian nerve control vasodilatation and glandular secretion. The parasympathetic co-transmitters are acetylcholine and vasoactive intestinal peptide. Axon reflexes can be powerful in the nasal mucosa, resulting in vasodilatation and transudation with thickening of the mucosa. These reflexes may be initiated by the effect of irritants and inflammatory mediators at sensory nerve endings and the transmitters include sensory neuropeptides, substance P, neurokinin A, and calcitonin gene-related peptide (CGRP). Additionally, sensory nerve activation can cause vasodilatation via neural connections from the trigeminal to the sphenopalatine ganglia and via central nervous reflexes. There are also nasobronchial reflexes which may be activated in asthmatics to promote reflex bronchoconstriction in response to nasal obstruction.

Control of mucus secretion

Mucus is secreted by goblet and serous cells in the epithelium, by submucosal serous glands, and by deep nasal glands. It is diluted by transudate from the blood vessels. Secretion is controlled by parasympathetic cholinergic nerves, but sympathetic stimulation and axon reflexes also enhance secretion.

Functions of the nose

Aside from the sense of smell, the nose provides 'air conditioning' of inspired air and filtration of potentially harmful particulate matter (Fig. 4. 8).The paranasal sinuses contribute high levels of nitric oxide which are toxic to bacteria, viruses , fungi and tumor cells. The nose has a remarkable capacity to humidify inspired air, raising the temperature of room air to 32°C, and humidifying it to 98% relative humidity before it reaches the lungs. This is affected by fluid shift across the highly vascular mucosa and increasing blood flow through the sinusoids.

The narrow, irregular shape of the nasal cavity promotes turbulent air flow, which contributes to impaction of inhaled particles in the upper airway, a protective function against the inhalation of potentially harmful particles into the bronchial tree. Pollen grains, which are around 10 μm in size, are largely deposited in the nose, whereas turbulent air flow is insufficient to deposit particles less than 2 μm in size, such as mold spores, in the nose. These particles will usually reach the distal airways. Particles trapped in the nose are moved into the pharynx by mucociliary transport within 10–30 minutes of impaction, and subsequently swallowed. Additionally, 99% of water-soluble gases, such as sulfur dioxide, are prevented from reaching the lower airways because of passage over the nasal mucosa.

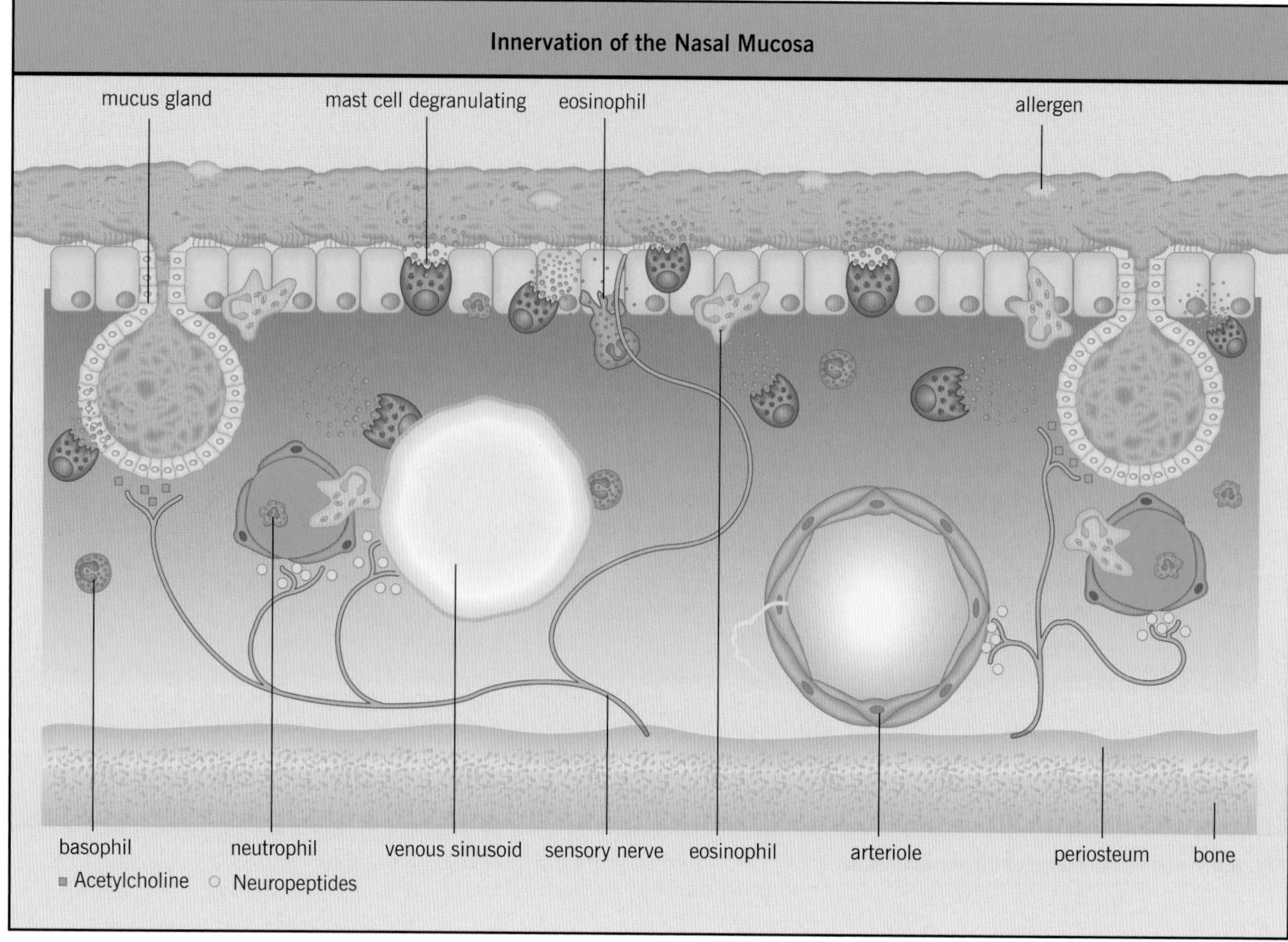

Fig. 4.7 The innervation of the nasal mucosa.

PATHOGENESIS OF ALLERGIC RHINITIS

Pathophysiology

Nasal responsiveness

Increased nasal responsiveness, which may be measured in terms of both symptoms and nasal airway resistance (NAR), can be demonstrated in rhinitics by the response to the inhalation of non-specific challenge agents such as histamine and methacholine. Although there is considerable overlap, measurements of NAR show significantly greater histamine responsiveness in rhinitics than in both atopic and non-atopic non-rhinitics (Fig. 4.9). Methacholine does not increase NAR and it causes a significant increase in nasal secretion only in rhinitics. This contrasts with bronchial hyperresponsiveness, in which there is a much closer association with symptomatic asthma and a strong correlation between the response to histamine and methacholine (Fig. 4.10). It is likely that the pathogenetic mechanisms of rhinitis and asthma are very similar, with hyperresponsiveness being a cardinal feature in both conditions. The difference in responsiveness of the upper and lower respiratory tracts may be explained by the absence of a smooth muscle response in the nose. The action of histamine on the vascular network thus remains effective in reducing airway patency by causing hyperemia and edema of the mucosa, whereas methacholine acts predominantly on glandular secretion, with a much less potent effect on vasodilatation because of the dominance of sympathetic vasoconstrictor nerves. The importance of vascular congestion as the mechanism of nasal obstruction is demonstrated by the rapid response to vasoconstrictor sprays, which is not a feature of bronchoconstriction in asthma.

Allergen provocation

Early and late-phase responses may be demonstrated in the nose after inhalation of allergen by sensitized individuals. Late-phase responses, with associated increases in symptoms and NAR, occur in approximately 50% of patients between 2 and 8 hours after allergen provocation. The physiologic changes of the late phase can be very subtle compared to the intense blockage and symptoms of the early phase (Fig. 4.11). Small increases in NAR during the late phase may be obscured by the nasal cycle. Recent research suggests that platelet activation factor (PAF) and other mediators can increase the nasal response to bradykinin (BK) and histamine.

Priming

During the pollen season, sensitized individuals are exposed to low levels of pollen for a prolonged period. This differs markedly from the artificial conditions of allergen challenge in

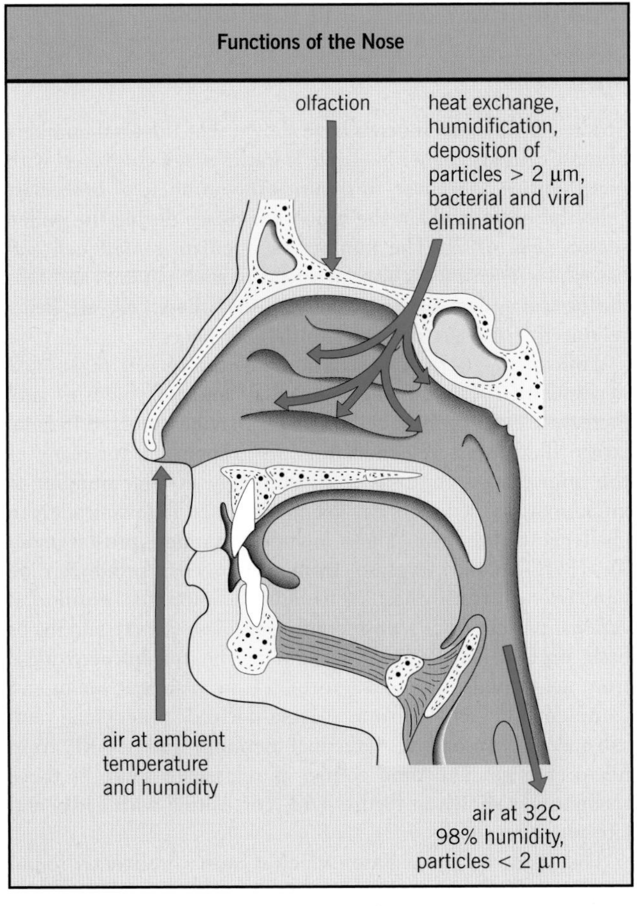

Fig. 4.8 Functions of the nose in warming, humidifying, and filtering inspired air.

the laboratory where large doses of allergen over a short period of time are usually required to evoke a response. Thus, during the pollen season, a sensitized person may become increasingly responsive to allergen, a process known as priming. This may be simulated in the laboratory by repeated allergen challenge after which the dose of allergen required to elicit a response may be reduced by up to 100 times.

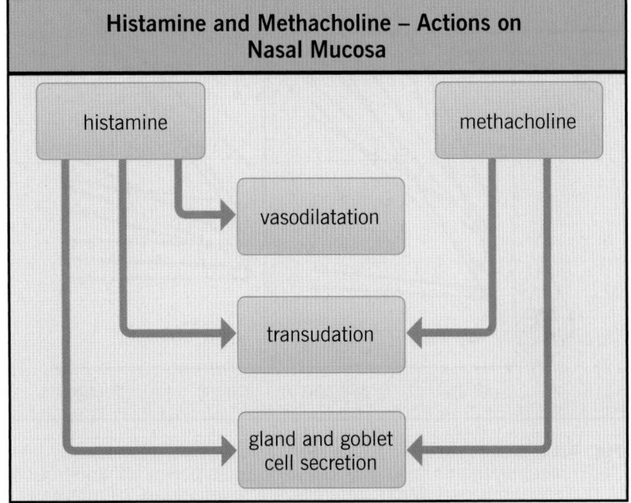

Fig. 4.10 Effects of histamine and methacholine on the nasal mucosa in rhinitis.

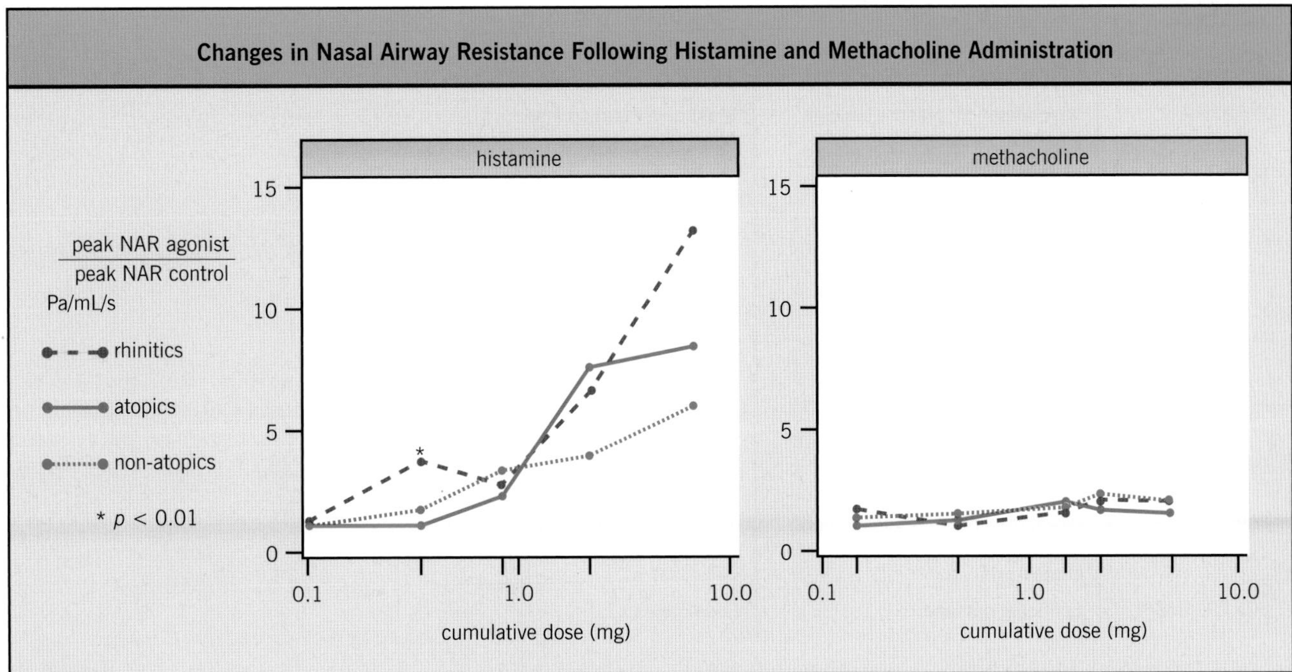

Fig. 4.9 Changes in nasal airway resistance (NAR) following the administration of histamine and methacholine (weighted geometric mean change).

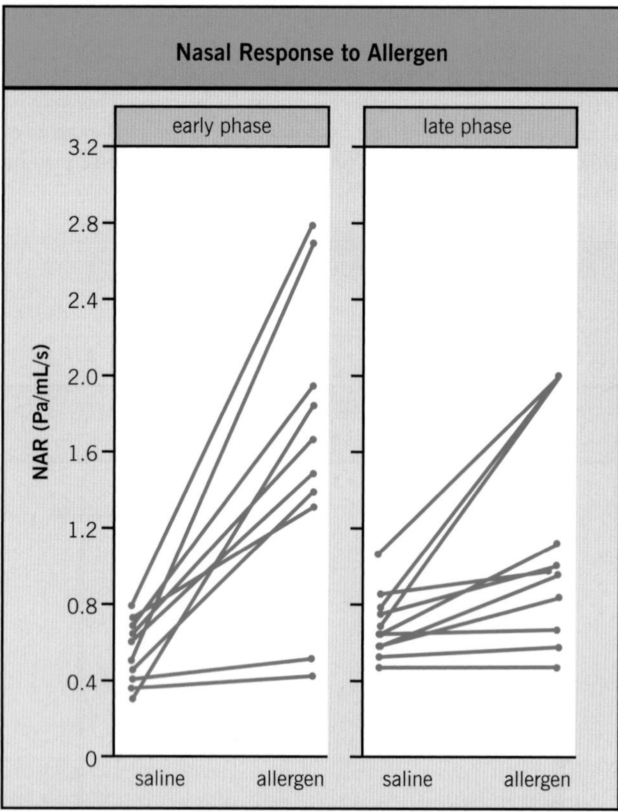

Fig. 4.11 Nasal response to allergen. Nasal airway resistance (NAR) measurements following saline or grass pollen administration to the nasal mucosa. Measurements are taken either 30 minutes after allergen challenge (early response) or 2–7 hours after challenge (late response).

Inflammatory cells and mediators

Mast cells

Studies of the nasal mucosa have shown that the total numbers of mast cells are higher in atopic rhinitics when compared with non-rhinitics. Moreover, in rhinitics the numbers of both mast cells and eosinophils in the mucosa increase during the pollen season (Fig. 4.12). The number of circulating mast cell and basophil progenitors is also increased in such patients and falls during the pollen season, suggesting that these cells are being recruited to the site of allergic inflammation.

Following allergen inhalation, evidence of mast cell degranulation can be seen in nasal mucosal biopsies and increased levels of mast cell products may be detected in nasal lavage fluid. Mast cell mediators are responsible for many of the immediate symptoms of nasal allergy. A large number of inflammatory mediators have been identified following allergen challenge of the nose. These include histamine, prostaglandin D_2 (PGD_2), and tryptase from mast cells; sulfidopeptide leukotrienes from mast cells and eosinophils; eosinophil cationic protein (ECP), eosinophil peroxidase (EPO), and major basic protein (MBP) from eosinophils; neutrophil peroxidase from neutrophils; PAF and serotonin from platelets; kinins and complement factors from plasma-derived precursors; and substance P, vasoactive intestinal peptide, and CGRP from nerve endings. The time course of release of some of these mediators is shown in Figure 4.13, correlating with early- and late-phase responses.

Histamine is the mediator which is most consistently found following allergen challenge. Administration of histamine, albeit at high doses, reproduces many of the symptoms of nasal

Table 4.3 Mediators which act on the nose, their action, and their source

The Effects of Mediators in the Nose

Mediator	Action	Source
Histamine	Vasodilatation, plasma leakage, glandular secretion	Mast cells, early phase; basophils, late phase
PGD_2	Vasodilatation	Mast cells; also platelets, fibroblasts
Tryptase	? activates Kallikrein	Mast cells
TAME-esterase	Vasodilatation	Plasma/glandular kallikrein; mast cell tryptase
LTB_4	Eosinophil chemotaxis, neutrophil activation	Mast cells; neutrophils in late phase
LTC_4 and LTD_4	Vasodilatation, increased blood flow	Mast cells; eosinophils; neutrophils
Kinins	Vasodilatation, increased capillary flow	Plasma
PAF	Vasoconstriction/vasodilatation, eosinophil and neutrophil chemotaxis	Macrophages; neutrophils; eosinophils; endothelial cells
ECP, EPO, MBP	Epithelial damage	Eosinophils

ECP, eosinophil cationic protein; EPO, eosinophil peroxidase; LTB_4, leukotriene B_4; LTC_4, leukotriene C_4; LTD_4, leukotriene D_4; MBP, major basic protein; PAF, platelet activation factor; PGD_2, prostaglandin D_2.

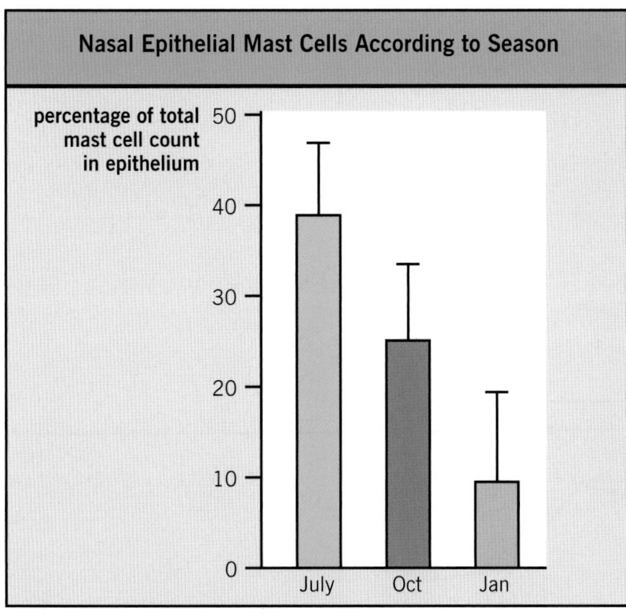

Fig. 4.12 Percentage of total mast cell numbers present in the nasal epithelium in July (in the grass pollen season), compared to October and January, in rhinitics sensitive to grass pollen.

allergy, while specific H_1 antagonists reduce such symptoms. The response to other mediators varies: for example, PAF causes an increase in nasal patency. None of the putative mediators have been shown to cause the ongoing inflammation of a late response. During the late phase, the presence of histamine, in the absence of PGD_2, is suggestive of basophil activation. This is supported by the demonstration of basophils in nasal lavage fluid during the late-phase response.

N-a-tosyl l-arginine methyl ester (TAME)-esterase is a non-specific marker of inflammation that consists of a mixture of plasma and glandular kallikrein activity and, to a lesser extent, mast cell tryptase activity. Levels of TAME-esterase parallel nasal symptomatology and pollen counts during the pollen season and it. TAME-esterase is found in nasal secretions following allergen challenge, indicating that plasma leakage is a major component of the allergic response in the nose (see Fig. 4.13). It is likely that kinins, and complement and coagulation factors derived from the plasma, augment the inflammatory response in the nose. The levels of TAME-esterase and histamine show the features of priming, with an increase following repeated allergen challenge within 24 hours of the initial challenge.

BK (Bradykinin), a nonapeptide derived from kallidin, has been shown to increase in seasonal allergic rhinitis and following nasal allergen challenge. BK challenge causes nasal blockage, rhinorrhea, and pain; BK_1-antagonists of BK do not block these symptoms. However, the recently developed BK_2-antagonist, icatibant, if given intranasally 2 minutes prior to house dust mite challenge, causes almost complete ablation of nasal obstruction (Fig. 4.14).

Nitric oxide (NO) is a colorless, odorless gas and is the final common pathway of many inflammatory reactions. It is derived from arginine via an enzyme, nitric oxide synthase, which exists in an inducible form in macrophages. The concentration of NO is seven times higher in paranasal sinuses than in the nose, which in turn shows concentrations higher than those in the lungs. The levels of the gas increase in the nose after nasal allergen challenge. Pretreatment with N^G-nitro-L-arginine methyl ester (L-NAME) – an inhibitor of nitric oxide synthase – partially blocks the nasal obstruction produced by BK and has interesting differential effects upon allergen-induced nasal reactions (Fig. 4.15).

Mast cell heterogeneity has been observed in nasal polyp tissue with tryptase-containing mast cells (MC_T) predominating in epithelium and the tryptase and chymase-containing mast cells (MT_{TC}) being dominant in the lamina propria. Unlike mast cells in the skin, those in the nose are sensitive to sodium cromoglycate, which explains the effectiveness of this drug in rhinitis. Mast cells migrate from the lamina propria to the epithelium in response to allergen exposure and differentiate in situ under the influence of cytokines derived from CD4+ T cells, fibroblasts, epithelial cells, and endothelial cells. In addition, the number of mast cells showing interleukin-4 (IL-4), IL-5, and IL-6 immunoreactivity is increased in the nasal mucosa in rhinitis.

Eosinophils

Eosinophil numbers are increased in rhinitics, and rise during the pollen season in pollen-sensitive individuals (Fig. 4.16). Eosinophils increase transiently in nasal mucosal biopsies from pollen-sensitive rhinitics 30 minutes after allergen challenge, but the numbers in nasal secretions are persistently raised, and peak at 7–10 hours. This suggests rapid migration from the mucosa into the secretions. The chemoattractants involved in this process remain to be identified, although they may include leukotriene B_4, PAF, eotaxin, and adhesion molecules (VCAM-1). The eosinophils are activated, with hypodense granules, and can damage nasal epithelial cells cultured in vitro, slowing and disorganizing the ciliary beat. The influx of activated eosinophils results in the release of toxic granule products, particularly EPO and MBP, which are toxic to cultured human nasal epithelial cells and cause lysis. Even at low concentrations, MBP can reduce ciliary beat frequency. Such damage may contribute to the inflammatory features of the late-phase response and subsequent nasal hyperresponsiveness.

Dendritic cells and T cells

The number of both dendritic (or Langerhans') cells and T cells at the surface of the nasal epithelium is increased in rhinitis. The interaction of dendritic cells (which process and present allergen) with T cells promotes differentiation of T cells towards the IL-4 and IL-5 producing the helper T cell type 2 (Th2) subtype, leading to IgE production by plasma cells and eosinophil activation respectively. In situ hybridization studies have shown increased numbers of T cells from atopic rhinitics expressing mRNA for IL-4 and IL-5.

Epithelial cells

Given the similarities between the pathogenesis of asthma and rhinitis, it might be expected that rhinitics would demonstrate evidence of epithelial damage. However, there is no difference between mean epithelial heights in pollen-sensitive rhinitics when mucosal biopsies are examined either during or outside the pollen season. The lamina reticularis is not thickened as it is in asthmatics. There is also no significant increase in numbers of epithelial cells in nasal lavage specimens following allergen challenge even during the late response. It is likely that epithelial

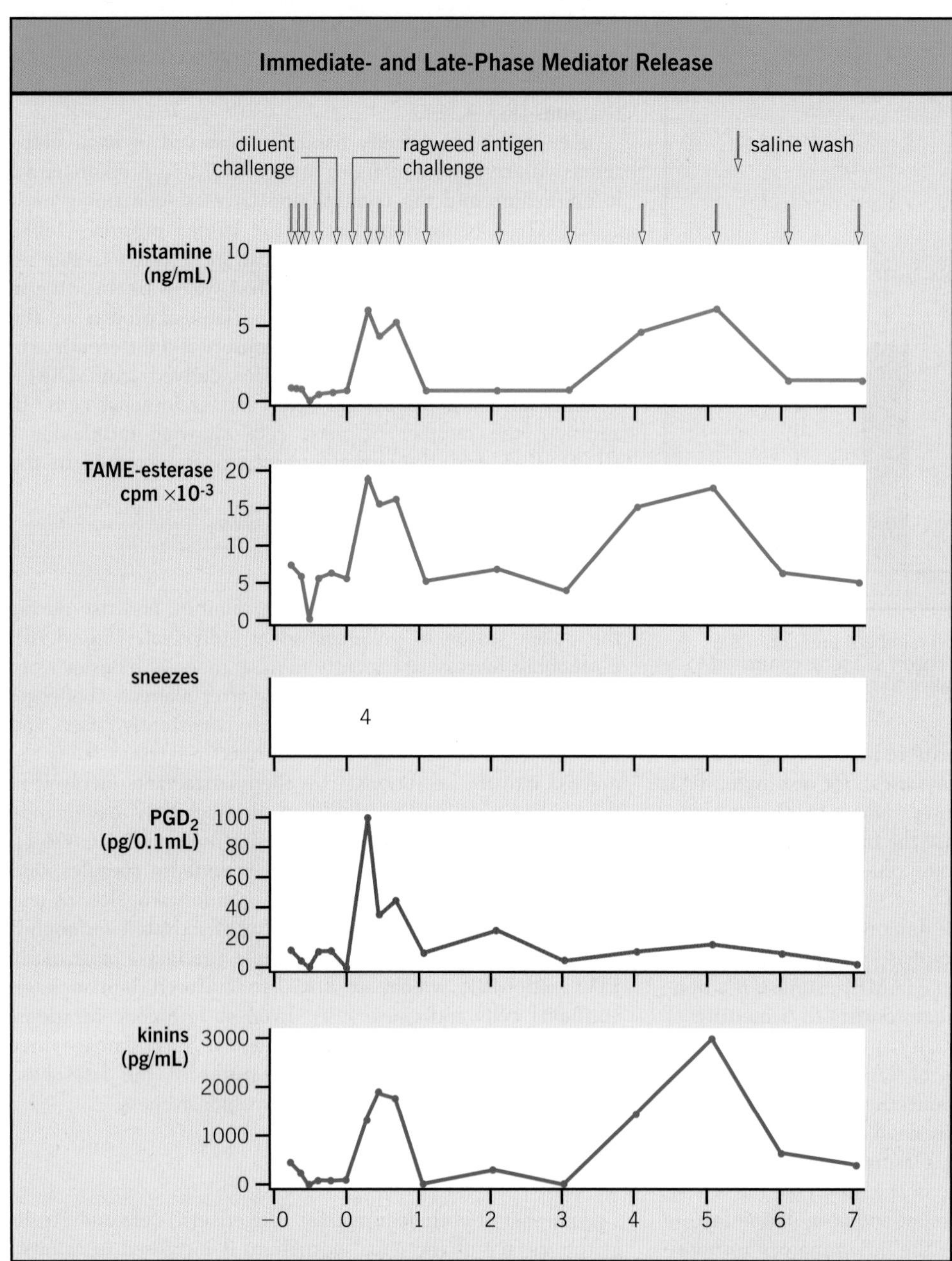

Fig. 4.13 Immediate- and late-phase mediator release following nasal provocation with allergen. [Adapted from Togias A, Naclerio RM, Proud D, et al. Mediator release during nasal provocation. A model to investigate the pathophysiology of rhinitis. Am J Med 1985; 79(6A):26–33, Excepta Medica Inc.]

damage only occurs in the context of prolonged inflammation, as with nasal polyps.

Pathogenesis of nasal polyps

The histologic features of nasal polyps are more similar to those of asthma than those of allergic rhinitis: frequently there is epithelial damage, epithelial cell shedding, and thickening of the lamina reticularis. There may be squamous metaplasia, and eosinophils and mast cells are present in increased numbers in the epithelium. The stroma of the polyp is grossly edematous with marked eosinophil infiltration and increased numbers of plasma cells, mast cells, and lymphocytes. Some patients with perennial rhinitis also demonstrate such features to a lesser degree, with evidence of squamous metaplasia, edema, and increased numbers of inflammatory cells.

Nasal polyp tissue has been used to study local hematopoietic mechanisms. Nasal polyp epithelial cells and fibroblasts are capable of stimulating eosinophil and basophil differentiation in blood from atopic individuals. Additionally, mononuclear cell colonies from nasal polyps yield mainly eosinophil and basophil precursors, indicating an advanced stage of differentiation. High levels of granulocyte–macrophage colony-stimulating factor (GM-CSF) and granulocyte colony-stimulating factor (G-CSF) are present, which contribute to this differentiation. Fibroblasts from nasal polyps also demonstrate increased growth in vitro.

In contrast to rhinitis, patients with nasal polyps predominantly demonstrate peripheral blood eosinophilia and the counts are further increased if asthma is also present. However, such eosinophilia occurs regardless of the presence of allergy. It is possible that secretion of GM-CSF from nasal tissue contributes

Effects of the Bradykinin Antagonist, Icatibant

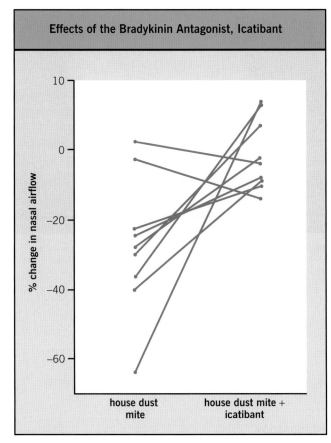

Fig. 4.14 Effects of bradykinin antagonist, icatibant, in intranasal challenge with house dust mite. (Adapted from Austin CE, Foreman JC, Scadding GK. Reduction by Hoe140, the B2 kinin receptor antagonist, of antigen-induced nasal blockage. Br J Pharmacol 1994; 111:969–971.)

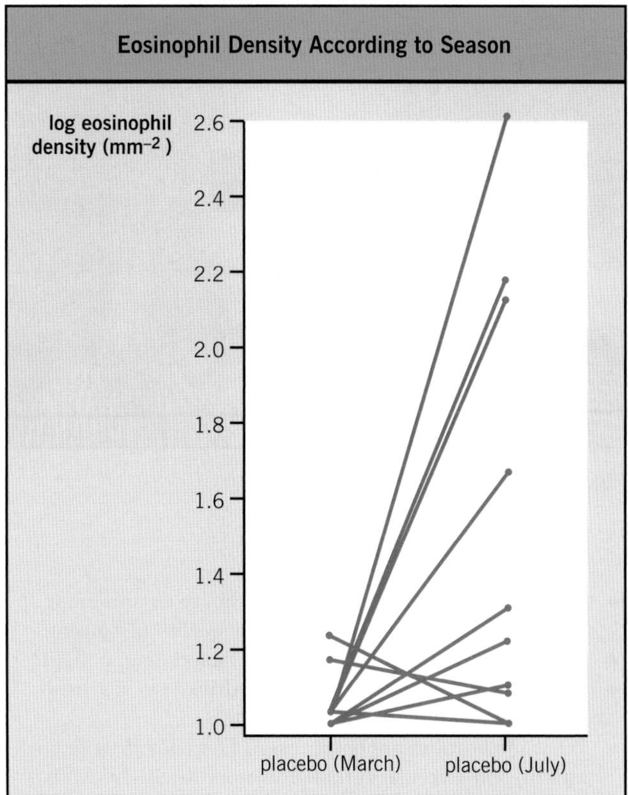

Fig. 4.16 Eosinophil density in rhinitics sensitive to grass pollen before (March) and during (July) the grass pollen season.

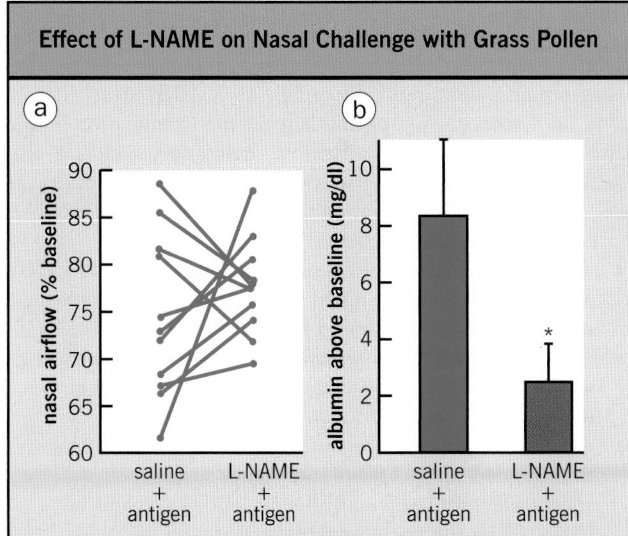

Fig. 4.15 Effect of saline or L-NAME on nasal challenge with grass pollen. L-NAME inhibits albumin release but has no effect on nasal blockage in response to allergen challenge. (Adapted from Dear JW, Scadding GK, Foreman JC. Reduction by NG-nitro-L -arginine methyl ester of antigen induced nasal airway plasma extravasation in human subjects in vivo. Br J Pharmacol 1995; 116:1720–1722.)

to differentiation of eosinophil–basophil colonies and to increased eosinophil survival locally or in the systemic circulation.

DIAGNOSIS OF RHINITIS

The diagnosis of rhinitis in a patient complaining of upper airway problems consists of obtaining a detailed history and performing a physical examination supplemented by critical tests. Further laboratory, radiologic, and morphologic examinations may also be performed if considered necessary.

History

A detailed history augmented with specific questions, presented in the form of either a structured oral interview or a written questionnaire, is essential to distinguish rhinitis from upper respiratory infections or other nasal complaints. Such a questionnaire should cover the following:

- Is there a family history of atopy?
- What is the symptom profile – is there a dominant nasal symptom, such as blockage, sneezes, or nasal secretions?
- Are the nasal problems isolated or are there more extensive symptoms?
- Are there concomitant signs from other parts of the upper airways, such as sinuses or ears?
- Is there a history of lower airway, ocular, or dermatologic disease?
- How would you describe the symptoms and what is the chronology of their onset?

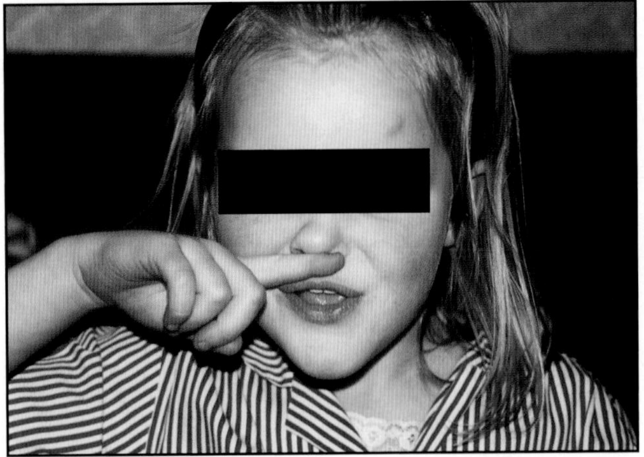

Fig. 4.17 The allergic salute.

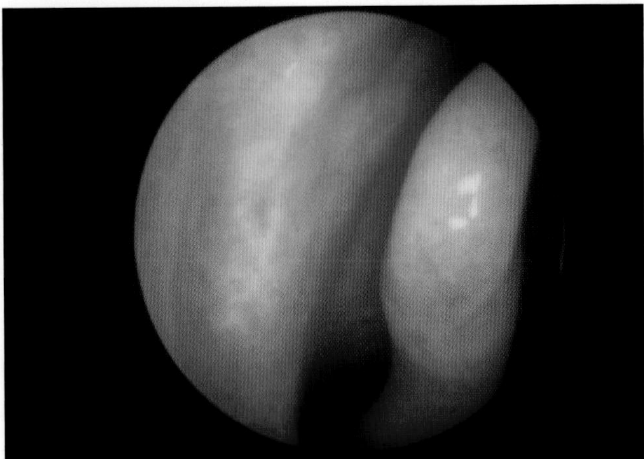

Fig. 4.18 A rigid rhinoscopic examination of a normal nose. The interior of the right nasal cavity is shown with the lateral nasal wall to the right and the middle turbinate on the left. (Courtesy of Jan Kumlien, MD.)

- Are there potential allergens in the house environment, e.g. bedding materials, any pets, low quality of housing?
- Are there any specific precipitating factors (e.g. pollen)?
- Is there any relationship to food or drink? Do any fresh fruits or vegetables cause oral itching?
- What medications are being taken? Does any drug [e.g. aspirin, non-steroidal antiinflammatory drugs (NSAIDs)] worsen symptoms?
- What are the occupation and leisure activities, particularly those which aggravate symptoms?
- What is the impact of problems on lifestyle?

Symptom presentation

The traditional symptoms are as follows: nasal blockage, itching, sneezing bouts, and increased nasal surface fluid, but the dominant symptom may differ from one patient to another. There is also wide individual variation in terms of the tolerability of nasal symptoms. Some people may find a few bouts of sneezing troublesome, while others do not seek medical advice even when their nasal passage is completely blocked. A detailed symptom score registration may well prove helpful when it comes to assessing the severity of rhinitis.

The variability of symptoms may be a result of the difference in the pathogenesis of the major nasal symptoms. Nasal blockage is the result of a decrease in the tone of the capacitance vessels and, to a minor degree, tissue edema. The increase in nasal surface liquid is the result of glandular activity, the leakage of plasma, and the increase in fluids from other sources, such as the conjunctiva. Conjunctival symptoms of itching and increase in tear fluid are also very common in association with allergic rhinitis: the term rhinoconjunctivitis is often more relevant.

Physical examination

Several facial features are associated with the various symptoms of the nasal and ocular disease (Fig. 4.17). These include:

- 'allergic shiners' – infraorbital dark circles, related to venous plexus engorgement;
- 'allergic gape' or continuous open-mouth breathing – a result of nasal blockage;
- 'transversal nasal crease'– a result of the frequent upward rubbing of the nose 'allergic salute'; and
- dental malocclusion and overbite resulting from long-standing upper airway problems.

Rhinoscopy

A rhinoscopy is essential in the clinical workup of nasal problems, especially since there are several possible explanations of nasal problems. Simple inspection will reveal any external nasal deformities, but there may also be inner septal deformities. The rhinoscopic examination can be made using the traditional light-mirror, and a nasal speculum to widen the nasal opening. The posterior rhinoscopy is performed with a mirror placed below the soft palate to permit the inspection of the epipharyngeal region. When possible this examination should be supplemented with an endoscopic examination of the nasal cavities and epipharyngeal region. This examination is performed using either a short rigid rhinoscope (Fig. 4.18) attached to a good light source – of specific help in the examination of the ostial regions – or a short flexible rhinoscope, which is also useful for examining the posterior parts of the nasal cavity, as well as permitting examination of the epipharynx and larynx.

The following findings should be noted:

- any structural deformities, such as septal deviations – the site of any deformity should be specified and the presence or absence of polyps should be recorded (Fig. 4.19);
- the amount and the condition of nasal surface liquids (e.g. watery, mucoid, or purulent), which can be useful in differentiating infection from other conditions;
- the condition of the mucous membranes and the color, texture, and signs of scars and lesions should be specifically evaluated – an allergic condition might be indicated by the traditional bluish tint; and
- unilateral nasal obstruction may also indicate a foreign body.

Since there are several causes for nasal symptoms, these steps are essential.

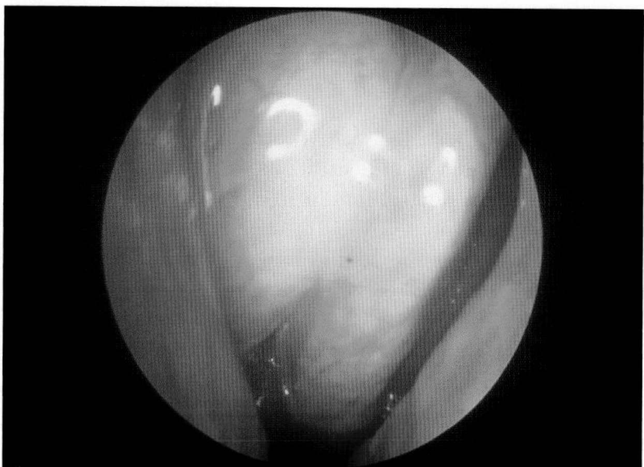

Fig. 4.19 A rigid rhinoscopic examination from a patient with a small nasal polyp in the right nasal cavity, immediately between the middle turbinate and the lateral nasal wall. (Courtesy of Jan Kumlien, MD.)

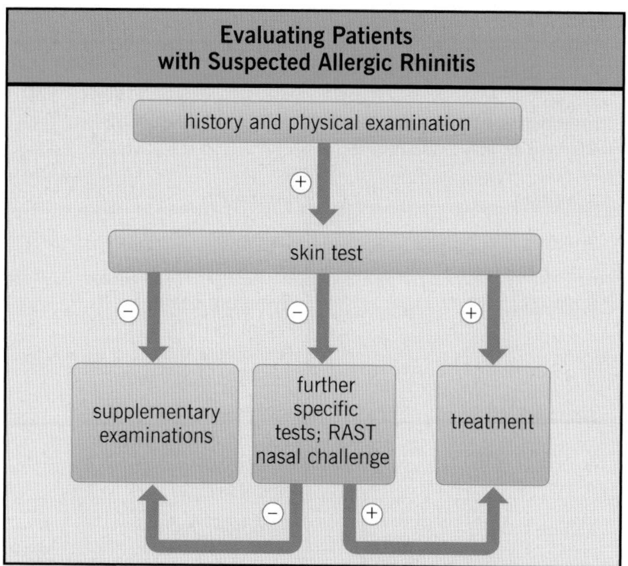

Fig. 4.20 A simplified scheme for evaluating patients with upper airway problems which are suspected of being allergic in origin. If the skin prick test confirms the history, treatment can be instituted. Otherwise, further examinations and tests are indicated. RAST, radioallergosorbent test.

Examination of extranasal regions

Other regions which should be assessed are the eyes, the ears, the chest, and the skin. The presence or absence of conjunctivitis, or watering with conjunctival injection, and edema should be noted.

All patients with persistent rhinitis should have a history taken looking for asthma, their chest should be examined and some form of lower respiratory tract functional measurement, such as peak flow or spirometry, should be made.

Since otitis media and middle ear effusions may occur with increased frequency in children with allergic rhinitis, the ears should be examined, looking especially for any middle ear pathology. This is best done using the otomicroscope. Tympanometric examination is also helpful. Atopic skin diseases also may occur with increased frequency, so the physician should check for urticaria or eczematous lesions.

Additional tests

Tests for the presence of allergy

The history and physical examination should be supplemented with an allergen reactivity test.

Skin tests

The routine test for allergy of the upper airways is the SPT. It should be carried out when there are no other obvious reasons for the nasal symptoms (Fig. 4.20). A clear-cut history of seasonal allergic rhinitis in an adult patient who responds favorably to symptomatic treatment does not necessarily require confirmation by an SPT. The SPT panel should include a positive and a negative control and the major airborne allergens for the area in question. The intracutaneous test is seldom used for the work-up of patients with upper airway problems and should be reserved for specific occasions, as indicated elsewhere.

Blood tests

The traditional test for allergy has been the determination of blood eosinophilia: high numbers indicate that atopy is present. To some degree the eosinophilia is dependent upon the size of the diseased organ and therefore the usefulness of this test for rhinitis is limited. The same applies to the determination of total IgE and this procedure cannot be used as a screening technique for the presence of an allergic condition.

An alternative procedure, a multi-RAST, which indicates the presence of a specific IgE to any of the more common airborne allergens, is useful for screening, however. This could be of value when there are no facilities for performing an SPT. The value of RAST procedures is discussed in Chapter 1. RAST is indicated in testing for the specific allergens that are not available for skin tests or when an SPT cannot be performed because a patient is taking treatment (e.g. histamine H_1 antagonists), which suppress the cutaneous response. The specific value of other procedures, such as the basophil histamine release test, is still uncertain.

Nasal challenge

A nasal challenge can be used to test for specific as well as non-specific reactivity. Non-specific reactivity may be tested using methacholine and histamine as the challenge agents. The test for specific reactivity involves the application of the specific allergens to the nasal mucosa. Some of the tests used to monitor the changes in the challenge situation (Table 4.4) may also be used to monitor the progression of disease.

Test for non-specific reactivity

The overlap in the upper airways between normal and hyper-reactive patients is greater than in the lower airways and the clinical usefulness of such tests for the assessment of the degree of non-specific reactivity is therefore limited. Methacholine, when given locally in the nasal cavity in the dose range of 0.1–10 mg, will generally produce a monosymptomatic secretory response. A simple way to determine the volume of the

Table 4.4 Methods for monitoring nasal symptoms during active disease or after challenge

Methods for Monitoring Nasal Symptoms During Active Disease or after Challenge	
Symptom	**Method**
Sneezes	Counting Symptom score
Blockage	Symptom score Nasal peak flow Rhinomanometry Acoustic rhinometry
Secretion	Symptom score Volume measurement Weight measurement Nasal lavage
Itching	Symptom score

rhinorrhea is to have the subject in a head-forwards position and collect the delivered volume of secretion in a funnel. Alternatively, preweighed tampons may be inserted into the nose to absorb exudate fluid, which may be reweighed.

Histamine has also been used to assess the degree of non-specific reactivity. When given locally in the dose range of 0.1–10 mg, histamine will produce all the nasal symptoms relevant to allergic rhinitis. The evaluation of this response is therefore more complex and may involve the same techniques that are used for the determination of specific reactivity. The clinical usefulness of the histamine challenge is similar to that of methacholine challenge.

Test for specific reactivity

There are some clinical situations that may call for a nasal allergen challenge. These include confirmation or rejection of a suspected allergen where the history and skin test are not completely in agreement. Furthermore, it may sometimes be of interest to see whether a local allergy is present. The bulk of nasal allergen challenges have, however, been performed primarily for research purposes in order to understand nasal pathophysiology and to test potentially beneficial drugs.

There is no generally accepted technique for performing a nasal allergen challenge or for monitoring the clinical response. In the clinical setting, a simple sneeze count and a score for the other symptoms may well be sufficient, but if a graded (quantitative) response is required for research purposes, more complicated techniques are needed. The risks involved in the nasal challenges are minimal and, even if total nasal blockage occurs, other organs are seldom affected especially if the patient holds their breath in inspiration as the allergen is administered.

Challenge of the nasal mucosa

The allergens used should be well characterized and standardized. An aqueous solution is the easiest way of introducing them into the nasal cavity and a widespread distribution of the allergens is obtained using a mechanical pump spray.

Monitoring the nasal reaction

The reaction to allergen comprises three main symptoms: sneezing, nasal blockage, and nasal secretions. All three are relevant and should be monitored.

Sneezing is the result of a central reflex elicited in the sensory nerve endings in the nasal mucosa. It is easy to grade by counting and is the most reproducible of the nasal symptoms in the challenge procedure.

Nasal blockage is the result of the pooling of blood in the capacitance vessels of the mucosa, and to some degree the result of tissue edema. Nasal blockage can be assessed subjectively by means of symptom scoring and there are several objective techniques which can be used for assessing the degree of nasal blockage:

- rhinomanometry, which is the determination of nasal air flow and pressure relationships (Fig. 4.21);
- nasal peak flow determination (Fig. 4.22); and
- acoustic rhinometry (Fig. 4.23) – a recently introduced technique.

Of the rhinomanometric procedures, the active anterior technique is preferred. In this technique, the patient's normal nasal breathing is assessed and the nasal cavities are assessed separately. The presence of a nasal cycle (alternating baseline nasal congestion and decongestion) may, however, give rise to problems in the interpretation of the results obtained. There is no uniformly accepted way of determining when a change in any of these parameters should be considered as positive, and they must still be considered to be mainly research instruments. The recently introduced acoustic rhinometry uses the reflection of sound to determine the cross-sectional area of the nasal cavity over its entire length. This is a promising technique which will permit the determination of the cross-sectional area in order to determine the site of a mucosal swelling. It is more reproducible than rhinomanometry and readings are obtainable even on patients with marked nasal obstruction.

Increase in nasal surface liquid or nasal secretions is the third main symptom. Weighing the blown secretion is a simple way to determine the amount of liquid produced. It may also be of interest to assess any changes in the specific composition of the nasal surface liquid. Lavage of the nasal cavity with saline solution before and after challenge with allergen and the subsequent analysis of various markers of specific cell activation have been performed (Fig. 4.24). It is important to wash out the nasal cavity at fixed time intervals, and a thorough cleansing of the nasal cavity is sometimes necessary before the lavage challenge procedure. As described earlier, histamine or tryptase may be used as markers of mast cell activation, and ECP, MBP, and eosinophil-derived neurotoxin are markers of eosinophil activation. In addition, IgA and lysozyme may be used as functional markers for glandular secretion, and albumin and fibrinogen for plasma leakage.

At present, these techniques are primarily useful for research and have contributed to our knowledge of the pathophysiology of upper airway allergic reactions. Their application in the clinical setting has still not been defined. The lavage technique has, however, also been used successfully to monitor the allergic inflammation of the upper airways during natural allergen exposure as well as the effect of therapeutic intervention. Increases similar to those seen in the challenge situation, namely increased surface levels of TAME-esterase, BK, albumin, and ECP have also been demonstrated during clinical disease.

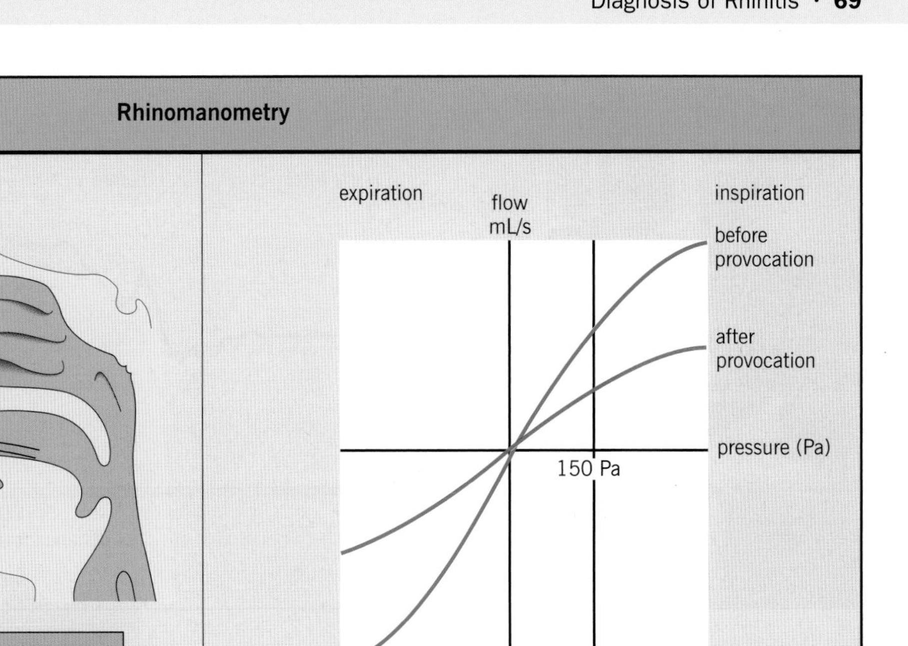

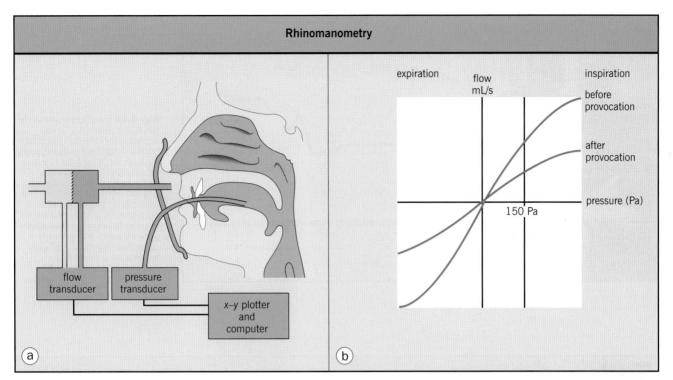

Fig. 4.21 The rhinomanometric examination. (a) The patient breathes through the nose via an anesthetic mask to which a flow transducer is attached. A further tube is introduced into the mouth and held tightly between the lips. This is attached to a pressure transducer to measure mouth pressure. (b) Pressure and flow are plotted on an x–y plotter. Resistance may be calculated by reading flow at a constant pressure, usually 150 Pa.

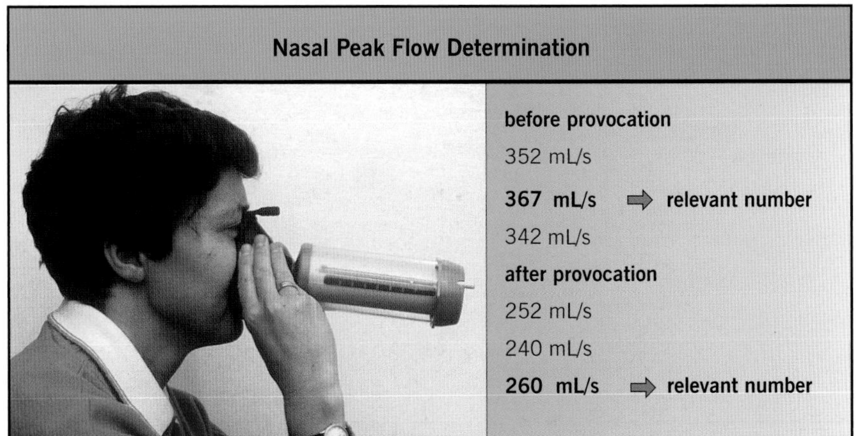

Nasal Peak Flow Determination
before provocation
352 mL/s
367 mL/s ⇨ relevant number
342 mL/s
after provocation
252 mL/s
240 mL/s
260 mL/s ⇨ relevant number

Fig. 4.22 The nasal peak flow determination can be made on expiration or inspiration. A maximum nasal breath is performed with the mask tightly fitted around the nose without influencing the nasal alii. The peak flow is determined at least three times and the highest value is noted. After an allergen challenge, lower values may be obtained.

Cytologic studies

To assess the severity of the disease, or to elucidate whether the upper airway disease is of allergic origin, examination of the cytology of the upper airway mucosa is required. The various cytologic techniques are relatively easy to perform, without major discomfort or risk to the patient. Biopsy should only be undertaken by someone who is very familiar with the nasal anatomy, and who is prepared to deal with the sometimes profuse post-biopsy bleeding. Until now, the main focus has been to demonstrate the presence or absence of eosinophils. The presence of eosinophils is a sign of active inflammatory disease of allergic origin and, in intermittent allergic rhinitis, there is a strong correlation between seasonal exposure to allergen and the local eosinophil density. A reduction in eosinophil numbers has also been taken as a sign of susceptibility to topical glucocorticoid therapy. The density of the mast cells or basophils is also of interest. The presence and density of mast cells on the mucosa or within the epithelium indicates the severity of the disease (Fig. 4.25).

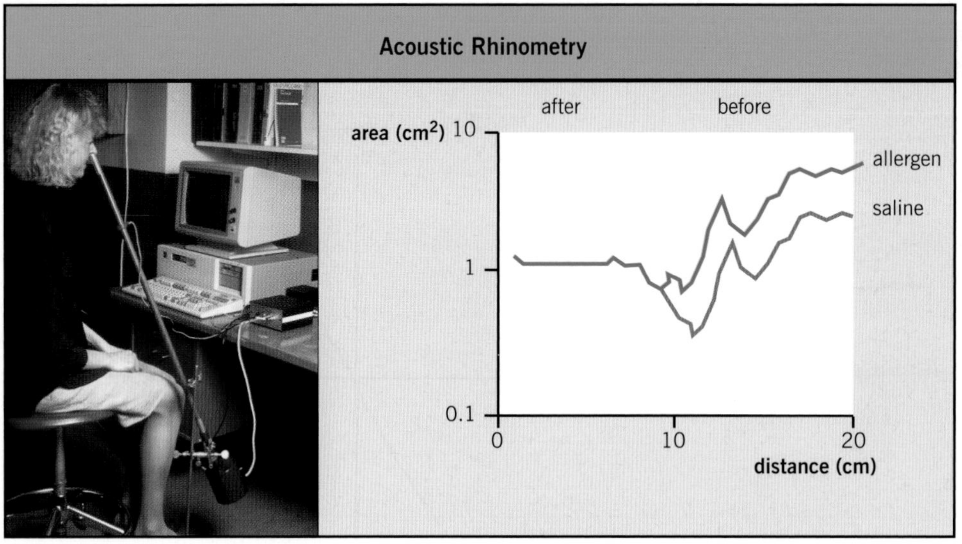

Fig. 4.23 The determination of the nasal geometry using acoustic rhinometry. The spark sound is led to the nasal cavity through the long tube where a microphone is fitted some distance from the nosepiece. The difference in the time and intensity of the sound is monitored and this information is used to compute the nasal geometry with the aid of the computer. Allergen challenge will induce a mucosal thickening, which can be determined using this method.

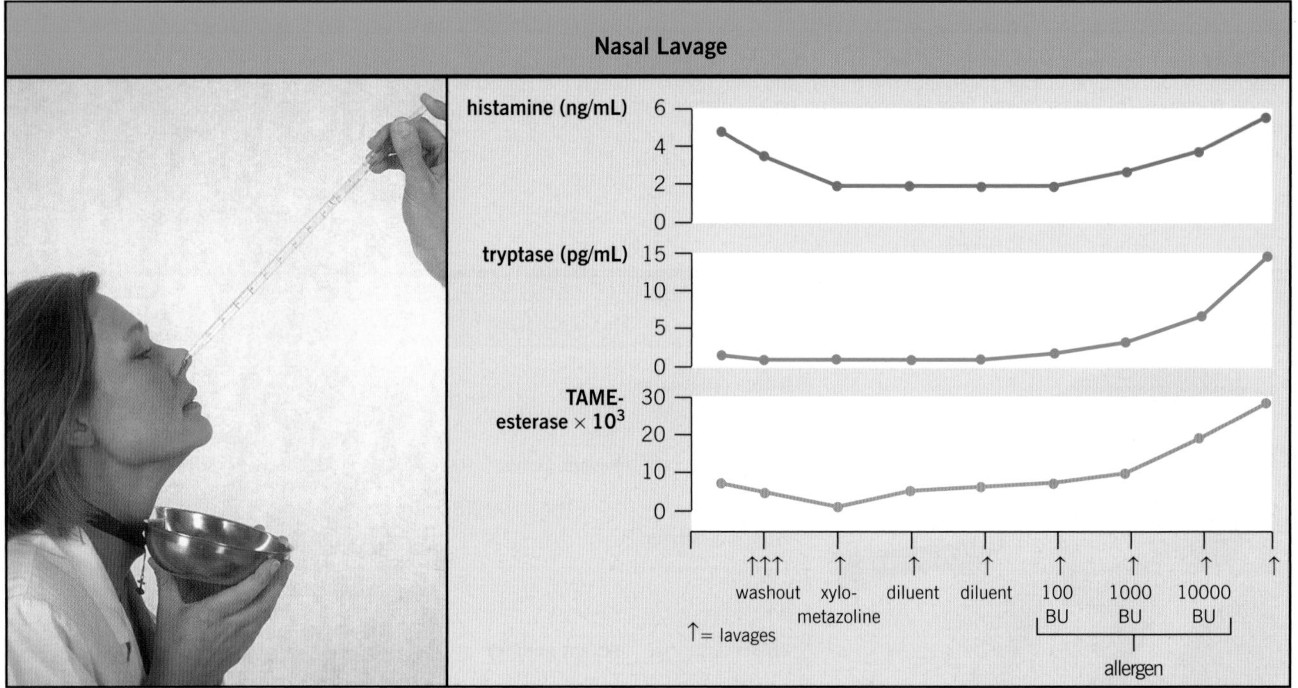

Fig. 4.24 A nasal lavage can be performed by administering normal saline solution (approximately 5 mL/nasal cavity) whilst simultaneously closing the epipharynx. A nasal-allergen challenge can be performed during a series of repeated lavages at a fixed time interval. Increasing doses of allergen in an allergic individual will produce increasing quantities of markers of mast-cell activation such as histamine, tryptase, TAME-esterase, and plasma proteins.

Monitoring the home allergen exposure

By using a specific device adapted to a vacuum cleaner, a sample of house dust can be obtained and can then be assessed for its content of mite allergens. Symptoms of upper airway allergy can thus be related to the degree of home exposure to this allergen.

Supplementary investigations

Radiology

It has been suggested that sinus disease is often associated with upper airway allergy but the predisposing factors are unclear. There are no specific studies which demonstrate an increase in

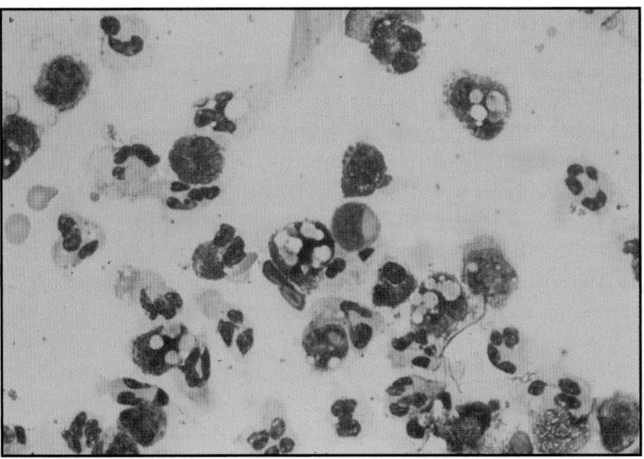

Fig. 4.25 Brush sample from a patient with seasonal allergic rhinitis during natural allergen exposure, showing a few neutrophils, some epithelial cells, and several eosinophils, some with vacuoles indicating ongoing secretory activity. (Giemsa stain, original × 400.)

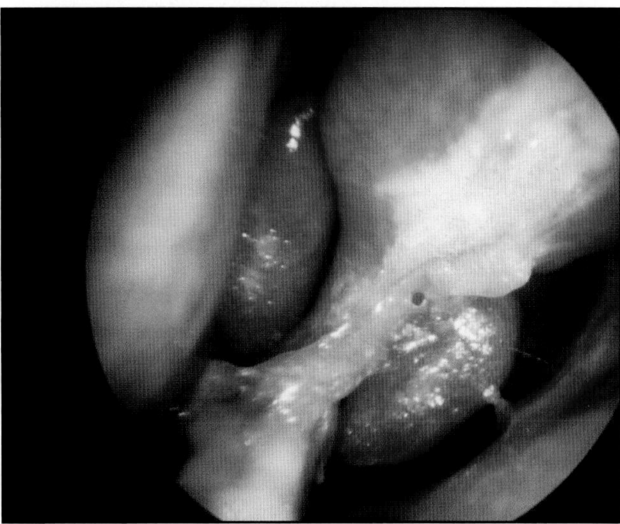

Fig. 4.27 Endoscopic appearances of the nasal mucosa in Wegener's granulomatosis. (Courtesy of Professor VJ Lund.)

acute sinusitis in patients with seasonal allergic rhinitis. On the other hand, it has also been claimed that there is an increase in the frequency of upper airway allergy in patients with 'chronic sinusitis'. A plain radiograph of the sinus regions is rarely useful since a minor degree of mucosal swelling in the maxillary sinuses in conjunction with the allergic ailment is not indicative of sinusitis, but should instead be interpreted as part of the overall allergic condition. Nevertheless, the presence of fluid in one or more of the sinuses, or their complete opacification, needs to be further evaluated by either sinus puncture or sinoscopy. Better visualization of the nasal cavity and the sinus region is obtained using a computed tomography (CT) scan specifically directed towards the ethmoidal and ostial regions where pathology is often present (Fig. 4.26). However, CT scans remain abnormal for several weeks following a common cold, therefore they should not be used for diagnosis of sinusitis

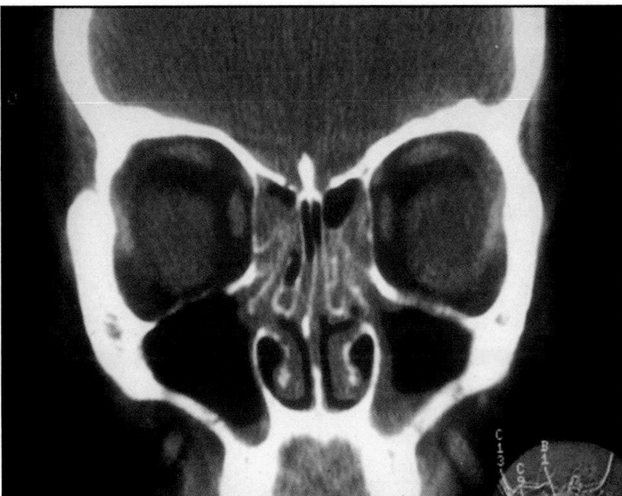

Fig. 4.26 Computed tomography (CT) scan showing ethmoiditis and obstruction of the osteomeatal complex.

but to provide a 'road map' for endoscopic surgery, or if malignancy is suspected.

Differential diagnosis

The most common differential diagnosis is perennial non-allergic rhinitis (see Fig.4.2). The clinical relevance of dividing this group into subgroups is limited except, perhaps, for the demonstration of cytologic changes such as the presence of eosinophils. However, the more common problems which the physician sees are endocrine disturbances, such as nasal congestion as a complication of pregnancy, oral contraceptives, or hypothyroidism, giving rise to a thickened and edematous nasal mucosa. Rhinitis medicamentosa with a rebound vasodilatation (the effect of overuse of topical nasal decongestants) often produces an edematous and red nasal mucosa which should not be confused with true rhinitis.

It is important to be aware of other diseases which may present with nasal symptoms. Uncharacteristic features, such as unilateral nasal blockage, bleeding, or pain, may suggest other pathologies (e.g. malignant tumors or Wegener's granulomatosis; Fig. 4.27). In infants, unilateral nasal blockage and discharge may also be caused by the presence of a foreign body or, rarely, congenital choanal atresia. Septal deviation, whether congenital or traumatic, may cause nasal blockage, but it is unlikely to be noticed for the first time in adulthood unless there is superadded rhinitis. Chronic infective rhinosinusitis can usually be differentiated by its predominantly greenish secretions and infective exacerbations, although it can occur in association with perennial rhinitis because of impaired drainage from the sinuses.

Recently a syndrome of allergic fungal sinusitis has been recognized, in which patients may have symptoms of rhinitis, sinusitis, and, sometimes, nasal polyps. The condition is similar to allergic bronchopulmonary aspergillosis and casts are sometimes blown from the nose during exacerbations. Classically, calcification is seen on the CT scan (Fig. 4.28). Removal of polyps containing fungal material from the nose and sinuses by endoscopic surgery should be undertaken and local corticosteroids used to decrease recurrence.

TREATMENT OF RHINITIS

Information

The most important element in the treatment is information to the patient and, if the patient is a child, the parent should be the target for this. It cannot be overstressed that successful treatment depends on the patient understanding the nature of the disease, and that it may be a life-long ailment in which the symptoms respond with a success rate that is largely dependent on the cooperation of the patient. Books or pamphlets can be helpful.

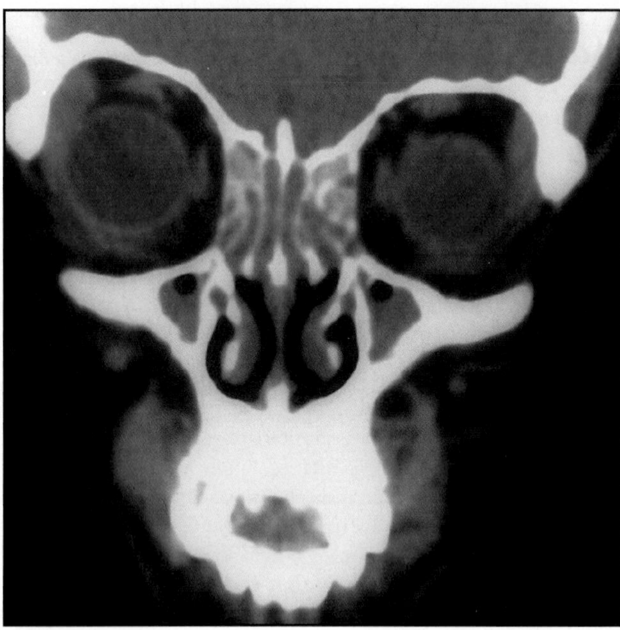

Fig. 4.28 Computed tomography (CT) scan showing calcification in allergic aspergillus sinusitis.

Allergen avoidance

Avoidance regimens improve symptoms by decreasing the exposure to allergens which trigger the allergic reactions. This approach should be strictly enforced when there is an allergic reaction to foods, drugs, or animals. Because seasonal pollens and molds have a widespread airborne distribution, complete avoidance of these allergens is difficult if not impossible. Sometimes a total change of environment might be of value.

Measures designed to reduce the degree of mite exposure in the home include covering mattresses, boxsprings, duvets, and pillows in vinyl or synthetic materials. Breathable allergen-proof covers are now available for mattresses, pillows, and duvets. More extreme measures include the removal of upholstered furniture, stuffed animals, carpeting, and wall hangings to eliminate dust traps. Superheated steam cleaners remove or denature house dust mite, mold, and pet allergens. However, the cost:benefit ratio of taking more drastic measures, such as major house renovation, is poor. Careful and regular cleaning with a damp mop is important. The benefit of local air filtration is limited, and calls for careful maintenance of the filters if it is to be useful. The effects of animal dander can be reduced by washing the animal once a week.

In the case of mold allergy, the local environment should be kept dry and dense vegetation around the house eliminated. It might also be useful to avoid raking leaves and other similar activities.

It is also important to try to eliminate other local irritants as much as possible. The importance of a non-smoking environment cannot be stressed enough.

Drug treatment

Several pharmacologic agents are available for the treatment of rhinitis symptoms, most of which have different efficacy profiles, as is shown in Table 4.5. A combination of drugs with different effect profiles can be productive. The conjunctivitis which is often present, and as troublesome as the nasal symptoms, should also be treated.

Table 4.5 Efficacy profile of the various drugs used to treat allergic rhinitis. Some of the drugs inhibit only one nasal symptom (e.g. decongestants only work on nasal blockage), while others have more widespread activity (e.g. topical glucocorticoids)

Efficacy Profile of the Various Drugs Used to Treat Allergic Rhinitis

Drug	Sneezing	Discharge	Blockage	Anosmia
Cromolyn	+ +	+	+	–
Decongestant	–	–	+ + +	–
Antihistamine	+ + +	+ +	+/-	–
Ipratropium	–	+ +	–	–
Topical steroids	+ + +	+ +	+ +	+
Oral steroids	+ +	+ +	+ + +	+ +
Anti-leukotriene	–	+ +	+	+

After Mygind N. Pharmacological management of perennial rhinitis. Rhinol Suppl 1991; 11:21–26, International Rhinologic Society.

α-Adrenoceptor stimulant drugs (decongestants)

Vasoconstrictors are used by millions of rhinitis sufferers, both as topical preparations and as tablets. All the nasal vasoconstrictors which are available commercially possess α-adrenoceptor stimulant properties to a greater or lesser degree and cause contraction of the smooth muscle of the venous erectile tissue, thereby increasing reactive hyperemia and rebound congestion. The most popular topical preparations contain xylometazoline or oxymetazoline, which have a long duration of action. Prolonged use can be associated with the risk of rebound congestion, so they can be recommended for occasional limited use for a few days only. The risk of rhinitis medicamentosa, in which nasal obstruction becomes unresponsive to venoconstrictive agents, is even lower when the decongestant is administered orally. However, this route is associated with several disturbing and undesirable side-effects including bladder dysfunction, restlessness, nausea, vomiting, insomnia, headache, tachycardia, dysrhythmias, hypertension, and angina, and is contraindicated in patients with cardiovascular disease, thyrotoxicosis, glaucoma, and in those taking monoamine oxidase inhibitors. As many of these receptor-blocking drugs are available without prescription, patients at risk should be warned of their possible harmful effects. Patients with hypertension and glaucoma are at particular risk and should avoid oral decongestants.

Histamine H_1-receptor antagonists (antihistamines)

Many drugs with antihistaminic activity are available for use in clinical practice. The older antihistamines, including chlorphenamine, triprolidine, and promethazine, all exhibit competitive H_1-receptor antagonism, but their therapeutic index is low, and the large doses needed for therapeutic efficacy lead to the unwanted effects of sedation and blockade of cholinergic and α-adrenergic receptors. The more recent introduction of antihistamines, such as loratadine and cetirizine, which have little or no sedative or anticholinergic effect, has re-awakened interest in the use of antihistamines in the treatment of hayfever. The increased potency of these newer antihistamines, together with their lack of sedation resulting from their relative inability to cross the blood–brain barrier, allows the administration of doses with good therapeutic benefit. Their greatest therapeutic benefit is on rhinorrhea, and they also have a beneficial effect on sneezing and itching, but little effect on nasal blockage. Two most recent additions are desloratadine and levocetirizine which do unblock the nose to some extent.

Terfenadine and astemizole, which have now been withdrawn from the market in many countries, at high blood levels can block potassium channels and cause cardiac arrhythmias (torsades de pointes) (Fig. 4.29) which have proved fatal in a few patients. Both drugs are hepatically metabolized and this is competitively inhibited by concomitant use of erythromycin or related antibiotics, ketoconazole and related antifungals, and by grapefruit juice. Thus these combinations must be avoided as should excessive dosage or the use of terfenadine or astemizole in patients with cardiac or hepatic disease or with a known prolongation of the Q–T interval. Safer alternatives are cetirizine, levocetirizine and desloratadine which are not hepatically metabolized and have no effect on calcium channels; loratadine, which is partially hepatically metabolized but has no effect on the Q–T interval at high concentrations; or fexofenadine, which is the active metabolite of terfenadine and has no cardiac effects.

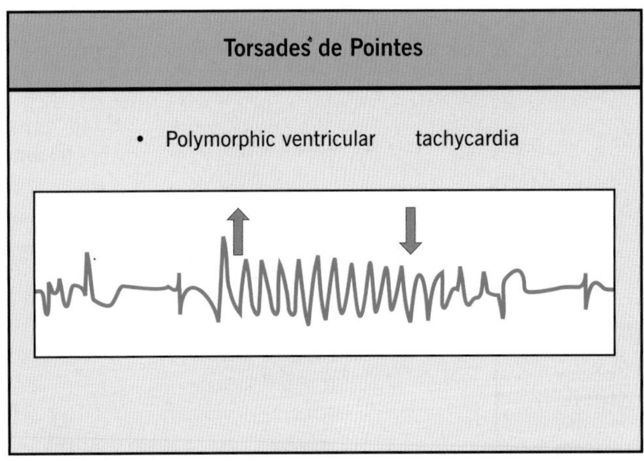

Fig. 4.29 Torsades de pointes. This cardiac arrhythmia can occur with high blood levels of terfenadine and astemizole, due to blockage of potassium channels.

The side-effects of antihistamines may be minimized by administering them as nasal sprays; thus far azelastine and levacobastine sprays are available. Although the putative sensitizing effect of topically applied antihistamines has been questioned, the risk of such unwanted effects appears to be minimal when it comes to application onto mucous membranes.

Since the effect of antihistamines on nasal obstruction is limited, a logical step would therefore be to combine these drugs with an α-adrenoceptor antagonist which only affects nasal obstruction. These combinations, which are now being introduced with the newer non-sedating antihistamines, represent an alternative therapy. However, these combinations also carry the side-effects and precautions associated with the oral vasoconstrictor agents. The combination of H_1- and H_2-receptor antagonists has also been suggested to be more effective than H_1 blockers alone in reducing nasal congestion, suggesting that H_2 receptors may be present on nasal blood vessels. However, histamine H_2-receptor blockade in isolation has no demonstrable therapeutic value.

Anticholinergics

From a theoretical point of view, atropine ought to be of considerable benefit in the control of watery rhinorrhea. The basis of this assumption is the fact that the rhinorrhea is primarily the result of glandular hypersecretion. However, its presumed efficacy has only been tested to a limited degree largely because of the undesirable anticholinergic effects occurring in other organs, such as dryness of the mouth and blurred vision. Topical administration would be of interest but, since atropine is readily absorbed, it is likely to carry systemic effects prior to any topical efficacy. However, an atropine derivative, ipratropium bromide, is poorly absorbed from mucous membranes, and patients whose predominant symptom is that of profuse nasal discharge benefit from this drug. This is also relevant for patients with a perennial non-allergic, autonomic rhinitis in which the main symptom is watery hypersecretion.

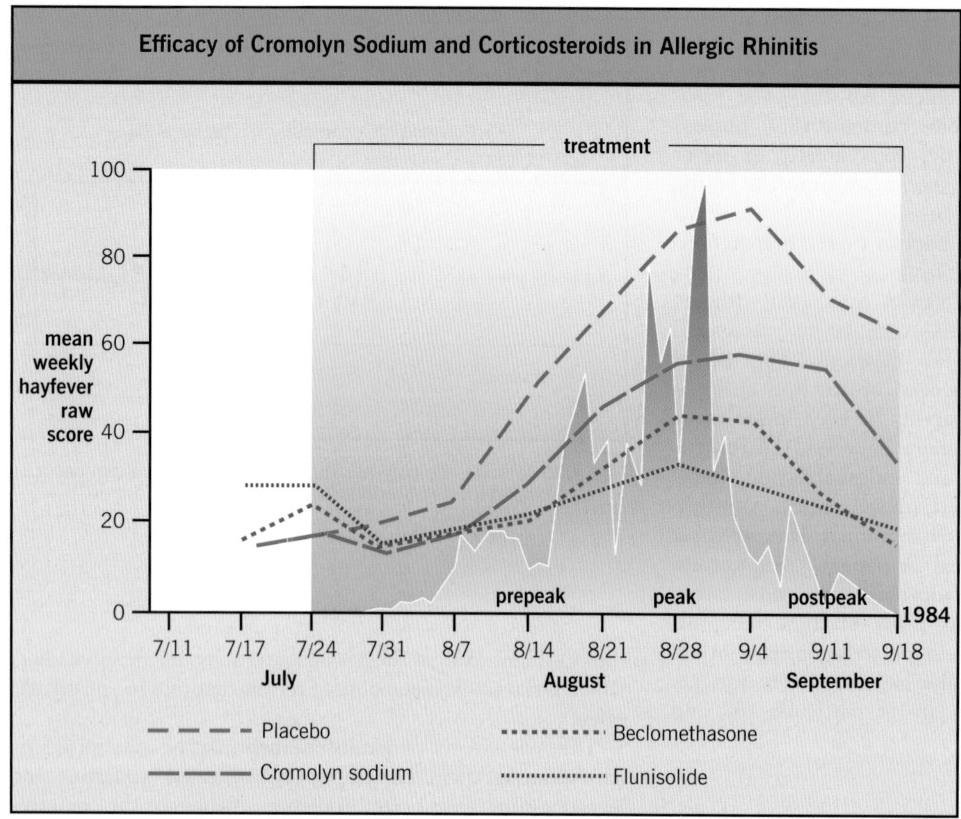

Fig. 4.30 Relative clinical efficacy of cromolin sodium and topical corticosteroids in allergic rhinitis. Cromolyn sodium is approximately as efficacious as antihistamines; topical nasal corticosteroids are more effective against most symptoms. [Adapted from Welsh PW, Stricker WE, Chu CP, et al. Efficacy of beclomethasone nasal solution, flunisolide, and cromolin in relieving symptoms of ragweed allergy. Mayo Clin Proc 1987; 62(2):125–134.]

Cromolyn sodium and nedocromil sodium

Cromolyn sodium, introduced in the 1960s, is a drug whose mode of action remains controversial. Traditionally, it is considered to act by stabilizing mast cells and, if this were indeed a mode of action, this drug would be particularly useful for the treatment of allergic rhinitis. More recent evidence suggests additional mechanisms of action pertinent to mucosal inflammation, including inhibitory effects on eosinophils, platelets, and macrophages. However, the clinical efficacy of cromolin sodium in allergic rhinitis is less than that of the topical glucocorticoids, but more or less equal to that of antihistamines (Fig. 4.30). Cromolyn sodium is also especially useful for the treatment of ocular problems which often accompany rhinitis. The administration of cromolin sodium is safe, and minimal or no side-effects have been reported: it is particularly suitable for small children for whom topical corticosteroids are not available. Patient compliance is hampered by its short duration of action, necessitating topical administration up to six times daily.

Nedocromil sodium is an addition to the family of chromones. It is effective when used twice daily and is useful in seasonal allergic conjunctivitis. Its potential antiinflammatory effects are evident from its ability to reduce the accumulation of mast cells in the nasal mucosa during the pollen season. Like cromolin sodium, nedocromil sodium has an excellent safety profile, making it particularly popular among pediatricians.

Antileukotrienes

These exist in two forms: drugs which inhibit leukotriene formation such as zileuton, and leukotriene receptor antagonists (LTRAs) such as montelukast, zafirlukast, and pranlukast. These have been shown to be effective in asthma and more recently in rhinitis, both in allergic rhinitis and in nasal polyposis. In the former, antileukotrienes have an efficacy similar to that of antihistamines; combination with an antihistamine results in very little additional benefit and is not superior to use of a topical corticosteroid alone. In nasal polyposis approximately 60% of patients derive some benefit, with no significant difference between aspirin-tolerant and aspirin-sensitive patients. There is a wide variation in patient responsiveness to the LTRAs, with around 10% of patients deriving marked benefit. Since nasal polyposis is frequently accompanied by asthma, which can be severe, the antileukotrienes are likely to be of most use in such patients, where they may be steroid-sparing.

Topical corticosteroids

The introduction in the 1970s of topical glucocorticoids – now including beclometasone dipropionate, budesonide, triamcinolone acetonide, flunisolone acetonide, fluticasone propionate, and mometasone furoate – for nasal use has provided several effective treatment alternatives for allergic rhinitis. They are more efficacious than antihistamines and cromolin sodium, and can be administered conveniently once or twice daily. It should, however, be explained clearly to patients that the maximal benefit of glucocorticoids is not immediate but may take several days to be apparent. Furthermore, it should be explained that if the drugs are to be effective they must reach the target organ. This means that if symptoms are already present it may be necessary to open up the nasal cavity with a topical decongestant prior to glucocorticoid aerosol adminis-

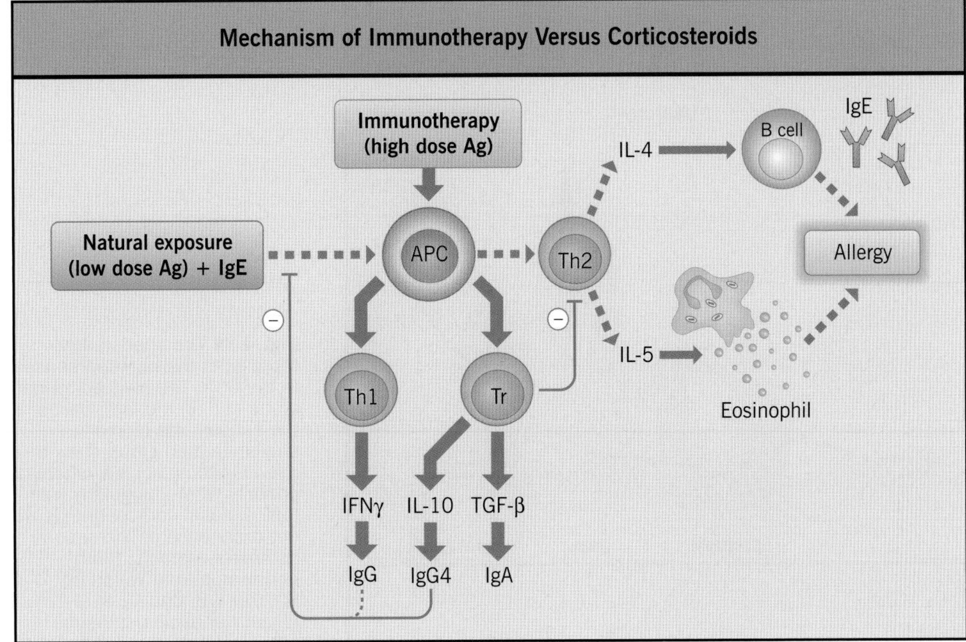

Fig. 4.31 The mechanism of immunotherapy is complex. There is evidence of switching from a Th2 to a Th1 reaction with consequent IgG production. T regulatory cells may be involved: these produce IL-10, which promotes a switch to IgG4 which is then capable of blocking IgE facilitated antigen presentation by B cells, and also TGF beta which switches IgE to IgA production. In contrast corticosteroids reduce Th2 without augmenting Th1 responses. (Adapted from Robinson DS, Larche ML, and Durham SR. J Clin Invest 2004; 114: 1389–1397.)

tration. Sometimes a short course of oral glucocorticoids may be necessary to open up the nasal cavity.

The use of topical glucocorticoids during the last decade has provided a great deal of information about their safety. They have limited local and systemic side-effects and may be used even for long-term treatment in adults. In the case of long-term treatment, rhinoscopy is recommended once or twice a year. One should not hesitate to use topical glucocorticoids for seasonal disease in children over 4 years old. Long-term treatment should not be instituted without careful individual evaluation, as is the case with all drugs. Some patients may suffer from local irritation from the spray, with blood spotting. Septal perforation is a very rare side-effect, probably due to maladministration of spray directly on the septum.

Systemic corticosteroids

Systemic corticosteroids are highly effective in all forms of rhinitis. However, they all have systemic side-effects, whether given as depot injections or orally, and the benefit/risk ratio should be considered. Depot injections are simple but have been linked to disfiguring muscle atrophy after repeated injection and the timing of release does not coincide with maximal effects of seasonal allergen. In cases of severe seasonal allergic disease, the administration of oral prednisolone or prednisone to cover some peak days may be considered. If, however, more regular treatment fails then specific hyposensitization should be considered.

Immunotherapy

Immunotherapy is an alternative which should be considered if patients do not respond to any allergen avoidance measures combined with traditional pharmacologic therapy. Classic immunotherapy involves repeated injection of the allergen at regular intervals and the treatment has been shown to be effective in allergic rhinoconjunctivitis with clear-cut allergens like pollens, mites, and animal dander. Before it is started, a careful explanation must be given to the patient, outlining the details and commitment required as it is a long-term program involving frequent injections of allergenic extracts for at least 3 years. Also, immunotherapy carries with it the risk of a systemic anaphylactic reaction should an allergen penetrate directly into the bloodstream. Consequently, facilities for resuscitation must be available, and procedures using highly potent allergens should be avoided. Because of the possible risks associated with immunotherapy, some countries have introduced guidelines to govern the use of this form of therapy. The mechanism probably involves a switch from Th2 to Th1 or Th0 type immune responses (Fig. 4.31).

Immunotherapy for allergic rhinitis in children has been shown to reduce the progression to asthma.

Newer methods of immunotherapy are under investigation: these include peptides, local (nasal) application of allergen, and the use of interferon γ (IFNγ) stimulators such as *Mycobacterium vaccae*.

Relationships to other organs

The eye

In any of the treatment programs for upper airway allergy, the ocular symptoms must not be neglected since they may well be as severe as the nasal symptoms. The eye should, therefore, also be treated either locally with a vasoconstrictor or antihistamine, or systemically with antihistamine. Corticosteroid drops should only be used under ophthalmologic supervision.

Upper–lower airway interactions

One of the main organs that may be affected indirectly by upper airway disease, or by the dysfunction of the upper airways, is the lung. It has been suggested that the failure of the upper airways to humidify and clean the inspired air effectively

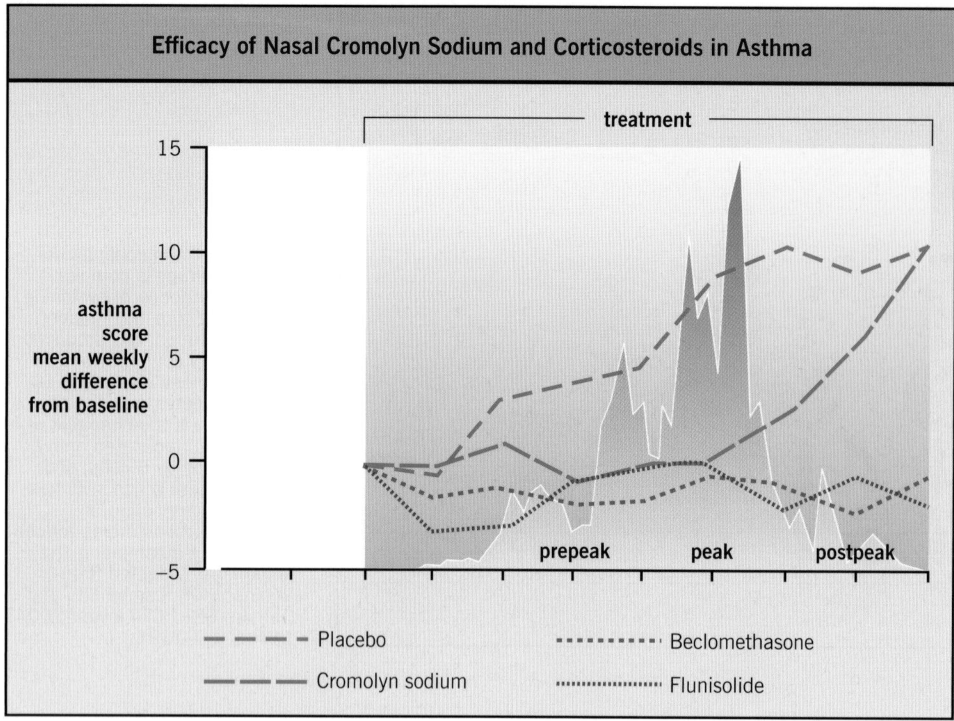

Fig. 4.32 The shaded area represents the ragweed season in the USA. The placebo-treated group and, in the later part of the season, the cromolin sodium-treated group show a rise in asthma scores, whereas patients treated regularly with topical nasal corticosteroids do not experience an increase in asthma symptoms. [With permission from Welsh PW, Stricker WE, Chu CP, et al. Efficacy of beclomethasone nasal solution, flunisolide, and cromolin in relieving symptoms of ragweed allergy. Mayo Clin Proc 1987; 62(2):125–134.]

might precipitate or aggravate asthma. Asthma is often associated with upper airway disease, with up to 80% of the adult population with asthma also suffering from upper airway symptoms. These symptoms often precede the onset of asthma. It is not known whether early intervention in terms of the nasal symptoms will affect the onset of lower airway problems. However, since asthma is considered to be a more serious disease, the frequently associated upper airway problems are often overlooked and under treated. Active and successful treatment of the upper airways has been shown not only to reduce nasal symptoms but also to benefit the lower airways (Fig. 4.32), including reduction of asthma emergency visits and hospitalization.

Sinus–nose–ear interaction

Sinus afflictions are common among asthmatic hayfever sufferers and should generally be considered to be part of the airways disease and treated as such. A careful diagnostic examination is necessary. The possibility of polyps, perhaps possibly provoked by aspirin and other NSAIDs, should also be considered. The sinus disease may call for surgical intervention which may include a functional endoscopic surgical procedure. However a recent prospective study has demonstrated that medical intervention is equally efficacious. Ear disease has been linked to allergy in children in particular and treatment directed towards rhinitis may be effective in reducing recurrences of otitis media with effusion.

Nasal polyps

Nasal polyps have sometimes been linked to allergic disease, partly because they often contain eosinophils. The clinical finding is often one of mucosal bags filled with fluid lying in the nasal cavity (see Fig. 4.19). There is, however, very little evidence of a clear-cut allergic origin for these polyps. When lower airway problems are present, the link to NSAID sensitivity should be considered. Smaller polyps may shrink on topical glucocorticoid treatment, while larger polyps may require surgical intervention. The endoscopic approach may be productive. Topical glucocorticoids used regularly in the long term decrease the recurrence rate. Antileukotrienes should be tried in unresponsive nasal polyps, especially where asthma is also present.

FURTHER READING

Bousquet J and the ARIA workshop. Allergic rhinitis and its impact on asthma. J Allergy Clin Immunol 2001; 108:S147–S334.

Jones AS, Phillips DE, Hilgers FJM. Diseases of the head and neck, nose and throat, Part 3. London: Arnold; 1998.

Raeburn D, Giembycz MA, eds. Rhinitis: immunopathology and pharmacotherapy. Basel: Birkhauser Verlag; 1997.

Scadding GK, Lund VJ. Investigative Rhinology. London: Taylor & Francis; 2004.

Chapter 5

Definition:

Conjunctivitis is inflammation of the conjunctiva, the mucous membrane lining the anterior sclera and the inner eyelid surfaces, seen in a broad spectrum of conditions, including allergy.

Conjunctivitis

Melanie Hingorani, Virginia L Calder, Roger J Buckley, and Susan Lightman

INTRODUCTION

Allergic inflammation of the ocular surface (the lid margins, conjunctiva and cornea; Fig. 5.1) is one of the commonest ocular disorders, affecting 21% of the adult population of the UK. In its mildest form, the conjunctiva becomes inflamed in response to a transient allergen (e.g. pollen in seasonal allergic conjunctivitis), or a persistent allergen (e.g. house dust mite in perennial allergic conjunctivitis), producing unpleasant symptoms but not threatening sight. At the other end of the spectrum are disorders such as vernal keratoconjunctivitis and atopic keratoconjunctivitis that can have blinding complications when the cornea is involved, and for which current therapeutic agents are only partially effective.

CLASSIFICATION OF ALLERGIC CONJUNCTIVITIS

Allergic conjunctivitis can be classified into five main disorders:

- seasonal allergic conjunctivitis (SAC);
- perennial allergic conjunctivitis (PAC);
- atopic keratoconjunctivitis (AKC);
- vernal keratoconjunctivitis (VKC); and
- giant papillary conjunctivitis (GPC).

Seasonal and perennial allergic conjunctivitis

These disorders are the commonest forms of allergic conjunctivitis and are similar except in their time course, which is determined purely by the duration of exposure to the causative allergen. In SAC (hayfever), the offending allergens are plant pollens and spores, and clinical manifestations occur only during the seasons in which high atmospheric concentrations of these allergens are reached (Fig. 5.2). In PAC, the allergens (most commonly house dust mite, but also animal dander, mold, etc.) and, therefore, the symptoms and signs, are present year-round (Fig. 5.3). In both conditions the eyes are itchy, watery, sticky and red but any visual disturbance is mild, caused by excessive tearing and production of mucus. Contact lens wearers may find that their lens tolerance decreases while the condition is active. The clinical appearance is of a mild conjunctival inflammation and clinical signs may be very slight. The bulbar and tarsal conjunctivae show mild to moderate hyperemia, edema, and infiltration (loss of transparency and thickening resulting from inflammatory infiltration). Small papillae may be seen on the tarsal conjunctiva. There may be more dramatic chemosis (gross edema of the bulbar conjunctiva) and some swelling of the eyelids after a particularly intense or acute allergen exposure. Differences between the two conditions relate to chronicity, and more infiltration and a greater papillary response are seen in PAC whereas chemosis is more suggestive of SAC. The cornea

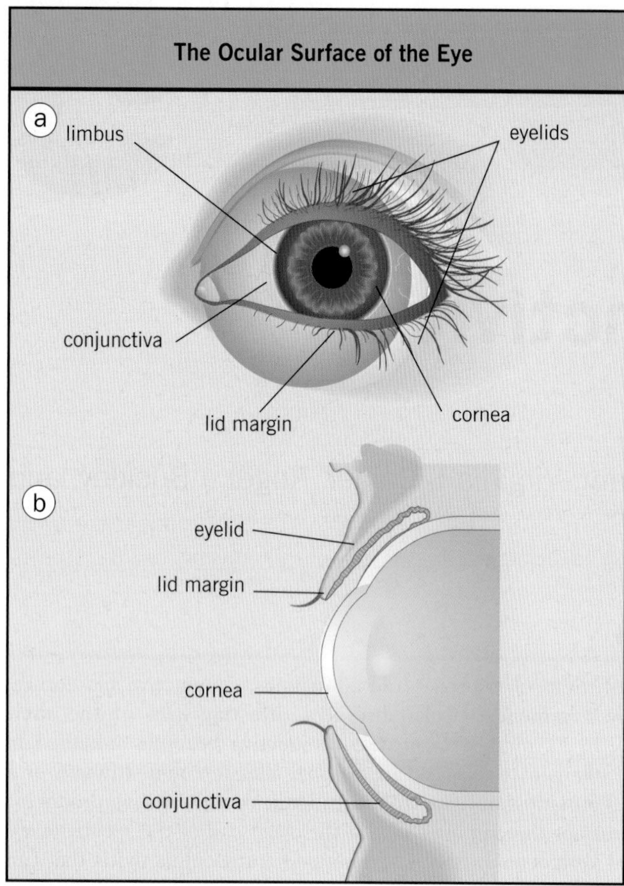

Fig. 5.1 The ocular surface. (a) Anterior view. (b) Cross-sectional view.

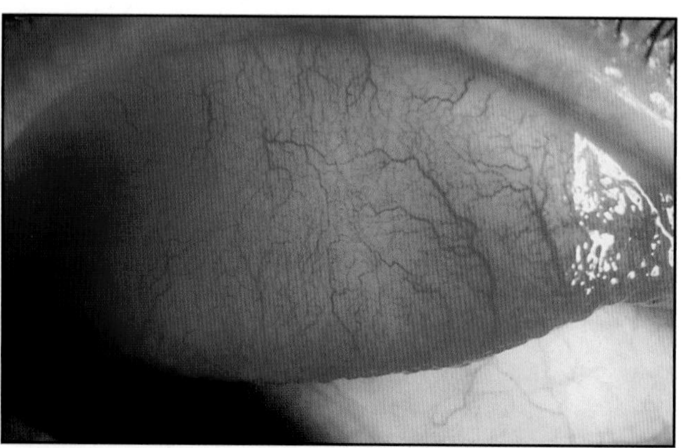

Fig. 5.2 The upper tarsal surface in seasonal allergic conjunctivitis.

and limbus are not affected, nor is there any scarring of the conjunctival surface – therefore there is no serious visual threat. There is usually a good response to topical therapy using antihistamines and mast cell inhibitors or to systemic antihistamines. Topical steroids are usually not appropriate as their unwanted effects can be far more serious than those of the conditions themselves. These disorders usually affect teenagers and young adults and tend to lessen in severity and eventually resolve with increasing age.

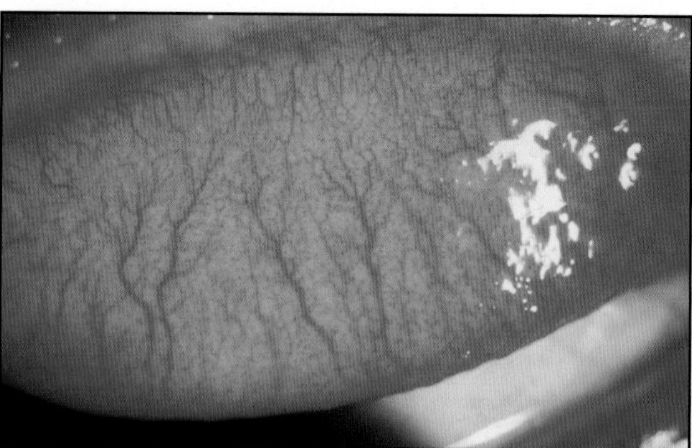

Fig. 5.3 The upper tarsal surface in perennial allergic conjunctivitis.

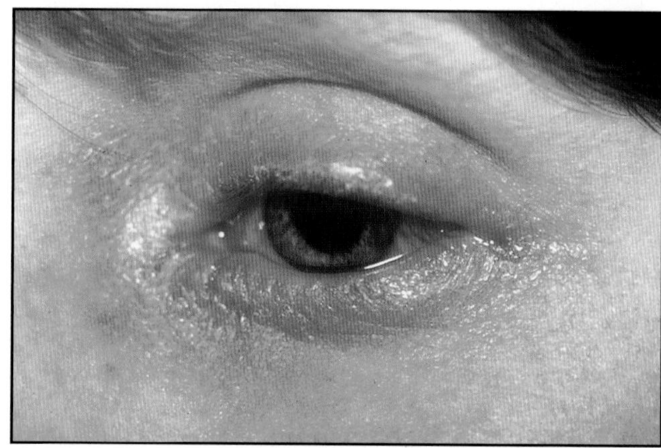

Fig. 5.4 The eyelids in atopic keratoconjunctivitis.

Atopic keratoconjunctivitis

AKC is a rare, life-long, sight-threatening condition that affects adults who have systemic atopic disease, particularly atopic dermatitis. AKC is a highly symptomatic disorder with severe itching, watering, stickiness and redness of the eyelids and eye, and sometimes causes ocular pain. There is usually facial eczema involving the eyelids (Fig. 5.4) and the lid margins show blepharitis (chronic inflammation of the lash follicles and meibomian glands) and often carry large numbers of *Staphylococcus epidermidis* or *S. aureus* organisms. The lid margins are thickened and hyperemic, posteriorly rounded, sometimes keratinized and the lid anatomy may be distorted with ectropion (outwardly turning eyelid), entropion (inwardly turning eyelid), trichiasis (in-turning lashes) and notching. The whole conjunctiva is affected and shows intense infiltration, papillae (which may be giant, i.e. >1 mm in diameter), linear and stellate scars and often shrinkage (Fig. 5.5). Marked limbal inflammation may develop. The cornea is subject to epithelial defects and progressive scarring, and neovascularization (Fig. 5.6); thinning and secondary corneal infections (herpetic, bacterial, and fungal) may occur. Alterations in the volume or quality of the tear film may cause dry eye. Corneal plaque similar to that of VKC is sometimes seen. Associations between AKC and eye rubbing, keratoconus, atopic cataract and retinal detachment are recognized.

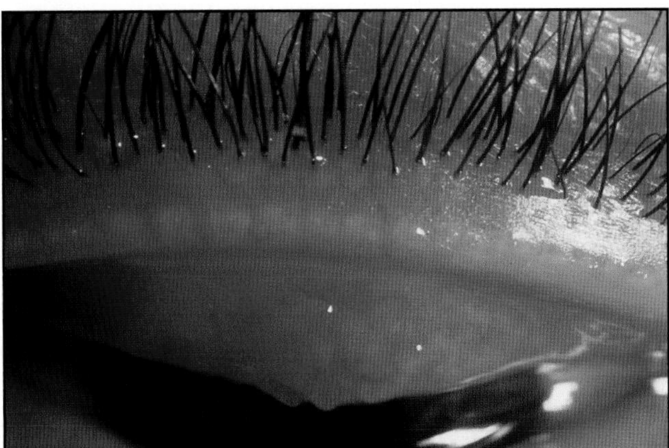

Fig. 5.5 The upper tarsal surface in atopic keratoconjunctivitis.

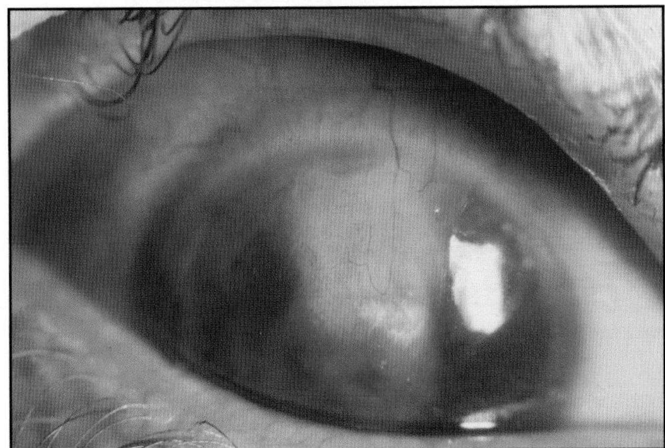

Fig. 5.6 Corneal scarring and neovascularization in atopic keratoconjunctivitis.

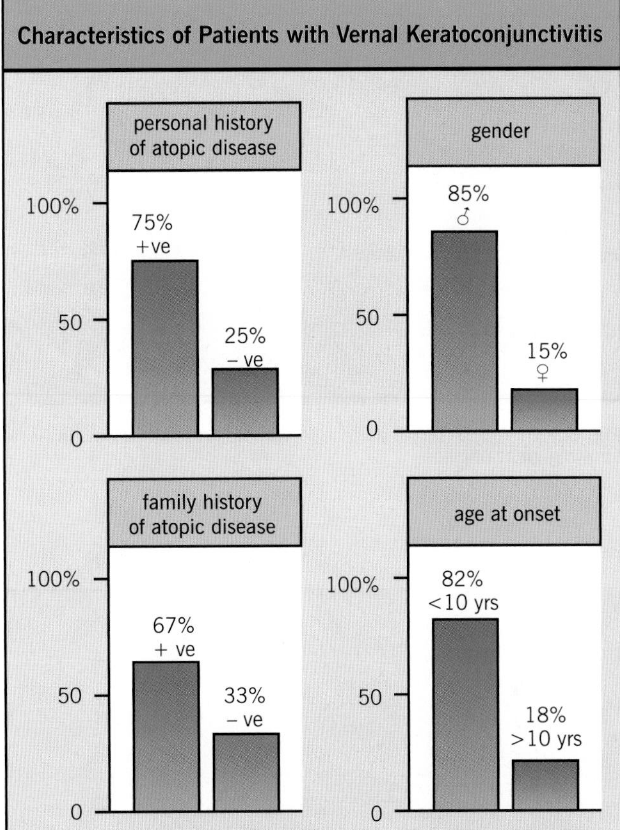

Fig. 5.7 The characteristics of vernal keratoconjunctivitis patients from a series of 100. (Data modified from Buckley RJ. Long-term experience with sodium cromolin in the management of vernal keratoconjunctivitis. In: Pepys J, Edwards AM, eds. The mast cell. London: Pitman Medical, 1980:518–523.)

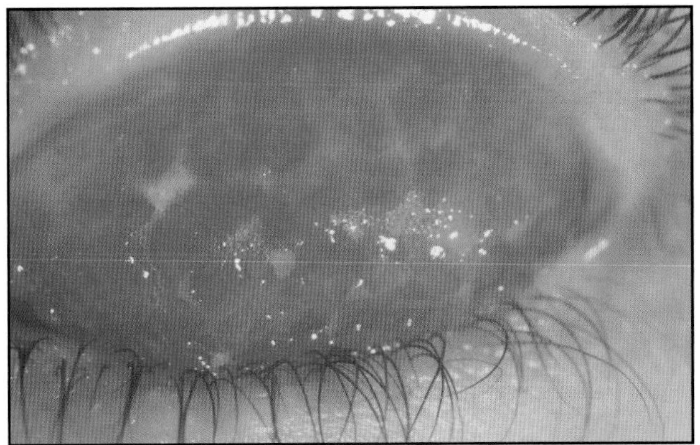

Fig. 5.8 Active vernal conjunctivitis.

The management of AKC is difficult and patients cannot be cured. It is crucial to control the facial eczema and lid margin inflammation as much as possible. Topical mast cell inhibitors are used chronically but the application of topical steroids is often necessary. A number of these patients require corneal surgery which, in the presence of AKC, is a high-risk procedure.

Vernal keratoconjunctivitis

In the UK, VKC is an unusual, self-limiting, often seasonal ocular allergy that affects children and young adults, males in particular, many of whom have a personal or family history of atopy (Fig. 5.7). The condition is a common and serious cause of ocular morbidity in parts of the Mediterranean basin, the Middle East, the Far East, Africa, and South America, where the disease is perennial and the association with atopy is less consistent.

The symptoms are marked itching, discomfort, photophobia, blepharospasm, stringy inflammatory exudate, blurred vision, and 'morning misery' – an inability to open the eyes in the morning. The superior tarsal conjunctiva and the limbus are the most markedly affected areas and other conjunctival areas show less specific signs of inflammation. When the disease is active, the conjunctival surfaces are hyperemic, edematous and infiltrated, and a tenacious mucus is present (Fig. 5.8). The tarsal conjunctiva is densely infiltrated, with papillae that are often giant (>1 mm in diameter, also known as cobblestone papillae) (Fig. 5.9). In the later stages, fine subepithelial scarring is also seen but conjunctival shrinkage and distortion does not

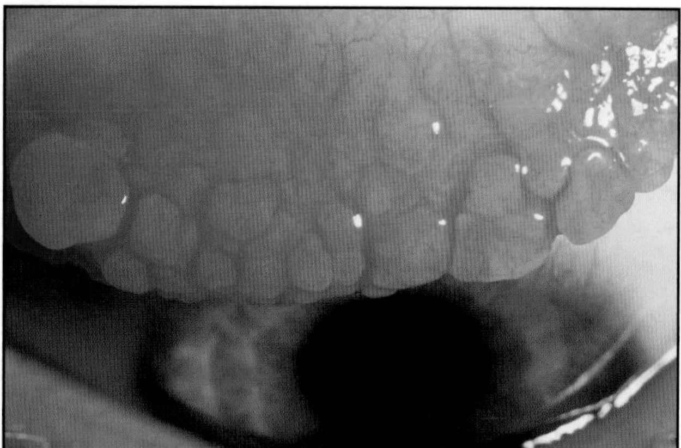

Fig. 5.9 The upper tarsal surface in vernal keratoconjunctivitis showing giant papillae.

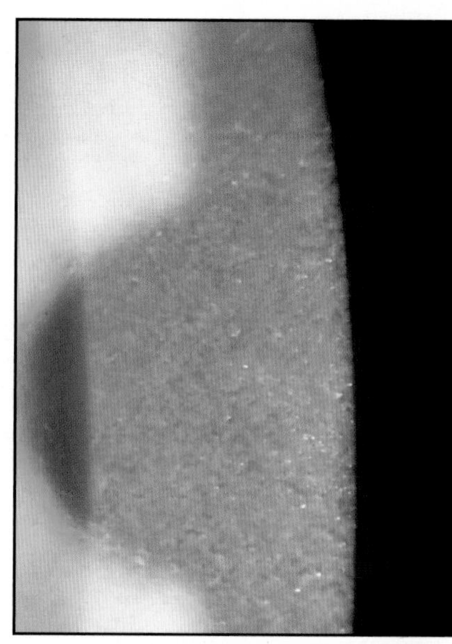

Fig. 5.11 Punctate epithelial keratitis in vernal keratoconjunctivitis.

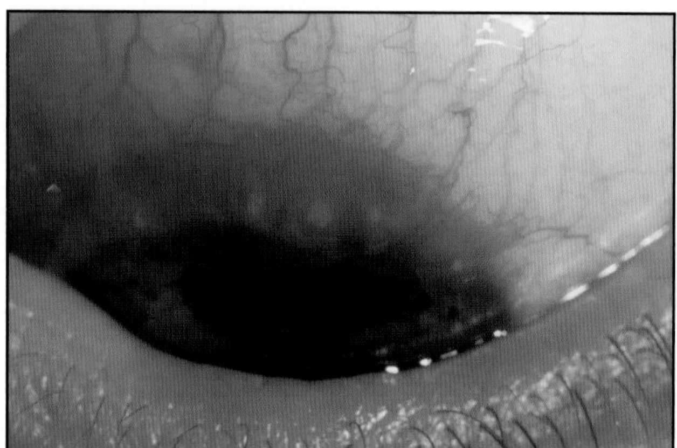

Fig. 5.10 Trantas' dots at the limbus in vernal keratoconjunctivitis.

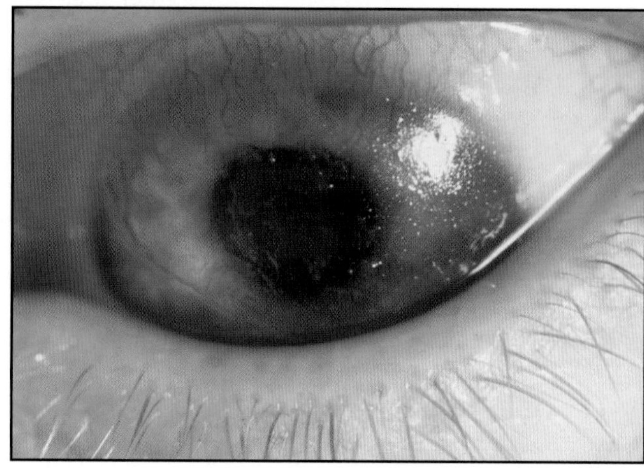

Fig. 5.12 Macroerosion in vernal keratoconjunctivitis.

occur. The limbus may show hyperemia and infiltration, and discrete swellings may be present. The presence of small white dots, first described by Trantas, is typical of vernal limbitis (Fig. 5.10).

The most serious aspect of the condition is the corneal involvement. At its mildest, there is a punctate disturbance of the epithelium (Fig. 5.11). If not treated the lesions coalesce to form a macroerosion (Fig. 5.12); deposition of mucus, fibrin, and inflammatory debris can then result in the formation of plaque (Fig. 5.13). In VKC the signs can be remarkably different in severity between the two eyes, a phenomenon that has not been satisfactorily explained.

Treatment is generally in the hands of the ophthalmologist, because so many cases require topical corticosteroids at some point. For the majority some benefit is obtained from topical mast cell inhibitors which also act as steroid-sparing agents. Additional relief may be provided by mucolytic drops. When the corneal epithelium is breached by a macroerosion or by plaque, topical antibiotic drops are required for antibacterial prophylaxis.

When corneal plaque is present, medical therapy is aimed at quietening the conjunctival inflammation as rapidly as possible

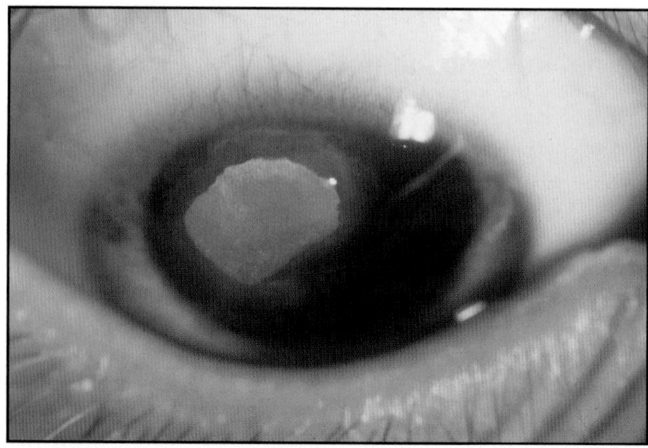

Fig. 5.13 Corneal plaque in vernal keratoconjunctivitis.

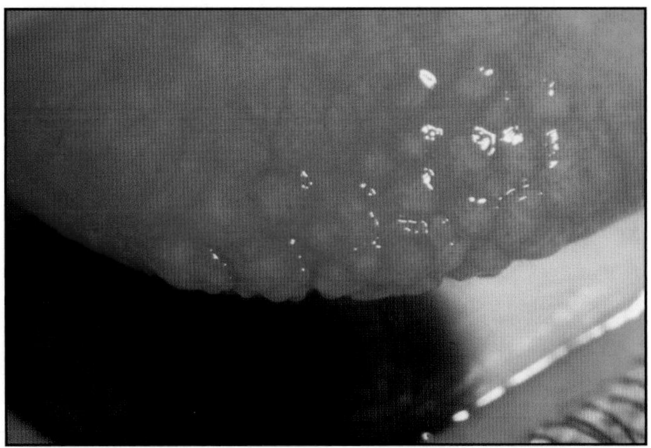
Fig. 5.14 The upper tarsal surface in giant papillary conjunctivitis.

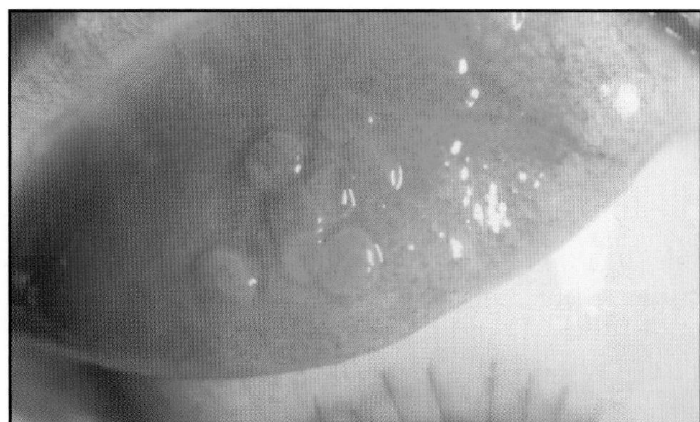
Fig. 5.15 Suture-induced giant papillary conjunctivitis: the offending corneal sutures and the tarsal surface showing giant papillae.

so that plaque can be surgically removed. This is achieved by lamellar dissection using the operating microscope, usually under general anesthesia, as most patients are children. Re-epithelialization usually takes place in a few days after this procedure.

VKC usually resolves spontaneously at or after puberty, but it may develop into AKC.

Giant papillary conjunctivitis

Foreign body-associated papillary conjunctivitis, as it should properly be called, was first reported in wearers of soft contact lenses in 1974. It is now recognized that it may occur in wearers of all types of lenses and also in association with the use of ocular prostheses and the presence of other foreign bodies and material, such as protruding sutures, extruded scleral buckles and cyanoacrylate glue, on the ocular surface. Although associations with atopy have been reported, this is not a consistent finding.

The onset of symptoms may occur a few weeks to years after contact lens or prosthesis wear has begun. There is no seasonal variation and GPC occurs in both sexes and at all ages. There is discomfort and accumulation of mucus on the lens. Patients complain of ocular itching when the lens is removed. The tolerance of the lens, as measured by the daily wearing time, is reduced and there is a tendency for the lens to displace upward under the upper eyelid. The patient may notice that the symptoms are alleviated if a brand new lens is worn.

The distribution and nature of conjunctival signs are very similar to those of VKC (Fig. 5.14); however, the limbus is less often involved. Despite the name of the condition, papillae are not always giant. The cornea is not involved.

GPC is managed by careful attention to lens hygiene, by improvement of the fit and surface quality of the lenses or prosthesis, by minimizing the wearing time, and, as a last resort, by administration of drugs. There is a place for the use of disposable contact lenses. In the case of other foreign bodies (e.g. suture GPC; Fig. 5.15) removal of the offending cause will cure the condition. Mast cell inhibitors have been shown to be effective in the management of GPC. Topical steroid preparations should not be used as they can be very much more sight-threatening than the condition itself, except in the case of ocular prosthesis wearers.

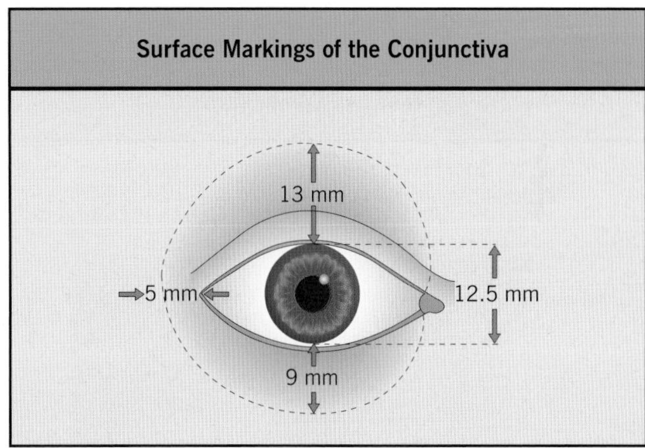

Fig. 5.16 The surface markings of the conjunctiva.

ANATOMY AND PHYSIOLOGY OF THE EYE

The conjunctiva is a thin, transparent, vascular mucous membrane investing the inner lid surfaces and the anterior sclera (Fig. 5.16). It runs in continuity with the corneal epithelium at the limbus (the transition zone between sclera and cornea) and with the skin at the gray line on the lid margin (Fig. 5.17). There are three major zones of the conjunctiva (Fig. 5.18) – the tarsal portion (lining the inner eyelid and firmly adherent to underlying fibrous tissue), the bulbar conjunctiva (lying over the anterior sclera and loosely attached to underlying tissue) and the forniceal conjunctiva (upper and lower) that joins the other two portions and where conjunctiva lies in loose folds.

The normal conjunctiva consists of a non-keratinizing squamous epithelium two to ten cell layers thick, resting on the substantia propria, which is composed of loose vascular connective tissue. The conjunctival epithelium is continuous with the squamous epithelium of the cornea (which is five cell layers thick and covered with microvilli, which interact with tear-film mucus; Fig. 5.19) and with the keratinized stratified squamous epithelium of the epidermis of the skin at the lid margin, along the posterior margin of the openings of the meibomian glands.

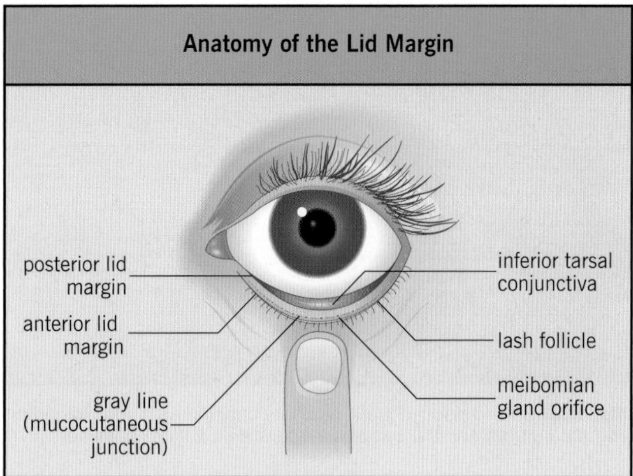

Fig. 5.17 Anatomy of the eyelid margin.

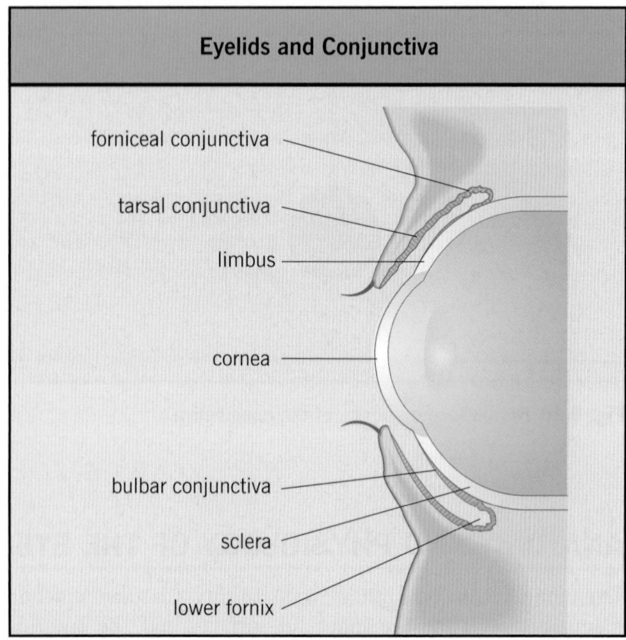

Fig. 5.18 The eyelids and the conjunctiva (forniceal cavities shown are virtual spaces in vivo).

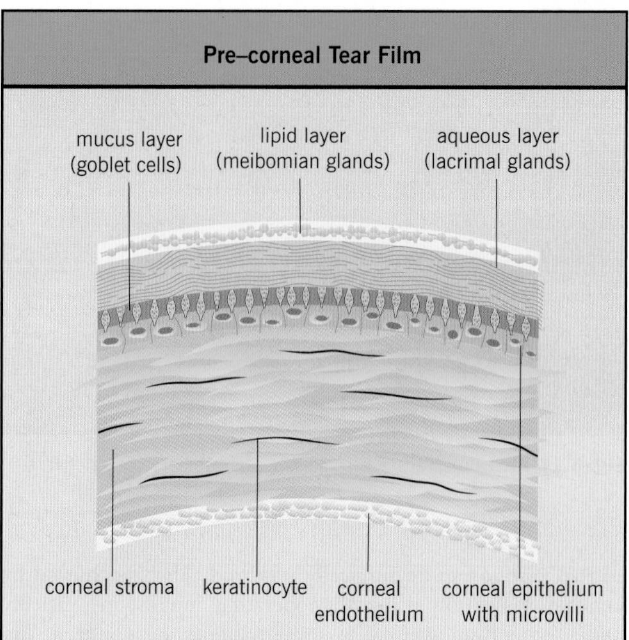

Fig. 5.19 The pre-corneal tear film.

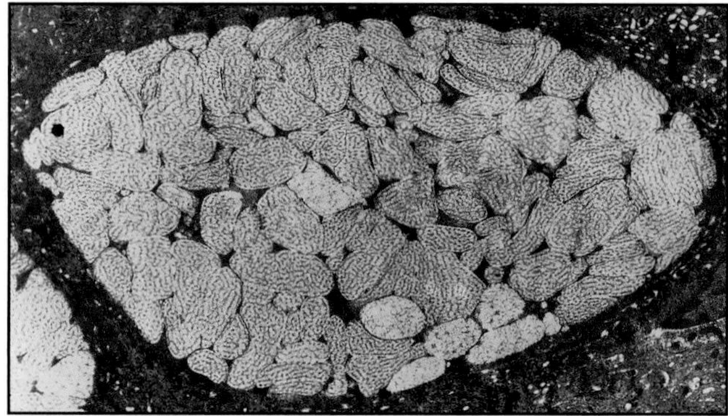

Fig. 5.20 Transmission electron micrograph showing microvilli of conjunctival epithelium above a goblet cell (× 12 500).

Goblet cells along the surface of the conjunctiva produce mucin, which allows moisturization of the hydrophobic ocular surface by the aqueous layer of the tear film. The conjunctival accessory glands (of Wolfring and Krause) lie scattered in the substantia propria and their ducts open directly on to the free surface of the conjunctiva. Their secretions supplement the aqueous tear film, which is mainly produced by the lacrimal gland.

At the ultrastructural level, the surface conjunctival cells are hexagonal and completely covered in microvilli, which can be seen by transmission electron microscopy (Fig. 5.20). These microvilli are thought to enlarge the resorbent area of the epithelium and to stabilize and anchor the tear film.

The arterial supply of the tarsal and forniceal conjunctiva is provided by the marginal and peripheral palpebral arcades arising from the lateral and medial palpebral arteries, in turn supplied by the ophthalmic artery. The bulbar conjunctiva contains a superficial and a deep arterial plexus derived from the anterior ciliary artery. The veins accompany the arteries and drain into the palpebral veins or directly into the superior and inferior ophthalmic veins. Lymph drains to the submandibular and the preauricular nodes. The conjunctiva is a very vascular organ with all areas having an extensive vascular bed.

Innervation

The sensory innervation of the superior conjunctiva derives mostly from the nasociliary (via the long ciliary nerves), frontal and lacrimal branches of the ophthalmic division of the trigeminal nerve, and that of the inferior conjunctiva from the infraorbital branch of the maxillary division of the trigeminal nerve. Reflex lacrimation secondary to irritation or inflammation

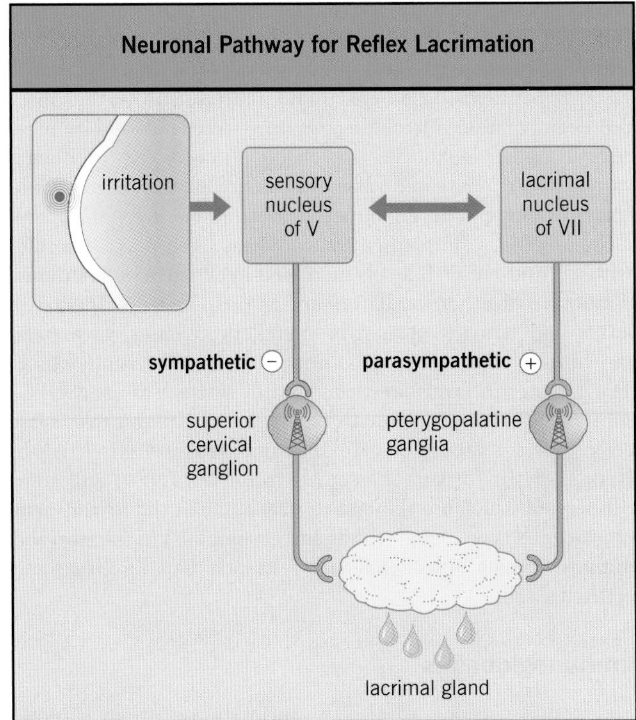

Fig. 5.21 The neuronal pathway for reflex lacrimation. The parasympathetic pathway stimulates the lacrimal gland to produce tears, while the sympathetic route acts to reduce the blood supply which modulates tear formation.

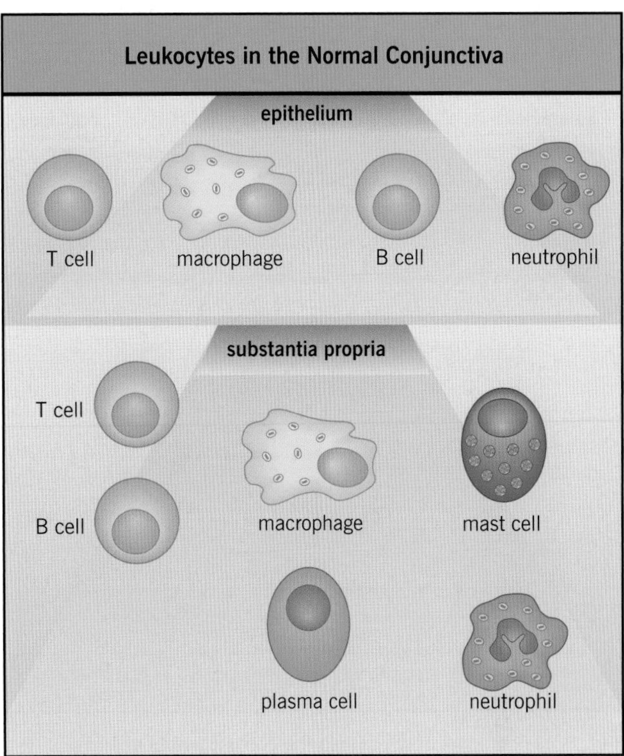

Fig. 5.22 Leukocytes in the normal conjunctiva.

of the cornea and conjunctiva occurs as a result of the connections of the sensory nucleus of the Vth cranial nerve (trigeminal nerve) with the lacrimal nucleus of the VIIth cranial nerve (facial nerve) in the brainstem (Fig. 5.21), with parasympathetic effector nerves passing via the pterygopalatine ganglion and zygomatic nerve to the lacrimal gland. Sympathetic nerve supply to the conjunctiva derives from the superior cervical ganglion and vasomotor parasympathetic fibers from the pterygopalatine ganglion.

Functions

The conjunctiva is important in maintaining a suitable environment for the cornea, particularly via its role in the stabilization of the tear film. It is also crucial for defence of the eye against infection and trauma. There are multiple non-specific mechanisms involved in the defence of the ocular mucosal surface, including:

- the mechanical protection of the bony orbit, eyelids and lashes;
- the flushing action and chemical composition of the aqueous tears;
- the tear-film mucus; and
- the presence of neutrophils, natural killer cells and macrophages in the conjunctiva.

Many leukocytes are present in the normal human conjunctiva (Fig. 5.22) and their numbers vary between the different regions of the conjunctiva and with the age of the individual. T cells, macrophages, and occasional B cells and neutrophils are present in the normal conjunctival epithelium. T cells, B cells, macrophages, plasma cells, natural killer cells, mast cells, and neutrophils are present in the normal substantia propria, concentrated in the subepithelial 'adenoid' layer. Eosinophils and basophils are not normally seen. Mast cells are concentrated around blood and lymphatic vessels and glands, and the vast majority is of the MC_{TC} type (containing both tryptase and chymase in their secretory granules). T cells are the most common cell type, and macrophages the second most common. In the epithelium the majority of T cells are CD8+ and in the substantia propria the numbers of CD4+ and CD8+ cells are nearly equal. The conjunctival lymphocytes and plasma cells constitute the conjunctival-associated lymphoid tissue (CALT), part of the mucosal-associated lymphoid tissue (MALT). The CALT can be divided into three components: intraepithelial lymphocytes (mainly CD8+ and HML-1+); scattered substantia propria lymphocytes; and CALT aggregates lying just under specialized, flattened conjunctival epithelium containing M (microfold) cells.

IgA plasma cells heavily outnumber other plasma cell types in the substantia propria. Dimeric IgA is secreted and is transported across the epithelial cells, where a secretory component is added (Fig. 5.23). Many dendritic cells in the epithelium and macrophages in the substantia propria express class II HLA antigens and act as antigen-presenting cells to T cells in the CALT and in local lymph nodes.

PATHOGENESIS OF ALLERGIC CONJUNCTIVITIS

Pathophysiology

SAC and PAC are type I hypersensitivity reactions to specific allergens in sensitized individuals. In VKC and AKC the allergen

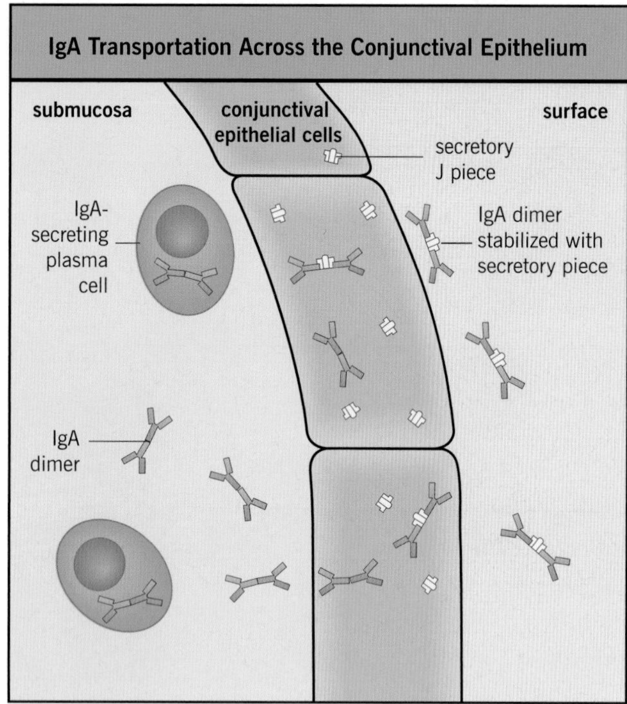

Fig. 5.23 Transport of IgA across the conjunctival epithelium.

sensitivity is not well defined and the pathogenesis is believed to involve complex interactions of type I hypersensitivity, T-cell mediated inflammation and other mechanisms. Colonization of the lid margins by staphylococci may play a role in the pathogenesis of AKC. In GPC, chronic mechanical irritation of the conjunctiva is thought to promote a hypersensitivity reaction to allergenic deposits that are held in prolonged contact with an eroded conjunctival surface by an ocular surface foreign body. GPC shows many histopathologic and pathophysiologic similarities with VKC and AKC but the reason why the cornea is not damaged in GPC is unknown. The interrelationship between different cell types and, in particular, between different cellular sources of cytokines in VKC, AKC and GPC is still very poorly understood.

Inflammatory cells and mediators

Mediators

Mast cells release histamine in allergic conjunctivitis, which acts via both H_1 and H_2 receptors in the conjunctiva to produce vasodilatation, increased vascular permeability, chemokinesis of granulocytes and neuropeptide release (via antidromic nerve stimulation) (Fig. 5.24). Itch is mediated primarily by H_1 receptors. In addition, in VKC histaminase activity is reduced in the serum and in the tears.

Conjunctival mast cells also release tryptase in allergic conjunctivitis and its relevant actions may include:

- proteolysis of basement membrane and connective tissue material (facilitating leukocyte infiltration);
- activation of growth factors and neuropeptides;
- activation of kinin, complement and fibrinogen cascades; and
- stimulation of chemotaxis and degranulation of eosinophils and mast cells.

Prostaglandins, leukotrienes, and hydroxyeicosatetraenoic acids (HETEs) are released by mast cells and other leukocytes in allergic conjunctivitis and produce vasodilatation, increased vascular permeability, an eosinophil infiltrate and further mast cell degranulation. Platelet aggregating factor released by mast cells and other leukocytes is probably also involved, producing vasodilatation, increased vasopermeability, platelet aggregation, and monocyte and granulocyte infiltration, activation, and degranulation. Complement activation is likely to play a role, with C3 and factor B levels increased in allergic conjunctivitis. A number of other mediators are of early interest. Increased levels and activity of matrix metalloproteinases have been shown in VKC which may be important in tissue remodelling. Tear lactoferrin levels are decreased in active VKC and GPC; substance P and nerve growth factor may also play a role. Mast cells secrete a variety of cytokines [interleukin-4 (IL-4), IL-5, IL-6, IL-8, IL-13, tumor necrosis factor α (TNFα) and stem cell factor] which are thought to play a role in the recruitment of other cell types (neutrophils and eosinophils) to the site, and in the activation of local resident cells including fibroblasts and epithelial cells.

Immunoglobulins

Elevated levels of total IgE antibody occur in allergic conjunctivitis in both the serum and the tears, mainly as a reflection of the presence of systemic atopy. Allergen-specific IgE is frequently found in the tears in SAC, PAC, and VKC, and at least some of this is produced locally by conjunctival and lacrimal gland plasma cells. Patients with SAC also have low levels of pollen-specific IgG in the tears.

Histopathology

A single application of allergen to the conjunctiva produces a biphasic clinical response, with an early-phase response at 0–1 hours and, in some patients, a late-phase response at 6–24 hours. The early-phase response is associated with a conjunctival neutrophilia and the late-phase response with infiltration by eosinophils, mast cells, neutrophils, lymphocytes, and macrophages. In comparison, in active SAC and PAC the most dramatic change is an increase in mast cell and eosinophil numbers with migration of these cells into the epithelium, along with the development of some edema of the conjunctiva. In AKC (Fig. 5.25), VKC and GPC there is a dense mixed cellular infiltrate in the substantia propria (least dense in GPC) consisting of eosinophils, mast cells, neutrophils, lymphocytes, basophils, plasma cells, and macrophages, accompanied by extensive mast cell degranulation. The conjunctival epithelium contains mast cells, eosinophils, basophils, plasma cells, lymphocytes, macrophages, and increased numbers of dendritic cells. AKC, GPC and VKC are differentiated from SAC and PAC by the heavy predominance of T cells, particularly of the CD4+ type, and macrophages are the second most common infiltrating cell type. Occasionally, lymphocytes can be seen grouped into immature lymphoid follicles in these disorders (Fig. 5.26).

In VKC, GPC, and AKC the conjunctiva is edematous and thrown up into large papillae. The epithelium is thickened with downgrowths into the substantia propria and occasional keratinization. There is mucinous degeneration of the epithelial cells at the tips of papillae and a goblet cell hyperplasia, most marked in the interpapillary zones. Extensive collagen deposition

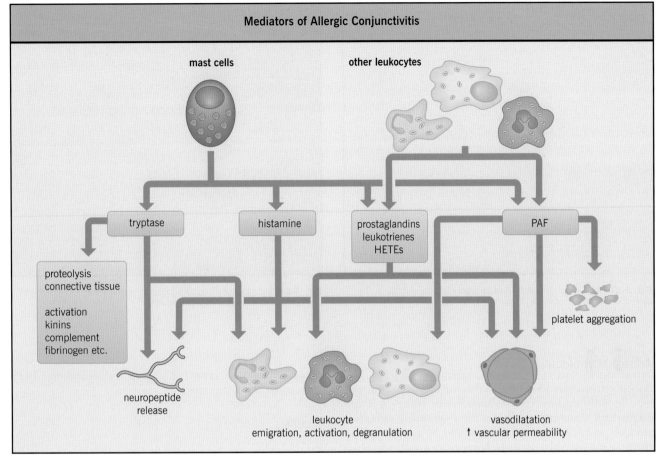

Fig. 5.24 Mediators of allergic conjunctivitis. HETEs, hydroxyeicosatetraenoic acids; PAF, platelet activating factor.

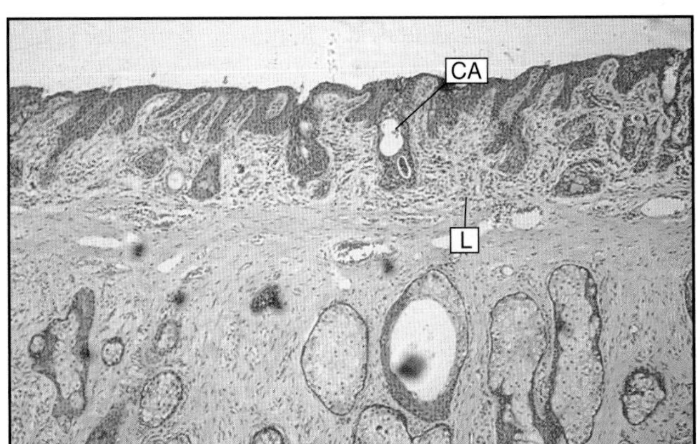

Fig. 5.25 In atopic keratoconjunctivitis, crypt abscesses (CA) are present in the epithelium and there is a band-like lymphocytic infiltrate (L). (Hematoxylin and eosin, × 40).

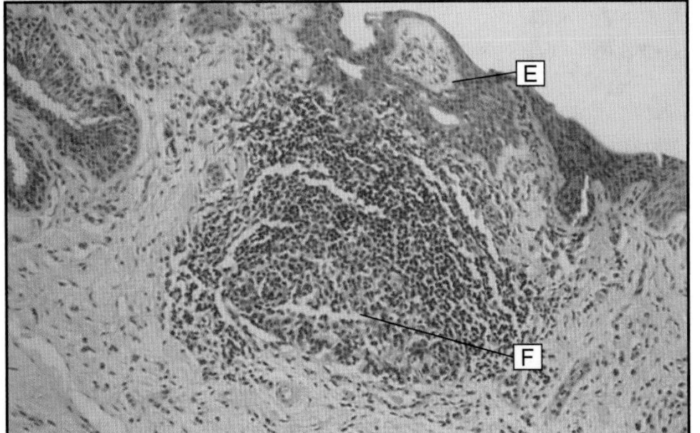

Fig. 5.26 Lymphoid follicle in submucosa in giant papillary conjunctivitis. (Hematoxylin and eosin, × 65). E, epithelium; F, follicle.

in the substantia propria is seen in AKC and VKC, but this is less marked in GPC and only seen in advanced disease. In VKC, blood vessel endothelial cell swelling and death occur, with extravasation of red blood cells and fibrin.

Corneal plaque, which may develop in VKC and less often in AKC, has a laminated structure, is tightly adherent to the underlying corneal stroma and consists of a mixture of mucopolysaccharides, immunoglobulins, complement, fibrin, necrotic epithelial cells, cell debris, eosinophil granule proteins and a few inflammatory cells.

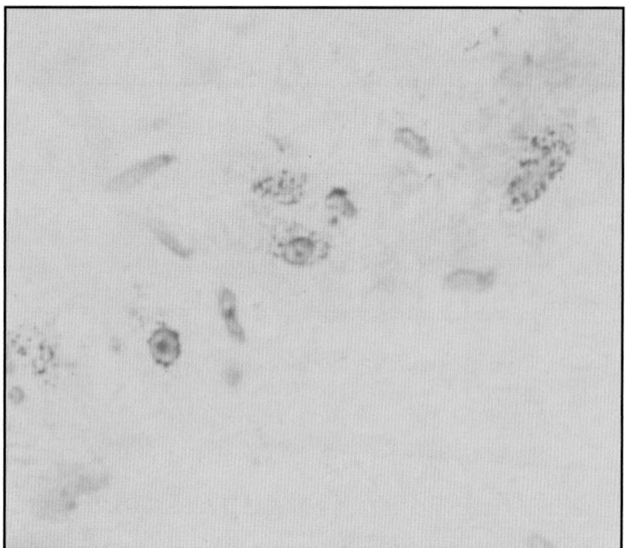

Fig. 5.27 Mast cells demonstrated immunohistochemically in the epithelium and submucosa. (Courtesy of Dr Puman.)

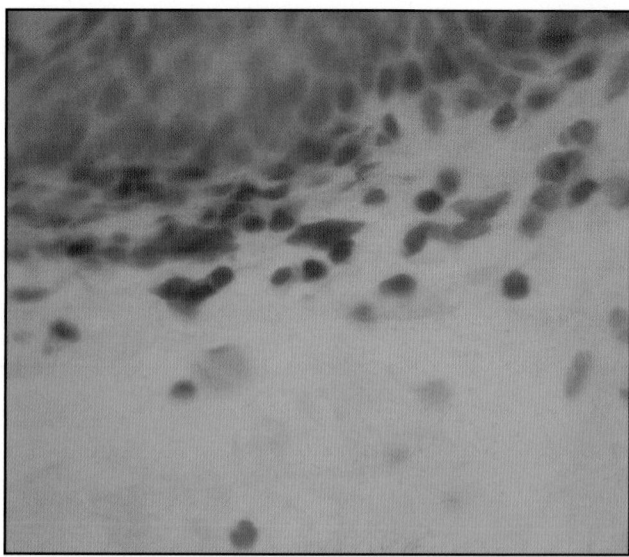

Fig. 5.28 Submucosal T lymphocytes in vernal keratoconjunctivitis demonstrated immunohistochemically.

Adhesion molecules

Adhesion molecules are central in determining the degree and type of inflammatory cell infiltration into tissue. A single conjunctival exposure to allergen in a sensitized individual produces an upregulation of E-selectin by 30 minutes and of ICAM-1 and VCAM-1 by 4–24 hours on vascular endothelial cells. Vascular endothelial cell expression of E-selectin, ICAM-1 and VCAM-1 is upregulated in all types of allergic conjunctivitis and correlates with the degree of cellular infiltration. The VLA-4/VCAM-1 interaction probably underlies selective eosinophil recruitment, and conjunctival vascular VCAM-1 concentration correlates very closely with tissue eosinophil numbers.

ICAM-1 is also expressed by conjunctival epithelial cells after allergen challenge and in all forms of active allergic conjunctivitis, correlating with disease severity and eosinophil numbers. This expression is modifiable by drop therapy. Corneal epithelial cells express ICAM-1 in allergic corneal disease and this may play a role in directing inflammatory cells to attack the corneal epithelium.

Mast cells

In the normal human conjunctiva there are no mast cells in the epithelium and the vast majority of mast cells in the substantia propria are MC_{TC} (Fig. 5.27). In allergic conjunctivitis, mast cells migrate into the epithelium and there is an increase in the proportion of MC_T cells, particularly in the epithelium (although still fewer in number than MC_{TC} cells). The degree of these changes, and alterations in other mast cell proteases (e.g. carboxypeptidase A), differ for each clinical syndrome. Mast cells can synthesize, store and release proallergic cytokines, and conjunctival mast cells contain IL-4, IL-5, IL-6, and TNFα in normal and VKC patients and after allergen challenge. Mast cell IL-4 is upregulated and IL-8 is induced in active SAC. Release of stored mast cell cytokine may be important in orchestrating the early-phase response and may form a link between the events surrounding the initial allergen exposure and the onset of chronic inflammation, T-cell stimulation and differentiation.

T cells

In GPC, VKC, and AKC, T cells dominate the cellular infiltrate (Fig. 5.28) and the CD4:CD8 ratio is markedly increased. T cells in these disorders are activated with increased expression of IL-2R and HLA-DR and there are also increased numbers of memory T cells (CD45RO+). There is evidence that Th2-like cytokines, which promote IgE synthesis and eosinophilic inflammation, are important in allergic conjunctivitis. IL-4 levels are increased in the serum in SAC and in the tears in SAC and VKC. IL-5 is increased in the tears in VKC and RANTES in the tears in SAC, PAC and VKC, but there are a number of potential non-T cell sources for these cytokines. Protein and mRNA for Th2-like cytokines (IL-3, IL-4, and IL-5) have been localized to T cells in GPC, VKC and AKC, but in AKC there is evidence for a more mixed Th population with increased production of IFNγ and IL-2. More recent work suggests that Th subtype variation in the different allergic conjunctival disorders is even more complex than this.

Eosinophils

Conjunctival eosinophils are particularly characteristic of allergic conjunctivitis in contrast to other forms of ocular inflammation. Eosinophils produce multiple proinflammatory mediators (Fig. 5.29) but it is believed that differences in eosinophil function, via their release of granule proteins (e.g. major basic protein, eosinophil cationic protein), may be important in allergic corneal damage and may explain why corneal damage is not seen in GPC. Eosinophils show increased activation in the disorders affecting the cornea, and granule proteins are deposited in the conjunctiva and the tears in these disorders, their levels correlating with disease severity. Eosinophil granule proteins have been shown to be toxic to the

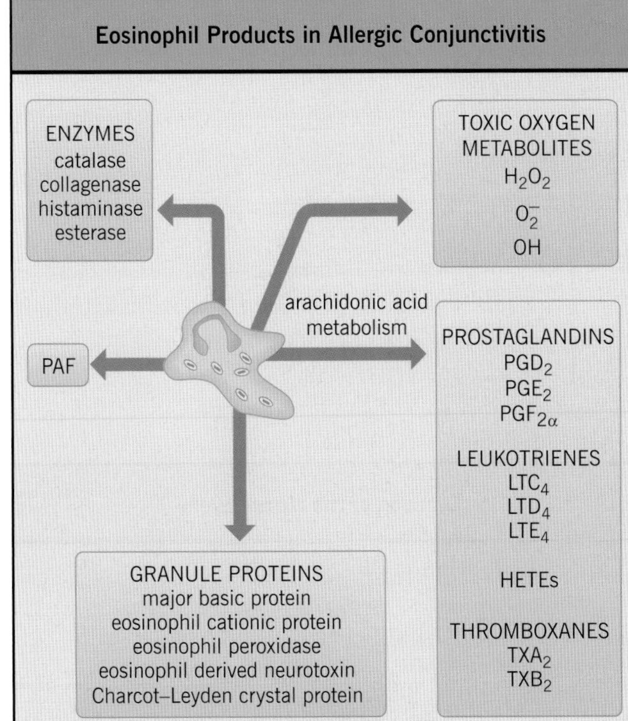

Fig. 5.29 Eosinophil products in allergic conjunctivitis. HETEs, hydroxyeicosatetraenoic acids.

corneal epithelium and they can be found deposited over areas of allergic corneal damage.

Eosinophils can also store and release cytokines, and conjunctival eosinophils express IL-8 in AKC and VKC that parallels neutrophil infiltration. Conjunctival eosinophils in allergic conjunctivitis express a wide range of other cytokine proteins [including granulocyte–macrophage colony-stimulating factor (GM-CSF), RANTES, TNFα and TGFβ] and there are characteristic differences in this expression in the different disorders (e.g. IL-3, IL-5, IL-6 are prominent in VKC, IL-4 in AKC).

Resident conjunctival cells

In the conjunctiva, epithelial cells and fibroblasts appear to play an active role in the allergic inflammatory process, as they do in other allergic disorders such as asthma. Epithelial cell expression of adhesion molecules is altered in ocular allergic disease (see above) and epithelial cells are also likely to be involved through their increased expression of HLA class II antigens and their ability to produce proinflammatory cytokines (e.g. IL-8, GM-CSF and RANTES) in these conditions. Fibroblasts are activated and have altered functions in the chronic ocular allergic conditions, being directly influenced by cytokines such as TGFβ and IL-13 from mast cells, eosinophils and T cells. They may be involved not only in fibrosis and tissue remodeling but also in the inflammatory process through their expression of surface-bound cytokines (e.g. stem cell factor and GM-CSF) and the production of soluble eotaxin, which in turn modulate the functions of mast cells and eosinophils.

DIAGNOSIS OF ALLERGIC CONJUNCTIVITIS

History

The history is a vital component of the diagnosis of allergic eye disease. Most patients have a personal or family history of other atopic diseases such as asthma, eczema, and hayfever. Because the allergic eye diseases, apart from seasonal conjunctivitis, are much rarer than non-ocular atopic disorders, they are unlikely to feature in the family history.

The timing of symptom onset is important. Allergic eye disease appears before the age of 30 years in more than 80% of patients. Seasonal allergic conjunctivitis will appear at the same time as its causative pollen (e.g. spring in birch pollen sensitivity, fall in ragweed sensitivity) whereas perennial allergens such as *Dermatophagoides* provoke year-round disease. VKC usually worsens in the spring and summer, and if severe will persist all year round. AKC and PAC may also show seasonal exacerbations. Diurnal variation can also occur and in PAC, symptoms may be at their worst at night and in the early morning, as a result of heavy exposure to house dust mite in the bedroom.

Allergic eye diseases can be as sensitive to geographic location as other manifestations of the atopic state. Parents of children with vernal keratoconjunctivitis usually know of locations where the symptoms improve and others that can be relied upon to worsen them. Those children with pollen sensitivity tend to feel better indoors, particularly with air-conditioning. Those with animal dander sensitivity are likely to feel worse at home.

Provoking factors should be explored. Non-specific ocular irritants such as smoke may aggravate the symptoms of allergic eye disease, as may exposure to reactive chemicals such as isocyanates, and to other environmental or occupational factors. Certain foods and food additives, such as tartrazine, occasionally exacerbate ocular allergies. If the patient wears contact lenses, a full contact lens history, including the hygiene routine, should be taken.

Symptom presentation

Characteristic symptom complexes are usually found. Tearing, discomfort and photophobia are common, but not specific to allergy. Specific symptoms include itching, which is very common and causes much distress, and eye rubbing. Mucus discharge is often troublesome and the mucus is unlike normal conjunctival mucus, being profuse, sticky and stringy. Blepharospasm is a particular problem in AKC and VKC. Conjunctival edema and hyperemia cause the bulbar surface to take on a 'glassy' appearance, which is often pink rather than red. 'Morning misery' is characteristic of VKC: the child is unable to open the eyes on waking, because of a combination of sticky mucus, photophobia, and blepharospasm. Attempts to open and clear the eyes often take an hour or more, often causing the child to arrive late for school.

Physical examination

Before a diagnosis of allergic eye disease can be entertained, the surfaces of the eye must be examined. This can be done with the naked eye, using a bright pen torch for illumination,

Table 5.1 Clinical involvement of the ocular tissues in allergic eye disorders

Tissues Involved in Allergic Eye Disorders				
Disorder	**Tarsal conjunctiva**	**Limbus**	**Cornea**	**Lid margin**
Seasonal allergic conjunctivitis	+	–	–	–
Perennial allergic conjunctivitis	+	–	–	–
Vernal keratoconjunctivitis	+ +	+ +	+ +	+
Atopic keratoconjunctivitis	+ +	+ +	+ +	+ +
Giant papillary conjunctivitis	+ +	–	–	–

although a magnifying glass, a watchmaker's eyeglass, or a pair of spectacle loupes will help. Ophthalmologists use a slit-lamp biomicroscope, which provides a range of illuminations, i.e. slits, spots, broad beams at a variable intensity, and which can magnify the surface of the eye up to 16-fold.

Table 5.1 shows the various tissues involved in the different allergic eye diseases.

The eyelids and lid margins

Swelling or discoloration of the eyelids, indicative of inflammation, should be noted, as should drooping of the upper eyelids (known as ptosis) which, in allergic eye conditions, can signify active disease. The lid skin should be examined for signs of active dermatitis or changes such as induration, scaling, and lichenification. Blinking should also be checked; 'flick blinking' – incomplete closure of the eyelids – is quite often seen in contact lens wearers. Blepharospasm – spasm of the muscles of lid closure – occurs in corneal and conjunctival inflammation and is often accompanied by photophobia. Any obvious distortion of the lid anatomy, such as entropion (inwardly turning eyelid) or ectropion (outwardly turning eyelid) should be noted.

On examination of the lid margins, observe the eyelashes and note whether they are in-turned (trichiasis) and whether their bases are crusted. Crusting, redness and swelling of the anterior lid margin indicate anterior blepharitis. The posterior lid margins are seen if the eyelid is partially everted. Determine whether the posterior lid margins are squared (normal) or rounded (indicating chronic disease). In chronic lid margin disease, the meibomian gland orifices are unevenly dilated and their secretion is yellow and semi-solid, or even forms a solid wax, in contrast to the clear fluid normally produced.

The conjunctival surfaces

All areas of the conjunctiva may be inflamed in allergic processes, but it is the tarsal conjunctiva in particular that is involved. The bulbar conjunctiva is examined by looking directly at the eye, and if the patient is asked to look up and then down while the eyelids are gently retracted the whole of the bulbar surface can be seen.

The tarsal conjunctiva is examined by everting the eyelids. The lower tarsal surface and forniceal conjunctiva (between which no junction is visible) are seen when the lower eyelid is drawn downward using a finger. The upper tarsal surface is seen when the upper eyelid is everted over a cotton bud, a glass rod, or another narrow object (Fig. 5.30). This will not hurt if the patient looks down. The upper forniceal conjunctiva can only be examined with the aid of a retractor such as Desmarre's while the patient looks down to as great an extent as possible (Fig. 5.31); this is the area where follicles typical of viral and chlamydial infection are commonly seen.

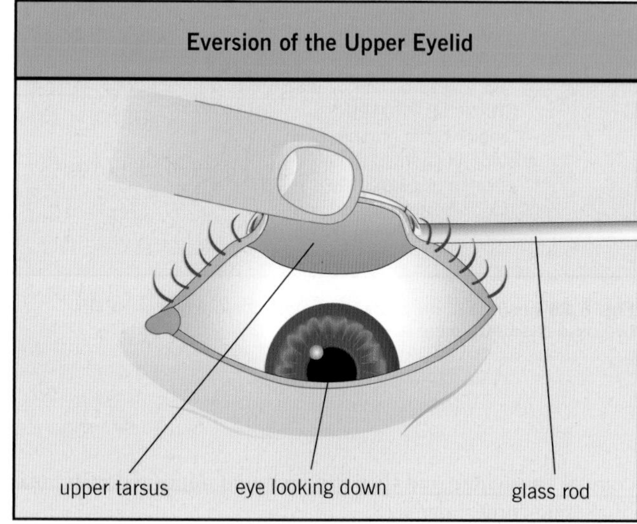

Fig. 5.30 Eversion of the upper eyelid to allow examination of the upper tarsal conjunctiva.

When examining the conjunctiva, which is normally smooth and transparent, the following points should be checked. Hyperemia shows as an enhanced pinkness or redness of the surfaces. Edema produces a filmy or glassy appearance and an apparently jelly-like consistency. If the surfaces are infiltrated, it will generally be impossible to see the normal vascular pattern through the conjunctiva. Follicles and papillae show as elevations of the tarsal conjunctival surface; if such elevations are pale and glistening they are probably follicles (Fig. 5.32), if flat and pink with a central vessel they are likely to be papillae (see Figs 5.9, 5.14 and 5.15). Papillae are designated normal when not greater than 0.3 mm in diameter (micropapillae). Papillae larger than 0.3 mm in diameter (macropapillae) or larger than 1 mm in diameter (giant papillae) are designated abnormal. Scarring shows as pallor of the surface in a reticular, linear or sheet pattern. Cicatrization (shrinkage) of the

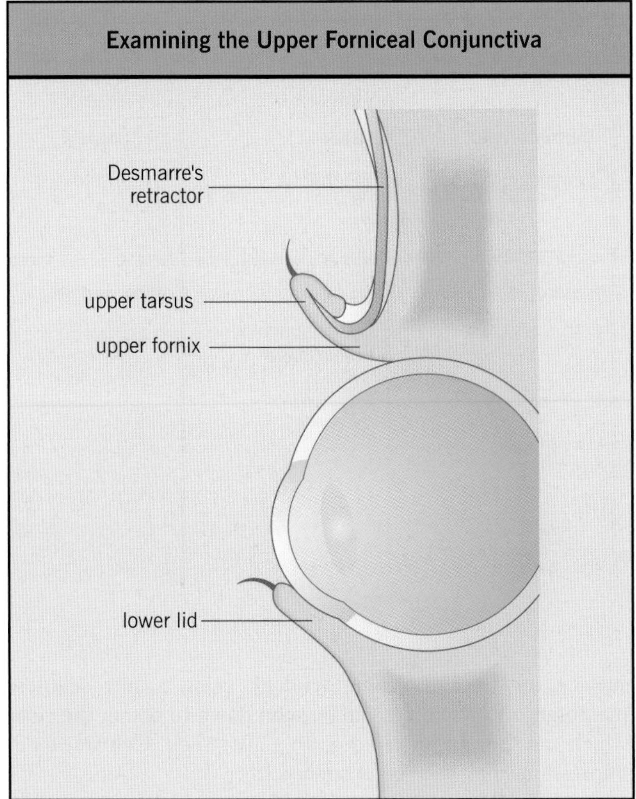

Fig. 5.31 Eversion of the upper eyelid using a Desmarre's retractor.

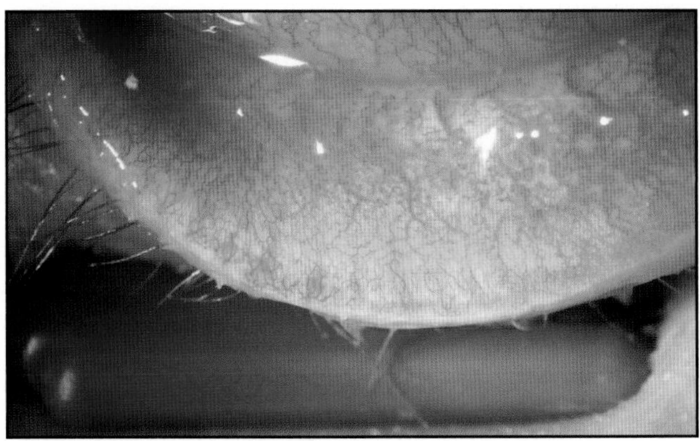

Fig. 5.32 Follicles in the inferior tarsal and forniceal conjunctiva.

conjunctival surface produces shortening of the tarsal surfaces and entropion (in-turning) of the lid margins. A thin thread of mucus in the lower fornix is normal; a larger quantity and flecks of mucus in the tear film are abnormal.

The cornea and limbus

The cornea and limbus are best examined with the slit lamp biomicroscope. However, some features can be seen with the naked eye.

Cornea

The cornea should be perfectly smooth and transparent and have a spherical profile at its center, flattening gently toward its edges. Any imperfection on its surface will be shown as a disturbance of the normal bright (specular) reflex of a light source such as a pen torch. Surface lesions are seen more easily if a little fluorescein is placed in the tear film (by dipping the end of a fluorescein-impregnated paper strip into the marginal tear meniscus) and the cornea is examined with a cobalt blue light. (Medical pen torches are often supplied with a blue filter that can be placed over the beam.) It should be possible to decide whether the corneal surface appears perfectly clear, as is normal, or whether there are opacities present – these may be either infiltrates or scars. The nature of any surface disturbance should be noted: a fine dusting indicates punctate epithelial keratitis; a localized epithelial defect indicates a macroerosion or an ulcer; a surface disturbance white or yellowish and dry in appearance indicates the possible presence of corneal plaque. Mucus adherent to the corneal surface is always pathologic.

Limbus

The limbus is the zone immediately surrounding the cornea and is normally invisible to the naked eye, but when it is inflamed it becomes visible; it may appear pale or pink, and swollen in an annular pattern. Discrete swellings may indicate limbal papillae. The presence of small white dots (Trantas' dots) is diagnostic of vernal keratoconjunctivitis.

Examination of extraocular regions

The facial skin is closely examined for atopic dermatitis. The non-ocular examination generally concentrates on confirming the presence of other atopic disease, and therefore examination of the skin and other mucous membranes and a respiratory examination are performed. However, the number of disorders that may cause a red eye or otherwise mimic allergic conjunctivitis is large (Table 5.2), and further examination is guided by what the history and ocular findings suggest.

Additional tests

Total serum IgE antibody level can be measured but this test is neither sensitive nor specific for allergic conjunctivitis. These levels can fluctuate widely in one individual with time; a high level may indicate the presence of atopy. Levels of allergen-specific IgE in the serum can be measured [e.g. by radioallergosorbent test (RAST)] but often this is only performed when skin prick testing is not feasible. Skin prick testing to determine the presence and approximate levels of specific serum IgE is performed by introducing aero-allergens intradermally and examining the wheal and flare response within 20 minutes. However, the results may be misleading when investigating allergic conjunctivitis as allergens that produce a positive result in the skin of an individual do not correlate well with those which do so in the eye and vice versa. Therefore, this test is not performed routinely in allergic conjunctivitis.

Levels of total and allergen-specific IgE in the tears can also be measured by collecting the tears from the inferior fornix with a cellulose sponge or a capillary tube, although this is not a frequently used clinical investigation. High levels of total tear IgE are possibly the most sensitive indicator of allergic

Table 5.2 The main non-allergic causes of a red eye

The Main Non-allergic Causes of a Red Eye					
Trauma	**Infection**	**Inflammatory**	**Dermatologic**	**Other**	**Secondary**
Corneal abrasion	Conjunctivitis: viral, bacterial, chlamydial	Uveitis	Pemphigoid	Blepharitis	Dysthyroid eye disease
Foreign body	Corneal infection:	Reiter's syndrome	Stevens–Johnson syndrome	Acute glaucoma	Lid abnormalities
Blunt injury	adenoviral herpetic bacterial chlamydial, fungal, acanthamoebal	Dry eye		Subconjunctival hemorrhage	
Penetrating injury		Episcleritis			
Chemical injury		Scleritis		Stye	
Ultraviolet light					

conjunctivitis and measurements of >16 IU/mL are very suggestive, but such results can also be seen in atopy without ocular involvement. Measurement of specific tear IgE (e.g. by RAST) can help to identify the offending allergen.

Detection of blood eosinophilia may indicate atopy but again the result is variable and is not indicative of ocular allergic disease.

Ocular challenge

Ocular challenge involves the instillation of pharmacologic agents (to test for non-specific reactivity) or soluble allergen (to test for specific reactivity) into the conjunctival sac. A positive response consists of itching, tearing and conjunctival hyperemia (sometimes with edema). Symptoms usually begin within 5 minutes and conjunctival changes are detectable after 20–30 minutes. The response can be graded by comparing the ocular signs with standardized clinical photographs and by scoring symptoms. Tear sampling, cytology, and conjunctival biopsy can be performed after the challenge for more detailed analysis. Pharmacologic challenge using histamine or compound 48/80 (producing non-immunologic mast cell degranulation) is used for research into the cells and mediators involved in allergic conjunctivitis. Allergen challenge using standardized dilutions of aero-allergens elicits an early-phase response and, in some patients at higher allergen concentrations, a late-phase reaction. This can occasionally be useful for identifying an allergen and is more reliable (although more unpleasant) than skin testing, but is still mainly an experimental tool for use in specialized centers.

Cytologic studies

Specimens for cytology can be obtained directly from the conjunctival surface or indirectly by collecting tears (see above). In allergic conjunctivitis the upper eyelid should be everted for the direct collection of cells from the superior tarsal conjunctiva; this can be performed by scraping, using a disposable spatula to produce a smear on a glass slide, by brushing the conjunctival surface, or by impression cytology using a nitrocellulose membrane. Tear samples can be spun down to obtain the cells, which can then be smeared on to a glass slide. Cell smears or impressions may then be examined for:

- eosinophils, free eosinophil granules or granule proteins (all diagnostic);
- mast cells (in particular, those degranulated: suggestive); and
- other cells such as lymphocytes (non-specific).

Cytologic staining with, for example, Giemsa, is simple, quick and very specific but poorly sensitive. This is partly because eosinophils and mast cells may lose their characteristic light microscopic morphology during degranulation. This can be circumvented by the use of immunohistochemistry and electron microscopy with, consequently, greater sensitivity.

Supplementary investigations

Tear mediator levels (for example, histamine, tryptase, or eosinophil granule proteins) can be measured in active disease or after conjunctival challenge, but this is usually reserved for research purposes. Levels of eosinophil granule proteins in the tears and serum have been shown to correlate with disease activity and the response to treatment, and may in future be used for clinical monitoring. Conjunctival biopsy may be performed and is very sensitive and specific but is invasive and seldom indicated.

MANAGEMENT OF ALLERGIC CONJUNCTIVITIS

Information

The nature of allergic conjunctivitis and, in particular, the ability to treat but not to cure the disease, should be explained to the patient. The likely time course of the condition should also be outlined. In patients with:

Table 5.3 Summary of therapy for allergic conjunctivitis

Therapy of Allergic Eye Disease			
Non-drug	**Non-specific drug**	**Specific drug**	**Surgical**
Allergen avoidance	Lubricants	Antihistamines	Plaque removal
Cold compress	Mucolytics	Vasoconstrictors	Lamellar keratoplasty
Desensitization	Antibiotics	Mast cell inhibitors	Penetrating keratoplasty
	Rx eczema	Ciclosporin	Excimer laser
	Rx lid margins	Non-steroidal antiinflammatories	Tissue glue
			Therapeutic contact lenses

- VCK, a spontaneous resolution is probable by puberty or adulthood;
- SAC and PAC, a reduction in severity or resolution can also be expected with time;
- GPC, the disease is usually rapidly reversible if the cause is eliminated;
- AKC, however, the disease can be life-long.

Realistic treatment possibilities and aims should be agreed upon early and this depends upon the balance of the risks of therapy with the risks of the disease (Table 5.3). Heavy steroid treatment can often reduce or eliminate symptoms but the side-effects are sight-threatening and therefore it may be necessary to accept less complete symptom control but safer treatment, particularly in those disorders that do not themselves cause any significant visual reduction. For example, the aim in VKC is to get the child through the active disease years, gaining sufficient control over the disease to prevent long-term ocular sequelae, and to allow a good quality of life and regular school attendance without creating iatrogenic problems that may persist once the disease has resolved.

Making information pamphlets and contact addresses available to allergy groups may be helpful.

Allergen avoidance

Where an allergen can be identified, reducing exposure often decreases symptoms. In the case of pollen sensitivity, grassy fields, trees and flowers are to be avoided, car and bedroom windows must remain shut during the pollen season, and patients should ideally attempt to remain indoors on high pollen-count days. A reduction in exposure to house dust mite may be achieved by:

- zealous household cleaning (regular dusting, use of a special vacuum cleaner on mattresses, carpets and curtains);
- removal of bedroom carpet and curtains;
- laundering bed linen above 60°C;
- the use of mite-impermeable mattress and pillow covers;
- killing mites with acaricides.

In mold sensitivity, dehumidifying devices may be used and in dander sensitivity elimination of a pet is of help. For any allergen, the employment of high-efficiency filters may be useful and, in more serious cases, moving to a new location, wearing occlusive goggles, performance of tarsorrhaphy (iatrogenic ptosis by surgery or botulinum toxin) or even admission to hospital may be necessary to reduce the allergen load.

Immunotherapy, via parenteral and oral routes, has been shown to be effective in SAC and PAC. Its use has been confined to severe cases because of the potential risk and the prolonged duration of treatment. Immunotherapy has not been shown to be effective in the other ocular allergies in which a specific causative allergen is difficult to identify.

In GPC, it may be possible to remove the allergen completely, e.g. by removal of an exposed suture or by ceasing to wear contact lenses. However, many patients are contact lens or ocular prosthesis wearers who wish to continue use of their device. In this case, a reduction in the wearing time, either temporarily or permanently, is often advisable and provision of a new (non-deposited) lens or device is helpful. The surface quality and edge profile of the lens are optimized, including elimination of any irregularities or scratches, and the fit and lens shape may be changed if necessary, as may the lens material (e.g. from soft to rigid). Lens hygiene must be regular and thorough, with avoidance of preserved solutions where possible and frequent enzymatic protein removal. The use of disposable lenses also has a place in the management of GPC.

Drug treatment

Non-specific medical therapy

Cold compresses may be all that is required in mild SAC and PAC and may reduce the need for pharmacotherapy. The use of topical normal saline or lubricants (artificial tears) will reduce symptoms and may help dilute or flush away allergen and inflammatory mediators. They should be used in AKC if there is dry eye. Additional relief is provided by mucolytic drops, which dissolve the abnormal mucus (e.g. acetyl cysteine 5, 10 or 20%) and may speed the resolution of early corneal plaque. Whenever there is a serious breach of the corneal epithelium (macroerosion or plaque), the use of topical antibiotics should be considered.

In AKC, facial and lid eczema are treated – preferably in conjunction with a dermatologist – with emollients, topical steroids and occasionally systemic therapy. It is important to control the lid margin disease with lid margin hygiene (using cotton buds soaked in weak sodium bicarbonate solution), application of topical antibiotic (and occasionally steroid) ointment, and systemic antibiotic therapy with a long-term low-dose regime (e.g. doxycycline100 mg daily for 3 to 6 months).

Antihistamines

Topical antihistamines

These are commonly prescribed in combination with a sympathomimetic vasoconstrictor (e.g. antazoline–naphazoline) for SAC and PAC, the combination being more effective than either component used alone. They have a rapid onset of action but no preventive effect and prolonged use of these preparations may cause contact blepharoconjunctivitis.

Levocabastine, azelastine and emedastine are selective and potent topical H_1 receptor antagonists available in eye drop formulations. They have proved effective in decreasing the symptoms and signs of SAC and PAC and have also been used as adjunctive therapy in the management of the chronic ocular allergic disorders.

Oral antihistamines

These drugs, particularly those with less sedative and anticholinergic side-effects (e.g. cetirizine, fexofenadine), are widely used in SAC and PAC. They are occasionally also used in AKC and VKC as an adjunct to break the itch–scratch cycle, particularly at night. They have the added advantage of controlling associated non-ocular atopic manifestations such as rhinitis, but unwanted effects, such as drying of the mucous membranes, may be uncomfortable.

Mast cell inhibitors

These compounds are used topically to reduce mast cell degranulation but also have a wide range of other antiinflammatory effects that may be relevant. These drugs are used extensively in all forms of allergic conjunctivitis, are generally well tolerated and have no serious ocular side-effects. They offer a preventive action and are most effective if used before the onset of symptoms, where possible (e.g. at the beginning of the pollen season), or early in the disease process. As their onset of action is relatively slow (5–7 days) and stinging upon instillation can occur, particularly in the presence of active inflammation, patients should be warned that their eyes may initially feel worse. In VKC and AKC, mast cell inhibitors act as steroid-sparing agents.

Cromolyn sodium is the longest established of these drugs and both 2% (UK) and 4% (USA) drops are available for use up to four times daily. Nedocromil sodium is a newer, higher potency mast cell stabilizer that compares favorably to cromolin and can be used twice daily in SAC and PAC. Lodoxamide tromethamine is another more recently introduced mast cell stabilizer which may evoke less stinging than other preparations. Both nedocromil and lodoxamide are said to have a more rapid onset of action than cromoglycate.

Olopatadine and ketotifen are agents that combine high potency anti-H_1 receptor effect with inhibition of mast cell degranulation and, particularly for ketotifen, inhibition of eosinophil functions. They are useful in SAC and PAC and probably also have a role in the treatment of VKC and AKC. They may avoid the initial worsening of symptoms sometimes seen with the use of conventional mast cell inhibitors.

Steroids

Topical steroids are very powerful in controlling allergic conjunctivitis but have potentially sight-threatening side-effects, including glaucoma, cataract, and the potentiation of herpetic, bacterial, and fungal corneal infections. Therefore steroids are generally contraindicated in SAC and PAC, and in GPC (except with an ocular prosthesis where there is no visual potential) as the severity of the side-effects outweighs that of the condition. In AKC and VKC, steroids are frequently required, but should be used in as low a concentration and for as short a time as possible to minimize side-effects. The use of surface-acting steroids (fluorometholone, rimexolone) may also reduce adverse effects. They are most helpful in periods of increased disease activity or corneal involvement. Other treatment, mast cell inhibitors in particular, should be continued during steroid use. Supratarsal injection of short- or long-acting steroids (e.g. triamcinolone) is occasionally used in refractory cases. In a small number of cases systemic steroids are required in AKC and VKC. As well as considering the serious side-effects, it should be remembered that the reduction in and cessation of use of systemic steroids after the ocular disease has been suppressed can create new difficulties in the management of asthma and eczema by causing rebound activation.

Ciclosporin

Ciclosporin is a potent immunosuppressive which acts by inhibiting CD4+ T-cell proliferation and IL-2 production. Topical preparations of 2% ciclosporin have been shown to provide a marked reduction in the symptoms and signs of VKC, and ciclosporin is particularly helpful as a steroid-sparing agent. More recently, a similar effect has been shown in AKC. An instilled ciclosporin eye drop often causes intense stinging. Also, because of its lipophilic nature, ciclosporin has to be dissolved in oil (e.g. maize) to achieve the therapeutic concentration of 2%, and the oily drops can cause subjective visual blurring for up to 3 hours after instillation. This means that ciclosporin drops, although highly effective, can be very difficult for patients to tolerate. Topical ciclosporin does not produce the serious ocular side-effects seen with steroids but may cause a reversible punctate corneal epitheliopathy and mild lid-skin maceration. Systemic absorption occurs but serum levels are substantially lower than those required for therapeutic action or systemic side-effects, which have not been reported even in prolonged use.

The role for a new, lower concentration (0.05%) but better tolerated ciclosporin ophthalmic emulsion, licensed for use in dry eye, remains to be established, but early research suggests it may have a beneficial effect in steroid-resistant AKC. The unlicensed use of a veterinary ophthalmic ointment containing 0.2% ciclosporin has however proved beneficial for many patients with VKC and AKC.

Non-steroidal antiinflammatory agents

Topical non-steroidal antiinflammatory drugs (NSAIDs) appear to have some beneficial effect in allergic conjunctivitis. Reports of a reduction in symptoms and signs have been published for suprofen in VKC and GPC, tolmetin sodium in VKC and ketorolac tromethamine in SAC. Oral aspirin, as an adjunct to topical therapy, may speed resolution of allergic keratopathy. Topical NSAIDs are not as potent as steroids but have the advantage of a good ocular safety profile and are probably most helpful in treating non-sight-threatening allergic conjunctivitis where antihistamines and mast cell inhibitors are not sufficiently effective.

Surgery

Surgery is usually limited to the treatment of sight-reducing corneal disease in AKC and VKC. For corneal plaque, medical therapy is used to minimize inflammation rapidly and surgical removal of the plaque allows early re-epithelialization. Procedures including lamellar or penetrating keratoplasty, cyanoacrylate glue application or therapeutic contact lens use may be indicated if corneal scarring is reducing visual acuity or if there is extensive thinning or perforation of the cornea; penetrating keratoplasty carries a higher risk of complications in these patients, partly because of the presence of atopy and partly resulting from the compromised ocular environment.

Conjunctival surgical procedures that attempt to influence active inflammation, such as excision of papillae, mucous membrane, or whole tarsus, may provide short-term relief but have long-term adverse effects and are therefore best avoided.

New approaches to therapy

Medical

Potential therapeutic agents, such as leukotriene antagonists, lipoxygenase inhibitors, anti-IgE antibodies and platelet activating factor (PAF) antagonists, are likely to arise from research into the treatment of non-ocular atopic disease. Other potential therapeutic interventions include antieosinophil granule protein compounds, adhesion molecule antagonists and drugs that influence cytokine production and action, such as the anti-IL-4 and -5 monoclonal antibodies in development for use in asthma. Topical tacrolimus shows promise for the treatment of lid skin dermatitis in AKC.

Surgical

The use of excimer laser phototherapeutic keratectomy for the treatment of corneal plaque has been reported and this procedure may have other applications in the treatment of patients with allergic corneal complications. The increased use of collaborative multispecialist teams in combination with medical intervention to control allergic disease and prevent graft rejection (involving both topical and systemic therapies) and the use of modern surgical and allied techniques is likely markedly to improve the outcome of corneal surgery in these patients.

FURTHER READING

Bonini S, Lambiase A, Sgrulletta R, et al. Allergic chronic inflammation of the ocular surface in vernal keratoconjnctivitis. Curr Opin Allergy Clin Immunol 2003; 3:381–387.

Buckley RJ. Vernal keratoconjunctivitis. Int Ophthalmol Clin 1989, 29:303–308.

Butrus SI, Abelson MB. Laboratory evaluation of ocular allergy. Int Ophthalmol Clin 1988; 28:324–328.

Calder VL. Cellular mechanisms of chronic cell-mediated allergic conjunctivitis. Clin Exp Allergy 2002; 32:814–817.

Dart JKG, Buckley RJ, Monnickendam M, et al. Perennial allergic conjunctivitis: definition, clinical characteristics and prevalence. A comparison with seasonal conjunctivitis. Trans Ophthalmol Soc UK 1986; 105:513–520.

Foster CS, Rice BA, Dutt JE. Immunopathology of atopic keratoconjunctivitis. Ophthalmology 1991; 98:1190–1196.

Friedlaender M. Overview of ocular allergy treatment. Curr Allergy Asthma Rep 2001; 1:375–379.

Hingorani M, Lightman S. Therapeutic options in ocular allergic disease. Drugs 1995; 50:208–221.

Leonardi A, Jose PJ, Zhan H, et al. Tear and mucus eotaxin-1 and eotaxin-2 in allergic keratoconjunctivitis. Ophthalmology 2003; 110:487–492.

Strauss EC, Foster CS. Atopic ocular disease. Ophthalmol Clin North Am 2002; 15:1–5.

Suchecki JK, Donshik P, Ehlers WH. Contact lens complications. Ophthalmol Clin North Am 2003; 16:471–484.

Tabbara KF. Immunopathogenesis of chronic allergic conjunctivitis. Int Ophthalmol Clin 2003; 43:1–7.

Trocme SD, Sra KK. Spectrum of ocular allergy. Curr Opin Allergy Clin Immunol 2002; 2:423–427.

Tuft SJ, Kemeny MD, Dart JKG, et al. Clinical features of atopic keratoconjunctivitis. Ophthalmology 1991; 98:150–158.

Zhan H, Towler HM, Calder VL. The immunomodulatory role of human conjunctival epithelial cells. Invest Ophthalmol Vis Sci 2003; 44:3906–3910.

Chapter 6

Definition:
Urticaria is characterized by transient swellings anywhere on the skin surface. Wheals are usually itchy with raised pale centers and are surrounded by a red flare. Deeper swellings, known as angioedema, are most often found in the mouth, eyelids, or genitalia, but may occur anywhere.

Urticaria

Clive E Grattan and Ernest N Charlesworth

INTRODUCTION

Urticaria is also known as nettle rash or hives. Even though it may be difficult to find a specific cause it is nearly always possible to define clinical groups and identify aggravating factors that help management. The clinical presentation may vary widely from occasional localized wheals to generalized urticaria with systemic features. Urticarial wheals arise in the upper dermis, ranging in size from a few millimeters to many centimeters across. The duration of individual lesions may be as little as 30 minutes in the physical urticarias to several days in urticarial vasculitis. Attacks may be daily or infrequent. Affected patients usually feel well but may experience systemic symptoms with severe episodes, such as lassitude, shivering, and indigestion. Progression of urticaria to anaphylaxis is rare. Angioedema is part of the spectrum of urticaria and it presents with deeper swellings of the subcutis and submucosa which may be painful and resolve more slowly than wheals. Urticaria should be distinguished from other forms of urticarial eruption, such as toxic urticated drug reactions and papular urticaria, where plasma leakage is only one component of the inflammatory reaction.

CLASSIFICATION OF URTICARIA

It is more useful to classify urticaria clinically from the history, supported by examination and physical challenge tests where appropriate (Table 6.1) than by etiology since many cases remain unexplained after full evaluation. Laboratory investigations are usually unhelpful except in urticarial vasculitis and angioedema due to C1 esterase inhibitor (C1 inh) deficiency. More than one type of urticaria may occur at the same time. For instance, delayed-pressure urticaria may accompany chronic ordinary urticaria and there may be overlap between the physical urticarias (e.g. dermographism with cholinergic urticaria). Angioedema may accompany wheals in most patterns of urticaria but may, less commonly, occur without wheals, as in hereditary angioedema. Urticaria may be acute, chronic or episodic depending on its duration. Continuous urticaria resolving in less than 6 weeks is acute by definition but becomes chronic if it continues longer than this. A few patients have episodic attacks lasting a few days that recur intermittently for years. Physical and vasculitic urticarias nearly always follow a chronic course.

Ordinary urticaria

This is the commonest presentation of urticaria to specialist clinics. The diagnosis is suggested by a history of daily, or almost daily, wheals anywhere on the body lasting up to 24 hours and may be associated with angioedema (Fig. 6.1), especially when severe. Acute ordinary urticaria is more likely to follow a mild viral infection than an allergy although many cases remain unexplained and some will become chronic. Histamine-releasing autoantibodies have been found in at least 30% of patients with

Table 6.1 Classification of urticaria

Clinical Classification of Urticaria	
Classification	**Type**
Ordinary urticaria	Acute, chronic and episodic
Physical urticarias	Dermographism Delayed-pressure urticaria Cholinergic urticaria Cold urticaria Solar urticaria Aquagenic urticaria
Urticarial vasculitis	
Angioedema (without wheals)	C1 inhibitor deficiency (hereditary and acquired) Normal C1 inhibitor
Contact urticaria	
Autoinflammatory syndromes	e.g. Muckle–Wells syndrome

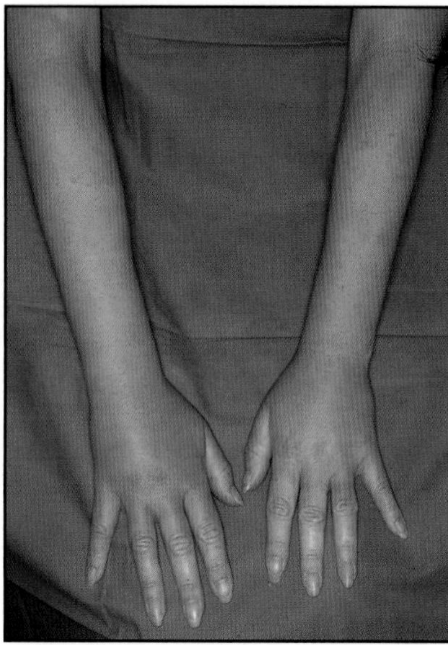

Fig. 6.1 Urticarial wheals of chronic ordinary urticaria by the elbows occurring simultaneously with angioedema of the hands.

chronic ordinary urticaria and the term 'autoimmune urticaria' is increasingly being used for this subgroup. Immediate hypersensitivity reactions are almost never a cause of chronic urticaria in adults but have sometimes been implicated as a cause of chronic urticaria in very young children. If there is no evidence of functional autoantibodies, allergy or pseudoallergic reactions as a cause of chronic ordinary urticaria it may be called 'idiopathic'. Episodic urticaria may be due to drug or dietary exposures but often remains unexplained. Ordinary urticaria can remit but then relapse months or years later.

Physical urticarias

These are defined by the initiating physical stimulus. Typically, wheals erupt within minutes of the stimulus and resolve within an hour, except in delayed-pressure urticaria which has a delayed onset and resolution. Wheal and flare morphology can be of some value in distinguishing between the types. Simple challenge tests in the clinic can be used to confirm the diagnosis. When urticaria is provoked by more than one physical stimulus (summation urticaria) the triggers may be less easy to define.

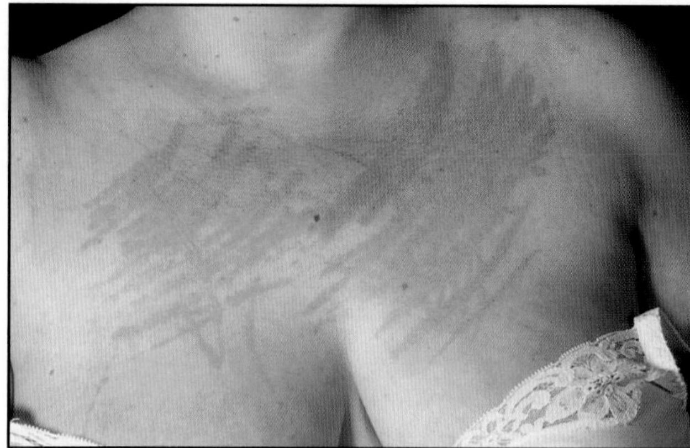

Fig. 6.2 Linear wheals of dermographism caused by scratching.

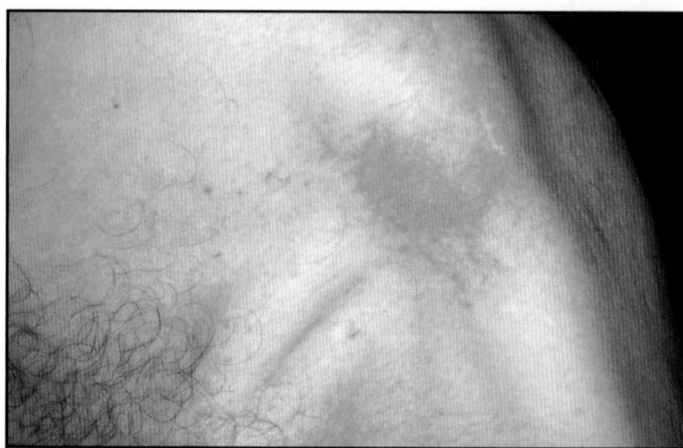

Fig. 6.3 Delayed-pressure urticaria on the shoulder induced by carrying a heavy pipe 6 hours earlier.

Symptomatic dermographism

Scratching or stroking the skin will bring out wheals which are linear and may coalesce (Fig. 6.2). A calibrated spring-loaded instrument called a dermographometer is valuable for clinical studies but it is usually sufficient in the clinic to stroke the upper back lightly with a smooth edge to demonstrate an inappropriate wheal and flare response. Lesser degrees of dermographic response may be present in a minority of the general population (known as simple dermographism).

Delayed-pressure urticaria

Triggered by sustained local pressure, delayed-pressure urticaria is completely different from immediate dermographism. Urticaria does not come up for several hours after the pressure stimulus and may take 24 hours or more to resolve. Morphologically, the wheals resemble ordinary urticaria (Fig. 6.3) but may be deeper and painful rather than itchy,

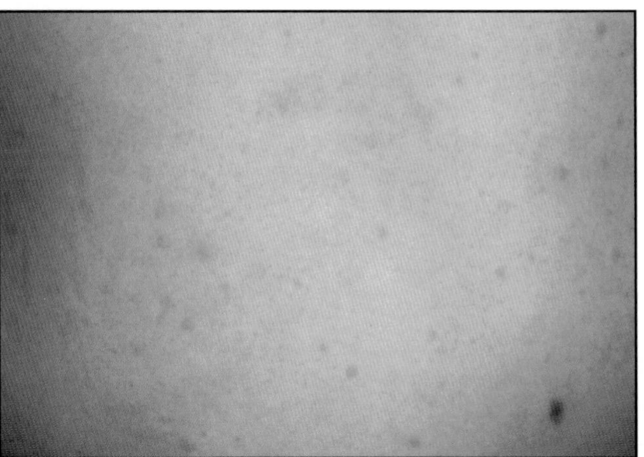

Fig. 6.4 Cholinergic urticaria, induced by sweating, presenting with numerous papular wheals surrounded by a flare.

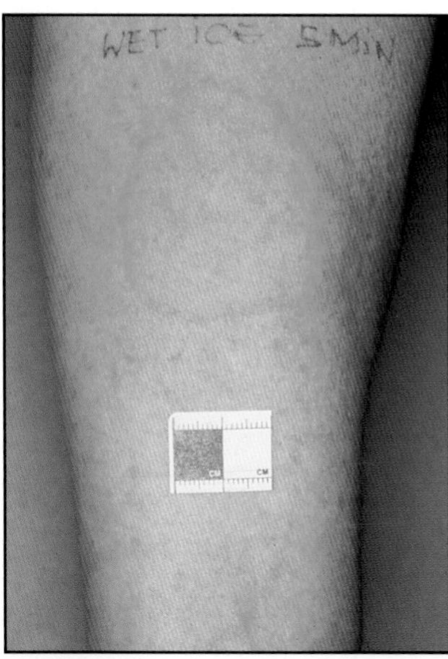

Fig. 6.5 Cold urticaria induced by ice application to forearm skin for 5 minutes.

especially on the hands and feet. Patients may feel unwell with severe attacks. Hanging a heavy weight from a narrow band over the forearm or thigh for 15 minutes may be sufficient to elicit whealing but reproducible testing can be difficult in the clinic.

Cholinergic urticaria

Urticaria triggered by sweating is termed cholinergic as the sweat glands are activated by acetylcholine released from sympathetic nerve fiber endings. A rise of core temperature after exercise, very hot baths, or emotional stress, can initiate numerous small papular wheals on the trunk surrounded by a flare (Fig. 6.4).

Cold urticaria

Localized cooling of the skin by exposure to cold wind or water or generalized chilling may elicit urticaria in susceptible individuals. Cold contact urticaria can be demonstrated by applying an ice cube to forearm skin for up to 20 minutes although whealing may occur after much shorter exposures in highly sensitive individuals. Localized whealing occurs as the skin rewarms (Fig. 6.5).

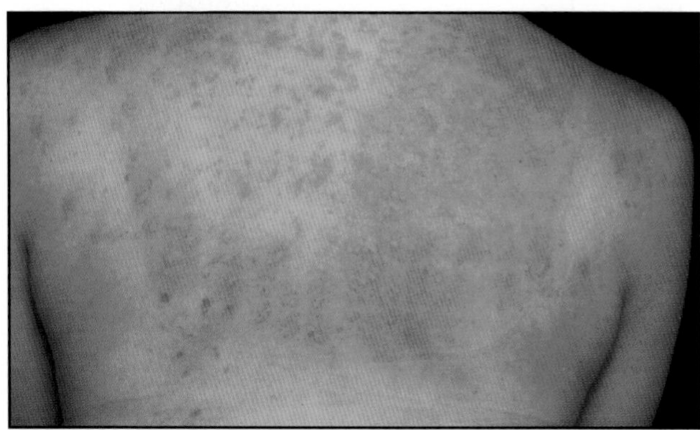

Fig. 6.6 Confluent and papular wheals of solar urticaria appearing on light-exposed skin within minutes of sun exposure. (Courtesy of Dr JLM Hawk, Institute of Dermatology, St Thomas's Hospital, London, UK.)

Solar urticaria

Urticaria triggered by ultraviolet (UV) radiation in sunlight (Fig. 6.6) is uncommon. A history of immediate whealing in sunlight should differentiate it from the much more common condition known as polymorphic light eruption, or 'heat bumps', which appears hours later and persists for days. Solar urticaria can be confirmed by phototesting. A broad spectrum of wavelengths from visible to UVA and UVB may be implicated so the use of window-glass as a filtering agent is unlikely to offer adequate protection.

Aquagenic urticaria

Water contact, at any temperature, may trigger this very rare form of urticaria. Typically, a few papular wheals surrounded by a large irregular flare occur on the trunk (Fig. 6.7).

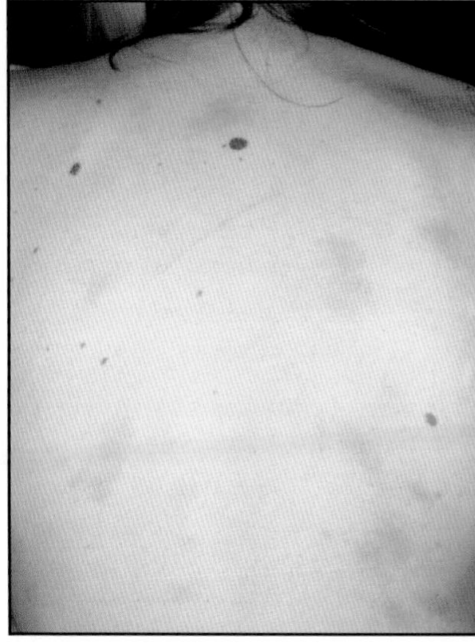

Fig. 6.7 Widely separated papular wheals surrounded by wide irregular flares, induced by swimming, typical of aquagenic urticaria.

Urticarial vasculitis

Best regarded as a presentation of cutaneous small vessel vasculitis with urticarial skin lesions, rather than urticaria, urticarial vasculitis is often included in classifications of urticaria because it may present with wheals and angioedema morphologically indistinguishable from ordinary urticaria but is rare by comparison. The underlying problem is small blood vessel damage rather than temporary permeability. The diagnosis should be suspected if urticarial lesions last more than 3 days or show bruising (Fig. 6.8). They may burn rather than itch and are often accompanied by other symptoms of this systemic disorder, including malaise and arthralgia. It may be associated with an underlying connective tissue disease, viral hepatitis or drugs but many cases are idiopathic. A skin biopsy is essential to confirm the diagnosis. A raised erythrocyte sedimentation rate (ESR) is the most consistent blood abnormality but may be normal. A precipitating IgG autoantibody against C1q may be present in more severe cases with hypocomplementemia. Hypocomplementemic urticarial vasculitis is associated with a more severe clinical course. Patients with chronic urticaria, fever, arthralgic or bone pain, and an IgM gammopathy are diagnosed as having Schnitzler's syndrome. About 50% of them show vasculitis histologically in spontaneous wheals.

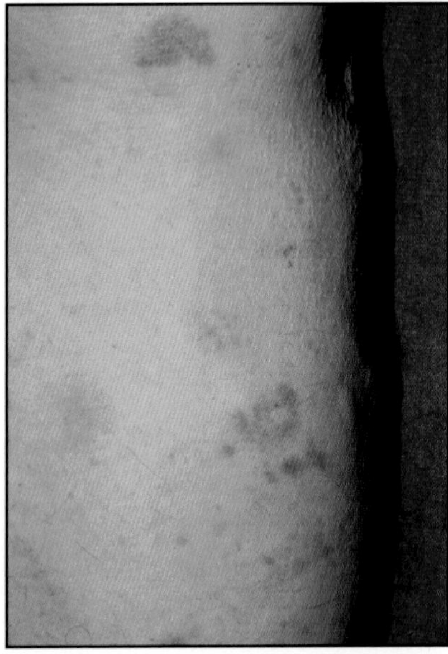

Fig. 6.8 Wheals of urticarial vasculitis, lasting over 24 hours and resolving with bruises.

Angioedema (without wheals)

The presence or absence of wheals is a key point in the diagnosis of angioedema (Fig. 6.9). If wheals are not associated with angioedema, it is very important to exclude C1 inh deficiency. This small subgroup of patients with angioedema due to hereditary and acquired C1 inh deficiency needs to be clearly separated from the angioedema seen with urticaria because the pathogenesis, prognosis, and management are completely different. The deficiency may be due to reduced production of C1 inh (type 1 disease) or the production of normal amounts of dysfunctional inhibitor (type 2 disease). Hereditary angioedema is an autosomal dominant condition. Large painful subcutaneous (Fig. 6.10) or submucosal swellings

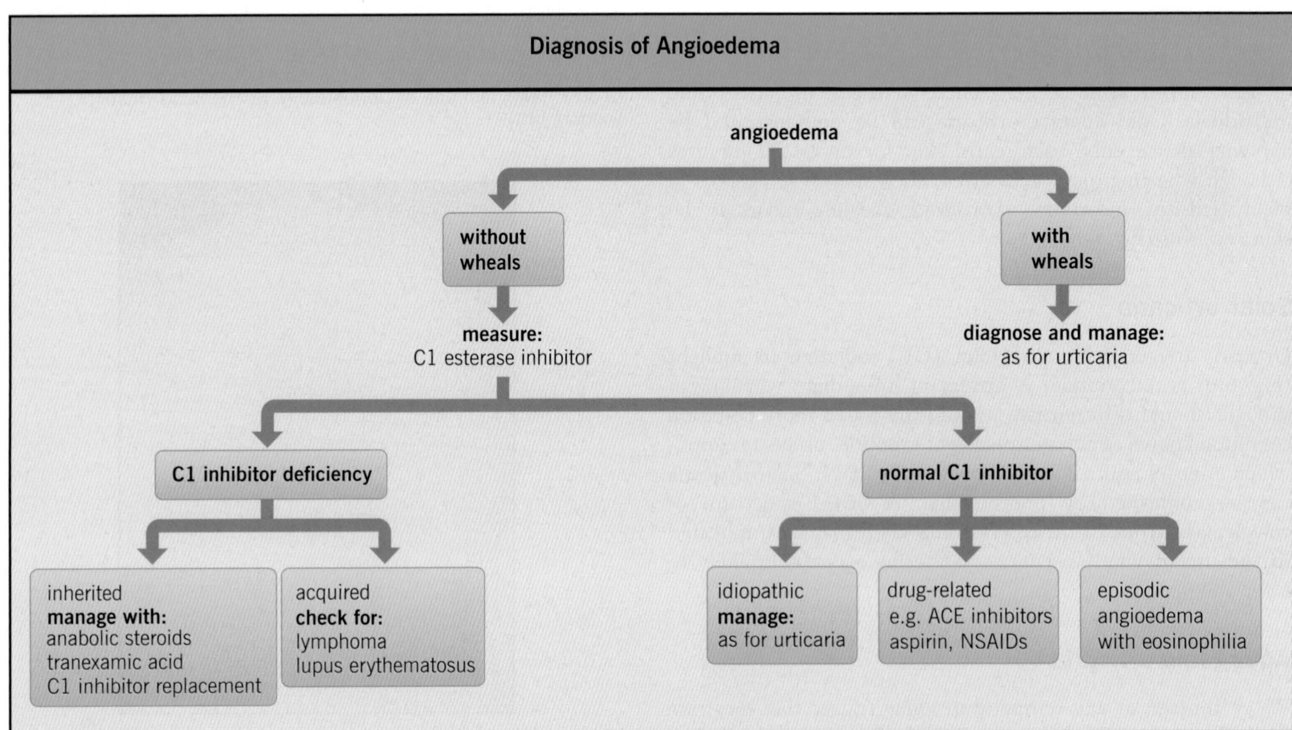

Fig. 6.9 Diagnosis of angioedema. ACE, angiotensin-converting enzyme; NSAIDs, non-steroidal antiinflammatory drugs.

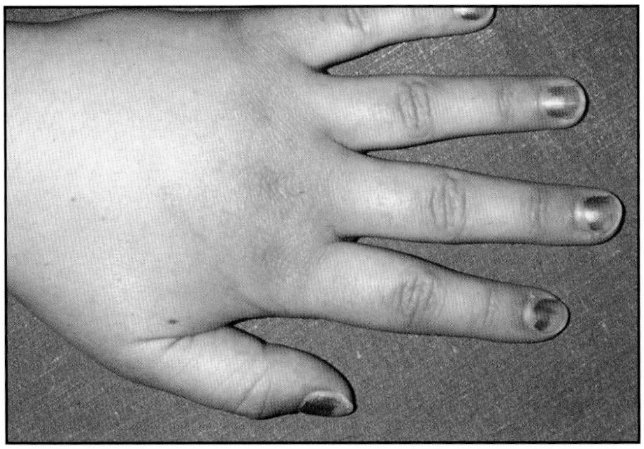

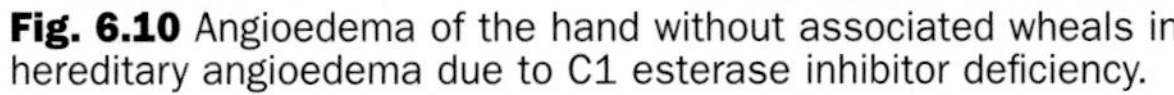

Fig. 6.10 Angioedema of the hand without associated wheals in hereditary angioedema due to C1 esterase inhibitor deficiency.

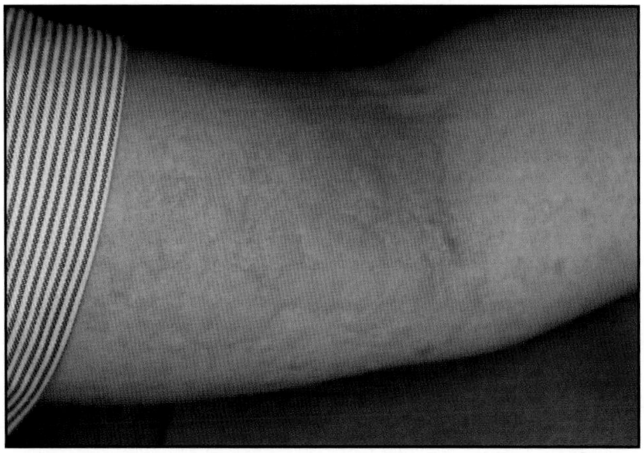

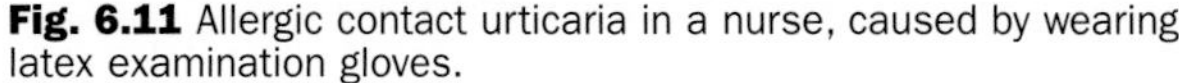

Fig. 6.11 Allergic contact urticaria in a nurse, caused by wearing latex examination gloves.

may be initiated by trauma, including dental extraction or intubation, and persist for days without treatment. Bowel edema presents with colic, and laryngeal involvement may cause suffocation.

Angioedema results from uninhibited activation of the early components of complement leading to the generation of vasoactive kinin-like peptides and the formation of bradykinin. Minor trauma activates Hageman factor (XII), which promotes the formation of plasmin and kallikrein: plasmin activates C1 with formation of a C2 kinin-like peptide and kallikrein generates bradykinin from kininogen. The C_4 component of complement is always reduced during and nearly always reduced between attacks with both forms and is, therefore, a good screening blood test. A very rare acquired form of C1 inh deficiency may be associated with autoimmune disease or lymphoma.

Recurrent angioedema with normal C1 inh levels is usually idiopathic. However, it is important not to overlook the possibility of a drug-induced cause. Angioedema is a well recognized side-effect of angiotensin-converting enzyme (ACE) inhibitors and may occur with aspirin and non-steroidal antiinflammatories.

Contact urticaria

Localized contact urticarial reactions are very common but are not often a reason for presentation to specialist clinics. The cause is usually obvious because urticaria follows the stimulus within minutes. Wheals tend to be short-lived but may have a delayed phase if severe. Allergic IgE-mediated contact urticaria to allergens, such as peanuts, animal dander, or latex (Fig. 6.11), are particularly common in atopic individuals. Non-allergic contact urticaria can occur with a wide range of chemicals in common use in the cosmetics and food industries, such as cinnamic aldehyde (a food flavoring) and benzoic acid (a food preservative).

ANATOMY AND PHYSIOLOGY OF THE SKIN

The skin is the largest organ in the body, and is more than a simple barrier to dehydration, external insults, and allergens. The epidermis is composed predominantly of keratinocytes. Langerhans' cells comprise 2–6% of the total epidermal structure and play a critical role as antigen-presenting cells, thus providing a link for the processing of foreign antigens introduced into the skin. The dermis contains the small blood vessels, lymphatics, mast cells, and sensory nerve fibers in a framework of collagen and elastin, which are involved in urticaria pathogenesis.

Innervation

Sensory nerve endings in the dermis are innervated by afferent neurons to the central nervous system. Signals from mechanoreceptors are mainly conveyed by myelinated A fibers whereas those generated by painful stimulation of nociceptors are transmitted more slowly by unmyelinated C fibers with some A fiber involvement. Antidromic stimulation of sensory C fiber twigs is responsible for the flare reaction seen in the triple response of Lewis to injection or release of histamine. There is now good evidence that capillary dilatation in the flare is due to the release of neuropeptides from sensory nerve endings rather than histamine which mediates the central wheal. Autonomic sympathetic innervation of sweat glands is mediated by release of acetylcholine rather than norepinephrine.

Functions

The complex interplay between Langerhans' cells, cytokine-producing keratinocytes, and skin-targeting lymphocytes has been referred to as the skin-associated lymphoid tissue (SALT) system and appears to be analogous to the gastrointestinal-associated lymphoid tissue (GALT) system. Although mast cells have been considered to be the primary effector cells in urticaria, lymphocytes may play an integral role by the production of various histamine-releasing factors, including cytokines and autoantibodies. Investigation into the T-cell subsets in the dermis of patients with urticaria shows a predominance of CD4+ cells over CD8+ cells. The cytokine products of lymphocytes and other cutaneous cells, including mast cells, may then result in an upregulation of vascular adhesion molecules. Vascular endothelial activation occurs early as a response to pressure in delayed-pressure urticaria with a significant upregulation of

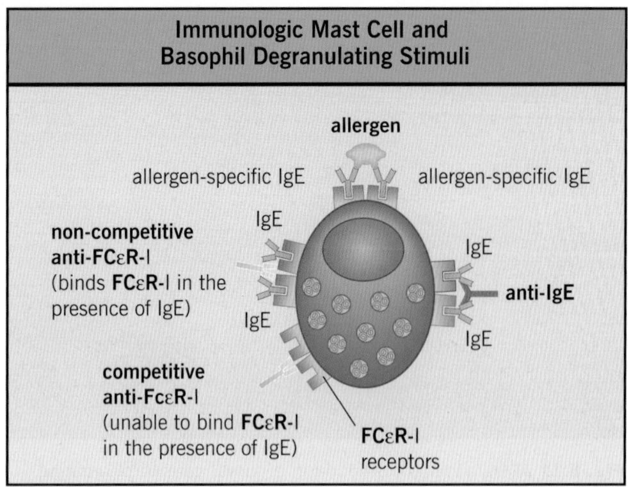

Fig. 6.12 Immunologic mast cell and basophil degranulating stimuli.

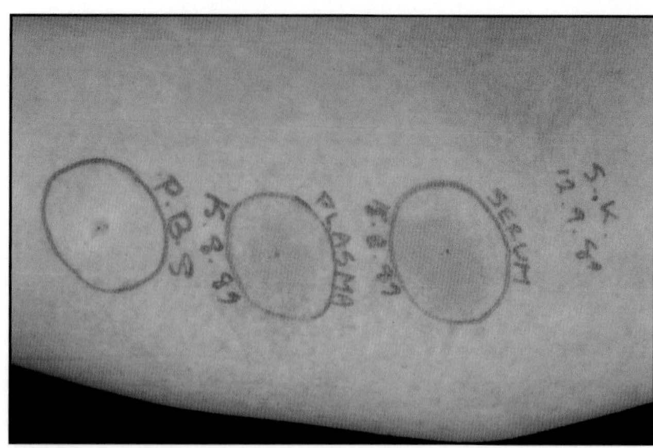

Fig. 6.13 Wheal-and-flare response at 60 minutes to intradermal injection of autologous serum and plasma in a chronic urticaria patient. Note there is no reaction to a control skin test of phosphate-buffered saline (PBS).

E-selectin and of vascular adhesion molecule-1 (VCAM-1) at 24 hours.

PATHOGENESIS OF URTICARIA

Pathophysiology

Mast cells play an important role in both immediate hypersensitivity reactions and urticaria/angioedema. In allergic disease they are activated by the cross-linking of specific IgE bound to the high-affinity IgE receptor (FcεRI) on tissue mast cells and on peripheral blood basophils. This activation of mast cells, through the FcεRI receptor, ultimately results in an influx of inflammatory cells including eosinophils, neutrophils, lymphocytes, and basophils into the surrounding tissue, thus ushering in the late-phase response (LPR). It is the LPR of IgE-mediated allergic disease which sets this cascade of events in place.

Some potential mechanisms for FcεRI-mediated degranulation of mast cells and basophils are illustrated in Figure 6.12. Urticaria due to allergen exposure, as seen with certain foods and latex, results from cross-linking of receptor-bound IgE. Histamine-releasing IgG autoantibodies, with properties of anti-IgE and anti-FcεRI, have been found in the serum of about 30% of patients with chronic 'idiopathic' urticaria referred to specialist clinics. These functional autoantibodies appear to be directed against FcεRI in about 85% of the positive patients and, in many cases, histamine release is complement dependent. The majority binds FcεRI with or without the presence of IgE on the receptor (i.e. they do not compete with IgE for the binding site). Others can only bind unoccupied receptors (i.e. they compete with IgE for the binding site). Functional assays for histamine-releasing activity are not straightforward and are only available in a few specialist research centers. Intradermal injection of the patient's own serum (the autologous serum skin test, ASST) can be used as a simple screening test for histamine-releasing activity in blood. The development of a wheal and flare over 30–60 minutes at the site of skin testing (Fig. 6.13) provides a fairly sensitive, but not very specific, indication of histamine-releasing activity on basophil assays. Preliminary work indicates that a low molecular weight 'mast cell-specific' factor in some sera, causing a positive ASST but no release from healthy donor basophils, may nevertheless cause release of histamine from skin mast cells.

Non-functional autoantibodies against IgE and FcεRI have also been detected by immunoassay in chronic urticaria patients and in other groups of control patients and even healthy subjects. The importance of these autoantibodies is less certain. Non-functional anti-IgE autoantibodies may be detectable in atopic syndromes and healthy subjects. Immunoassays, based on enzyme-linked immunosorbent assay (ELISA) and Western blotting, have been developed for detecting anti-FcεRI autoantibodies but are not yet commercially available. Non-functional autoantibodies against FcεRI have been found in dermatomyositis, systemic lupus erythematosus, pemphigus vulgaris, and bullous pemphigoid.

The role of the skin mast cell in the evolution of the urticarial wheal in patients with chronic urticaria was first appreciated by Juhlin in 1967. The findings were confirmed by a study in which almost all of the patients with chronic urticaria displayed increased histamine release into skin blisters overlying lesions of urticaria. Similar results have been found with cold urticaria. Furthermore, total histamine was elevated in both lesional and non-lesional skin of patients with chronic urticaria when compared with patients without urticaria. The time kinetics for mast cell histamine release from the cutaneous mast cells in patients with cold urticaria is interesting in that it is not simply lowering of skin temperature that causes the mast cells to release histamine, as the skin must be rewarmed before the mast cells will undergo release.

Analysis of the release of histamine into blister fluid overlying non-lesional skin in patients with chronic urticaria has shown an increase in both spontaneous release of histamine and an increase in the histamine release induced by the non-specific mast cell degranulator, compound 48/80, when compared to non-urticaria controls. The hypothesis of increased mast cell releasability in urticaria patients was subsequently confirmed by codeine skin testing. It is unlikely that the early histamine release in chronic urticaria is secondary to the recruitment and stimulation of blood basophils, which are also a possible source

Table 6.2 Agents capable of causing mast cell histamine release

Agents Capable of Causing Mast Cell Histamine Release	
Agents	**Group**
Non-cytotoxic stimuli Immunologic	Allergen cross-link of specific, mast cell bound IgE (e.g. latex, nuts, fish) Autoantibodies which cross-link the Fc portion of IgE or the FcεRI directly C3a and C5a anaphylatoxins
Physiologic	Substance P Vasoactive intestinal polypeptide (VIP)
Therapeutic	Morphine Codeine Tubocurarine, atracurium
Experimental	Compound 48/80 Calcium ionophore A23187
Cytotoxic stimuli	C5a, C3a Surfactants
Anaphylactoid-causing agents	Dextran Endotoxin Radiocontrast material

of histamine, but they probably contribute to prolongation of the wheals. The fact that the mast cell, not the basophil, is the source of spontaneously released histamine observed in patients with urticaria is further corroborated by increased levels of tryptase in suction blister fluid. Table 6.2 reviews the multiplicity of agents capable of causing the skin mast cell to release histamine. There is also a degree of mast cell heterogeneity in that many of the non-cytotoxic agents, such as compound 48/80 and codeine, cause release only in the skin mast cell and not in mast cells located in the gut or the respiratory tree. The role of neuropeptides in causing the skin mast cell to release histamine is unclear. In one study, substance P and the vasoactive intestinal peptide (VIP), in venous blood draining from challenged skin in urticaria patients, was not found to be elevated. In another study, somatostatin was increased and VIP was decreased. It may very well be that the microenvironment of the skin mast cell in patients with urticaria uniquely enhances the liberation of cytokines, chemokines, or histamine-releasing factors that then lower the release threshold for the cutaneous mast cell, thus resulting in an urticarial lesion.

Inflammatory cells and mediators

The wide diversity of mast cell mediators including histamine, tryptase, chymase, and cytokines upregulate E-selectin and VCAMs. This upregulation of adhesion molecules promotes the influx of lymphocytes and granulocytes into the site of the urticarial skin reaction.

The role of eosinophils in urticaria

Eosinophils frequently play a role when there is an allergic etiology to the urticaria, such as a reaction to a drug, food, or

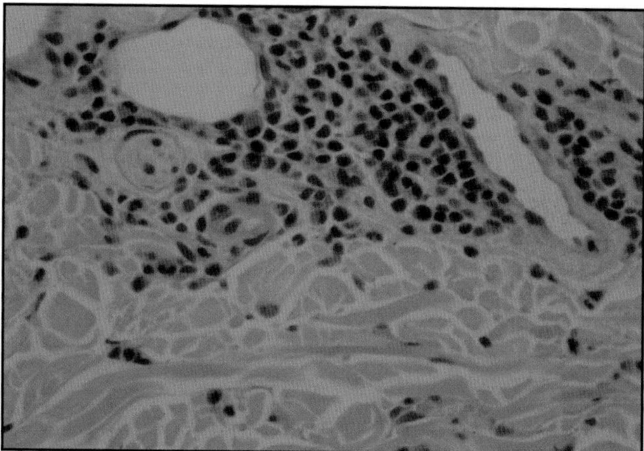

Fig. 6.14 Histology of the late-phase reaction in skin showing perivascular polymorphonuclear cells and eosinophils with no evidence of vasculitis.

exogenous antigen. Eosinophils may also comprise a portion of the inflammatory cell infiltrate, along with neutrophils, in delayed-pressure urticaria. Eosinophils are predominantly tissue cells: for every one eosinophil observed in the peripheral blood, there are 300 eosinophils in the tissues. A specific syndrome, referred to as episodic angioedema associated with eosinophilia (EAAE), has been described in which patients have cyclic angioedema associated with significant weight gain (15% of body weight), fever, urticaria, and leukocytosis with marked peripheral and tissue eosinophilia. These patients do not have internal organ involvement and have a benign course in contradistinction to hypereosinophilic syndrome.

Exactly how eosinophils effect an urticarial reaction is not fully understood. However, eosinophils are the major site of leukotriene C_4 (LTC_4) production in allergic inflammation. With the advent of leukotriene-receptor antagonists, the contribution of LTC_4 to the symptoms of chronic urticaria is now becoming apparent. The cationic proteins of the eosinophil have also been shown to elicit a wheal-and-flare when directly injected into the skin. The potential role of the eosinophil is further supported by the demonstration of eosinophil degranulation in addition to the degranulation of mast cells.

There have been reports of patients with chronic urticaria in whom there is a predominance of polymorphonuclear cells and eosinophils in lesional skin without evidence for a vasculitis. The histology in these patients is identical to that observed in patients with an IgE-mediated LPR (Fig. 6.14). Suspects in whom the histology resembles a cutaneous LPR usually have lesions which last longer than 24 hours and frequently burn or sting, in addition to itching. Unlike an urticarial vasculitis, these patients do not display purpura and there is no evidence for an urticarial vasculitis when biopsied.

The role of basophils in urticaria

Peripheral blood basophils of chronic urticaria patients are reduced or absent in patients with strong serum histamine-releasing activity. This may be due to spontaneous degranulation which, in turn, contributes to the urticarial reaction. However, more likely explanations are that these basophils migrate into skin lesions or are removed from the circulation by macrophages

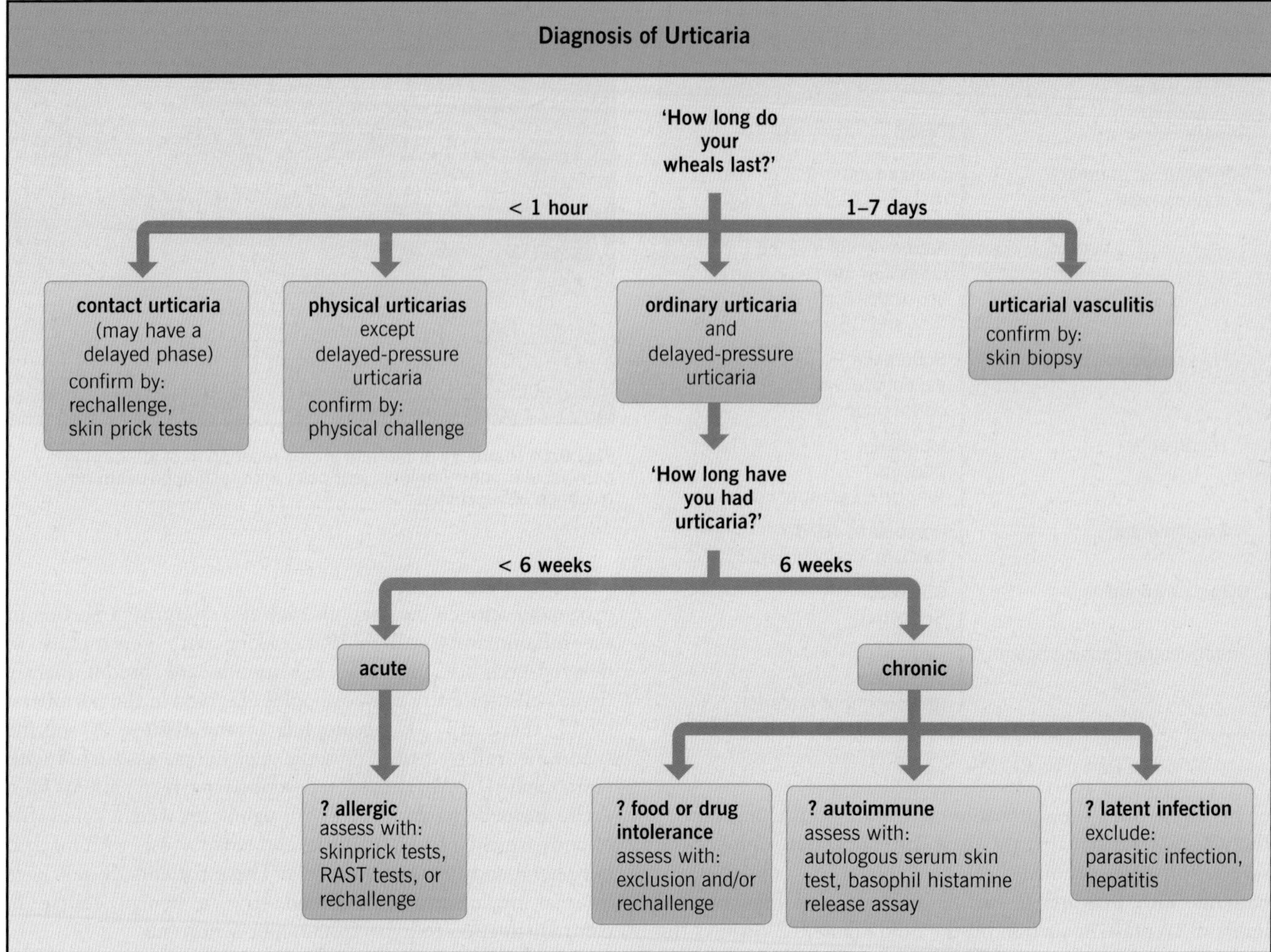

Fig. 6.15 Diagnosis of urticaria. RAST, radioallergosorbent test.

after partial degranulation. Previous work has shown that basophils from urticaria release less histamine when stimulated with anti-IgE than those from healthy controls, possibly due to being in a state of desensitization from prior exposure to histamine-releasing autoantibodies in the blood. Charlesworth and colleagues have clearly demonstrated a role for the basophil in the LPR in which the late rise in cutaneous histamine is related to the influx of basophils and not to a mast cell origin. Nevertheless, basophils are not easily identified in the tissues, a technical problem which has only recently been overcome with the development of antibasophil antibodies. Preliminary studies with these demonstrate an influx of basophils into the skin 6 hours after allergen provocation.

DIAGNOSIS OF URTICARIA

History

The history is of great importance in the diagnosis of urticaria and the duration of wheals can also be very helpful (Fig. 6.15). Wheals lasting less than 1 hour are probably due to a physical urticaria with the exception of delayed-pressure urticaria which characteristically takes 2–6 hours to develop and about 24 hours to clear. Contact urticaria is usually short-lived but may last hours if severe enough to elicit an LPR. Ordinary urticaria wheals may last up to 24 hours, whereas the lesions of urticarial vasculitis typically last for up to a week. It is important to ask for details of preceding infections, drugs, infusions, immunizations, and unusual foods although the precipitating factor for chronic urticaria usually remains uncertain. It is common for patients with established urticaria to observe that their symptoms are worse with heat, stress, and, sometimes, alcohol. A family history of angioedema should alert the clinician to the possibility of C1 inh deficiency.

The two most common causes for acute ordinary urticaria are drugs and infections (e.g. viral infections of the upper respiratory tract). We live in a time of polypharmacy in which many patients receive a multiplicity of medications, both prescribed and over the counter, in addition to non-regulated natural products. It may take quite a medical sleuth to sort out the ingested culprit from the chemical morass introduced into the alimentary tract.

Drugs as aggravating factors in urticaria

Drugs may cause or aggravate urticaria by stimulating mast cell degranulation or influencing eicosanoid synthesis at the time of degranulation. Opiates, curare, radiocontrast media, and some antibiotics (e.g. polymyxin B) can cause non-immunologic degranulation from cutaneous mast cells (Table 6.2) but very rarely cause urticaria when administered at therapeutic concentrations in healthy subjects. Nevertheless, chronic urticaria patients might be at risk of exacerbation from these drugs during disease activity and should avoid them if possible. Immunologic hypersensitivity to dietary penicillins has been suggested as a cause of chronic urticaria but remains unproven. The non-selective cyclooxygenase inhibitors, aspirin and non-steroidal antiinflammatory drugs occasionally cause urticaria or anaphylactoid reactions in healthy subjects. They also aggravate urticaria non-specifically in about one-third of patients with established disease. They inhibit prostaglandin formation by cyclooxygenase on arachidonic acid at the time of degranulation but it is unclear how this exacerbates urticaria. Diversion of arachidonic acid metabolites to leukotrienes may, perhaps, facilitate cellular infiltration into the wheals with prolongation of the response. Reduction in PGE_2 has been shown in an animal model to augment immunologically stimulated mast cell degranulation. A smaller proportion of aspirin-sensitive chronic urticaria patients react similarly to dietary salicylates, azo dyes (including tartrazine), and benzoates in foods. ACE inhibitors may also be a cause of angioedema by inhibiting breakdown of kinin. There have been preliminary reports of angioedema with angiotensin-II receptor antagonists too although the reason for this is uncertain because kinin levels are not affected.

Foods can result in an acute allergic urticaria. This is related to the ingestion within 30–90 minutes of a particular food, and may be associated with other symptoms of an IgE-mediated reaction such as abdominal cramping, diarrhea, and nausea, or even bronchospasm, nasal congestion, or vascular instability. The role of food additives as a cause of urticaria is uncertain but some authorities believe that benzoate preservatives and azo dyes (e.g. tartrazine) may aggravate pre-existing chronic urticaria.

Symptom presentation and differential diagnosis

The clinical recognition of the usual urticarial lesion is not difficult. It usually presents as a raised erythematous wheal associated with varying degrees of pruritus, ranging from mild itching to an intense and unrelenting itch that interferes with daytime work and night-time sleep. When angioedema occurs with urticaria, the disease appears to have a worse prognosis than in the majority of urticaria patients, sometimes lasting longer than 5 years. In addition to the persistent urticaria associated with urticarial vasculitis, there are several dermatologic conditions that may have urticarial-like lesions as part of their clinical spectrum, including erythema multiforme, pruritic urticarial plaques and papules of pregnancy (PUPPP syndrome), bullous pemphigoid, dermatitis herpetiformis, and papular urticaria.

Physical examination

Cutaneous examination should be used to assess the activity of urticaria, the morphology and distribution of wheals and angioedema, evidence of purpura, generalized skin edema (sometimes seen with very severe urticaria), and connective tissue disorders. Attention should be paid to possible associated systemic disorders including thyroid dysfunction, arthritis, and jaundice.

Additional tests

Tests for the presence of allergy and serum histamine releasing factors

Allergy suspected from the history can often be confirmed by skin prick testing in vivo, radioallergosorbent tests (RASTs) or the equivalent test in vitro, and rechallenge where clinically appropriate. Skin prick and RAST testing will only yield information on immediate hypersensitivity reactions and would not, for instance, be informative for urticarial vasculitis, which is believed to be an immune-complex reaction, cytotoxic reactions seen after certain drugs or blood transfusions or autoantibody-mediated histamine release. The techniques of skin prick and RAST testing are covered in Chapter 1.

Allergy testing is most likely to be informative for acute urticaria, especially when presenting as a symptom of anaphylaxis. The cause of contact urticaria may be obvious from the history. Other forms of food and drug intolerance which are not mediated by IgE-allergen interactions are more likely to present with chronic ordinary urticaria. Intradermal injection of 50 μL of the patient's own serum to look for an immediate localized wheal response (the autologous serum skin test) is a simple screening test for circulating vasoactive factors, including histamine-releasing autoantibodies, in the blood.

Provocation studies

Physical challenge tests are very helpful for defining the physical urticarias. Provocation (rechallenge) may be appropriate to confirm the cause of other types of urticaria when allergy tests have been inconclusive or negative. Considerable care must be taken to ensure the safety of the patient, by having appropriate facilities and expertise available for resuscitation, if there is a history of anaphylaxis or anaphylactoid reactions. Rubbing the allergen, such as a latex glove, or fruit, onto forearm skin may be sufficient to demonstrate contact urticaria. Oral rechallenge may be necessary to demonstrate reactions to certain drugs and foods. Some specialist centers use a series of challenge capsules containing food preservatives, colors, and small doses of acetylsalicylic acid which are alternated with placebo capsules. Challenge tests of this sort are difficult to interpret unless urticaria is quiescent and the patient is off medication. They therefore tend to be used, if and when the urticaria has subsided, on strict exclusion diets prior to reintroduction of food groups least likely to have caused the reaction.

Biopsy studies

The 4 mm lesional punch biopsy is a useful diagnostic procedure to confirm a clinical suspicion of urticarial vasculitis (Fig. 6.16), which is characterized by damage to small blood vessels but does not, in itself, provide information on etiology. The histopathology of urticaria covers a wide spectrum, from a sparse mixed or lymphocytic cellular infiltrate with dermal edema to a prominent dermal edema with a moderately dense mixed cellular infiltrate of neutrophils, lymphocytes, and eosinophils – the latter being seen in allergic urticaria.

Supplementary studies

Routine blood tests are usually uninformative in ordinary and physical urticarias unless there is clinical suspicion of associated

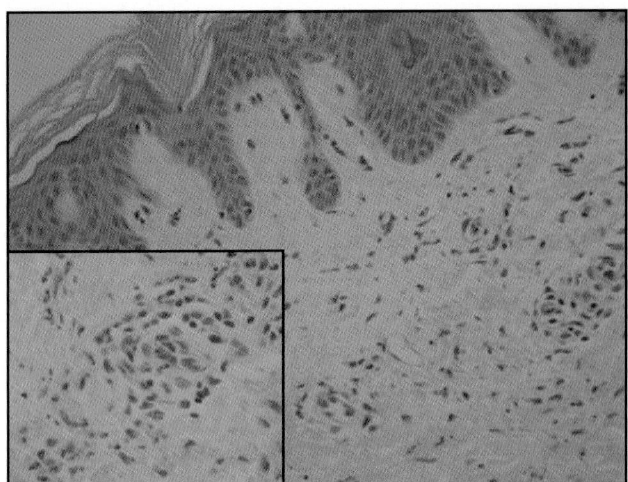

Fig. 6.16 Histology of urticarial vasculitis showing some leukocytoclasia, red cell leakage and a moderately dense perivascular infiltrate containing eosinophils with swollen venules (inset) but no fibrin deposition in this case. (Courtesy of Dr B McCann, Department of Histopathology, Norfolk and Norwich University Hospital, UK.)

disease, such as thyroid autoimmunity. A full blood count and ESR may be of value as a screen for associated helminthic infection or urticarial vasculitis. Further tests of complement, non-organ specific autoantibodies, serum electrophoresis, and renal and liver function with urinalysis would be appropriate for confirmed urticarial vasculitis. Immunochemical and functional assays of C1 inh are essential at the first assessment of patients with recurrent angioedema without wheals, and with low C4 blood complement.

MANAGEMENT OF URTICARIA

Information

Providing information concerning the type of urticaria, cause (if known), simple measures to alleviate symptoms, available drug treatments, and future outlook can be of great importance to individual patients who may have to live with their condition for months or years.

Avoidance of causes and triggers

The first priority in treatment of urticaria is the elimination of the causative agent, stimulus, or antigen, although this is often much easier said than done. Avoidance of allergens identified as the cause of contact urticaria or anaphylaxis should prevent the problem. Food and drug intolerance that is not due to IgE-mediated allergy needs to be considered in chronic ordinary urticaria patients responding poorly to antihistamines. These patients may benefit from avoidance of dietary salicylates, azo dyes, benzoates, and other food preservatives, including sorbic acid, especially when confirmed by double-blind challenge.

Drug treatment

A suggested management scheme for urticaria is summarized in Figure 6.17.

First-line therapies (antihistamines)

For the majority of chronic urticaria patients, symptomatic treatment with classic H_1 antihistamines is the mainstay of management for their disease. The success of the classic antihistamines is somewhat limited by undesirable side-effects such as daytime sedation and anticholinergic-induced dry mouth. Since it is well documented that the skin mast cell is triggered by unknown stimuli to release preformed mediators – primarily histamine and tryptase – it is logical that antihistamines function best when taken as a prophylactic measure rather than just at the time of a flare of urticaria. Until the recent introduction of the newer, low- and non-sedating antihistamines, physicians were reluctant to prescribe antihistamines for daytime use.

Non-sedating antihistamines currently in use for urticaria include acrivastine; cetirizine and its enantiomer cetirizine; loratadine and its major metabolite desloratadine; fexofenadine, the non-cardiotoxic replacement for terfenadine and mizolastine. Clinical experience indicates little variation between the drugs in their effect on chronic urticaria although individual patients may prefer one over another. The kinetics of all non-sedating H_1 antihistamines, except acrivastine, allow for once-a-day dosing, a single oral dose being effective within a few hours and lasting 1–48 hours. Acrivastine is distinguished from other non-sedating antihistamines by its short plasma half-life and three-times-daily dosing. Acrivastine and mizolastine are not available in the USA. Cetirizine, the carboxylic acid metabolite of hydroxyzine, is classed as a low-sedating antihistamine and has been shown to significantly reduce the incidence of erythema, wheals, and pruritus in both spontaneous and provoked urticaria in double-blind cross-over trials. Several investigators have demonstrated a decrease in the influx of eosinophils to the site of the antigen-induced cutaneous LPR following treatment with cetirizine. This antiinflammatory property, combined with its excellent H_1-receptor blockade, is unique to cetirizine and may offer certain benefits in patients in whom the histologic picture demonstrates a mixed cellular inflammatory infiltrate.

While little evidence exists that H_2 blockers on their own have any therapeutic effect in the treatment of chronic urticaria, there are some studies that support the effectiveness of a combination of H_1 and H_2 blocking antihistamines (e.g. hydroxyzine and cimetidine or fexofenadine with ranitidine) in selected instances of urticaria. Although the combined treatments may be disappointing for urticaria, H_2 antagonists are often helpful for the indigestion which sometimes accompanies severe attacks.

Second-line therapies

Although antihistamines can control the symptoms of urticaria in many patients, they may be so severe in others as to require oral glucocorticosteroids. Prior to committing a patient to frequent courses or alternate-day doses of steroids, a skin biopsy should be done to better classify the urticaria histologically. Because prolonged use of steroids is associated with many side-effects, steroid-sparing drugs should be introduced where possible. Pulses of high-dose oral corticosteroids (e.g. prednisolone 60 mg daily) for 3–5 days can be given for particularly severe and disabling urticaria in addition to regular antihistamines. Adrenaline by the intramuscular, subcutaneous, or inhaled route can be of great value for the acute manage-

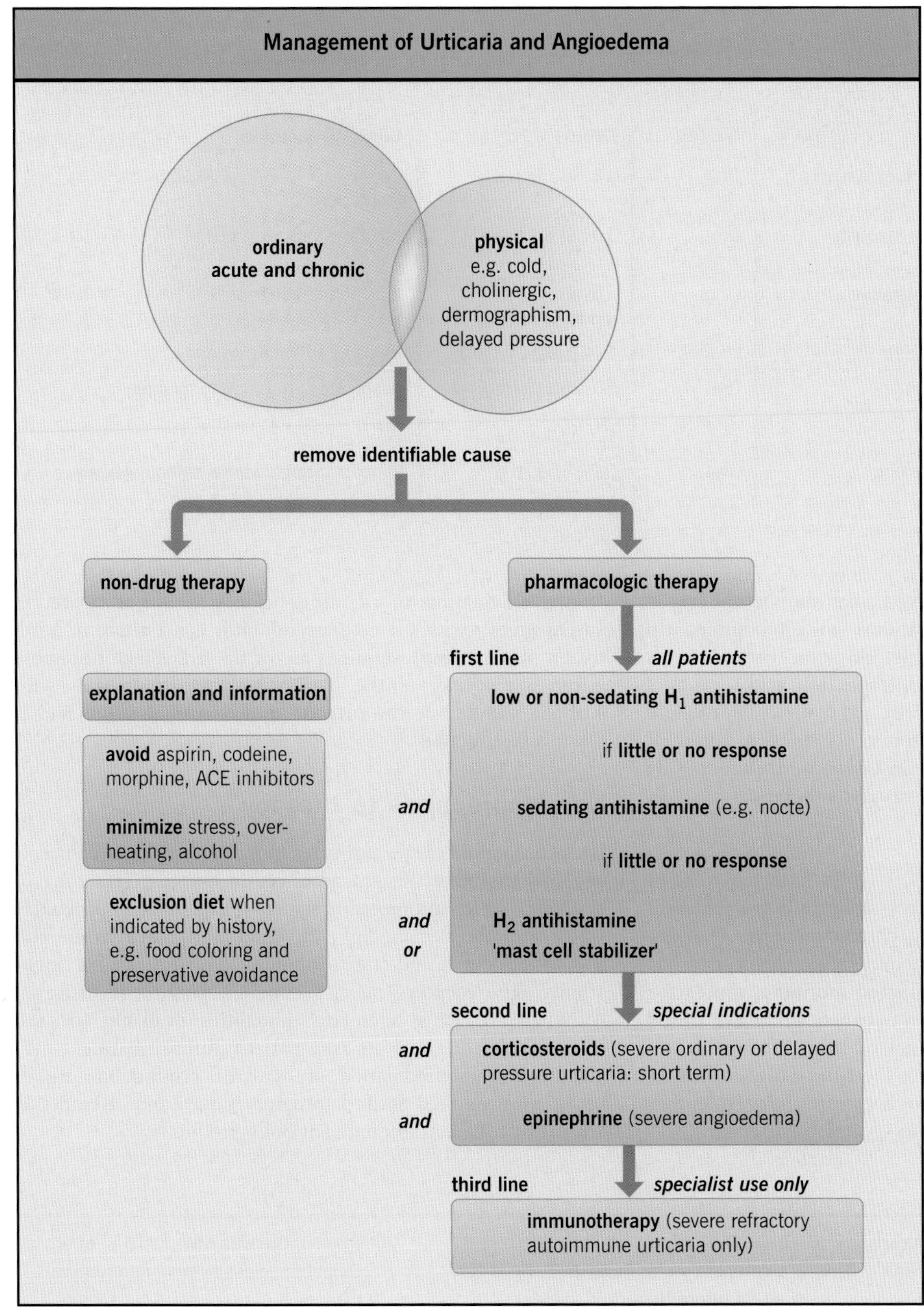

Fig. 6.17 Management scheme summary for urticaria.

ment of severe angioedema in all types of urticaria except C1 inhibitor deficiency.

The aim of using second-line therapies is to target specific clinical problems and thereby reduce the requirement for corticosteroids and adrenaline. A number of drugs have been reported for different situations (Table 6.3) but the evidence for using them is often poor and the response of individual patients is unpredictable. Tricyclic antidepressants, such as doxepin, possess potent H_1-receptor blockade properties that are several orders of magnitude greater than those observed with the classic antihistamines but anticholinergic and soporific side-effects can be dose-limiting. There is no mood-elevating effect when doxepin is used in this clinical context. There is an increasing literature on the use of leukotriene receptor antagonists in ordinary urticaria. Montelukast appears to be more effective than zafirlukast although a direct comparison has not been done. Clinical experience suggests that montelukast is more likely to be effective in aspirin-sensitive urticaria than other patterns. Drugs which have a theoretic mast cell stabilizing action, such as nifedipine, have been shown to be beneficial in some studies of chronic urticaria. However, in practice, the effect is small and it is probably best reserved for the urticaria patient who also needs treatment for coincidental hypertension. Reports of thyroxine helping urticaria in patients with positive

Table 6.3 Summary of second-line therapies for urticaria

Second-Line Therapies				
Generic name	**Drug Class**	**Route**	**Dose**	**Clinical indication**
Doxepin	Tricyclic antidepressant	Oral	10–30 mg nocte	Consider if response to antihistamines insufficient
Montelukast	Leukotriene receptor antagonist	Oral	10 mg nocte	Aspirin-sensitive urticaria
Nifedipine	Calcium antagonist	Oral	10–40 mg/day modified release	Associated hypertension
Sulfasalazine	Aminosalicylate	Oral	1–4 g/day	Delayed pressure urticaria
Thyroxine	Thyroid hormone	Oral	50–250 μg/day (aim for 1.7 μg/kg/day)	Associated thyroid autoimmunity
Tranexamic acid	Plasmin inhibitor	Oral	0.5–4.5 g/day	Idiopathic angioedema without wheals

thyroid autoantibodies have involved small numbers. Clinical experience of sulfasalazine in patients with predominantly pressure urticaria may be favorable and some patients with idiopathic angioedema do well with tranexamic acid.

Colchicine, dapsone, indomethacin, and hydroxychloroquine have all been reported in the literature as showing potential effectiveness in reducing the amount or frequency of corticosteroid needed in urticarial vasculitis therapy.

Third-line therapies

Plasmapheresis has been used successfully in a few patients with severe unremitting ordinary chronic urticaria showing evidence of histamine-releasing autoantibodies. Ciclosporin has been the most thoroughly evaluated immunosuppressive therapy to date and has been shown to benefit up to two-thirds of patients with evidence of histamine releasing autoantibodies. Other promising immunosuppressive therapies under evaluation are intravenous immunoglobulin, methotrexate and azathioprine but their use should be restricted to specialist centers.

Angioedema due to C1 inh deficiency should be treated in an emergency with C1 esterase inhibitor concentrate or fresh frozen plasma. Antihistamines are of no value since histamine is not a mediator of the plasma leakage. Prophylaxis with anabolic steroids or the plasmin inhibitor tranexamic acid is often very effective.

New approaches to therapy

Urticaria, and its causes and cures, remain a puzzle for clinicians and patients alike. Recent advances in our understanding of cytokines which promote mast cell releasability, interleukins which promote eosinophil activation and block eosinophil apoptotic death, and autoantibodies directed against high-affinity IgE receptors paint a complex picture of urticaria. Although we have adequate modalities available for the treatment of the usual urticaria patient, future treatment may include immunomodulation of cytokine production, use of better non-steroidal antiinflammatory drugs, and attempts at downregulating autoimmune antibody production.

FURTHER READING

Charlesworth EN. The spectrum of urticaria. All that urticates may not be urticaria. In: Charlesworth EN, ed. Urticaria. Immunology and allergy clinics of North America. Philadelphia: WB Saunders Co; 1995:15:641–657.

Charlesworth EN. Cutaneous allergy. Cambridge, MA: Blackwell Science; 1996.

Grattan CEH. Chronic urticaria. In: Lichtenstein LM, Busse WW, Geha RS, eds. Current therapy in allergy, immunology and rheumatology. Philadelphia: Mosby; 2003:72–76.

Grattan CEH. Autoimmune urticaria. In: Dreskin S, ed. Urticaria. Immunology and allergy clinics of North America. New York: Elsevier; 2004:163–182.

Zuberbier T, Greaves MW, Juhlin L, et al. Definition, classification and routine diagnosis of urticaria: a consensus report. J Invest Dermatol Symp Proc 2001; 6:123–127.

Chapter 7

Atopic Dermatitis and Allergic Contact Dermatitis

Thomas Werfel and Alexander Kapp

Definition:
Atopic dermatitis is a common inflammatory skin disorder, characterized by severe pruritus, chronically relapsing course, a distinctive distribution of eczematous skin lesions and often a personal or family history of atopic diseases. Allergic contact dermatitis, which is not linked to atopy, is the prototype of a delayed type hypersensitivity reaction (so-called type IV reaction), which is mediated largely by lymphocytes preciously sensitized to low molecular weight allergens causing inflammation and edema in the skin.

INTRODUCTION

Eczema is a pattern of inflammatory responses of the skin which can be defined either clinically or histologically. Clinically, acute eczema is associated with marked erythema, superficial papulae, and vesiculae which easily excoriate and lead to crusts. Chronic eczema is composed of rather faint erythema, infiltration, and scaling (Fig. 7.1). Histologically, eczema is characterized by edema and spongiosis of the epidermis, edema of the papillary dermis, and a mononuclear infiltrate in the dermis which extends into the epidermis (Fig. 7. 2).

Eczema accounts for a large proportion of all skin diseases and is the most common cause for consultation with a dermatologist. The condition may be induced by a range of external and internal factors acting singly or in combination. The individual classification of the clinical form may be difficult because multiple causative factors may be implicated and more than one form of eczema may be present in the same patient simultaneously. Table 7.1 gives a classification of the most common forms of eczematous skin diseases. Since allergic mechanisms play a major role in only the atopic and allergic contact forms of dermatitis, this chapter will concentrate on these diseases. The reader is referred to dermatological textbooks to learn more about the other forms of eczematous skin diseases. Generally, the terms eczema and dermatitis are synonymous but the term dermatitis will be used preferentially in this chapter to describe all forms of diseases which involve the eczematous process.

CLASSIFICATION OF ATOPIC DERMATITIS

Atopic dermatitis is an inflammatory skin disorder which is increasing in incidence, and is characterized by severe pruritus, a chronically relapsing course, a distinctive distribution of eczematous skin lesions, and a personal or family history of atopic diseases. It often begins in early infancy and follows a course of remissions and exacerbations. The role of exogenous and endogenous factors in the pathophysiology of atopic dermatitis has been intensively discussed in recent years. There is increasing evidence that T-cell responses to environmental or food allergens are important for the pathogenesis of atopic dermatitis. In patients with atopic dermatitis the skin disease is most often associated with the existence of environmental or food allergen-specific IgE. This variant of the disease, which is also associated with environmental allergen-specific IgE, is usually called the 'extrinsic' form of atopic dermatitis. The 'intrinsic' variant is found in 20% of diseases with the typical clinical appearance of atopic dermatitis but without specific IgE. In this respect, atopic dermatitis resembles

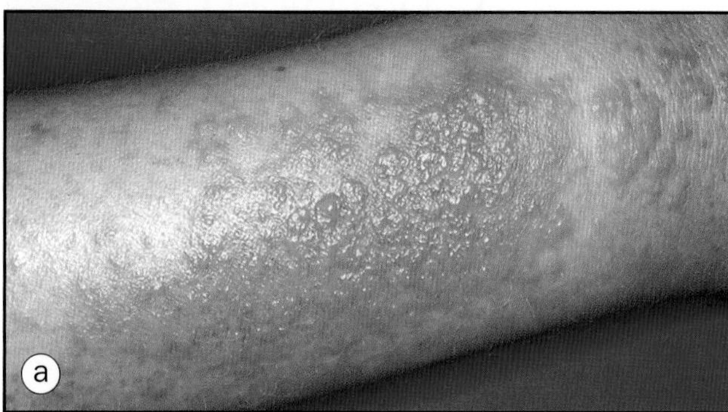

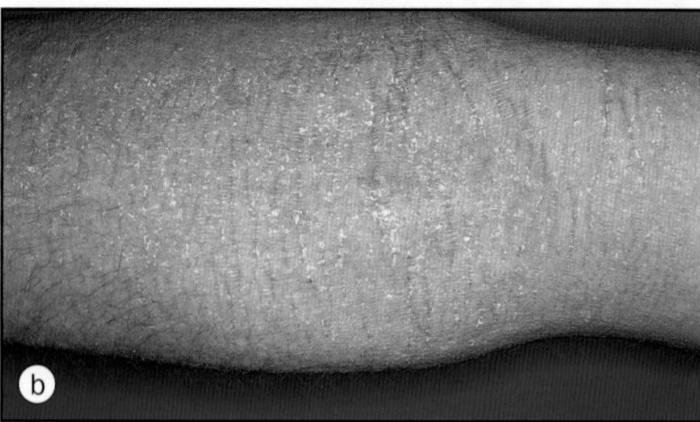

Fig. 7.1 Morphology of acute versus chronic eczema. (a) Acute eczema characterized by marked erythema, superficial papulae, and vesiculae. (b) Chronic eczema characterized by faint erythema, infiltration, and scaling (chronic atopic dermatitis).

Table 7.1 Classification of eczematous skin diseases

Classification of Eczematous Skin Diseases

Disease	Feature
Allergic contact dermatitis	Provoked by local contact with allergen Hematogenous/drug induction possibly with allergen
Photoallergic dermatitis	Provoked by local contact plus UV radiation Hematogenous/drug induction possibly
Atopic dermatitis/ neurodermatitis	Extrinsic type (i.e. atopic dermatitis) Intrinsic type (i.e. neurodermatitis)
Irritant contact dermatitis	Provoked by local contact
Phototoxic dermatitis	Provoked by local contact plus UV radiation
Seborrheic dermatitis	Provoked by *Malassezia sympodialis* plus endocrine factors
Nummular dermatitis/ discoid eczema	Provoked by inflammatory focus
Varicosis dermatitis/ stasis eczema	Provoked by a state of chronic venous insufficiency

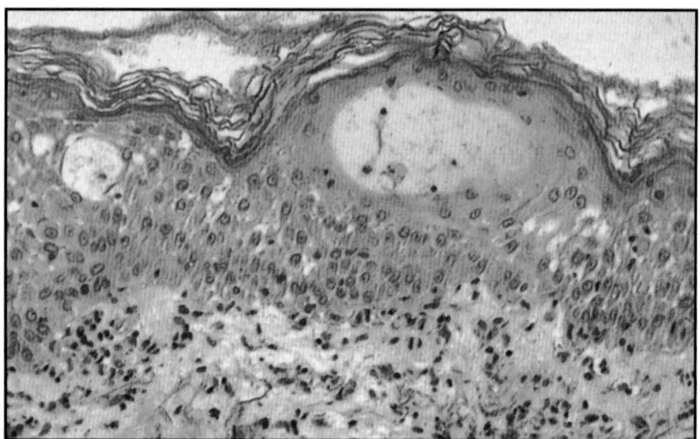

Fig. 7.2 Histologic appearance of allergic contact dermatitis. The epidermis is edematous with microvesicle formation and mononuclear cells have infiltrated the dermis and epidermis (× 130).

bronchial asthma, which also has an extrinsic and an intrinsic variant (Fig. 7.3). Perhaps the old term neurodermatitis might be reintroduced to differentiate the intrinsic form from atopic dermatitis associated with specific IgE to food or inhalant allergens.

PATHOGENESIS OF ATOPIC DERMATITIS

Histologic examination of the skin in acute atopic dermatitis reveals a picture similar to that of allergic contact dermatitis, with microvesiculation in the epidermis and a lymphohistiocytic infiltrate in the dermis.

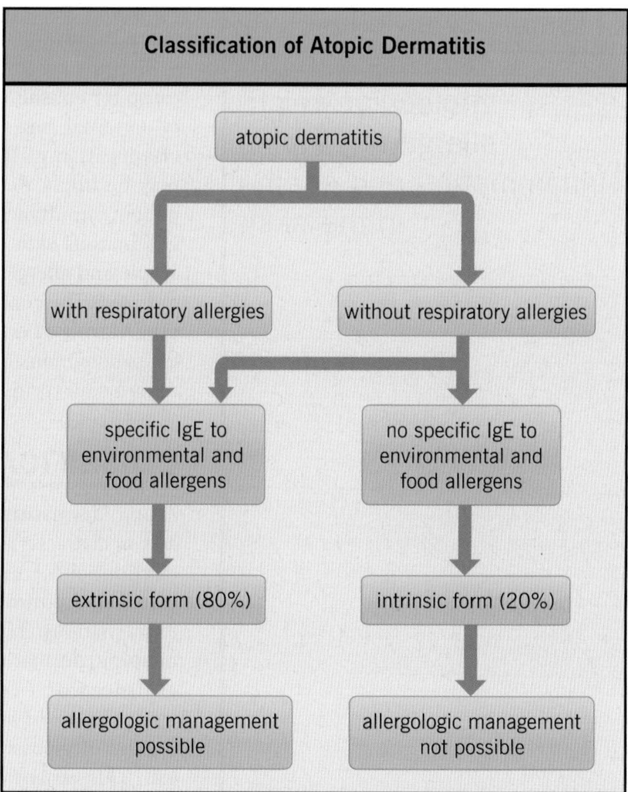

Fig. 7.3 Classification of atopic dermatitis. [Modified from Wüthrich B. Atopic dermatitis flare provoked by inhalant allergens. Dermatologica 1989; 178(1):51–53.]

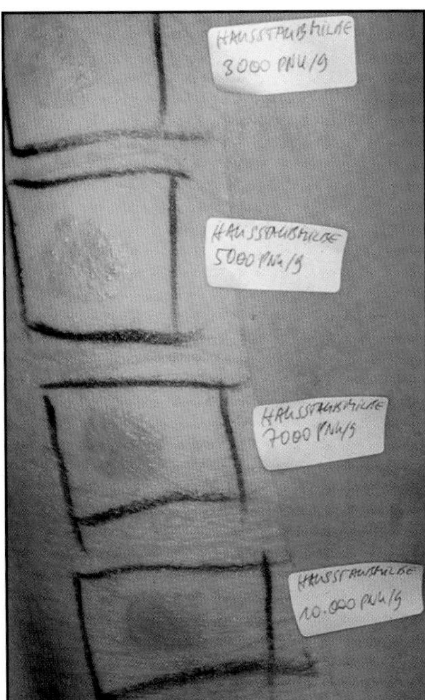

Fig. 7.4 Patch-test reactions to house dust mite allergens provoked on the back of a highly sensitized patient with atopic dermatitis. Note the dose-dependent strength of the reactions.

Pathophysiology

Many studies addressing the pathophysiology of atopic dermatitis have focused on processes potentially involving the regulation of IgE, which is higher than normal in 80% of all patients. Although IgE has a half-life of only 5–7 days there are no marked intra-individual fluctuations in the serum levels between exacerbations and remissions of atopic dermatitis. Specific IgE is commonly associated with food or environmental allergens. Those allergens may be directly involved in the eczematous skin reaction since eczematous patch-test reactions to house dust mites, pollen, animal dander, or foods are frequently observed in sensitized patients (Fig. 7.4). These tests have led to new and stimulating results relating to the pathophysiologic role of different hematopoietic cell populations in the early eczematous reaction (Fig. 7.5). Antigen-bearing dendritic cells, binding IgE mainly via the high-affinity Fc receptor FcεRI, are found in the epidermis after 6 hours and mainly in the dermis after 24–48 hours. A model has been proposed in which the delayed hypersensitivity to protein allergens is thought to be IgE mediated with the binding of allergens to IgE-bearing epidermal Langerhans' cells. Allergens can mainly bind to uncomplexed IgE attached to dendritic cells, via FcεRI, and further preformed IgE-allergen complexes can bind to the low-affinity FcεRII/CD23. A significant migration of eosinophils into the skin is detected 2–6 hours after the application of allergens to the skin in atopic dermatitis. After 24 hours of allergen challenge, eosinophils can be detected even in the epidermis and many activated eosinophils are seen in spongiotic epidermal lesions. Later, secretory proteins, such as major basic protein or eosinophil cationic protein, from the eosinophils, can be detected but no intact cells can be found in the lesional dermis.

Proliferative responses to inhalant allergens, including mites and pollen, and to food antigens can be elicited in blood lymphocytes. In sensitized patients with atopic dermatitis such responses are high in the circulating T-lymphocyte subpopulation expressing the skin-homing molecule cutaneous lymphocyte antigen (CLA). In contrast, in sensitized patients with allergic bronchial asthma, allergen-dependent proliferation is found in the CLA-negative subset. This observation points to an allergen-dependent mechanism which targets specific T cells to the skin in atopic dermatitis.

The first direct evidence for the presence of skin-infiltrating, inhalant allergen-specific T cells came from the analysis of T-cell clones generated from biopsies of patch-test lesions in atopic dermatitis. The majority of allergen-specific T cells derived from skin lesions that have been provoked by the epicutaneous application of inhalant allergens in patients with atopic dermatitis, produce predominantly type 2 cytokines such as interleukin-4 (IL-4), or IL-13. These cytokines have important effector functions in the perpetuation of the local inflammatory reaction, such as upregulation of adhesion molecules and stimulation of lymphocytes or eosinophils. A polarized type 2 cytokine pattern was previously regarded as a specific feature reflecting immune dysregulation in atopic dermatitis. Later, it became clear that it is confined to early atopy patch-test reactions and allergen-specific T cells from the blood, or from spontaneous skin lesions, secreting both type 1 and type 2 cytokines. Moreover, IL-4 is found both at the mRNA level and as a protein in nickel-induced patch-test reactions. Local IL-4 production, therefore, is related to the type of skin lesion (i.e. acute eczema) but not to atopy. At present, epidermal and dermal milieu factors are being investigated; this may influence the different cytokine pattern of infiltrating T cells (Fig. 7.6)

Inflammatory cells and mediators

Genetic and expression factors of atopic dermatitis

Specific genetic components appear to be involved in the manifestation of atopic dermatitis. The risk of this skin disease is higher in families where other members are affected with atopic dermatitis than in families with members suffering exclusively from respiratory allergy. A number of certain allotypes or mutations of functionally relevant molecules (e.g. mast-cell chymase, FcεRI, Toll-like receptors) are currently felt to be involved in the manifestation of atopic dermatitis.

During the last five decades a marked increase in the frequency of atopic dermatitis has been observed and it is now the most frequent inflammatory skin disease, with a prevalence of more than 10% in children aged 6–7 years in Northern Europe and in the USA. There is still no satisfactory explanation for this increase and a number of possible expression factors are currently being considered (Fig. 7.7).

Some studies point to a higher prevalence of atopic dermatitis in children who live in areas with a greater degree of air pollution. The comparison of genetically similar populations who have been exposed to different types of air pollution (i.e. children from former East and West Germany shortly after the reunification) did not, however, reveal marked differences in the prevalence of atopic dermatitis.

The manifestation of atopic dermatitis in childhood appears to be greater in families with a higher income and a more

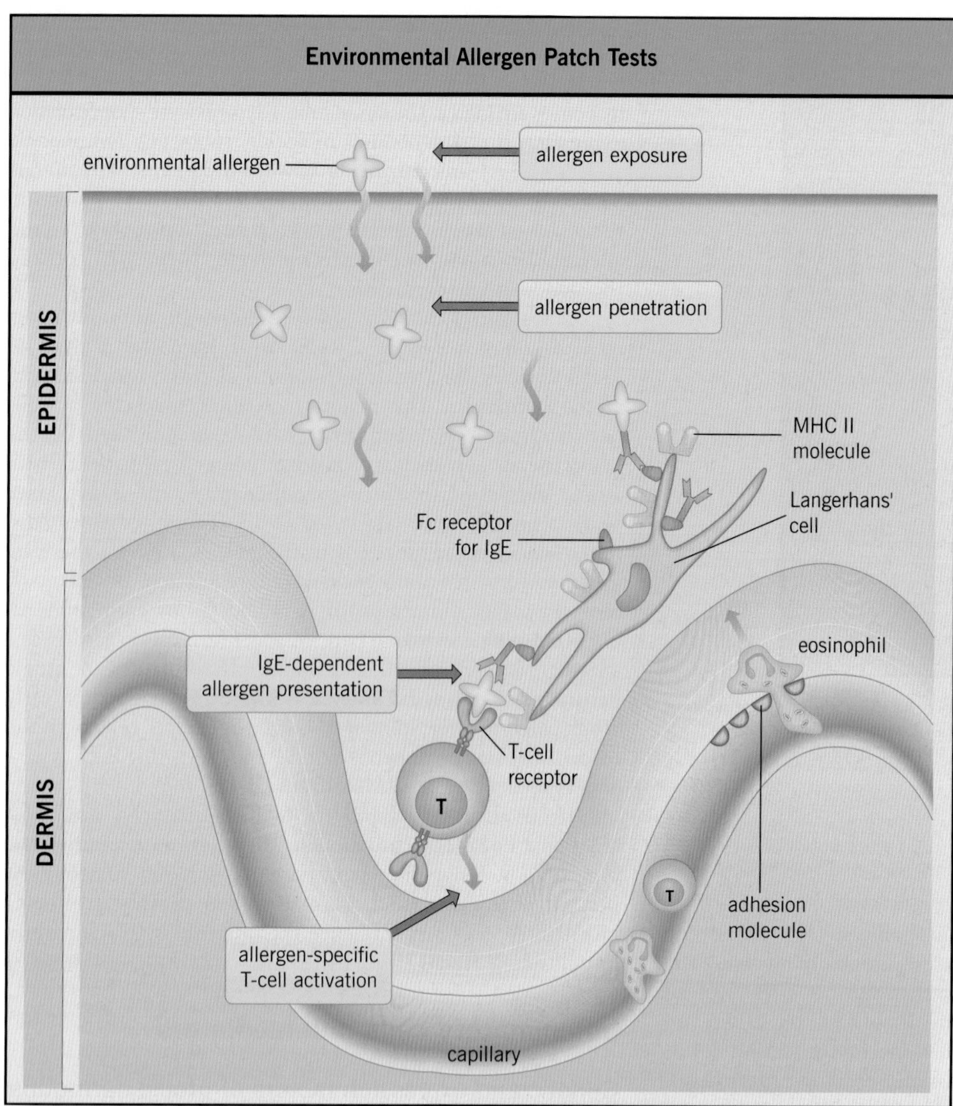

Fig. 7.5 Scenario in patch tests with environmental allergens. Environmental allergens (e.g. house dust mite extracts, cat epithelia or grass pollen extracts) are applied onto uninvolved skin of the back for at least 24 hours. This allows allergens to penetrate into the skin and bind to the epidermal Langerhans' cells. These cells can present allergens either via molecules of the major histocompatibility complex (MHC II) or via IgE bound to Fc receptors for IgE for skin-infiltrating T lymphocytes.

privileged lifestyle. The reduced incidence of infection observed in early childhood and reduced contact with agents that elicit cellular immune responses associated with a type 1 cytokine pattern of T lymphocytes (i.e. vaccination responses) are currently felt to be associated with manifestations of atopic diseases. However, differences of prevalences of respiratory allergic diseases often do not parallel prevalences of atopic dermatitis in larger epidemiologic studies, which points to independent risk and manifestation factors being critical for the atopic skin disease. Changes in the quality and quantity of food and environmental antigens which have contact with the immune system may be involved in the increased prevalence as well.

Provocation factors in atopic dermatitis

A number of different trigger factors of atopic dermatitis are well established (Fig. 7.8). Although there is still no consensus about the relative importance of these factors, the points given below should be considered in the management of individual patients.

Hormonal and emotional factors

Intra-individual fluctuations in the severity of atopic dermatitis are frequently observed in women. This points to hormonal influences with menstruation, pregnancy, birth, and menopause as possible trigger factors. However, more recent data suggest that hormonal factors may also play a role in male patients. Many studies emphasize the importance of psychologic factors, such as personality traits or psychosocial stress, in the exacerbation and maintenance of skin symptoms. Stressful life events may be associated with an increase in itching which leads to scratching and, by this mechanism, to a deterioration of the skin condition. The action of neuropeptides and the increasing number of nerve fibers which have close contact with mast cells may be possible links between the nervous system and the skin condition in atopic dermatitis.

Seasonal and climatic factors

Individual patients show a seasonal variation in the severity of their problems; most patients tend to experience a flare in the autumn and winter months while few are affected in the spring

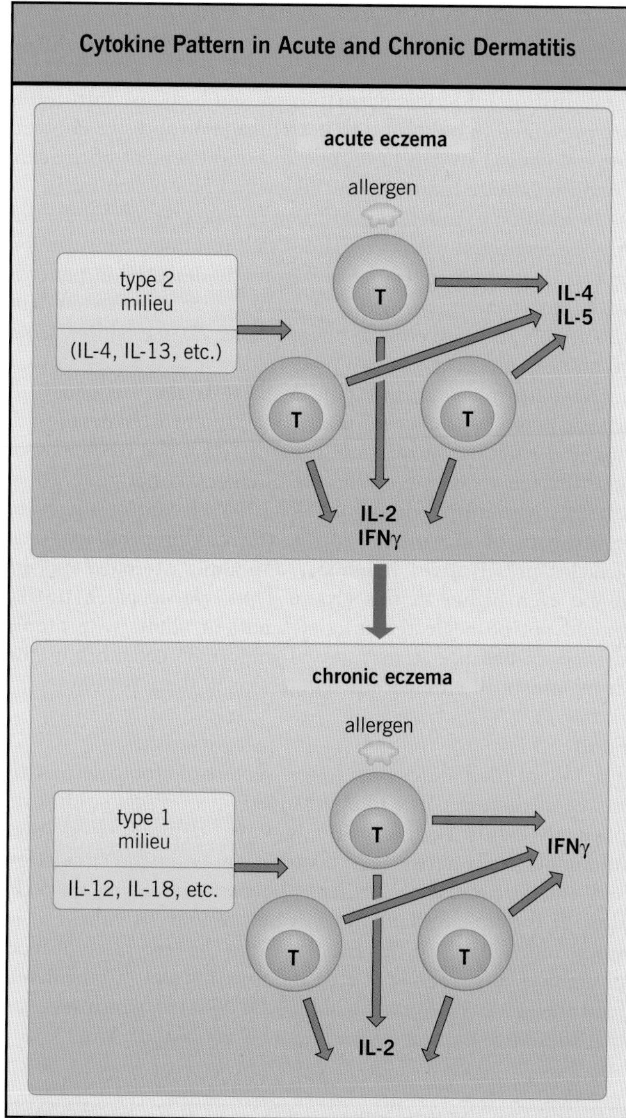

Fig. 7.6 Switch of cytokine pattern in acute versus chronic dermatitis.

and summer. Those who experience problems in the spring and summer may be sensitized to pollen allergens or belong to the small group of patients whose skin deteriorates upon exposure to ultraviolet (UV) radiation. Large temperature fluctuations and continental climates also lead to a worsening of the skin condition. This is one reason why those patients not sensitive to UV radiation are encouraged to spend some weeks every year at the seaside if possible.

Irritating factors

The most consistent perturbators of atopic skin conditions are irritants. The skin response to sodium lauryl sulfate is increased in atopic individuals with or without apparent dermatitis. Occupational substances have particular clinical and social relevance and it appears that a history of atopic dermatitis, rather than of respiratory allergies, is a better prognostic factor of future work-related dermatitis. Intolerance to wool is based on its irritating effect on atopic skin, and cigarette smoke may elicit irritating eczema on the eyelids in atopic dermatitis. It is speculated that an altered composition of the epidermal lipids,

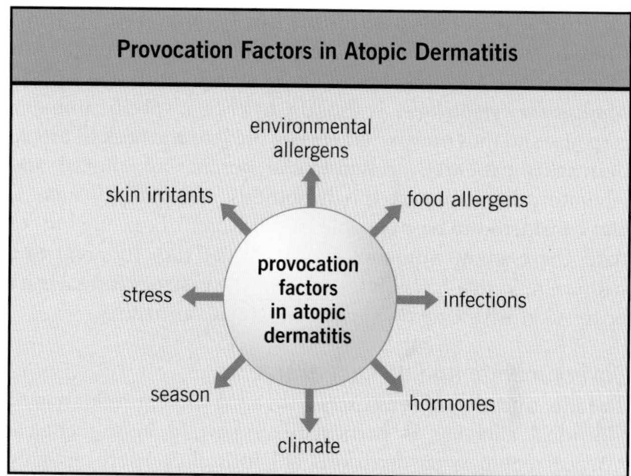

Fig. 7.8 Common provocation factors in atopic dermatitis.

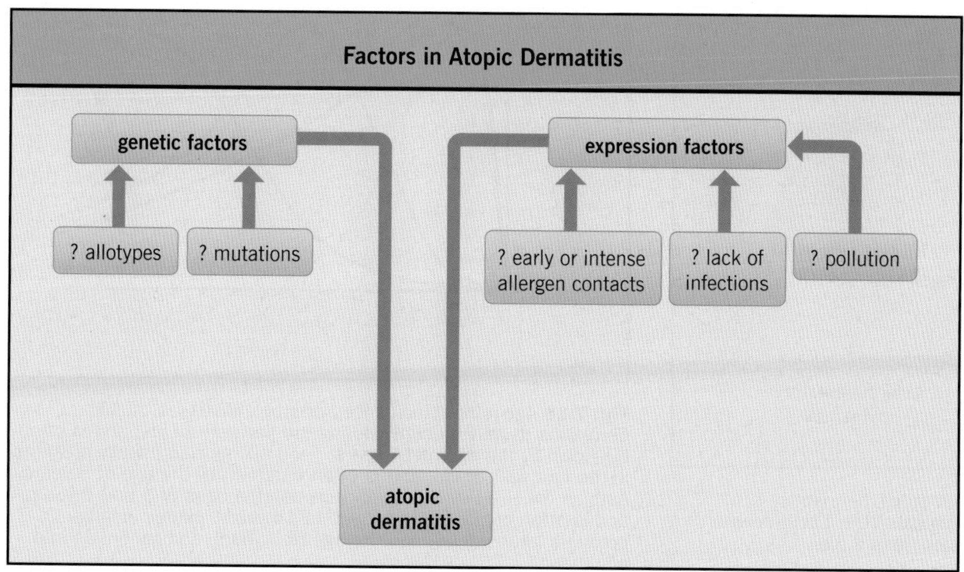

Fig. 7.7 Genetic and expression factors in atopic dermatitis.

an enhanced release of histamine, or a latent, subclinical inflammatory reaction in the skin may play a role in the enhanced vulnerability of the atopic skin.

Infections

Both systemic and local infections can trigger the eczematous response in atopic dermatitis. *Staphylococcus aureus* has been studied extensively as a possible trigger factor. It is detected on the skin in more than 90% of all atopic dermatitis patients, which may at least in part be due to the decreased expression of antimicrobial peptides in the atopic skin. Cell wall components from *S. aureus* may directly stimulate inflammatory cells via Toll-like receptors. In addition, exotoxins are detectable in more than 50% of all cultures containing *S. aureus* which have been generated from skin swabs in atopic dermatitis. They may function as superantigens which can bind to major histocompatibility complex class II (MHC II) molecules of monocytes and dendritic cells and release a number of proinflammatory molecules such as IL-1 or tumor necrosis factor α (TNFα). Moreover, T cells which express reactive T-cell receptor Vβ chains can be stimulated to proliferate and secrete cytokines in response to superantigens, which may maintain the eczematous skin response (Fig. 7.9). It is well established in clinical experience that atopic dermatitis can be improved, in many cases, by systemic antibiotics or by topical antiseptic compounds (e.g. triclosan). In addition to *S. aureus*, the saprophyte *Malassezia sympodiales* is thought to elicit a specific immune response and thus provoke eczema on the face and neck of atopic dermatitis patients – a substantial number of clinical and laboratory data support this hypothesis. *Candida albicans* is also considered to be a possible trigger factor of eczema but, to date, there are no immunologic data which directly point to a pathogenetic role for an infestation of the gastrointestinal tract or the skin with *Candida* species in atopic dermatitis.

Environmental and contact allergens

The identification of sensitizers with a subsequent reduction of individual allergens is particularly important in the clinical management of atopic dermatitis, although allergens are certainly not the only trigger factors in this condition.

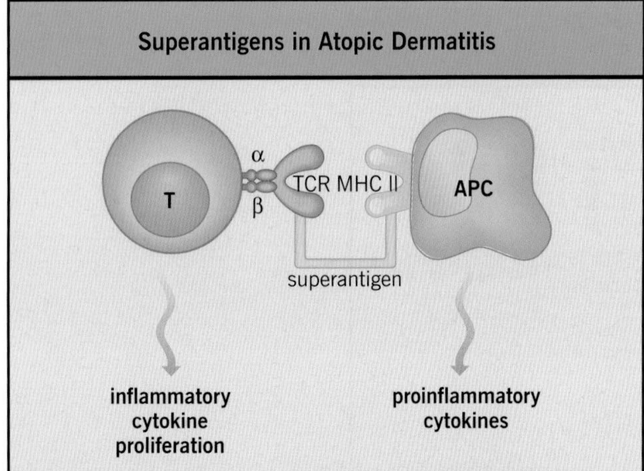

Fig. 7.9 The action of superantigens in atopic dermatitis. T, T lymphocyte; APC, antigen-presenting cell; TCR, T-cell receptor; MHC II, major histocompatibility complex class II (i.e. HLA-DR, -DQ, -DP).

Hypersensitivity to house dust mite antigens is found in 5% of all people in Western nations whereas it is found in up to 90% of adolescents or adults suffering from atopic dermatitis. Exacerbations of atopic dermatitis caused by house dust mites are presumed to be related to both inhalation and skin contact. Several clinical studies have reported improvement of the skin condition after a reduction in the level of house dust mites.

In addition to mites, sensitization to pollen or animal dander may be associated with eczematous skin reactions. Sensitization to cat, dog, or horse dander is frequently detected in patients with atopic dermatitis, and repeated contact with animals should be avoided even if the patients do not suffer from respiratory symptoms.

An issue that remains controversial is the frequency of 'classic' allergic contact dermatitis to haptens in patients with atopic dermatitis. Most studies indicate that the frequency of sensitization to common contact allergens is not reduced in patients with atopic dermatitis. The risk of contact allergy to ingredients of commonly applied topical preparations (e.g. vehicles, preservatives, fragrances, antibiotics, steroids) appears to be even higher in this group. Thus, classic patch testing should not be neglected in adolescents or adults with atopic dermatitis because it may reveal important cofactors in the development of eczematous skin lesions in these patients.

Food

The role of food antigens as trigger factors of atopic dermatitis has been discussed for more than 60 years. Early studies on passively sensitized individuals have demonstrated that immunologically active food proteins can enter the circulation and are distributed throughout the body, including the skin sites. It is possible that intestinal permeability is enhanced in atopic individuals and this may facilitate the resorption of food proteins. The incidence of atopic dermatitis and IgE-mediated food allergies peaks in early childhood (Fig. 7.10), which suggests that these two clinical entities may be associated.

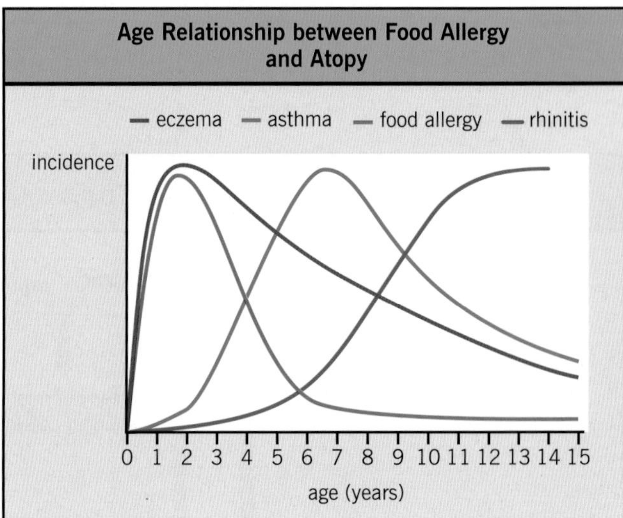

Fig. 7.10 Age-related incidences of atopic diseases. Atopic dermatitis usually presents during the first year of life, and is often outgrown by the age of 14 years. Food allergy also usually presents in the first year of life, and is often outgrown by the age of 5 years. Asthma develops later, usually between the ages of 3 and 7 years, and is often outgrown by the age of 14 years. Allergic rhinitis presents later still, around the age of 7 years, and continues into adulthood.

Most young patients with atopic dermatitis (or their parents) suspect that certain foods trigger their skin abnormalities. The tendency to try restrictive diets which have uncertain benefits may lead to a risk of malnutrition or additional psychologic stress. Placebo-controlled oral food challenges represent the 'gold standard' for the diagnosis of food allergy. Many food-inducible symptoms are immediate, occurring within 15 minutes of food ingestion, but a subpopulation of patients suffer from late symptoms, such as pruritus and worsening of their eczema, 8–24 hours later. In some patients the late symptoms follow directly on from the immediate manifestations (e.g. erythematous flush of the face leading to eczema of the face), a situation analogous to the dual reaction in asthma (Fig. 7.11). Immediate reactions are easily related to the suspected foodstuff in most cases (Fig. 7.12). The causes of isolated late eczematous reactions – which are also observable to pollen associated foods in adolescent and adult patients with atopic dermatitis – are difficult to identify, and repeated provocation by the same foodstuff, on at least 2 subsequent days, is proposed as an aid to identification.

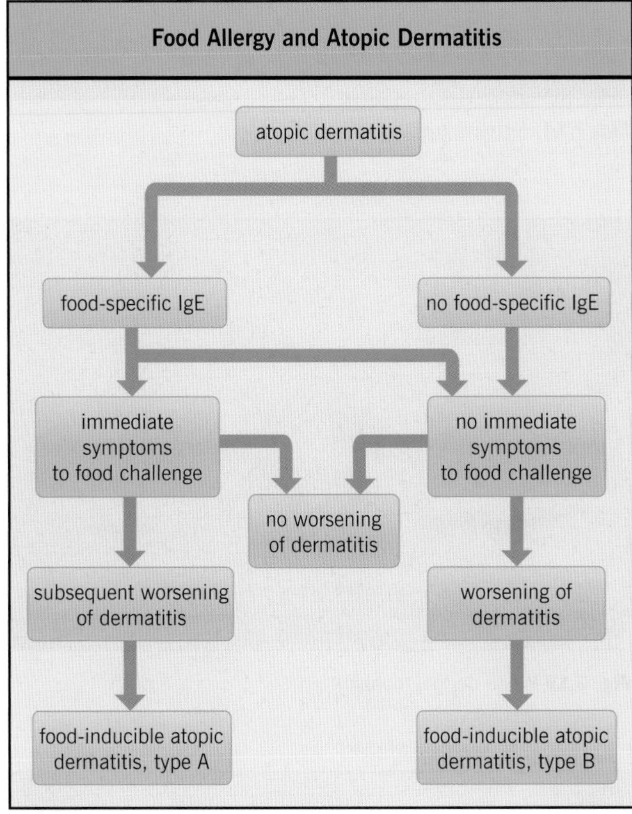

Fig. 7.11 Association between food allergy and atopic dermatitis.

A high proportion of children with food intolerance will outgrow the problem – particularly cows' milk allergy – and the controlled reintroduction of the previously offending foodstuffs 12 months after the first problem occurred will not be associated with further deterioration. However, IgE-mediated food allergy is not the whole story so far as food intolerance is concerned. A lack of correlation between specific IgE and the clinical response to food has been reported for food-responsive atopic dermatitis in several studies and this may point to the relative importance of allergen-specific T lymphocytes in these reactions. Moreover, many patients assert that consumption of citrus fruits exacerbates their eczema and adult patients observe that alcoholic beverages (particularly in excess!) cause worsening of their eczema on the day following the consumption of alcohol. It seems, therefore, that both food allergy and food intolerance due to non-immunologic mechanisms are complicating factors in atopic dermatitis.

DIAGNOSIS OF ATOPIC DERMATITIS

History

The highest incidence of atopic dermatitis is found within the first 2 years of life although the disease can begin virtually at any age (see Fig. 7.10). A small proportion of patients present with atopic dermatitis before the age of 6 months and, in this situation, it is important to exclude the common dermatologic problem of infantile seborrheic dermatitis. In the young infant

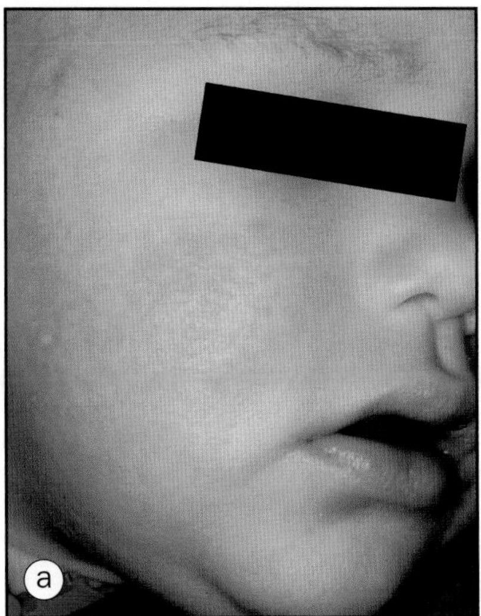

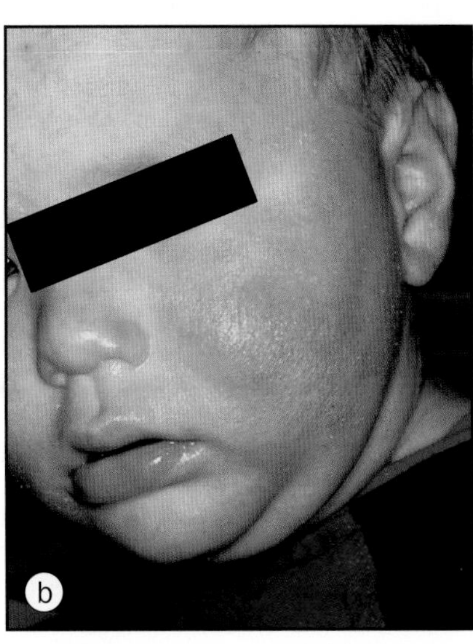

Fig. 7.12 Clinical presentation of an 18-month-old boy with atopic dermatitis sensitized to cows' milk casein 1 day before (a) and 30 minutes after (b) provocation with 30 mL cows' milk. The erythematous flush led to a late-phase dermatitis during the following days.

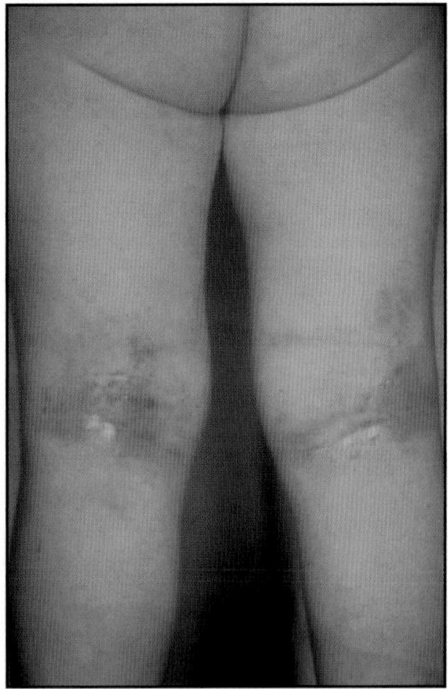

Fig. 7.13 Child with flexural (mild) atopic dermatitis.

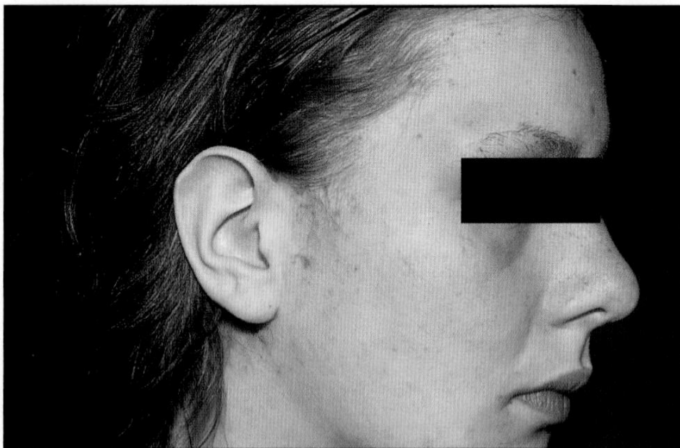

Fig. 7.14 Hertoghe's sign.

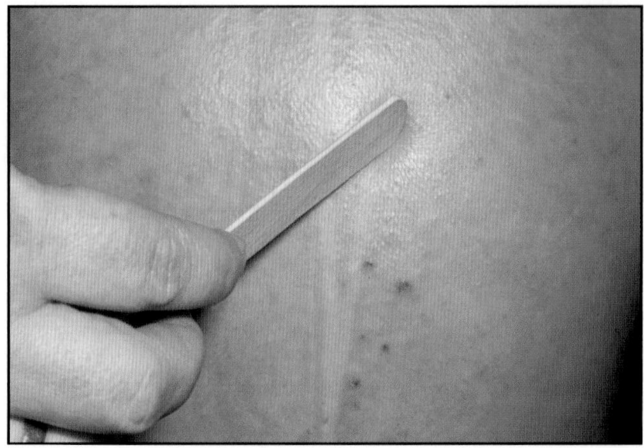

Fig. 7.15 White dermographism.

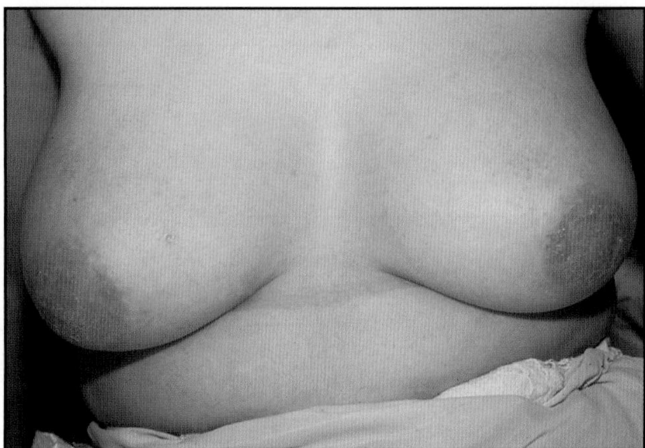

Fig. 7.16 Nipple dermatitis.

the trunk, cheeks, and the extensor sites of the extremities are frequently involved and, as the infant develops, the limbs also become affected.

Symptom presentation

Many infants with atopic dermatitis have erythematous oozing lesions, predominantly on the cheeks. As the child grows, the affected sites tend to be the hands, the neck area, and the feet, particularly under the straps of footwear. The older child has predominant involvement behind the knees (Fig. 7.13), in the elbow folds, and frequently also on the face. The adult patient has a more generalized distribution, commonly with diffuse involvement on the trunk and upper thigh area.

With continual rubbing and excoriation, the skin becomes lichenified and develops a thickened, coarse appearance. A clinical variant found in adolescents and adults is the pruriginous form of atopic dermatitis, which is probably caused by repeated localized scratching.

The facial appearance of a patient with chronic atopic dermatitis is characteristic, with premature small wrinkles underneath both eyes – Dennie–Morgan folds – and, frequently, the loss of the outer third of the eyebrow through rubbing the face on the pillow while sleeping. This is referred to as Hertoghe's sign (Fig. 7.14). The characteristic white dermographism (Fig. 7.15) of the atopic patient gives rise to an unhealthy pallor. Although most patients with atopic dermatitis are encouraged to keep their nails cut very short to avoid excoriation of the skin by scratching, many patients buff or rub at their skin using the flat surface of the nail, which gives the nails a highly polished appearance.

Young women with atopic dermatitis may develop persistent and, at times, severe dermatitis around the nipple and periareolar area (Fig. 7.16). In a proportion of patients with hand dermatitis their condition is associated with atopy. This should be considered particularly with regard to hairdressers, nurses, and others whose work involves persistent exposure of the skin to detergents, soaps, and other degreasing materials.

A large proportion of patients with chronic atopic dermatitis have an associated dry skin, which is frequently hypersensitive and mildly pruritic, and its control may help to alleviate the pruritus of atopic dermatitis.

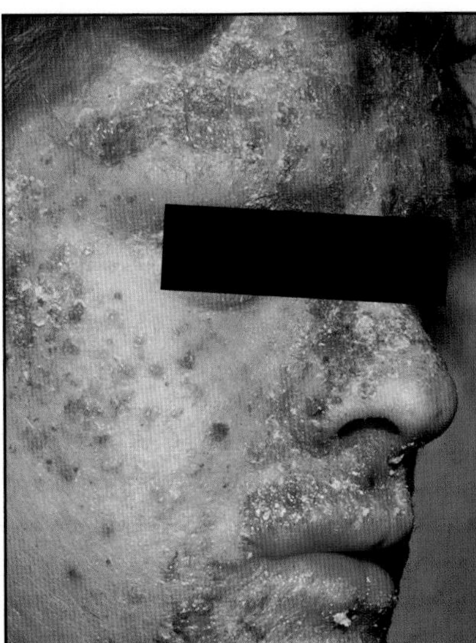

Fig. 7.17 Atopic dermatitis with obvious secondary infection and impetiginization on the face.

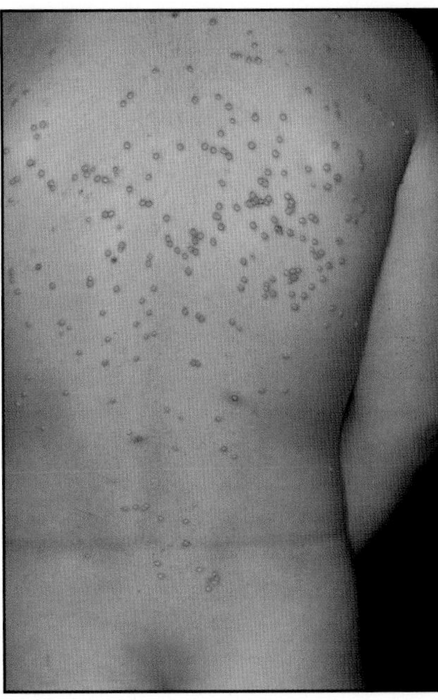

Fig. 7.18 Infection with molluscum contagiosum virus as a stigma for atopic children.

Some patients with atopic dermatitis do not develop their first lesions until later childhood, adolescence, or even adulthood. Individual case reports are recorded of patients who develop atopic dermatitis for the first time after acute intercurrent infection, such as infectious mononucleosis, and after successful marrow transplantation for leukemia.

Patients with atopic dermatitis are unusually susceptible to certain cutaneous viral and bacterial infections and, of these, colonization with *S. aureus* is most common (Fig. 7.17). As outlined above there is now evidence of a causative relationship between *S. aureus* colonization and the severity of the disease.

Patients with atopic dermatitis have a higher than expected incidence of warts caused by human papilloma virus or infections by molluscum contagiosum virus (Fig. 7.18). They are also susceptible to severe infection when exposed to the herpes simplex virus type I, which may spread and cause eczema herpeticum (Fig. 7.19). In a patient with severe excoriations caused by pre-existing dermatitis, it may be difficult to identify these new vesicles. Herpes simplex infection is an important, and at times severe, complication of atopic dermatitis and if it is not identified and treated appropriately it can prove lethal.

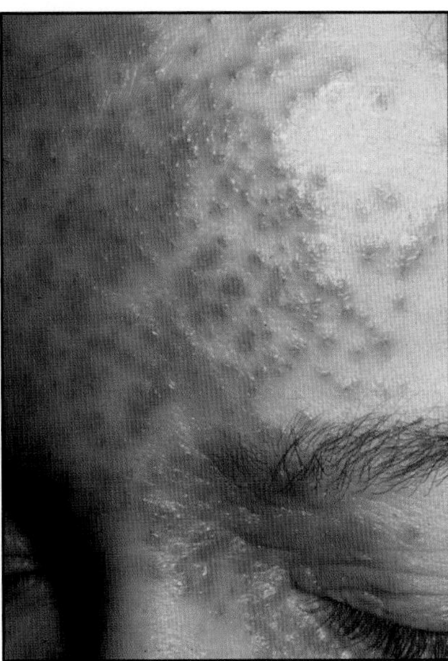

Fig. 7.19 Eczema herpeticum.

Additional tests

The diagnosis of atopic dermatitis is usually made by evaluation of anamnestic data and clinical presentation. According to Hanifin and Rajka, three of their major and three of their minor criteria (Table 7.2) must be fulfilled to classify a skin disease as atopic dermatitis. Since this list is too long to be evaluated in daily practice, easier diagnostic criteria have been subsequently defined. Table 7.3 displays a simplified proposal, which was evaluated by a multicenter study group from the UK.

Laboratory data may sometimes be helpful in the diagnosis of atopic dermatitis. Patients with atopic dermatitis frequently have eosinophilia and approximately 80% of patients have abnormally high serum levels of IgE, the highest levels being recorded in those patients with additional respiratory symptoms and in those with apparently associated food allergy. However, up to 15% of the normal population has serum IgE levels above the normal range and a number of other diseases (e.g. helminthic infestations, cutaneous T-cell lymphoma) are also associated with high serum IgE levels. Thus, total serum IgE levels are not specific markers of the atopic dermatitis patient.

Radioallergosorbent (RAST) or skin prick tests to identify IgE levels specific to allergens have a higher specificity in the diagnosis of atopy than total serum IgE. In the young child, the bulk of IgE is directed against ingested foodstuffs; however, later in life, a large proportion of IgE appears to be directed against inhalant allergens. It is important to note that these tests show a sensitization but often do not prove that the patient has a clinically relevant allergy.

Table 7.2 Diagnostic criteria of atopic dermatitis according to Hanifin and Rajka

Guidelines for the Diagnosis of Atopic Dermatitis
Major features (at least three must be fulfilled):
Pruritus Typical morphology and distribution: flexural lichenification or linearity in adults facial and extensor involvement in infants and children Chronic or chronically relapsing dermatitis Personal or family history of atopy (asthma, allergic rhinitis, atopic dermatitis)
Minor features (at least three must be fulfilled):
Xerosis Ichthyosis/palmar hyperlinearity/keratosis pilaris Immediate (type 1) skin-test reactivity Elevated serum IgE Early age of onset Tendency towards cutaneous infections (esp. *Staphylococcus aureus* and *Herpes simplex*) or impaired cell-mediated immunity Tendency towards non-specific hand or foot dermatitis Nipple eczema Cheilitis Recurrent conjunctivitis Dennie–Morgan infraorbital fold Keratoconus Anterior subcapsular cataracts Orbital darkening Facial pallor/facial erythema Pityriasis alba Anterior neck folds Itch when sweating Intolerance to wool and lipid solvents Perifollicular accentuation Food intolerance Course influenced by environment/emotional factors White dermographism/delayed blanch

From Hanifin JM, Rajka G. Diagnostic features of atopic dermatitis. Acta Derm Venereol 1980; 92:44.

Table 7.3 Simplified diagnostic criteria of atopic dermatitis according to the UK Working Party's diagnostic criteria for atopic dermatitis

Simplified Diagnostic Criteria of Atopic Dermatitis
Itchy skin condition (obligatory)
Plus three of more of the following: History of flexural involvement History of asthma/hay fever History of generalized dry skin Onset of rash under the age of 2 years Visible flexural dermatitis

According to Williams HC, Burney PG, Pembroke AC, et al. Validation of the UK diagnostic criteria for atopic dermatitis in a population setting. UK Diagnostic Criteria for Atopic Dermatitis Working Party. Br J Dermatol 1996; 135(1):12–17. © Blackwell Science Ltd.

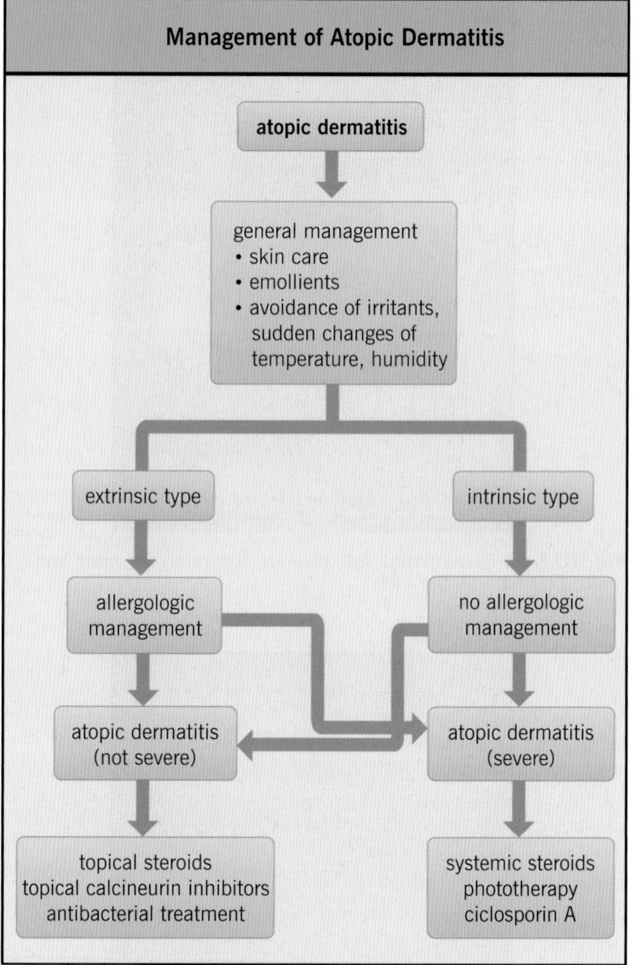

Fig. 7.20 Management of atopic dermatitis.

MANAGEMENT OF ATOPIC DERMATITIS

General management

General management of atopic patients usually begins with control of the commonly associated dry skin (Fig. 7.20). If this is treated, the need for topical steroid therapy will be greatly reduced. Most patients benefit from an emollient, either added to a bath, used after a bath, or applied continuously to the skin. The use of soap should be restricted in favor of a syndet, and an emollient substituted. Most patients will learn by trial and error which specific emollient preparations best suit their skin. A structured patient education performed with groups of approximately 10 patients or with 10 parents of young patients suffering from atopic dermatitis has recently been evaluated in a controlled multicenter trial. It proved to be effective in the management of atopic dermatitis with respect to sustained improvement of the skin condition and of quality of life.

Avoidance of skin irritants

Patients with atopic dermatitis should avoid materials which irritate the skin. These frequently include both natural products, such as wool, and synthetic fibers. The majority of patients find that pure cotton is the most comfortable clothing. Moving rapidly from one environmental extreme to another should also be avoided as large changes in ambient temperature, particularly from cold to hot, and changes in humidity, are associated with deterioration of the skin condition.

Allergen avoidance

Reasonable steps to reduce the environmental exposure to allergens should be taken. This can be difficult with some allergens, but with others the precautions are obvious (e.g. households with a severely atopic child should not keep a cat). Although the house dust mite is ubiquitous and difficult to control, every effort should be made to reduce the prevalence of the mite in the environment, particularly in the sleeping area. The established and recommended avoidance procedures include removal of the carpet and curtains from the bedroom, encasing mattresses, pillows, and blankets in impermeable synthetic material, and hot washing of all bedding once a week.

Drug treatment

Antiinflammatory and antimicrobial agents

The mainstay of control in atopic dermatitis is the appropriate use of topical corticosteroid creams or topical antiinflammatory calcineurin-inhibitors. Topical steroids must be handled with care and under regular supervision since they may be absorbed through the skin and the inappropriate use of potent steroids may lead to unwanted topical and systemic effects. In Europe, topical steroids are divided into four classes, with increasing potency ranging from grade I, containing hydrocortisone, to grade IV (Table 7.4). It is important to note that this classification differs from that in the USA (seven classes) and that there is no direct link between these classes and prednisone-equivalent doses calculated for systemic applications of steroids. It is normal dermatologic practice to use a topical steroid no more potent than grade I on the face, and then only for a short time, and only moderately potent steroids (grade II) on other body sites. As preparations vary widely throughout the world, current national formularies should be consulted. Topical calcineurin-inhibitors such as tacrolimus or pimecrolimus are also effective in atopic dermatitis. Since they do not have the same local side-effects as topical steroids, such as the induction of skin atrophy, their use may be particularly favorable at sensitive skin regions such as the face or intertriginous areas. Severe chronic atopic dermatitis will benefit from the use of systemic corticosteroids; however, long-term treatment must be reserved for exceptionally stubborn cases because of the side-effects.

Ciclosporin, a polypeptide of fungal origin, is a potent inhibitor of T lymphocyte-dependent immune responses and was originally introduced as an immunosuppressive agent to facilitate allogenic organ transplantation; it is also very effective in patients with atopic dermatitis in doses from 2.5 to 5 mg/kg per day. Clearing of acute eczematous skin lesions is usually observed after 4–6 weeks of therapy but, as with steroids, improvement is only temporary and frequent flares occur after discontinuation of the drug therapy.

Many dermatologists find that the addition of a topical antibacterial agent (such as triclosan) to the steroid preparation will apparently improve atopic dermatitis and for many this is routine practice. Others prefer to use intermittent short courses of systemic antibiotics and the most useful are those which have an antistaphylococcal action (e.g. clindamycin, cephalosporin derivates, or flucloxacillin).

Management of eczema herpeticum requires systemic acyclovir or related derivates which are given either orally or intravenously depending on the severity of the exacerbation and on the need to obtain a rapid response.

Table 7.4 Classification of external corticosteroids

European Classification of the External Corticosteroids		
Group	**Substance (examples)**	**Concentration (%)**
I (Low)	Hydrocortisone Hydrocortisone acetate Prednisolone	0.500; 1.000 0.250; 1.000 0.400
II (Medium)	Hydrocortisone butyrate Triamcinolone acetonide Prednicarbate	0.100 0.100 0.250
III (Strong)	Betamethasone valerate Flucinolone acetonide Mometasone furoate	0.100 0.025 0.100
IV (Very strong)	Clobetasol	0.050

Antihistamines

Systemic histamine H_1-receptor antagonists are frequently prescribed for patients with atopic dermatitis, but their value is disputed. It is found that these antihistamines are initially of some benefit to individual patients, particularly with regard to pruritus at night and loss of sleep. Newer non-sedating histamine H_1 antagonists are suitable for daytime use, but many patients with chronic severe atopic dermatitis will find the older antihistamines of more value, possibly because of the sedative effect rather than the specific antihistaminic actions of the drugs.

Other procedures

Phototherapy

Phototherapy – including UVB (290–320 nm), UVA (320–400 nm), and combinations of UVA and UVB – and photochemotherapy (PUVA) have long been used to treat atopic dermatitis. The recent development of specific emission spectra has resulted in a re-evaluation of the efficacy of phototherapy for atopic dermatitis. Compared with conventional UVB, narrow band UVB (311 nm) radiation is less erythemogenic and causes fewer side-effects and, according to recent studies, atopic dermatitis appears to respond well to the therapy. High-dose UVA (UVA1, 340–400 nm) is used successfully for the treatment of an acute exacerbation of atopic dermatitis: it is less erythemogenic than conventional UVA and allows irradiation of 130 J/cm^2. However, long-term side-effects, such as premature skin aging and carcinogenesis, must be considered.

Dietary measures

Two differing approaches, preventive and curative, can be adopted. The preventive approach involves the delayed introduction of mixed feeding, and the exclusive breastfeeding of infants known to be at high risk. A lower incidence of atopic dermatitis has been found in children who have been breastfed, or fed with extensively hydrolyzed milk formula for at least 4 months. After 4 years, however, there are no differences in the prevalence of atopic diseases between the diet and control groups. An additional maternal diet during the last trimester of pregnancy and into lactation probably has no further protective effect on the manifestation of atopic dermatitis. Although elimination diets during early childhood are not sufficient to generally prevent the manifestation of atopic dermatitis, breast-feeding or the feeding of hypoallergenic formula during the first 4 months of life should be recommended for high-risk infants.

The curative approach concerns dietary control of the established disease. This may either be by exclusion of an item of food that the patient or parent has noticed specifically exacerbates the disease or by non-specific exclusion of foods (e.g. dairy foods and other protein sources). The first approach is logical but identification of provoking foods can be difficult, particularly if there is a 48-hour gap between ingestion and the onset of symptoms.

Exclusion of dairy products is a very popular move with parents of affected children. However, this should only be recommended for a prolonged period after a positive oral provocation test since there is a very real danger of malnutrition and only about 10% of all patients notice a benefit. A very small number of patients with severe and intractable disease derive benefit from an elemental diet.

New approaches to therapy

Interferon

Interferon α (IFNα) and IFNγ appear to be of potential therapeutic value in the treatment of acute eczema associated with a predominance of type 2 cytokines and several clinical trials have been performed with these cytokines for the treatment of atopic dermatitis. Although in some patients slight clearing of eczema is observed, the overall response rate is not encouraging and most patients have a relapse shortly after discontinuation of the therapy.

Specific desensitization

Specific desensitization with extracts of airborne allergens that attenuate the cutaneous late-phase response to aero-allergens appears to be a promising treatment. Allergen desensitization has been shown to be effective in open therapeutic trials in patients who have a history of exacerbation after exposure to the suspected allergens. A recent controlled study showed a dose-dependent beneficial effect of specific immunotherapy with house dust mite allergens on eczema in patients who were sensitized to house dust mite via IgE to a high degree.

Unsaturated fatty acids

Oral ingestion of unsaturated fatty acids – such as evening primrose oil – has been found, in open studies, to benefit some aspects of atopic dermatitis in adults. The postulated mechanism suggests that by raising the levels of dihomogammalinolenic acid a defect in δ-6-desaturase activity is bypassed. This theoretic mode of action has not yet been proven, and not all studies of the use of evening primrose oil or marine fish oil are positive.

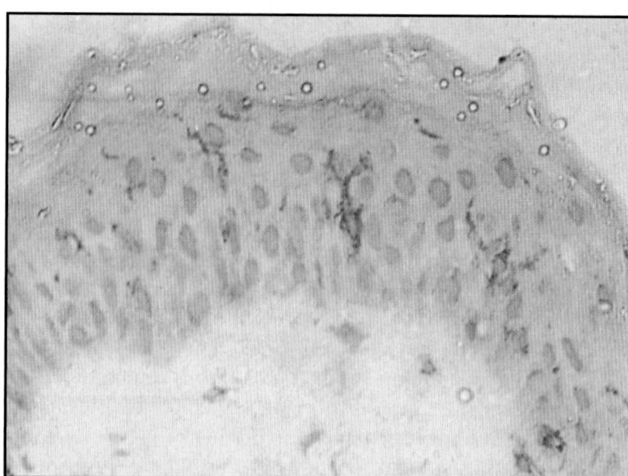

Fig. 7.21 Langerhans' cells in a skin section stained using a monoclonal antibody to CD1a. These dendritic cells comprise 3% of epidermal cells (× 312).

CLASSIFICATION OF ALLERGIC CONTACT DERMATITIS

In this type of dermatitis, prior exposure to the allergen responsible is necessary – either briefly or over many years. This last point is often difficult for patients to understand.

Allergic contact dermatitis is not linked to atopy. It is the prototype of a delayed-type hypersensitivity reaction (so-called type IV reaction), mediated largely by previously sensitized lymphocytes, that causes inflammation and edema in the skin.

PATHOGENESIS

Pathophysiology

Most allergens in allergic contact dermatitis are of low molecular weight (less than 1 kDa) and, though many of them have a complicated structure, they are often called simple chemicals. Contact allergens are haptens and need to link with proteins (so-called carriers) in the skin before they become antigenic. Haptens may be readily absorbed transcutaneously: the hapten dinitrochlorobenzene has been shown to penetrate the epidermis within 30 minutes of epicutaneous application. Of clinical interest, humidity and warmer ambient temperature increase allergen penetration. An intact skin surface decreases penetrability, while maceration by sweating, occlusion, or water immersion increases the accessibility of antigens and irritants. A dry or inflamed skin presents a broken barrier and a greater vulnerability.

Once in the extravascular spaces, most haptens bind in a covalent fashion to their carrier proteins – usually serum proteins – or to the cell membranes of antigen-presenting cells. For example, nickel binds, through its interaction with the amino acid histidine, to peptides present in the specialized peptide-binding groove of MHC class II molecules.

The most potent cells which are able to present antigens to T lymphocytes in the skin are epidermal Langerhans' cells and dermal dendritic cells. Langerhans' cells form an extensive network in the epidermis to trap and process epicutaneously applied antigens (Fig. 7.21). Langerhans' cells are dendritic cells derived from bone marrow and characterized by the membrane expression of CD1a and MHC class II antigens and by containing a unique organelle, the Birbeck granule, which is seen on electromicroscopic examination. In the corium, dermal dendritic cells – composed of at least three subpopulations – and certain types of macrophages are available for antigen presentation, which is the key event in delayed hypersensitivity.

The development of contact hypersensitivity usually occurs in only a minority of individuals exposed to potential allergens, although certain substances have a greater likelihood of inducing sensitivity. For example, dinitrochlorobenzene will sensitize over 90% of normal individuals upon repeated skin contact. Recent studies suggest that the allergeneity of a molecule may be associated with its potential to induce intracellular activation steps with the subsequent release of proinflammatory cytokines – such as IL-1β – from antigen-presenting cells. This reaction may perhaps serve as an indicator in future predictive test systems that estimate the allergenic potency of newly developed substances.

Sensitization takes 10–14 days to develop. If examined prospectively, it is characterized clinically on about the 10th day by an eczematous flare reaction at the site of the sensitizing application. Most epicutaneously applied allergens which attach to the Langerhans' cell membrane are internalized. Some of the fragments which result from the processing of the antigen are expressed on the surface of the Langerhans' cell in association with MHC class II molecules. Activated Langerhans' cells upregulate certain chemokine receptors (particularly CCR7) and follow a gradient of the respective receptor ligands in the dermis and draining lymphatics after they have moved out of the epidermis until they reach the regional lymph nodes. There they congregate in the paracortical areas of the regional lymph nodes and have the opportunity to present the processed antigen (associated with MHC class II molecules) to a large number of T lymphocytes (Fig. 7.22). If sensitization develops, a population of antigen-specific sensitized CD4+ T lymphocytes is produced.

Inflammatory cells and mediators

Figure 7.23 illustrates that an antigen applied epicutaneously to the skin of a sensitized individual is again processed by Langerhans' cells and expressed on the cell surfaces in association with MHC class II molecules. Langerhans' cells then present antigens not only in the lymph nodes but also in the skin to specific memory T lymphocytes. T cells become activated both by the direct contact of antigen receptors to the antigen–MHC complex and by cytokines secreted from antigen-presenting cells, from bystander cells (e.g. keratinocytes), and from other skin-infiltrating T cells. The latter appear to produce a mixed cytokine pattern – including IL-4 and IFNγ – in acute allergic contact dermatitis and a more pronounced type 1 cytokine pattern in the chronic phase of dermatitis. The production of cytokines and chemokines results, through a variety of mechanisms, in the accumulation of antigen-specific and non-antigen-specific effector T cells and in the expression of adhesion molecules and MHC class II molecules on the cell membranes in the skin (Fig. 7.24). Less than 10% of T cells in allergic contact dermatitis are allergen specific. Endothelial cells are stimulated early by cytokines to express molecules involved in lymphocyte adhesion such as the intercellular adhesion molecule (ICAM-1) or E-selectin. Circulating T lymphocytes, through their expression of corresponding ligands such as leukocyte function antigens (LFA) or CLA, recognize adhesion molecules on the surface membranes of endothelial cells and can bind to these cells. This further increases the trafficking of mononuclear cells through the skin.

The main histologic findings of contact dermatitis have been summarized earlier and Figure 7.2 shows some of these. The earliest histologic change, seen about 4 hours after epicutaneous challenge with an antigen, is a periappendageal and perivascular mononuclear cell infiltrate. By 8 hours, mononuclear cells begin to infiltrate the epidermis. The infiltrates increase to a maximum at 48–72 hours – by which time there is edema of the epidermis – after which the reaction subsides. The majority of infiltrating cells are CD4+ although the quantity of CD8+ T cells can be as high as 50%. Basophils are also observed in the early infiltrate of allergic contact dermatitis. The numbers of Langerhans' cells increase in the epidermis at 24–48 hours, and CD1a+ cells are found in the dermal infiltrate as well. Macrophages invade the dermis at 48 hours.

Spontaneous resolution occurs after the antigen is removed and the T-cell mediators disappear. A number of mechanisms are involved in the downregulation of the inflammatory response. Macrophages and keratinocytes produce prostaglandins of the E series which inhibit the production of (proinflammatory) cytokines. Other mediators, such as leukotriene B_4, transforming growth factor, or IL-10, may be involved in downregulation of the eczematous reaction as well. In addition, T-regulatory cells expressing the transcription factor fox p3 inhibit T-cell proliferation by cell-to-cell contacts. The role of skin-infiltrating CD8+ T cells is not clear yet but they may function as suppressor cells which dampen down the reaction.

DIAGNOSIS OF ALLERGIC CONTACT DERMATITIS

History

Women present more commonly than men with allergic contact dermatitis, and there is an increase in incidence with advancing age. The clinical features of allergic contact dermatitis depend on the type of allergen responsible (Fig. 7.25). Usually, dermatitis occurs at the site of allergen application but a spreading of the dermatitis is also possible. The important points in the clinical identification and management of allergic contact dermatitis are given in Figure 7.26. In taking the patient's history, it is important to consider occupational, household, and recreational exposure to possible allergens.

Symptom presentation

A battery of common allergens has been defined in several parts of the world, and they differ from continent to continent. In some areas of North America, plants – particularly poison oak and poison ivy – are the most common cause of allergic contact dermatitis. Worldwide, however, nickel sulfate is now the leading cause of allergic contact dermatitis.

Common sources of allergens in Europe and North America are shown in Table 7.5. Many patients find it difficult to understand that material handled for many years can suddenly give rise to an allergic contact dermatitis; similarly, allergy to a regular cosmetic or washing powder may not be regarded by the patient as a possible cause of their problems. In such cases

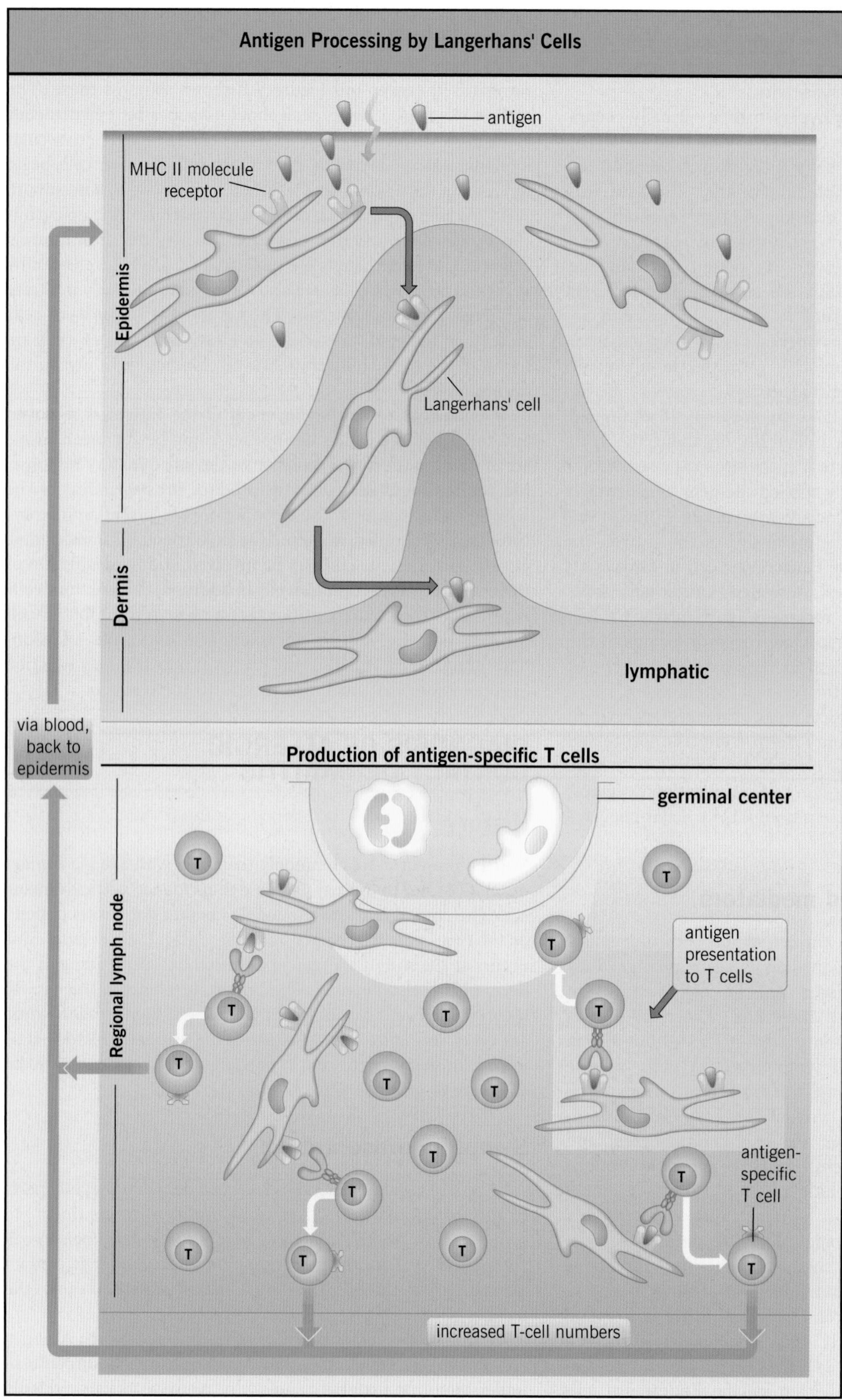

Fig. 7.22 Antigen-bearing Langerhans' cells migrate, via the lymphatics, to the regional lymph nodes. In the paracortical area they interdigitate with CD4+ T lymphocytes resulting in the generation of antigen-specific memory T cells.

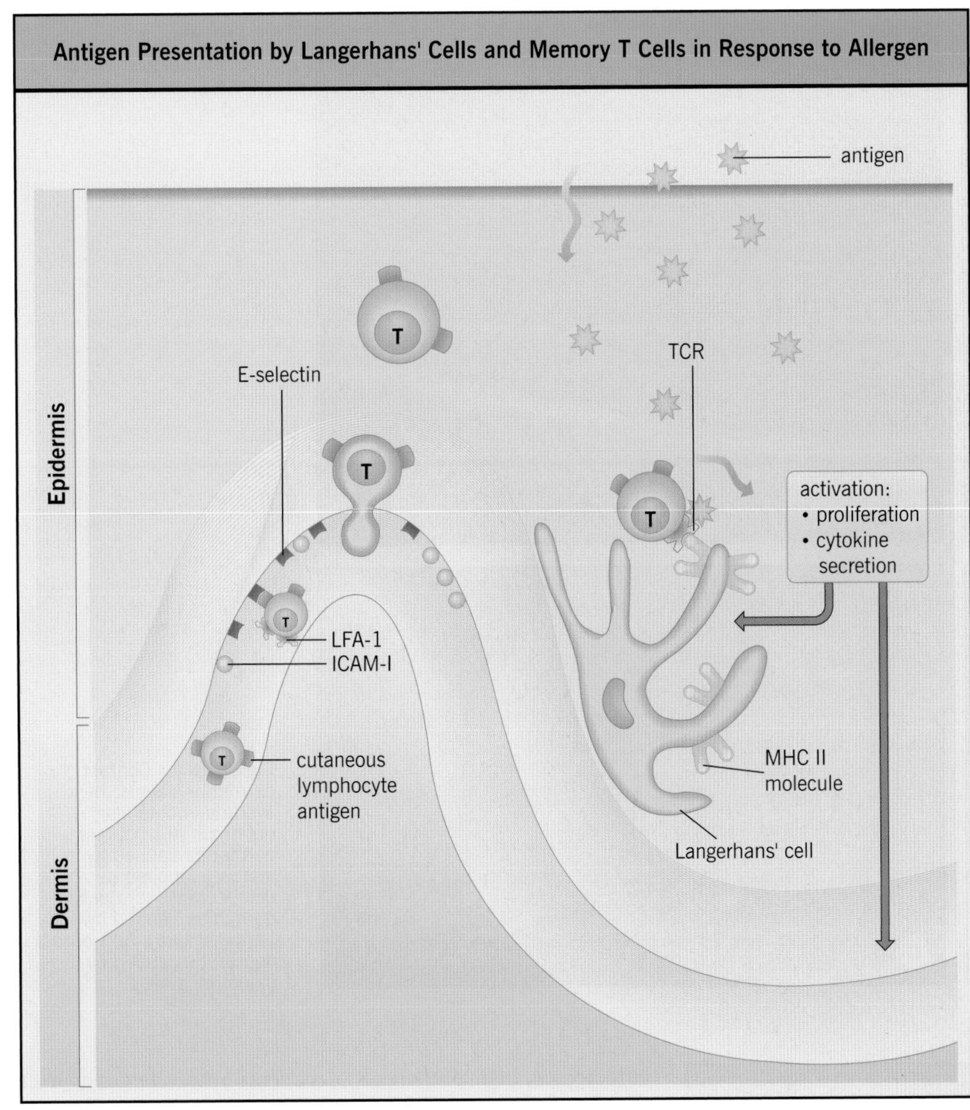

Fig. 7.23 The presentation by Langerhans' cells of processed antigen to T cells results in a cascade of events leading to the influx of mononuclear cells into the dermis and epidermis and the development of dermatitis. For the purpose of clarity most constitutional cutaneous cells are deleted from the scheme. LFA-1, leukocyte function associated antigen 1; ICAM-1, intercellular adhesion molecule 1; T, T lymphocyte; MHC II, major histocompatibility complex class II; TCR, T cell receptor.

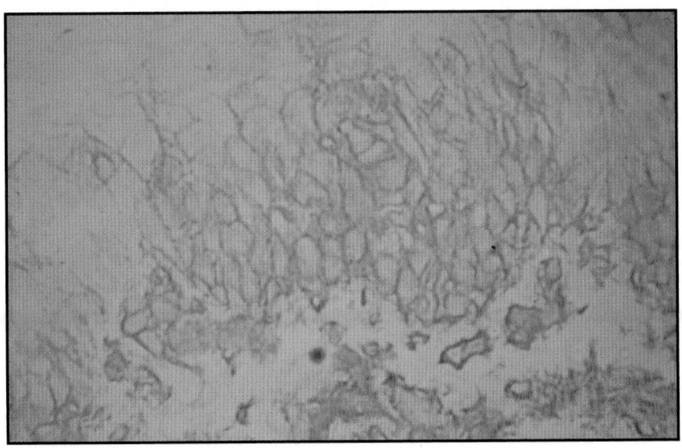

Fig. 7.24 MHC class II antigen expression by keratinocytes in allergic contact dermatitis (× 400).

it must be remembered that new, improved formulations are continually being introduced and also that it is often the preservative – rather than the main ingredient of such preparations – which gives rise to problems.

Contact dermatitis caused by an allergy to airborne material may be difficult to identify, but this can occur (e.g. with plants, volatile preservatives in wall colors or with fine particles of rubber dust in cars). If a contact allergen is ingested or inhaled it can lead to hematogenous allergic contact dermatitis. Due to the common involvement of the buttocks this particular characteristic is called baboon syndrome by some authors (Fig. 7.27). The basic battery of standard antigens is helpful in the great majority (80%) of cases. Substances that commonly cause allergic contact dermatitis include rubber, cosmetics, preservatives, fragrances, dyes, chemicals, topical medicaments, and metal salts.

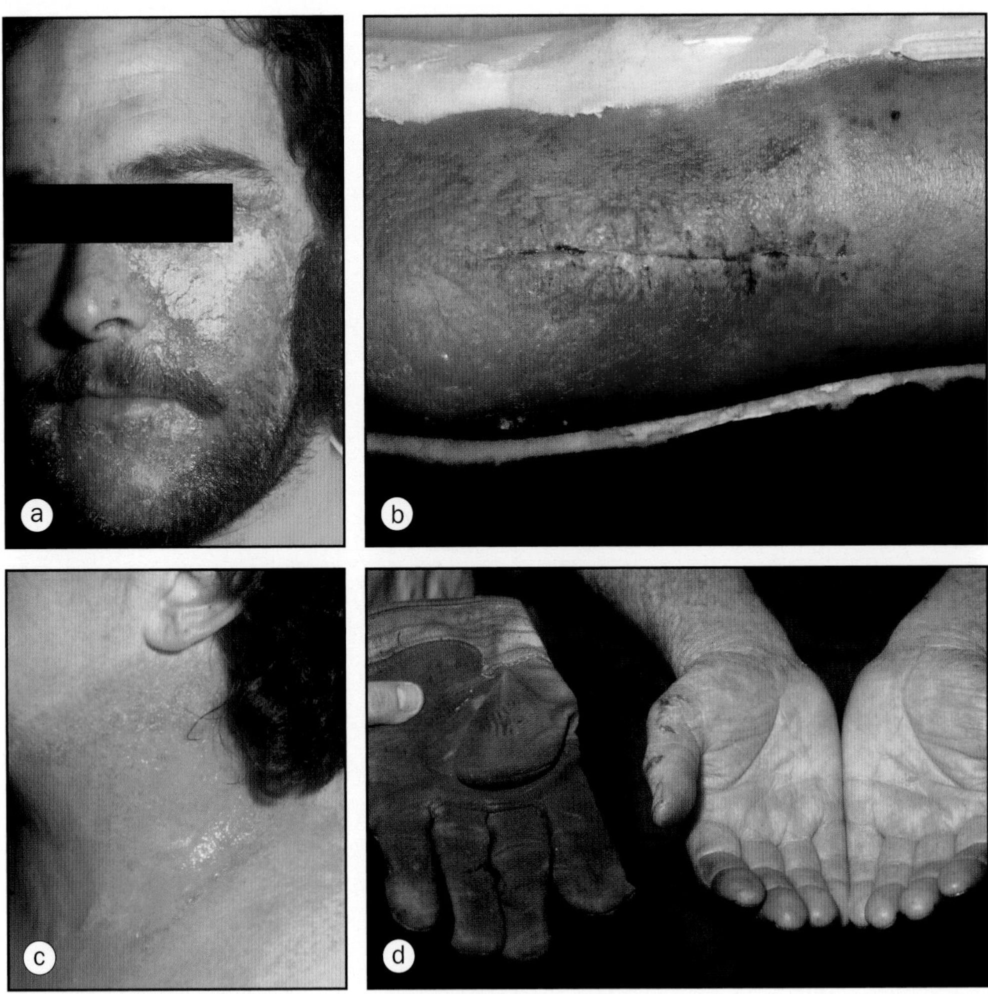

Fig. 7.25 (a) Contact dermatitis caused by eyedrops containing neomycin. (b) Contact dermatitis caused by mercury (applied as disinfectant). (c) Contact dermatitis caused by perfume spray. (d) Contact dermatitis caused by industrial gloves.

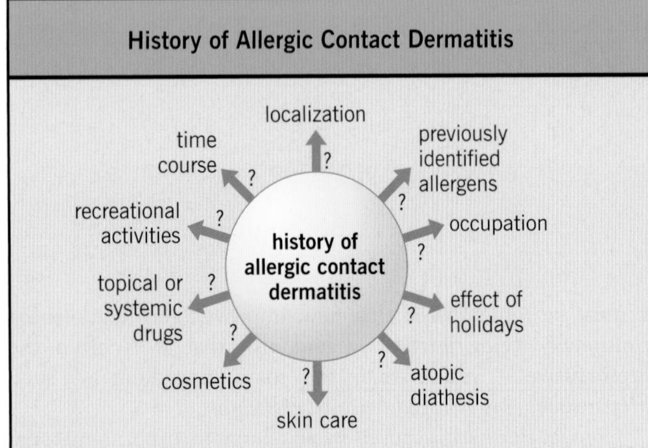

Fig. 7.26 Important points of the patient's history of allergic contact dermatitis.

Common allergen sources and special clinical features of allergic contact dermatitis

Metal allergies

Nickel dermatitis is extremely common in women, and in North Europe more than 10% of the female population is affected. A high proportion of patients with allergic contact dermatitis first develop their problem after ear piercing. The frequency of nickel dermatitis has increased in the male population during the last decade, and this may be due to an increased popularity of piercing in this group. In the European Union, it is now illegal to sell earrings and other items of jewellery which release a high concentration of nickel. Obvious areas of involvement are under rings, watches, bracelets, spectacle frames, coins in pockets, jeans studs, and other sites of direct contact with metal (Figs 7.28 and 7.29). Less obvious areas are the eyelids and the nape of the neck. A serious problem in occupational dermatology is the well-known induction of hand dermatitis in individuals sensitized to nickel who have to work in a wet environment. This may be due to additional effects of continuing skin irritation and contact with low concentrations of nickel ions in fluids.

To determine whether a metal contains nickel, a spot test can be carried out using dimethylglyoxime – a pink color develops if nickel is present in the material tested. There is continuing controversy as to whether the nickel content of a normal diet can provoke or aggravate pre-existing nickel dermatitis. Such a diet may be beneficial to those patients who clearly respond to oral provocation with 2–20 mg nickel sulfate within 24–48 hours with a dyshidrosiform eruption on the hands and feet but the rate of nickel allergic patients who respond to nickel upon oral provocation is less than 3%.

Table 7.5 Common agents causing allergic contact dermatitis and their sources

Agents causing Allergic Contact Dermatitis	
Agent	**Found in**
Nickel	Clothing clasps, earrings, spectacle frames, jewellery, coins, household utensils
Chromate	Leather, bleaches, matches, cement
Formaldehyde	Preservatives, cosmetics, cigarettes, newsprint, fabric softeners, wrinkle-resistant clothes
Chloroisothiazolinone	Preservatives in creams and technical fluids
Dibromocyanobutane	Preservatives in creams and cosmetics
Mercaptobenzothiazole	Rubber products (especially boots and gloves), catheters
Thiurams	Rubber products, fungicide in paint and soap, paraphenylenediamine hair dye, clothing dye, stockings and tights
Plants	*Primula obconica* (Europe), *Rhus*, (poison ivy – North America), Compositae, tulips

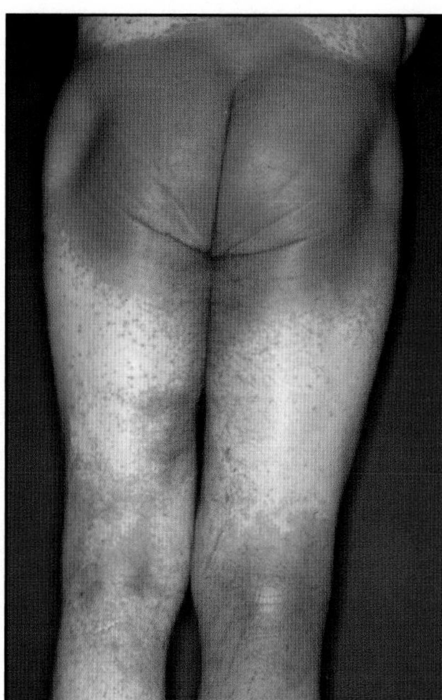

Fig. 7.27 Hematogenous contact dermatitis (baboon syndrome).

Dry lichenified hand or foot dermatitis is frequently caused by chromates (Fig. 7.30). Hexavalent metal salts of chromate are among the most important causes of contact reactions (see Fig. 7.30). They are found in cement, detergents, bleaches, and match heads and are used in tanning leather. In some countries

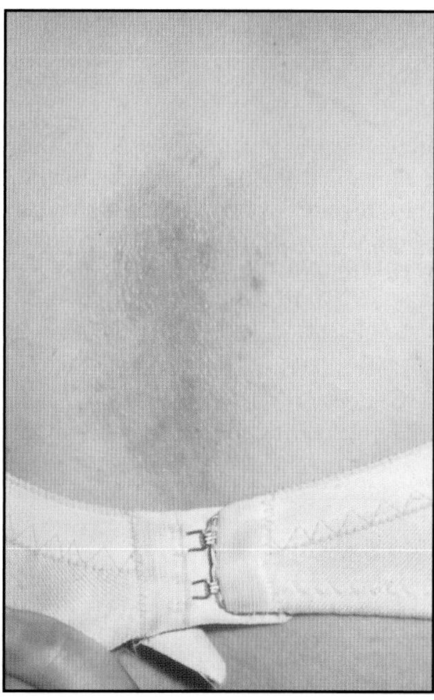

Fig. 7.28 Nickel sensitivity to metal clips in underwear.

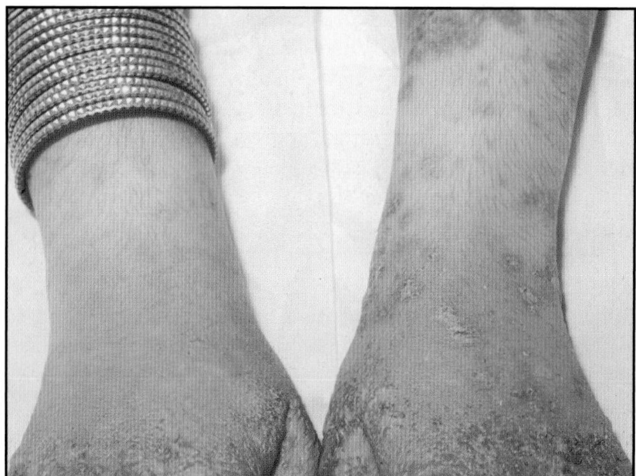

Fig. 7.29 Nickel sensitivity to bracelets.

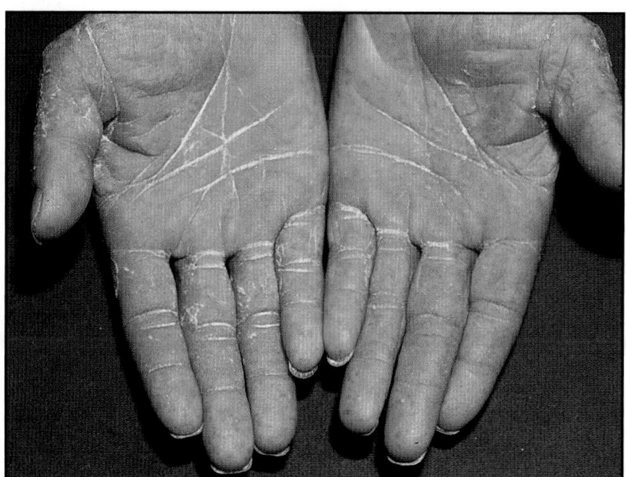

Fig. 7.30 Hand dermatitis caused by chromates.

chromate is removed from cement because of its association with contact dermatitis.

Preservatives

These are ubiquitous antibacterials used in the industry to prevent contamination. Cosmetic products with a high water content (lotions) require more preservatives than pure ointments (petroleum jelly), which can be preservative-free. Formaldehyde, quaternium-15, imidazolidinyl urea, dimethyloldimethyl hydantoin, dibromocyanobutane, methylchloroisothiazolinone, and parabens are common sensitizers. Quaternium-15, imidazolidinyl urea, and dimethyloldimethyl hydantoin are potential formaldehyde releasers and may therefore cause problems with formaldehyde-sensitive patients. Each preservative can be identified by a vast number of synonyms and the clinician must be familiar with these when reading product labeling.

Rubber ingredients

Patients with hand, foot, waistband, and chest rashes should be suspected of being allergic to rubber ingredients in gloves, shoes, and bra straps respectively. Knee braces, elbow braces, and other prostheses are also common culprits. Shoes present a particular challenge in these patients as virtually every commercially available shoe contains some rubber.

Rubber allergies are common among those involved in rubber manufacturing and the possible allergens include the thiurams, mercaptobenzothiazole, and *p*-phenylenediamine (PPD). Mercaptobenzothiazole and thiurams are accelerators used in the manufacture of both natural and synthetic rubber and PPD derivates are found in dark rubber. They are also major components of most hair dyes and also of dyes for some stockings and tights.

Plant dermatitis

While common, plant dermatitis is not evaluated by standard patch testing. The most common plant dermatitis in the USA is caused by poison ivy and/or poison oak and their allergenicity is due to the antigen urushiol. There is also cross-reactivity to other related plants such as cashew, mango skin, and ginko (tree leaves). Patients with acute perioral dermatitis due to these foods are usually unaware of the cross-relationship. Sesquiterpene lactones are found in members of the Compositae family (chrysanthemum, ragweed, artichoke, chamomile, daisy, dandelion, etc.) but also in unrelated plants and, in North Europe, *Primula obconica* is a common cause of problems (Fig. 7.31). The allergen involved is primin, which is airborne and can cause an acute reaction. Tulip bulb handlers may also develop a problem with a dry cracked dermatitis on the fingertips, caused by handling bulbs.

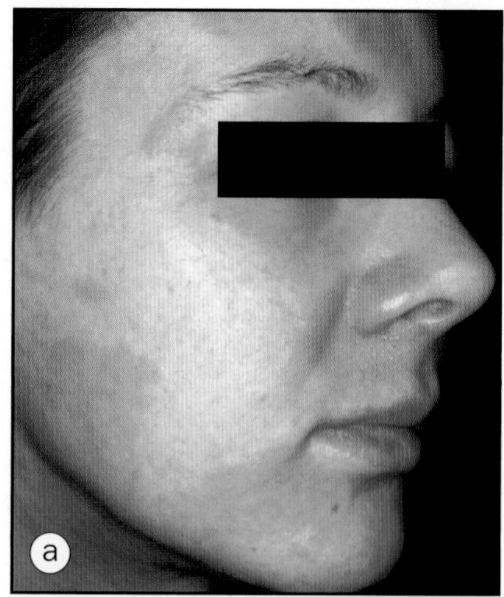

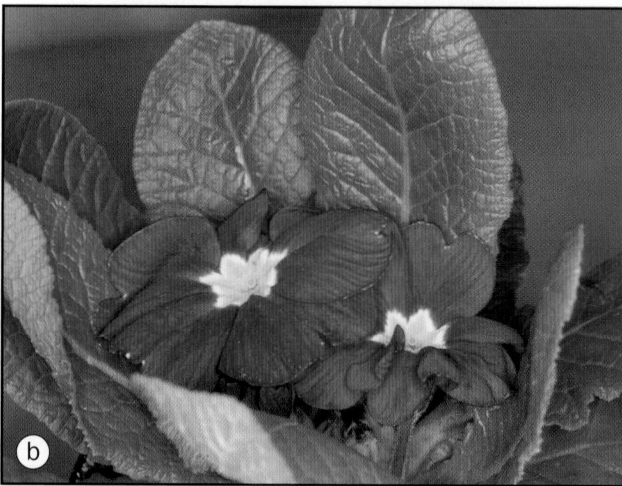

Fig. 7.31 Plant dermatitis. Facial dermatitis eruption (a) (with the characteristic patchy distribution) caused by *Primula* (b).

Photosensitizers

The most frequent sites of allergic photocontact dermatitis are exposed areas (e.g. face, neck, back of the hands, etc.), but any skin area receiving sufficient light and a photosensitizing chemical may manifest a reaction (Fig. 7.32). The most important differential diagnoses are airborne or phototoxic contact dermatitis, the latter being based on a non-immunologic mechanism and often manifested clinically as exaggerated sunburn reactions. The most common phototoxins and photoallergens are activated by UVA radiation (320–400 nm). Paradoxically, sunscreen agents have become the most common causative substances of photo allergic contact dermatitis. *p*-Aminobenzoic acid (PABA) – and its esters – and oxybenzone are the most frequent sensitizers. Other frequent photoallergens are fragrances, chlorpromazine, and phenothiazine and its derivatives.

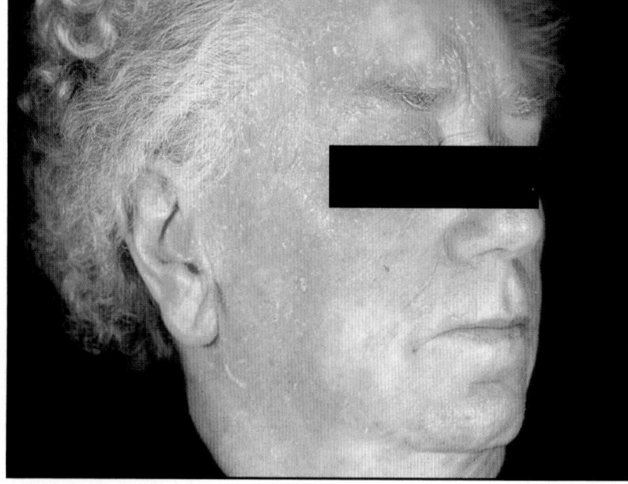

Fig. 7.32 Photoallergic contact dermatitis.

The latter substances are used as sedatives in veterinary medicine, as insecticides, and as antipsychotic agents.

Some individuals who develop a photoallergic contact dermatitis will retain a persistent reactivity to light long after the exposure to photosensitizing compounds. The mechanism of this reaction remains obscure. A plausible theory may be that the patient has become autophotosensitized to a carrier protein that absorbs photons in the UV range thereby producing an eczematous response.

Additional tests

Once there is a suspicion of allergic contact dermatitis, patch testing is warranted. The selection of test batteries for patch tests is highly dependent on the clinical presentation of the disease and on anamnestic data. It has been estimated that 2800 of more than 6 million chemicals which are in the environment have contact-sensitizing properties, which underlines the need for a rational selection of substances for individual tests. It is crucial, however, to realize that many patients are unaware of any relevant exposures, despite a careful history. Done appropriately, patch tests always provide useful information whether the results are positive or negative.

False-positive reactions may be due to patch testing too soon after treatment of acute dermatitis and false negatives may be due to prior UV radiation, or the use of steroids or other immunosuppressant drugs. Systemic antihistamines have no effect on eczematous patch-test results. The technique of patch testing is deceptively simple. The European standard battery of allergens, shown in Table 7.6, is a collection of the allergens which most often lead to epicutaneous sensitization and a similar battery is available for North America. In addition to the European standard battery, additional batteries are available for certain body sites and for certain occupations.

The allergens are prepared in appropriate concentrations in an appropriate diluent – usually white soft paraffin – and are applied to the skin on inert metal disks, such as Finn chambers (Fig. 7.33). After 24–48 hours, the battery of chambers is removed and areas of erythema or induration are noted (Fig. 7.34 and Table 7.7). A similar reading is taken 24 hours after removal of the chambers (i.e. 48–72 hours after application of the prepared allergens).

Antigen selection and patch-test interpretation can be difficult and a well-demarcated, red, raised area is in most cases not due to an allergic contact dermatitis but to an irritant reaction. Adverse reactions during patch testing include a severe irritant reaction which may cause blistering, sensitization to material which previously produced no response, the development of a Koebner reaction if the patient has a tendency to psoriasis or lichen planus, and a flare of pre-existing dermatitis.

The sensitivity of patch tests depends on individual contact allergens and, on the whole, it is about 60–80% in different studies. On the other hand, around 10% of healthy people in populations who have no skin disease will have unexpected, apparently irrelevant, positive results.

In the case of some potential allergens, the classic 48-hour closed patch test is inappropriate as it does not give a true reflection of the contact with the allergen in normal daily life. Consequently, some alternatives have been introduced, the most important being the open patch test, which is recommended for the investigation of irritating substances.

Table 7.6 The European standard contact dermatitis testing battery

European Standard Contact Dermatitis Testing Battery	
Compound concentration/vehicle	**%(w/w)**
1. Potassium dichromate	0.5 pet
2. 4-Phenylenediamine base	1.0 pet
3. Thiuram mix	1.0 pet
4. Neomycin sulfate	20.0 pet
5. Cobalt(II) chloride hexahydrate	1.0 pet
6. Benzocaine	5.0 pet
7. Nickel sulfate hexahydrate	5.0 pet
8. Clioquinol	5.0 pet
9. Colophony	20 pet
10. Paraben mix	16.0 pet
11. *N*-Isopropyl-*N*-phenyl-4-phenylenediamine	0.1 pet
12. Wool alcohols	30.0 pet
13. Mercapto mix	2.0 pet
14. Epoxy resin	1.0 pet
15. Balsam Peru	25.0 pet
16. 4-tert-Butylphenolformaldehyde resin	1.0 pet
17. 2-Mercaptobenzothiazole	2.0 pet
18. Formaldehyde	1.0 aq
19. Fragrance mix	8.0 pet
20. Sesquiterpene lactone mix	0.1 pet
21. 1-(3-Chloroallyl)-3,5,7-triaza-1-azoniaadamantane chloride (Quaternium 15)	1.0 pet
22. 2-Methoxy-6-n-pentyl-4-benzoquinone (Primin)	0.01 pet
23. 5-Chloro-2-methyl-4-isothiazolin-3-one	0.01 aq
24. Budesonide	0.01 pet
25. Tixocortol-21-pivalate	0.1 pet

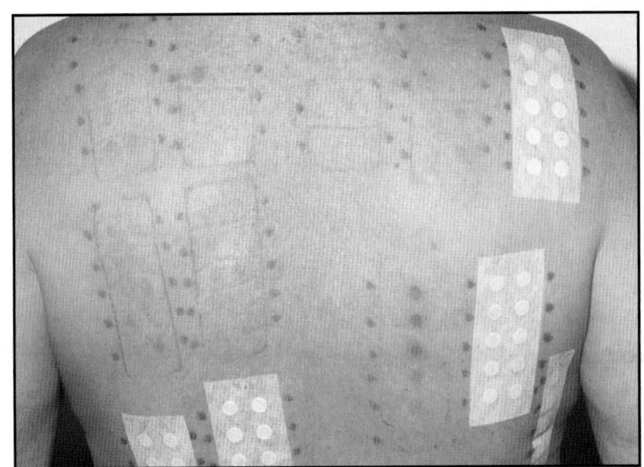

Fig. 7.33 Patch testing. General view showing the number of allergens which can be tested for at any one time.

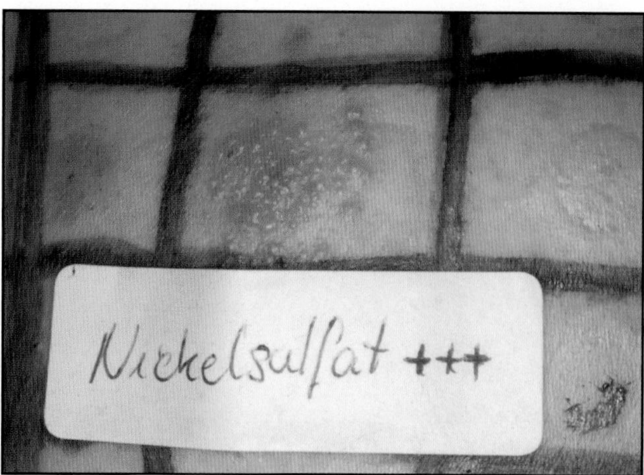

Fig. 7.34 Patch testing showing 48 hours' positive reaction to nickel sulfate.

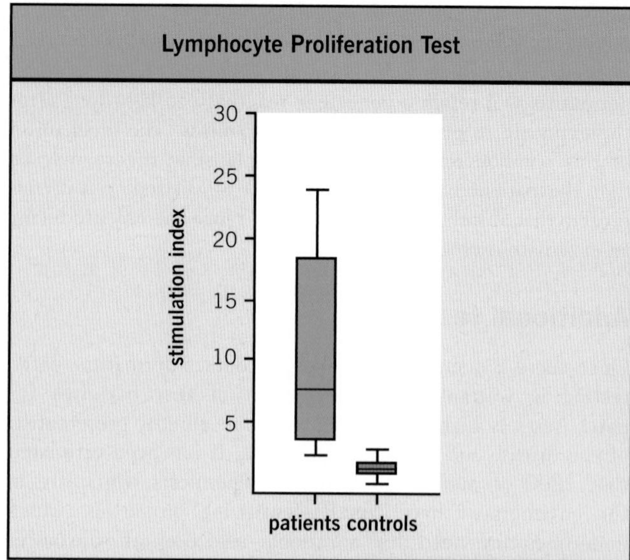

Fig. 7.35 Lymphocyte proliferation (transformation) test with nickel sulfate. The incorporation of labeled thymidine is significantly higher in mononuclear blood leukocytes from patients with a positive patch-test reaction to nickel as compared to cells from control individuals.

Table 7.7 Interpretation of patch-test reactions

Interpretation of Patch-Test Reactions	
?	Doubtful reaction, faint macular erythema only
+	Weak (non-vesicular) positive reaction; erythema, infiltration, possibly papules
+ +	Strong (vesicular) positive reaction; erythema, infiltration, papules, vesicles
+ + +	Extreme positive reaction; bullous reaction
–	Negative reaction
IR	Irritant reaction of different types
NT	Not tested

The identification of a photosensitizer is performed with the photopatch test. Each substance has to be applied at two symmetric sites on the back, as in classic patch-test procedures. One set of the duplicate patches will be irradiated with UVA light whereas the non-irradiated set serves as a control.

For many years there have been efforts to develop more sensitive in vitro tests. Most attention has been paid to the use of lymphocyte stimulation tests to predict cell-mediated hypersensitivity. The sensitivities and specificities of these tests vary with different allergens and technologies. Encouraging results have been published for nickel (Fig. 7.35), chromate, and methylchloroisothiazolinone using sensitive thymidine incorporation assays in some studies. Modified in vitro techniques with a higher specificity and sensitivity are now under study in many laboratories.

MANAGEMENT OF ALLERGIC CONTACT DERMATITIS

General principles

The initial management of all types of suspected allergic contact dermatitis consists of reduction or, if possible, elimination of all suspected allergens and the use of an appropriate-potency topical steroid or – particularly in the face – a topical calcineurin inhibitor to return the skin to a normal state. The use of systemic steroid, such as prednisone in doses of 30 mg or greater daily, will be necessary in the treatment of allergic contact dermatitis which involves more than 30% of the body surface. Once the likely causes of the patient's dermatologic problems have been determined by patch testing, it is very important to communicate this information to the patient in a way that is easy to understand. This involves careful explanation of the material or materials which contain the offending allergen. In some countries the patient gets an 'allergy passport' which usually contains both the designation and information about identified allergens. This information should also be given to other physicians involved as their support will be needed.

Allergen avoidance

Allergen avoidance can be rather simple at times (e.g. topical antibiotics), whilst it can also be virtually impossible at other times (e.g. chromate or nickel). A visit to a patient's place of employment may be necessary to identify an occupational causative substance. Skin protection from chemicals known to cause allergic contact dermatitis is sometimes difficult and barrier creams or gloves should be used whenever possible. The prognosis of allergic contact dermatitis varies depending on the individual's sensitization pattern. Unfortunately, 70% of patients sensitized to ubiquitous allergens will still have some degree of dermatitis after some years, in spite of avoiding substances containing high concentrations of such allergens.

FURTHER READING

Akdis CA, Akdis M, Bieber T, et al. AAAAI/EAACI RACTALL Consensus report. Diagnosis and treatment of atopic dermatitis in children and adults. J Allergy Clin Immunol 2006 (in press).

Akhavan A, Cohen SR. The relationship between atopic dermatitis and contact dermatitis. Clin Dermatol 2003; 21:158–162.

Beltrani VS. Occupational dermatoses. Curr Opin Allergy Clin Immunol 2003; 3:115–123.

Breuer K, Kapp A, Werfel T. Bacterial infections and atopic dermatitis. Allergy 2001; 56:1034–1041.

Breuer K, Werfel T, Kapp A. Safety and efficacy of topical immunomodulators in the treatment of childhood eczema. Am J Clin Dermatol 2005; 6:65–70.

Bruckner AL, Weston WL. Allergic contact dermatitis in children: a practical approach to management. Skin Therapy Lett 2002; 7:3–5.

Cohen DE. Contact dermatitis: a quarter century perspective. J Am Acad Dermatol 2004; 51(suppl 1):S60–63.

Dearman RJ, Kimber I. Factors influencing the induction phase of skin sensitization. Am J Contact Dermatol 2003; 14:188–194.

Fonacier L, Charlesworth EN. Patch testing for allergic contact dermatitis in the allergist office. Curr Allergy Asthma Rep 2003; 3:283–290.

Leung DY, Boguniewicz M, Howell MD, et al. New insights into atopic dermatitis. J Clin Invest 2004; 113:65165–65167.

Nicolas JF. Allergic contact dermatitis. Eur J Dermatol 2004; 14:284–295.

Novak N, Bieber T, Leung DY. Immune mechanisms leading to atopic dermatitis. J Allergy Clin Immunol 2003; 112(suppl 6):S128–139.

Rietschel RL, Fowler JF. Fisher's contact dermatitis. 5th edn. Philadelphia: Lippincott Williams & Wilkins; 2001.

Rycroft RJG, Menne T, Frosch PJ, et al. Textbook of contact dermatitis. 3rd edn. Berlin: Springer; 2001.

Saint–Mezard P, Rosieres A, Krasteva M, et al. Evidence-based diagnosis in patch testing. Contact Dermatitis 2003; 48:121–125.

Schnuch A, Uter W. Decrease in nickel allergy in Germany and regulatory interventions. Contact Dermatitis 2003; 49:107–108.

Werfel T, Breuer B. Role of food allergy in atopic dermatitis. Curr Opin Allergy Clin Immunol 2004; 4:379–385.

Werfel T, Kapp A. Environmental and other major provocation factors in atopic dermatitis. Allergy 1998; 53:731–739.

Werfel T, Kapp A. T-cells in atopic dermatitis. In: Leung D, Bieber T. Atopic dermatitis. St Louis: Marcel Decker; 2002:241–266.

Chapter 8

Gastrointestinal Allergy

Stephan C Bischoff

Definition:
'Gastrointestinal allergy' is a non-toxic, immune-mediated, abnormal reaction of the gastrointestinal tract in response to ingested food protein or any other exogenous antigen causing variable gastrointestinal symptoms such as pharyngeal pruritus, vomiting, abdominal pain, diarrhea, flatulence and malassimilation.

INTRODUCTION

The gastrointestinal (GI) tract as an organ of shock in allergic disease has been studied less extensively than have other organs, such as the respiratory tract, the skin, or the eye. However, there are several lines of evidence suggesting that the GI tract may be of particular relevance for allergic disease, since it may function not only as a shock organ but also as a site of antigen uptake and primary immune response. The mucosal surfaces are more susceptible to antigen penetration than the skin, the keratin layer of which forms an effective barrier for most exogenous antigens. The GI mucosa is challenged daily with thousands of potential allergens, such as food proteins, bacteria, chemicals, and even pollens, which are not only inhaled but also swallowed into the GI tract. In contrast to other mucosal surfaces, the GI mucosa is specialized for the uptake of nutrients and, therefore, the risk of pathologic immune reactions is high. In this chapter, the current knowledge on the mechanism and the clinical management of GI allergy is presented.

CLASSIFICATION OF GASTROINTESTINAL ALLERGY

GI allergy can be classified according to the triggering antigen, the mechanism of immune reaction, or the anatomic site of reaction.

GI allergy may be triggered by food components (e.g. food proteins or glycoproteins), and by other antigens (e.g. bacterial, viral, fungal, and worm antigen), drugs and chemicals, inhaled antigens such as pollens or house dust mites, and any other protein entering the GI tract (Fig. 8.1). Whereas GI food allergy has been studied by several laboratories in the past, our knowledge is limited concerning GI allergy of other agents. For example, only anecdotal information is available on GI allergy induced by allergens derived from infectious agents or inhaled allergens. The GI tract contains bacteria (approximately 100 times more than the skin), pollens, and other inhaled antigens that are usually swallowed in large amounts and persist during their passage through the GI tract. Since most studies on GI allergy are concerned with food allergy, this chapter will focus mainly on this aspect.

GI allergy is defined as an immune-mediated pathologic reaction toward food or other antigens (Fig. 8.2) and it must be distinguished from other forms of adverse reaction to food. In general, adverse reactions to food are divided into toxic and non-toxic reactions. Toxic reactions (e.g. in response to food contaminants such as bacterial toxins or chemicals) will occur in any exposed individual provided that the dose is high enough. The occurrence of non-toxic food reactions depends on individual susceptibility to a certain food. The non-toxic adverse reactions to food are either immune-mediated (food allergy) or not (food intolerance). Food intolerance is subdivided into enzymatic, pharmacologic, and undefined food intolerance. The most important enzymatic food intolerance, which affects large numbers of the adult world population, is the acquired lactose intolerance due to lactase deficiency. Pharmacologic food intolerance is present in individuals who are abnormally reactive to substances, such as vasoactive amines present in some foods. Undefined food intolerance reactions may include reactions to food that induce endogenous histamine release, or to food additives such as dyes, tartrazine, sulfites, benzoates, parabens, antioxidants, salicylates, and glutamate. Such reactions may be based on immune-mediated and non-immune-mediated responses (unspecific mediator release, enzyme inhibition), the mechanisms of which are poorly defined.

GI allergy may affect different sites of the GI tract, leading to a range of clinical symptoms (Table 8.1). Some clinical entities, obviously related to food-induced GI allergy, have been described, such as oral allergy syndrome (OAS) which affects the lips and the mucosa of the pharynx, gluten enteropathy which leads to villus atrophy in the duodenum, and malassimilation, or eosinophilic proctitis in children, which causes stool incontinency and pain. In principle, all sites of the GI tract may be affected by allergy. The factors determining the site of allergy, which is not necessarily the site of antigen uptake, are unknown.

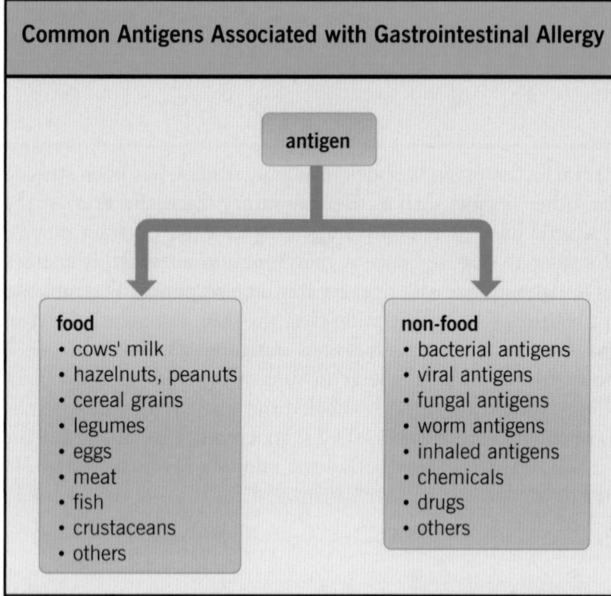

Fig. 8.1 Common antigens associated with gastrointestinal allergy.

ANATOMY AND PHYSIOLOGY OF THE INTESTINE

Anatomy

In general, the GI tract is composed of four concentric layers, which, from the lumen outward, are the mucosa, submucosa, muscularis propria, and serosa (Fig. 8.3). The mucosa consists of the epithelium and the lamina propria, a loose connective tissue rich in immune-competent cells, and the circular muscularis mucosae. The epithelium may invaginate to form

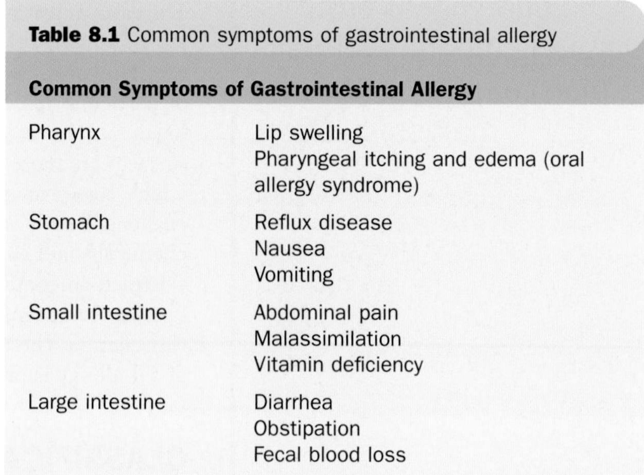

Table 8.1 Common symptoms of gastrointestinal allergy

Common Symptoms of Gastrointestinal Allergy	
Pharynx	Lip swelling Pharyngeal itching and edema (oral allergy syndrome)
Stomach	Reflux disease Nausea Vomiting
Small intestine	Abdominal pain Malassimilation Vitamin deficiency
Large intestine	Diarrhea Obstipation Fecal blood loss

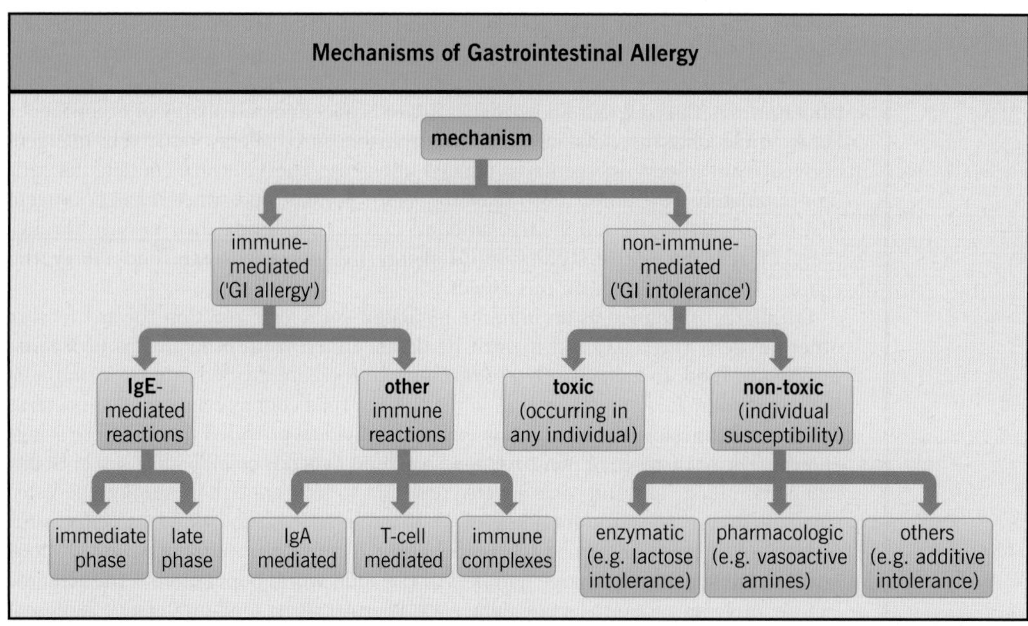

Fig. 8.2 Mechanisms of gastrointestinal allergy.

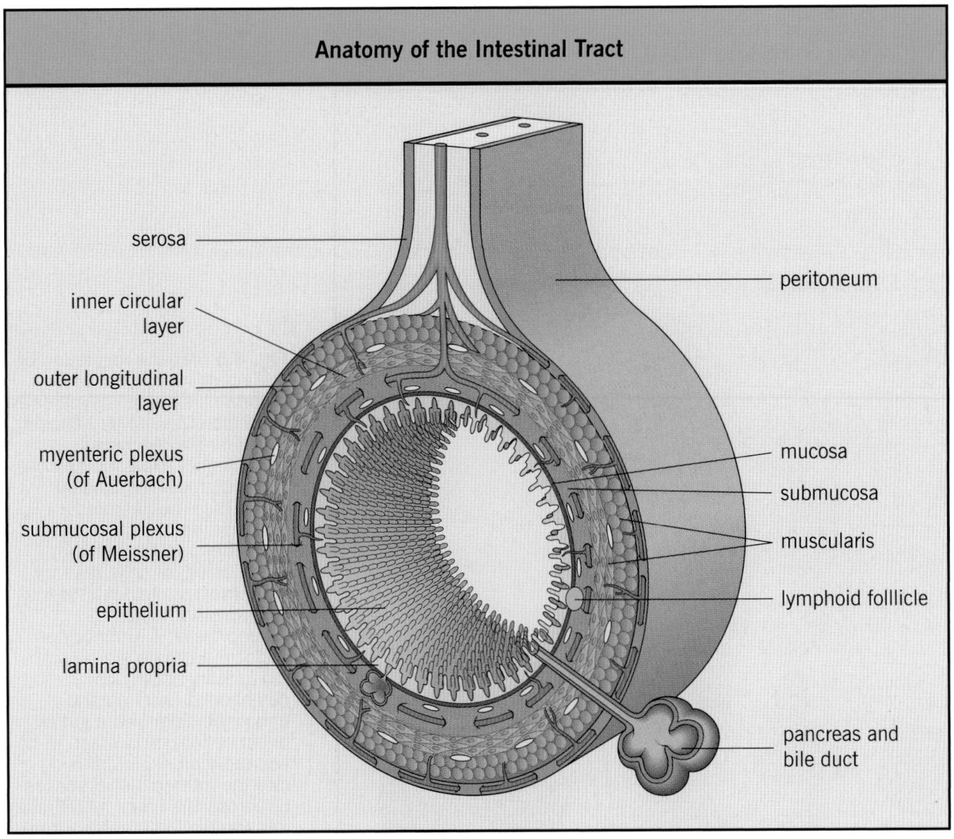

Fig. 8.3 Anatomy of the intestinal wall. The histological anatomy of the small intestine is shown. A similar architecture of the bowel layers is found at other sites of the gastrointestinal tract.

glands or ducts that extend to organs outside the GI tract, such as the pancreas or the liver. The mucosa (and submucosa) may also project into the GI lumen as folds (plicae) or villi. The submucosa is a more densely collagenous, less cellular structure than the mucosa, and contains major blood vessels, lymphatics, nerves, ganglia, and occasionally lymphoid collections. The tunica muscularis consists of at least two muscular layers, the inner circular layer and the outer longitudinal layer. The tunica serosa consists of loose, connective tissue with fat, collagen, and elastic fibers.

Lymphoid tissue

The gut-associated lymphoid tissue (GALT) is primarily located in the lamina propria (Fig. 8.4). It may be present diffusely or as solitary or aggregated nodules, known as Peyer's patches, in the small intestine. Lymphoid follicles surrounded by a plexus of blood vessels and lymphatic capillaries are found in all sections of the GI tract, and contain both B and T lymphocytes. The lymphoid cells form part of the mucosal immune system and secrete IgA as well as other immunoglobulins and cytokines. Lymphocytes are found in the lamina propria [mostly CD4+ helper T cells (Th cells)] and between the epithelial cells (mostly CD8+ T cells). It is believed that both T and B lymphocytes migrate out of the epithelium to the lymphoid follicles where Th cells aid in the differentiation of B cells to antibody-producing plasma cells. T cells also migrate to mesenteric lymph nodes where they proliferate and enter the systemic circulation, returning back to the mucosa as memory T cells. Antigen-presenting cells are predominantly found in Peyer's patches or as scattered cells in the lamina propria. The most efficient antigen sampling occurs in the flattened epithelial cells overlying lymphoid aggregates.

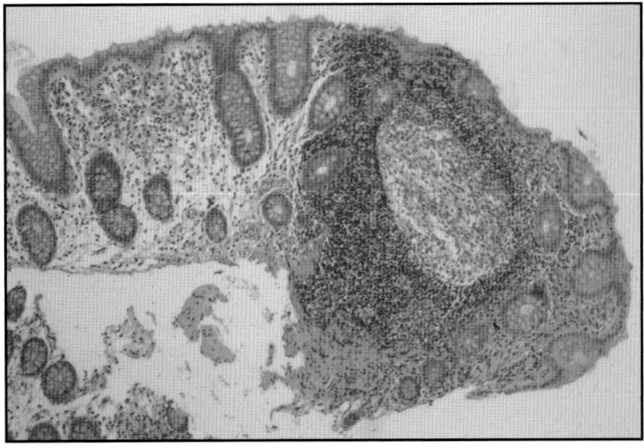

Fig. 8.4 Gut-associated lymphoid tissue. A large lymphoid follicle can be seen in the mucosa of the cecum. (Hematoxylin and eosin stain, original magnification × 100.)

The M cell, which is an epithelial cell with microfolds, endocytoses macromolecules and transports them to the basolaterally located intraepithelial lymphocytes. Mucosal plasma cells produce predominantly IgA and IgM antibodies. The Ig monomers are linked by J chains to dimeric secretory IgA or pentameric IgM, which bind to the secretory component, a

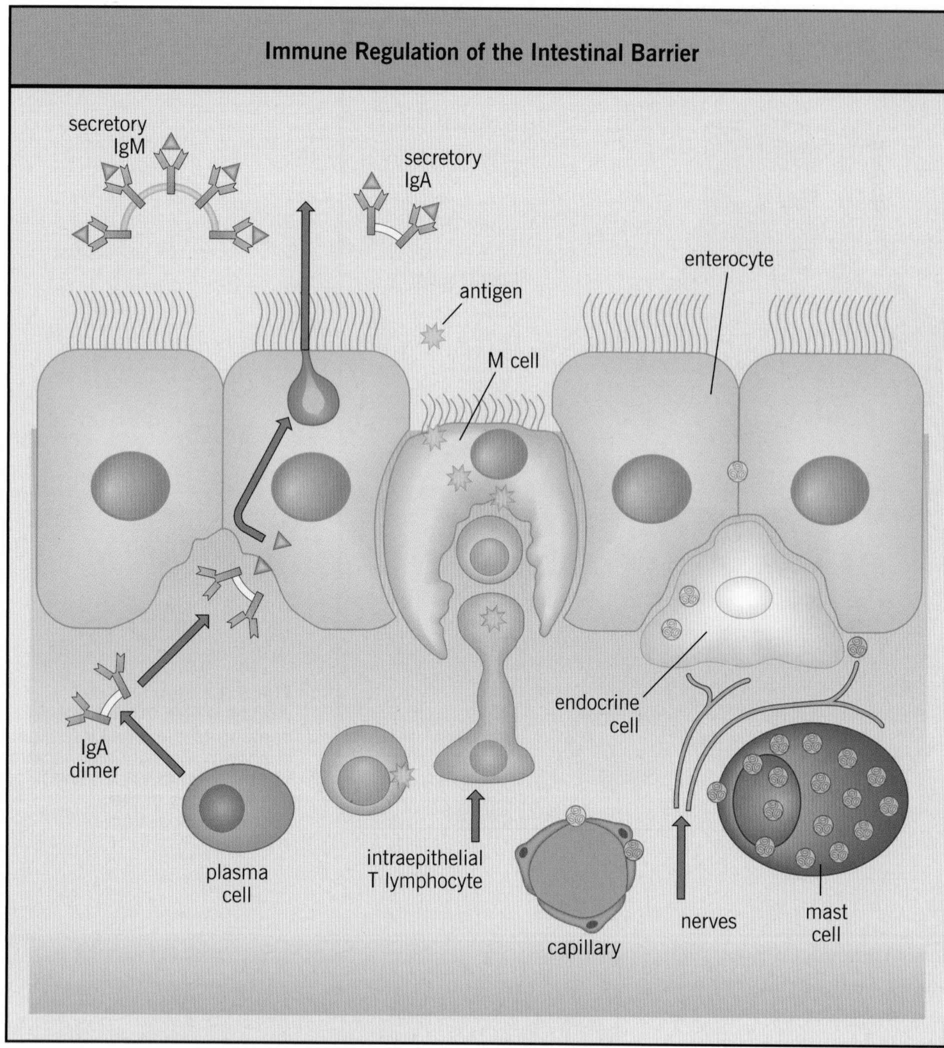

Fig. 8.5 Immune regulation of the intestinal barrier. Lamina propria plasma cells synthesize IgA dimers (linked by J chains), which bind to secretory components expressed on the basal surface of epithelial cells. They are secreted together into the gut lumen. Pentameric IgM is similarly transported. M cells take up and process luminal antigens for presentation to intraepithelial T lymphocytes. Endocrine cells exert a local modulatory activity on neighboring exocrine and endocrine cells of the gut by direct cell-to-cell contact, or by secretory products diffusing into the interepithelial spaces or across the basal membrane into the lamina propria, where they affect nerve endings, blood vessels, and smooth muscles. Mast-cell-release mediators, such as histamine, cause contraction of the muscularis mucosae and blood vessels, modulation of lymphocyte function, and increase of mucus secretion and permeability.

receptor on glandular epithelial cells that mediates the transport of IgA and IgM to the lumen. IgG and IgE are secreted into the lumen as monomers and the majority diffuse directly into the lymphatics. Apart from lymphocytes, other hematopoietic cells found in the GI tissue, particularly in the small and large bowel, are eosinophil granulocytes (4–6% of the lamina propria cells), neutrophil granulocytes (rare in non-inflamed GI tissue), monocytes, mast cells (2–3% of lamina propria cells), and various types of endocrine cells producing hormones and neurotransmitters, such as somatostatin, vasoactive intestinal polypeptide, serotonin, motilin, and substance P (Fig. 8.5).

Innervation

The enteric nervous system (ENS) is the most complex portion of the peripheral nervous system. It differs from the sympathetic and parasympathetic division of the autonomous nervous system because most of its component neurons do not receive direct input from the brain or the spinal cord. Therefore, it can mediate reflex activity independently of the central nervous system (Fig. 8.6). The ENS contains integrative circuiting, consisting of interneurons within the ganglia that process information from intramural and mucosal sensory receptors (e.g. fluidity, volume, chemical composition, and temperature of luminal contents) and, via the motoneurons, programs the appropriate behavior of the effector system. The majority of the neurons from the submucosal ganglia project into the mucosa. Sympathetic ganglia are external to the gut wall lying in the celiac plexus as well as in the superior and inferior mesenteric plexus.

Neurons of the parasympathetic ganglia are located in the submucosal plexus (Meissner's plexus) and in the myenteric plexus (Auerbach's plexus) lying between the circular and longitudinal layers of the tunica muscularis propria. The myenteric plexus generates the basic electrical rhythm of the gut, but it is not necessary for propagation of the interdigestive myoelectric complex. However, Meissner's and Auerbach's plexuses are interconnected into a single functional system. Stimulation of the parasympathetic neurons usually increases circulation, secretion, and muscular activity, whereas stimulation of the sympathetic system has the reverse effects.

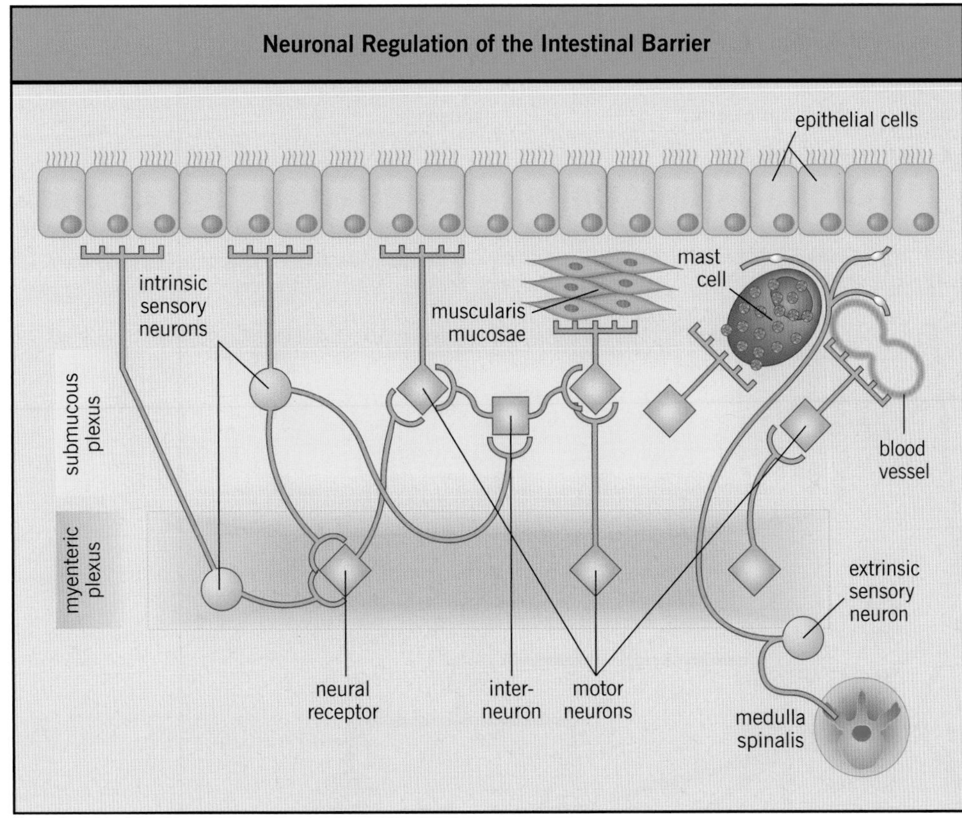

Fig. 8.6 Neuronal regulation of the intestinal barrier. Diagram showing the presence of intrinsic (within the gut wall) and extrinsic (paravertebral neuronal cell bodies) sensory neurons and motor neurons regulating the function of epithelial cells, smooth muscles, blood vessels, and mast cells. Motor neurons are interconnected by interneurons forming a largely autonomous enteric nervous system.

PATHOGENESIS OF GASTROINTESTINAL ALLERGY

Pathophysiology

The exact mechanisms of GI allergy are not clear at present. However, evidence comes from clinical and basic science studies suggesting that both IgE-dependent and IgE-independent mechanisms may be involved in the pathophysiology of GI hypersensitivity reactions.

Two phases of IgE-mediated allergic reactions have been distinguished:

- the sensitization phase, characterized by the induction of specific IgE against particular antigens in genetically predisposed individuals; and
- the effector phase, often occurring months or years later.

The effector phase is initiated by re-exposure to antigen and, like other allergic reactions, consists of an immediate and a late-phase response. In the immediate reaction, mediated by tissue mast cell mediators including histamine and leukotrienes, there is an increase in vascular permeability, muscle contraction, edema, and electrolyte secretion. These result in clinical symptoms such as nausea, cramps, or diarrhea, but no significant histologic changes. The immediate reaction may be followed by a late-phase reaction occurring approximately 4–24 hours later. This is characterized by tissue infiltration with inflammatory cells including eosinophils and mononuclear cells. In other tissues it has been recognized that the late-phase reaction is of particular relevance to tissue damage, organ dysfunction, and perpetuation of clinical symptoms. It is tempting to speculate that similar mechanisms occur in the GI mucosa, although cytotoxic tissue damage caused by allergy remains to be confirmed in vivo.

GI allergy and food allergy may be recognized as a breakdown of natural oral tolerance against food and other self or non-self antigens. The pathogenesis of oral tolerance is not well understood. However, several mechanisms have been implicated in oral tolerance induction, such as antigen-driven suppression, clonal anergy, and clonal deletion. Antigen-specific oral tolerance may depend on a genetic background, the means and amount of antigen administration, and the way the antigen is processed and presented to immune-competent cells. It is known that minor amounts of protein antigen reach the circulation in an undegraded state. Achlorhydria and reduced mucosal barrier function have been found to increase macromolecular absorption without clear evidence of an increased risk of developing GI allergy. According to Strobel, pathologic immune responses can be prevented by immune exclusion (mucus layer, secretory IgA, and IgM), by immune elimination (innate immune defense mechanisms, such as complement and phagocytosis), and by immune regulation (adaptive immune defense and oral tolerance). Oral tolerance may be related to the following hypothetical mechanism: luminal antigen is usually processed by GI epithelial cells and presented directly to T cells via the T-cell receptor (TCR)/CD3 complex. A secondary co-stimulatory signal via the CD28/CD8 or the CD40/CD40 receptor ligand complexes is not provided, and, therefore, the T cell receives a tolerogenic signal. Alternatively, antigen that bypasses processing by the enterocytes will be presented by conventional antigen-presenting cells (e.g. macrophages, dendritic cells) to T cells in association with class II major

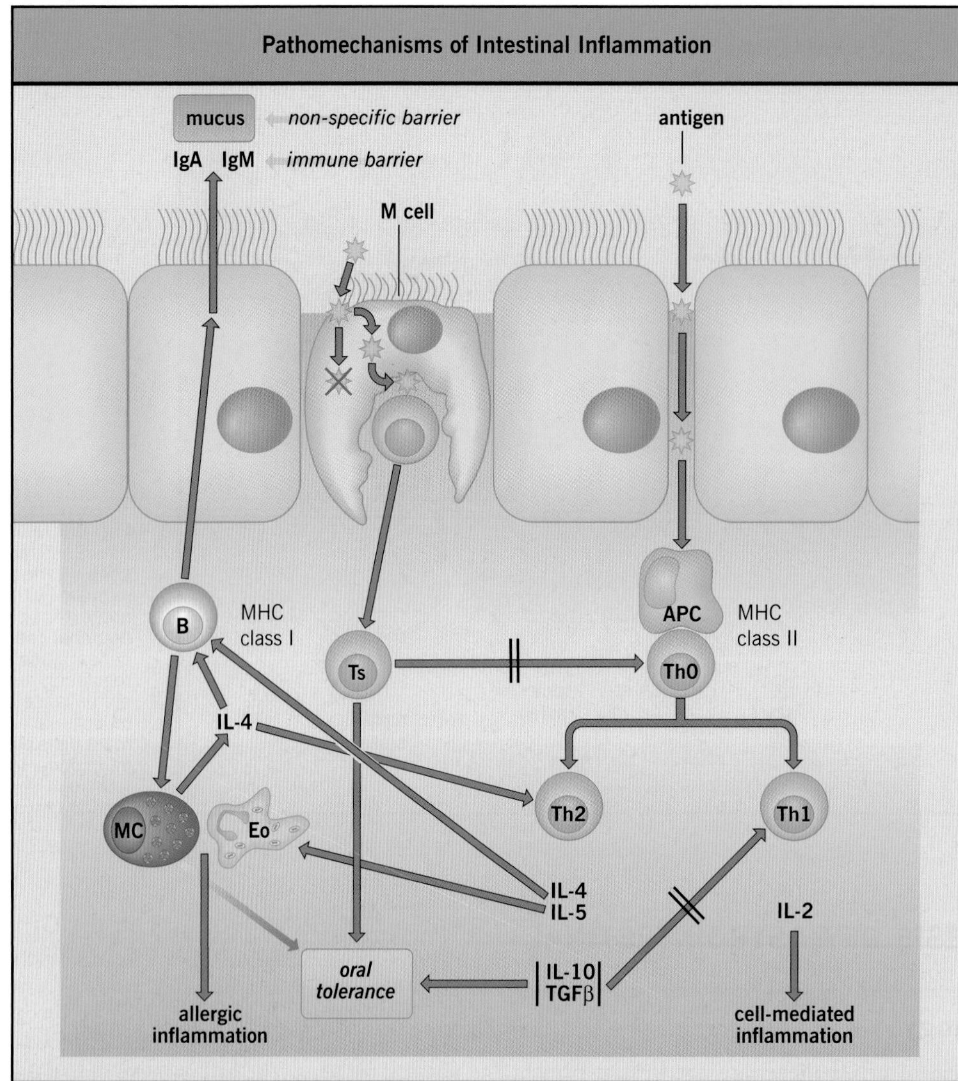

Fig. 8.7 Pathomechanisms of intestinal inflammation (hypothesis). Possible mechanisms of allergic inflammation in the gastrointestinal tract are based on current hypotheses on hypersensitivity reactions and oral tolerance. In a normal situation, luminal proteins (antigens) are digested and hardly enter the tissue due to non-specific (e.g. mucus) and immune (e.g. luminal IgA and IgM) barriers; or, after uptake by M cells, processing, and presentation to intraepithelial cells and CD8+ lamina propria T-suppressor cells (Ts), oral tolerance results. However, the immune response can be polarized if antigens bypass the epithelial processing and are presented by conventional antigen-presenting cells (APC) to CD4+ lamina propria helper T cells (Th0). After activation, T-helper cells may predominantly release either interleukin-2 (IL-2) and interferon γ (INFγ) (Th1), or IL-4 and IL-5 (Th2). Th1 cells induce cell-mediated hypersensitivity and inflammation. Cytokines of Th2 cells induce IgE synthesis and eosinophil infiltration leading to IgE-mediated hypersensitivity and inflammation. On the other hand, Th2 cell-derived cytokines, such as IL-10, may be involved in downregulation of Th1 responses and inflammation, and, by the release of transforming growth factor β (TGFβ) may support the development of oral tolerance.

histocompatibility complex (MHC) molecules. The latter may cause local or systemic immune responses rather than suppression, and finally lead to GI allergy. T cells with suppressive activity have been identified in the intestinal mucosa, mesenteric lymph nodes, and spleen after ingesting an antigen. Such T cells are of CD8+ phenotype; they secrete transforming growth factor β (TGFβ) (which may act on other immune cells and induce bystander suppression in naive cells) and interleukin-10 (IL-10) (which downregulates inflammatory reactions), and they can transfer oral tolerance from one organism to another. These findings, derived mainly from animal models, have to be confirmed for humans. The current hypotheses on the pathomechanisms of allergic inflammation and the induction of oral tolerance are summarized in Figure 8.7.

Several risk factors for the breakdown of oral tolerance and development of GI allergy have been suggested, such as genetic predisposition (e.g. predominance of Th type 2 (Th2) lymphocytes, increased production of IL-4 and IL-5, or enhanced mast cell releasability), lack of protective factors (e.g. IgA deficiency, decreased suppressive factors, or suppressive CD8+ lymphocytes), and increased antigen resorption (e.g. increased intestinal permeability and loss of mucosal integrity caused by intestinal infections or inflammatory bowel disease (IBD), drugs, or nutrients such as alcohol, nicotine, and spices).

Inflammatory cells and mediators

The most relevant effector cells of GI allergy, as in immediate allergic reactions at other mucosal membranes, are mast cells and eosinophil granulocytes. The biology and mediator generation of these cells is described in Chapter 21. Of particular relevance to GI allergies is exposure of mast cells in the intestinal mucosa to relatively high levels of food, bacterial, or other antigens. Furthermore, suggestions have been made that the function of intestinal mast cells, in particular, may be influenced by neuronal reflexes. With the eosinophil, the presence of extracellular secretory IgA may influence the cell in two ways. First, it provides a source of IgA to arm the eosinophil for activation. Second, the secretory chain of IgA is capable of binding IL-8, causing conversion from a cytokine which primarily attracts neutrophils, to one which attracts eosinophils.

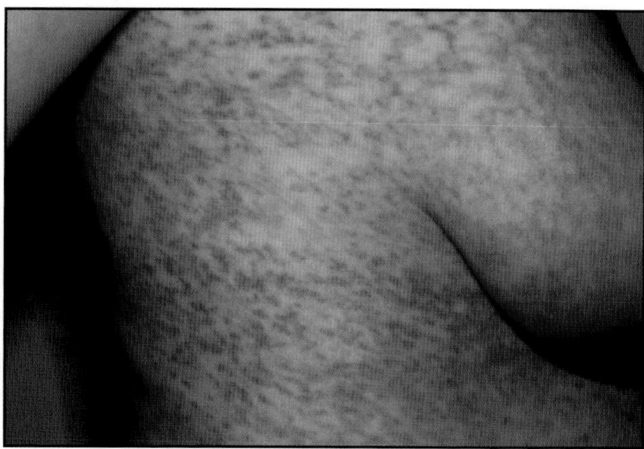

Fig. 8.8 Mastocytosis. Cutaneous manifestation of systemic mastocytosis (urticaria pigmentosa). The patient also suffered from gastrointestinal mastocytosis and hypersensitivity reactions against multiple food allergens.

DIAGNOSIS OF GASTROINTESTINAL ALLERGY AND FOOD INTOLERANCE

History

The first scientific report on the ability to transfer allergy in the serum involved the use of a food allergen. A small amount of serum was transferred from a Dr C Küstner, a fish-allergic individual, to the non-allergic Dr H Prausnitz. Subsequent challenge of Dr Prausnitz resulted in a wheal-and-flare reaction at the site of serum injection. This study, the Prausnitz–Küstner or PK-reaction, was published in 1921.

During the next three decades increasing numbers of cases of allergic reactions to foods were described, and the spectrum of clinical abnormalities in these cases was broadened to include reactions that were often slower in onset and involved solely the GI tract, skin, or respiratory system. However, the diagnoses were usually based on the case history alone and improvement in the condition was made subsequent to elimination of the suspected allergen from the diet. Gruskay and Cooke found, in 1955, that particularly high levels of unaltered food protein could be found in the blood of children recovering from diarrhea and, to a lesser extent, in healthy individuals. The discovery of IgA in 1953 by Heremans, secretory IgA in 1961 by Hanson, and IgE in 1969 by Ishizaka, Johansson, and their co-workers formed the basis of modern allergology and immunology. In the 1970s the pivotal role of human intestinal lymphocytes (belonging to the GALT) in mucosal immunity was recognized. During the last decade, many functions of intestinal T cells and B cells, monocytes, and epithelial cells, as well as their regulation by a complex network of cytokines, adhesion molecules, and neuroimmune interactions, have been unraveled. However, the function of other intestinal cells such as mast cells and eosinophils is still largely unknown and our knowledge of the mechanisms of GI allergy and oral tolerance is mostly hypothetical. Subsequently, the means for clinical management, diagnosis, and treatment of patients suffering from GI food allergy and other forms of GI hypersensitivity are still unsatisfactory.

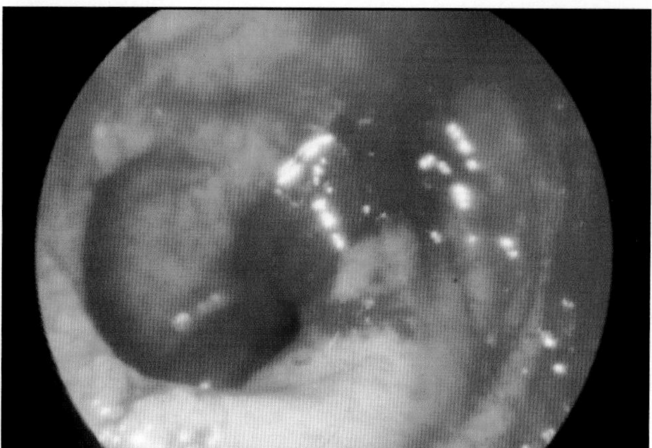

Fig. 8.9 Eosinophilic enterocolitis: macroscopic findings. Endoscopic view of the mucosa of the small intestine (ileum). Note the severe mucosal inflammation with mucosal thickening, loss of normal mucosal surface, and spontaneous bleeding of the mucosa. The photograph was taken from a patient with eosinophilic enterocolitis due to intestinal hypersensitivity reactions toward multiple food allergens.

Symptom presentation

The symptoms of food allergy manifesting in the GI tract are variable and, to a large extent, unspecific. Depending on the site of mucosal reaction and the type of allergic reaction, the patient may suffer from: swelling of the lips, pharyngeal itching, and laryngeal edema (oral allergy syndrome); reflux, nausea, and vomiting (gastric reactions); abdominal pain, malassimilation, and vitamin deficiency (small intestine); and diarrhea, obstipation, and fecal blood loss (colon and rectum). Macroscopic or histologic evidence for inflammatory infiltration and tissue destruction is facultative and may be related to late-phase or delayed-type hypersensitivity reactions. In some cases, intestinal food allergy is accompanied by histologic findings typical for intestinal mastocytosis, eosinophilic gastroenteritis, or celiac disease (Figs 8.8–8.12). Typically, the lamina propria is infiltrated with high numbers of eosinophils in patients with active GI allergy (see Fig. 8.10). In rare cases, GI allergy may cause a total loss of intact intestinal mucosa and, therefore, severe malassimilation, thus making oral nutrition almost impossible (see Fig. 8.11).

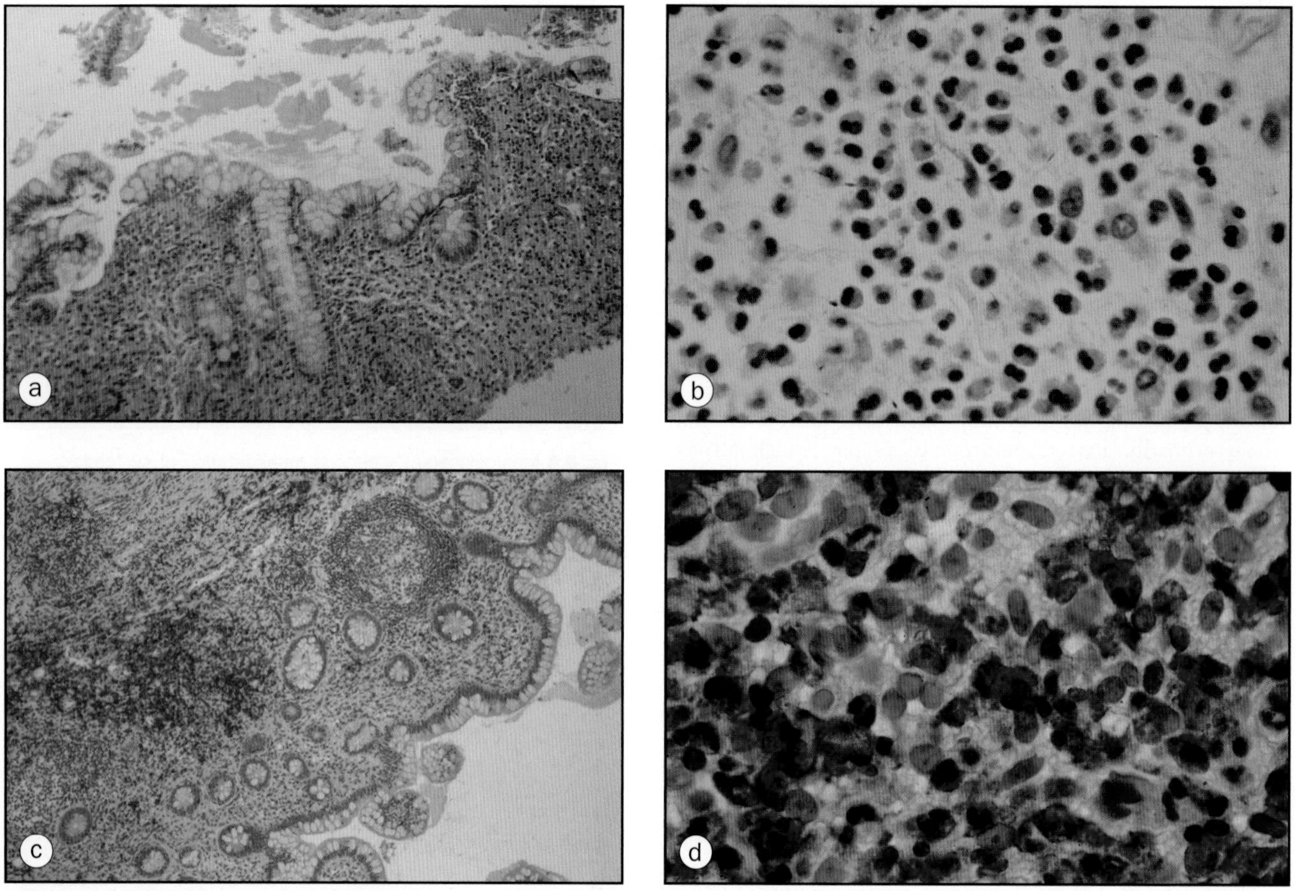

Fig. 8.10 Eosinophilic enterocolitis: histologic findings. Large bowel sections (same patient as in Fig. 8.9). (a) Mucosal destruction and cell infiltration (hematoxylin and eosin stain, × 100). (b) Eosinophilia in the submucosa (hematoxylin and eosin stain, × 500). (c) Immunohistochemical staining using an antibody directed against eosinophil cationic protein stored in the granules of eosinophils (EG2 monoclonal antibody stain, × 100). (d) Same as (c) (× 1000).

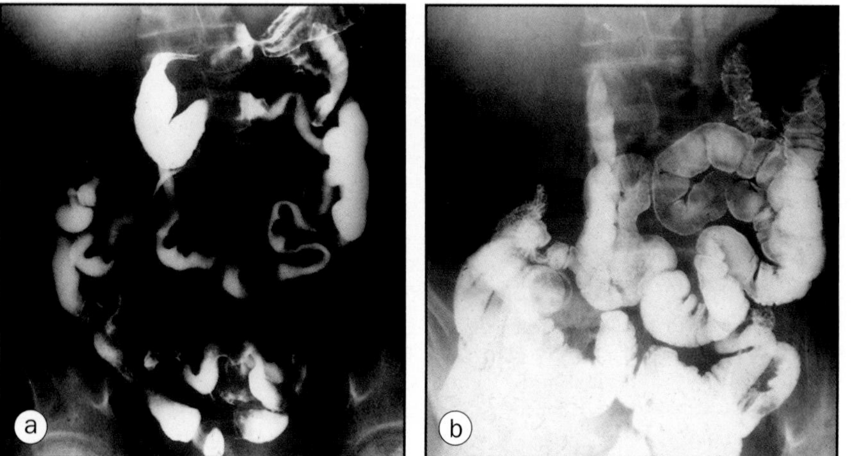

Fig. 8.11 Eosinophilic enterocolitis: radiologic findings. X-ray photographs of the small intestine after barium contrast filling (same patient as in Fig. 8.9). (a) Complete loss of normal intestinal mucosa. At that time, the patient suffered from malassimilation syndrome, excessive weight loss, and anemia. (b) Almost normal mucosa after 8 months of total food allergen avoidance (home-parenteral nutrition). At that time, the patient started to eat following an individual elimination diet without recurrence of the initial symptoms.

The time interval between food challenge and onset of clinical symptoms may vary from a few minutes to many hours. In general, early reactions, occurring within minutes, involve the upper part of the GI tract (e.g. lips, pharynx, stomach, duodenum), whereas late reactions starting after several hours (or days) are often related to the small or large intestine. Early reactions are more frequently IgE-mediated (type I hypersensitivity reactions) and can be readily diagnosed by skin tests or measurements of specific serum IgE. In contrast, delayed reactions are often based on other mechanisms and are much more difficult to confirm on an objective basis. Early IgE-mediated reactions, but not delayed reactions, are frequently associated with atopy (allergic rhinoconjunctivitis, extrinsic asthma, atopic relatives etc.). The relationship between GI

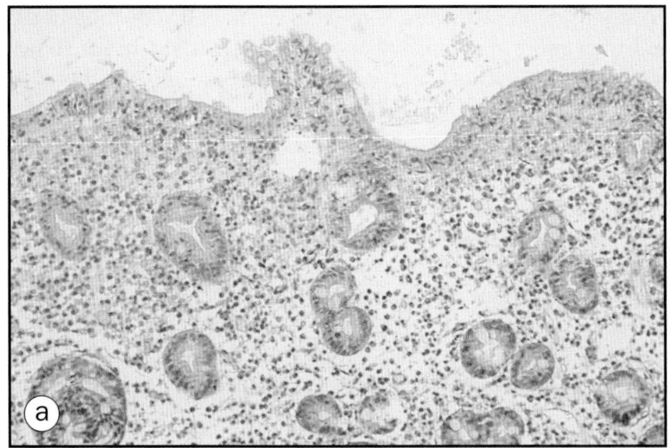

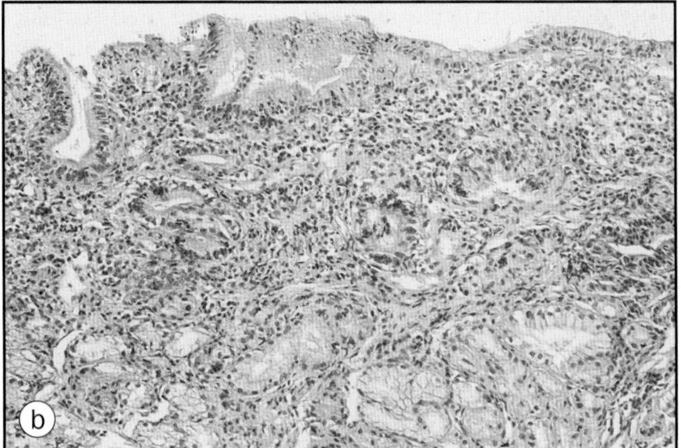

Fig. 8.12 Celiac disease. Two examples of duodenal tissue sections derived from patients with active celiac disease (a), (b). See the complete loss of mucosal villi and dense infiltration of the lamina propria with mononuclear cells and eosinophils. (Courtesy of Rolf Rüdiger Meliβ, Institute of Pathology, Medical School of Hannover, Germany.)

allergy and other chronic idiopathic diseases of the gut, such as eosinophilic enterocolitis (see Figs 8.9–8.11), celiac disease (see Fig. 8.12), IBD, and irritable bowel syndrome (IBS), is unclear at present. Evidence comes from clinical and pathophysiologic observations that such a relationship may exist, at least in subsets of afflicted individuals, and, therefore, GI allergy should be considered in the differential diagnosis of chronic inflammatory or functional GI diseases of unclear origin.

The prevalence of food allergy is largely unknown. It has been estimated that, depending on the methods used for diagnosis, 1–4% of the general population suffer from food allergy or food intolerance reactions. A population study of food intolerance in adults, published by Young et al in 1994, reported a prevalence of 1.4% based on a questionnaire involving 20 000 individuals who had taken oral-food-challenge tests. Of the individuals testing positive in the food-challenge test 28% had intestinal symptoms. In children, during their first 3 years, the prevalence of GI food allergy may be somewhat higher (2–4%). On the other hand, it has been repeatedly reported that 20–45% of the general population believe that they suffer from adverse reactions to food, indicating the necessity of objective diagnostic means.

Physical examination

The patient's history (in particular the onset of disease, the type of symptoms, the time interval between food ingestion and onset of symptoms, the dietetic regimens, and history of atopy) as well as the patient's physical examination must be recorded carefully. This is particularly important because of the lack of specific clinical symptoms and laboratory tests indicating GI allergy and, therefore, the diagnosis of GI allergy to foods or other antigens is largely based on the exclusion of other diseases. Physical examination includes a general examination of major body functions as well as specific examinations, such as inspection of the skin, the oral cavity, and the pharynx, the palpation and percussion of the abdomen, and the digital examination of the rectum. However, normal findings in physical examinations do not exclude GI (food) allergy.

Additional tests

In order to exclude other GI diseases, additional apparative diagnostic means are required, such as endoscopy of the upper and lower GI tract; histologic examinations of GI biopsies; radiologic examinations; laboratory tests; microbiologic examinations of serum, intestinal liquids, biopsies, and feces; and stool analyses for parameters of malassimilation. In principle, infectious diseases, IBDs (e.g. Crohn's disease, ulcerative colitis), celiac disease, and tumor disease of the GI tract have to be excluded. Therefore, classic gastroenterologic means and tests for the presence of GI allergy have to be combined to confirm GI allergy on an objective basis (Table 8.2).

Tests for the presence of gastrointestinal allergy

Laboratory parameters indicating GI (food) allergy are lacking and skin tests are known to be of limited value in confirming or excluding the diagnosis. The measurement of total IgE in serum may predict atopy, but it has no value in the confirmation of allergic disease. Negative skin tests and absence of specific serum IgE against food protein [negative radioallergosorbent (RAST) or similar test systems] may confirm the absence of IgE-mediated reactions, but the positive predictive accuracy of these tests is low. The clinical value of these tests is further limited by the fact that IgE-mediated sensitivity is frequently not detected with commercially prepared reagents, because of the lability of the allergen responsible. Moreover, it has been suggested in several studies that allergic reactions to food are not necessarily IgE-mediated. For example, it has been shown that patients with food allergy, confirmed by oral challenges, had intestinal mast cells that released histamine when challenged with food antigen in vitro or in vivo, but skin tests and RASTs were positive in only about 50% of these patients. This implies that local IgE production may explain some GI hypersensitivities not generally considered to be IgE-mediated. Nevertheless, skin tests and RAST should be performed in patients with suspected GI food allergy for two purposes: they may raise evidence for atopy or atopic diseases within or outside the GI tract, and they may be useful in patients suffering from IgE-mediated, immediate-type GI allergy. In patients testing positive for particular food allergens, the skin test and RAST may aid selection of relevant allergens for further testing (e.g. by provocation tests).

Laboratory tests other than skin tests and RAST have been developed, although most of them have not been thoroughly

Table 8.2 Diagnosis of gastrointestinal allergy

Diagnosis of Gastrointestinal Allergy	
History	Symptoms Atopy Other disease
Gastroenterological examination	Endoscopy (gastroduodenoscopy, colonoscopy) Sonograph of the abdomen X-ray examinations of the gastrointestinal tract Malassimilation tests Histology of biopsy specimens
Laboratory studies	Routine laboratory parameters Microbiologic examinations (serum, titers, feces) Serum IgE and specific IgE (RAST) Eosinophil-derived cationic proteins in serum and feces (EPX) Basophil histamine-release test (BHR) Cellular allergen stimulation test (CAST)
Provocation tests	Skin prick tests Elimination diet and stepwise rechallenge Double-blind placebo-controlled food challenges (DBPCFC) Colonoscopic allergen provocation test (COLAP)
Probative treatment	Disodium cromoglycate Enteral nutrition (chemically defined tube feeling) Total parenteral nutrition

EPX, eosinophil protein X; RAST, radioallergosorbent test.

validated for clinical sensitivity and specificity. For example, IgE, IgA, and IgG4 have been quantified in serum and feces, but a pathogenic role for these antibodies has not been conclusively demonstrated. Tests such as the basophil histamine release (BHR) test and the cellular allergen stimulation test (CAST) may be used. In both assays, peripheral blood leukocytes containing basophils are challenged with allergen extracts and subsequently histamine (BHR) or leukotrienes (CAST) are quantified in the cell supernatants. The sensitivity and specificity of both tests compared to controlled-food challenges are comparable to the skin prick test and RAST. A major advantage of BHR and CAST is that freshly prepared extracts of labile foods can be used, but it has to be considered that 5–10% of the population have circulating basophils unresponsive to in vitro challenges. Intestinal mast cell histamine release (IMCHR), performed by adding food antigen to dispersed mast cells, was shown to correlate most closely with oral food challenge results in patients experiencing only GI symptoms when compared with skin prick tests, RAST, and BHR test.

Another approach is to diagnose or monitor GI allergy independently of IgE using the measurement of eosinophil-derived cationic proteins, such as eosinophil cationic protein (ECP) and eosinophil protein X (EPX). Increased serum ECP levels were found in children with food hypersensitivity. Even more interesting could be the quantification of ECP and EPX in stool samples, because it reflects eosinophil activation in the GI tract more accurately than serum measurements, as shown recently by Bischoff and colleagues. In search of additional parameters indicating GI allergy, or at least a predisposition for developing GI hypersensitivity reactions, different groups have demonstrated increased permeability of the GI tract to probes of various sizes, such as polyethylene glycol or ratios of sugars, such as mannitol and lactulose or rhamnose. Unfortunately, intestinal permeability varies widely among healthy individuals as well as among food-sensitive patients, resulting in large overlaps between the groups. However, changes in intestinal permeability before or after challenge have repeatedly been demonstrated to correlate with the results of challenge tests.

Provocation studies

The double-blind placebo-controlled oral-food-challenge (DBPCFC) test and the methods of exclusion diet and rechallenge have been proposed as gold standards for the confirmation of food allergy. The diagnostic dietetic regimens cover allergen avoidance (e.g. water–rice diet, hydrolyzed proteins, elemental diet, or total parenteral nutrition) and allergen search diets in which the patient is first put on an allergen-free diet (e.g. water–rice diet) and then challenged stepwise (8–12 steps, each for 2–3 days) with different groups of food proteins. An example is shown in Table 8.3. Together with the diet, patients record their symptoms in a diary booklet. The allergen search diet has several disadvantages, such as the risk of anaphylaxis (therefore the patient must generally be hospitalized), the time requirements (16–36 days), and the lack of controlled studies indicating the sensitivity and specificity of the test procedure. The DBPCFC has been used successfully by a number of investigators, in both children and adults, to examine a variety of food-related complaints. However, the test is limited because:

- only one or a few allergens can be tested;
- the test has the risk of systemic anaphylactic reactions;
- underlying pathogenic mechanisms cannot be studied by this test; and, most importantly,
- the interpretation of results may be difficult depending on the kind and the time course of occurrence of symptoms.

In particular for GI manifestations of food allergy, the interpretation of the DBPCFC is difficult, because the read-out system is poorly defined and it is dependent on the patients' subjectivity of their symptoms following oral challenge.

To overcome the limitations of the DBPCFC, Bischoff and co-workers developed a new diagnostic approach for intestinal food allergy, the colonoscopic allergen provocation test (COLAP test). Local provocation tests are established for the nasal, conjunctival, and bronchial mucosa, their value in confirming the diagnosis of allergic disease and in identifying relevant allergens being well-recognized. A few attempts have been made to develop similar tests for the GI mucosa [e.g. intragastral provocation under endoscopic control (IPEC) proposed by Reimann et al], but they could not be established for clinical practice. In the COLAP test, the cecal mucosa is challenged endoscopically with three food antigen extracts selected according to patient history, skin tests, and RAST (Fig. 8.13). The mucosal wheal-and-flare reaction is registered semiquantitatively 20 minutes after challenge. The COLAP test has been performed in adult patients with abdominal symptoms suspected to be related to food allergy, and in healthy volunteers.

Table 8.3 Allergen search diet

Step	Principle	Examples
Allergen Search Diet		
1	Allergen-free diet	Rice, potatoes, sunflower oil, salt, white sugar, water
2	Milk and milk products	Milk, butter, cheese, cottage cheese, yoghurt
3	Cereals	Wheat (bread, rolls, noodles), oats, maize, honey, yeast
4	Vegetables and legumes	Tomatoes, carrots, broccoli, celery, peanuts, soya, garlic
5	Eggs and poultry	Eggs, omelette, chicken, turkey
6	Meat	Pork, beef, lamb
7	Fruit and nuts	Apple, strawberry, peach, cherry, kiwi fruit, hazelnut, walnut
8	Fish and shellfish	Codfish, shrimps
9	Spices and herbs	Pepper, paprika, oregano, curry, caraway, mustard
10	Additives, preservatives	Ready-to-serve meals, frozen foods, wine, beer, coffee

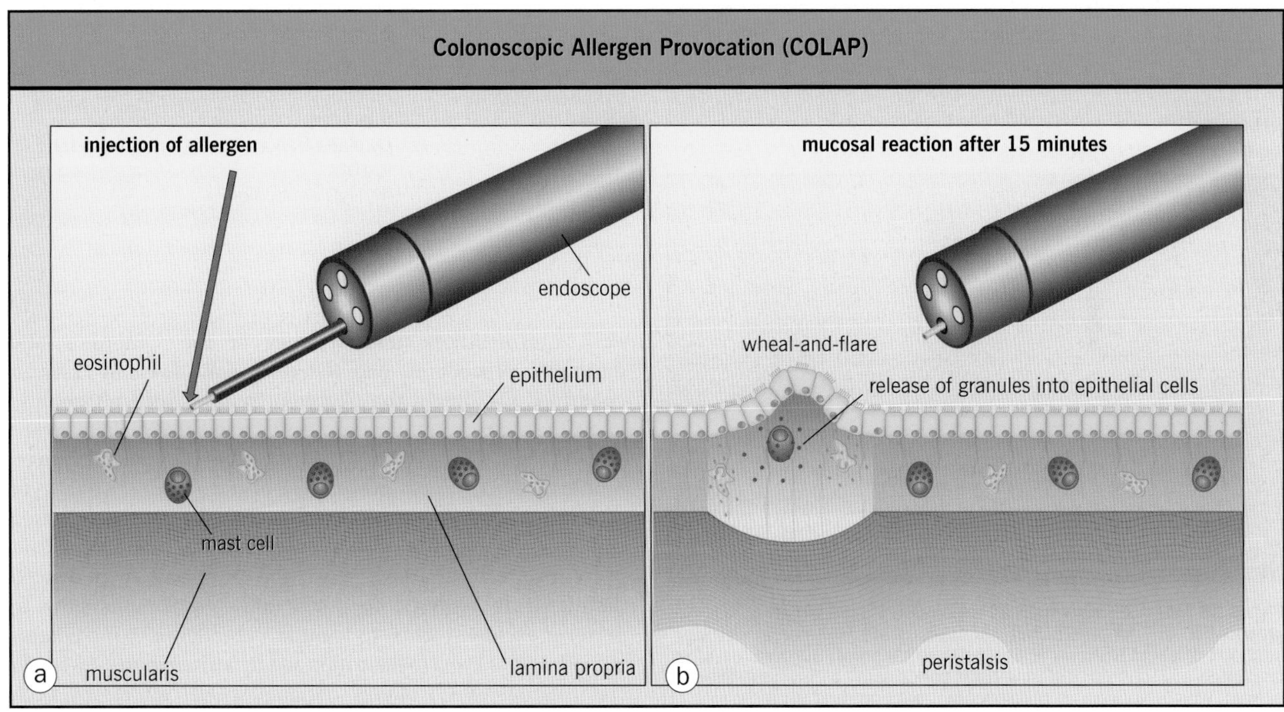

Fig. 8.13 (a) Technique of colonoscopic allergen provocation. Allergen extracts are injected into the intestinal mucosa by a fine needle during colonoscopy. (b) After 15 minutes, a mucosal wheal-and-flare reaction, accompanied by mast cell and eosinophil degranulation and increased peristalsis, can be observed in cases reacting positively toward the administered allergen.

Half of the selected antigens cause a significant wheal-and-flare reaction of the mucosa in patients, whereas no reaction in response to antigen is observed in healthy volunteers (Fig. 8.14). Antigen-induced wheal-and-flare reactions are related to the patient's history of adverse reactions to food, but not to serum levels of specific IgE or skin test results. No severe systemic anaphylactic reactions have been observed in response to intestinal challenge. It has been found that antigen-induced wheal-and-flare reactions are closely correlated with intestinal mast cell and eosinophil activation (Fig. 8.15). The studies suggest that the COLAP test may be a useful diagnostic means in patients with suspected intestinal food allergy and a new tool for the study of the mechanisms of GI allergy and oral tolerance.

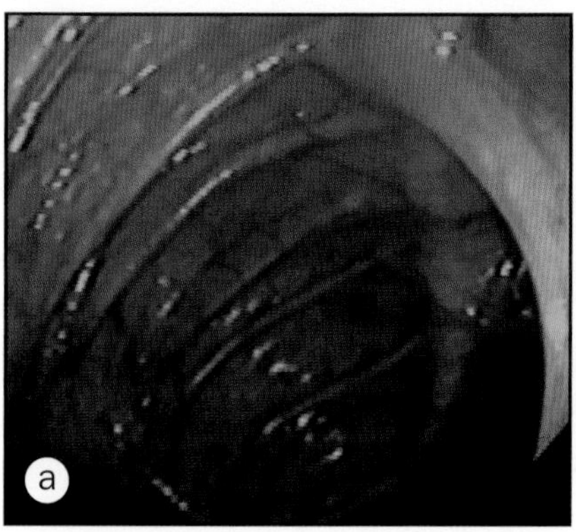

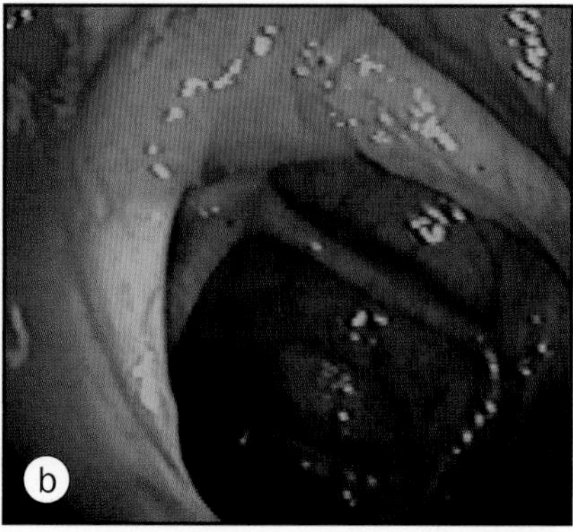

Fig. 8.14 Mucosal reaction after colonoscopic allergen provocation. (a) Normal mucosa before challenge. (b) Mucosal reaction 15 minutes after administration of milk allergen extract.

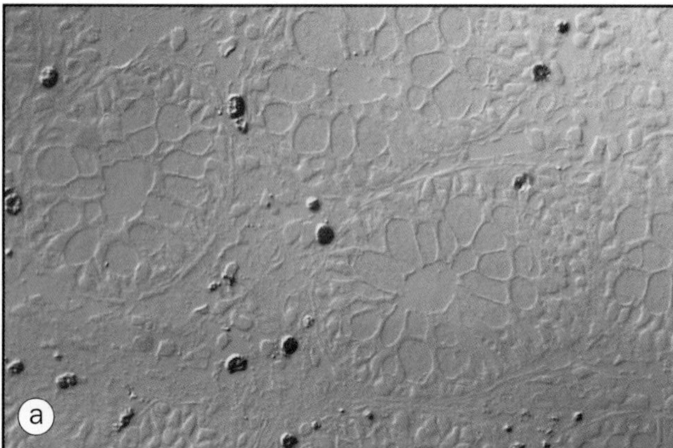

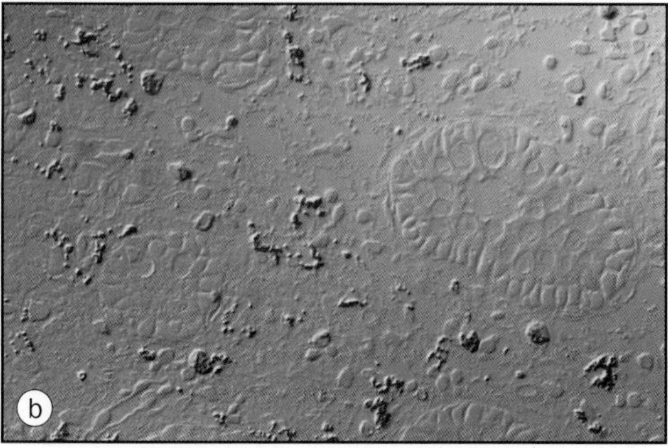

Fig. 8.15 Mast cell activation after colonoscopic allergen provocation. Immunohistochemical staining of histamine in tissue sections of cecal mucosa. Biopsies were taken (a) 20 minutes after challenge of a patient suffering from pork allergy with wheat antigen extract, which induced no macroscopic reaction, and (b) after challenge with pork antigen extract, which induced a significant wheal-and-flare reaction of the mucosa. Note the more widespread distribution of histamine, which is black (× 400).

Table 8.4 Treatment of gastrointestinal allergy

Treatment of Gastrointestinal Allergy	
Allergen avoidance	Hypoallergenic diet Elimination diet according to history and test results (Total parental nutritional)
Drug treatment	Cromolyn sodium Corticosteroids (local or systemic administration) H_1 blockers? Leukotriene antagonists?
Future concepts	Immunotherapy (induction of oral tolerance) Cytokine treatment (e.g.interleukin-10; IL-10)? Anti-IgE antibodies?

MANAGEMENT OF GASTROINTESTINAL ALLERGY

Information

The diagnosis of GI food allergy is difficult, time consuming, and sometimes even hazardous for the patient. Therefore, afflicted patients need intimate care by a competent specialist with a sympathetic understanding of the symptoms, the diagnostic procedures, and the treatment. Even in cases of confirmed GI allergy, the treatment remains difficult because allergen avoidance requires a high degree of discipline by the patient, and drug treatment options are limited. Moreover, immune therapy and prevention of GI allergy is not yet established. Only breastfeeding of babies, who have an increased risk of developing atopic disease, was shown to have a significant preventive effect. Apart from the physician, experienced dietitians are required to advise afflicted patients how to perform exclusion diets, to identify potential risky ingredients in food, and to avoid malnutrition and hypovitaminosis. Although confirmation of GI allergy requires special efforts by both patient and physician, the diagnosis offers multiple treatment options, such as allergen avoidance, drug treatment, and, in the future, possibly immune modulation (Table 8.4).

Allergen avoidance

The best strategy in the management of confirmed GI allergy is avoidance of the triggering allergen or allergens. However, this approach requires that the allergen responsible can be clearly identified, and that it is possible to exclude the allergen completely from the diet. The success of allergen avoidance depends on the patient's compliance, the quality of advice, the number of allergens to be avoided, and the kind of allergens. The 10 foods most commonly implicated in GI food allergy are milk, hazelnut, peanut, wheat, soya, apple, pork, fish, shellfish, and egg. Some allergens, such as nuts and apple, are relatively easy to avoid whereas others, such as milk, egg, and wheat, require enormous efforts to eliminate them completely from the diet. Patients have to be selected for their capacity to follow sophisticated dietary regimens and to be advised by experienced personnel. They should be cautioned to read the ingredient labels on all foods they consume, and they need educating in how to read the labels, to understand the technical names and abbreviations, and to appreciate that some ingredients are not necessarily indicated. They need instructions about the effects of cooking on the allergenicity of food proteins, and about eating away from home. They must be informed about the cross-reactivities within different food allergens and between some food allergens and pollens. Finally, patients who follow an extensive exclusion diet need surveillance of body weight, body composition, vitamin status, electrolytes, and bone density.

Drug treatment

Controlled reports on medical treatment of GI allergy are not available. Therefore, the recommendations for drug therapy of food allergy in general should be followed. One must distinguish between treatment of acute reactions and chronic or recurrent symptoms. Some patients, particularly those with a history of systemic anaphylaxis, should be equipped with an emergency set of drugs consisting of adrenaline [automatic syringe for intramuscular or subcutaneous injection or inhaler (0.3 mg)], prednisolone (100 mg) and H_1 blockers, such as clemastine (2 mg). In children, half the doses indicated here should be used.

Long-term drug therapy of GI allergy is required in patients who cannot, for whatever reason, achieve a complete avoidance of food allergen independently. Drug treatment and dietetic regimen are not mutually exclusive, since partial exclusion of relevant allergens may help to reduce the doses of drugs required to become free of symptoms. In our experience, H_1 blockers are in most cases not effective for the treatment of chronic GI symptoms except for itching in patients suffering from OAS. Cromolyn administered orally (200 mg four times a day) may be useful in cases with mild reactions. The advantages of this drug are that it is well tolerated by most individuals and that no relevant side-effects have been reported. In moderate to severe cases, additional treatment with oral corticosteroids (e.g. prednisolone 5–40 mg per day, or budesonide 3–12 mg per day) may be useful. Only anecdotal reports of successful use of other long-term treatments, such as non-steroidal immunosuppressants and cytokines, exist at present. In extremely severe cases, treatment by higher doses of corticosteroids and total parenteral nutrition may be indicated for a limited time period. If such cases are accompanied by symptoms of systemic anaphylaxis, the general recommendations of management of anaphylaxis must be taken into account.

New approaches to therapy

Controlled studies on empirically established and newly developed treatment options for GI allergy are lacking. The most effective long-term treatment of GI allergy is, apart from allergen avoidance, the treatment with corticosteroids, which includes well-characterized side-effects. Therefore, there is an urgent need for new therapeutic strategies and concepts for prevention of GI allergy. One of the most elegant approaches is suggested by nature, i.e. the induction of oral tolerance. However, the mechanisms of oral tolerance are not well understood, and the clinical application is not established. Moreover, evidence for classic allergen immunotherapy by parenteral administration of food allergen extracts being an appropriate treatment option in GI allergy is lacking. To date, many laboratories have put in huge efforts to unravel the mechanisms of oral tolerance and to apply them for clinical therapy. Therefore, other treatment options (e.g. leukotriene antagonists, or cytokines such as IL-10) still have to be evaluated in patients with GI allergy.

FURTHER READING

Bindslev-Jensen C, Poulsen LK. In vitro diagnostic methods in the evaluation of food hypersensitivity. In: Metcalfe DD, Sampson HA, Simon RA, eds. Food allergy: adverse reactions to food and food additives. 2nd edn. Cambridge: Blackwell Science; 1997:137–150.

Bischoff S, Crowe SE. Gastrointestinal food allergy: new insights into pathophysiology and clinical perspectives. Gastroenterology. 2005; 128(4):1089–1113.

Bischoff SC, Mayer J, Wedemeyer J, et al. Colonoscopic allergen provocation (COLAP): a new diagnostic approach for gastro-intestinal food allergy. Gut 1997; 40:745–753.

Bischoff SC. Mucosal allergy: role of mast cells and eosinophil granulocytes in the gut. Baillières Clin Gastroenterol 1996; 10(3):443–459.

Bock SA, Sampson HA, Atkins FM, et al. Double-blind placebo-controlled food challenge (DBPCFC) as an office procedure: a manual. J Allergy Clin Immunol 1988; 82:986–997.

Brandtzaeg P, Halstensen TS, Kett K, et al. Immunobiology and immunopathology of human gut mucosa: humoral immunity and intraepithelial lymphocytes. Gastroenterology 1989; 97:1562–1584.

Bruijnzeel-Koomen C, Ortolani C, Aas K, et al. Adverse reactions to food. Allergy 1995; 50:623–635.

Crowe SE, Perdue MH. Gastro-intestinal food hypersensitivity: basic mechanisms of pathophysiology. Gastroenterology 1992; 103:1075–1095.

Goldman AS, Kantal AG, Ham Pong AJ, et al. Food hypersensitivities: historical perspectives, diagnosis, and clinical presentation. In: Brostoff J, Challacombe SJ, eds. Food allergy and intolerance. London: WB Saunders; 1987:797–805.

Strobel S. Development of oral tolerance. In: De Weck AL, Sampson HA, eds. Intestinal immunology and food allergy. New York: Raven Press; 1995:155–168.

Young E, Stoneham MD, Petruckevitch A, et al. A population study of food intolerance. Lancet 1994; 343:1127–1130.

Chapter 9

Occupational Allergy

Piero Maestrelli, Leonardo M Fabbri, and Jean-Luc Malo

Definition:

Occupational allergy is defined as allergy caused by exposure to a product that is present in the workplace. Both elements of the definition are important as the agent should be specific to the workplace and be causally related to the disease.

INTRODUCTION

The recognition of occupational allergy goes back to Olaus Magnus who, in 1555, wrote

> 'When sifting the chaff from the wheat, one must carefully consider the time when a suitable wind is available that sweeps away the harmful dust. This fine-grained material readily makes its way into the mouth, congests in the throat, and threatens the life organs of the threshing men. If one does not seek instant remedy by drinking one's beer, one may never more, or only for a short time, be able to enjoy what one has threshed.'

Since then, many agents encountered at the workplace have been associated with allergic reactions in various organs. These include high-molecular-weight agents in, for example, castor beans and vegetal gums, low-molecular-weight agents in wood dust, and inorganic materials such as platinum salts and diisocyanates, the latter agent currently being, with flour, the most common cause of occupational asthma. Reactions can lead to permanent impairment and disability. Due to its significant medical, social, and possibly, legal consequences, a definitive diagnosis of occupational allergy, including identification of the causative agent, is imperative. Whenever possible, prevention programs should be set up in high-risk workplaces.

Occupational allergy can affect many target organs, including the lungs, nose, eyes, and skin. This chapter focuses on occupational allergy affecting the bronchi, i.e. occupational asthma, which is often accompanied by symptomatic manifestations in other target organs, especially the nose and the eyes.

DEFINITION AND CLASSIFICATION OF OCCUPATIONAL ASTHMA

Occupational asthma (OA) is defined as a type of asthma that is caused by exposure to a product present in the workplace. To fulfill this definition, the causative agent(s) should be almost exclusive to the workplace, hence this definition excludes asthma triggered by physical agents such as cold air or exercise. A previous history of asthma does not exclude the diagnosis of OA.

Figure 9.1 summarizes the various ways in which asthma can be induced or exacerbated at work. Besides OA with a latency period for which an allergic mechanism can be identified or is highly probable, another form of work-related airflow obstruction and bronchial hyperresponsiveness has also been described, i.e. irritant-induced asthma or reactive airway dysfunction syndrome (RADS), which may be developed after acute exposure to high concentrations of irritant gases or fumes. RADS therefore develops without a latency period of exposure and, although its functional characteristics resemble those of OA, its symptoms cannot be reproduced by re-exposure of the affected patients to non-irritant amounts of the offending agent. Also,

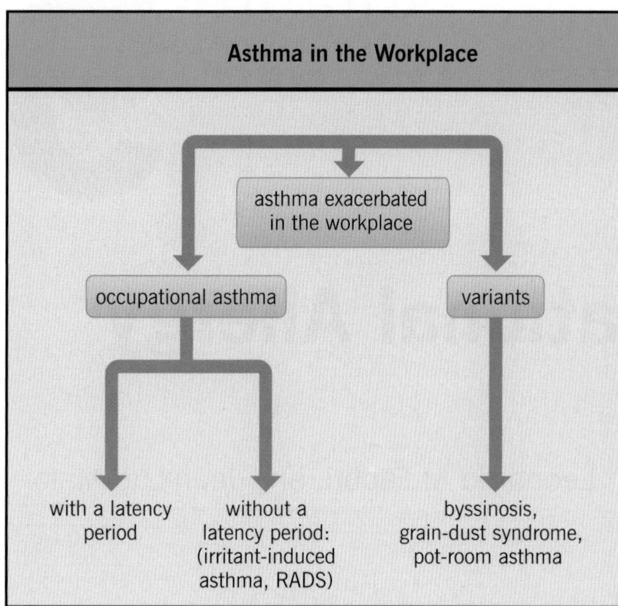

Fig. 9.1 Occupational asthma and asthma-like occupational variants. RADS, reactive airway dysfunction syndrome.

Table 9.1 Classification and major causes of occupational asthma

Classification and Major Causes of Occupational Asthma
High-molecular-weight compounds
Plant products
Animal products
Enzymes
Seafood proteins
Low-molecular-weight compounds
IgE-dependent causes:
Acid anhydrides
Metals
Non-IgE-dependent causes:
Diisocyanates
Wood dust
Amines
Colophony
Pharmaceutical products
Glutaradehyde
Formaldehyde
Pot-room aluminum-induced asthma

the airway pathology of RADS is different. The bronchial epithelial damage and subepithelial fibrosis are more pronounced, while inflammatory cell infiltration in the bronchial wall is generally less evident than in asthma, and the presence of eosinophils is inconsistent. The basic difference in pathophysiology can be explained by OA with a latency period incorporating a process of 'sensitization' to the offending agent (and presumably being immunologic in origin), with RADS relating to direct injury of the airways by a reactive chemical. Also occurring in the workplace are a number of asthma-like conditions including byssinosis (which is related to exposure to natural textile fiber dust), aluminum pot-room 'asthma', and grain-dust-induced syndrome.

OA may be induced by several different mechanisms. Immunologic mechanisms are generally implicated when OA occurs upon exposure to an agent after a latent period of sensitization. These mechanisms can be further divided into those that induce asthma through either an IgE-dependent or an apparently non-IgE-dependent mechanism. In the latter, specific IgE antibodies are not detectable or are found only in a small proportion of the patients with proven disease, even though the clinical picture is compatible with an 'allergic' reaction (i.e. sensitization and an exaggerated tissue damaging response upon re-exposure). The identity of the causative agents for such immunologic mechanism(s) is still unknown. Non-immunologic mechanisms are implicated when OA occurs without a latency period of exposure, i.e. RADS or irritant-induced asthma.

The causes of OA can be classified into high- and low-molecular-weight compounds. High-molecular-weight compounds, which are often from biological sources, generally induce asthma through an IgE-dependent mechanism, whereas the majority of low-molecular-weight compounds, which are usually highly reactive, induce asthma through non-IgE-dependent mechanisms. A list of etiologic agents according to industries, jobs, or work processes where the exposure can be found has recently been prepared (see Chang-Yeung and Malo in Further Reading) or available on web sites (asmanet.com; asthme.csst.qc.ca).

Table 9.1 summarizes the most important causes of OA.

EPIDEMIOLOGY

Asthma is becoming a common occupational ailment (more frequent than pneumoconioses such as asbestosis and silicosis), as based on the number of cases referred or accepted for medicolegal compensation and on the number of cases reported by sentinel physicians. The causes of this increase are unknown but may reflect heightened recognition of the problem as well as a broader range of environmental exposure. Besides medicolegal and sentinel-based program statistics, the frequency of OA can be assessed in general populations and in specific at-risk workplaces. It has been estimated that 23.4% of the US total workforce (7.8 million out of 33.4 million) is exposed to at least one of the 367 potentially asthmogenic products in the workplace. The most extensive survey in a general population was carried out in the course of the European Community Respiratory Health Survey. This study reached the conclusion that approximately 5–10% of adult-onset asthma can be attributed to the workplace. When the occupations associated with increased risk of asthma were evaluated, the job of 'cleaner' was the fourth occupation associated with excess risk of asthma. The finding was unexpected since these workers are not obviously exposed to well-recognized causes of occupational asthma. Repeated inhalations of irritants may play a role in cleaners who are exposed to mixtures of irritants, including chlorine compounds, acidic, and alkaline solutions. In a meta-analysis of publications using various study designs, Blanc and colleagues have proposed a figure close to 10% as a reasonable estimate of occupational contribution to the population burden of adult-onset asthma.

Table 9.2 Frequency of occupational asthma

Study population	Number of subjects	Participation (%)	Prevalence or Incidence
Frequency of Occupational Asthma			
Population-based:			
European-Community	2646	61	50–7.7%
Respiratory Health Survey	1609	64	1.9–3.1%
Sentinel-based:			
UK	554	Not relevant	22/million/year
Quebec	287	Not relevant	60/million/year
British Columbia	124	Not relevant	92/million/year
Sweden	1010	Not relevant	80/million/year
High-risk workplaces from cross-sectional studies			
High-molecular-weight agents:			
Snow crab processors	303	97	15%
Clam/shrimp	57	93	4%
Psyllium (pharm.)	130	93	4%
Psyllium (nursing)	194	91	4%
Guar gum	151	96	3%
Low-molecular-weight agents:			
Isocyanates	51	100	12%
Spiramycin	51	100	8%
White cedar	31	94	10%
Medicolegal:			
Quebec	~60/year	Not relevant	~20/million/year
Finland	352	Not relevant	~156/million/year
High-risk workforces from longitudinal studies			
Animal health	395	> 85%	2.7%
Pastry making	186	> 85%	1.6%
Dental hygiene	109	> 85%	4.5%

Most epidemiologic surveys of OA in specific workplaces have been cross-sectional and have, therefore, assessed the prevalence of the condition. The main pitfall of this approach is that it is likely to be influenced by the 'healthy worker effect'. It is to be suspected that this bias is more pronounced in the case of OA than for slowly progressing conditions such as pneumoconiosis. Asthma symptoms can be very troublesome and even life threatening, so it is likely that many subjects will leave the workplace before a survey can be conducted. The other difficulty lies in the diagnostic tools available for assessing the prevalence. Surveys rely on questionnaires, immunologic testing, assessment of airway caliber and bronchial responsiveness, and peak expiratory flow (PEF) monitoring, used alone and in combination. Only rarely are surveys performed in a stepwise fashion leading to the identification of cases which are then confirmed either by PEF monitoring or specific inhalation challenge. When assessed in case-identification studies, the prevalence of OA due to high-molecular-weight agents varies from 2 to 5%, whereas it is more in the order of 5 to 10% with low-molecular-weight agents (Table 9.2). Some recent epidemiological surveys conducted by Gautrin and co-workers from 1993 onwards have used a prospective design in apprentices who started being exposed. Figures of incident skin sensitization to a program-specific allergen expressed as rate by person-year were 7.9% in the case of animal-health technicians, 4.2% for pastry making and 2.5% in dental hygiene. The incidence of probable OA was 2.7% in animal-health technicians, 1.6% in apprentice pastry makers and 4.5% in dental hygienists.

PATHOGENESIS

Clinical, functional, and pathologic alterations in OA are similar to those found in non-OA. Airway smooth muscle contraction and mucosal edema are the main causes of acute airflow obstruction. Chronic airflow obstruction may be due to an increase in the airway wall thickness caused by any of the following:

- the accumulation of inflammatory cells;
- edema;
- hypertrophy of airway smooth muscle;
- subepithelial fibrosis;
- obstruction of the airway lumen by exudate or mucus;
- changes in the mechanical properties of the airway wall.

As in other types of asthma, airway hyperresponsiveness, i.e. an excessive reaction to bronchoconstrictor stimuli, is the hallmark of both occupational and non-OA. The pathogenesis of this hyperresponsiveness, which is generally long lasting and poorly

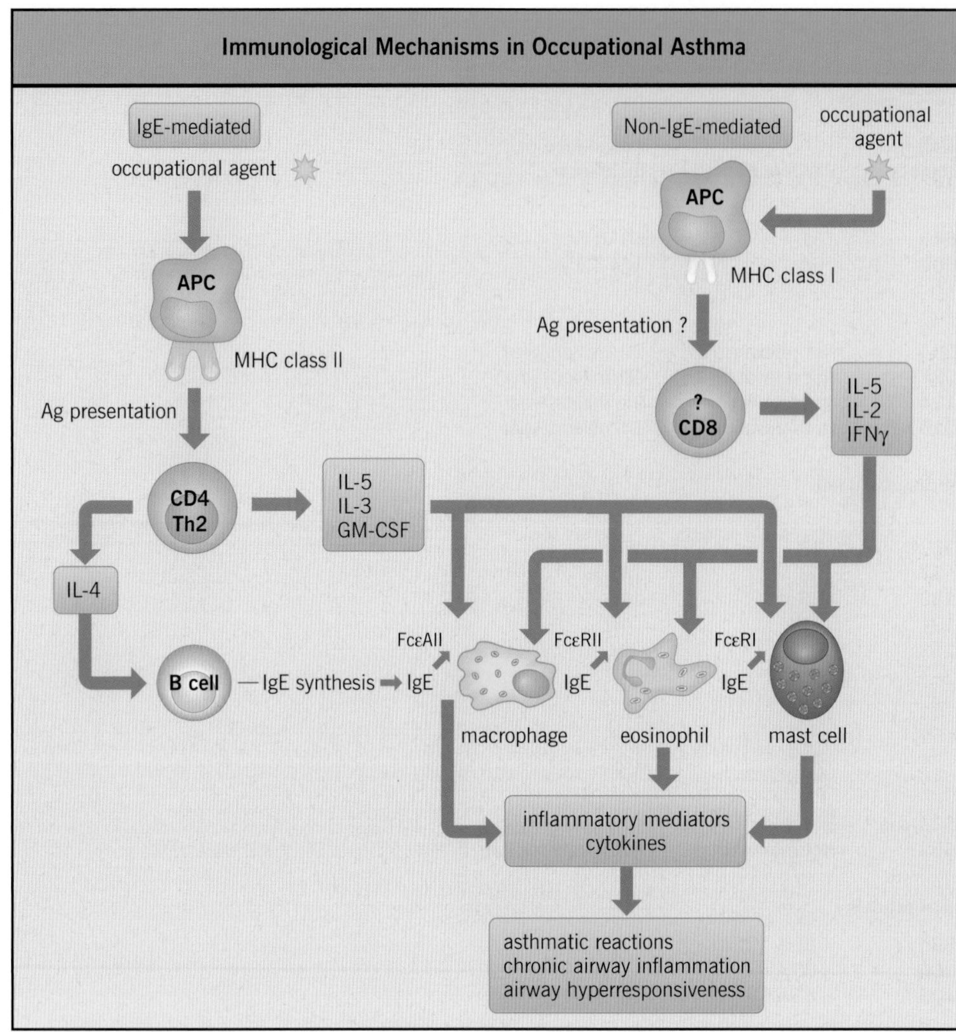

Fig. 9.2 Postulated immunologic pathways in occupational asthma with IgE-mediated mechanism (a) and non-IgE-mediated mechanism (b). IgE, immunoglobulin E; APC, antigen-presenting cell; MHC, major histocompatibility complex; Ag, antigen; Th, helper T cell lymphocyte; IL, interleukin; GM-CSF, granulocyte–macrophage colony-stimulating factor; IFNγ, interferon γ; FcεRI and FcεRII, high-and low-affinity IgE receptors.

reversible, remains unknown. By contrast, the transient increase of airway responsiveness observed in exacerbations of OA seems to be associated with an acute inflammatory reaction in the airways. The pathologic alterations of the airways in OA are characterized by infiltration of inflammatory cells, including eosinophils, activation of lymphocytes, and an increased thickness of subepithelial collagen. However, the relationship of pathologic alterations to clinical and functional features of the disease remains largely undetermined.

The mechanisms of 'induction' or sensitization, by which many occupational agents induce asthma, are believed to be mainly related to immunologic sensitization.

Immunologic mechanisms

An immunologic mechanism does not necessarily imply an IgE-mediated immunity but possibly also cell-mediated and mixed reactions. Some occupational agents, particularly high-molecular-weight sensitizers, act through an IgE-mediated mechanism. According to this mechanism, inhaled sensitizing agents bind to specific IgE on the surface of mast cells, basophils, dendritic cells and probably also macrophages, eosinophils, and platelets. High-molecular-weight sensitizing agents may act as complete antigens. By contrast, low-molecular-weight sensitizers probably need to react with autologous or heterologous proteins to produce a 'complete' antigen.

The reaction between antigen and IgE causes the cascade of events which is responsible for the activation of inflammatory cells (mast cells, eosinophils, macrophages, and T cells) and for the synthesis and release of a wide variety of preformed and newly generated inflammatory mediators which interact with target cells in the airway to cause the asthma syndrome (Fig. 9.2).

Many low-molecular-weight agents, such as diisocyanates and plicatic acid, cause OA that has the clinical and pathologic features of immunologic asthma, but do not generally and consistently induce specific IgE antibodies. It has been suggested that, when specific antibodies to plicatic acid are present, they may be markers of exposure and not causes of disease. In contrast, the presence of IgE to diisocyanates exhibits high specificity, but is insensitive in detecting occupational asthma. An increased number of activated T lymphocytes [i.e. lymphocytes expressing the interleukin-2 (IL-2) receptor, CD25, or very late antigen-1 (VLA-1)], of activated eosinophils, and of mast cells have been observed in patients with OA induced by toluene diisocyanate (TDI) (Fig. 9.3 and Table 9.3) and other low-molecular-weight sensitizers. This suggests that similar immunologic mechanisms may be involved in asthma of occupational as well as non-occupational origin. The presence of activated lymphocytes and eosinophils in bronchial biopsies indicates that a T-lymphocyte–eosinophil interaction may be important in asthma of different origins, a view further supported by the finding of cells expressing IL-5 in bronchial biopsies of atopic, intrinsic, and occupational asthmatics. Along

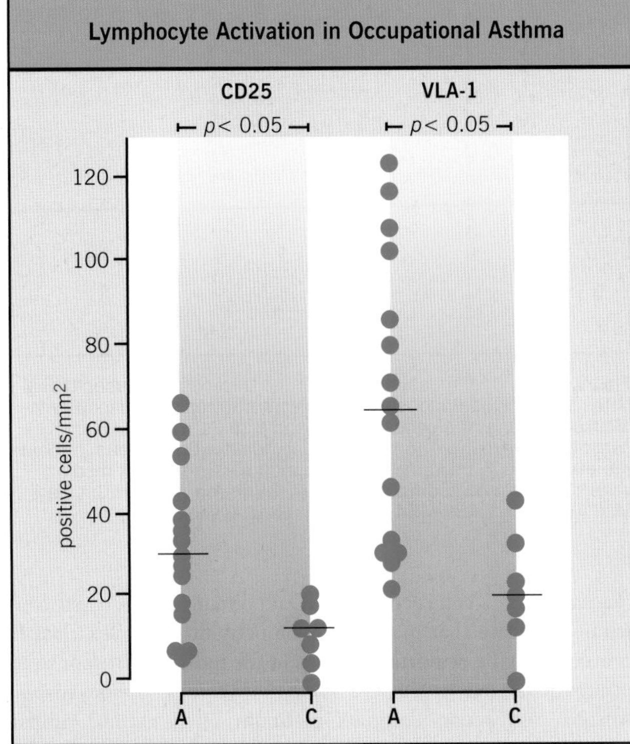

Fig. 9.3 Lymphocyte activation in occupational asthma. Individual counts for CD25- and VLA-1-positive cells in the submucosa of subjects with toluene-diisocyanate-induced asthma, A, and normal control subjects, C. The results are expressed as the number of positive cells per mm^2 of submucosa. Horizontal bars represent median values. VLA-1, very late antigen-1. (Data modified from Maestrelli et al. Am J Respir Crit Care Med 1995; 151:607–612, American Lung Association.)

with the increased expression of lymphocyte activation markers, in asthma induced by low-molecular-weight agents (e.g., diisocyanates) an increased number of cells producing proinflammatory cytokines has been reported. These proinflammatory cytokines, produced primarily by mononuclear phagocytes, may contribute to airway inflammation by several mechanisms, including increased expression of adhesion molecules, chemotaxis, and stimulation of inflammatory leukocytes. The observation that monocyte chemoattractant protein-1 (MCP-1) is specifically produced by peripheral blood mononuclear cells upon stimulation with diisocyanate–protein conjugates in subjects with diisocyanate OA, supports the hypothesis of an immunologic mechanism in this form of OA.

It has been suggested that CD8+ cells are key cells in OA with an IgE-independent mechanism (e.g. diisocyanate-induced asthma), since it was found that the majority of T cells obtained from bronchial biopsy specimens of subjects with diisocyanate-induced asthma showed the CD8 phenotype and produced interferon γ (IFNγ) and IL-5, with few clones producing IL-4. These T cells may represent a CD3+/CD4-/CD8+ population expressing the γ/δ T-cell receptor specific for the diisocyanate. Thus, CD4+ helper T cell type 2 (Th2)-like T cells may play a central role in determining the nature of the inflammatory response seen in the bronchial mucosa of asthmatic atopic patients through the induction of both allergen-specific IgE (via IL-4) and eosinophilia (via IL-5), because of their pattern of cytokine production. At the same time, CD8+ T cells may play a similar role in non-atopic subjects with TDI-induced asthma by directly causing bronchial eosinophilia via the local production of IL-5 (see Fig. 9.2). However, in a mouse model, it has been shown that the lung inflammatory response to inhaled hexamethylene diisocyanate (HDI) depends primarily on the effective generation of a CD4+ Th2 response, as in the case of atopic asthma. CD4+ and not CD8+ T cells mediate the airway eosinophilic response in HDI-sensitized mice. The authors suggested that the type of response induced after exposure to diisocyanates might be genetically influenced and that the generation of an HDI-specific CD4+ T-cell response must occur for the development of airway disease. Much research in humans and

Table 9.3 Inflammatory cell numbers in the submucosa of TDI-induced asthma subjects and control subjects. Results are expressed as a median (range)

Inflammatory Cell Numbers			
Cell type	**TDI asthma (cells/mm²)**	**Control subjects (cells/mm²)**	***p* Value***
CD45	1069 (526–3383)	414 (27–839)	< 0.005
Eosinophils	38 (0–1940)	3 (0–18)	< 0.005
Mast cells	131 (11–466)	18 (4–17)	< 0.005
Neutrophils	18 (0–293)	250 (87–295)	< 0.005
Macrophages	182 (36–1184)	404 (5–764)	NS
CD3	716 (124–1435)	433 (206–682)	NS

* Mann-Whitney U test. TDI, toluene diisocyanate. Data modified from Maestrelli P, Di Stefano A, Occari P, et al. Am J Respir Crit Care Med 1995; 151:607–612, American Lung Association.

with different diisocyanates remains to be performed to validate this hypothesis. Among the several animal models of OA, a mouse model developed using TDI showed a role for matrix metalloproteinase (MMP) activity in the development of airway inflammation and the inhibition of most of the inflammatory changes by administration of an MMP inhibitor.

Airway pathology

Bronchoalveolar lavage (BAL) – obtained during or after late asthmatic reactions induced by occupational sensitizers – shows a significant increase of inflammatory cells, i.e. eosinophils in the case of high-molecular-weight agents and both neutrophils and eosinophils in the case of isocyanates, and a marked increase in albumin concentration in lavage supernatant. By contrast, although early asthmatic reactions induced by occupational agents are associated with increased histamine, leukotrienes, and other mediators in BAL fluid, they are not followed by a marked increase of inflammatory cells. After challenge with isocyanates, leukotriene B_4 levels are increased, which may contribute to the leukocyte infiltration present in the airways; macrophages, epithelial cells, or neutrophils may be the source of this mediator. In BAL fluid obtained during late asthmatic reactions induced by exposure to an occupational stimulating agent, there is an increased concentration of albumin when compared to levels obtained from normal controls or during an early asthmatic reaction, indicative of microvascular leakage and mucosal edema. Evaluation of changes in induced sputum cell counts after exposure to both low- and high-molecular-weight occupational agents consistently showed airway eosinophilia. The time course of the influx of eosinophils into the airway lumen was more prolonged (up to 24 hours) than bronchoconstriction, and in some instances airway eosinophilia preceded bronchoconstriction. An increase in sputum neutrophils and neutrophil activation has been observed by some investigators after exposure to isocyanates.

OA may be fatal. In a sensitized subject who died in the workplace after re-exposure to isocyanates, histologic examination of the airways showed denudation of the airway epithelium and thickening of the basement membrane with infiltration of the lamina propria by leukocytes (mainly eosinophils) and diffuse mucous plugging of the bronchioles. Bronchial smooth muscle appeared hyperplastic and disarrayed, and lung parenchyma showed focal areas of alveolar destruction adjacent to areas of intact alveolar walls.

An increase in the thickness of the reticular layer of the basement membrane is considered a histopathologic feature of asthma; this subepithelial fibrosis has also been observed in OA. In subjects sensitized to isocyanates then examined after removal from exposure to the allergen for a period of 6–21 months, the subepithelial fibrosis (Fig. 9.4), the number of mast cells and fibroblasts, and the sensitivity to TDI are significantly reduced, while eosinophils, mononuclear cells, and airway responsiveness to methacholine do not change. Persistence of airway inflammation assessed by induced sputum has nevertheless also been documented in about one-third of workers removed from exposure for a mean period of 10 years.

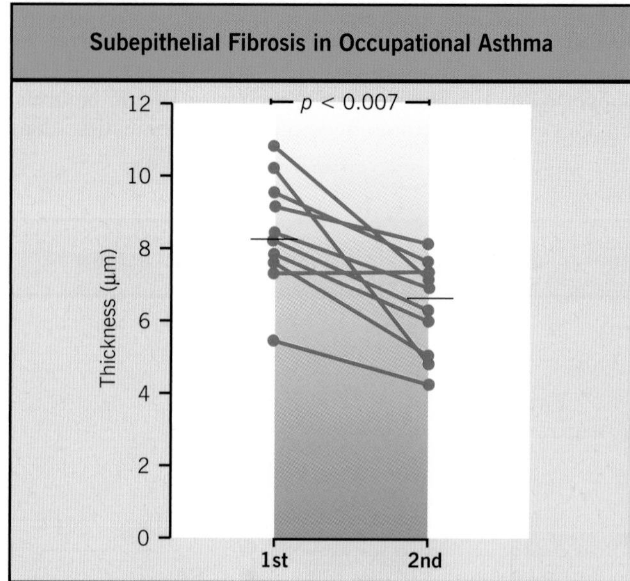

Fig. 9.4 Individual measurements of the thickness of subepithelial fibrosis in bronchial biopsies of subjects with toluene-diisocyanate-induced asthma at diagnosis (1st), and 6 to 21 months after cessation of exposure to toluene diisocyanate (2nd). Measurements are expressed in micrometers; horizontal bars represent median values. (Data modified from Saetta M, et al. Am J Respir Crit Care Med 1995; 151:489–494, American Lung Association.)

Genetic mechanisms

Individual differences in HLA class II molecules may alter the ability of the molecules to bind peptides and thereby change the nature of T-cell recognition. Data obtained in occupational studies indicate that major histocompatibility complex class II proteins may be important factors in the individual response to occupational agents such as acid anhydrides, diisocyanates, western red cedar, complex platinum salts, natural rubber latex, and animal proteins. An association of HLA molecules with specific symptoms and sensitization to rat lipocalin allergens has been demonstrated in a large study. In this investigation, approximately 40% of OA in the population examined could be attributed to an HLA-DRβ1*07 phenotype, while the attributable proportions for atopy and daily work in an animal housing facility were 58 and 74%, respectively. Associations with HLA might be found for other major animal allergens in light of the similarities among lipocalin animal allergens.

Specific HLA class II alleles are related to the susceptibility or resistance to isocyanate-induced asthma, with critical involvement of the hypervariable amino acid residue in position 57 of HLA-DQβ1 (Fig. 9.5).

The exact nature of the antigen related to sensitization to isocyanates is unknown. Isocyanates themselves may be involved in antibody binding or in the induction of structural changes in an unidentified protein. It has been proposed that the mechanism of low responsiveness to foreign antigens is linked to DQ alleles, whereas DR haplotypes are implicated in the upregulation of the immune response. Allelic variations at the same locus could be associated either with resistance or with susceptibility in isocyanate-induced asthma, such as occurs in autoimmune disorders where associations between the disease and allelic variations in the HLA region have been described. HLA class II associations with individual susceptibility to asthma induced by low-molecular-weight agents, for which the absence of specific IgE might challenge the immunologic mechanism, provide evidence for a specific immunologic response.

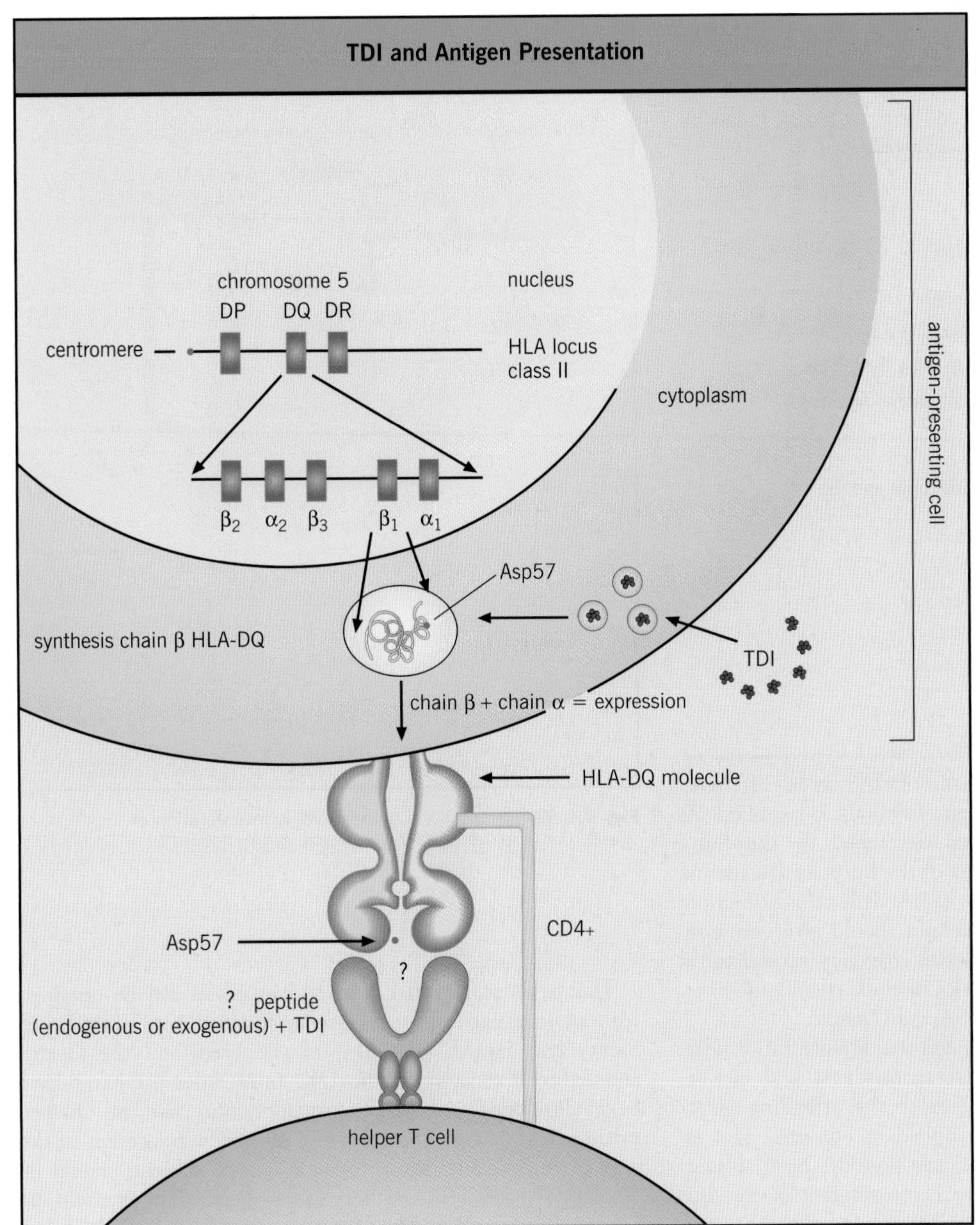

Fig. 9.5 The hypothetical interaction of toluene diisocyanate (TDI) with an antigen-presenting cell containing HLA-DQβ1-Asp57. The substitution of a single amino acid could affect a correct peptide antigen presentation. TDI could modify the structure of MHC class II molecules or the specificity of the T-cell receptor. MHC, major histocompatibility complex.

For the high-molecular-weight occupational agents, such as natural rubber latex, HLA associations confirm the importance of T cells in the regulation of IgE responses. However, genetic associations are not sufficiently strong to be used for selecting susceptible individuals. Indeed, while HLA phenotype is a significant determinant of sensitization to complex platinum salts, the association is looser in subjects with high intensity of exposure to the sensitizing agent. This implies that exposure-control measures remain the first option to prevent occupational sensitization.

A second pool of genes that could be involved in OA is the superfamily of glutathione S-transferase (GST), a family that is critical for protecting cells from oxidative stress products. A study of GST genotypes in workers exposed to various diisocyanates showed no significant association between GSTP1 genotype and overall risk of asthma. However, other investigators showed that in subjects who were exposed to TDI for 10 years or more the frequency of the GSTP1 Val/Val genotype was lower in those who had asthma and in those with more severe airway hyperresponsiveness. A possible explanation for the discrepancies among studies is that a protective effect of GSTP1 Val/Val genotype might be observed only in subjects exposed to diisocyanates for longer periods of time. Since the magnitude of protection associated with homozygosity for the GSTP1* Val allele increases in proportion to the duration of exposure to TDI, one might argue that the role of the GST and its allelic variants could lie in determining which subjects will have persistent asthma. More recently, a genetic variation in *N*-acetyltransferase, another antioxidant enzyme system, was shown to be associated with the risk of diisocyanate asthma, with slow acetylators being more susceptible.

Table 9.4 Tools generally used in the diagnosis of occupational asthma. This table summarizes the recommendations of the European Academy of Allergy and Clinical Immunology (1992)

Tools Used for the Diagnosis of Occupational Asthma
History
Confirmation of asthma: reversibility of bronchial obstruction non-specific bronchial challenges serial measurements of airway caliber
Confirmation of work-related bronchoconstriction: serial measurements of peak expiratory flow rates
Confirmation of sensitization to occupational agents: skin testing in vitro tests (specific IgE or IgG)
Confirmation of causal role of occupational agents: specific bronchial challenges

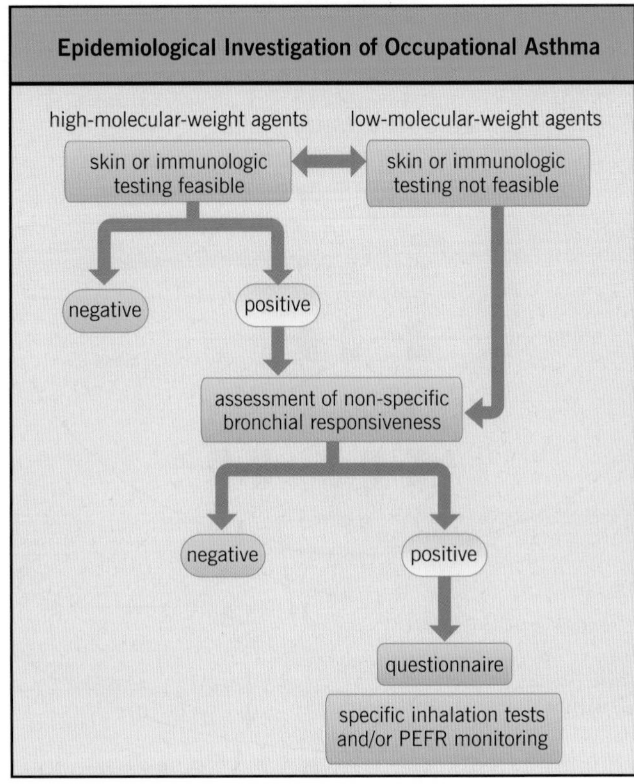

Fig. 9.6 Algorithm for the epidemiologic investigation of occupational asthma. PEFR, peak expiratory flow rate.

DIAGNOSIS

Since causative agents and mechanisms of OA may be different, a single detailed protocol for diagnosis cannot be applied. A general logical approach has been developed by the Subcommittee on Occupational Allergy of the European Academy of Allergy and Clinical Immunology (EAACI) for the evaluation of individual patients. These guidelines should give common diagnostic criteria, although the details may vary according to the features of each case (Table 9.4). Other excellent guidelines have also been published in the USA and Canada.

The confirmation of the disease and the demonstration that bronchoconstriction, airway hyperresponsiveness and airway inflammation are related to exposure to the offending agent require criteria similar to those applied in non-OA. This is justified by the findings that OA and non-OA have similar functional and pathologic features. These similarities are also found in types of asthma in which an IgE-mediated mechanism is not demonstrated, i.e. between intrinsic asthma and OA induced by many low-molecular-weight chemicals.

Clinical assessment

A scheme summarizing a proposed approach in the investigation of OA is shown in Figure 9.6. Every subject with asthma should be questioned about his or her current and past workplaces as persistent asthma can be attributed to past exposure. This holds for OA with a latency period as well as for RADS (see below). Two clues in the patient's history should point to the possibility of OA: the symptoms, and the job and products at work.

First, the subject may have a clear-cut history of exacerbations of respiratory symptoms at work. Secondly, the job and product at work can suggest the diagnosis. For example, if the medical history reveals that an asthmatic patient is a nurse, possible exposure to a sensitizing product such as latex should be considered. Being an asthmatic and exposed to polyurethane at work should also suggest the possibility of OA.

Databases of high-risk jobs and products can be obtained from national agencies, e.g. National Institute for Occupational Safety and Health (NIOSH) in the USA and the Health and Safety Executive in the UK. Interesting databases have been developed in France (asmanet.com) and in Québec (asthme.csst.qc.ca). The nature of all products present in the workplace, not only those handled by the subject, should be obtained by requesting safety data sheets. There could be products present that have not been listed as known causes of OA (but this does not preclude the possibility of their being so).

Besides chest symptoms, those related to ocular and nasal involvement should be investigated. These symptoms are more common in cases of OA due to high-molecular-weight rather than low-molecular-weight agents, and they precede those of asthma in the case of high-molecular-weight agents. Chest symptoms can be atypical, as for asthma. There are instances of cough and bronchitis of unknown etiology before the diagnosis of asthma was made.

At the onset of symptoms, improvement at weekends and when on vacation is generally the rule, although eventually the symptoms will persist through these short periods away from work. Therefore, improvement over weekends and when on vacation as the only criteria is not a satisfactory way to determine the presence of OA. Also, the regular use of potent antiinflammatory preparations, sometimes at high doses, can mask the symptoms. It must be remembered that, as with other medical conditions, questionnaires are sensitive but they are not specific tools, when results are compared with the final diagnosis.

Environmental assessment

Although air sampling can be undertaken at the workplace, the most important information is whether or not a product is actually present. In many instances, a causal agent can be released into the air in minute amounts, which makes its detection difficult even with sophisticated instruments. Product information is often difficult to obtain, so a good relationship should be established with the employer and the manufacturers of suspect products, as well as with local, regional, and national health and safety agencies. It is not mandatory for safety data sheets to give information on products present at concentrations below 1%, despite such concentrations being sufficient to cause OA.

A recent study showed that the total dose of the product (in this instance, isocyanate) is more significant than either the concentration or the duration of exposure in causing an asthmatic reaction. So a time-weighted average exposure may be more important once symptoms appear, whereas peak levels are probably more important in causing sensitization to the product. The level that provokes symptoms in already sensitized workers is lower than that which would cause sensitization. Many instruments cannot detect low levels of an agent, particularly the minute amounts that can cause asthmatic symptoms in some subjects, although air sampling at the workplace can serve several purposes; for example it can:

- confirm exposure as the cause of the disease;
- be used to investigate a plant where OA has been found;
- be part of a longitudinal monitoring of the worksite or of an investigation into the spread of an allergen from the plant to the community;
- establish risk levels; and
- make sure workers are not exposed to irritant concentrations of a product, i.e. those above the threshold limit values.

Exposure to irritant concentrations of a product (above threshold limit values) can cause RADS if the levels of gas or aerosol or particles are very high, or it can cause non-specific worsening of pre-existing asthma, if the level of exposure is not sufficiently high to cause RADS itself. General air sampling in a workplace does not usually provide an accurate reflection of what workers are exposed to, particularly if they are at any distance from the sampling apparatus. However, personal samplers have been developed to overcome this problem. With such apparatus, aerosols, mists, and dusts are sampled on filters or membranes that are then examined through various radioimmunoassay methods (for protein-derived materials) or through analytical chemical methods such as gas chromatography or high-performance liquid chromatography (for low-molecular-weight agents such as diisocyanates, acid anhydrides, formaldehyde, colophony, and metals).

Immunologic assessment

Specific IgE or IgG antibodies against an occupational sensitizer have been detected mainly for high-molecular-weight agents. The value of in vivo or in vitro tests in establishing a sensitization to low-molecular-weight chemicals has proved limited. In addition, the presence of immediate skin reactivity or increased specific IgE or IgG may reflect exposure or sensitization but it does not imply that the target organ is involved. This has been shown for common allergens and occupational sensitizers. With high-molecular-weight allergens, negative skin tests to such allergens almost completely exclude the possibility of OA. The worker may still be sensitized to another agent found in the workplace or to another component of the offending agent. With low-molecular-weight allergens, such as isocyanates and red cedar, negative skin tests or specific IgE or IgG do not refute or confirm the diagnosis of OA; skin tests are also usually unavailable.

Skin tests

If the offending agent has been identified and is known to induce asthma through an IgE-mediated mechanism and the appropriate antigen is available, a conventional diagnostic skin test can be used to confirm sensitization. Suitable preparations of antigens (extracts, complete allergens, or protein conjugates) are necessary that contain the biologically active substance and give a positive skin reaction in sensitized subjects, whereas the same preparations should give negative results in non-exposed subjects. Since commercial preparations of occupational agents are not usually available, the quality control of 'home-made' antigens is particularly important. Assessment of the relative sensitivity and specificity of prick tests is recommended for each preparation of antigen. Skin prick tests are quick, inexpensive, simple to perform, and safe. An allergy skin test with common inhalants should be performed in order to define the atopic status of the patients and to check for non-occupational etiologic factors. Skin prick tests can also be carried out in patients with impairment of lung function. There are limitations – they are not applicable for most of the low-molecular-weight agents, when the mechanism of asthma is not IgE mediated, and when the offending agent is unknown.

In vitro tests

Specific antibodies to allergens may be demonstrated in biological fluids using a variety of tests. They confirm a sensitization demonstrated by skin test but are often less sensitive. They represent an alternative to the skin test when the preparations of antigens have irritant, toxic, or mutagenic effects, and in patients under pharmacologic treatment that blunts normal skin reactivity. Control for specificity is required, especially when protein conjugates are used. Different factors, such as total IgE level, characteristics of the conjugate, carrier specificity, and cross-reactivity with other antigens, may affect the results. Assessment of the chemokine MCP-1 produced in vitro by diisocyanate-stimulated blood mononuclear cells exhibited higher test efficiency than specific antibodies for identification of isocyanate asthma.

Other in vitro tests, such as histamine release from basophils, are less standardized but may be useful occasionally.

Physiologic assessment

The presence of airway obstruction with demonstrable reversibility after inhaling a bronchodilator is a well-recognized confirmatory step for asthma. If there is no significant airway obstruction, the demonstration of increased bronchial responsiveness is suggestive of asthma, not necessarily of OA.

Pre- and post-workshift assessments of forced expiratory volume in 1 second (FEV_1) are not sensitive or specific enough to be useful in the investigation of OA. Serial PEF monitoring

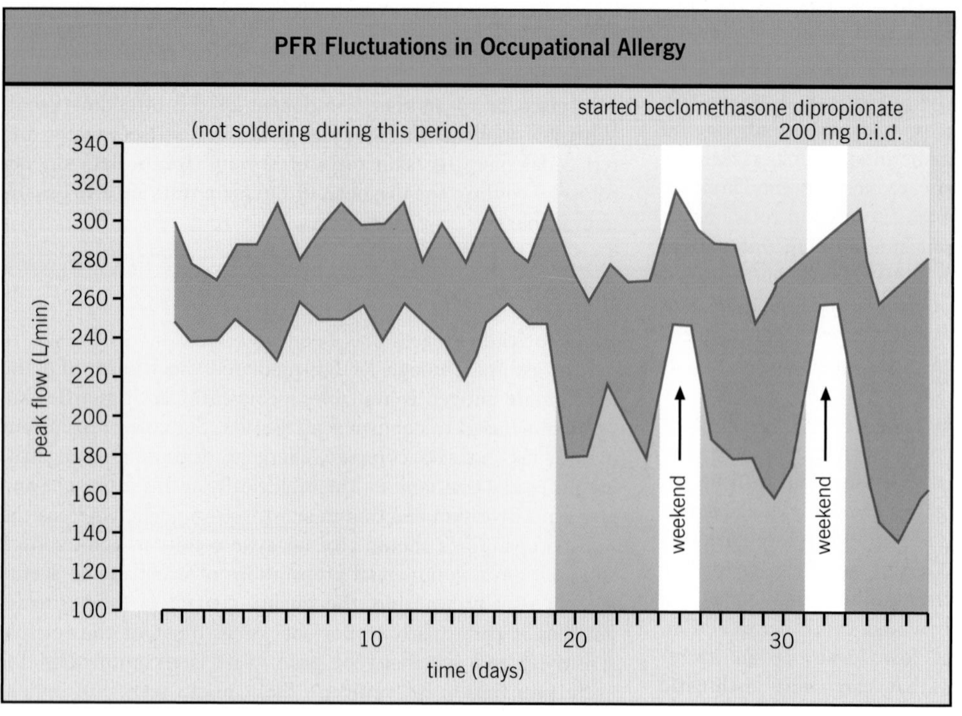

Fig. 9.7 Peak expiratory flows in occupational asthma. Plot of daily maximum (top line) and minimum (bottom line) peak flow in an asthmatic electronics worker who was exposed to colophony fumes. The days at work have a blue background, the days away from work a pale yellow background. There is definite occupational asthma with deterioration on return to work, and improvement each weekend. (Data modified from Burge PS. Physiologic assessment of occupational asthma. In: Bernstein IL, Chang-Yeung M, Malo J-L, et al, eds. Asthma in the workplace. New York: Marcel Dekker; 1993.)

has been proposed for both the investigation and assessment of asthma. The sensitivity and specificity of PEF monitoring, as compared with the 'gold standard' specific inhalation challenges, varies from 72 to 89% depending on the study. PEF graphs can be generated by plotting individual values or maximum, mean, and minimum values (Fig. 9.7). Recording the PEF twice a day is clearly not sufficient when compared to four or six times a day.

There are several problems associated with PEF monitoring:

- it requires good collaboration and honesty on the part of the subject;
- re-exposure of the subject to the same environment may be not feasible if he left work or may be dangerous;
- the interpretation requires specific expertise; and
- the interpretation is generally based on a visual reading (although automated reading programs have been recently proposed).

At times it is difficult to distinguish between a non-specific irritant exacerbation of asthma at work and OA. It has been found that compliance is unsatisfactory and that a substantial number of data are falsified, which may affect the interpretation. Combining PEF and the assessment of bronchial responsiveness for periods at work and away from work may, at times, improve the diagnostic yield although, in a more general way, it does not seem to add anything to monitoring of PEF alone. Laboratory and workplace monitoring of FEV_1 and clinical and functional parameters under close supervision of a technician is still regarded as the best way of confirming OA. The use of non-invasive tools to assess airway inflammation (induced sputum, exhaled nitric oxide, breath condensate) needs to be better defined. At present, evaluation of sputum eosinophils is the most promising tool in the investigation of OA.

Laboratory challenges in small cubicles were proposed by Pepys in the 1970s in an effort to reproduce the workplace environment. Improvement in the methodology of the test has been put forward using closed-circuit apparatus for dry particles and vapors, including diisocyanates. After exposure, various temporal patterns of reactions can occur, including those of typical (immediate, late, and dual) and atypical reactions (progressive, square waved, and prolonged immediate). Inhalation provocation testing with suspected sensitizers is not without risk and should only be undertaken in a laboratory properly equipped and by trained staff.

MANAGEMENT

Natural history

The natural history of OA is illustrated in Figure 9.8. Atopy is a well-known predisposing factor to asthma and OA due to high-molecular-weight agents. Smoking is not a predisposing factor in OA due to plicatic acid, which is the active agent in western red cedar, but it is a risk factor in subjects exposed to platinum salts, snow crab, and acid anhydrides. Anecdotal reports have suggested an association between spills of diisocyanates and the likelihood of developing asthma symptoms.

The total dose (i.e. duration of exposure × concentration) seems to be fundamental in the development of OA. In cross-sectional studies, an association has been found between the concentration of colophony, western red cedar, and flour on the one hand and the presence of symptoms on exposure to the causal agent on the other. The nature of the occupational agent can play a role in the rate of development of symptoms. More subjects exposed to western red cedar and diisocyanates develop work-related symptoms in the first 2 years of exposure when compared with subjects exposed to high-molecular-weight agents. After 5 years of exposure, the rate for developing symptoms is similar for high-molecular-weight agents and diisocyanates. Once sensitization has occurred, bronchial responsiveness is required to develop OA.

It is unlikely that asthma is a predisposing factor in the development of OA due to low-molecular-weight agents.

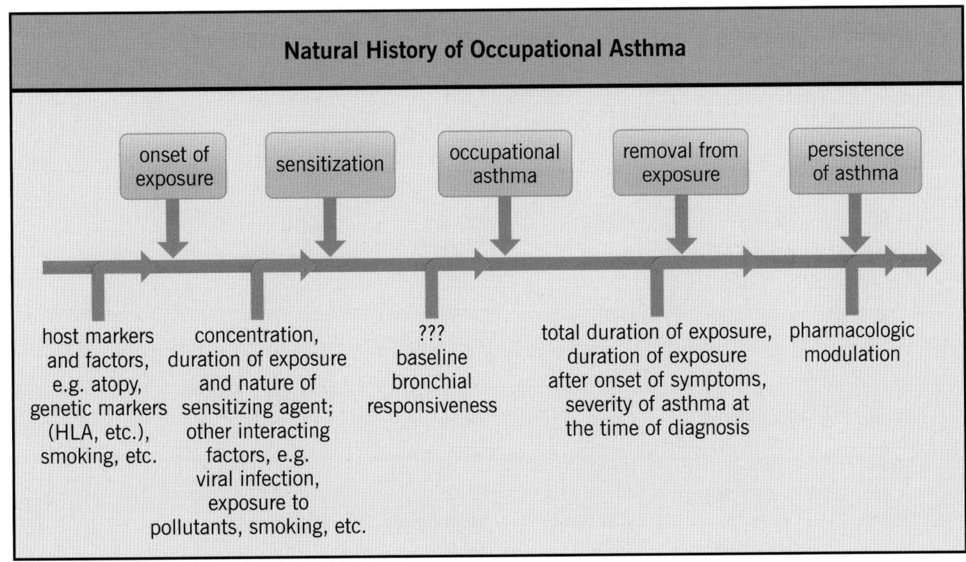

Fig. 9.8 The natural history of occupational asthma.

Although this information was gathered retrospectively in all studies, most subjects who developed OA did not have a history of asthma (before exposure began), though having enhanced bronchial reactivity may be a factor that is associated with the development of OA.

The outcome of OA after diagnosis is often poor. Removal from the occupational exposure is associated with recovery from asthma in about 50% of subjects. Many retrospective studies have unanimously demonstrated a persistence of asthmatic symptoms, bronchial obstruction, and hyperresponsiveness in subjects with OA after being removed from exposure. Most studies also showed that the total duration of exposure, the duration of exposure after the onset of symptoms, and the severity of the asthma at the time of diagnosis are all determinants of the prognosis. Improvement in bronchial responsiveness occurs predominantly in the first 2 years after cessation of exposure and continues, though at a slower rate, later on. If exposure continues, there is overall deterioration in the asthmatic condition.

Prevention

Primary prevention

Elimination of the sensitizing agent(s) is the most effective way of primary prevention, although this is often not practicable. In 1989 the European Community (EC) published a directive for the promotion of the improvement of the safety and health of workers in the workplace, which contains several general concepts that may be particularly relevant to the prevention of OA. The requirements which the member states have to meet in their legal regulations include the elimination of the risk or its reduction by substitution of hazardous agents, and the priority to adopt general protective measures to decrease environmental exposure to the causative substances, rather than providing personal protective devices. Moreover, the importance of adequate worker health and safety education is emphasized. Exclusion of atopic subjects from exposure to high-molecular-weight agents is considered inappropriate as 40–50% of young adults are atopic. Excluding them would exclude a large proportion of the workforce without effectively preventing OA since the predictive value of atopy is low. For instance, in laboratory-animal workers, the risk of developing symptoms is approximately 33%, i.e. not sufficiently high to justify excluding atopic subjects. Dissuading employees from smoking in industries where smoking has been identified as a significant risk factor appears reasonable.

Secondary prevention

The early detection of workers with established disease, and their subsequent removal from exposure, is the most effective way to prevent progression to moderate or severe disease with its associated morbidity and disability. Therefore, adequate worker medical surveillance has to be ensured, as recommended by the EC directive mentioned above. This can be done by routine skin testing with high-molecular-weight occupational agents; it is feasible and can identify subjects who have become immunologically sensitized and who should be followed more closely in terms of the development of bronchial hyperresponsiveness and asthma symptoms. In addition, rhinoconjunctivitis may be considered a predictor of the later development of OA due to these agents. In subjects exposed to low-molecular-weight agents, routine questionnaires coupled with an assessment of bronchial responsiveness could prove useful in detecting the disease at an early stage.

Tertiary prevention

Once the diagnosis of OA is made, it is important to remove the subject from exposure as soon as possible. If this is done, it is less likely that the subject will be left with the permanent sequelae of asthma and bronchial responsiveness requiring medication. The longer an individual with OA is exposed to the offending agent then the more likely it is that symptoms and impaired lung function will persist after withdrawal from the workplace. Relocation to jobs with less exposure may be successful in some workplaces. For instance, reduction of exposure to natural rubber latex was associated with clinical improvement and fewer negative social-economic consequences

Table 9.5 American Thoracic Society guidelines for assessing impairment and disability in asthma and occupational asthma

Assessing Impairment and Disability in Asthma and Occupational Asthma – American Thoracic Society Guidelines

	Score					
	0	1	2	3	4	5
FEV_1 (% pred.)	> 80	79–79	60-69	50–59	< 50	
Reversibility of airway obstruction (% change in FEV_1)	< 10	10–19	20-29	> 30		
Hyperresponsiveness $PC_{20}FEV_1$ (mg/mL)	> 8	2–8	0.25–2	< 0.25		
Medication needed:						
Bronchodilators	None	Occasional (not daily)	Daily	Daily		
Cromolin	None	Courses (1–3/year)	Daily	–		
Inhaled steroid	None	Courses (1–3/year)	Low dose daily	High dose daily	High dose daily	
Systemic steroid	None	None	None	Courses (1–3/year)	Daily	
Summary rating class:						
Class	0	I	II	III	IV	V
Total score	0	1–3	4–6	7–9	10–.11	Uncontrolled

FEV_1, forced expiratory volume in the first second; $PC_{20}FEV_1$, provocative concentration of histamine or methacholine producing a 20% fall in FEV_1.

than cessation of exposure. Respiratory protection has only been shown to be partially effective in reducing the consequences of exposure in a few selected cases of OA. Note that in western red cedar asthma, wearing a conventional face-mask while continuing to work does not reduce the risk. In some subjects, it may be worthwhile to consider wearing a helmet respirator whenever short periods of exposure to a sensitizer occur.

Drug treatment

Drug therapy of OA does not differ from that indicated in national and international guidelines for other forms of asthma. It is known that taking antiinflammatory inhaled corticosteroid preparations accelerates clinical, functional, and pathologic improvement once removal from exposure has been carried out. The long-term effects of inhaled steroids on OA have seldom been evaluated but it appears that these drugs have little effect on the long-term outcome in established disease. Antiasthma drugs are generally not sufficient to prevent asthma attacks upon re-exposure to the offending agent at work, although they can reduce the severity.

MEDICOLEGAL ASPECTS – ASSESSMENT OF DISABILITY AND COMPENSATION

As OA can lead to permanent asthma, even after removal from exposure, it has been proposed that affected workers should be offered compensation for the permanent impairment of lung function and disability. The principles of impairment assessment valid for chronic lung diseases (such as pneumoconiosis or chronic obstructive pulmonary disease), which are associated with a stable functional impairment and abnormalities of gas exchange and mechanical parenchymal properties, are inappropriate for subjects with asthma.

OA, like other forms of the disease, is characterized by variable airflow obstruction, amenability to therapy, no radiologic abnormalities, no clear relationship with the level of exposure to the offending agent, and triggering by multiple factors in the presence of bronchial hyperresponsiveness. A scaling system that includes some of these variables has been proposed by a committee appointed by the American Thoracic Society (Table 9.5). The long-term assessment of impairment should be performed for 2 years after the cessation of exposure, since the maximum rate of improvement occurs within this period of time. It is clear that the methods for reporting, recognizing, and paying compensation for occupational diseases are far from uniform from one country to the next.

Medicolegal requirements for the diagnosis of OA have not been uniform among countries, and also in respect of the clinical diagnosis of OA. In 1994 the EC published a bulletin containing guidelines for the medicolegal diagnosis of occupational diseases prepared by the Unit of Occupational Health and Hygiene (Table 9.6). The diagnostic criteria include the objective assessment of asthma. However, the confirmation that asthma is occupationally caused is based only on anamnesis, whereas bronchial provocation tests are not suggested and peak flow measurements are indicated as optional; this may lead to an incorrect diagnosis of OA. It appears obvious that nasal provocation tests can demonstrate rhinitis but they have no value when the lower airways are the target organ.

There are several reasons why it is important to confirm the diagnosis of OA both medically and medicolegally. Missing the diagnosis may well result in a worker's continued exposure to the asthma-provoking agent with all the medical consequences that implies. A diagnosis of OA also has significant social and

Table 9.6 Diagnostic criteria for the medicolegal diagnosis of occupationally caused asthma as given by the Commission of the European Community (1994)

Medicolegal Diagnosis of Occupationally Caused Asthma – Diagnostic Criteria
Clinical certification of asthma must be confirmed by an examination of respiratory function showing either:
bronchial obstruction reversible by bronchodilators; or
bronchial obstruction triggered by non-specific bronchodilators (methacholine test) when basic functional tests are normal
Anamnesis:
occupational exposure to a substance known to trigger occupational asthma
sequence of attacks is directly related to work schedule – attacks may begin several hours after exposure
recurrence of disorders following re-exposure to the same agent
Optional supportive evidence may be provided for certain allergens by:
serial peak flow rate
rhinomanometric study with nasal provocation tests
IgE-dependent immediate immune reactions:
skin (prick test)
raised levels of serum IgE specific to the occupational allergen
histamine release
basophil degranulation test

financial consequences. Unlike pneumoconiosis, OA frequently affects young people. Leaving the job on a physician's advice has a major impact, as it implies retraining for a new occupation. Although it is of the utmost importance to offer retraining programs or early retirement with financial compensation, the efficacy and cost of these programs should also be considered.

In most countries, OA is on the increase. Since all cases are avoidable, policies related to primary prevention must be encouraged, especially since the long-term prognosis for this type of disease is not good. Increasing concern by employers over compensation will provide a powerful lever for improved occupational hygiene. However, it is education of the workforce and employers on the dangers of this form of asthma that, in the long term, will produce change and a lowering of its incidence.

FURTHER READING

American Thoracic Society. American Thoracic Society Statement: Occupational contribution to the burden of airway disease. Am J Respir Crit Care Med 2003; 167:787–797.

Bernstein DI. Clinical assessment and management of occupational asthma. In: Bernstein IL, Chang-Yeung M, Malo J-L, et al, eds. Asthma in the workplace. New York: Marcel Dekker, Inc; 1999:145–157.

Bernstein IL, Chang-Yeung M, Malo J-L, et al. Definition and classification of asthma. In: Bernstein IL, Chang-Yeung M, Malo J-L, et al, eds. Asthma in the workplace. New York: Marcel Dekker, Inc; 1999:1–4.

Canadian Thoracic Society. Ad Hoc Committee on Occupational Asthma of the Standards Committee, Occupational Asthma: recommendations for diagnosis, management, and assessment of impairment. Can Med Ass J 1989; 140:1029–1032.

Chang-Yeung M, Malo J-L. Aetiological agents in occupational asthma. Eur Respir J 1994; 7:346–371.

Chang-Yeung M, Malo J-L. Occupational asthma. N Engl J Med 1995; 333:107–112.

European Commission. Information notices on diagnosis of occupational diseases. Health and Safety 1994; EUR 14768 EN.

Maestrelli P, Baur X, Bessot JC, et al. Subcommittee on Occupational Allergy of EAACI. Guidelines for the diagnosis of occupational asthma. Clin Exp Allergy 1992; 22:103–108.

Maestrelli P, Saetta M, Mapp C, et al. Mechanisms of occupational asthma. Clin Exp Allergy 1997; 27(suppl 1): 47–54.

Moscato G, Godnic-Cvar J, Maestrelli P, et al. Statement on self-monitoring of peak expiratory flows in the investigation of occupational asthma. J Allergy Clin Immunol 1995; 96:295–301.

Siracusa A, Desrosiers M, Marabini A. Epidemiology of occupational rhinitis: prevalence, aetiology and determinants. Clin Exp Allergy 2000; 30:1519–1534.

Venables KM, Chang-Yeung M. Occupational asthma. Lancet 1997; 349:1465–1469.

Chapter 10

Definition:
Drug allergy is an immunologically mediated adverse drug reaction. It consists of two phases: the indication of a specific immune response on initial exposure followed by the elicitation of symptoms upon subsequent exposure to the drug.

Drug Allergy

N Franklin Adkinson, Peter S Friedmann, and Jacqueline A Pongracic

INTRODUCTION

Adverse drug reactions (ADR) are a significant cause of morbidity and even mortality. The majority of ADR (called type A) are dose-related and predictable from the pharmacologic effects of the drug. Examples include tachycardia with theophylline and sedation with hydroxyzine. Many of the so-called idiosyncratic ADR are a significant cause of morbidity and even mortality. The majority of reactions (type B) have a much less obvious dose relationship, are due to individual susceptibility, and some may involve immune responses against the drug or a metabolite. Since drug molecules (xenobiotics) are too small to be recognized by the immune system, it is hypothesized that the native drug, or more likely, a metabolite acts as a hapten, binds to a protein carrier and the hapten–carrier complex is then recognized by T cells. Some drugs like β-lactams spontaneously form covalent haptens with macromolecules under physiologic conditions. But many drugs are detoxified through two phases: phase 1 performed by cytochrome P450 enzymes, involves oxygen addition reactions which generate reactive intermediates; phase 2 detoxification is performed by enzymes that add groups such as acetyl, glucuronyl or glutathione to the reactive phase 1 product. Slow acetylators are susceptible to drug-induced lupus syndromes – probably because the reactive intermediate persists, becomes a protein-bound hapten and elicits an immune response. In the case of halothane-induced hepatitis, the hepatic CYP2E1 involved in converting halothane to the trifluoroacetyl metabolite appears to end up with the trifluoroacetyl compound covalently bound to it. This forms the multivalent hapten–carrier complex recognized by the immune system. Subsequently, T cells and IgG are generated against this complex with resulting hepatitic liver damage.

Frequently, drug interactions occur where one drug modifies the detoxification or excretion of another. This can lead to situations in which a previously 'safe' drug manifests toxicity when used in conjunction with another. Obvious examples include the inhibition of cytochrome P450 by erythromycin or ketoconazole, precipitating cardiotoxicity of terfenadine and astemizole – resulting in a type A ADR. Similarly, ADRs to anticonvulsants may develop when a second drug is added that 'overloads' the detoxification processes that were just coping with the anticonvulsant alone. It is important to identify allergic reactions when they occur, since specific diagnostic and therapeutic options are available.

CLASSIFICATION OF IMMUNE REACTIONS UNDERLYING DRUG ALLERGY

Allergic drug reactions may be classified, at least theoretically, according to one of four implicated immunologic mechanisms, according to the scheme of Gell and Coombs (Table 10.1).

Table 10.1 The Gell and Coombs classification of allergic responses, types I–IV

Gell and Coombs Classification of Immune-mediated Allergic Responses		
Type	**Mechanism**	**Manifestations**
I	IgE-dependent	Anaphylaxis, urticaria
II	Cell surface antigens – cytotoxity	Cytopenias, other cellular damage
III	Immune complex deposition	Vasculitis/nephritis/drug fever
IV	Delayed-type hypersensitivity	Dermatitis or hepatitis

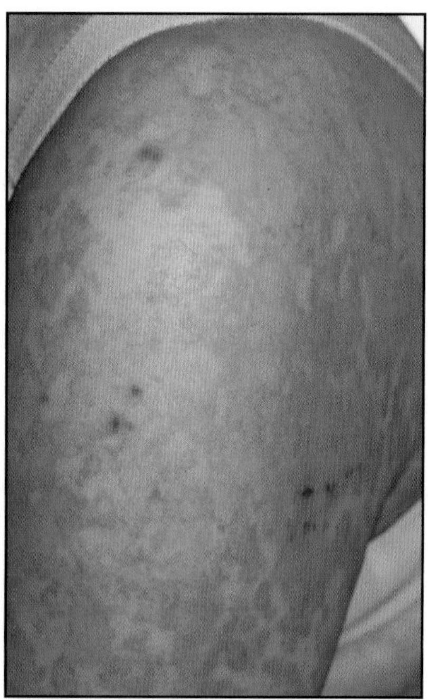

Fig. 10.1 Urticarial reaction to penicillin. This is an example of a Gell and Coombs type I reaction, resulting in a wheal-and-flare response. (Courtesy of Prof. Peter Friedmann.)

Type I reactions

Type I reactions are the result of an IgE antibody response, which induces immediate-type hypersensitivity reactions. With subsequent drug exposure following sensitization, the multivalent antigen–hapten complex cross-links IgE bound to mast cells and basophils, leading to the release of preformed mediators (such as histamine) and the production of newly generated mediators (such as the leukotrienes). Systemic anaphylaxis, angioedema, bronchospasm, or urticaria due to penicillin allergy are the best understood responses in this category (Fig. 10.1).

Type II reactions

Type II reactions are mediated by IgG, or possibly IgM, antibodies directed against drug-modified cell surface antigens, which elicit complement-mediated cytotoxicity. Such responses induce cytopenias, such as Coombs' positive hemolytic anemia where the drug or its metabolite binds to the erythrocyte membrane. Antibody, directed against the drug or altered cell membrane antigens, binds to its target, resulting in complement fixation and subsequent cell lysis. Similar reactions may occur in many tissues including the skin (Fig. 10.2). Alternatively, drug–antibody immune complexes may form and adhere to cell membranes, again leading to complement fixation and cell lysis (Fig. 10.3).

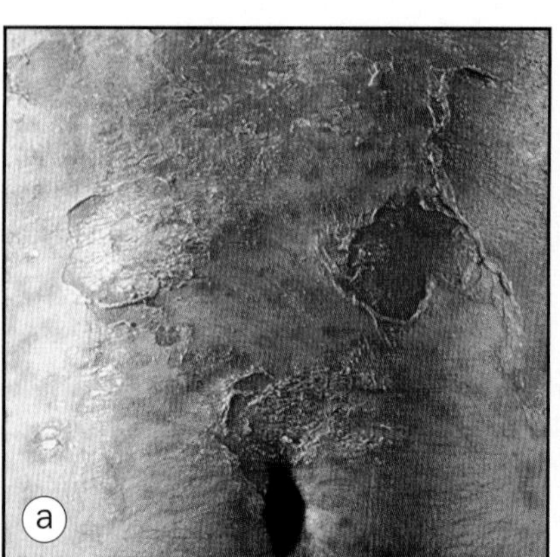

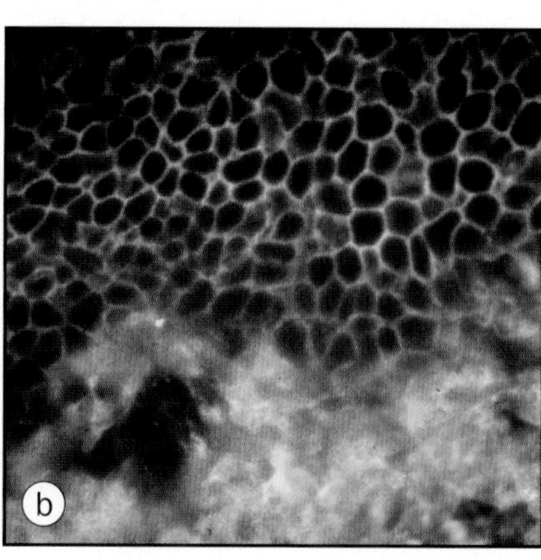

Fig. 10.2 (a) Penicillamine-induced pemphigus foliaceus. An autoantibody against epidermal cell surface proteins is generated, causing the separation of epidermal keratinocytes with the formation of superficial blisters. This is an example of a Gell and Coombs type II reaction. (b) Direct immunofluorescence of a skin biopsy from the same patient as in (a). This shows the autoantibody around the edge of every epidermal cell ('chicken wire' appearance).

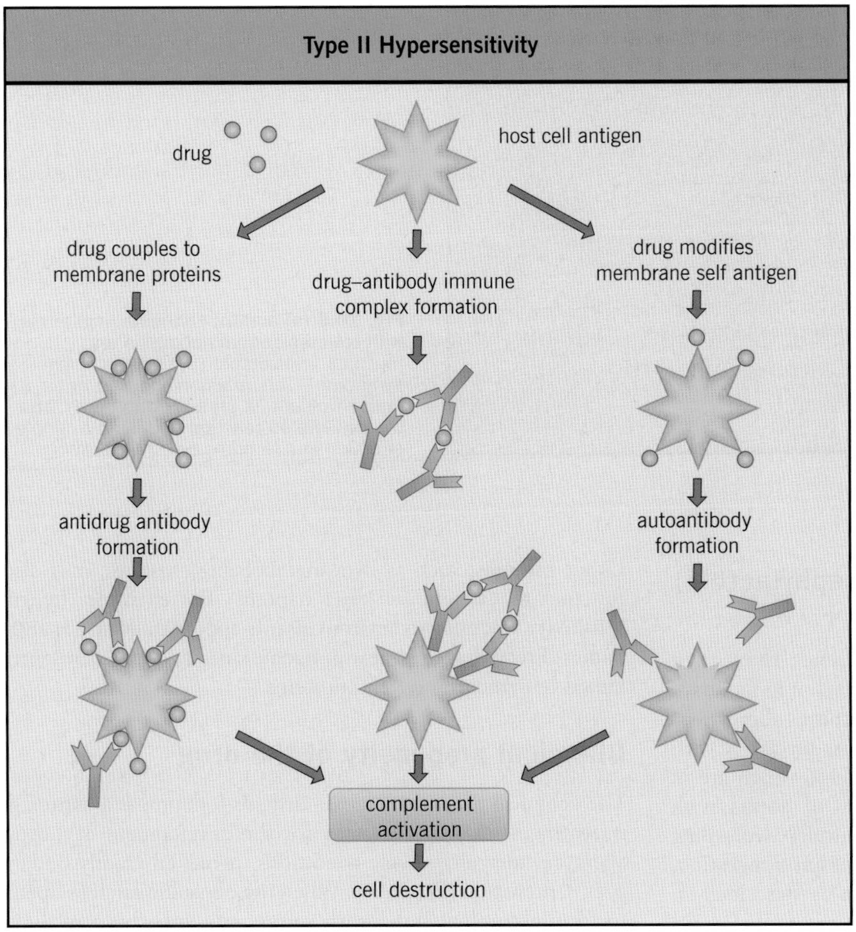

Type II Hypersensitivity

drug

host cell antigen

drug couples to membrane proteins

drug–antibody immune complex formation

drug modifies membrane self antigen

antidrug antibody formation

autoantibody formation

complement activation

cell destruction

Fig. 10.3 Mechanisms of type II drug hypersensitivity. Complement-mediated cell destruction may occur via several mechanisms. (i) The drug is covalently linked to the host cell membrane. Antidrug IgG then binds to the drug and activates the complement, e.g. penicillin. (ii) The circulating drug and antibody form immune complexes which affix to cell membranes and trigger the complement cascade (e.g. quinidine). (iii) The drug binds to the cell membrane but the immune response is directed against the altered host cell. Autoantibodies are produced, bind to the cell (even in the absence of the drug) and may activate complement (e.g. α-methyldopa).

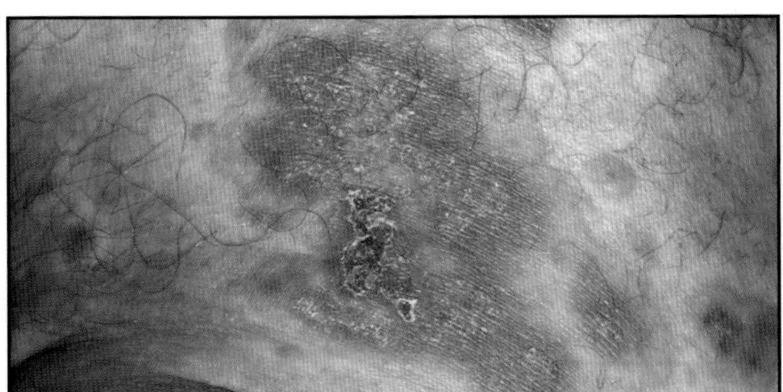

Fig. 10.4 Vasculitic rash induced by an oral hypoglycemic agent. This is an example of a Gell and Coombs type III reaction. Such purpuric eruptions tend to affect the extremities. (Courtesy of Prof. Peter Friedmann.)

Type III reactions

Type III reactions occur via immune complex formation. The size of the immune complex determines its site of tissue deposition and the resultant immune injury. The classic example is serum sickness, with involvement of the skin, joints, and lymphoid system, though drug fever is also commonly seen. An example of type III vasculitic rash is shown in Figure 10.4.

Type IV reactions

Type IV reactions, also known as delayed-type hypersensitivity, are cell mediated through T- lymphocyte responses to drug antigens. These may occur either as contact dermatitis associated with topically applied medications or as one of a variety of reaction patterns with systemic drug exposure. In contact sensitization, the drug forms a hapten and combines with self proteins to form an antigenic complex. Langerhans' cells internalize the complex and travel via the lymphatics to regional lymph nodes where the 'antigen' is presented to T lymphocytes. After clonal T-cell expansion, the T cells are redistributed in the skin. Once antigen is re-encountered, the T cells are activated, resulting in cytokine release and mononuclear cell recruitment, vesicle formation, and edema. Systemic drug exposure may generate maculopapular skin eruptions, eczematous or exfoliative dermatoses or erythema multiforme with or without mucosal involvement (Stevens–Johnson syndrome) (Fig. 10.5) or toxic epidermal necrolysis (TEN). While type IV contact hypersensitivity reactions to topical medications are relatively infrequent, nurses, pharmacists, and other personnel in the pharmaceutical industry are at the greatest risk of developing such an occupational allergy.

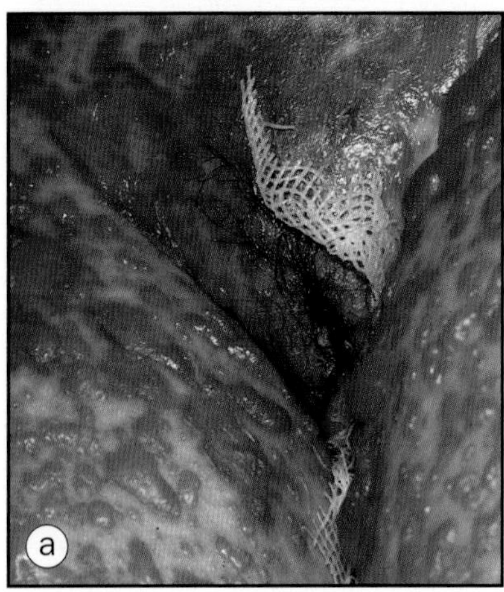

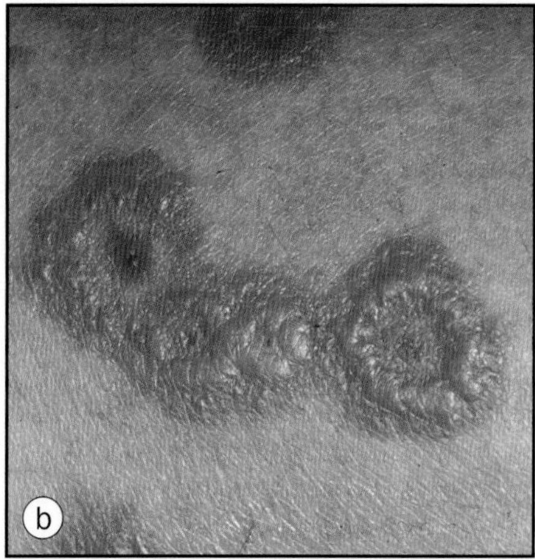

Fig. 10.5 (a) and (b) Erythema multiforme with toxic epidermal necrolysis and mucosal involvement (Stevens–Johnson syndrome). This reaction, induced by an anticonvulsant, is presumed to be a CD8+ T-cell-mediated reaction and is an example of a Gell and Coombs type IV reaction.

Drug-induced pseudoallergic (anaphylactoid) reactions

These reactions deserve a special mention since they often appear clinically to manifest as type I reactions, but in fact have no immunologic basis. The problem of aspirin allergy has become important due to the high rate of cross-reactivity with non-steroidal antiinflammatory drugs (NSAIDs), which are in common use. It is estimated that 20–30% of adults with asthma, nasal polyps, or chronic urticaria develop worsening rhinitis, bronchospasm, or urticaria following aspirin ingestion. The postulated mechanism of this reaction is described in Chapter 24. Radiocontrast media (RCM) induce anaphylactoid reactions that are caused by mast cell and basophil mediator release, but not through an IgE-dependent mechanism. The hypertonicity of RCM is probably the major cause of cellular degranulation and mediator release, since the newer non-ionic agents of lower osmolarity produce many fewer reactions. Angiotensin converting enzyme (ACE) inhibitors are known to cause cough and angioedema. As many as 25% of patients on ACE inhibitors experience cough, while angioedema is much less common, occurring at a rate of 0.2%.

PATHOGENESIS OF DRUG ALLERGY

Hapten–carrier complexes

Some drugs, such as insulin and chymopapain, are large protein molecules capable of eliciting an immune response in their own right. These 'complete' antigens are recognized as foreign and are taken up and processed by antigen-presenting cells. Most drugs, however, are small molecules which are not directly recognized by the immune system. In order to become immunogenic, such drugs or their reactive metabolites must first undergo the process of haptenation by covalently binding to macromolecular carriers, usually serum or cell surface proteins. The resultant hapten–carrier complexes are multivalent and relatively allergenic, capable of eliciting either a humoral or cellular response or both, e.g. with penicillin. Anaphylaxis is IgE dependent while many skin reactions are lymphocyte mediated. Immune responses may be directed against a variety of epitopes including the drug (hapten), the hapten–carrier complex (neoantigen), or the carrier protein (self antigen). Other proteins, such as liver-metabolizing enzymes, may also function as carriers for drug haptens. For example, hypersensitivity reactions to anticonvulsants appear to occur via antibodies directed against new antigenic drug epitopes covalently linked to cytochrome P450 proteins.

Chemical propensity of the drug

The chemical propensity of the drug to function as a hapten is a treatment-related risk factor for the development of a drug allergy. Under physiologic conditions, penicillin readily undergoes haptenation (Fig. 10.6). When the penicillin nucleus opens to form a covalent bond with serum proteins, the penicilloyl determinant is created. This neoantigen is designated the major determinant of penicillin allergy since more than 95% of penicillin antibodies recognize this determinant. Other chemical interactions are involved in the generation of minor penicillin determinants.

Unlike penicillin, most drugs are not inherently reactive and require metabolic activation before haptenation can occur. For example, sulfamethoxazole in co-trimoxazole undergoes bioactivation to yield an immunologically reactive hydroxylamine metabolite. Other treatment-related risk factors include the dose and duration of treatment as follows:

- Drug-induced serum sickness, interstitial nephritis, and cytopenias are more frequent with high-dose, long-term therapy.
- Long courses of treatment increase the length of exposure and therefore extend the risk period.
- The more often a drug is used, the greater is the likelihood of developing an allergic reaction.
- The route of administration may also affect the risk for allergy.
- Delayed-type hypersensitivity is frequently associated with topical drug delivery.
- Comparable doses of parenteral and oral penicillin have similar rates of allergic reaction, although the intramuscular administration of repository drugs (e.g. benzathine penicillin) appears to induce reactions more frequently, even at lower doses.

Risk factors may also relate to patient factors such as age. Hypersensitivity reactions to penicillin are more frequent in

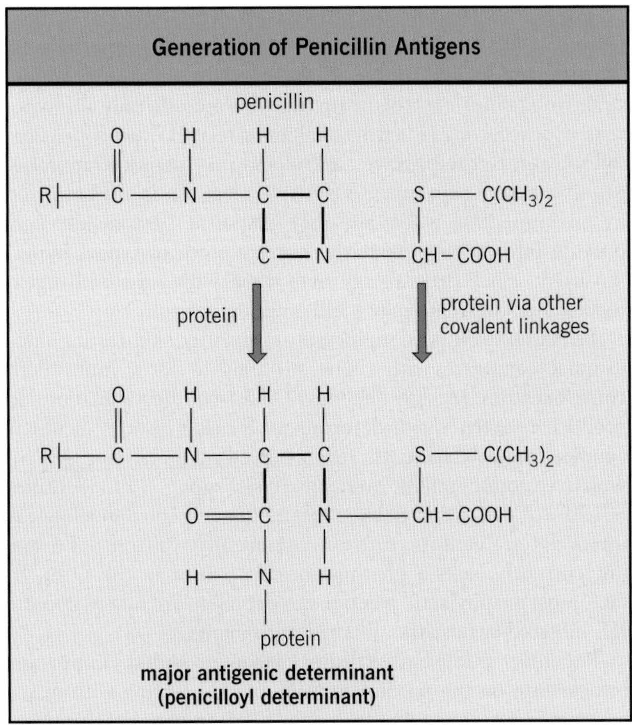

Fig. 10.6 The generation of penicillin antigens under physiologic conditions in vivo. The β-lactam ring spontaneously opens to form a covalent bond with serum proteins. This neoantigen is known as the penicilloyl determinant. Other covalent linkages may also occur, creating minor antigenic determinants.

Table 10.2 Drugs in everyday use that most commonly cause allergic reactions. Antibiotics account for the vast majority of these drugs

Allergenic Drugs in Common Use	
Haptenic drugs	**Complete antigens**
Penicillins	Insulin and other recombinant proteins
Cephalosporins	Enzymes (chymopapain, asparaginase)
Sulfonamide antimicrobials	Foreign antitoxins
Muscle relaxants	Organ extracts (ACTH, hormones)
Antituberculous drugs	Vaccines
Anticonvulsants	
Thiopental	
Quinidine	
cis-Platinum	

ACTH, adrenocorticotropic hormone.

adults than children. Genetic factors, such as slow acetylator phenotype or propensity to mount an antibody response, are predisposing factors for drug allergy; underlying host factors may also play a role. Examples include the high incidence of sulfonamide allergy in HIV-infected individuals and the frequency of antibiotic allergy in patients with chronic diseases for which antimicrobials are often needed, such as cystic fibrosis.

DIAGNOSIS OF DRUG ALLERGY

History

A carefully elicited history is often sufficient to identify hypersensitivity reactions. All medications taken should be thoroughly reviewed, whether or not they were previously well tolerated. The routes and frequency of administration along with a history of prior exposures may be useful as well, since intermittent parenteral administration is a risk factor for allergic reactions. The length of time between the introduction of medications and the onset of symptoms is very helpful information since a primary immune response generally requires 10–14 days. In contrast, the rapid onset of symptoms following initial drug administration suggests an idiosyncratic reaction. With prior sensitization, however, immune-mediated responses can and often do occur soon after the first dose. As previously mentioned, knowledge of the sensitizing potential of commonly used drugs is also helpful (Table 10.2).

Symptom presentation and physical examination

Clinical features, including symptom presentation, physical examination, and laboratory abnormalities, may also aid in the diagnosis of drug allergy. The rapid onset of symptoms such as urticaria, angioedema, bronchospasm, or hypotension is characteristic of type I hypersensitivity. Since type II reactions are associated with cytotoxicity, hematologic derangements are seen, including immune-mediated thrombocytopenia, Coombs' positive hemolytic anemia and granulocytopenia.

Although fever is a frequent manifestation of type III hypersensitivity, lymphadenopathy, rash, purpura, arthralgias, joint swelling, hepatitis, and interstitial nephritis may occur. Type IV hypersensitivity often involves the skin and mucous membranes with manifestations including 'toxic erythema' such as ampicillin rash, eczematous or exfoliative dermatitis and erythema multiforme. More severe reactions such as Stevens–Johnson syndrome or toxic epidermal necrolysis usually include fever and multisystem involvement reflected by leuko- and thrombocytopenias, rise in hepatic enzymes, and sometimes reduced renal function.

Taking the spectrum of potential manifestations into account, the physical examination of the patient with suspected drug allergy should include the evaluation of the patient's vital signs, along with the skin and joints, mucous membranes, respiratory tract, and cardiovascular and lymphoid systems.

Additional tests

Laboratory considerations may include a complete blood count with differential and platelet enumeration, Coombs' test, assays for the detection of circulating immune complexes, liver transaminase assessment, and urinalysis for the evaluation of proteinuria. Measurement of serum tryptase, because of its longer half-life, is preferred over quantification of serum histamine in the evaluation of anaphylaxis.

Tests for the presence of allergy

A variety of immunologic tests for the diagnosis of drug allergy are available, but only intradermal skin testing for IgE antibody has been demonstrated to have a strong predictive value. Skin testing has enjoyed an important role in the assessment of type I penicillin allergy. Since most patients experience a decline in drug-specific IgE over time, the identification of skin-test-negative individuals allows for the safe readministration of penicillin when β-lactam antibiotics are required.

When carefully performed, skin testing is quite safe and provides valuable information relatively quickly. For penicillin, adverse reactions to properly performed skin tests are rare (less than 1%) and most of these reactions are mild and resolve spontaneously. Skin testing also may be employed in the assessment of IgE-mediated allergy to other drugs (Table 10.3). Skin tests have no predictive value for non-IgE-mediated reactions, including drug fever, maculopapular exanthems, exfoliative dermatitis, interstitial nephritis, or hemolytic anemia.

Table 10.3 Drugs for which intradermal testing is used in the evaluation of allergy. Penicillin skin tests have proved useful; testing with other agents must be carefully interpreted

Drugs for which Intradermal Skin Testing may be Useful	
Penicillin	Foreign antitoxins
Cephalosporins	Antituberculous drugs
Insulin	Anticonvulsants
Chymopapain	Quinidine
Local anesthetics	*cis*-Platinum
Muscle relaxants	Penicillamine
Thiopental	Vaccines

The methodology of skin testing begins with prick or puncture testing. If this test is negative, intradermal testing is performed. Skin testing should always include positive (histamine) and negative (saline) controls. Patients who are critically ill, hypotensive or receiving H_1 antihistamines or related drugs sometimes fail to react to the positive control and may demonstrate false-negative type I skin tests. A positive response is characterized by an immediate wheal-and-flare response. Test results only provide information about the current state of type I hypersensitivity since drug allergy may wane with time and repeat testing at a later date may yield a negative result.

Penicillin itself is an inefficient reagent for skin testing since it must conjugate with tissue proteins to form multivalent complexes to elicit IgE-dependent mast-cell degranulation. To produce an active major determinant for skin tests, penicillin is coupled to polylysine to form penicilloyl-polylysine (PPL), which is commercially available. Used alone, PPL identifies 80–90% of patients at risk for IgE-mediated penicillin allergy. A minor determinant mixture is commercially available in Europe but currently lacks a pharmaceutical sponsor in the USA. In fact, most anaphylactic reactions to penicillin are due to specific IgE directed against the minor determinants.

Recently published studies have provided important information on the predictive value of skin testing with major and minor determinants (Table 10.4). When both determinants are used, skin tests have a high negative predictive value. Approximately 1% of patients with positive histories but negative skin tests develop mild transient urticaria with or without pruritus following β-lactam administration. There are no reports of penicillin anaphylaxis in individuals with negative skin tests. When benzylpenicillin G (10 000 U/mL) is used as a representative minor determinant for skin testing along with PPL, sensitivity approaches 90–95%. In such cases, graded provocative challenge may be helpful to safely establish whether sensitivity persists.

Alternative immunologic tests for the evaluation of drug allergy exist, but are less reliable, more time consuming, and often more costly. Penicilloyl-specific IgE antibody can be measured by radioallergosorbent testing (RAST), which detects serum antibody. RAST is less sensitive than intradermal skin tests. Although they are not validated for routine clinical use, RAST tests have also been developed for other β-lactam antibiotics, sulfonamides, trimethoprim, isoniazid, and other drug

Table 10.4 The frequency of IgE-dependent reactions to penicillin therapy following skin testing in history-positive and history-negative subjects. Note the high predictive value for negative skin tests

The Predictive Value of Penicillin Skin Tests				
History of penicillin allergy	+		–	
Penicillin skin test status	+	–	+	–
Frequency of allergic reactions associated with penicillin administration	50–70%	1–3%	10%	0.5%

Table 10.5 Diagnostic tests employed in the evaluation of drug allergies

Tests for Evaluating Drug Allergy		
In Vivo	**Assessment of**	**Gell and Coombs**
Prick, intradermal skin tests	IgE to agent	Type I
Provocation (dose escalation)	Tolerance	All
Patch testing	DTH	Type IV
Biopsy	Immunohistopathology	Types III, IV
In Vitro	**Assessment of**	**Gell and Coombs**
RAST	IgE in serum	Type I
Leukocyte histamine release+	IgE	Type I
Lymphocyte proliferation	T-cell responsiveness	Type IV
Lymphocyte cytokine production	T-cell responsiveness	Type IV
Lymphocyte cytotoxicity	T-cell responsiveness	Type IV

+ Alternative: CD63 or CD202 marker expression on basophils using flow cytometry. DTH, delayed type hypersensitivity; RAST, radioallergosorbent test.

determinants (Table 10.5). Leukocyte histamine release can also detect specific IgE antibodies but it is not diagnostically reliable for the evaluation of IgE antibodies to haptenic drugs. Other cellular tests, such as lymphocyte proliferation and tests for cytokine production may be useful in establishing a drug-specific T-cell mediated immune response but the range of drugs for which they work reliably is small.

Provocation studies

When skin testing or RAST cannot be performed, provocative challenge or test dosing may be helpful. In this procedure, the drug is administered at initially low doses which are serially increased until full dose therapy is reached (Table 10.6). The time interval between rising doses depends upon the nature of the suspected reaction: 20–30 minutes is usually adequate when considering IgE-mediated reactions whereas 24–48 hours may be necessary for delayed-type hypersensitivity reactions.

Table 10.6 A protocol for test dosing with local anesthetics

Protocol for Test Dosing with Local Anesthetics

Proceed in order, advancing to the next step every 15 minutes

1. Skin prick test with undiluted anesthetic (do not use epinephrine-containing agents)
2. If negative, 0.1 mL of 1 in 100 dilution is given subcutaneously (s.c.)
3. If no reaction, 0.1 mL of 1 in 10 dilution is given s.c.
4. If no reaction, administer 1 mL undiluted anesthetic s.c.
5. If no reaction, administer 2 mL undiluted anesthetic s.c.

Test dosing is useful when the likelihood of a true allergy is low. Because of the potential risks, provocative challenge should be performed with informed consent and careful monitoring by experienced physicians.

Patch testing is a diagnostic modality in which the skin is directly challenged with the suspected drug allergen. It may be employed when considering delayed type hypersensitivity (DTH) to topically applied medications, preservatives, or industrially contacted agents. For systemic drug reactions, patch testing can be a reliable form of in vivo challenge. The key point is that it works for type IV reaction patterns such as erythema multiforme or eczema, but does not work for non-lymphocyte mediated reactions. Non-irritating concentrations of the suspected contact sensitizer or 1 and 5% concentrations of systemic drugs are applied to the skin. Responses are evaluated 48–72 hours later for evidence of vesicles or localized dermatitis.

MANAGEMENT OF DRUG ALLERGY

Drug treatment

The proper assessment and management of drug hypersensitivity is important, not only because of the potential morbidity and mortality but also because of the subsequent restriction in therapeutic options for the patient. In an acute drug reaction, the offending drug should be discontinued. If the patient is on multiple medications, those drugs that are known to be most sensitizing and least necessary to the patient should be stopped empirically until the reaction abates. Symptomatic therapy may be instituted, depending upon the nature of the reaction. It is critical to institute treatment/management that relates to the immunologic reaction involved in the hypersensitivity. Thus, antihistamine therapy is helpful to relieve pruritus and the rash of type 1 reactions. However, histamine is not involved in lymphocyte-mediated cutaneous eruptions and hence,

Table 10.7 Recommended guidelines for penicillin desensitization in allergic subjects

Penicillin Desensitization Protocol				
Oral: penicillin V every 15 min		**Parenteral: penicillin G every 20 min**		
Step	**Dose (units)**	**Dose (units/mL)**	**Volume (mL)**	**Route**
1	100	100	0.1	i.d.
2	200	100	0.2	s.c.
3	400	100	0.4	s.c.
4	800	100	0.8	s.c.
5	1600	1000	0.1	i.d.
6	3200	1000	0.3	s.c.
7	6400	1000	0.6	s.c
8	12 000	10 000	0.1	i.d.
9	24 000	10 000	0.2	s.c.
10	48 000	10 000	0.4	s.c.
11	80 000	10 000	0.8	s.c.
12	160 000	100 000	0.1	i.d.
13	320 000	100 000	0.3	s.c.
14	640 000	100 000	0.6	s.c.
Change to i.v. penicillin G				
15	125 000	1 000 000	0.1	i.d.
16	250 000	1 000 000	0.2	s.c.
17	500 000	1 000 000	0.2	i.m.
18	1 125 000	1 000 000	0.4	i.m.
19		1 000 000	continuous i.v. infusion	

antihistamines are of no help in eczematous or erythema multiforme reactions. Corticosteroids may be necessary for the relief of severe urticaria and other extensive exanthems, as well as for severe systemic reactions, including nephritis and serum sickness. Steroid use in erythema multiforme syndromes (toxic epidermal necrolysis and Stevens–Johnson syndrome) is controversial. In the event of anaphylaxis (see Ch. 11), treatment includes aqueous epinephrine (1:1000 w/v) intramuscularly, diphenhydramine, and corticosteroids (to prevent or minimize late-phase allergic reactions). Systemic anaphylaxis may also require aggressive cardiovascular support with intravenous fluids and vasopressor agents. Hospital admission with overnight observation is indicated for severe anaphylaxis.

Allergen avoidance

As with hypersensitivity of any type, allergen avoidance is an integral component of long-term management of drug allergy. In the majority of clinical situations, appropriate alternative drugs exist and may be used without concern for adverse outcomes. For example, for penicillin-allergic patients, one or more non-beta lactam antibiotics are often acceptable for most infectious diseases. Drugs of similar structure may often be cross-reactive immunologically and clinically. However, such cross-reactivity is incomplete: in insulin allergy for example, insulin derived from animal sources may often be substituted with recombinant human insulin, even though partial cross-reactivity exists. Similarly, many subjects with penicillin allergies will tolerate cephalosporins despite the common β-lactam nuclear structure which penicillins and cephalosporins share. Immunologic cross-reactivity between penicillins and cephalosporins is as high as 15–25% for first generation cephalosporins but appears to be much lower for third generation agents, about 1–2%. Even so, severe life-threatening cross-reactions (e.g. anaphylaxis) have been reported. In contrast, a history of maculopapular rash due to amoxicillin or ampicillin is not associated with increased risk of a life-threatening reaction to penicillin.

Other approaches to therapy

Infrequently, certain medical conditions cannot be successfully treated with alternative therapy. For example, there is no acceptable substitute for penicillin in pregnant patients with syphilis. In these circumstances, drug desensitization is necessary. Standard protocols have been developed for penicillin, co-trimoxazole, dapsone, sulfasalazine, and insulin desensitization which, though risking mild systemic reactions, are usually effective in achieving clinical tolerance. These procedures require informed consent and close physician supervision. An

Table 10.8 Guidelines for pretreatment to prevent anaphylactoid reactions to radiocontrast media (RCM) for elective procedures. In emergency situations, hydrocortisone and diphenhydramine are given intravenously

Pretreatment Guidelines for the Prevention of Anaphylactoid RCM Reactions

Drug (dose)	Route	Instructions
Prednisone (50 mg)	Oral or i.m.	Administer 13, 7,and 1 hour before RCM procedure
Diphenhydramine (50 mg)	Oral or i.m.	Administer 1 hour before RCM procedure
Ephedrine sulfate (25 mg)*	Oral	Administer 1 hour before RCM procedure

* Withhold if there is a history of coronary artery disease or arrhythmia

intensive-care setting should be used whenever possible and rescue drugs, such as epinephrine, should be readily available. Desensitization is based upon the principle of administering gradually increasing doses of drug beginning with a very small dose and aiming toward a full therapeutic dose. Dose increments may be introduced as frequently as every 15–30 minutes so that full therapeutic doses are generally achieved within 24 hours (Table 10.7).

The mechanism by which desensitization induces tolerance is generally attributed to the induction of a desensitized state in IgE-primed cells by low-dose antigen. As a result, a higher antigen threshold is necessary for mediator release. Regardless of the mechanism, the state of tolerance is transient and must be actively maintained by continuous drug administration once achieved. If the patient needs the sensitizing drug in the future and repeat skin tests are still positive, desensitization must be performed again.

Additional treatment protocols have been developed for certain drug-induced anaphylactoid reactions. Patients with a history of RCM reaction are at an increased risk for reactions with future exposures; since these reactions are not IgE mediated, skin testing is not useful for the identification of those persons at risk. Prevention strategies have been devised which reduce reaction rates to 10% for hypertonic contrast media and 1% for non-ionic agents. The recommendations include the use of non-ionic contrast media and premedication with corticosteroids and antihistamines, as outlined in Table 10.8.

For the patient with aspirin or NSAID sensitivity, substitutes which generally are not cross-reactive, such as acetaminophen or choline magnesium trisalicylate, may be effective. If not, oral desensitization may be considered, in which initially small and gradually increasing doses may be administered, following a protocol such as that given in Table 10.9. Such an approach is somewhat similar to the desensitization protocol previously discussed and should be performed with informed consent and physician supervision. Once a full therapeutic dose is achieved, daily dosing is required in order to maintain tolerance. Although COX-2 inhibitors appear to be well tolerated in almost all individuals with NSAID sensitivity, a few cases of urticaria and angioedema have been reported.

Table 10.9 Oral aspirin challenge. The patient is gradually desensitized to aspirin. Initially small doses are administered, which are gradually increased over time

Oral Aspirin Challenge

Day	8 a.m.	11 a.m.	2 p.m.
1	Placebo	Placebo	Placebo
2	30 mg	60 mg	100 mg
3	150 mg	325 mg	650 mg

CONCLUSION

Drug hypersensitivity may occur through a variety of immunologic and non-immune pathways. Host- and drug-related risk factors are useful in considering the likelihood of drug allergy. Advances in our understanding of bioactivation and drug metabolism have led to the identification of immunogenic determinants of several drugs. The application of other immunologic and pharmacologic techniques should further advance the study of drug hypersensitivity with the result that additional diagnostic and therapeutic agents may be developed.

FURTHER READING

Adkinson NF. Drug allergy. In: Adkinson NF, Yunginger JW, Busse WW, et al, eds. Allergy: principles and practice. 6th edn. Philadelphia: CV Mosby; 2003:1679–1694.

Bernstein I, Gruchalla R, Lee R, et al. Disease management of drug hypersensitivity: a practice parameter. Joint Task Force on Practice Parameters, the American Academy of Allergy, Asthma and Immunology, and the Joint Council of Allergy, Asthma and Immunology. Ann Allergy Asthma Immunol 1999; 83:665–700.

DeShazo RD, Kemp SF. Allergic reactions to drugs and biologic agents. JAMA 1997; 278:1895–1906.

Friedmann PS, Lee M-S, Friedmann, AC, et al. Mechanisms in cutaneous drug hypersensitivity reactions. Clin Exp Allergy 2003; 33:1–12.

Gadde J, Spence M, Wheeler B, et al. Clinical experience with penicillin skin testing in a large inner-city STD clinic. JAMA 1993; 270:2456–2463.

Gruchalla RS. Drug allergy. J Allergy Clin Immunol 2003; 111:S548–459.

Kelkar PS, Li JT-C. Cephalosporin allergy. N Engl J Med 2001; 345(11):804–809.

Sogn DD, Evans R, Shepherd GM, et al. Results of the NIAID collaborative clinical trial to test the predictive value of skin testing with major and minor penicillin derivatives in hospitalized adults. Arch Intern Med 1992; 152:1025–1032.

Chapter 11

Anaphylaxis

Albert L Sheffer, Anna Feldweg, and Mariana Castells

Definition:
Anaphylaxis is a potentially life-threatening systemic allergic reaction, often explosive in onset, with symptoms ranging from mild flushing to upper respiratory obstruction with or without vascular collapse.

INTRODUCTION

Anaphylaxis is the most emergent clinical manifestation encountered in an allergy practice. Often abrupt in onset, symptoms are usually consequent to the effects of potent chemical mediators released upon antigen binding from previously sensitized mast cells or basophils. Symptoms may range from mild pruritus to life-threatening respiratory and/or cardiovascular collapse. Although there is a hieroglyphic depiction of anaphylactic death from a Hymenoptera sting dating to 4000 years ago, the mechanism for such reactions has only recently been clarified. The term anaphylaxis describes an explosive, often life-threatening response to the reintroduction of minute quantities of antigen, in direct opposition to tolerance.

While true anaphylaxis is mediated by the binding of antigen to specific IgE on the surface of the mast cells and basophils, similar symptoms may be precipitated by non-IgE mechanisms. Such reactions are described as anaphylactoid, and occur when agents such as radiocontrast media (RCM), codeine, vancomycin and aspirin or other non-steroidal antiinflammatory drugs (NSAIDs) induce mast cell degranulation.

The risk for an anaphylactic event in the USA ranges from 1 to 3%. Surveys have revealed that 1/1000 adult and 1/170 children experience at least one episode of anaphylaxis; 1/12 patients who experienced anaphylaxis suffered a recurrence. Compliance with carrying and the utilization of epinephrine was poor, although 1/50 required epinephrine. Other data indicate that 1/1500 emergency room visits are attributable to anaphylaxis. Evidence suggests the incidence of acute anaphylaxis is increasing, although the exact figure is not well established. Recent studies indicate that the incidence may be increasing from 5.6 cases per 100 000 hospital discharges in 1991–1992 to 10.2 in 1994–1995.

The most common causes for anaphylaxis are foods (61%), Hymenoptera stings (20.4%), and drugs (8.3%). Fatal anaphylaxis consequent to penicillin administration occurs with an incidence of 0.002% and accounts for 500 penicillin-related anaphylactic deaths annually in the USA. Non-fatal reactions occur in 0.7–1.0% of penicillin recipients. RCM agents are associated with a rate of anaphylactoid reactions of 0.4%. Aspirin and NSAIDs induce anaphylactic reactions at a rate of 0.9%. Peanut-induced anaphylaxis has significantly increased during the past decade. In UK and US studies, the incidence is approximately 0.5%. Natural latex was an increasing cause of anaphylaxis, particularly in nursing personnel and patients with spina bifida who had undergone multiple surgical interventions, until the recognition of the problem and introduction of latex alternatives. Hymenoptera anaphylaxis is associated with at least 40 fatalities annually in the USA.

Table 11.1 Risk factors for anaphylaxis

Risk Factors for Anaphylaxis
Age (adults > children)
Gender (females > males)
Route of administration (parenteral > oral)
Exposure to allergen (recent > remote)
Atopy
Systemic mastocytosis
Asthma

RISK FACTORS FOR ANAPHYLAXIS (Table 11.1)

Adults appear to be more susceptible to anaphylaxis than children. Race and geographic location do not appear to affect the incidence of anaphylaxis. However, gender is a factor for reactions to quaternary ammonium muscle relaxants, RCM reactions, aspirin, and latex, which occur more frequently in women, whereas stinging insect reactions occur more frequently in men. Route of antigen introduction impacts anaphylaxis: parenteral administration increases the severity and frequency of anaphylactic reactions. The duration of time between the original anaphylactic reaction and readministration of the antigen is important. A lower incidence of reactions occurs when the drug inducing the adverse reaction is re-administered 10 years or more after the adverse event. Constant antigenic exposure also affects the frequency of anaphylactic events. For example, insulin-induced anaphylaxis is rare, unless insulin therapy is repeatedly interrupted for a time period sufficient for clearance from the body and then re-administered. Repeat adverse reactions to allergens previously encountered occur in 24% of the patients presenting to emergency rooms.

There are also subsets of patients who are at elevated risk for anaphylaxis as well as adverse outcomes because of related disease states. The presence of atopy increases the risk of anaphylaxis from certain triggers, including insect stings and latex exposure, but not medications or RCM. Atopic patients also experience more exercise induced and idiopathic anaphylaxis. Pollen-allergic patients on immunotherapy may experience adverse reactions during their allergy season, even when they are administered the appropriate allergen in the usual dosage. Patients with mastocytosis may experience massive mediator release during an anaphylactic event, with subsequent symptoms so severe that they are unresponsive to therapy. This has been observed following Hymenoptera stings. Asthma sufferers are predisposed to respiratory failure during anaphylaxis, particularly if epinephrine therapy is delayed.

Certain pharmacologic therapies interfere with optimal therapeutic response in anaphylaxis. Patients receiving β-blocking agents are not at increased risk for anaphylaxis, but when an anaphylactic event occurs it may be more severe and refractory to therapy. Likewise, angiotensin converting enzyme inhibitors may interfere with the effectiveness of the renin angiotensin system, which may be activated during anaphylaxis to counter hypotension.

PATHOPHYSIOLOGY OF ANAPHYLAXIS

Systemic anaphylaxis is a clinical syndrome defined by its symptomatology and etiology. Its precise pathophysiology remains incompletely defined. Human studies are yielding more knowledge of the chemical mediators generated and their biologic effects. A pathophysiologic classification has been derived from studies and provides a framework for addressing the clinical entity in regards to its pathogenesis (see Table 11.2).

Anatomical changes occurring in patients with anaphylaxis include upper airway obstruction due to pharyngeal and laryngeal edema, acute pulmonary hyperinflation, pulmonary edema, parenchymal hemorrhage, and visceral congestion. A pathologic examination of the upper airway reveals non-inflammatory edema. Diffuse histologic changes of the airways include mucus accumulation, submucosal edema, and eosinophilic infiltration with vascular congestion. The pulmonary parenchyma may reveal hemorrhage, edema and atelectasis. The most significant cardiovascular event associated with anaphylaxis is consequent to postcapillary venule leakage, which can result in hypovolemia and shock. Myocardial necrosis occurs, and congestion of the liver, spleen, and other vital organs has also been described. Rarely, disseminated intravascular coagulation may occur. Significant pathologic changes may not be observed at the time of postmortem examination. Upper respiratory tract edema with airway obstruction is observed in two-thirds of the fatal cases and acute pulmonary hyperinflation in just half.

CLASSIFICATION OF ANAPHYLACTIC REACTIONS (Table 11.2)

IgE-mediated anaphylactic event

The most common and best-understood mechanism of anaphylaxis is IgE-dependent immediate-type hypersensitivity. This type of reaction is termed anaphylactic to distinguish such from non-IgE related reactions termed anaphylactoid. Tissue mast cells and circulating basophils become coated with IgE molecules specific for antigen, a process termed sensitization. If an antigen to which a subset of IgE molecule binds is introduced in sufficient quantity, it will result in cross-linking of those IgE molecules and intracellular signaling, which then triggers degranulation of the mast cell or basophil. The chemical mediators released rapidly from sensitized tissue mast cells and circulating basophils upon antigen challenge may include histamine, prostaglandin D_2 (PGD_2), leukotriene C_4 (LTC_4) and tryptase. Basophils in the peripheral circulation can be reached by soluble allergens administered intravenously and mast cells at mucosal membranes, by allergens ingested or inhaled. Those mediators relevant to the anaphylactic reaction are listed in Table 11.3.

Histamine can be measured in plasma within minutes of an anaphylactic event. As a consequence, the histamine receptors (H_1 and H_2) are stimulated, producing vasodilatation with postcapillary venule leakage, reduced vascular resistance with consequent hypotension, flushing, bronchial and smooth muscle contraction, and glandular secretion. Assay for histamine can best be accomplished by 24 hour urine assessment because of the short serum half-life of serum histamine.

Mast cell serum tryptase, which has a half-life of 60 minutes post anaphylaxis, can be measured by immunoassay. During an anaphylactic event, mature tryptase levels correlate linearly

Table 11.2 Common forms of anaphylaxis and their associated causes

Mechanisms			
IgE-Mediated (Anaphylaxis)	**Non-IgE-Mediated (Anaphylactoid)**		
	Complement-mediated	**5-Lipoxygenase-mediated**	**Mast cell-mediated**
Proteins: Foods, e.g. peanuts, seafood, eggs, milk Allergen extracts Inhalant allergens, e.g. pollen, cat dander Hymenoptera venom, e.g. bee stings Vaccines Antisera Hormones, enzymes Haptens: Antibiotics, e.g. penicillin Exercise-induced anaphylaxis	IgA deficiency (immune complex) Cuprophane dialysis membrane	Aspirin Non steroidal antiinflammatory drugs	Radiocontrast media Opiates Anesthetics: curare derivates Vancomycin (red man syndrome)

Table 11.3 Mediators of anaphylaxis

Mediators of Anaphylaxis	
Mast cell and basophil-derived mediators	**Other mediators**
Histamine	Complement:
Proteoglycans:	C3a, C5a anaphylatoxins
Heparin, condroitin sulfates	Kinin/kallikrein
Neutral proteases:	Nitric oxide
Tryptase α and β (mature) forms	Neuropeptides
Leukotrienes: LTC_4, LTD_4	(examples: vasoactive intestinal peptide VIP; platelet activating factor, PAF)
Prostaglandins: PGD_2	

with histamine concentration as well as the severity of clinical symptoms (Fig. 11.1). Following release into the circulation, tryptase rapidly inactivates fibrinogen, prolonging coagulation with possible disseminated intravascular coagulopathy, a rare clinical manifestation of anaphylaxis. This is further accentuated by the release of heparin, which is closely associated with tryptase in the mast cell granule. Tryptase also reduces the bronchodilatory effects of such neuropeptides as vasoactive intestinal peptide, inducing bronchoconstriction. A study of the postmortem tryptase levels in the serum of patients who died of unidentified causes has demonstrated that at least 20% exhibited a tryptase elevation that was demonstrable and consistent with an anaphylactic event. Elevated serum tryptase has been observed in 12% of the sudden death and 40% of sudden infant death syndrome. Elevations of tryptase in food-induced anaphylaxis are lower than in adverse drug reactions (ADR).

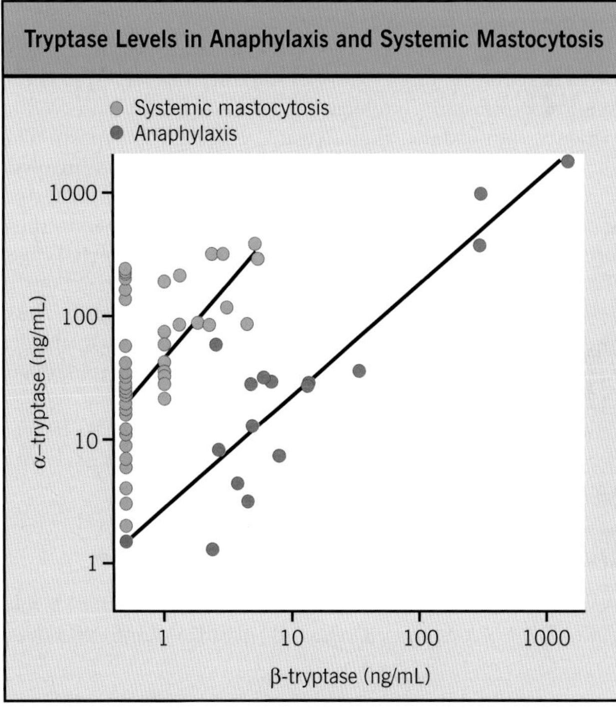

Fig. 11.1 Tryptase levels in anaphylaxis and systemic mastocytosis. In allergic responses including anaphylaxis, the β-tryptase form is released. In systemic mastocytosis α-tryptase is the predominant form. (Data from Schwartz LB, et al. The alpha form of human tryptase is the predominant type present in blood, is baseline in normal subjects, and is elevated in those with systemic mastocytosis. J Clin Invest 1995; 96:2702.)

Non-IgE-mediated anaphylactoid events

Complement-mediated anaphylaxis

The mechanisms for non-IgE-mediated anaphylaxis are not as well elucidated as IgE-mediated reactions. Immune complex complement-mediated anaphylaxis occurs during transfusions and administration of intravenous Ig. In such reactions, pre-existing IgG (and rarely IgE) anti-IgA antibodies recognize IgA in blood products and Ig form, immune complexes, and activate the classical complement pathway. Another type of complement-mediated anaphylactoid reaction involves the alternative complement pathway. Cuprophane membrane dialysis is an example of such a reaction. Activation of the alternative pathway results in the generation of anaphylatoxins C3a and C5a, which increase vascular permeability, enhance smooth muscle contraction, and induce the release of histamine from dermal mast cells.

Aspirin and NSAID-induced anaphylaxis

Multiple types of reactions are observed in response to ingestion of aspirin and NSAIDs, including anaphylaxis, urticaria/angioedema, rhinosinusitis/asthma, and hypersensitivity pneumonitis. Only those reactions which involve anaphylactic symptoms are discussed here. Urticaria, angioedema, and anaphylaxis can develop in response to a single, specific COX-1 inhibitor. This is usually seen in patients without underlying chronic urticaria/angioedema. Cross-reactivity with other NSAIDs is not predictable. The mechanism is not elucidated, but is proposed to be IgE-mediated.

Aspirin and other inhibitors of COX-1 can also cause severe bronchospasm by exacerbating respiratory disease. This is the syndrome of aspirin intolerance, and is classically observed in patients with asthma, rhinosinusitis, and nasal polyposis. The biochemical basis for reactions in such patients involves disordered leukotriene synthesis and/or regulation. Affected individuals excrete excessive amounts of leukotrienes in their urine at baseline, and this is exaggerated after aspirin challenge. The potency of such drugs in eliciting respiratory reactions is related to their ability to block prostaglandin synthesis. Thus, the likely mechanism is an acute reduction in the prostaglandin G_2 (PGE_2) brake on leukotriene synthesis with underlying excessive production of leukotrienes.

Chronic urticaria can be exacerbated by NSAIDs. Recent work suggests that this too is due to inhibition of COX-1 with consequent overproduction of leukotrienes.

Direct mast cell/basophil mediator release

Anaphylaxis consequent to the administration of opiates, highly cationic antibiotics, muscle relaxants, plasma volume expanders, vancomycin, and RCM results from the release of histamine directly from skin mast cells. The mechanism appears to involve G-protein stimulation, resulting in degranulation and release of preformed mediators such as histamine, tryptase, and heparin, but not the generation of arachidonic acid products or cytokines. Such reactions may occur upon first exposure to such agents. RCM reactions are of the greatest clinical significance in this regard, with highest risk for reaction because of their high ionic strength. Anaphylaxis may occur in 1–2% patients administered RCM intravenously; such affected individuals have a 35% risk of anaphylaxis upon re-exposure.

Exercise-induced anaphylaxis (and other physical allergies)

Exercise-induced anaphylaxis (EIA) is a form of physical allergy with episodic presentation of pruritus, urticaria, erythema, and upper respiratory obstruction with or without vascular collapse. Unlike other forms of physical allergy, such reactions do not occur predictably with every exertion. In some patients with this disorder, it is critical for exercise to occur in relation to ingestion of a specific food, particularly wheat. In others, such reactions occur in relation to IgE-mediated inhalant allergy. Exercise in the postprandial state, regardless of the food ingested, precipitates a reaction in many affected patients. In others, exercising in the postprandial state, following aspirin or NSAIDs, precipitates a reaction. Menstrual status may also influence the occurrence of exercise-induced anaphylaxis. The mechanism for this reaction has not been fully appreciated.

In the wheat-associated form of EIA, a more specific mechanism has been proposed. The intestinal enzyme tissue transglutaminase has been found to trigger aggregation of a peptic fraction of omega-5 gliadin, and enhance IgE reactivity in patients with wheat-dependent, exercise-induced anaphylaxis.

Elevations in plasma histamine and associated ultrastructural changes support mast cell degranulation in such affected individuals following exercise challenge (Fig. 11.2).

A few physical urticarial reactions may progress to anaphylaxis. Cold-induced urticaria, usually IgE-mediated, may be associated with monoclonal gammopathy. Such affected individuals may exhibit cryoglobulins, cryofibrinogen, immune complexes and complement mediated processes. Affected patients may experience life-threatening anaphylactic symptoms upon sudden cold exposure, i.e. cold-water immersion. Cholinergic urticaria occurring with an increase in core-body

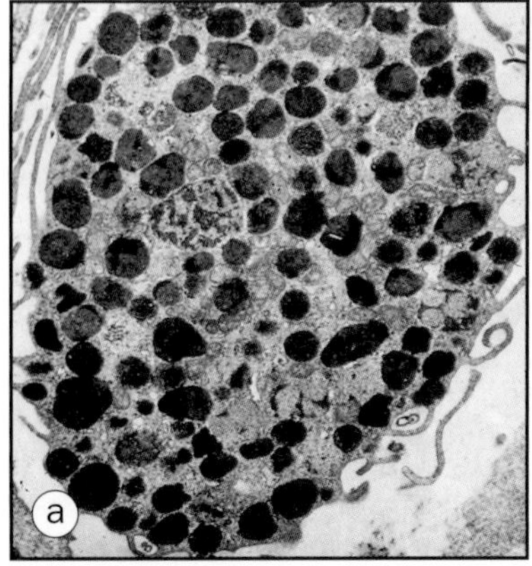

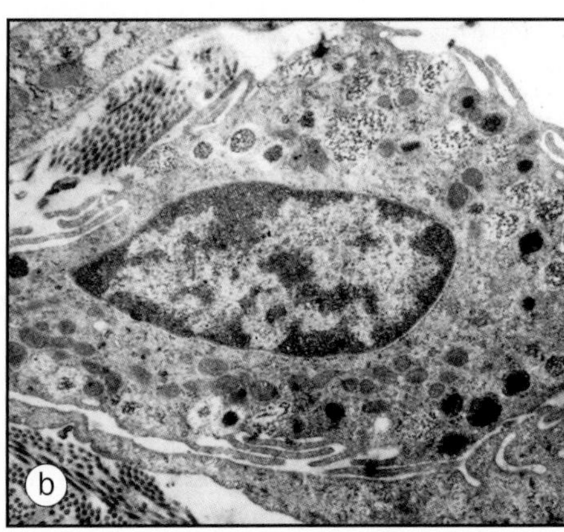

Fig. 11.2 Cutaneous mast cell. (a) Prior to exercise, (b) post exercise (anaphylaxis).

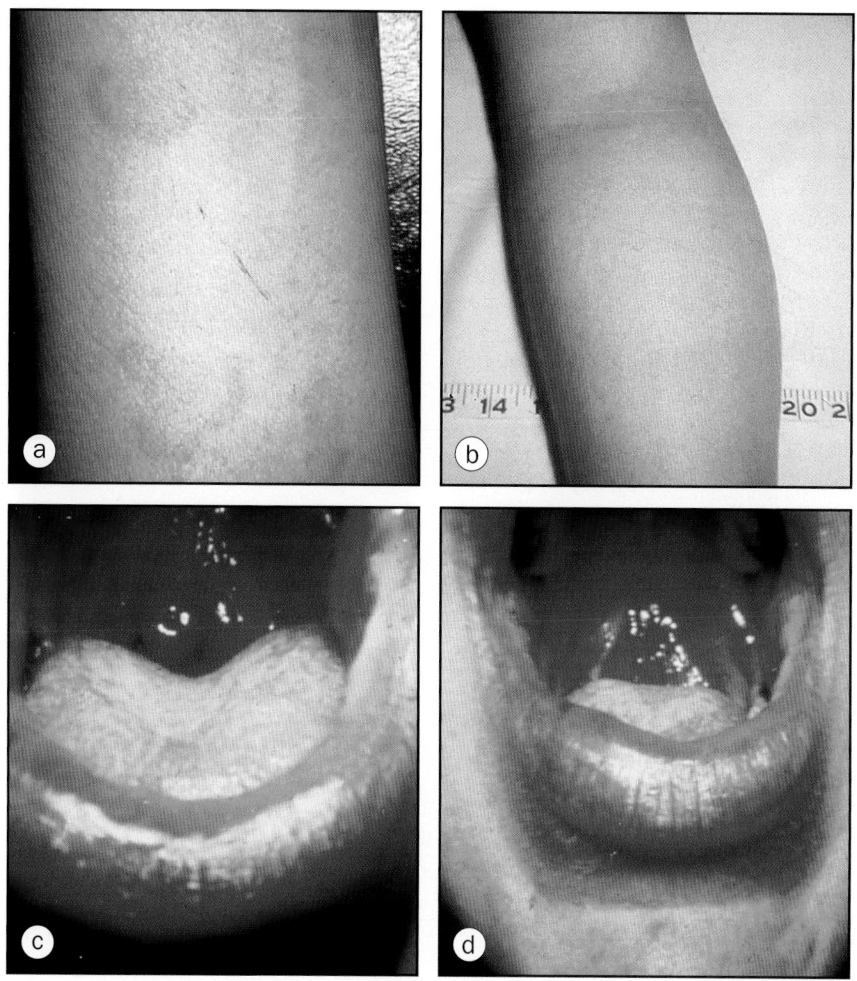

Fig. 11.3 (a) Urticaria, (b) angioedema of the skin, (c and d) upper respiratory angioedema.

temperature is characterized by punctate, pruritic, erythematous lesions that rarely progress to true anaphylaxis, but such lesions are associated with mast cell degranulation.

Idiopathic anaphylaxis

Despite intensive investigation, there remain many cases of anaphylaxis for which no etiology can be confidently established. Thus idiopathic anaphylaxis can be diagnosed only after extensive investigation fails to reveal precipitants. Clinical evaluation and laboratory assessment must exclude any underlying systemic disorder such as mastocytosis. The self-administration of an allergenic or pharmacologic substance must be considered. Selective skin tests and radioallergosorbent tests (RAST) may be helpful in establishing an etiology. Nearly half such affected individuals are atopic. Many have recurrent anaphylactic episodes that are refractory to the usual therapeutic interventions.

DIAGNOSIS OF ANAPHYLAXIS

Systemic anaphylaxis is a potentially fatal syndrome, which requires prompt recognition and immediate institution of therapy. Other clinical entities with similar signs and symptoms must be excluded. Obtaining an accurate history is central to establishing the diagnosis and instituting appropriate therapy.

Symptom presentation

Anaphylactic reactions are rapid in onset (usually within minutes following exposure to the precipitant) and may progress rapidly, usually over 10–20 minutes. The speed of onset and the clinical features vary with allergen concentration and the patient's sensitivity to the allergen. There may be a spectrum of presentations. Drugs administered intravenously can produce cardiovascular effects, whereas ingested antigens, such as foods, induce respiratory difficulty and asphyxia. The earliest symptoms include flushing and pruritus with intense erythema, urticaria (Fig. 11.3a) and angioedema (Fig.11.3b).

Food-induced reactions are associated with upper respiratory angioedema (Fig. 11.3c) and urticaria. Itching and edema of the oral mucosa with upper airway tightening may be the earliest indication of laryngeal edema. These symptoms may progress quickly to throat constriction, respiratory difficulty, cyanosis and asphyxia. Tachycardia, hypotension, upper or lower airway obstruction, and gastrointestinal colic may develop. Symptoms may be prolonged or may be delayed for several hours after the initial event.

Differential diagnosis

All causes for respiratory obstruction (Table 11.4) and vascular collapse, i.e. pulmonary embolism, cardiac arrhythmias, cardiac

Table 11.4 Differential diagnosis of anaphylaxis

Differential Diagnosis of Anaphylaxis	
Condition	**Clinical differentiation from anaphylaxis**
Vasovagal syndrome	Bradycardia not tachycardia Pallor rather than flushing No pruritus, urticaria, angioedema, upper respiratory obstruction, or bronchospasm Nausea but no abdominal pain
Angioedema and C1 inh deficiency	Prior history of C1 inh deficiency No flushing, pruritus, urticaria, bronchospasm, or hypotension More gradual onset of episodes
Serum sickness	No upper respiratory obstruction, bronchospasm or hypotension Fever, arthralgia, lymphadenopathy present Slower onset
Mastocytosis	No upper respiratory obstruction; bronchospasm uncommon Urticaria pigmentosa often present Slower onset of attacks; chronic low-grade symptomatology between attacks
Carcinoid syndrome	No upper respiratory obstruction, urticaria, or angioedema Slower onset of attacks May have cutaneous stigmata including telangiectases on the upper trunk
Scombroid syndrome	History of antecedent ingestion of suspect fish Oral burning, tingling, blistering, or peppery taste after ingestion Emesis common Episode may last days (though more commonly hours)
Globus hystericus	No clinical or radiologic evidence of upper respiratory obstruction No flushing, pruritus, urticaria, angioedema, bronchospasm, abdominal pain or hypotension

C1 inh, C1 esterase inhibitor.

tamponade, myocardial infarction, sepsis, seizure disorder, and insulin reactions must be excluded in addressing an anaphylactic event. While most of such reactions can be immediately excluded, others may require further consideration.

Vasovagal reactions

Vasovagal reactions are the most common mimic of anaphylaxis. There is often a rapid development of pallor, sweating, presyncope or even loss of consciousness due to hypotension. In contrast to anaphylaxis, which is usually accompanied by tachycardia, vasovagal reactions are usually associated with bradycardia. Upper respiratory obstruction and bronchospasm do not occur with vasovagal reactions. Nausea may be experienced during such episodes, but pruritus, abdominal pain, urticaria, and angioedema do not occur. Blood tryptase levels are not elevated.

Angioedema associated with a deficiency of C1 esterase inhibitor

Upper respiratory obstruction and angioedema due to C1 inhibitor deficiency may be confused with anaphylactic manifestations, but hereditary angioedema is not associated with pruritus, urticaria, flushing, rhinitis, and vascular collapse. The evolution of cutaneous angioedema and/or upper respiratory or abdominal symptoms during attacks in patients with angioedema associated with C1 inhibitor deficiency usually is slower than in patients with anaphylaxis. Biochemical confirmation of the absent C1 inhibitor (20% of the patients with hereditary angioedema blood levels appear normal, functional C1 inhibitor levels are reduced) and reduction in C4 are confirmatory of C1 inhibitor deficiency. A normal C4 level excludes the diagnosis of hereditary angioedema. Rarely, a reduced C4 may reflect an anaphylactic phenomenon consequent to a complement-mediated process or a hereditary deficiency of C4. Serum tryptase is not affected.

Serum sickness

Serum sickness may be accompanied by immune-complex-induced urticaria and angioedema. However, serum sickness is not associated with upper respiratory obstruction, bronchospasm or vascular collapse. Fever lymphadenopathy, arthralgia and purpuric skin lesions may occur with serum sickness, but are not features of anaphylaxis. Serum tryptase is not elevated.

Systemic mastocytosis

Systemic mastocytosis resembles idiopathic anaphylaxis with recurrent episodes of flushing, urticaria, rhinitis and gastrointestinal symptoms. Upper respiratory obstruction does not occur as a manifestation of the mastocytosis syndrome. Bronchospasm is infrequent and usually transient. Urticaria pigmentosa is associated with systemic mastocytosis and should alert any physician of the possible relationship. Patients with systemic mastocytosis demonstrate mast cell hyperplasia in the bone marrow and other organs. Plasma levels of histamine and serum total tryptase as well as mature tryptase may be elevated when anaphylaxis occurs. However, in mastocytosis the baseline tryptase may be elevated above the normal baseline total tryptase of 20 ng/mL.

Carcinoid syndrome

Carcinoid syndrome should be considered in the differential diagnosis of idiopathic anaphylaxis. Flushing, gastrointestinal symptoms and bronchospasm may occur in both entities. However, urticaria, angioedema, and upper respiratory obstruction do not occur as part of the carcinoid syndrome. The occurrence of elevated plasma serotonin or increased urinary levels of 5-hydroxyindoleacetic acid (5-HIAA) suggests the diagnosis, which is confirmed with the demonstration of the carcinoid tumor. Tryptase levels are not affected.

Scombroid poisoning

Scombroid poisoning results from the ingestion of partially decomposed fish containing histamine that has been generated by the action of histidine decarboxylase (a bacterial enzyme). Symptoms resemble anaphylaxis. Serum tryptase is not elevated.

Psychologic and non-organic syndromes

Syndromes such as globus hystericus, vocal cord dysfunction, and Munchausen stridor may also mimic anaphylaxis and must be excluded. Globus hystericus may be considered since a patient experiencing anaphylaxis may experience a subjective sensation of upper respiratory obstruction even without development of other clinical manifestations. Careful assessment of patients with globus hystericus requires laryngoscopic and possibly radiologic evaluation. In patients with globus hystericus and vocal cord dysfunction, pruritus, urticaria, angioedema, flushing, gastrointestinal colic, and hypotension do not occur. Serum tryptase levels are not elevated.

EVALUATION OF THE PATIENT

History of anaphylaxis event(s)

Central to the successful long-term management of anaphylaxis is a detailed historical assessment of the original anaphylactic event. This should include specific information regarding the events immediately preceding the onset of symptoms, such as foods ingested, insect stings, exercise (any exertion), drugs taken, and contact with latex. Known or suspected allergies should be revealed to the investigator. Hypotension is common in reactions to parenteral drugs and following insect (Hymenoptera) stings, less common in food-induced anaphylaxis. Adults may complain of lightheadedness or weakness, whereas young children become lethargic. In most sting reactions, some flushing or urticaria may precede systemic symptoms. There are instances when there are few prodromal symptoms and collapse or loss of consciousness may occur within 5 minutes of the sting.

Food allergy

Allergies to foods may occur at any age, but usually develop early in life. Over half the potential sufferers with peanut and nut allergy exhibit reactions by 2 years, and more than 90% by the age of 7 years. Peanuts and tree nuts are the most frequent cause of food-induced anaphylaxis, regardless of age. Nut-specific IgE is present in 7.8%, but may not be symptomatic. Oral food challenge can only validate a comprehensive clinical history in less than 50% of the patients. Positive peanut skin prick test wheal diameters of 8 mm or greater predict peanut allergy with 95% confidence. Threshold value of 14 kUA/L has been established for a positive predictive RAST value of 95%. However the magnitude of the skin test or CAP (RAST) does not predict clinical severity, further emphasizing the importance of clinical history in establishing the role of food allergy in the genesis of anaphylaxis.

Latex allergy

Allergy to natural latex (gloves, etc.) may induce adverse reactions upon contact in healthcare workers or laboratory staff, as well as in patients undergoing repeated surgical or other procedures such as vaginal examination and dental work. The onset of latex anaphylaxis may be longer than for other etiologies for anaphylaxis because the allergen is absorbed relatively slowly. Latex induced reactions may take up to 30 minutes from first contact until symptoms develop. In contrast to anesthetic agents, which may induce immediate reactions following exposure, the onset of latex allergy during surgery is slower. Atopy, asthma, and food allergy occur more frequently in patients with latex allergy.

Semen anaphylaxis

An unusual cause of anaphylaxis, adverse reactions to semen, occurs upon contact, usually after coitus. Pruritus of the vaginal area associated with localized angioedema and lower abdominal discomfort may develop prior to systemic manifestations of anaphylaxis.

Table 11.5 Levels of β-tryptase in serum or plasma measured by the G5 monoclonal antibody

Tryptase Levels in Serum	Total (α- + β-tryptases)	β-Tryptase	Ratio Total: β-Tryptase*
Sensitivity	0.5 ng/mL	1 ng/mL	na
Normal	1–15 ng/mL	<1 ng/mL	na
Systemic anaphylaxis	↑↑	↑↑	≤10 ng/mL
Systemic mastocytosis	↑↑	±↑	≥20 ng/mL

*When β-tryptase ≥ 1
↑↑ = marked increase; ±↑ = occasional small increase; na = not applicable.
[From Schwartz LB and Irani AM. Serum tryptase and the laboratory diagnosis of systemic mastocytosis. Hematol Oncol Clin North Am 2000; 14:641–657.]

Vaccine associated anaphylaxis

Vaccines, such as measles, mumps, and rubella (MMR) (containing egg and gelatin), have been associated with anaphylaxis. Studies reveal that egg-sensitive and gelatin-sensitized patients who experience anaphylaxis upon egg or gelatin ingestion may have positive skin reactions to MMR vaccine. A quarter of patients with reported anaphylaxis after MMR appear to have hypersensitivity to gelatin.

Perioperative anaphylaxis

The most common cause of perioperative anaphylaxis was neuromuscular blocking agents (NMBA) (58.2%), latex (16.7%), and antibiotics (15.1%). Cross-reactivity between NMBAs occurred in 75.1% of cases of anaphylaxis due to NMBA.

LABORATORY TESTS FOR ANAPHYLAXIS

A tryptase level obtained at the onset of symptoms is the most useful test for confirming the occurrence of anaphylaxis. Mast cell proteases include beta and alpha tryptase (Fig. 11.1). β-Tryptase is released during anaphylaxis and is measured by immunoassay as mature tryptase. α-Tryptase and β-tryptase are measured as total tryptase and are elevated higher than 20 ng/mL in systemic mastocytosis (Table 11.5). Elevations of total tryptase are seen in anaphylaxis depending on the extent and the severity of the symptoms. This test should be obtained in all instances of suspected anaphylaxis. An elevated serum tryptase level indicates mast cell activation with mediator release. Blood (serum) should be obtained within 1 hour after the reaction. Tryptase concentrations peak at 45–60 minutes and may remain elevated for several hours before gradually decreasing. In severe anaphylactic reactions, tryptase levels may remain elevated for several hours or even, in rare instances, for several days. The short half-life of histamine and the release of further histamine from basophil degranulation during blood taking make the assay for plasma histamine less useful. However, 24 hour urine collection for histamine assay may be helpful, particularly if collected shortly after the anaphylactic event.

Specific IgE antibodies may be elevated in association with most anaphylactic reactions. Their presence may assist in defining the precipitating etiology of the reaction. This can be demonstrated by skin prick test (SPT) or by detecting serum specific IgE by RAST or similar assays. SPTs are superior, although it is preferable to perform in vitro tests first when extreme hypersensitivity is suspected. Scratch or prick skin tests should be executed in preference to intradermal tests to avoid systemic reactions. In the case of individual foods, fresh fruits, for example, can be tested by pricking directly through the fresh fruit, rather than utilizing a commercial extract. Increasing attention has been directed to the size of the SPT reaction and the concentration of the RAST results. In all instances, these results must be interpreted in regard to the patient's allergy history.

Provocative tests may be performed if a cause is suspected and the RAST and SPT are negative. In most instances, this applies to foods, but such an approach has been developed for the treatment of adverse drug reactions, termed graded challenge. The principle of challenge tests is that the starting dose is very dilute, for example, 1:100 000, with incremental increases until the desired single dosage is attained. The aim of a provocation test is to induce only a minor reaction and interrupt the challenge upon the occurrence of a definitive response, a cutaneous wheal or generalized pruritus. Placebo challenges are required as control tests. Double blind testing would be most appropriate. Due to possible anaphylaxis, challenges should be performed under the direction of allergy specialists in settings where appropriate drugs to treat anaphylaxis, such as epinephrine, are available.

MANAGEMENT OF ANAPHYLAXIS

Therapy of anaphylaxis can be considered in two parts, including management of the acute episode with subsequent evaluation and prophylaxis.

Acute management

The acute management of systemic anaphylaxis requires the prompt recognition of the earliest symptoms since successful outcomes are contingent upon the institution of immediate aggressive treatment. Initial therapy is directed to the preservation of airway function, reversal of bronchospasm, and

Table 11.6 Acute management of anaphylaxis

Acute Management of Anaphylaxis in Adults
1. Assess vital signs
2. Administer cardiopulmonary resuscitation if necessary
3. Administer 0.3–0.5 mL 1/1000 epinephrine i.m.
4. If cardiovascular shock, infuse 10 mL 1/100 000 epinephrine over 10 min (1/100 dilution of 1/1000)
5. Preserve airway function: endotracheal intubation or tracheostomy and artificial respiration if necessary
6. Maintenance of circulating volume: infuse 500–2000 mL/h 5% dextrose add plasma expander if appropriate
7. Maintenance of blood pressure: initially infuse dopamine (2–20 μg/kg/min) or norepinephrine (4–8 μg/min) then titrate to maintain adequate blood pressure
8. Administer antihistamines (optional): H_1 antagonist, e.g. diphenhydramine 25–50 mg i.v. over 5–10 min H_2 antagonist, e.g. cimetidine i.m. after H_1 blockage initiated
9. Treat bronchospasm if present: inhaled or nebulized β_2-agonists e.g. albuterol theophylline 4–7 mg/kg by i.v. infusion
10. Glucocorticoids: hydrocortisone 100 mg i.v. or i.m.
11. Reduce allergen adsorption with oral charcoal
12. If β blockade is present use glucagon 5–15 μg/min i.v. continuous infusion
13. Observation for a minimum of 4–5 hours
14. At discharge, educate patient to avoid further episodes

maintenance of blood pressure and oxygenation. Such a management program is shown in Table 11.6. The prompt administration of epinephrine is the most important treatment since it inhibits mast cell mediator release, enhances bronchodilation, stimulates the cardiovascular system, and reduces postcapillary venule leakage. It is absorbed optimally when administered intramuscularly. In one study, those patients who were administered epinephrine early in the course of anaphylaxis survived, whereas those in whom epinephrine administration was delayed for several hours after the onset of symptoms succumbed. Epinephrine was administered in only 62% of fatal anaphylaxis and, prior to arrest, in 14%.

Prompt intramuscular injection (into the lateral aspect of the thigh) is critical to a successful therapeutic outcome (Tables 11.6 and 11.7). The dosage can be repeated every 5–10 minutes as required unless tachycardia or hypertension occurs. Because it may be dangerous and may induce myocardial ischemia, infarction, or arrhythmia, intravenous epinephrine should be reserved for profoundly hypotensive patients with life-threatening circulatory collapse. Under such circumstances, epinephrine may be infused slowly (1–10 mL diluted 1/10 000 over 10 minutes) with close cardiac monitoring, preferably in a cardiac care unit. Currently available epinephrine by inhalation is not a substitute for epinephrine by injection. Significant efforts are being exerted to develop a non-injectable delivery system by aerosol via large porous particles and sublingual administration.

The administration of an H_1 antihistamine, such as diphenhydramine 25–50 mg or chlorpheniramine 10 mg i.v. may be beneficial. The addition of an H_2 antagonist, although not well documented as beneficial, appears warranted, as hypotension and cardiac arrhythmias appear to be secondary to effects mediated by both $H_1$and H_2 types of histamine receptors.

Table 11.7 Drug doses for anaphylaxis in children

Drug Doses for Anaphylaxis (Pediatrics)
Follow the steps for acute management given in Table 11.6 but substitute the following doses at the relevant stages:
3. 0.01 mg/kg epinephrine i.m.
4. 0.1–1.5 μg/kg/min epinephrine
6. 30 mL/kg/h 5% dextrose
8. 12.5–25 mg diphenhydramine
10. 10–100 mg hydrocortisone i.v. or i.m.

The use of nebulized β-agonist therapy (albuterol) should be instituted promptly when treating an acute asthma episode associated with anaphylaxis.

Hydrocortisone, 0.5–1.0 mg/kg intramuscularly or intravenously, may be administered to all patients with serious anaphylaxis to reduce the occurrence of a prolonged (biphasic) response because of its established efficacy in the treatment of idiopathic anaphylaxis.

Antigen adsorption may be reduced by applying a tourniquet proximal to the sting or injection site. The injection of an

Table 11.8 Prevention and control of recurrent anaphylaxis

Prevention and Control of Recurrent Anaphylaxis
Careful history for the identification of precipitants, supplemented by radioallergosorbent (RAST) or skin test
Avoidance of identification precipitants:
Medications: avoidance of implicated drug and cross-reacting agents
Foods: avoidance of implicated food and cross-reacting/related foods
Latex: avoidance of contact with latex and exposure to aerosolized latex antigen during dental and medical procedures; may require occupational adjustments
Exercise-induced anaphylaxis: discontinuation of exercise with earliest premonitory symptoms; avoidance of exercise in postprandial state, or if aspirin or non-steroidal antiinflammatory agents have been recently utilized. Exercise with a companion
Immunotherapy: currently clinical indication is limited to Hymenoptera venom anaphylaxis
Patients should carry material for emergency self-administration of intramuscular epinephrine

additional dose of epinephrine into the sting or immunotherapy injection site may further reduce antigen adsorption. If administered early in the course of an anaphylactic event, the aforementioned therapeutic schedule may be adequate to reverse the reaction. Further supportive treatment may be necessary if there is persistent shock or respiratory distress.

Hypotension and shock not responsive to intramuscular epinephrine should be treated with intravascular volume repletion with crystalloid or colloid because of the profound vasopermeability consequent to the postcapillary venule leakage associated with anaphylaxis. Persistent hypotension may require the utilization of β-adrenergic agents. The occurrence of bradycardia associated with severe hypotension should alert the clinician to the possibility of β-adrenergic blockade. The prompt use of glucagon to overcome this effect is always recommended, although such maneuvers have not been consistently effective.

Patients must be observed for at least 4 hours in the advent of a prolonged anaphylactic response (biphasic) during which aggressive therapy should be administered. More delayed reactions associated with anaphylaxis make such observation mandatory.

Long-term management (prevention)

Anyone who has sustained an anaphylactic event should be referred to an allergy specialist for definition of the cause with advice regarding the management and institution of measures to prevent future anaphylactic reactions (Table 11.8). The primary care physician should be informed regarding possible sensitivities, including the advice and medications given to the patient by the allergy consultant. It is critical that anaphylaxis-prone individuals appreciate that, despite the institution of preventive measures, anaphylactic events may continue to occur. Therefore such affected people must be educated to recognize the earliest manifestations of anaphylaxis with rapid institution of appropriate therapy. The emergency plan, which should be written in an easily understandable format individualized for each patient, should anticipate possible future reactions and appropriate measures utilized to reverse the symptoms. Ideally, such a plan could define treatment options based upon the severity of the anaphylactic reaction. For example, such a plan might include manifestations such as cutaneous symptoms, moderate with some wheezing, or severe with marked respiratory impairment and possible hypotension. It should include instructions on when and how to seek medical attention.

All patients who have experienced an anaphylactic event, which may recur, should be provided with epinephrine in a preloaded syringe for intramuscular injection (e.g. EpiPen, available in child and adult volumes). Patients should be thoroughly trained in its use on repeated occasions, and be reminded that there is an expiration date printed on the barrel of the syringe. Education must include the patient's closest companion, or in the case of children, siblings and parents. Also for children, the emergency medication must be made available to a responsible and appropriately trained person at the child's school. A Medic-alert bracelet should indicate the patient's allergic reaction(s).

All individuals susceptible to anaphylactic events must avoid β-adrenergic blocking agents and probably angiotensin converting enzyme (ACE) inhibitors, which increase the risk of severe or refractory anaphylaxis.

Central to the prevention of anaphylaxis is the avoidance of factors known to precipitate the patient's anaphylaxis. All prior episodes of anaphylaxis must be reviewed in detail to ascertain the etiology. Specific tests, as enumerated, should be performed to help define the causes of past anaphylactic events. In this way, defined etiologies can be avoided. It is critical to review all ingestants, injectants, and substances inhaled just prior to the episode to further clarify the cause. Monoclonal humanized IgG anti-IgE (Xolair) may provide protection from these aforementioned allergens. Long-term studies are required to confirm this observation.

Food

Food-associated anaphylaxis requires identification of the specific food inducing the reaction and its avoidance. In the case of food additives, such as peanuts or preservatives, it may be helpful to provide the patients with a list of food products which contain the allergen(s). Patients must read labels carefully and avoid those foods whose contents are allergens.

Similarly, patients must be capable of convincing restaurateurs, chefs, and shopkeepers that even trace amounts of ingested allergen may result in a serious reaction. Utensils used to serve one dish may contaminate another. Patients allergic to nuts, including peanuts, should avoid all nuts.

Drugs

Drug-allergic individuals must be thoroughly educated regarding the drugs to which they are sensitive, wear a Medic-alert bracelet, and recognize cross-reacting substances, e.g. aspirin intolerant patients must also avoid non-steroidal anti-inflammatory agents.

Latex

Allergy to natural rubber latex, increasingly recognized, creates two problems. The first involves exposure in the home or workplace. Latex-sensitive healthcare workers and patients may be exposed to latex present in surgical gloves, anesthetic facemasks, sphygmomanometer tubing, and bottle stoppers. In the home, rubber is a content of many products including elasticized garments, nipples, balloons, bicycle tires, elastic bands, mattresses, condoms and diaphragms. Education is central to the successful elimination of these products. Hospitals are utilizing non-latex rubber substitutes more frequently. The second problem relates to the passive exposure to latex, e.g. latex sensitive patients undergoing medical evaluation and examination. The patient must alert the examiner, physician, nurse, or dentist of their latex sensitivity prior to the procedure. In this way, a non-latex environment can be provided, etc. Such affected individuals should wear a Medic-alert bracelet describing their latex sensitivity. Most hospitals are aware of latex sensitivity and have instituted programs to avoid exposure, e.g. avoiding balloons and utilizing non-latex gloves routinely.

Insect stings

Hymenoptera, i.e. bee, yellow jacket, hornet, wasp, and fire ant may precipitate life-threatening reactions. Such affected individuals with systemic manifestations due to stings of Hymenoptera must be educated to recognize such insects and avoid situations where the insects may be present. These individuals should always carry epinephrine (EpiPen) and be adept at its self-administration. They should also be aware how to apply a tourniquet proximal to the sting site on a limb to diminish venom (allergen) adsorption. Immunotherapy for such patients, after confirmation of specific venom IgE, greatly reduces the frequency of serious adverse reactions following further stings.

Semen

Seminal plasma anaphylaxis is rarely encountered and is best managed by avoiding contact with the ejaculate. Spontaneous improvement usually occurs, but desensitization may facilitate and accelerate the induction of tolerance.

Exercise

Patients with exercise anaphylaxis should avoid food ingestion for at least 4–6 hours prior to exercise. Those whose attacks occur with exercise following specific food ingestion, e.g. wheat, should avoid the specific food for at least 6 hours and preferably a day prior to exercise. In general, patients should discontinue exercise at the slightest provocation of an attack such as faintness, flushing, or even unusual warmth or pruritus. Early administration of H_1 antihistamines may blunt further evolution of an attack, but has not been shown to provide reliable prophylactic protection. Such affected individuals may experience anaphylaxis when exercising during the allergy season to which they have exhibited allergen sensitivity. Patients should carry epinephrine for serious or life-threatening episodes and seek medical attention if utilized. Such affected patients should always wear medical identification. Since exercise during the patient's inhalant allergy season may be associated with exercise-induced anaphylactic symptoms, exercise at that time should be severely limited, preferably avoided.

Cold

Cold exposure in individuals with cold-induced urticaria must be severely limited. When sudden cold exposure over a large area of the skin occurs, life-threatening hypotension may occur. Thus, boating, swimming, taking a cold shower or even sudden exposure to ambient freezing temperatures must be avoided. Epinephrine should be provided for such patients.

Idiopathic anaphylaxis

Patients with idiopathic anaphylaxis are usually refracting to maintenance H_1 and H_2 antihistamines, and may only be controlled with daily or alternate day steroids. Occasionally, the avoidance of aspirin or NSAIDs as well as food preservatives and dye-containing foods may be beneficial.

IMMUNOTHERAPY

Patients with high-risk antigen-specific IgE-dependent anaphylaxis may benefit from the administration of specific immunotherapy. Immunoprophylaxis for Hymenoptera venom allergy is effective, but severe adverse reactions, including rare fatalities, may occur.

Drug desensitization

Desensitization is being utilized with increasing frequency to induce tolerance to essential drugs. It is a process of rapid gradual reintroduction of a drug which has previously induced anaphylaxis in a sensitized patient. Intravenous and oral administration has successfully rendered patients tolerant to acetylsalicyclic acid (ASA), insulin, antibiotic and chemotherapeutic agents.

CONCLUSION

The outcome of an anaphylactic event is contingent upon early recognition of symptoms and prompt institution of effective therapy. The route of antigen administration, the recipient's sensitivity, and coexistent conditions all contribute to an individual's prognosis. Delay in epinephrine administration is a critical factor in determining outcome and every effort must be made to ensure that this treatment is administered promptly.

However, patients have succumbed despite the availability of optimal therapy, and anaphylaxis remains a frequently devastating event. Patients who have survived anaphylaxis must be appropriately instructed in the self-administration of epinephrine and counseled to avoid further exposure to the precipitating factors (allergen).

FURTHER READING

Austen KF. Allergies, anaphylaxis, and systemic mastocytosis. Disorders of immune-mediated injury. In: Harrison's principles of internal medicine. 16th edn. New York: McGraw-Hill; 2005; 298:1947–1956.

Bosso JR, Schwartz LB, Stevenson DD. Tryptase and histamine release during aspirin-induced respiratory reactions. J Allergy Clin Immunol 1991; 18:830–937.

Haeberli G, Brennimann M, Hunsiker T, et al. Elevated basal serum tryptase and hymenoptera venom allergy: relation to severity of sting reactions and to safety and efficacy of venom immunotherapy. Clin Exp Allergy 2003; 33(9):1216–1220.

Hepner DL, Castells MC. Anaphylaxis during the perioperative period. Anesth Analg 2003; 4:859–864.

Horan RF, DuBuske LM, Sheffer AL. Exercise-induced anaphylaxis. In: Anaphylaxis: immunology and allergy clinics of North America 2001; 21: 769–782.

Morisset M, Moneret-Vautrin DA, Kanay G, et al. Thresholds of clinical reactivity to milk, egg, peanut and sesame in immunoglobulin E dependent allergies: evaluation by double-blind placebo-controlled oral challenges. Clin Exp Allergy 2003; 33:1046–1051.

Mullins RJ. Anaphylaxis: risk factors for recurrence. Clin Exp Allergy 2003; 33(8):1033–1040.

Pumphrey RSH. Lessons for management of anaphylaxis from a study of fatal reactions. Clin Exp Allergy 2001; 30:1144–1150.

Sampson HA, Mendelson L, Rosen JP. Fatal and nonfatal anaphylactic reactions to food in children and adolescents. N Engl J Med 1992; 327:380–384.

Stewart AG, Ewan PW. The incidence, etiology and management of anaphylaxis presenting to an accident and emergency department. Q J Med 1996; 89:859–864.

Chapter 12

Definition:

Specific immunotherapy (SIT) is the administration of progressively increasing doses of an allergen to alter the immunologic and clinical response to that allergen, and thereby to ameliorate clinical allergic disease.

Immunotherapy

Anthony J Frew, M Thirumal Krishna, David BK Golden, and Thomas B Casale

INTRODUCTION

It is now almost a century since the pioneering work of Noon and Freeman was used to successfully treat hayfever patients using a low-dose incremental schedule of pollen injections. Noon based his doses of pollen extract on a pollen weight unit that remained in use for over 70 years; the basic principles of their work remain recognizable in the specific immunotherapy schedules used today. During the 1920s and 1930s, interest in allergy developed rapidly, especially in the USA. Desensitizing injections, with varying dosage schedules, were administered to a wide range of patients and showed varying success rates. Gradually, it became clear that patient selection and proper attention to detail were vital in achieving successful desensitization; more recently, improvements to the preparation and standardization of allergen extracts have made the whole process more reliable and predictable.

In addition, our understanding of the immunologic basis of immunotherapy has dramatically increased. Our improving knowledge of immunoregulatory pathways is leading to novel approaches to immunotherapy which target more directly the determinants of allergen tolerance. In the near future, new ways of administering immunotherapy, either using different delivery systems or giving it together with other immunomodulating agents, will likely result in new and better immunotherapy regimens that lead to long-lasting allergen-specific tolerance and better clinical outcomes.

CURRENT INDICATIONS FOR SPECIFIC IMMUNOTHERAPY (SIT)

The main indications for SIT are in the treatment of patients who have experienced life-threatening allergic reactions to Hymenoptera stings, and those with allergic rhinitis due to pollen, dust mite and animal dander allergies. As per the current international guidelines, venom immunotherapy for Hymenoptera stings is not indicated for patients who have only had local reactions, but those with non-life-threatening systemic reactions should also be considered for allergen immunotherapy, taking into account the risk of future stings and underlying medical conditions before reaching a decision regarding suitability for SIT.

In patients with seasonal allergic rhinitis, SIT is currently offered to those with intractable symptoms that are either unresponsive or only partially responsive to conventional pharmacotherapy. A similar approach is taken for patients with perennial rhinitis that is predominantly driven by dust mite allergy. In those with troublesome reactions to animal dander, in particular where avoidance measures cannot be undertaken for occupational reasons, SIT is appropriate. Although a number of studies have shown SIT to be efficacious in asthma (discussed below), the role of SIT in the current asthma management guidelines is unclear.

Table 12.1 Dosage schedule for conventional specific immunotherapy (SIT). After reaching the maintenance dose, the next injection is given after 2 weeks, then at 4-weekly intervals

Dosage Schedule for Conventional SIT

Injection number	Allergen concentration (SQU)	Volume (mL)	Dose (SQU)
1	100	0.1	10
2	1 000	0.1	100
3	10 000	0.1	1 000
4	100 000	0.02	2 000
5	100 000	0.05	5 000
6	100 000	0.1	10 000
7	100 000	0.2	20 000
8	100 000	0.4	40 000
9	100 000	0.6	60 000
10	100 000	0.8	80 000
11	100 000	1.0	100 000
Maintenance	100 000	1.0	100 000

SQU, standardized quality unit. Data modified from Varney VA, Edwards J, Tabbah K, et al. Clinical efficacy of specific immunotherapy to cat dander: a double-blind placebo-controlled trial. Clin Exp Allergy1997; 27(8):860–867 © Blackwell Science Ltd.

CONTRAINDICATIONS TO SPECIFIC IMMUNOTHERAPY

Although, asthma per se is not a contraindication, uncontrolled or brittle asthma substantially increases the risk of side-effects from SIT, and is therefore a contraindication for SIT. Other contraindications include concurrent treatment with β-blockers, angiotensin converting enzyme inhibitors, corticosteroid and immunosuppressive drugs. Underlying active autoimmune disease and malignancy also constitute a contraindication for SIT. SIT should not be initiated in pregnant women or in those who intend to conceive in the near future. However, SIT can be continued in women who become pregnant while on maintenance treatment provided they have tolerated the treatment well up to that point.

CONVENTIONAL SPECIFIC IMMUNOTHERAPY

Conventional SIT involves a series of subcutaneous injections of progressively more and more allergen, until a maintenance dose is reached. Typically, the incremental phase will be given as weekly or biweekly injections (Table 12.1) over a period of 10–24 weeks (typically 10–13 in Europe, 12–24 in USA). In a 'clustered dose' regimen, maintenance dose is achieved within 7 weeks and the safety profile of this regimen has been shown to match the conventional dosing approach of 12 weeks. Maintenance injections are then given at intervals of 4–6 weeks over a total period of 3 years or more. Several variations have been proposed, including 'rush' and 'semirush' protocols, in which the incremental phase of the regime is compressed by giving several injections on the same day. The principal drawback to these protocols is the increased likelihood of adverse side-effects, but this must be weighed against the ability to achieve protection within a few days or weeks, which may be particularly useful in patients with Hymenoptera allergy.

SUBLINGUAL IMMUNOTHERAPY

A number of alternative routes of administration have been used, the most promising of which is sublingual immunotherapy (SLIT). Many studies have demonstrated that high dose SLIT is an effective alternative to subcutaneous immunotherapy for both adults and children. SLIT can be administered by patients at home, unsupervised, which may result in greater compliance. Despite these positive attributes, much needs to be examined before recommending SLIT as a replacement for subcutaneous immunotherapy. There are very limited data comparing SLIT with subcutaneous immunotherapy, and those which do exist suggest that the overall efficacy of SLIT is less than for subcutaneous SIT. We also do not know the long-term effects of SLIT or what immunologic changes are evoked by this form of therapy. Finally, although the safety profile appears good with SLIT, long-term studies, similar to those done with subcutaneous SIT, are ultimately needed to define the true risk/benefit ratio with SLIT in comparison with subcutaneous immunotherapy. As more SLIT studies are published, some of these issues will be resolved and we will become clearer about its place as an alternative to traditional subcutaneous immunotherapy.

Several other non-conventional approaches are in current use. Oral and local nasal immunotherapy are less effective than

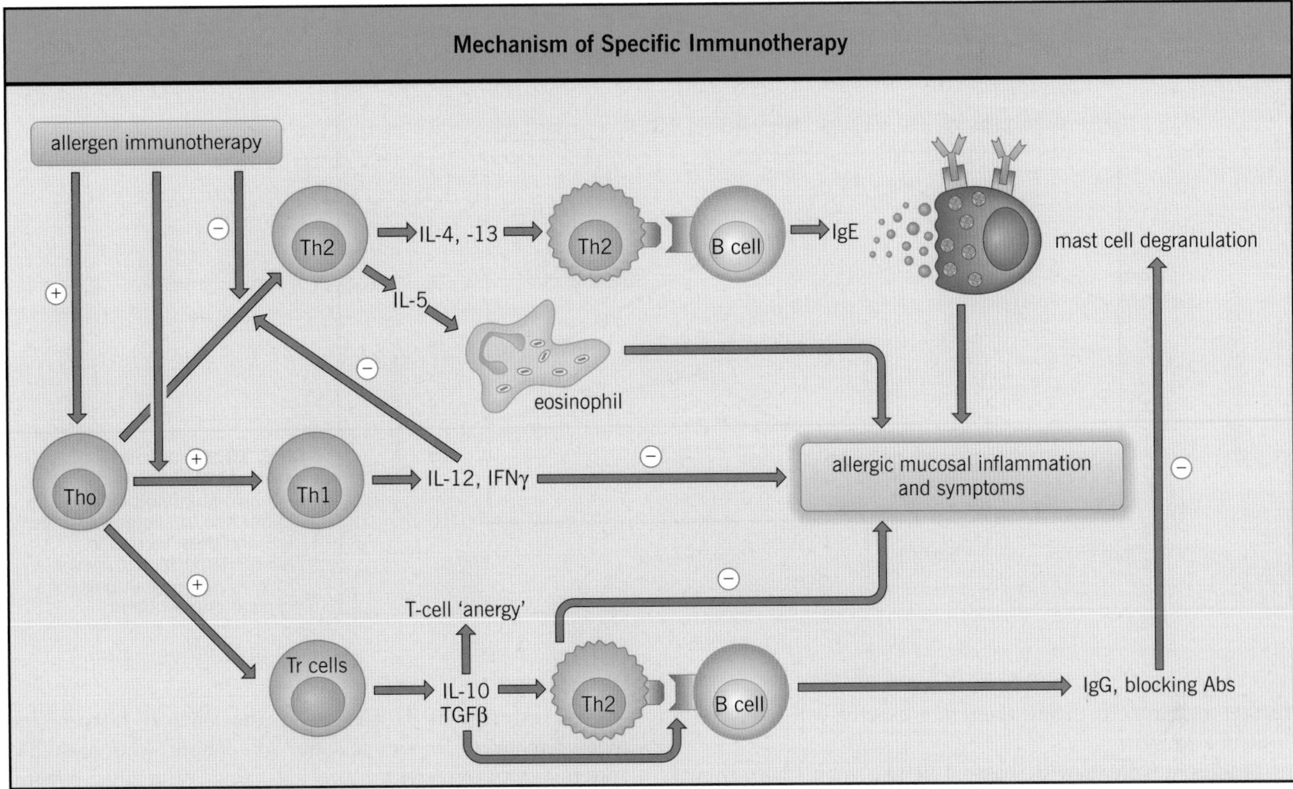

Fig. 12.1 Mechanisms underlying the action of specific immunotherapy (SIT): There is helper T cell type 2 (Th2) predominance in allergic diseases and this is characterized by secretion of interleukin-4 (IL-4), -5 and -13. IL-5 is involved in eosinophil survival, activation and maturation and IL-4 and -13 are important in class switching of B cells for IgE production. Th1 response induces IL-12 and interferon γ (IFNγ) production and this dampens the Th2 response. SIT induces Th1 response, dampens Th2 response and induces T regulatory cells (Tr cells) to secrete IL-10 and transforming growth factor (TGFβ) and recent studies have shown that IL-10 induces T-cell 'anergy' or 'unresponsiveness' and has other 'anti-allergic properties'. Abs, antibodies.

SLIT and cannot be recommended. Homeopathic immunotherapy, using ultralow doses of pollen, has not been shown to have any convincing activity, and is not recommended by mainstream allergists or allergy societies.

MECHANISMS OF IMMUNOTHERAPY (Fig. 12.1)

The precise mechanisms underlying the effects of SIT are not well understood but several studies have shown that SIT inhibits both early and late responses to allergen exposure.

Recently, there have been many studies aimed at elucidating the mechanisms by which allergen-specific immunotherapy works. Indeed, there are very impressive data defining the immunologic changes and long-lasting immunotolerogenic effects of immunotherapy. Allergen immunotherapy is the only antigen-specific immunomodulatory treatment routinely available. It has been shown to provide long-lasting benefits and to modify the natural history of allergic diseases, preventing the development of neosensitization and asthma in children.

It has long been known that immunotherapy blunts seasonal increases in IgE levels and results in increases in allergen-specific IgG levels (i.e. blocking antibodies), especially of the IgG4 subclass (Fig. 12.2). This results in decreased IgE-mediated histamine release and inhibition of IgE-mediated antigen presentation to T cells. Recent studies have also demonstrated the importance of examining the affinity and specificity of IgG subsequent to immunotherapy. The binding capacity of IgG4 increased, whereas that for IgE decreased after long-term immunotherapy. However, there is a weak correlation between IgG concentration and clinical response to treatment.

In addition to the effects of immunotherapy on immunoglobulins, its effects on lymphocytes have been intensely studied. Some peripheral blood studies have indicated a shift in the balance of T-lymphocyte subsets away from the helper T cell type 2 (Th2) phenotype and toward a Th1 phenotype on the basis of preferential production of interferon γ (IFNγ) and decreased production of interleukin-4 (IL-4) and IL-5. However, these findings are not consistent. What is consistent is the demonstration of increased allergen-specific IL-10 during the early stages of immunotherapy. IL-10 has also been shown to be increased in the respiratory mucosa and is produced by a number of cells, including Th1 cells, Th2 cells, regulatory T cells, monocytes–macrophages, dendritic cells, mast cells and eosinophils. IL-10 has a number of biologic consequences that could be important in mediating the immunotolerogenic effects of immunotherapy. These effects include modulation of IL4-induced B-cell IgE production in favor of IgG4, inhibition of IgE-dependent mast cell activation, inhibition of human eosinophil cytokine production and survival, suppression of IL-5, and induction of antigen-specific anergy.

The importance of IL-10, regulatory T cells (Tr cells) and dendritic cells cannot be overemphasized. These cells appear to be critical in the therapeutic effects of immunotherapy and

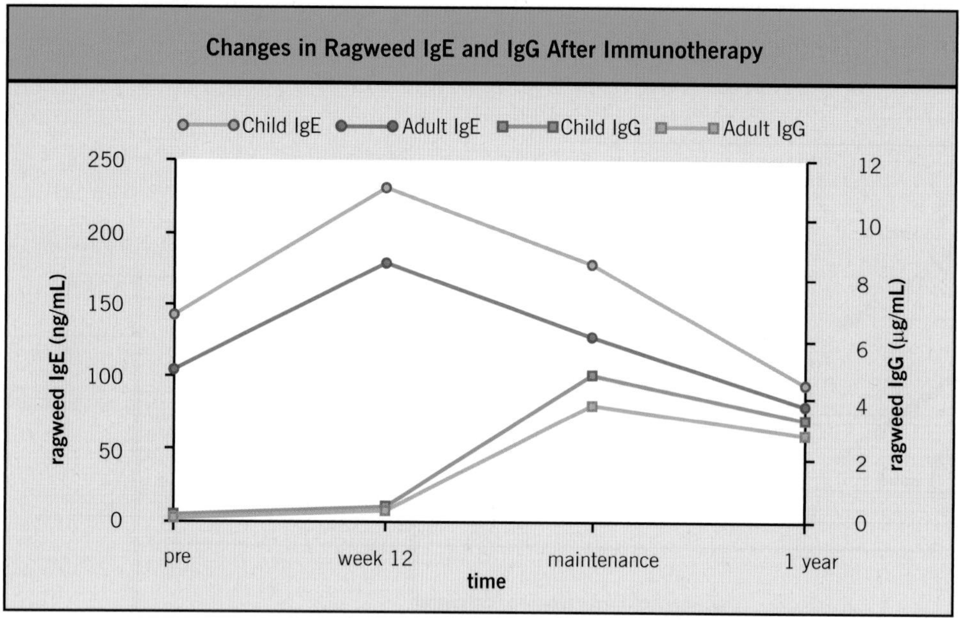

Fig. 12.2 Timecourse of serological changes during specific immunotherapy. Note initial rise in allergen-specific IgE and delayed rise in allergen-specific IgG, which follows rather than precedes clinical improvement.

further research to define their role exactly will likely be a fruitful area.

Studies in patients with seasonal allergic rhinitis have shown that SIT attenuates the seasonal influx of eosinophils, basophils and T cells in the nasal mucosa. There is now little doubt that there is Th2 predominance in allergic diseases and SIT has been shown to modulate the Th2/Th1 balance. SIT induces a Th1 response as evidenced by an increase in IFNγ production within nasal mucosa. Similar response is seen in patients undergoing venom immunotherapy where there is a reduction in IL-4 production and an increase in IFNγ production by peripheral blood lymphocytes. Recent studies have focused attention on Tr cells that are identified by their CD4+CD25+ phenotype. It has been shown that Tr cells are induced by SIT, leading to IL-10 and transforming growth factor β (TGFβ) production that may have a number of anti-allergic effects including modulation of IL-4-induced B-cell IgE production in favor of IgG4, inhibition of IgE-dependent mast cell activation and inhibition of human eosinophil cytokine production and survival. IL-10 also suppresses production of 'proallergic' cytokines, such as IL-5, and is able to induce a state of T-cell unresponsiveness or 'anergy' that might occur as a result of IL-10 receptor-dependent blockade of the B7/CD28 co-stimulatory pathway.

EFFICACY OF IMMUNOTHERAPY

Hymenoptera venom allergy

Anaphylactic reactions to Hymenoptera venom are relatively uncommon but can be life-threatening: venom immunotherapy is the treatment of choice. The primary allergen in honeybee venom is phospholipase A2 (Api m 1) and that of the vespid venoms (yellow jacket, hornet, wasp) is antigen 5 (Ves v 5). Another clinically important insect is the imported fire ant (also a member of the Hymenoptera family). Allergy to the imported fire ant is being reported increasingly often from the USA, Australia and South East Asia.

Risk assessment is based on the clinical history and measurement of venom-specific IgE. Those who have had systemic symptoms with a previous sting are at much greater risk of anaphylaxis than those who have only had large local reactions. The magnitude of the IgE response is not consistently correlated with the severity or pattern of reaction to a sting, since some patients who experience large local reactions have extremely high venom IgE levels, while other patients who suffer rapid vascular collapse and anaphylactic shock may have barely detectable levels of venom IgE. The frequency of systemic reactions in children and adults with a history of large local reactions and positive venom skin tests is in the range of 5–10%. The reported risk of another systemic reaction occurring in a patient with a previous systemic reaction varies from 30 to 60%, with lower risks in children and patients with milder reactions. The risk of systemic reaction in adults diminishes over 10–20 years towards 15–30% but does not seem to return to the background 3% prevalence in the general population. Children with a history of cutaneous systemic reactions had less than 5% risk of anaphylaxis during observation for 10–20 years. There is no test that accurately predicts the outcome of the next sting. Live sting challenge is a useful research procedure, but is generally not acceptable for clinical practice, not least because some patients who do not react to a first challenge sting may react to a subsequent sting.

The induction phase of venom SIT may be given weekly for 10 weeks, as a 'semirush' over 2–3 weeks, or as a 'rush induction' in hospital over 2–3 days. Once the maintenance dose is achieved, 95–98% of patients will have no systemic symptoms upon wasp-sting challenge (80–85% for honeybee venom SIT). Patients not fully protected by the conventional dose of 100 µg may be more effectively treated with a 200 µg maintenance dose. Protection is well maintained during subsequent maintenance therapy; maintenance injections are usually given every 4–6 weeks, but sometimes the interval is up to 8 weeks, especially in long-term maintenance therapy for venom allergy. Maintenance therapy is usually recommended for 3–5 years, with growing evidence that 5 years' treatment provides more lasting benefit, although this has to be balanced against the inconvenience of extended duration of SIT. More prolonged treatment is offered to those with more severe previous reactions, those who had systemic reactions during venom SIT, and those allergic to honeybees (as opposed to wasps). The decision to stop therapy may also be based on a reduction in the skin test response to venom or a reduction in venom-specific IgE. Venom-specific IgG rises in all patients as a result of therapy and a level of ≥ 3 μg/mL has been shown to be protective.

A low risk of systemic reaction to stings (10%) appears to remain for many years after discontinuing venom immunotherapy (VIT). Although post-SIT systemic reactions to stings have rarely been severe, a few fatalities have been reported, usually in patients with other risk factors (e.g. mastocytosis, severe previous reactions, systemic reactions during VIT, honeybee allergy). In children who have received venom SIT, the chance of systemic reaction to a sting is lower, remaining below 5% for up to 20 years after discontinuing therapy. How much of this is due to SIT and how much to natural resolution of the sensitivity is uncertain, but the clinical message is clear: treatment is effective in the short term and patients are then at relatively low risk of reactions for many years thereafter.

Specific immunotherapy in allergic rhinitis

Specific immunotherapy has been widely used to treat allergic rhinitis. As with any other form of SIT, careful patient selection is crucial. The diagnosis of allergic rhinitis needs to be secure, especially in those with perennial symptoms, and should be based on a careful clinical history supported by documentation of IgE-mediated sensitivity by skin or blood tests.

The efficacy of SIT in seasonal allergic rhinitis has been confirmed in a number of carefully controlled clinical studies involving pollens from grass, ragweed, birch, and mountain cedar. These studies have clearly demonstrated significant improvement in symptoms, medication use (Fig. 12.3), and quality of life and these changes are paralleled by a reduction in skin prick test reactivity, inflammatory cell influx in the nasal mucosa and induction of Th1 response. Furthermore, it has been shown that the therapeutic benefit lasts for at least 3–6 years after completion of a 3 year course of treatment.

Although drug treatment for perennial rhinitis may be effective, the use of multiple topical or oral preparations throughout the year is inconvenient and treatment adherence is often poor. Also, in up to 30% of patients with perennial allergic rhinitis, the condition cannot be controlled by topical corticosteroid therapy. For these reasons SIT retains a place in treatment for perennial allergic rhinitis due to house dust mite or animals, although its effects have been less well studied than for seasonal pollenosis. Recent studies have also shown that house dust mite SIT significantly reduced the development of sensitization to new, previously tolerated allergens in children. Formal evaluation is complicated by the heterogeneous and multifactorial nature of perennial rhinitis symptoms, in which non-allergic factors are frequently involved. The efficacy of SIT in treating perennial rhinitis due to domestic pet allergy is more difficult to assess because of the intermittent and variable allergen exposure. Nevertheless, double-blind, placebo-controlled trials of cat dander SIT have shown that patients' specific responsiveness to cat can be attenuated after only 3 months' treatment, along with an elevated conjunctival provocation threshold, reduced skin test reaction to cat dander (Fig. 12.4), reduction in bronchial sensitivity, and markedly reduced clinical response to field exposure to cats.

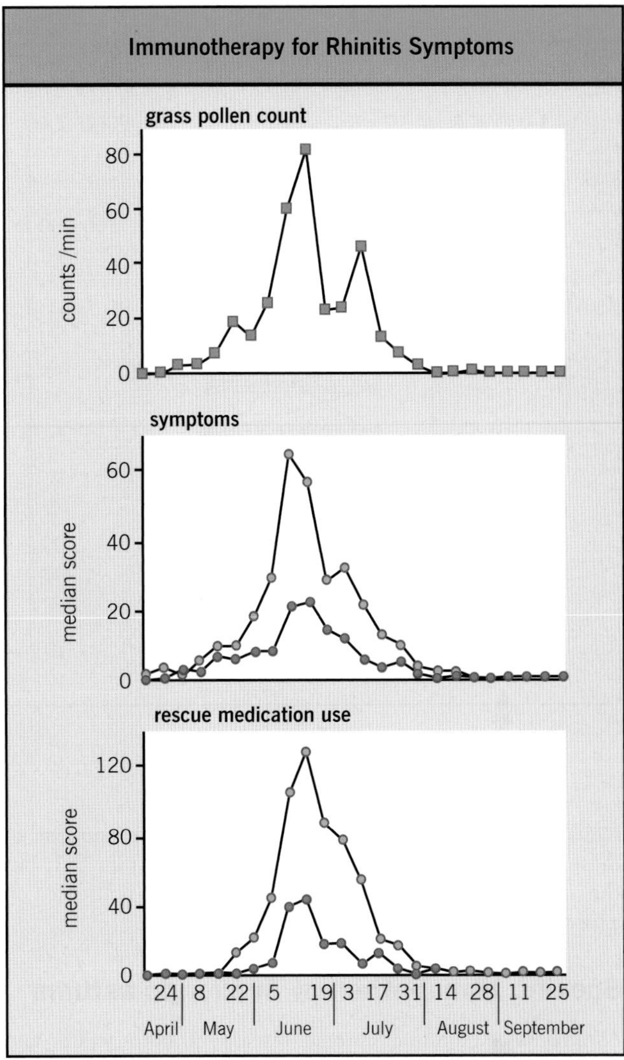

Fig. 12.3 Symptoms and drug scores following immunotherapy with a depot pollen extract or a placebo injection. Note the significant decrease in symptoms and the use of rescue medication after receiving immunotherapy. Green, weekly grass pollen counts for comparison; blue, placebo; red, depot pollen extract. (Data modified from Varney VA, Gaga M, Frew AJ, et al. Usefulness of immunotherapy in patients with severe summer hay fever uncontrolled by anti-allergic drugs. BMJ 1991; 302:265–269.)

At present, the accepted indications for SIT for the treatment of allergic rhinitis and perennial rhinitis vary between countries and largely reflect existing clinical practice. With the increasing costs of health care and the increasing sophistication of the healthcare market, questions of effectiveness and value for money are being asked more frequently. On the other hand, we are now more aware of the adverse effects of rhinitis on the quality of life. Thus the benefit, side-effects, cost, and duration of SIT have to be balanced against those of symptomatic treatment. A significant proportion of rhinitis patients experience side-effects from their drug therapy (nose bleeds in up to 10% of those receiving nasal steroid sprays, and drowsiness in many who receive oral antihistamines) or may find the daily

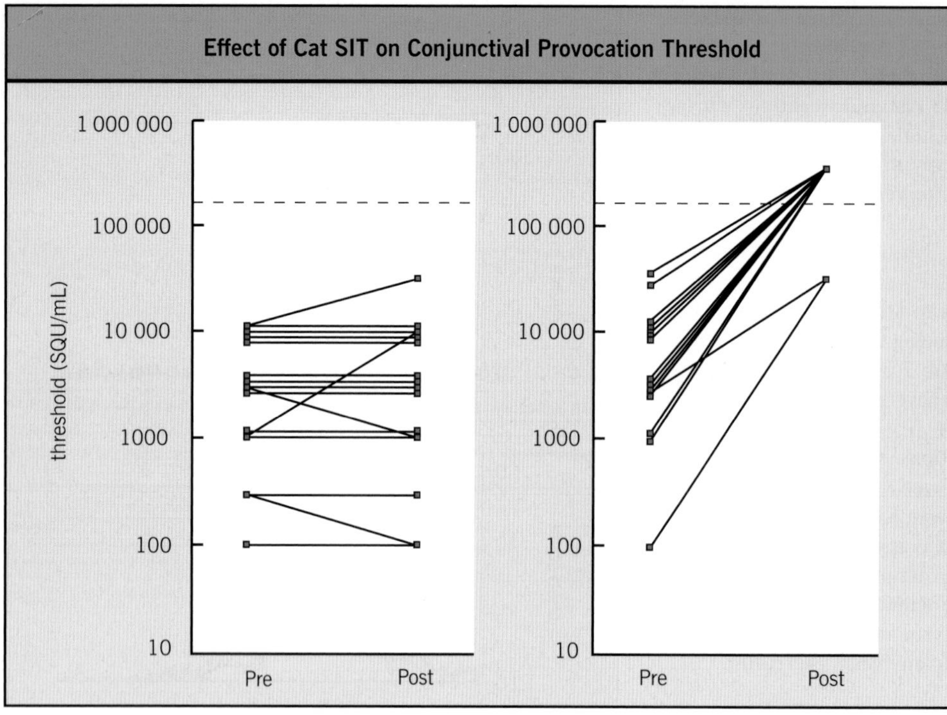

Fig. 12.4 Conjunctival provocation thresholds for cat dander before and after treatment in each group. Dotted line represents the threshold limit. Scores above this line represent no reaction at the maximum concentration tested. SIT, specific immunotherapy. [Data modified from Varney VA, Edwards J, Tabbah K, et al. Clinical efficacy of specific immunotherapy to cat dander: a double-blind placebo-controlled trial. Clin Exp Allergy 1997; 27(8):860–867 © Blackwell Science Ltd.]

rigmarole of using their drugs unsatisfactory. A proportion of these 'non-compliant' patients may also profit from SIT, but the risk/benefit and cost/benefit ratios need to be addressed on a case-by-case basis.

Specific immunotherapy in allergic asthma

Asthma is a common chronic disease of both adults and children, with a considerable amount of morbidity. The efficacy of SIT in adult asthma has been assessed in many trials over the last 40 years but the studies have sometimes been difficult to interpret, either because poor-quality allergen extracts were used or because of poor study design. Many trials were not placebo controlled and only small numbers of patients were treated. Moreover, the extracts used in older trials bear little relationship to those currently marketed and it seems wisest to concentrate on evidence from recent trials using current extracts and orthodox double-blind, placebo-controlled methodology.

The risk/benefit ratio of allergen-specific immunotherapy for asthma has been a controversial area for many years. This is largely due to the potential risk of severe and sometimes fatal adverse events in patients with asthma. This has led to professional societies recommending that patients with asthma and FEV_1 values < 70% (forced expiratory volume in 1 second) should not receive SIT. Furthermore, it can be difficult to demonstrate improvements in physiologic measurements, because most patients with mild asthma have an FEV_1 close to their predicted value, leaving little room for improvement in this parameter.

Because of this controversy, a Cochrane review was undertaken to define the role of allergen immunotherapy for asthma. Published in 2004, this review considered 75 trials published up to June 2001, including all randomized controlled trials using various forms of allergen-specific immunotherapy to treat asthma and reporting at least one clinical outcome. These trials included a total of 3506 participants, 3188 of whom had asthma. The review included 36 trials of immunotherapy for house mite allergy; 20 pollen allergy trials; 10 animal dander allergy trials; 2 *Cladosporium* mold allergy trials; 1 latex and 6 trials looking at multiple allergens. Unfortunately treatment allocation was adequately concealed in only 15 of these trials. There was also significant heterogeneity in the number of comparisons. Nonetheless, the review found a significant reduction in asthma symptoms and medication and improvement in bronchial hyperreactivity following SIT. The review calculated that in order to prevent one patient showing deterioration in asthma symptoms it would have been necessary to treat four (95% CI 3–5) patients with SIT. Overall, it would have been necessary to treat five (95% CI 4–6) patients with SIT to prevent one from requiring increased anti-asthma medication. SIT significantly reduced allergen-specific bronchial hyperreactivity, but had only marginal effects on non-specific bronchial hyperreactivity. No consistent effect on lung function was determined. The reviewers concluded that SIT was effective in asthma, and interestingly, one trial found that the size of the benefit was possibly comparable to inhaled corticosteroids.

In summary, SIT may be beneficial in mild asthma but is not employed as a first-line treatment because of the availability of other effective and safer options. There is no place for SIT for the treatment of moderate and severe asthmatics, due to the potential risk of severe adverse reactions.

SIT for food or drug-induced anaphylaxis

Many causes of anaphylaxis have been recognized, including food allergens (especially nuts and shellfish), latex, and a variety of drugs including penicillin and anesthetic agents. Although these reactions involve IgE and ought, in theory, to be amenable

Table 12.2 Factors associated with adverse reactions to specific immunotherapy (SIT)

Factors Associated with Adverse Reactions to SIT
Early months treatment (induction course)
Dosage errors
Intravenous injection of dose (inadvertent)
History of previous systemic reaction
Extreme sensitivity to allergen
Vigorous exercise before injection
Change of vial
Febrile illness
Uncontrolled asthma
Environmental exposure to allergen, e.g. during the pollen season
Administration of β-blocker drugs

to SIT, thus far few suitable extracts or preparations have been developed or field tested. Perhaps the most promising of these is desensitization for latex allergy, which has been shown to have moderate efficacy in a small preliminary study. A trial of SIT for peanut allergy gave limited protection but caused many severe reactions. For some drug allergies it is possible to perform rapid desensitization to ablate the allergic response to specific drugs but this is not comparable to SIT in either technique or the mechanism of action.

SAFETY OF CONVENTIONAL SPECIFIC IMMUNOTHERAPY

In the UK between 1957 and 1986, 26 fatal reactions associated with SIT were reported to the Committee on Safety of Medicines. In 17 of these, the indication for SIT was documented; 16 of the 17 patients were receiving SIT to treat their asthma. A 12 year survey of fatal reactions to allergen immunotherapy injections between 1990 and 2001 in the USA concluded that fatal reactions occurred at a rate of 1 per 2.5 million injections, with an average of 3.4 deaths per year. This rate of fatalities per immunotherapy injection has not changed much over the last 15 years. The vast majority of fatalities occurred in patients with asthma, most of whom were poorly controlled (Table 12.2). Interestingly, some of these reactions occurred more than 30 minutes after the injections (i.e. at a time exceeding the current recommended waiting time for allergen immunotherapy injections in the USA). In many of the fatalities, there was either a substantial delay in starting epinephrine or epinephrine was not administered at all.

Several studies have shown that pretreatment with antihistamines can reduce the frequency and severity of local and systemic reactions during SIT, but this is not yet standard practice. Efforts to standardize immunotherapy forms and vial labeling will decrease patient and dosing errors. However, clinicians involved in the practice of immunotherapy must constantly assess their patients' current medical status, avoiding the administration of injections to inappropriate candidates, especially patients with poorly controlled asthma. Furthermore, the appropriate and timely administration of epinephrine to treat anaphylaxis is essential.

FUTURE DIRECTIONS

Effects on the natural history of allergic disease

The annual rate of progression to asthma among patients with rhinitis has been estimated at 5% in US college students. A number of long-term epidemiologic studies are now in progress, which could shed light on the current rate of progression to asthma at different ages and the extent of regional and international variation. It is clear that there is a link between allergic rhinitis and asthma, and more than 70% of asthma patients report nasal symptoms. Approximately 20% of all allergic rhinitis patients develop asthma later in life. Different studies have reported that between 11 and 73% of rhinitic patients show bronchial hyperresponsiveness outside the pollen season, with about half of those with normal bronchial reactivity outside the pollen season showing hyperresponsiveness during the season. Preventing the development of full blown asthma in patients with allergic rhinitis is thus a valid and worthwhile objective. A recent study, (the PAT-study) has shown that pollen immunotherapy can reduce the development of asthma in children with seasonal rhinoconjunctivitis. A total of 205 children aged 6–14 years with grass and/or birch pollen allergy, but without any other clinically important allergy, were randomized either to receive specific immunotherapy for 3 years or to an open control group. Of those children who did not have any symptoms of asthma at the start of the study, the actively treated children had significantly fewer asthma symptoms after 3 years as evaluated by clinical diagnosis (odds ratio, 2.52). Methacholine bronchial provocation test results improved significantly in the active group as well. This study demonstrated that a 3 year course of specific immunotherapy in children with allergic rhinoconjunctivitis significantly reduced the risk of developing clinical asthma and improved bronchial hyperresponsiveness.

Peptide immunotherapy

Peptide immunotherapy is based on the concept that SIT works by altering the function of allergen-specific T cells. To be seen by T cells, the injected allergen has to be presented to Th cells as short peptide fragments held in major histocompatibility complex (MHC) class II molecules on antigen-presenting cells. Since T-cell epitopes are different from the B-cell epitopes seen by antibodies (Fig. 12.5), it should be possible to give T-cell peptides to target T cells, without risking IgE-mediated anaphylaxis. The candidate peptides are identified on the basis of their ability to induce proliferation in lymphocyte lines from a group of patients with specific allergy. Peptide vaccines based on Fel d 1 and Amb a 1 have been tested in patients with cat and ragweed allergy respectively and have shown modest benefit. Up to a third of patients experienced mild systemic reactions between 1 and 3 hours after injection but these reactions reduced in frequency with continuation of therapy. Occasional immediate reactions were also noted in these studies, suggesting that sensitization to these peptides was possible. At present peptide immunotherapy remains

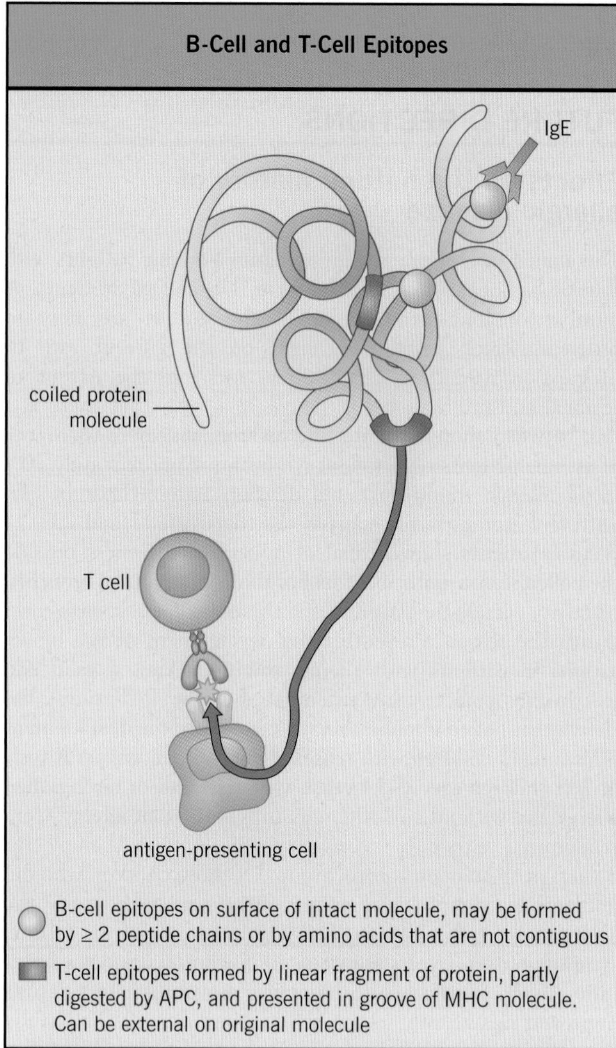
B-Cell and T-Cell Epitopes
IgE
coiled protein molecule
T cell
antigen-presenting cell
B-cell epitopes on surface of intact molecule, may be formed by ≥ 2 peptide chains or by amino acids that are not contiguous
T-cell epitopes formed by linear fragment of protein, partly digested by APC, and presented in groove of MHC molecule. Can be external on original molecule

Fig. 12.5 Schematic representation of B-cell and T-cell epitopes. Note that T-cell epitopes are linear peptides, derived by partial degradation of the allergen, while B-cell epitopes are 3-dimensional or 'configurational' and may involve portions from quite separate parts of the primary structure, which are brought together by pleating and folding of the allergenic molecules. APC, antigen-presenting cell; MHC, major histocompatibility complex.

experimental but there are ongoing studies examining its efficacy and safety.

Antiimmunoglobulin E

The anti-IgE monoclonal antibody omalizumab (Xolair®) is a recombinant humanized antibody, consisting of IgE-binding regions derived from a murine anti-human-IgE attached to a human IgG1 framework. Thus it retains the antigen-binding domain of the original murine antibody (comprising about 5% of the hybrid antibody) while approximately 95% of the sequence is human, which prevents the recipient from seeing it as foreign. Omalizumab binds only to circulating free IgE: after several weeks' treatment it attenuates allergic responses, downregulates expression of IgE receptors on mast cells and basophils, and is clinically effective in allergic disorders. Omalizumab has recently been approved by the US Food and Drug Administration for moderate to severe allergic asthma. Omalizumab has been shown to reduce asthma exacerbations, improve asthma symptom scores, reduce rescue medication use, improve lung function and quality of life and has a steroid sparing effect. It has also been shown to be effective in the treatment of ragweed- and birch pollen-induced seasonal allergic rhinitis. Apart from mild–moderate urticaria in a minority of patients no serious adverse effects have been reported.

Most recently, omalizumab has been studied as an add-on therapy to immunotherapy in young patients aged 6–17 years. Subjects allergic to birch and grass pollen were treated by specific immunotherapy and then omalizumab was added after the maintenance phase of allergen immunotherapy was reached. The combination of omalizumab plus immunotherapy showed superior efficacy with good safety and tolerability. Omalizumab is also being used to try to reduce systemic adverse effects of immunotherapy: formal results are yet to be published, but preliminary data indicate that omalizumab has a protective effect against immunotherapy-induced systemic reactions, and improved efficacy over immunotherapy alone.

Immunostimulatory DNA

Studies in animal models have identified bacterial DNA, and in particular specific palindromic DNA motifs containing unmethylated cytosine residues in the sequence CpG, as potent adjuvants of the Th1 response. CpG DNA exerts its effects via the Toll-like receptor 9 (TLR9) on dendritic cells. DNA hexamers based on the general formula of 5′purine-purine-CG-pyrimidine-pyrimidine-3′ are considered optimal. When protein antigens were mixed with these immunostimulatory oligodeoxynucleotide sequences (ISS-ODN) and injected into mice, they induced a Th1 immune response characterized by IgG2 formation and IFNγ-secreting CD4+ T cells. When ISS-ODN are covalently conjugated to allergen, a novel type of allergoid for SIT is produced that has several potential advantages: first, this conjugate delivers the ISS-ODN and the allergen to the same antigen presenting cell; second, no free ISS-ODN reaches bystander cells to produce excess mediators that could cause adverse reactions; and third, the conjugate allergoid probably presents fewer B-cell epitopes, reducing the risks of side-effects.

This strategy has yielded some encouraging observations in a study of 28 patients with ragweed-induced hayfever. In this study there was no improvement in symptoms during the first post-immunotherapy season, which started 3 weeks after the last injection. However, when challenged 4–5 months after therapy (i.e. after the ragweed pollen season), fewer eosinophils and IL-4 mRNA positive cells and increased numbers of IFNγ-positive cells were noted in patients who received active therapy. A modest symptomatic improvement was noted in the following pollen season, without the subjects receiving any further treatment. These results are encouraging but clearly further studies are required to study the safety and efficacy of these vaccines.

It is not clear whether CpG admixed with multiple allergens as in traditional immunotherapy would also be more effective than allergen immunotherapy alone. Furthermore, although CpG works least well in animal models when given as mono-therapy, the effects of CpG administered either before or during a pollen season with natural high dose exposure are also worthy of consideration. The prospect of invoking profound and long-lasting tolerance to allergens with much less intensive immunotherapy regimens makes this approach intriguing.

CONCLUSION

SIT is the only available treatment that alters the natural course of allergic disease, offering sustained relief of symptoms, and limiting progression of rhinitis to asthma. Although there are some risks, these can be minimized when SIT is given in a controlled environment to carefully selected patients. SIT in conjunction with anti-IgE offers a great prospect not only to reduce the incidence of serious systemic reactions but also to enhance efficacy, although further data are needed to address this important issue. Combining allergens with CpG-DNA or other adjuvants may also improve the efficacy and safety profile of SIT. SIT is thus a valuable therapy for allergic disease, with the potential for further improvement and wider application in the future.

FURTHER READING

Abramson MJ, Puy RM, Weiner JM. Allergen immunotherapy for asthma (Cochrane Review). In: The Cochrane Library. Issue 2. Chichester: John Wiley; 2004.

Canonica GW, Passalacqua G. Noninjection routes for immunotherapy. J Allergy Clin Immunol 2003; 111:437–448.

Des Roches A, Paradis L, Menardo JL, et al. Immunotherapy with a standardised *D. pteronyssinus* extract. VI. Specific immunotherapy prevents the onset of new sensitisations in children. J Allergy Clin Immunol 1997; 99:450–453.

Durham SR, Ying S, Varney VA, et al. Grass pollen immunotherapy inhibits allergen-induced infiltration of CD4+ T-lymphocytes and eosinophils in the nasal mucosa and increases the number of cells expressing mRNA for interferon-gamma. J Allergy Clin Immunol 1996; 97:1356–1365.

Golden DB, Kagey-Sobotka A, Norman PS, et al. Outcomes of allergy to insect stings in children, with and without venom immunotherapy. N Engl J Med 2004; 351:668–674.

Lerch E, Muller U. Long-term protection after stopping venom immunotherapy. J Allergy Clin Immunol 1998; 101:606–612.

Li JT, Lockey IL, Bernstein JM, et al. Allergen immunotherapy: a practice parameter. Ann Allergy Asthma Immunol 2003; 90:1–40.

Moller C, Dreborg S, Ferdousi HA, et al. Pollen immunotherapy reduces the development of asthma in children with seasonal rhinoconjunctivitis (the PAT-Study). J Allergy Clin Immunol 2002; 109:251–256.

Spiegelberg HL, Horner AA, Takabayashi K, et al. Allergen-immunostimulatory oligonucleotide conjugate: a novel allergoid for immunotherapy. Curr Opin Allergy Clin Immunol 2002; 2:547–551.

Till SJ, Francis JN, Nouri-Aria K, et al. Mechanisms of immunotherapy. J Allergy Clin Immunol 2004; 113:1025–1034.

Varney VA, Gaga M, Frew AJ, et al. Usefulness of immunotherapy in patients with severe summer hay fever uncontrolled by anti-allergic drugs. BMJ 1991; 302:265–269.

Chapter 13

Pediatric Allergy

Ulrich Wahn and Estelle Simons

Definition:

This chapter covers the prevalence and natural history of allergic diseases in the pediatric population, as well as the diagnosis and treatment of these diseases in this population. The possibility of primary and secondary prevention of allergic diseases in children is also discussed.

INTRODUCTION

Over the last decade, atopic diseases in childhood have become increasingly prevalent in many parts of the world and they now represent a major public health problem in almost all industrialized countries. Atopic diseases are understood as those allergic conditions that tend to cluster in families and are associated with the production of specific IgE antibodies to common environmental allergens. The most prevalent clinical manifestations are allergic rhinitis, asthma, atopic dermatitis and food allergy, which have the highest incidence during infancy, childhood or adolescence.

The term 'atopic march' refers to the natural history of atopic manifestations, which is characterized by a typical sequence of IgE antibody responses and clinical symptoms that appear during a certain age period, persist over years and decades, and often show a tendency for spontaneous remission with age. Several prospective longitudinal birth cohort studies have become valuable for our current understanding of the development and outcome of allergy and asthma in childhood.

PREVALENCE AND NATURAL HISTORY OF ALLERGIC DISEASES IN THE PEDIATRIC POPULATION

Longitudinal follow-up studies with birth cohorts have been designed to describe the natural history of various atopic phenotypes. Although wide individual variations may be observed, the manifestation of atopic diseases tends to be related to the first two decades of life (Fig. 13.1).

The production of IgE starts in the 11th week of gestation. Total IgE levels are mostly below 0.35 kU/L, but these levels increase steadily during the first decade of life (Table 13.1).

Current studies suggest that the immune responses of newborns to ubiquitous injected and inhaled proteins are helper T cell type 2 (Th2)-biased. No specific sensitization to food or inhalant allergens, as measured by elevated serum IgE antibodies, can be detected in cord blood with standard methods. Postnatally, repeated encounters with these common allergenic proteins leads to the development of mature immune responses. While IgG antibodies to food proteins are detectable in sera of nearly all infants, indicating that the infantile immune system sees and responds to commonly ingested proteins, allergen specific IgE (to hens' eggs and cows' milk proteins) is detectable in only a minority of subjects. Low level IgE responses to food allergens may be transient and may occur before the introduction of food into the diet. In children who develop clinical allergic conditions, however, higher levels and persistence of food allergen-specific IgE are typical.

Levels of allergen-specific serum IgE antibody to indoor or outdoor allergens (pollen, pets, dust mites) increase in prevalence with age to approximately 20% by the age of six.

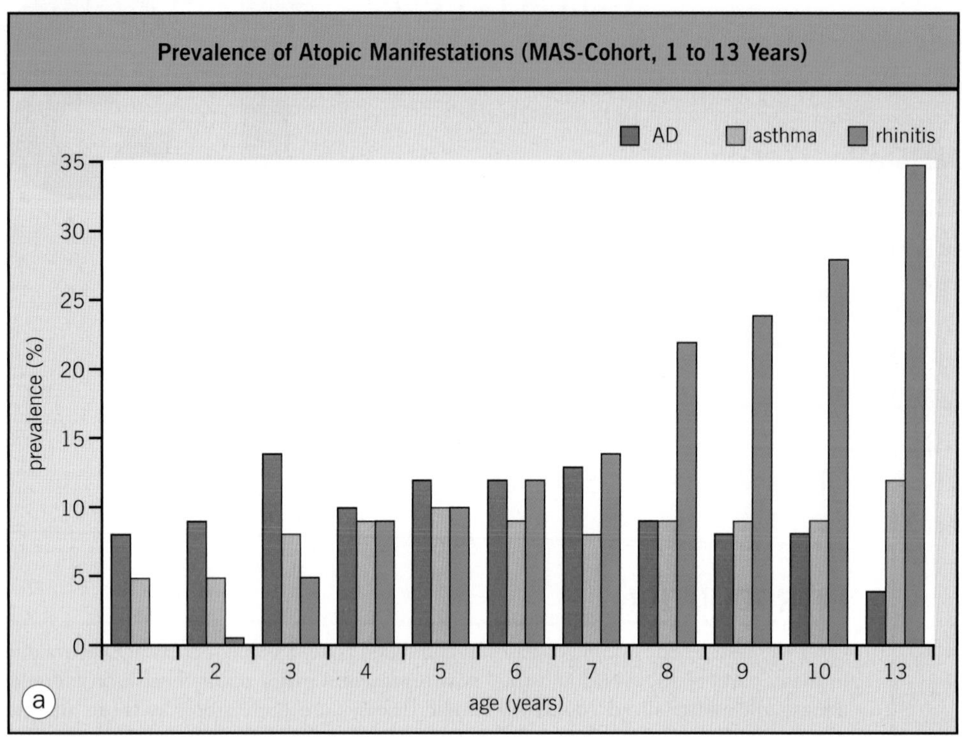

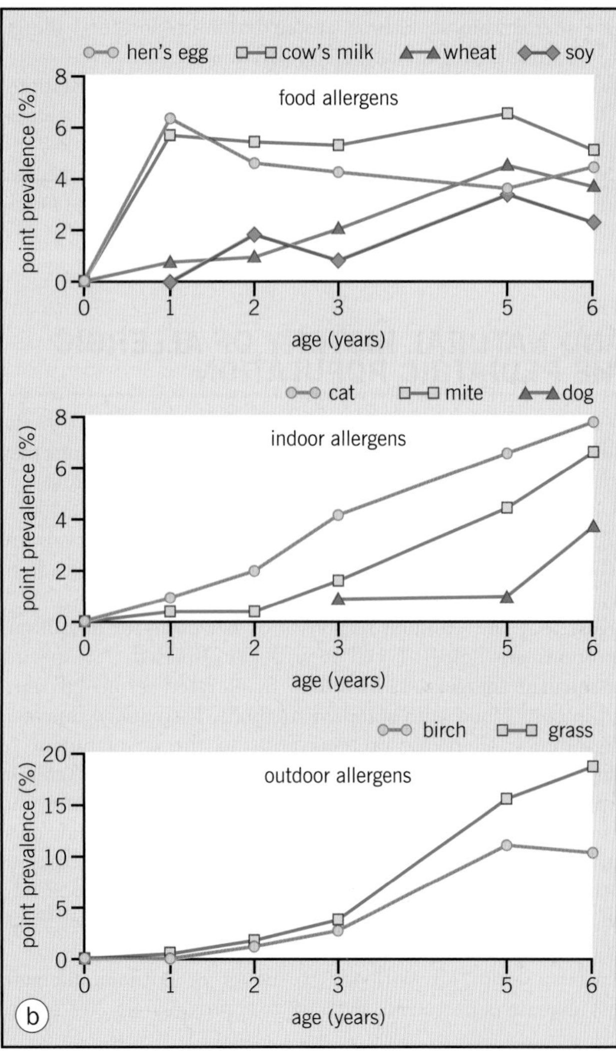

Fig. 13.1 Allergic march of early childhood. Prevalence of allergic diseases, asthma, and allergen sensitization in a large birth cohort study (Multicentre Allergy Study, Germany). (a) Period prevalence of atopic dermatitis, asthma, and allergic rhinoconjunctivitis at different ages. (b) Point prevalence of sensitization to common food allergens, indoor allergens, and outdoor allergens. Based on serum allergen-specific IgE (cutoff level 0.7 kU/L). [(a) from Wahn U. What drives the allergic march? Allergy 2000; 55(7):591–599 and (b) from Kulig M, Bergmann R, Klettke U, et al. Natural course of sensitization to food and inhalant allergens during the first 6 years of life. J Allergy Clin Immunol 1999; 103(6):1173–1179.]

Table 13.1 Percentiles for total serum IgE concentrations in German children at 1, 2, 3, 5 and 6 years of age (estimates for a population based sample)

Total Serum IgE (kU/L)					
Age (years)	1	2	3	5	6
25th Percentile	2	5	8	14	16
50th Percentile	5	15	20	34	42
75th Percentile	13	40	58	85	95
85th Percentile	26	75	111	150	170
90th Percentile	40	107	155	212	259
95th Percentile	78	226	261	372	428

[From Kulig M, et al. Serum IgE levels during the first 6 years of life. J Pediatr 1999, 134:453–458.]

Recent studies have indicated that children with higher serum IgE levels to food in infancy and a subsequent 'switch' to IgE antibodies directed to indoor or outdoor allergens are at risk of developing bronchial hyperresponsiveness and persistent allergic asthma.

Atopic dermatitis

Atopic dermatitis (AD) generally represents the first atopic manifestation with the highest incidence during the first 6 months of life and the highest period prevalence during the first 3 years of life. Parental history of AD is probably the most important risk factor for childhood AD. This heritability is also suggested by a high concordance rate of AD among monozygotic versus dizygotic twins (0.72 and 0.23, respectively). Whole genome-scan studies in large numbers of affected sib families with a well defined phenotype of infantile atopic dermatitis suggest that gene polymorphisms with linkage to atopic dermatitis are located on the long arm of chromosome 3.

According to birth cohort studies, a higher level of maternal education has to be considered a risk factor for early onset AD, while exclusive breastfeeding of infants with a family history of atopy for at least the first 3 months of life is associated with a lower likelihood of childhood AD. This protective effect, however, is not observed in children without a family history of atopy.

Natural history studies have reported a wide variation in disease persistence throughout childhood. In a recent cohort study it was demonstrated that more than 40% of cases of infants with atopic dermatitis result in complete remission after the age of 2, whereas almost one-fifth of all children with early atopic dermatitis had persistent symptoms at the age of 7 (Fig. 13.2). The strongest risk factor for a poor prognosis was initial severity in infancy and atopic sensitization to inhalant or food allergens as detected during infancy. Of adolescents with moderate to severe AD, 77–91% continue to have persistent disease in adulthood. Food allergen sensitization can contribute to AD development and is associated with disease severity. It also has to be considered as a predictor for persistence of dermatitis. Several cohort studies have demonstrated that atopic dermatitis in infancy and early childhood is associated with a high prevalence of sensitization to inhalant allergens and the subsequent development of childhood asthma.

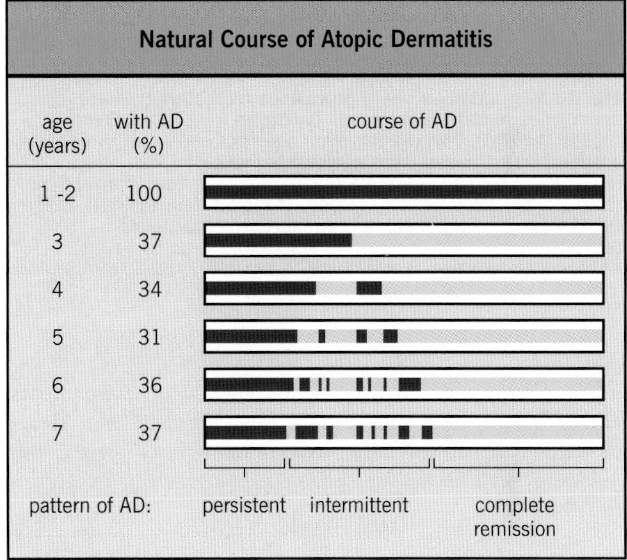

Fig. 13.2 Natural course of atopic dermatitis (AD) up to age 7 years in children with early manifestation of the disease (~2 years). Each symbol represents 1% of the children with early AD, and the natural course of each 1% subsample can be traced vertically. Filled squares represent AD in the respective time period. [From Illi S, von Mutius E, Lau S, et al. The natural course of atopic dermatitis from birth to age 7 years and the association with asthma. J Allergy Clin Immunol 2004; 113:925–931.]

In most cases the first clinical manifestations affect mainly the face, followed by the trunk, arms and legs. Flexural eczema is characteristic for preschool and school children. Chronic itch and disturbed sleep are the most troublesome symptoms, which profoundly affect the quality of life not only of the children, but also of their caregivers. From infancy onwards the skin is chronically affected by superantigen producing *Staphylococcus* A strains, which may enhance chronic inflammation via T-cell activation. They may also induce purulent superinfection of the skin, which is facilitated by scratch induced wounds.

Although food allergy should not be considered as the primary cause of atopic dermatitis, alimentary allergens have been shown to contribute to skin rashes and the degree of

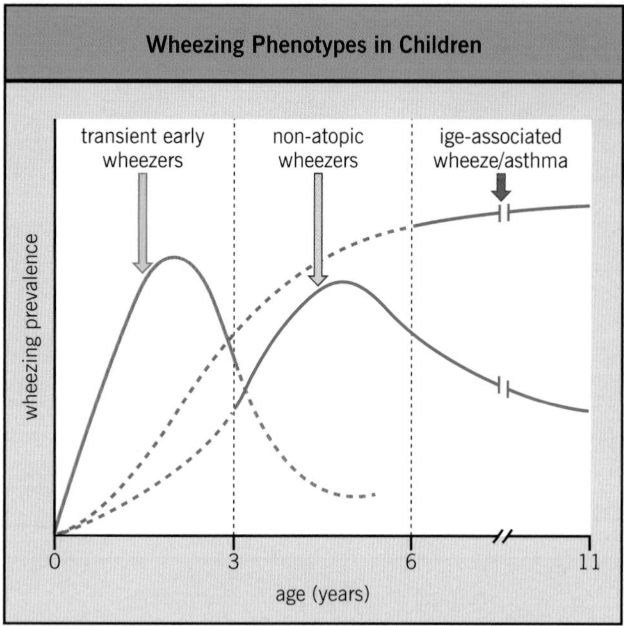

Fig. 13.3 Hypothetical yearly prevalence for recurrent wheezing phenotypes in childhood (Tucson Children's Respiratory Study, Tucson, Arizona). This classification does not imply that the groups are exclusive. Dashed lines suggest that wheezing can be represented by different curve shapes resulting from many different factors, including overlap of groups. [Adapted from Stein RT, Holberg CJ, Morgan WJ, et al. Peak flow variability, methacholine responsiveness and atopy as markers for detecting different wheezing phenotypes in childhood. Thorax 1997; 52(11):946–952.]

Table 13.2 Predictive Index for children (Tucson Children's Respiratory Study, Tucson, Arizona). Through a statistically optimized model for 2- to 3-year-old children with frequent wheezing in the past year, one major criterion or two minor criteria provided 77% positive predictive value and 97% specificity for asthma in later childhood (i.e. at 6, 8, 11 and/or 13 years of age

Major criteria	Minor criteria
Parent asthma	Allergic rhinitis
Eczema	Wheezing apart from colds
	Eosinophils > 4%

From Castro-Rodriguez JA, Holberg CJ, Wright AI, et al. Am J Respir Crit Care Med 2000; 162:1406.

inflammation, particularly in infancy. The role of environmental allergens in the manifestation, severity, and persistence of eczema is far less clear. Anecdotal reports suggest that indoor as well as outdoor allergen exposure can exacerbate the disease.

Childhood asthma

Asthmatic wheeze may already be observed during early infancy. The majority of early wheezers turn out to be only transiently symptomatic, whereas in a minority of children symptoms persist throughout school age and adolescence. Our understanding of the natural history of childhood asthma is still limited. Approximately 80% of asthmatic adults report disease onset before 6 years of age. Numerous data sets support the existences of various asthma subtypes (Fig. 13.3) in childhood.

During the first 3 years of life the manifestation of wheeze is not related to elevated serum IgE levels or specific sensitization, and positive parental history of atopy and asthma seems to be of minor importance during the first 2 years of life. These 'transient wheezers' are not at an increased risk of having asthma later in life. Transient wheezing is associated with airway viral infections, smaller airways and lungs, male gender, low birth weight and maternal prenatal environmental tobacco smoke exposure.

Persistent asthma commonly begins and coexists with a large population of transient wheezers. Those who have persistent wheezing show an increasing association with sensitization to aeroallergens with age. In addition the association with a positive family history of atopy and asthma in first degree relatives becomes more and more obvious. Severity of childhood asthma, determined clinically or by lung function impairment, also predicts asthma persistence into adulthood.

Natural history studies of asthma have identified biological, genetic, and environmental risk factors for persistent asthma. The Tucson Children's Respiratory Study uses a statistical optimization of the major risk factors for persistent asthma which allows prediction of persistent asthma with a high positive predicted value and specificity (Table 13.2).

Allergic rhinoconjunctivitis

The manifestation of seasonal or perennial allergic rhinoconjunctivitis is exceptionally rare during the first 2 years of life, although a minority of children will develop specific IgE antibodies during this early period (Fig. 13.1). Ordinarily, at least two seasons of pollen allergen exposure are required before classic symptoms become manifest. The prevalence of allergic rhinoconjunctivitis in children varies from country to country. In Europe, it reaches more than 20% in young adolescents. In the USA, in one study doctor-diagnosed allergic rhinitis was reported in more than 40% of 6 year-olds. Follow-up studies have provided evidence that without specific immunotherapy the risk of asthmatic wheeze during peak pollen allergen exposure in children with allergic rhinoconjunctivitis is 45%.

Allergic rhinitis persistence has not been thoroughly evaluated in children. From adult studies it is known that allergic rhinitis patients have a disease remission rate of 5–10% AFTER? 4 years and 23% AFTER 23 years. Onset of disease in early childhood was associated with a greater chance of improvement.

Urticaria

Both acute and chronic urticaria may already become manifest in infancy. Among children, the prevalence of urticaria/angioedema has been estimated to be about 6–7%. Acute urticaria with or without angioedema may be observed in the atopic population as a result of IgE-mediated reactions primarily to food proteins, whereas chronic urticaria (persistence of symptoms > 6 weeks) is mostly not related to identifiable allergic trigger factors. Understanding the course of chronic idiopathic urticaria remains a particular challenge, as one rarely finds a direct relationship between the disease and exposure to an external agent or infection. The cause of inflammatory changes with a typical non-necrotizing mononuclear cell infiltrate around small venules remains uncertain. According to recent studies a significant proportion of chronic urticaria cases in adults obviously has to be interpreted as the result of underlying autoimmune processes.

Food allergy

Adverse reactions to food in childhood include food hypersensitivity that is IgE mediated and manifests as classic allergic symptoms of immediate onset. Most reactions involve the skin (urticaria, eczematic rash), the gastrointestinal tract (vomiting, colic, diarrhea), and the airways (asthma).

The prevalence of food hypersensitivity is highest in the first few years of life affecting up to 5% of children in the first year of life. Whether or not children will 'outgrow' their food allergy and become tolerant may depend on the food allergen source.

During infancy and childhood, three distinct types of food allergy can be identified:

- The infantile type of food allergy, mostly directed to proteins from hens' eggs, cows' milk, wheat or soy, which leads to skin, airways or gastrointestinal symptoms during the first year of life, requires strict elimination diets for 2–8 years and has a benign long-term prognosis. In a prospective study of young children with milk allergy, most became non-allergic within a few years: 50% by 1 year of age, 70% by 2 years and 85% by 3 years.
- IgE-mediated, sometimes life-threatening reactions to allergens from peanuts or seafood, which may become manifest during the first 3 years of life and are unlikely to develop remission. Two recent long-term follow-up studies of peanut allergic children found that loss of clinical hypersensitivity was uncommon especially in children with anaphylactic symptoms in addition to urticaria and/or atopy dermatitis.
- Pollen-associated food allergy as a result of true immunologic cross-reactivity based on shared epitopes between allergenic molecules from pollen, or on proteins from fruit or vegetables. A classic clinical manifestation is the 'oral allergy syndrome'. It is rarely observed in infancy and commonly follows an established pollen allergy.

Other food allergic reactions such as eosinophilic gastroenteropathy have variable associations with foods and lack natural history studies.

Anaphylaxis

Anaphylaxis in infancy and childhood can be induced by numerous possible allergen sources like food, antibiotics, insulin, insect venoms, or latex. In general atopy is not considered as a risk factor for anaphylaxis to insect stings. Besides classical IgE-mediated reactions, anaphylactoid reactions induced by radio contrast media and aspirin/non-steroidal antiinflammatory drugs have to be considered. The natural history of anaphylactic reactions in children has only been studied prospectively for food and bee sting induced anaphylaxis.

Insect allergy

Demographic studies suggest that the incidence of insect sting allergy in the general population ranges between 0.4 and 3%. Approximately one-third of individuals who have insect sting anaphylaxis are atopic.

Older studies in children suggested that insect sting anaphylaxis is often self-limited in children with spontaneous remission, usually occurring in 4 years. Those at greatest risk of persistent hypersensitivity include those with severe anaphylactic episodes. Children with mild systemic reactions to bee stings are less likely to have an allergic reaction on another sting and any future anaphylactic episodes from bee stings are not likely to be severe. Recent surveys indicate that a large number of children do not outgrow allergic reactions to insect stings. Venom immunotherapy in children may lead to a significantly lower risk of systemic reaction to stings even 10–20 years after treatment is stopped and this prolonged benefit is greater than the benefit seen in adults.

DIAGNOSIS OF ALLERGIC DISEASE IN THE PEDIATRIC POPULATION

The first diagnostic step for children with a history of clinical manifestations is a careful family history. Atopic disease in first-degree relatives is an important factor which has to be taken into account. The seasonality of manifestations, recurrent symptoms upon exposure to specific environmental conditions, or food sources can be considered as most useful information.

Generally, skin tests as well as in vitro tests can be performed from early infancy on. For almost all clinical conditions a skin puncture test (prick test) with a steel lancet is sufficient. In some cases of food allergy it might be preferable to use fresh food, since allergen extracts of acceptable quality are not available (prick-prick-method). The wheal-and-flare reaction to skin puncture test should be evaluated after 10 minutes.

The atopy-patch-test has been studied in combination with the skin prick tests to determine whether the combination is more sensitive and specific for the diagnosis of food allergy in atopic dermatitis. It has been reported to be useful in the diagnosis of non-IgE-mediated food reactions, but further studies are necessary to determine its place in the diagnosis of food hypersensitivity.

Skin tests are not always acceptable in infants and younger children, but the determination of specific serum IgE antibody concentrations (immuno-cap-test) has been shown to be equally sensitive to identify specific sensitizations to food or inhalant allergens. For total serum IgE concentrations, percentiles have been established for preschool children (Table 13.1). For the diagnosis of allergic diseases in childhood, however, total IgE values are of limited diagnostic value, whereas in a number of other clinical conditions (immunodeficiencies etc.) extremely high elevated total IgE values can be found.

The precision of conjunctival, nasal, and bronchial challenge tests using specific allergens has been thoroughly evaluated. In doubtful cases with discrepancies between history, skin test, or in vitro test they might be useful in determining the clinical relevance of a specific sensitization.

In cases of suspected food allergy, oral challenge tests should be considered as the 'gold standard'. Several studies suggest that in many cases a clinical history of suspected food allergy in infants and children is unreliable and the identification of a

Table 13.3 Identification of children at high risk for fatal or near-fatal asthma episodes

- Previous near-fatal episodes, e.g. Intensive Care Unit admission, intubation, and/or mechanical ventilation
- Hospitalizations or Emergency Department or Urgent Care visit(s) during previous year
- Excessive use of short-acting β_2-adrenergic agonist (one canister per month, or equivalent)
- Concurrent use of, or withdrawal from, oral glucocorticoids
- Poor perception of asthma symptoms and delay in treatment
- History of non-adherence to asthma medications
- History of psychosocial problems or psychiatric disease in child or caregiver
- Sensitization to *Alternaria* (mold)*
- Passive smoke exposure
- Reduced access to health care, including living in a remote rural area, poor socioeconomic status
- Lack of formal education, language barrier, low income or overcrowded housing

* Best documented in North America

Table 13.4 Identification of children at high-risk for fatal or near-fatal anaphylaxis episodes

- Previous or near-fatal reaction*
- Concurrent diagnosis of asthma
- Previous reaction to peanut, tree nut, milk, egg, fish or seafood
- Poor access to emergency medical services (e.g. living or vacationing in a remote rural area)
- Dysfunctional or chaotic family situation
- No reliable transportation available

*Note, however, that absence of such a history does not eliminate the possibility of a near-fatal or fatal reaction in the future

specific sensitivity by either skin tests or specific serum IgE alone is not sufficient to justify elimination diets. In recent years a sufficient consensus has been reached on titrated oral challenge tests and their evaluation.

In children with asthma, spirometry and other pulmonary function testing is important for objectively documenting reversibility of obstruction to airflow and for monitoring response to treatment. In infants and very young children, however, age-appropriate pulmonary function tests are generally available only in pediatric hospitals or specialty clinics. Non-specific challenges with exercise, methacholine or histamine may be helpful in diagnosing asthma. Measurement of exhaled nitric oxide and assessment of eosinophilia in induced sputum are useful research tests. For diagnosis of allergic rhinitis, identification of eosinophils in blown nasal secretions is helpful. Inspiratory peak nasal flow monitoring is sometimes used in research. Quality-of-life scales for asthma and allergic rhinitis and rating scales for severity of disease, for example, atopic dermatitis/eczema, have proven to be useful in research but are infrequently used in clinical practice.

TREATMENT OF ALLERGIC DISEASES IN THE PEDIATRIC POPULATION

General overview

Treatment of allergic diseases in childhood presents unique challenges, as both the beneficial effects and the detrimental effects of intervention(s) may last for decades and even for a lifetime. Most allergic diseases are managed in a community setting by primary care physicians, rather than in a hospital setting by allergy specialists. Here, we describe outpatient treatment, which is focused on prevention and relief of morbidity from allergic diseases and on the identification of children at high risk of fatality from asthma (Table 13.3) or anaphylaxis (Table 13.4), who require regular, frequent monitoring.

The quantity and quality of evidence for the efficacy and safety of therapeutic approaches for allergic disease in the pediatric population varies greatly with: the age of the patients, the disease, and the treatment modality studied. The evidence base consisting of adequately powered, randomized, placebo-controlled, double-blind trials is largest for adolescents receiving pharmacologic interventions for asthma or allergic rhinoconjunctivitis. It is considerably smaller for young children and infants; for allergic diseases such as urticaria, atopic dermatitis/eczema, and anaphylaxis; and for non-pharmacologic interventions such as education, avoidance of environmental allergens, and allergen-specific immunotherapy. At this time, evidence-based international and national guidelines are available only for asthma treatment in the pediatric population.

Children often have allergic co-morbidities, that is, concomitant allergic diseases such as asthma, allergic rhinitis, atopic dermatitis/eczema, and food allergies. For such children

Table 13.5 Asthma education: objectives

- Improve child's and caregiver's understanding of asthma as a persistent disease with intermittent symptoms of variable severity
- Discuss short-term and long-term treatment goals, emphasizing the goal of being free from asthma symptoms
- Discuss the importance of avoiding trigger factors such as cigarette smoke and airborne allergens and using medications to prevent symptoms
- Improve ability to recognize and manage 'breakthrough' symptoms and acute asthma episodes
- Help parents and children to differentiate between preventer/controller/antiinflammatory medications and reliever medications
- Acknowledge and discuss parental fears and concerns, such as potential side-effects of medications
- Identify practical economic resources for the family: assistance with cost of medications, transport to healthcare facilities
- Discuss potential barriers to meeting treatment goals such as: lack of faith in conventional medical treatment, preference for complementary treatment, 'different' sociocultural beliefs
- Provide a list of websites that are a reliable source of relevant health information

and their families, it is therefore important to provide a comprehensive approach to management including: education about the long-term nature of allergic inflammation and the intermittent exacerbations that characterize allergic diseases, and the need to avoid triggers for symptoms where possible and to consider the potential benefits of allergen-specific immunotherapy. It is also important to have a systematic, stepwise approach to pharmacologic treatment and to keep the overall number of prescribed medications to a minimum, in order to facilitate adherence to treatment regimens. Healthcare professionals should recognize that the most common reason for apparent lack of response to treatment is lack of adherence. This is particularly true for glucocorticoid treatment, due to caregivers' concerns about potential adverse effects. Although many physicians respond to a child's apparent failure to improve on a medication by prescribing an increased dose, this is of little value if the medication is not being given or taken in the first place. Intensified efforts with regard to education, allergen avoidance, non-specific, non-medicinal approaches to treatment and, in some children, allergen specific immunotherapy, may be more helpful.

Education

Interactive educational partnerships with children and their caregivers are important. The persistent inflammatory nature of inflammatory diseases such as asthma, allergic rhinitis, and atopic dermatitis/eczema should be explained and the differing natural history of each disease should be outlined. The main goal in treatment should be clearly stated: complete freedom from symptoms such as wheezing, coughing, and shortness of breath in asthma; itching, sneezing, discharge and congestion in rhinitis; and itching in urticaria or atopic dermatitis/ eczema.

All education programs should be age appropriate. For infants and very young children, programs should be parent oriented. For school age children, programs involving both parents and children in separate, small groups are optimal. Teens should have sessions focused on their unique needs. Education programs should provide written, clearly focused information in an appropriate language and at an appropriate literacy level about: avoiding triggers for exacerbations (with the exception of exercise), understanding the differences between preventer/controller and reliever medications, and how to anticipate exacerbations and respond by intensifying treatment in a timely manner. Education programs should emphasize the importance of development and regular review of written action plans for recognition and management of exacerbations of allergic disease.

Many families are interested in non-specific, non-medicinal approaches to the treatment of allergic diseases. For a child with exercise-induced asthma, it may be appropriate to discuss selection of a sport such as swimming or distance running that is less likely to trigger symptoms than sprinting or skating, and to emphasize the importance of aerobic conditioning and warm-up. For a child with allergic rhinitis, nasal rinses with saline can be recommended. For a child with atopic dermatitis/ eczema, it is appropriate to discuss avoidance of exposure to hot, humid environmental conditions and wooly or rough-textured clothing and bedding, use of skin hydration and emollients to repair stratum corneum barrier function, and treatment of superinfections with antibiotics. For all children with allergic diseases, physicians should recommend a healthy diet including fresh fruits and vegetables, and optimal, age-appropriate rest and recreation.

Child and family asthma education programs (Table 13.5) have been documented to improve outcomes and are becoming widely available; however, for other allergic diseases, education programs are not yet as well developed. For asthmatics, enrollment in a formal asthma education program may begin at any time, but often follows a child's visit to the hospital emergency department, or a hospitalization for an exacerbation.

Table 13.6 Avoidance and control of allergens

House dust mites
• Avoid having carpet, rugs and upholstered furniture in the child's bedroom
• Encase the mattress and box spring with airtight, dustproof covers or plastic
• Use new, dust mite-free pillows. Dry on the hot cycle for 45 minutes every 2 weeks, and replace every few years
• Use cotton or synthetic bedding and mattress cover; wash weekly in hot water (55°C) and dry on the hot cycle
• Treat stuffed animals as described above for pillows or bedding
• Use a central vacuum system or a vacuum with a HEPA filter (e.g. Nilfisk). An upright vacuum or vacuum with a double-bag is also satisfactory. Damp-dust all surfaces weekly
Mold and mildew
• Repair water leaks and, if appropriate, check basement, attic, and crawlspace for standing water and mold
• Use a dehumidifier if the humidity in the home is > 60%; molds (and mites) thrive when humidity is high
• Do not use a humidifier
Cats, dogs, and other animals
• If a child is allergic to animal dander, do not have an animal in the home
• If it is impossible to remove the animal, keep it outside as much as possible and consider bathing it regularly
• **Never** allow the animal into the child's bedroom. (Keep the door closed!). Seal off or cover the room's heating vent with a filter. Use a portable heater if necessary
Pollen
• Keep windows closed in house/apartment/automobile. Use air conditioning if available
• Avoid going outdoors during times of peak pollen exposure, e.g. early morning
• Installation of portable high efficiency particulate air filters (HEPA filters*) may be helpful

*HEPA filters need to have a high air flow (250 cubic feet per minute or more). They may also be helpful in removing animal dander, but they will not be helpful in removing dust mites or dust mite fecal pellets

Avoidance of triggers

Avoidance of respiratory irritants such as environmental tobacco smoke, whether actively or passively inhaled, is universally recommended and is considered to be fundamentally important in the successful treatment of asthma and allergic rhinitis. Control of environmental airborne allergens such as house dust mites for prevention of asthma, allergic rhinitis, or atopic dermatitis/eczema symptoms is also widely recommended, although not supported by all studies. While it is recognized that children cannot completely avoid exposure to animal danders, reducing the dander 'load' in their home environments may help to prevent symptoms. Similarly, although it is impossible to avoid pollen exposure completely, such exposure can be minimized (Table 13.6).

In the treatment of atopic dermatitis/eczema, avoidance of specific food and inhalant allergens, although often overlooked, is helpful in many patients. For prevention of anaphylaxis (acute systemic allergic reaction) triggered by food, latex, or medication, total avoidance of an individual's specific trigger factor(s) is the fundamental treatment approach and may be life-saving. In all children for whom dietary restrictions are necessary, growth should be monitored, dietary supplements should be recommended where appropriate, and the involvement of a nutritionist may be required.

Allergen-specific immunotherapy

Allergen-specific immunotherapy aims to correct the underlying immune imbalance associated with allergic rhinitis, asthma, and systemic reactions to insect stings. Conventional allergen-specific immunotherapy has proven dose-related efficacy in these disorders; however most of the data supporting this therapeutic approach have been obtained in adolescents and adults rather than in young children or infants. Current allergen-specific immunotherapy is neither optimally convenient nor perfectly safe; therefore, considerable attention is being focused on alternative routes and dosing formulations such as sublingual immunotherapy and on the development of novel immunotherapy strategies, for example, those involving immunostimulatory DNA sequences which preferentially elicit Th1-dominated immunity and can inhibit developing or ongoing Th2 responses. Non-invasive forms of immunotherapy, particularly high dose sublingual immunotherapy, hold considerable promise for use in the pediatric population. Concurrent administration of allergen-specific immunotherapy along with non-specific immunomodulators such as anti-IgE antibody also appears to be promising.

Pharmacologic treatment

Prescription of medications is the most common approach to the treatment of allergic diseases. There have been major advances in this area of therapeutics during the past decade. Pharmacologic treatment should always be carried out in the context of an educational program providing information about avoidance of allergen triggers and general approaches to health and well-being. For mild intermittent asthma symptoms, occasional use of reliever medications (short-acting β_2-adrenergic agonists such as albuterol (salbutamol)) is appropriate. For mild, intermittent allergic rhinitis symptoms, occasional use of a second-generation H_1 antihistamine is appropriate. In all children with *persistent* asthma, allergic rhinitis, or atopic dermatitis/eczema, however, regular daily use of an antiinflammatory medication is the mainstay of management. The classes of medication that are used in asthma and/or allergic rhinoconjunctivitis will be discussed first, followed by those used in urticaria, atopic dermatitis/eczema, and anaphylaxis.

Glucocorticoids (inhaled for asthma, intranasal for allergic rhinitis)

Inhaled glucocorticoids for asthma and intranasal glucocorticoids for allergic rhinitis given daily on a regular basis, while not a cure, are the most effective antiinflammatory medications currently available for decreasing morbidity and reducing symptoms, exacerbations, and the need for reliever medications (Tables 13.7 and 13.8). Many of the delivery devices for inhaled and intranasal glucocorticoids have not been optimally tested in infants and very young children. These include pressurized metered-dose inhalers with holding chambers/spacer devices, dry powder inhalers, and nebulizers for asthma, and metered-dose inhalers, dry powder inhalers, and aqueous pump sprays for allergic rhinitis. Healthcare professionals should be able to demonstrate the optimal use of inhalation devices for inhaled or intranasal glucocorticoids to children and to their caregivers, and should provide regular coaching in the correct way to use these devices.

Inhalation of older glucocorticoids such as beclomethasone dipropionate or budesonide is potentially associated with a significant reduction in growth velocity during the first few months after starting treatment, but this effect is non-progressive and most affected children eventually attain expected adult height. Newer inhaled and intranasal glucocorticoids are promulgated as being safer than their predecessors, but prospective, controlled studies lasting several years are needed. In all children receiving daily glucocorticoid treatment, regardless of the formulation(s) being administered, use of the lowest doses that control symptoms, addition of glucocorticoid-sparing treatment, and regular monitoring of linear growth are important.

Leukotriene modifiers (for asthma, allergic rhinitis)

Montelukast, an oral leukotriene D_4 antagonist, has both anti-inflammatory and bronchodilator properties. It plays a role in the prevention of exercise-induced asthma, and in the treatment of mild–moderate persistent asthma, also as a glucocorticoid-sparing agent in moderate–severe persistent asthma (Fig. 13.4, Table 13.7). Administered orally once daily, it has a 24 hour duration of action, and tolerance does not develop to its effects when it is given regularly. It is safe for long-term use, even in very young children. In some countries montelukast is also indicated for allergic rhinitis and it therefore provides a user-friendly treatment option for the many children who have asthma and allergic rhinitis concurrently.

Long-acting β_2-adrenergic agonists (for asthma)

Salmeterol and formoterol are widely used as glucocorticoid-sparing agents in children with asthma; however, their glucocorticoid-sparing role is not as convincingly proven in young children as it is in adolescents and adults. The main pharmacologic differences between these agents is that salmeterol is a partial agonist of the β_2-receptor, with an onset of bronchodilation beginning 15–30 minutes after inhalation, and formoterol is a full β_2-adrenergic agonist, with onset of bronchodilation beginning 3 minutes after inhalation (Table 13.7).

Long-acting β_2-adrenergic agonists are useful in the prevention of exercise-induced asthma, although some tolerance to their effects may occur during regular daily use. Potential dose-related side-effects include tremor, palpitations, and headache. Although fixed-dose salmeterol/fluticasone combination formulations and fixed-dose formoterol/budesonide combinations are now commonly prescribed for patients of all ages, it is important to note that these formulations have not been optimally studied in children under the age of 12 years.

Short-acting β_2-adrenergic agonists (for asthma)

These rapidly-acting bronchodilators are used intermittently to prevent exercise-induced asthma and as 'rescue' treatment for breakthrough acute asthma symptoms (Table 13.7). They are not recommended for regular daily use. They should be given by inhalation rather than by the oral route.

Frequent use of and/or lack of effect of a short-acting β_2-adrenergic agonist indicates unsatisfactory asthma control and the need for regular use of a controller medication such as an inhaled glucocorticoid or a leukotriene modifier, or if the child is already taking a controller medication, the need for discussing adherence issues and for changing or combining controllers.

Oral glucocorticoids (for asthma)

The most effective medications available for the treatment of acute exacerbations of asthma in outpatients are oral glucocorticoids, which, when given daily for 5–7 days, decrease

Table 13.7 Medications for treatment of asthma*

Generic (Brand Name)
Inhaled glucocorticoids**
Beclomethasone dipropionate CFC (e.g. Beclovent, Vanceril) Beclomethasone dipropionate HFA (e.g. QVAR) Budesonide [e.g. Pulmicort (Turbuhaler; Respules)] Triamcinolone acetonide (Azmacort) Flunisolide (AeroBid, AeroBid-M) Fluticasone propionate (Flovent) Mometasone furoate (Azmacort) Ciclesonide (pending)
Leukotriene modifiers
Montelukast (Singulair) Zafirlukast (Accolate)
Inhaled long-acting β_2-adrenergic agonists alone and combined with a glucocorticoid**
Salmeterol (Serevent); salmeterol and fluticasone (Seretide, Advair) Formoterol (Foradil); formoterol and budesonide (Symbicort)
Inhaled short-acting β_2-adrenergic agonists**
Albuterol (salbutamol) (Ventolin HFA, Proventil HFA) Terbutaline (Bricanyl)
Oral glucocorticoids
Methylprednisolone (Medrol) Prednisolone (Prelone, Pediapred) Prednisone (Deltasone, Orasone, Liquid Pred) Omalizumab (Xolair)

*For correct doses and dose regimens, see product monographs. Leukotriene modifiers are also indicated for the treatment of allergic rhinitis in many countries

**Inhaled medications require assessment of a child's ability to use a particular inhalation device (metered-dose inhaler with spacer or metered-dose inhaler with spacer and face mask) or wet nebulization

Repeat assessment and coaching with regard to optimal use of inhaler device is fundamental for optimal prevention and control of asthma symptoms

symptoms and prevent relapse (Table 13.7). Long-term daily use of oral glucocorticoids should be avoided, as it is associated with glucose intolerance, weight gain, suppression of linear growth, increased blood pressure, mood disorder, cataract and immunosuppression. Alternate day use of oral glucocorticoids, which is occasionally necessary in children with extremely severe asthma, decreases the likelihood of these adverse effects.

Anti-IgE antibody (omalizumab, for asthma)

More than 90% of children with allergic disease have positive skin tests to common aeroallergens and increased specific IgE to these allergens, and many have raised levels of circulating IgE. Omalizumab is a recombinant humanized monoclonal anti-IgE antibody that binds to, and forms, complexes with circulating free IgE, preventing it from binding to high-affinity IgE receptors on mast cells and basophils. It does not induce the cross-linking of receptor-bound IgE on mast cells and basophils which leads to the release of mediators of inflammation, and therefore it does not trigger anaphylaxis.

Subcutaneous injections of omalizumab (weight-based dosing) every 2–4 weeks in children with moderate to severe allergic asthma reduce the requirement for inhaled and oral glucocorticoids (Fig. 13.5, Table 13.7) while preventing exacerbations and improving quality of life.

Omalizumab, injected before the pollen season, with or without allergen-specific immunotherapy, is also effective in preventing and relieving allergic rhinitis symptoms. In addition, it is currently being studied in patients who are highly allergic to peanut; a similar, although not identical, anti-IgE antibody was shown to improve the ability of such patients to tolerate ingestion of peanut.

H_1 antihistamines (for allergic rhinitis, urticaria)

First-generation, relatively sedating oral H_1 antihistamines such as diphenhydramine and chlorpheniramine have no role in the out-of-hospital management of children with allergic diseases. Most of the older H_1 antihistamines, although available in palatable liquid formulations, have not been optimally studied in infants or children.

Table 13.8 Medications for allergic rhinoconjunctivitis treatment*

Generic (Brand Name)
Intranasal glucocorticoids
Beclomethasone dipropionate (Beconase AQ)
Budesonide (Rhinocort)
Fluticasone propionate (Flonase)
Mometasone furoate (Nasonex)
Triamcinolone acetonide (Nasacort AQ)
H_1 antihistamines
Oral
Cetirizine (Zyrtec/Reactine)
Desloratadine (Clarinex)
Fexofenadine (Allegra)
Levocetirizine (Xyzal/Xusal)
Loratadine (Claritin)
Nasal Spray
Azelastine (Astelin; nasal spray)
Ophthalmic
Azelastine (Optimar)
Levocabastine (Livostin)
Ketotifen (Zaditor)
Olopatadine (Patanol)
Other
Leukotriene antagonist: montelukast (Singulair) (some countries)
Decongestant: pseudoephedrine (Sudafed)

*For correct doses and dose regimens, see product monographs. Leukotriene modifiers are also indicated for the treatment of allergic rhinitis in many countries

Second-generation, relatively non-sedating, H_1 antihistamines such as cetirizine, desloratadine, fexofenadine, levocetirizine, and loratadine have an improved safety profile compared to their predecessors. Long-term safety studies have been performed with cetirizine, levocetirizine, and loratadine. These medications are first-line treatment for the management of allergic rhinoconjunctivitis in children (Table 13.8). Topical intranasal or ophthalmic H_1 antihistamines have a more rapid onset of action than oral H_1 antihistamines, but require administration several times per day.

Second-generation oral H_1 antihistamines are also first-line medications for the treatment of acute and chronic urticaria in children (Table 13.9). They are not effective in asthma; however, when needed for the management of concurrent allergic disorders such as allergic rhinitis or urticaria, they do no harm in asthma and may contribute to symptom relief.

Other medications for asthma and allergic rhinitis

Sodium cromoglycate and nedocromil sodium, which have antiallergic effects when inhaled several times daily, now play only a minor role in the treatment of asthma and allergic rhinitis worldwide. They are significantly less effective than inhaled or intranasal glucocorticoids; however, they have an excellent safety record over long-term use.

Anticholinergic/antimuscarinic medications play no role in the outpatient management of persistent asthma in children, although ipratropium bromide remains in use for the treatment of acute asthma episodes in the Emergency Department and the hospital.

Theophylline and related methylxanthines are no longer widely used for children with asthma in most countries, having been supplanted by inhaled glucocorticoids which are more efficacious and safe.

In children with allergic rhinitis, orally-administered decongestants such as pseudoephedrine, and decongestants such as xylometazoline which are applied topically to the nasal mucosa, have not been optimally studied. These medications are more commonly used in North America than in other parts of the world.

Topical glucocorticoids (for atopic dermatitis/eczema)

Until recently, topical glucocorticoids were the mainstay of pharmacologic treatment in atopic dermatitis/eczema. They remain a cost-effective way of controlling inflammation in this disease. For maintenance treatment in any given child, the best topical glucocorticoid to recommend is the one with the lowest potency that is effective in reducing symptoms. Low-potency glucocorticoids such as hydrocortisone cream are safe for use on the face and intertrigenous areas. Medium-potency glucocorticoid creams such as mometasone furoate 0.1% and triamcinolone acetonide 0.1–0.5% may be needed to control acute inflammation (Table 13.10). Long-term use of medium- and high-potency glucocorticoids can lead to the development of striae and skin atrophy, or if used on the eyelids, to glaucoma and cataract. The potential for suppression of the hypothalamic pituitary adrenal axis or suppression of growth is greatest when medium- or high-potency glucocorticoids are used under occlusive dressings in infants and young children with widespread skin involvement who require long-term treatment.

Topical calcineuron inhibitors (for atopic dermatitis/eczema)

Pimecrolimus and tacrolimus, microbial-derived macrolactams which inhibit proinflammatory cytokines, are important new topical medications for the treatment of atopic dermatitis/ eczema. Unlike most other medications introduced for the treatment of allergic diseases, they are being extensively studied in infants and young children relatively early in drug development. They lead to a reduction in skin inflammation and itching within days of starting treatment and reduce or eliminate the need for topical glucocorticoid applications in most patients with mild or moderate atopic dermatitis/eczema (Fig. 13.6, Table 13.10). Tolerance to their beneficial effects does not develop over long-term treatment.

The most commonly reported adverse effect of pimecrolimus and tacrolimus is a feeling of burning or warmth at the site of application. Unlike topical glucocorticoids, these medications do not cause skin atrophy and are suitable for use on the face and the genital area. They do not appear to increase the likelihood of bacterial or viral skin infections. Their long-term safety is unknown.

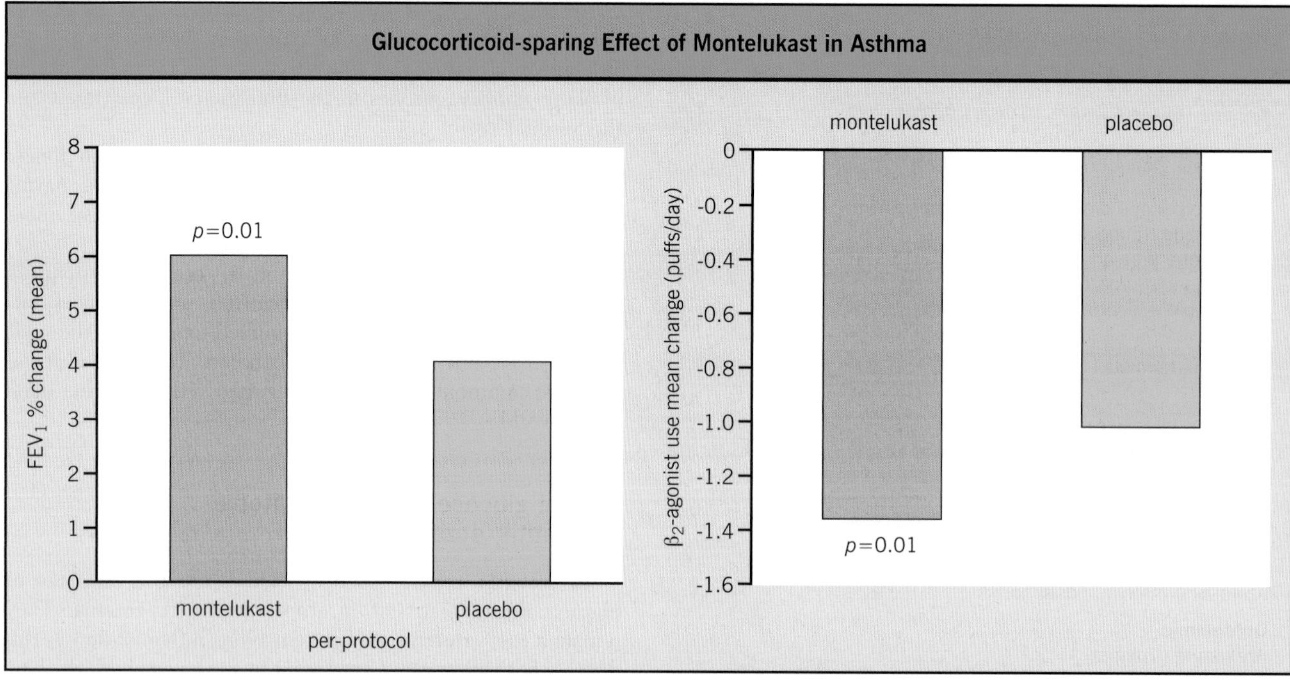

Fig. 13.4 Glucocorticoid-sparing effect of montelukast in asthma: mean percentage change in FEV_1 (forced expiratory volume in 1 second) in children treated with montelukast or placebo in addition to 200 Fg of budesonide twice daily. During montelukast add-on treatment, children had a greater mean increase in FEV_1 than during placebo treatment ($p = 0.01$, per protocol group), despite a greater mean decrease in β_2-adrenergic agonist use during montelukast treatment compared to placebo treatment ($p = 0.01$). In addition, asthma exacerbation days decreased by 23% ($p < 0.001$) (not shown). [From Simons FE, Villa JR, Lee BW, et al. Montelukast added to budesonide in children with persistent asthma: a randomized, double-blind, crossover study. J Pediatr 2001; 138(5):694–698, with permission.]

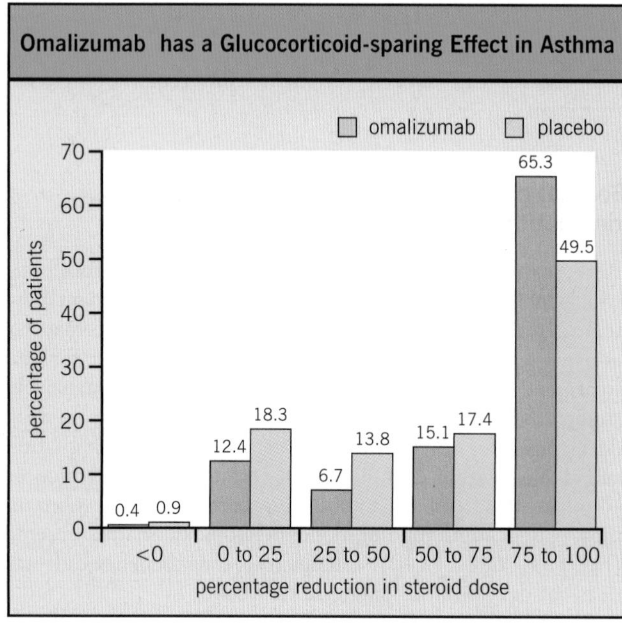

Fig. 13.5 Omalizumab has a glucocorticoid-sparing effect in asthma: percentage of children with reduction in dose of inhaled glucocorticoid at the end of treatment, shown as percentage reduction in glucocorticoid dose. The difference between the omalizumab group and the placebo group is statistically significant ($p = 0.002$). [From Milgrom H, Berger W, Nayak A, et al. Treatment of childhood asthma with anti-immunoglobulin E antibody (omalizumab). Pediatrics 2001; 108(2):E36, with permission.]

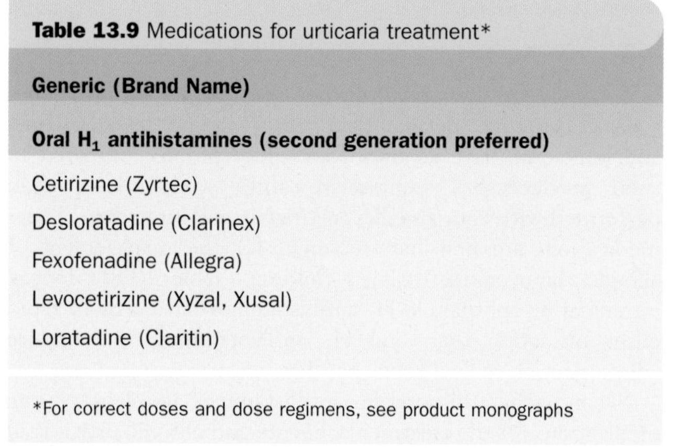

Table 13.9 Medications for urticaria treatment*

Generic (Brand Name)
Oral H_1 antihistamines (second generation preferred)
Cetirizine (Zyrtec)
Desloratadine (Clarinex)
Fexofenadine (Allegra)
Levocetirizine (Xyzal, Xusal)
Loratadine (Claritin)

*For correct doses and dose regimens, see product monographs

Epinephrine

When anaphylaxis (severe acute systemic allergic reaction) occurs in a community setting, epinephrine is the first-aid treatment of choice and should be injected intramuscularly into the lateral thigh (midpoint of the vastus lateralis muscle) from an auto-injector such as EpiPen Jr (0.15 mg) or EpiPen (0.3 mg) (Table 13.11). Instruction and repeated coaching with regard to when and how to use an epinephrine auto-injector is an important component of caring for children at risk for anaphylaxis. A wider range of epinephrine fixed doses in auto-injectors is needed. After epinephrine injection, for an acute allergic reaction, children should be taken to the nearest hospital Emergency Department for monitoring and additional treatment, if indicated.

Table 13.10 Medications for atopic dermatitis/eczema treatment*

Generic (Brand Name)
Topical glucocorticoids
Lowest potency – hydrocortisone 0.5%, 1%, 2.5% (cream, ointment and lotion)
Low potency – triamcinolone acetonide 0.025% (cream, lotion)
Medium potency – mometasone furoate (Elocom) (0.1% cream), triamcinolone acetonide cream 0.1% or 0.5%
High potency – mometasone 0.1% (Elocom ointment), triamcinolone acetonide
(Aristocort) 0.5% (ointment)
Topical calcineuron inhibitors
Pimecrolimus (Elidel cream) 1% cream
Tacrolimus (Protopic) 0.03% cream, 0.1% ointment

* For correct doses and dose regimens, see product monographs

PRIMARY AND SECONDARY PREVENTION OF ALLERGIC DISEASES IN CHILDREN – IS IT POSSIBLE?

Primary prevention

Primary prevention of asthma and other allergic diseases is defined as prevention of sensitization to aeroallergens and to foods which, along with exposure to environmental tobacco smoke early in life, constitute important risk factors for these diseases. Avoidance of food allergens and other individual risk factors has met with mixed success in the prevention of sensitization to allergens and prevention of asthma and other allergic diseases. For example, although a recent meta-analysis demonstrated that children who were breastfed for at least 3 months had a 20% decrease in risk for asthma, other epidemiologic data suggest that breastfeeding might actually lead to a higher prevalence of asthma in children at age 6 years.

Table 13.11 Medication for treatment of anaphylaxis

Generic (Brand Name)
Epinephrine (EpiPen Jr 0.15 mg, EpiPen 0.3 mg) (Fastjekt 0.3 mg)
(AnaPen 0.3 mg, AnaHelp)

Instruction and repeated coaching with regard to when and how to use an epinephrine auto-injector is extremely important

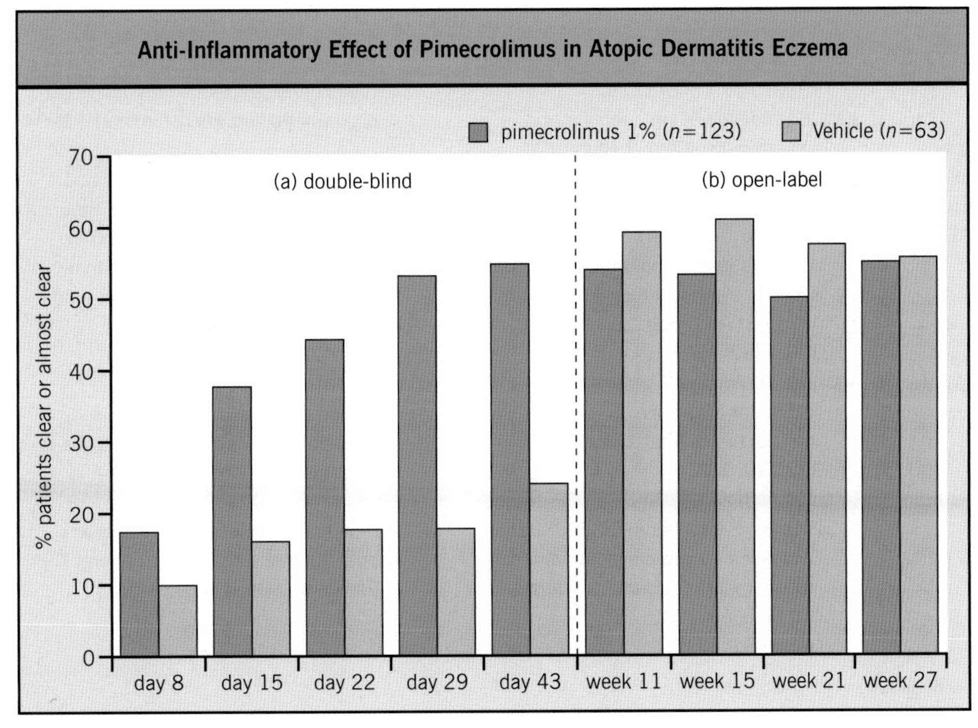

Fig. 13.6 Anti-inflammatory effect of pimecrolimus in atopic dermatitis/eczema. After treatment with pimecrolimus cream 1%, more infants had clear or almost clear skin than after treatment with vehicle ($p < 0.001$). After completion of the double-blind phase [day 43; (a)], infants in the 'vehicle' group were switched to pimecrolimus treatment in the open-label phase (b). [From Ho VC, Gupta A, Kaufmann R, et al. Safety and efficacy of non-steroid pimecrolimus cream 1% in the treatment of atopic dermatitis in infants. J Pediatr 2003; 142(2):155–162, with permission.]

In several cohorts of infants, extensive and multifaceted allergen avoidance interventions have been reported to lead to reduced allergen sensitization and/or reduced wheezing in early life, which may or may not be maintained.

Secondary prevention

Secondary prevention is defined as intervention(s) for infants and children who have one allergic disease, for example, atopic dermatitis/eczema (the harbinger of the 'allergic march'), but have not developed symptoms of asthma or other allergic diseases. Such children also often have a family history of allergy, positive allergy skin tests, elevated allergen-specific IgE and elevated total IgE levels, and/or blood eosinophilia.

Secondary prevention of asthma in high-risk young children has been attempted by using H_1 antihistamines such as cetirizine, with modest success. The potential role of other pharmacologic and immunologic interventions such as levocetirizine, montelukast, topical pimecrolimus, and of sublingual allergen-specific immunotherapy, is also of considerable interest in the secondary prevention of asthma.

SUMMARY

Allergic diseases are increasing in prevalence worldwide. To date, there has been modest progress in improving diagnostic capabilities for these diseases. A detailed history, including a description of the environments in which the child spends most of his/her time, is combined with physical examination and documentation of evidence of sensitization to relevant common allergens, either by epicutaneous testing or by measurement of allergen-specific IgE.

Challenge tests, although time-consuming, are useful not only in research but also in certain clinical situations; for example, specialist-supervised incremental, allergen-specific challenges in carefully selected children with food allergies may be helpful in identifying those who are outgrowing their food allergies, for example, to milk or egg.

During the past decade, major advances in the pharmacologic treatment of allergic diseases in children include: increasingly widespread acceptance of inhaled glucocorticoid treatment for asthma and intranasal glucocorticoid treatment for allergic rhinitis, and the introduction of montelukast, a safe leukotriene antagonist, and of second-generation, relatively non-sedating H_1 antihistamines which are safe for long-term use in the pediatric population. Atopic dermatitis/eczema treatment has been revolutionized by the availability of calcineuron inhibitors. Epinephrine remains the cornerstone of treatment of anaphylaxis; however, new pediatric formulations for outpatient use are urgently needed. Cost-effectiveness of some new immunomodulators, for example, anti-IgE antibody (omalizumab), remains to be proven.

Time spent by healthcare professionals in listening to the concerns of children and families and providing them with education and coaching will be rewarded by improved long-term management, fewer crises, and better adherence to recommended treatment regimens. Avoidance of relevant airborne allergens is recommended for children with asthma, allergic rhinitis and/or atopic dermatitis/eczema. Strict allergen avoidance remains fundamental to the successful treatment of food, latex, or medication-induced severe acute systemic allergic reactions (anaphylaxis). Permanent modification of disease severity by the use of allergen-specific immunotherapy remains an attractive goal, but appropriately controlled, randomized, double-blind studies are needed in very young children. New allergen-specific immunotherapy formulations with an improved benefit/risk ratio and involving fewer injections, and new routes of administration, for example, sublingual immunotherapy, hold promise for the future.

FURTHER READING

Abramowicz M, Zuccotti G, Rizack MA, et al. Drugs for allergic disorders. Treat Guidelines Med Letter 2003; 1:93–100.

Castro-Rodriguez JA, Holberg CJ, Wright AL, et al. A clinical index to define risk of asthma in young children with recurrent wheezing. Am J Respir Crit Care Med 2000; 162:1403–1406.

Gdalevich M, Mimouni D, David M, et al. Breast-feeding and the onset of atopic dermatitis in childhood: a systematic review and meta-analysis of prospective studies. J Am Acad Dermatol 2001; 45:520–527.

Illi S, von Mutius E, Lau S, et al. The natural course of atopic dermatitis from birth to age 7 years and the association with asthma. J Allergy Clin Immunol 2004; 113:925–931.

Kulig M, Bergmann R, Klettke U, et al. Natural course of sensitization to food and inhalant allergens during the first 6 years of life. J Allergy Clin Immunol 1999; 103:1173–1179.

Lack G. Pediatric allergic rhinitis and comorbid disorders. J Allergy Clin Immunol 2001; 108 (suppl 1):S9–S15.

Lau S, Illi S, Sommerfeld C, et al. Early exposure to house-dust mite and cat allergens and development of childhood asthma: a cohort study. Multicentre Allergy Study Group. Lancet 2000; 356:1392–1397.

Martinez FD, Wright AL, Taussig LM, et al. Asthma and wheezing in the first six years of life. N Engl J Med 1995; 332:133–138.

National Asthma Education and Prevention Program Expert Panel (NAEPP) Report. Guidelines for the diagnosis and management of asthma. J Allergy Clin Immunol 2002; 110 (suppl):S1–S219.

Niggemann B, Wahn U, Sampson HA. Proposals for standardization of oral food challenge tests in infants and children. Pediatr Allergy Immunol 1994; 5:11–13.

The International Study of Asthma and Allergies in Childhood (ISAAC) Steering Committee. Worldwide variation in prevalence of symptoms of asthma, allergic rhinoconjunctivitis, and atopic eczema: ISAAC. Lancet 1998; 351:1225–1232.

Warner JO, on behalf of the ETAC study group. A double-blind, randomized, placebo-controlled trial of cetirizine in preventing the onset of asthma in children with atopic dermatitis: 18 months' treatment and 18 months' post-treatment follow-up. J Allergy Clin Immunol 2001; 108:929–937.

SECTION TWO

BASIC MECHANISMS

Chapter 14

Definition:

Allergic diseases cluster in families indicating an important role for susceptibility genes. Multiple genes interact with environmental factors to generate the different allergic phenotypes.

The Genetic Basis of Allergic Disease

Stephen T Holgate

INTRODUCTION

Medical genetics comprises the study of human variability and heredity and its application to human disease. Heredity represents the transmission of information required for the formation and regulation of proteins. The questions that surround human genetics are concerned with the transmission of heritable traits. The study of human variation depends upon analysis of the outcomes of matings of individuals and the scientific study of definable differences.

Most cells contain 46 chromosomes (the diploid number), which can be arranged into 22 pairs of autosomes and a pair of sex chromosomes – XX in the female and XY in the male (Fig. 14.1). Each chromosome has a narrow waist, called the centromere, which has a constant position within a given chromosome. The short arm is labeled 'p' (for petit, French for 'small') and the long arm 'q', the tip of each arm being called the telomere.

During mitosis each chromosome replicates to form a pair of sister chromatids, which are held together at the centromere (Fig. 14.2). Reductive cell division, meiosis, results in cells with a half-set of 23 chromosomes (the haploid number). Meiosis only occurs in gonadal cells and consists of two sequential divisions in which the DNA replicates only once, before the first division (Fig. 14.3).

The chromosomes which have exchanged genetic material are called recombinants. On average there are about 52 crossovers per human male meiosis, and, with the exception of the short arms of chromosomes 13–15, 18, 21, and 22, there is at least one chiasma per chromosome arm. Therefore, few chromosomes are inherited intact from a parent and so cosegregation or linkage of genes on a chromosome will only occur if they are physically close.

INHERITANCE AND LINKAGE

Mendelian inheritance

Gregor Mendel (1822–1884) clearly defined pairs of contrasting characters and concluded that their inheritance (traits) must be particulate, with pairs of hereditary elements or genes and their variants (alleles) segregating at meiosis, one gene of a pair being assigned to one gamete and one to another gamete – this is Mendel's first law. Mendel's second law states that members of different gene pairs assort gametes independently of one another.

Modes of single gene inheritance

In autosomal dominant disorders the condition is produced by a mutation of one member of an autosomal gene pair. Thus, the affected individual has one normal gene

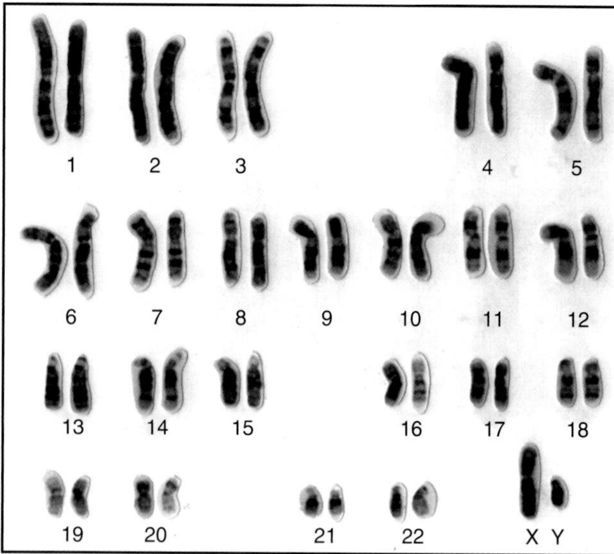

Fig. 14.1 Normal male human chromosomes (46,XY) stained by Giemsa banding.

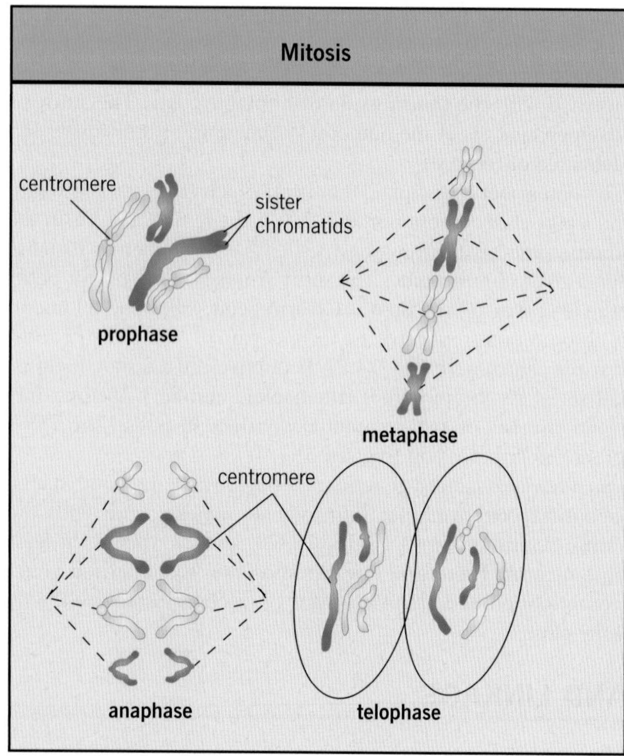

Fig. 14.2 Diagrammatic representation of mitosis (two chromosome pairs are shown). Note the distinctive centromere.

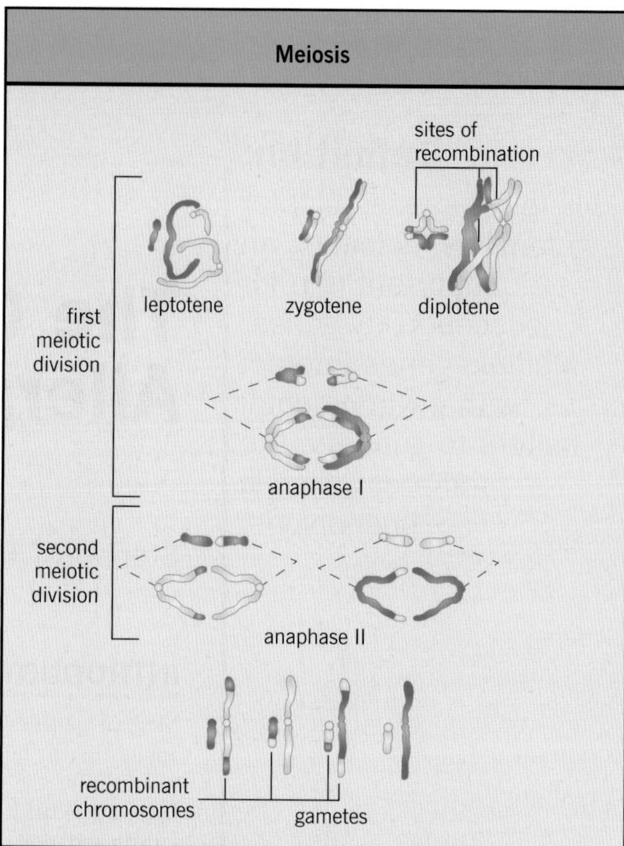

Fig. 14.3 Diagrammatic representation of meiosis (two chromosome pairs are shown).

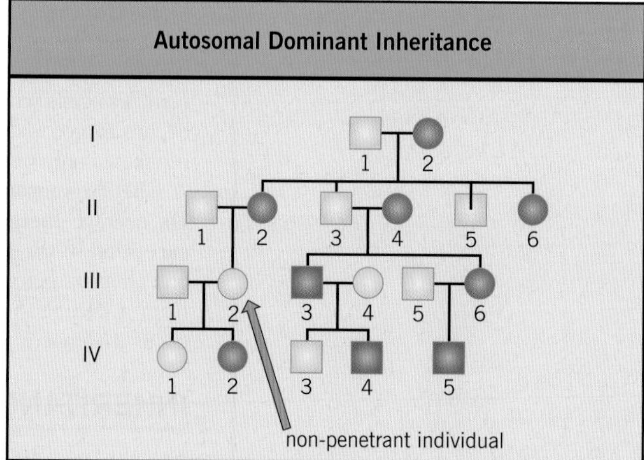

Fig. 14.4 Autosomal dominant inheritance. Vertical type of pedigree with both males and females affected.

and one mutant gene and is heterozygous at this locus (Fig. 14.4). Autosomal dominant traits show a vertical type of pedigree pattern with equal numbers of males and females affected. Many dominant traits exhibit variable expression, i.e. affected individuals in the same family vary in their clinical severity. The mechanisms for this are not clearly understood but seem to involve gene–gene interactions (epistasis).

In contrast to dominant disorders in which heterozygotes manifest the condition, in autosomal recessive disorders the affected individual has mutations in both members of a gene pair, i.e. the individual is homozygous at this locus (Fig. 14.5). The parents are commonly unaffected yet each has one defective gene which will only express itself if the two defective genes are combined in the offspring.

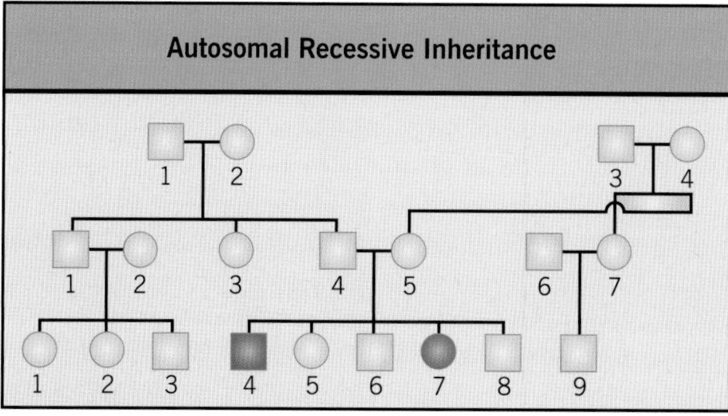

Fig. 14.5 Autosomal recessive inheritance. In this example, the parents are carriers of one defective gene each. Expression is only seen in offspring 4 and 7, who inherit both genes.

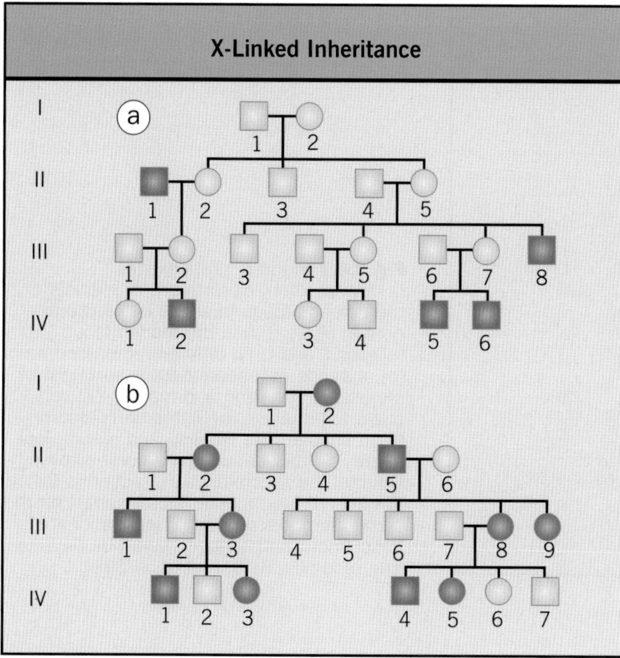

Fig. 14.6 (a) Pedigree showing X-linked recessive inheritance; (b) pedigree showing X-linked dominant inheritance.

Further complications are introduced in X-linked recessive and X-linked dominant disorders, which, on account of the uneven distribution of the sex chromosomes, result in a characteristic pattern of inheritance (Fig. 14.6).

Recombination and linkage

When two genes are close together, they are said to be linked. Therefore, alleles at such loci have a tendency to pass together into each gamete. Thus, any disturbance of independent assortment defined by Mendel's second law provides an important clue that two genes are linked. If the chromosomal location of one of the genes is known, then the other can be mapped to the same region.

If the disease and marker loci are on separate chromosomes, independent assortment will occur and the disease and markers should be found as often together as apart in the offspring (Fig. 14.7). If the disease and marker loci lie close together on the same chromosome, independent assortment will not occur and the disease and marker will occur together in each child unless they are separated by a crossover at meiosis. As the distance between the disease locus and a marker locus increases so the chance of recombination in the interval between them increases and the proportion of recombinant increases. If the disease and marker loci are separated by a considerable distance on the same chromosome, a crossover between the loci is highly likely and the disease and marker traits will occur separately in each recombinant but together in non-recombinants. Thus, for a distant marker trait, the number of recombinants will approximate to the number of non-recombinants and the number of recombinants divided by the total number of offspring (the recombination fraction, or q) will be 0.5, or 50%, which obeys the rule of independent assortment. As this distance decreases, q decreases from 50 to 0% when tight linkage occurs.

The relationship between q and the actual physical distance between loci depends upon several factors. A q of 0.1 (10%) corresponds to a map distance of 10 centimorgans (cM) but with increasing distance apart the apparent recombination fraction falls due to double crossovers. Secondly, crossovers for autosomes occur more frequently in females than in males and also vary in different parts of the chromosome. The total length of the genome is 3000 cM, which is equivalent to 3×10^9 base pairs. Thus, 1 cM is equivalent to one megabase of DNA.

Polygenic inheritance

Asthma and atopy are classified as multifactorial disorders in which both environmental and genetic factors are important (Fig. 14.8). Many genetic loci participate (Fig. 14.9). Thus, the risk of a polygenic disease in first degree relatives is generally 5–15%. Within a family the risk will be influenced by the severity of the disorder in the proband, the number of affected family members, and the contribution made by environmental factors.

GENETIC MODELING

Knowledge of the recurrence risk of a disease in relatives and curve fitting of disease measures between affected and non-affected families (commingling analysis) may point towards a mode of inheritance. Analysis of the segregation of a disease such as asthma within families (segregation analysis) using computer programs helps establish a possible mode of inheritance of a trait or partial phenotype.

GENETIC VARIATION AND SUSCEPTIBILITY

Variation in DNA sequences occurs once in approximately every 200–500 base pairs. This means that in every human population, most genes can be expected to show variation. Sequence variation (mutations) occurring in over 1% of the population are called polymorphisms and those that occur in less than 1% are rare alleles. Thus, the risk of developing a disease such as asthma depends upon a complex interaction among common alleles, each exerting a small effect, which together combine to give the end phenotype. The influence of rare alleles will be superimposed on the population distribution.

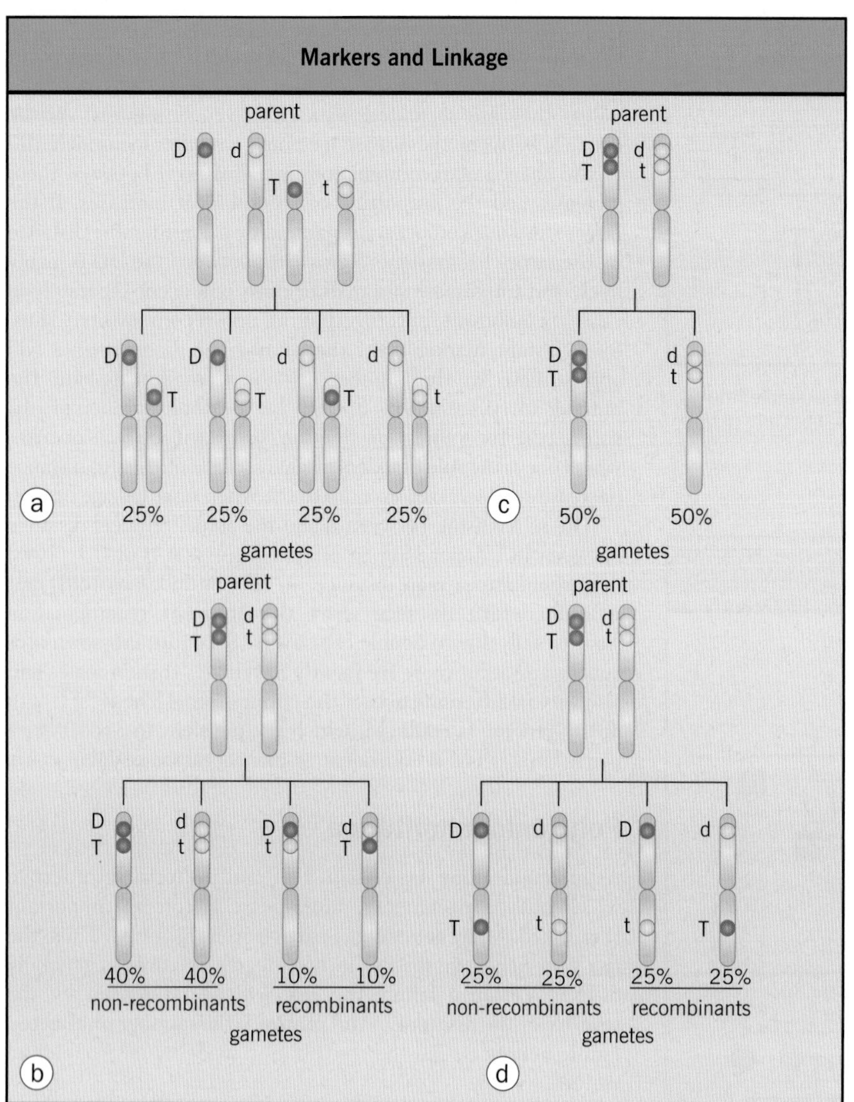

Fig. 14.7 Markers and linkage. (a) Independent assortment at meiosis of the disease locus (disease allele D and normal allele d) and the marker locus (alleles T and t) on different chromosomes; (b) absence of independent assortment at meiosis for disease and marker loci very close together on the same chromosome (tight linkage); (c) disease and marker loci nearby on the same chromosome showing linkage (the recombination fraction is 20%); (d) disease and marker loci far apart on the same chromosome mimic independent assortment and linkage cannot be detected (the recombination fraction is 50%).

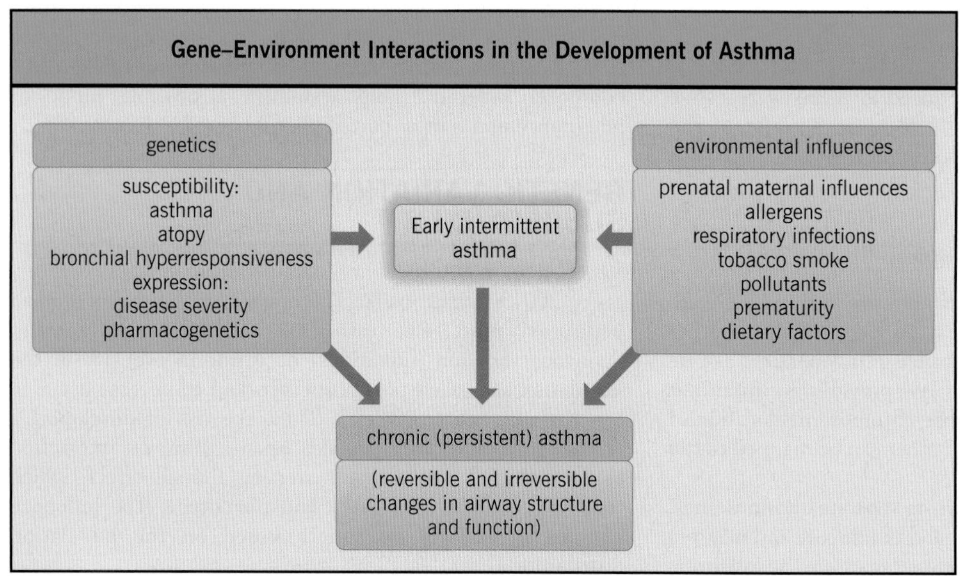

Fig. 14.8 Gene–environment interactions in the development of asthma.

Polymorphisms

Polymorphisms form the basis of human diversity, including our responses to environmental stimuli. Genetic epidemiology has provided statistical methods for measuring the effects of gene polymorphisms on a clinical phenotype. The term 'candidate' gene is used when a particular gene has a strong possibility of influencing a disease, based on an understanding of pathophysiology. In the case of allergic disorders, interleukin 4 (IL-4) represents such a candidate because it controls the switching of B cells to IgE synthesis and the maintenance of the helper T cell type 2 (Th2)–T cell phenotype – both essential features of allergic disorders. An alteration in the rate of IL-4 secretion (produced by an appropriate polymorphism of a transcription binding site in the IL-4 gene promoter) would provide the basis for a good candidate gene (Fig. 14.10 and Table 14.1). As shown in the example of the cytosine to thymidine exchange, the thymidine-containing polymorphism is associated with the following:

- a unique nuclear factor for activated T cells (NF-AT)-binding site separate from P0–P4 sites;
- higher NF-AT-binding affinity;
- increased levels of IgE in vivo.

This example explains the molecular basis of one mechanism of the IL-4-associated increase in IgE production.

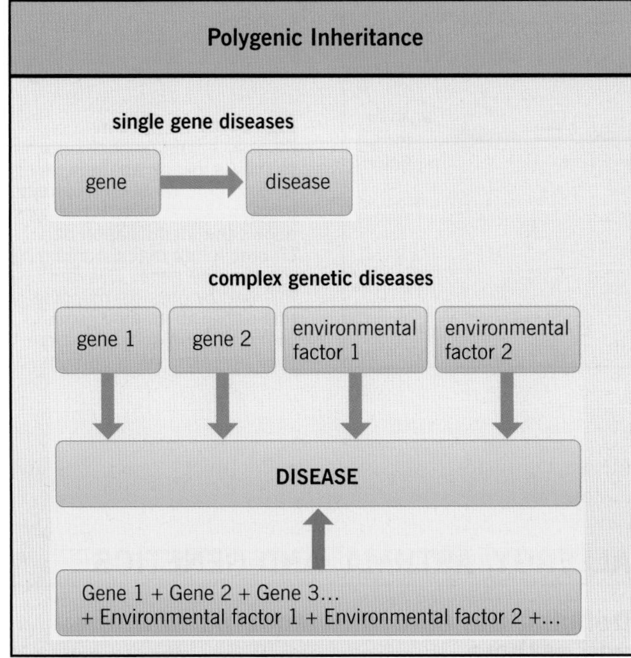

Fig. 14.9 In complex genetic disorders there are multiple interactions between individual genes and between genes and the environment. This is polygenic inheritance.

Table 14.1 The association of IgE production with C→T exchange

Association of IgE Production with C → T Exchange		
Subjects	**Affected**	**IgE (IU/dL)**
15	+ (~590, T)	146
29	– (~ 590, C)	39
44 Subjects, $p = 0.0028$		

IU, international unit

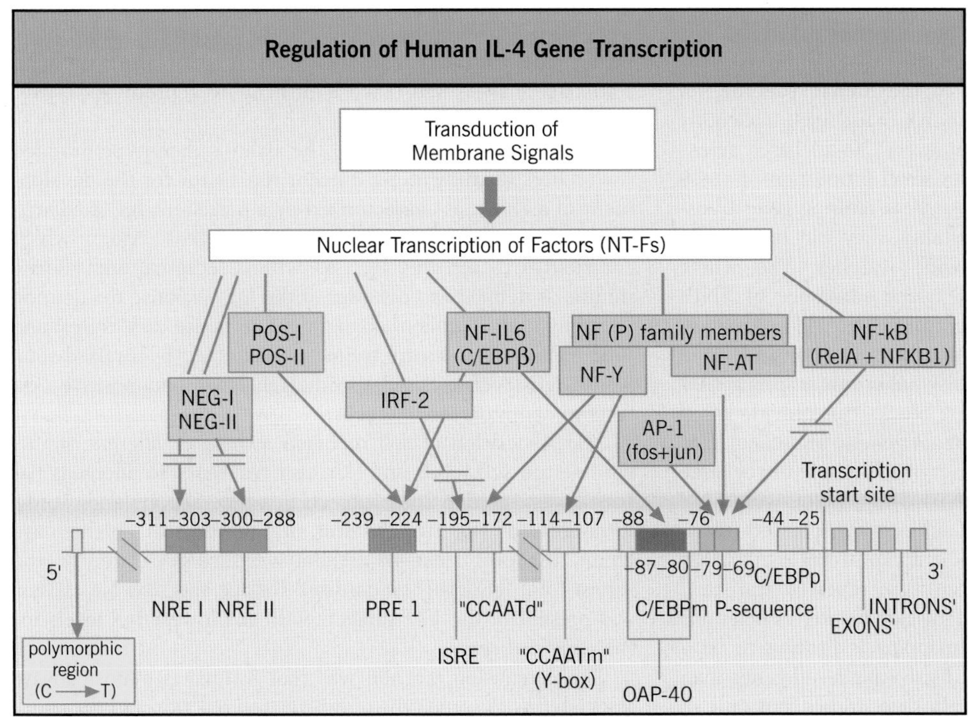

Fig. 14.10 The transcription factor binding site of the interleukin-4 (IL-4) gene is a good allergic disease candidate because of the pivotal role of IL-4 in maintaining the helper T cell type 2 (Th2) cytokine repertoire and B-cell switching to IgE. The promoter region is complex but at -589 a C→T exchange is associated with increased IgE production (see Table 14.1).

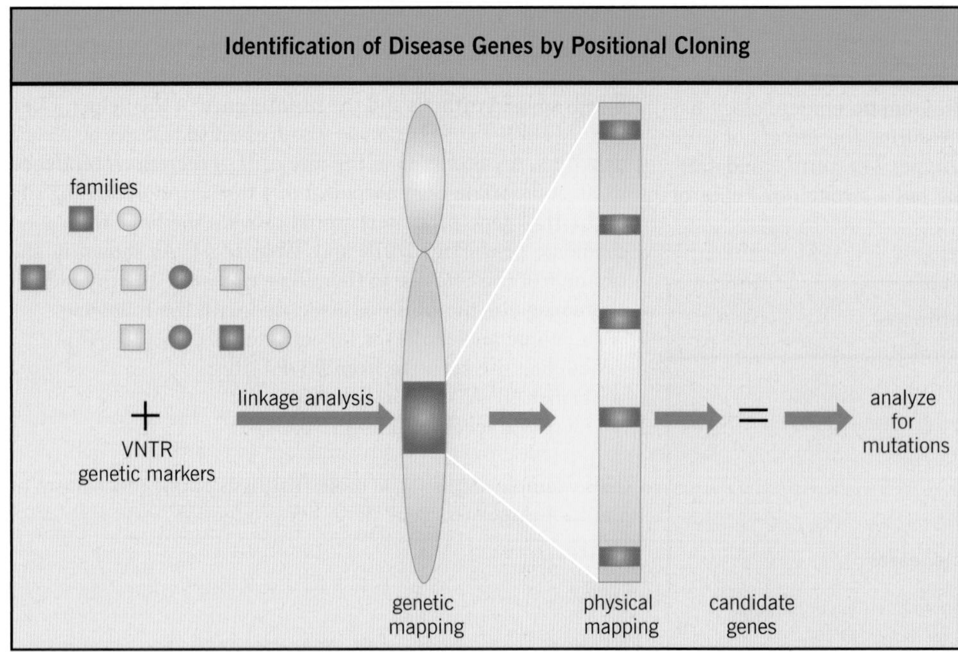

Fig. 14.11 Identification of disease genes by positional cloning. Linkage analysis using polymorphic variable nucleotide tandem repeat (VNTR) markers allows the identification of a chromosomal region containing the disease gene. This is followed by physical mapping of this region to identify genes within it; candidate genes are then screened for mutations.

New loci that contribute to a disease such as asthma can be identified by positional cloning (Fig. 14.11). If a disorder cannot be accounted for by alterations in known candidate genes, then it may be necessary to screen the entire human genome for linkage. This approach has been made easier by the identification of variable nucleotide tandem repeats (VNTR) and simple di-, tri-, and tetra-nucleotide repeats, which themselves are functionally inactive. With such highly polymorphic markers spaced at regular intervals across each chromosome (10–20 cM), it has been possible to deduce linkage to a locus that contains a gene that contributes to the clinical phenotype. This approach can be strengthened by information from classic genetic studies in which chromosome deletions or translocations may provide additional clues that help identify new disease-related loci.

Because the number of microsatellites that can be used for linkage studies leaves large gaps in the human genome, an alternative and highly effective approach is to use single nucleotide polymorphisms (SNPs) that occur every 30–50 bases across each stretch of DNA. While only a small proportion of these SNPs have identifiable functions such as altering gene transcription, induction, splicing or stability, they can be used in association studies for genome-wide searches. The whole procedure can be streamlined by taking advantage of SNPs present only in known genes, promoters, and adjacent silent 'dark' areas of the genome. As genes are often transmitted in blocks to the offspring, linkage disequilibrium mapping that takes advantage of these haplotype blocks can provide rapid and efficient access to small regions of genetic sequences that associate with specific disease phenotypes. Because of the large number of statistical tests that are used in genome-wide SNP associate studies, large numbers of subjects are required (often into the thousands) to ensure efficient capture of signals that are not purely the result of chance from repeated statistical testing. Thus, the detection of SNP disease marker associations and linkage disequilibrium (LD) mapping is proving to be a much more powerful approach in discovering novel genes than the more traditional microsatellite linkage studies, not only in identifying major novel asthma susceptibility genes, but also discovering those with small effects.

ALLERGY, ASTHMA, AND GENETICS

Defining the clinical phenotype of atopy and asthma

Asthma is a clinical diagnosis with no foolproof diagnostic test, so surrogate markers for the disease are used including atopy, bronchial hyperresponsiveness (BHR), and clinical history. Inevitably this leads to some disagreements between various research groups and an inability to compare results achieved using different definitions. Genetic heterogeneity, incomplete penetrance, and environmental factors may also confound statistical analysis and make it difficult to reproduce positive findings.

Problems with definition of the asthma phenotype have led researchers to study atopy, a major risk factor for the development of asthma, as characterized by a persistent IgE-mediated response to common environmental allergens. Atopy, which contributes to diseases such as asthma, eczema, and allergic rhinitis, is defined as a disorder of the IgE response to common allergens such as pollen, animal dander, house dust mites, and fungi. These diseases are frequently detected by a raised total serum IgE level, a raised specific IgE level, and positive skin tests to common aeroallergens.

The association of self-reported asthma or allergic rhinitis with serum IgE levels and skin test reactivity to allergens has been investigated in 2657 subjects in a general population study. Regardless of the atopic status of the subjects or their age group, the prevalence of asthma was closely related to the serum total IgE level standardized for age and sex. No asthma was present in the 177 subjects with the lowest IgE levels for their age and sex.

The conclusion reached was that asthma is almost always associated with some type of IgE-related reaction and therefore

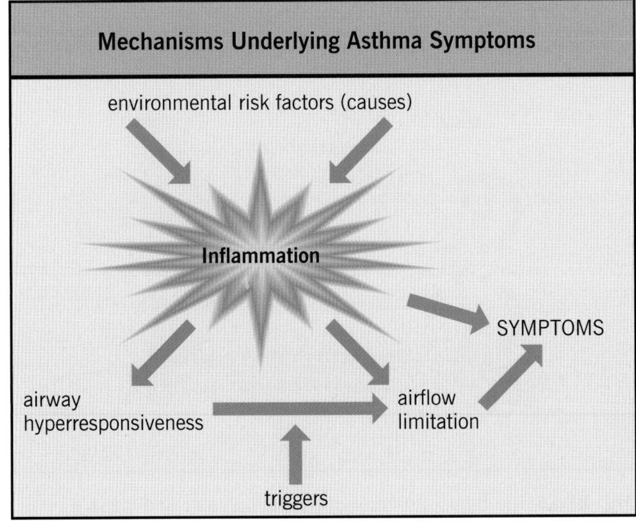

Fig. 14.12 The relationship between bronchial hyperresponsiveness and the expression of asthma symptoms.

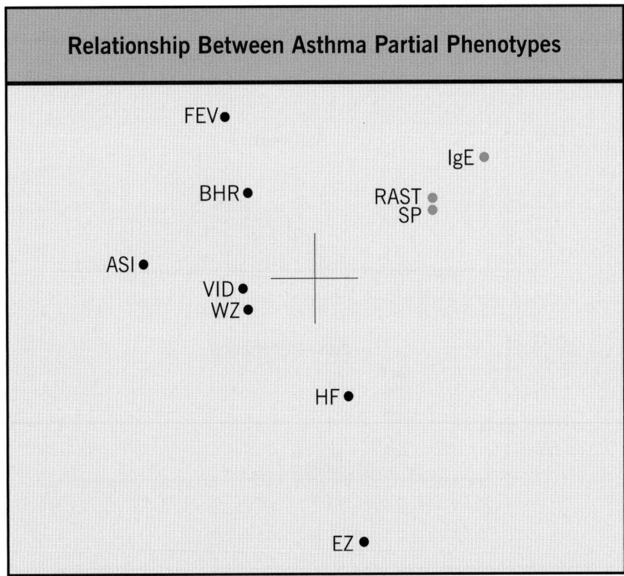

Fig. 14.13 Principal component regression analysis used to examine the relationship between various asthma partial phenotypes. The asthma index (ASI) represents the principal component derived from bronchial hyperresponsiveness (BHR) and the wheeze responses on a standardized questionnaire. The relationship between the ASI and the various partial phenotypes is displayed as an eigenvector plot. The close proximity of RAST, IgE and SP indicate their possible association. FEV(forced expiratory volume) and FEV1 (FEV in 1 second), % predicted; VID and WZ, responses to the video and written questionnaire on wheezing in the last year; IgE, total serum IgE level; SP, summated positive skin tests to common aeroallergens; RAST, summated radioallergosorbent test for specific IgE; HF, hayfever; EZ, eczema.

has an allergic basis. Further evidence for the relationship between IgE levels and asthma has been provided by Sears, who studied the relationship between serum total IgE levels and airway responsiveness to methacholine challenge in the presence or absence of asthma in a birth cohort of New Zealand children. The prevalence of diagnosed asthma was significantly related to the serum IgE level and airway hyperresponsiveness was still related to an allergic diathesis, as reflected by the serum total IgE level, even in children who had been asymptomatic throughout their lives and had no history of atopic disease.

Bronchial hyperresponsiveness, atopy, and asthma

Further work on the New Zealand cohort of children has looked at the relationship between airway hyperresponsiveness, asthma, and atopy. Airway hyperresponsiveness (methacholine PC_{20} FEV_1 < 8 mg/mL) (provocative concentration of methacholine causing a 20% fall in forced air expiratory volume in 1 second) was found to be strongly correlated with reported asthma and wheezing and with atopy as defined by a positive skin prick test, particularly to house dust mite and cat. Furthermore, all the children with diagnosed asthma and airway hyperresponsiveness were atopic. It was concluded that atopy was a major determinant of airway hyperresponsiveness in children, not only in those with a reported history of asthma and wheezing but also in those without any history suggestive of asthma and rhinitis.

There is clearly a link between atopy, airway hyperresponsiveness, and asthma, although the precise relationship remains a source of continued debate (Fig. 14.12). There is a tendency to dichotomize subjects as hyperresponsive or non-responsive on the basis of whether or not their FEV_1 falls by 20% at a given dose of inhaled histamine or methacholine; different cut-off doses have been used by different workers. On the basis of this, one would hope to be able to discriminate clearly between asthmatics and non-asthmatics. However, some atopic subjects with no evidence of symptomatic asthma will also demonstrate BHR according to the same criteria, as will a small percentage of normal subjects.

Enhanced bronchial responsiveness has a strong association with clinically defined asthma and the association appears to be stronger in those with more immediate and severe symptoms and with greater treatment requirements, although the overlap between groups is large. Moreover, there is documentation from longitudinal studies that BHR may not be present in some people at a time when they have unmistakable asthma symptoms and airway obstruction and, conversely, that greatly enhanced bronchial responsiveness may be present in the absence of symptoms, or may develop after symptoms have become manifest as occurs in seasonal asthma. Thus, although BHR and asthma are related, the two are not synonymous.

A further confounding factor is the discovery that measures of indirect BHR which rely on the activation of mediator secreting cells to cause bronchoconstriction e.g. exercise, hypertonic saline, and adenosine 5′-monophosphate appear to generate signals that relate more closely to the disease phenotype than either histamine or methacholine challenges. These have yet to be used as partial phenotypes in genetic studies.

A number of variables have been shown to affect both serum IgE levels and BHR. For example, smoking has been shown to lead to an increase in total serum IgE levels. As an alternative to studying asthma or surrogate markers (IgE or BHR) as the principal phenotype, the separate variables derived from the clinical and laboratory data can be combined to generate quantitative asthma and atopy scores. An eigenvector plot (Fig. 14.13) illustrates the separation of individual traits into

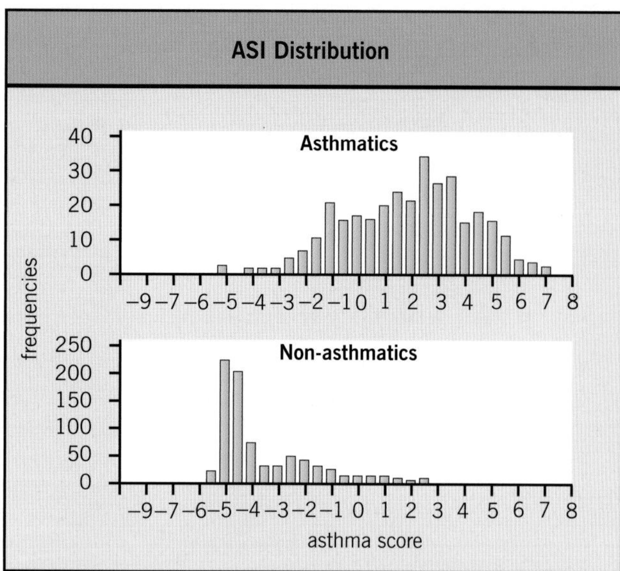

Fig. 14.14 Distribution of the asthma index (ASI) in a population of families with one or two affected children with asthma (top), compared to a normal population (bottom).

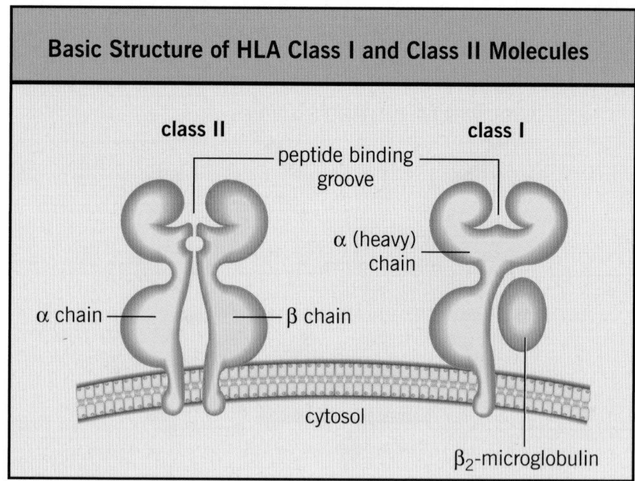

Fig. 14.15 The basic structure of the HLA class I and class II molecules.

clusters associated with asthma, atopy, and wheeze. Principal component and logistic regression analyses of eight traits (IgE, BHR, skin prick, atopy, asthma, wheeze, video questionnaire, and migraine) were used to define an asthma and atopy score. Using a physician-based diagnosis to define the presence of asthma, the asthma score distributions differ significantly between asthmatics and non-asthmatics from the combined random and multiplex populations (Fig. 14.14). A significant shift in atopy score distributions can also be seen between atopic and non-atopic individuals.

Evidence for candidate genes

Candidate genes (or regions) have now been investigated in all but two human chromosomes, although between studies, repeatability has proven problematic. Linkage and strong association has been detected to specific alleles on chromosomes 5 and 11. Several other studies provide strong evidence for these two regions, as well as for chromosomes 1, 2, 6, 7, 12, and 16. Each of these regions will be discussed in more detail, and the results available so far from genome screening projects will be briefly described.

Chromosome 5

The 5q31–34 region of the genome contains several candidate genes implicated in the pathogenesis of asthma and in the regulation of IgE, including the IL-4 cytokine cluster (IL-3, IL-4, IL-5, IL-9, IL-13 and the granulocyte–macrophage colony-stimulating factor) and the β_2-adrenergic receptor (ADRB2). Evidence of linkage for this region to total serum IgE, centered around the IL-4 locus, was first reported in 11 large Amish pedigrees. The linkage evidence was strongest when subjects with high specific IgE were excluded from the analysis, suggesting that specific IgE responsiveness is a confounding factor in the analysis of the genetics of total serum IgE. Using a similar phenotype a second study also reported linkage to total IgE in 92 Dutch families, as well as to a phenotype based on BHR. The strongest evidence for both phenotypes in the Dutch population was more distal than the IL-4 locus, centered around the ADRB2 gene. This makes ADRB2 a promising candidate, particularly as coding variants as well as SNPS in the intronic and promoter regions have been associated with hyper-responsiveness and total serum IgE. There is also evidence that these variants could have a functional significance. These studies on chromosome 5q do not have sufficient power to produce an accurate localization of the disease gene(s) and it is highly likely that more than one important locus exists in the region including CD14 (lipopolysaccharide receptor) and α-catenin (involved in epithelial homeostasis).

There is also much interest in chromosomal factors that influence the coordinate expression of genes encoded in the IL-4 cluster gene. These are involved in polarizing the T-cell response to a Th2-type phenotype as well as in the recruitment and activation of allergic inflammatory cells.

In at least 20 separate studies, there is now overwhelming evidence that genetic variation in the region encoding the IL-4 gene cluster is strongly associated with asthma. Specific attention has also been devoted to the related cytokine, IL-13, which is involved in IgE switching airway inflammation and airway wall remodeling (see chapter 23). Polymorphic variation in the IL-13 promoter that influences secretion of IL-13, in the IL-13 exon that alters the structure of the cytokine thereby influencing its interaction with its receptors, or changes in the expression of the IL-13 α_1- and α_2- receptors themselves influence pathways that are under IL-13 regulations. IL-13 is a strong candidate for the complex expression of asthma and is a new therapeutic target for this disease. In addition a newly identified gene encoded close to the IL-4 gene cluster – PCDH1 – has been identified that is involved in epithelial adhesion.

Chromosome 6

The major histocompatibility complex (MHC) on chromosome 6 includes genes that code for HLA class II molecules (designated DR, DP, and DQ) and also those that are central to the process of antigen recognition and presentation and, as a consequence, modulate the specificity of the immune response (Figs 14.15 and 14.16). Both population- and family-based

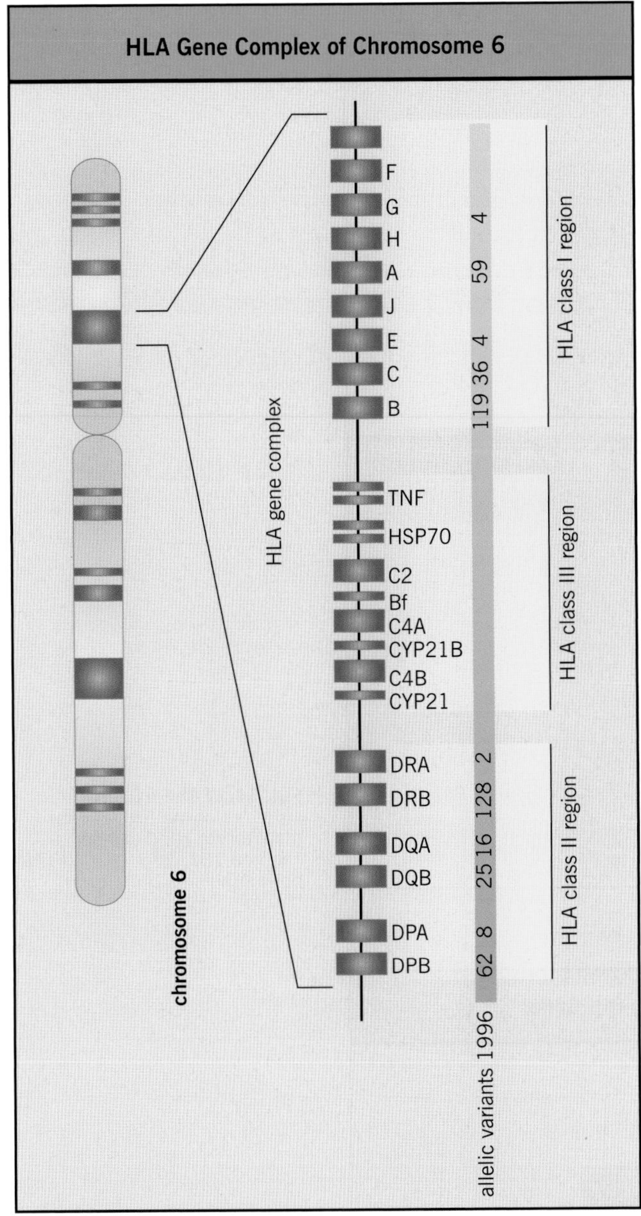

Fig. 14.16 The HLA gene complex on the short arm of chromosome 6. The number of alleles identified by 1996 is indicated. CYP, cytochrome P450 enzymes; HSP, heat shock protein; TNF, tumor necrosis factor.

studies have examined the relationship between HLA type and specific IgE responses and there is much evidence for association between certain haplotypes and individual responses to purified allergens.

The first demonstration was an association between HLA haplotypes and IgE responses to antigen E derived from ragweed (*Ambrosia artemisifolia*). This was subsequently shown to be due to a restriction of the response to a minor component of the ragweed antigen (Amb a V) by HLA-DR2.

Generally, significant associations have been found with highly purified simple allergens rather than with more complex common ones. Any comparisons between studies are complicated by differences in the ethnic origin of the study population, the phenotypic definitions used, and in the method of HLA typing used. Thus, the accumulated evidence associating HLA type with specific IgE responsiveness is inconsistent and appears insufficient to account for individual differences in reactivity to common allergens. Most recently HLA-G has been strongly associated with asthma, possibly through its effect in diverting T-cell polarization towards a Th2 phenotype. HLA-G is expressed strongly on airway epithelial cells. An additional factor contributing to positive association to MHC class I and II genes through linkage disequilibrium is the presence of additional candidates, e.g. heat shock protein-70 (HSP-70) and tumor necrosis factor α (TNFα), polymorphisms of which are associated with asthma.

Genetic association studies have made a strong case for the gene encoding TNFα and TNFβ (lymphotoxin) being of importance in asthma. Specific attention has focused on the -308 A→G SNP that, in a number of studies, has been found to be associated with both asthma and its severity. Although there is some evidence that this SNP alters gene transcription, prevailing opinion is that the -308 SNP is in disequilibrium with functional SNPs in TNFβ.

Chromosome 11

The Oxford, UK group first reported genetic linkage of atopy to chromosome 11q13 in extended and nuclear families with the 'atopy gene' preferentially active in maternally derived alleles. The gene encoding the β subunit of the high-affinity IgE receptor (FcεRIβ) was proposed as the candidate gene and determination of its coding sequence identified two amino acid substitutions within exon 6, designated Leu 181 and Leu 183, which were highly predictive of atopy when inherited maternally. An additional substitution, E237G, has now been identified in exon 7, which is also associated with asthma but with no maternal effect (Figs 14.17 and 14.18). This SNP is in linkage disequilibrium with other SNPs that result in a truncated form of FcεRIβ with impaired signaling functions.

The substitution of glutamic acid for glycine at residue 237 (E237G) has been demonstrated at frequencies of 5.3 and 6% in unselected Australian and Japanese populations. In both cases the presence of E237G is strongly associated with asthma ($p = 0.005$) and in the Australian population it is also associated with BHR ($p = 0.0009$). The substitution occurs at a frequency of around 3.5% in both random and asthma UK populations. Alterations in the wild type sequence of a gene can have biological and clinical significance, but clearly it is important to attribute functions to FcεRI in the expression of elevated IgE levels and to asthma if the clinical relevance of the polymorphisms within the β chain is to be demonstrated.

It is now known that that FcεRIβ variants are able to alter the activity of the high-affinity receptor of IgE through modulation of the level of expression of the receptor on the surface of mast cells, by generating an intracellular truncated decoy that lacks function. From the first association of asthma with SNPs in the β chain of FcεRI in 1989 to the precise sequence that produces the truncated version has required the application of molecular biological approaches coupled to genetic studies. It is clear that for the newly identified asthma genes, this combined approach is likely to reap success.

It is important to note that significant association between a gene polymorphism and a disease trait does not necessarily indicate a causative function but that the gene is in linkage disequilibrium with a neighboring relevant gene close by, e.g.

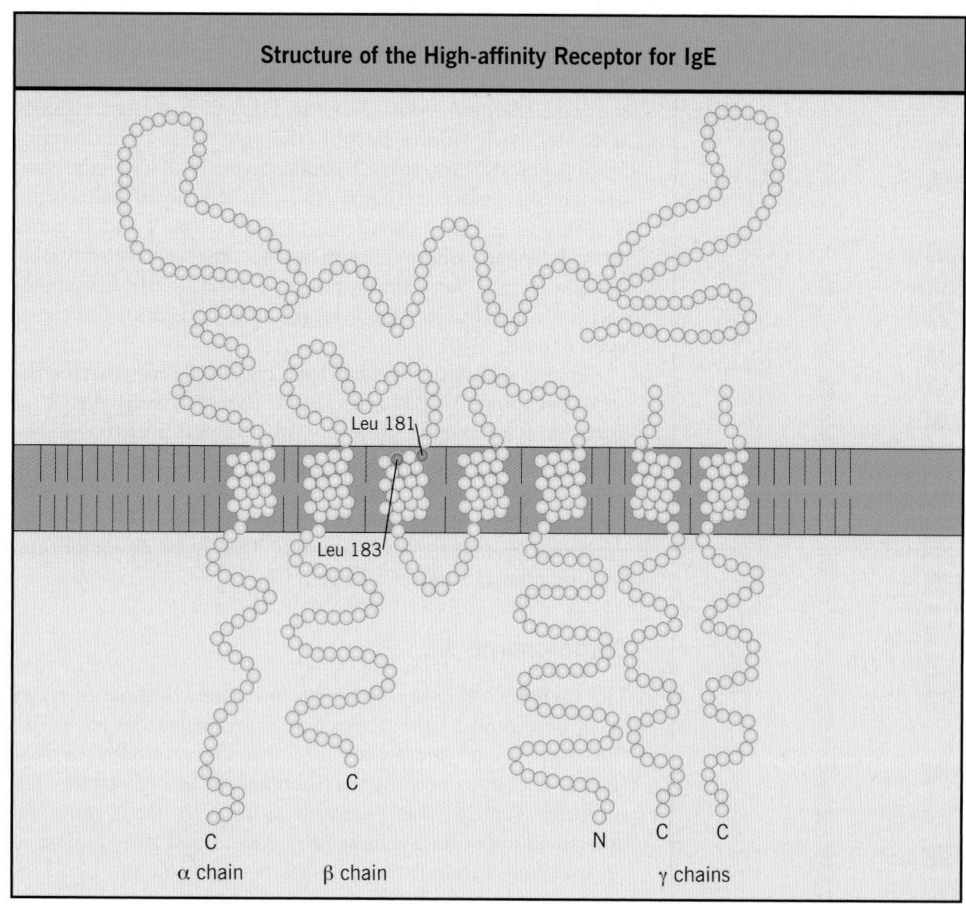

Fig. 14.17 The four-chain structure of the high-affinity receptor for IgE (FcεRIαβγ$_2$). The Leu 181, 183, and E237G polymorphisms are shown.

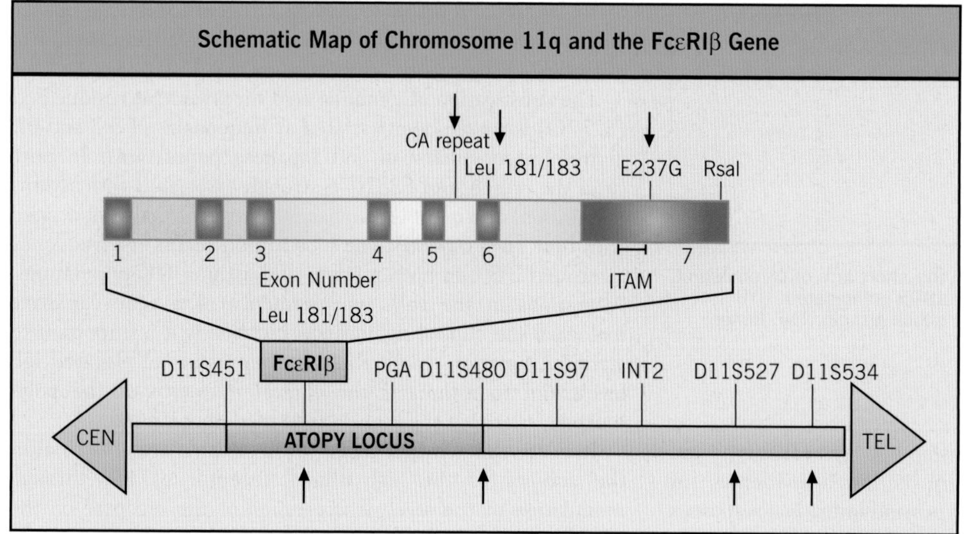

Fig. 14.18 Schematic map of chromosome 11q and the FcεRIβ gene.

the antiinflammatory protein, uteroglobin, secreted by Clara cells (CC10 or CC16) which has also been strongly associated with asthma.

Chromosome 14

Together with HLA, the T-cell receptor (TCR) proteins are central to the handling and recognition of foreign antigens. TCR complexes are usually made up of α and β chains, which are coded for by genes on chromosomes 14 and 7 respectively. An investigation of genetic linkage between specific IgE responses to common allergens and both the TCRα and TCRβ gene complexes identified no linkage to TCRβ serotypes. However, significant linkage of IgE responses to house dust mite allergens, cat, and total serum IgE was demonstrated in TCRα serotypes, implying that a gene in the TCRα region modifies specific IgE

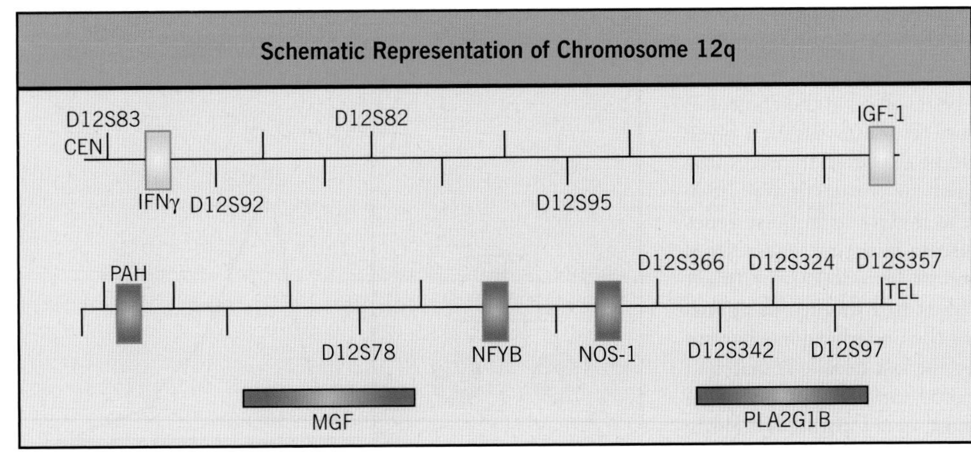

Fig. 14.19 Schematic representation of chromosome 12q where linkage to asthma has been found. (MGF, mast cell growth factor; PLA2G1B, phospholipase A_2 group 1 B.)

responses. Positive linkage has also been found in distinct sample populations, from the UK and Australia. Through an understanding of how the TCR generates immunologic signals at its 'synapse', it is highly likely the TCR variation will reflect more interactions with allergens specific to asthma e.g. dust mite, cat flea etc.

Chromosome 12

Linkage to chromosome 12 has been identified by genotyping a chromosome-12-specific marker set, together with additional 12q markers taken from published Genethon® sequences on the multiplex sample. Single-locus, non-parametric analysis revealed linkage evidence to several markers, with the strongest linkage evidence in distal 12q around the marker D12S97. Linkage to this marker was also replicated in the random sample to the atopy score, and analysis of the 12q data also identified two allelic associations in the same region – D12S366 and atopy and D12S78 and $\log_e$ IgE ($p = 0.001$). Multipoint locus testing has confirmed linkage to these regions (Fig. 14.19).

Guidelines for the interpretation of genetic linkage studies of complex traits have been proposed and, while the linkage values for chromosome 12 would be classed as significant by this convention ($p < 0.05$), they fall short of being highly significant ($p < 0.001$). However, positive linkage has been replicated in other populations, which is a strict criterion for the confirmation of a putative linkage signal. There are two further reasons to think that linkage to this region is genuine. Firstly, chromosome 12q contains several candidate genes including interferon γ, a mast cell growth factor (MGF-1), an insulin-like growth factor (IGF-1), the constitutive form of the nitric oxide synthase gene (NOS-1), and the β subunit of the nuclear factor Y involved in transcription of HLA genes (NFYB). Secondly, there is independent evidence for linkage to chromosome 12q from a genome screen in two populations (Afro-Caribbean and Caucasian Hutterite families), although the maximum linkage determined by multipoint analysis in this study was a considerable distance proximal to the D12S97 locus. Most recently, addition of a large number of further families to the original sample that identified chromosome 12q24 as a major focus for an asthma susceptibility gene has led to the isolation of the *MUC8* gene that encodes mucin8 as accounting for the majority of this association. Mucin8 shares with mucins5AC and 5B the property of being highly glycosylated and, therefore, of special relevance to asthma where the mucins secreted impart increased viscoelasticity to the sputum, making clearance from the airways difficult.

Genome screens

Recent advances in molecular technology and the availability of dense genetic maps have made it feasible to screen the whole genome. A number of these projects have been completed and others are underway. The first to be completed (in Oxford, UK) identified six positive linkages ($p < 0.001$) to chromosomes 4, 6, 7, 11, 13, and 16. Of these six regions, four also showed linkage in a second panel of markers (chromosomes 4, 11, 13, and 16). The chromosome 11q13 has been implicated in the pathogenesis of asthma and atopy and a polymorphism in the esterase D protein on chromosome 13 had previously been linked to total serum IgE. An additional whole genome screen includes the US CSGA study comprising three racial groups – Caucasians, Hispanics, and Afro-Caribbean. Due to this racial admixture, and relatively small numbers of families in each group, the level of significance achieved for linkage was low.

Candidate genes in allergic disease and their potential contribution to asthma severity

There have been at least 11 whole genome scans in asthma that are now in the public domain. These have revealed at least 10 regions of linkage that could be reproduced between scans and additionally four regions that, while being statistically significant, have not been replicated by others. Of interest is that a number of the regions of chromosomal linkage to asthma overlap with related disorders, especially atopic dermatitis and psoriasis, directing focus on the epithelium as an important site for the expression of asthma susceptibility genes.

Thus of the positionally cloned genes, PCDH1, ESE-3, DPP10, *MUC8*, HLA-G, and GPRA (GPR154) all are expressed in the epithelium. Equally the underlying mesenchyme also seems important as a site for expressing genetic disease susceptibility. Of particular significance in this compartment is ADAM33, a metalloprotease gene restricted in its expression of smooth muscle and fibroblasts, and GPRA that exists in two forms – GPRA-A and GPRA-B, the latter isoform being selectively expressed in airway smooth muscle. However, reviewing candidate genes with known mutations, which have been associated with allergic disease, it is clear that the majority of these genes will be expected to be involved in the control of IgE- and Th2-mediated inflammatory responses. As such, given that mutations in these genes would be expected to predispose to asthma per se, it is perhaps not surprising that positive results have been obtained looking at mutations in these genes using endpoints likely to identify disease-initiating genes. Novel genes influencing the immune response include PHF11 (plant homeodomain finger protein 11), identified through positional cloning. The explosive knowledge of the underlying mechanism of asthma that has taken place over the last decade is matched by an almost equal number of genetic variations in candidate molecules linked to asthma. Almost every pathophysiologic molecule has been shown to exist in a variant form associated with asthma so it has proven difficult to establish primacy. Some exciting and highly relevant molecules exhibiting disease-related polymorphic variation include CD14, Toll-like receptors (TLR) 2, 3 and 4, T- bet, transforming growth factor β (TGFβ), NOD1 and 2 (nucleotide binding oligomerization domains 1 and 2).

Of special significance were the genes identified by the Oxford Group involved in immune regulation and cytokine processing. PHF11 in chromosome 13q12 is expressed on a range of immune cells and encodes a nuclear receptor that is partly a complex that contains a histone methyl transferase (SET domain bifurcated 2; SET D B2) that regulates a histone deacetylase enzyme (HDAC) and karyopherin α3, a nuclear transporter protein 3, that are implicated in modifying the behaviour of the nucleoprotein histones that regulate gene transcription. DPP10 was positionally cloned as an asthma gene from a large UK population and was subsequently replicated in Australia as well as in other populations. DPP10 is selectively expressed in the airway epithelium and is involved in the processing of cytokines and chemokines. In addition, it has also been shown to control a specific K channel in the epithelium. These functional studies of asthma related genes are leading to a new vision of this disease. A good example of this is ADAM33, a novel gene disassociated with asthma that was reported in 2002.

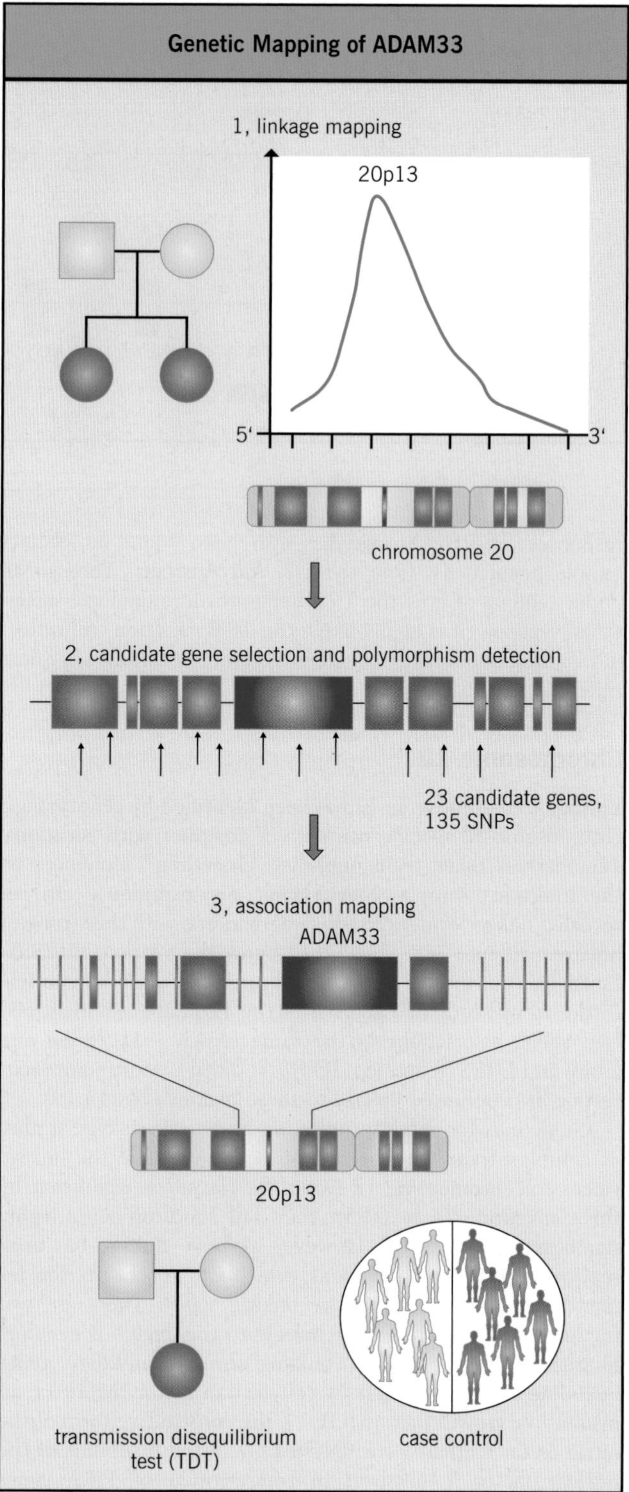

Fig. 14.20 Genetic mapping of *ADAM33*.

ADAM33 as an example of a new asthma gene

In 2002 *ADAM33* was the first susceptibility gene for asthma to be positionally cloned and is located to chromosome 20p13 (Fig. 14.20). The initial linkage study identified a greater linkage and association with asthma when the diagnosis was conditioned by the phenotype BHR (Fig. 14.21). The cellular provenance of ADAM33 mRNA also strengthened the initial view that this gene was involved in airway BHR and remodeling in that its transcription was limited to mesenchymal cells (e.g. muscle, fibroblast and myofibroblast). Following the initial study, a number of different populations and ethnic groups have been used to replicate the association between polymorphisms in *ADAM33* and asthma, but several have not. However, in a meta-analysis of studies that included those which individually failed to find a statistical association between *ADAM33* and asthma, analysis of the greatly expanded number of cases and controls yielded a positive association. This emphasizes the importance of study power to detect new genes in complex diseases such as asthma.

ADAM33 belongs to the family of a disintegrin and metalloproteases involved in fertility and in the regulation cytokine growth factor release. The structure of the gene and its putative function in relation to asthma are depicted in Figures 14.22 and 14.23.

Further studies of ADAM33 have established several facts:

- The majority of the mRNA transcripts and protein in airway fibroblasts and smooth muscle are expressed as alternative spliced molecules (Fig. 14.24).
- Six alternatively spliced ADAM33 variants have been described which fail to contain the ADAM metalloprotease domain.
- There are no significant differences in the levels of ADAM33 in mRNA or protein expression in asthmatic compared to normal airways.
- Polymorphic variation in ADAM33 predicts both an accelerated decline in lung function over time in asthma and chronic obstructive pulmonary disease (COPD) (Fig. 14.25).
- ADAM33 polymorphism is a predictor of reduced lung function in 3–5 year old children born of parents with asthma or allergy (Fig. 14.26).
- A soluble form of ADAM33 has been identified (55 Kda) in bronchoalveolar lavage from asthma.

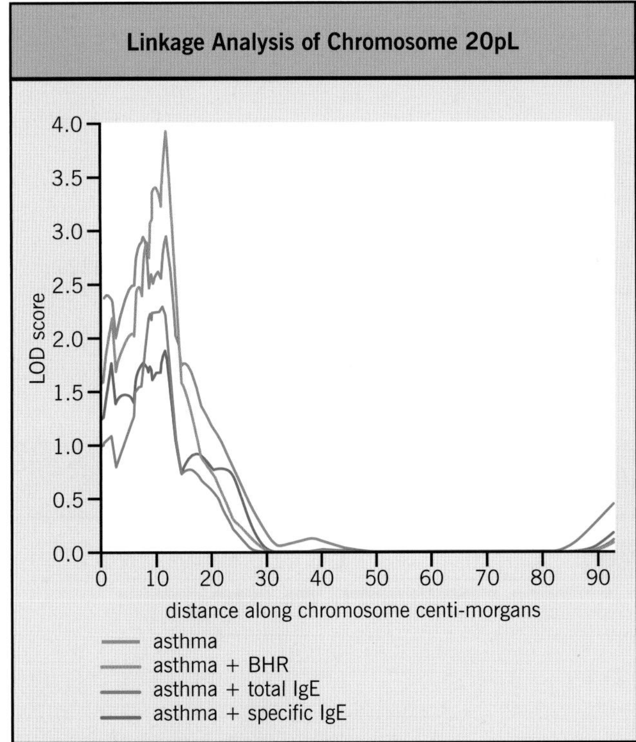

Fig. 14.21 Linkage analysis of chromosome 20.

Although we do not know how the ADAM33 molecule translates to increased asthma risk, it appears that it is involved both in airway remodeling associated with the progression of asthma and COPD and, also, in lung morphogenesis. The fact that the full length molecule which comprises 22 exons (Fig. 14.22) is expressed at a much lower level suggests that the non-enzymatic functions of ADAM33 are important in its association with lung disorders. Possible mechanisms that link ADAM33 with abnormalities in airway fibroblasts and/or smooth muscle are shown in Figure 14.23. The recent documentation that ADAM33 is preferentially expressed in primitive mesenchymal cells involved in lung development highlights the importance of relating morphogenetic genes with those involved in 'remodeling' of the airways (Fig. 14.27). Drawing from this experience, there are clearly complex issues that connect ADAM33 to asthma. What is important from this experience is to understand at the gene level how such a complex molecule translates its effect into asthma. There is likely to be a high level of subtlety in this that will have implications for other complex lung diseases. For example almost all the new genes identified by positional cloning (ADAM33, DPP10, PCDH1, PHF11 and GPRA) contain a high proportion of SNPs associated with disease (Fig. 14.28) and many of these occur in introns or in the 3′- non-coding region of the gene.

Pharmacogenetic studies

One obvious way in which gene factors may influence asthma severity is by determining treatment responses. This possibility has been specifically examined in asthmatics with respect to responses to corticosteroids and to β_2-adrenoceptor agonists to date. There is a small group of individuals who do not appear to respond to corticosteroids even at a high dose. Such patients have been labeled 'corticosteroid-resistant asthmatics'. In practice there appears to be a continuum of corticosteroid responsiveness and such patients may just represent one extreme

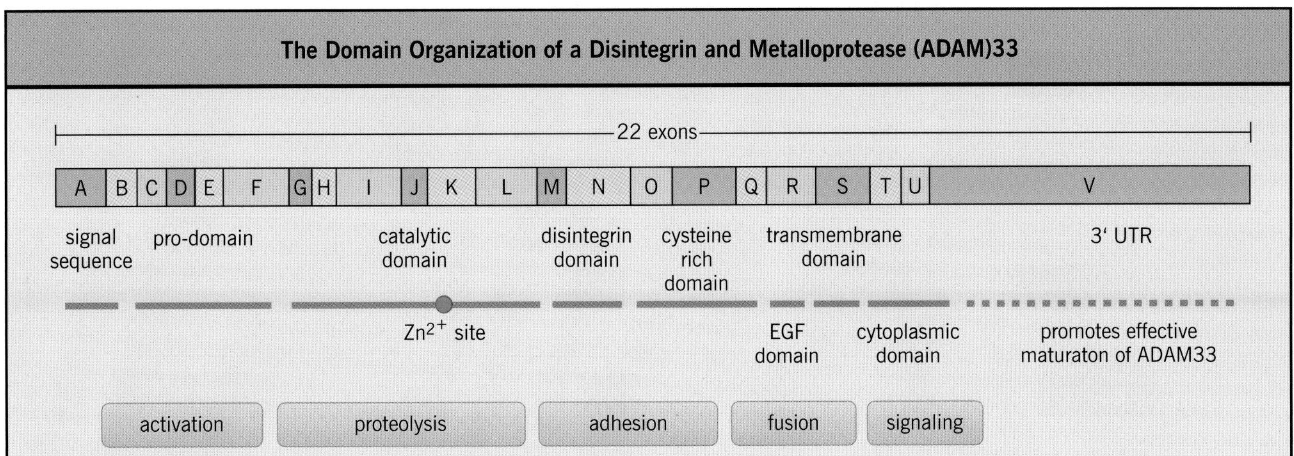

Fig. 14.22 The domain organization of a disintegrin and metalloprotease (ADAM)33.

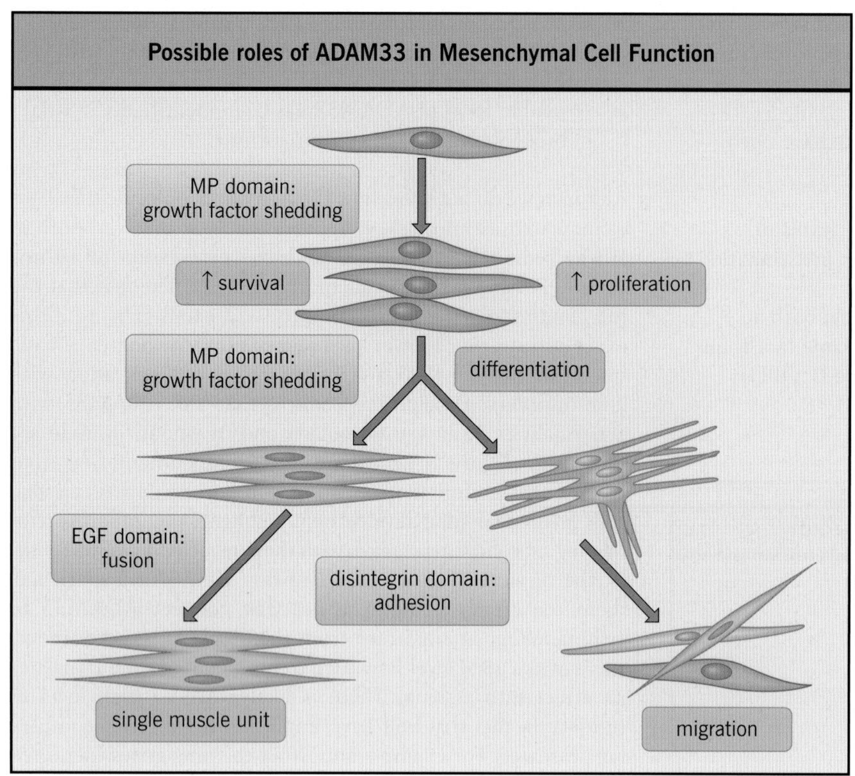

Fig. 14.23 Possible roles of ADAM33 in mesenchymal cell function.

Alternatively Spliced Variants of ADAM33

A B C D E F G H I J K L M N O P Q R S T U V

SS PRO- MMP domain disintegrin cysteine-rich EGF TM cytoplasmic

1 A B C P Q R S T U V

2 A B C R S T U V

3 A B C D G H O P Q R S T U V

4 A M N O P Q R S T U V

5 A B C D G H M N O P Q R S T U V

6 A B C D M N O P Q R S T U V

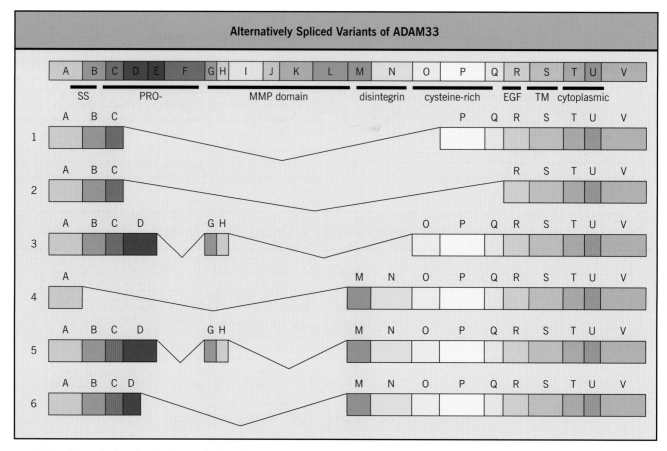

Fig. 14.24 Alternatively spliced variants of ADAM33. The letters represent the individual exons.

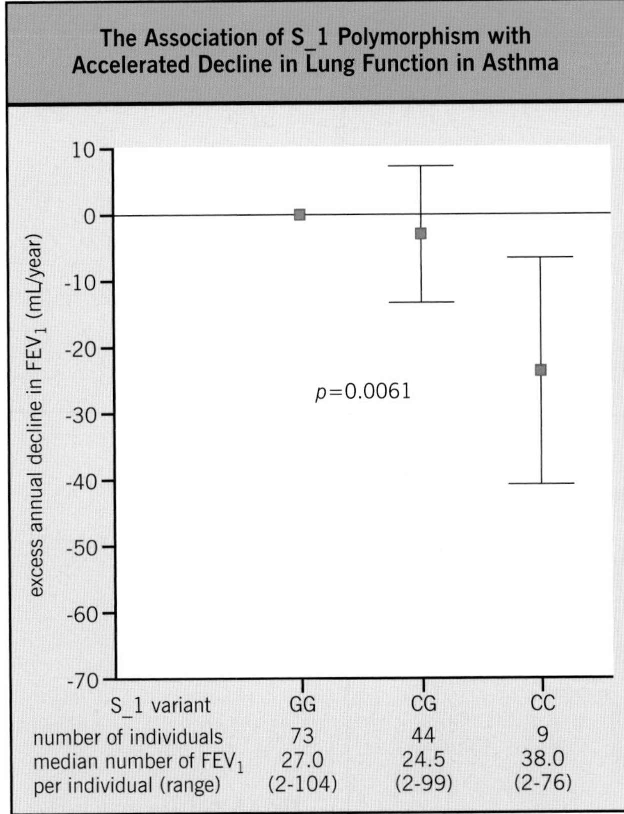

Fig. 14.25 Polymorphic variation in *ADAM33* predicts both an accelerated decline in lung function over time in asthma and chronic obstructive pulmonary disease (COPD). FEV_1, forced air expiratory volume in 1 second. [From Jongepier H, Boezen HM, Dijkstra A, et al. Polymorphisms of the ADAM33 gene are associated with accelerated lung function decline in asthma. Clin Exp Allergy 2004; 34(5):757–760.]

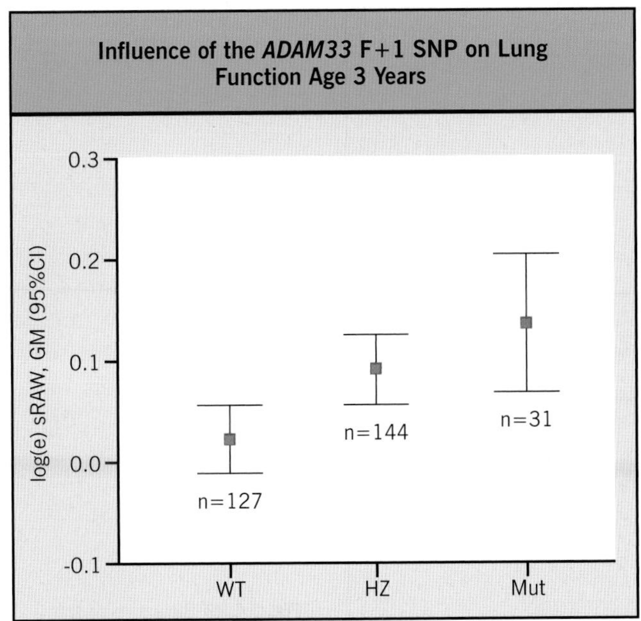

Fig. 14.26 Influence of the *ADAM33* F+1 SNP on lung function, age 3 years. SNP, single nucleotide polymorphism.

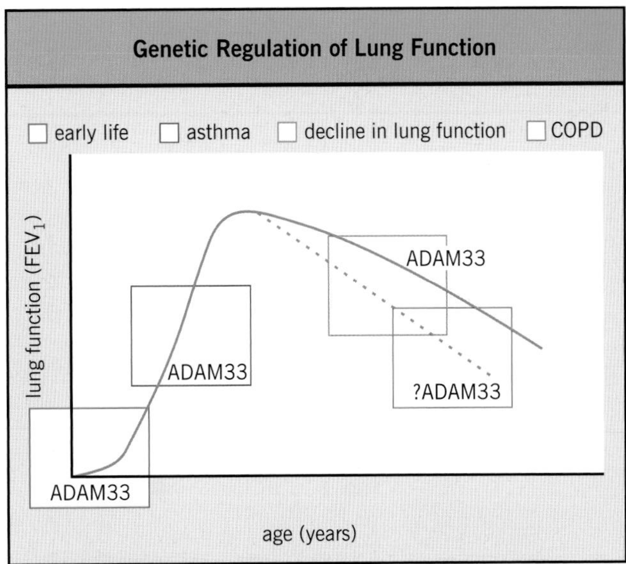

Fig. 14.27 Genetic regulation of lung function. COPD, chronic obstructive pulmonary disease; FEV1, forced air expiratory volume in 1 second.

end of the distribution. The recent discovery of polymorphic variations in the corticotrophin hormone releasing receptor (CRHRI) and the response of asthma to inhaled corticosteroids provides a rationale for predicting the therapeutic response to this drug class.

A number of attempts have been made to define the molecular basis of corticosteroid resistance including sequencing the glucocorticoid receptor from a number of such patients. To date, no specific mutations have been identified which determine steroid resistance although this work is ongoing. Obviously, relevant mutations do not have to be within the coding region of the glucocorticoid receptor gene itself but could be in genes for products in downstream signaling pathways.

Other researchers have concentrated on assessing the contribution of β_2-adrenoceptor polymorphism to allergic disease (Fig. 14.29). Initial studies demonstrated that the glutamate 27 β_2-adrenoceptor polymorphism was associated with lower IgE levels and less reactive airways in asthmatic subjects although it is possible that these findings are due to linkage disequilibrium with other genes close by on 5q31, given that both IgE and BHR have been linked to this region of 5q by other groups. More recently the response to long-acting β_2-adrenoceptor agonists of individuals who are homozygous for the glycine 16 β_2-adrenoceptor variant has been studied. In vitro, this polymorphism confers increased levels of down-regulation following agonist exposure. Subjects with this variant develop tachyphylaxis to the bronchodilator effects of long-acting β-agonists following chronic dosing with oral formoterol, although whether this effect occurs with clinically relevant doses of inhaled long-acting β_2-adrenoceptor agonists remains to be determined. The glycine 16 form of the receptor is also associated with a nocturnal fall in FEV_1.

One other study has been reported which is potentially relevant to asthma pharmacogenetics. The Boston, USA group has recently described a promoter polymorphism in the 5-lipoxygenase gene which alters transcription of this leukotriene generating enzyme in in vitro systems. With the development

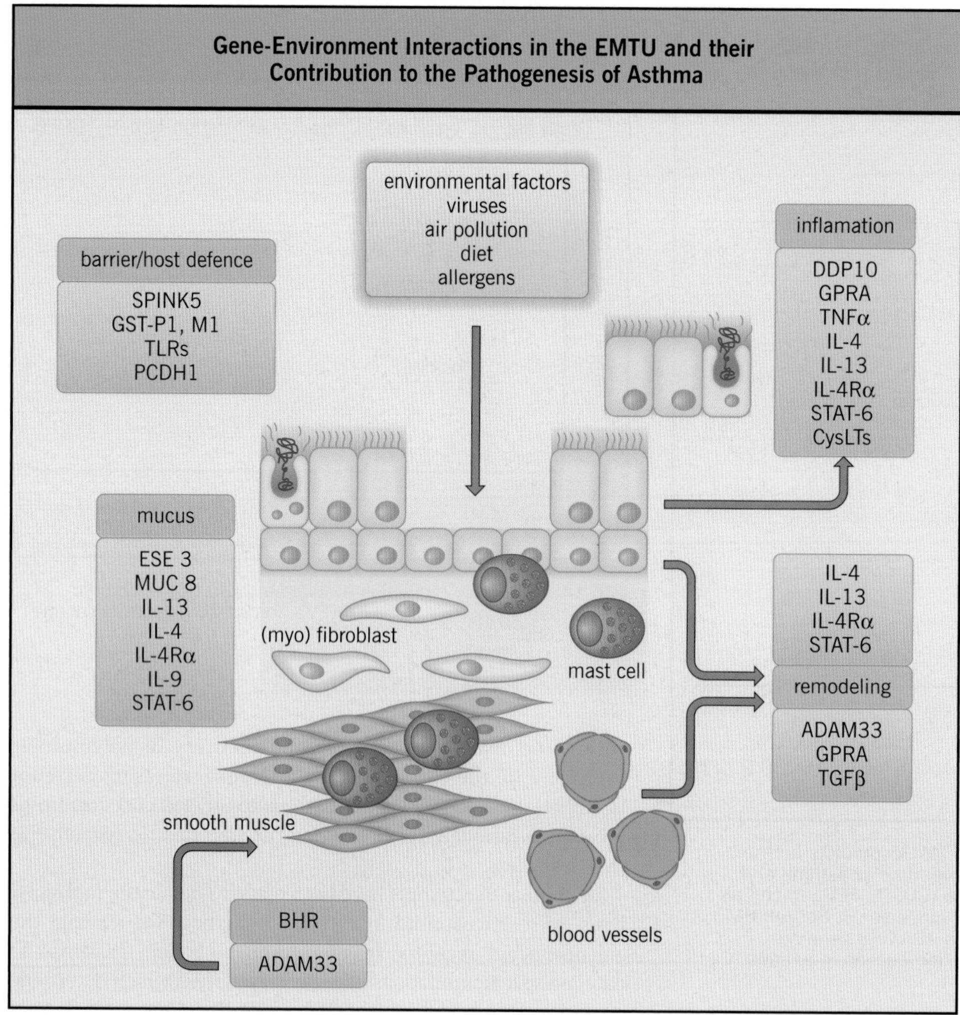

Fig. 14.28 Gene–environment interactions in the epithelial mesenchymal trophic unit (EMTU) and their contribution to the pathogenesis of asthma. CycLTs, cysteinyl leukotrienes; IL, interleukin; TGF, transforming growth factor, TLR, Toll-like receptors; TNF, tumor necrosis factor.

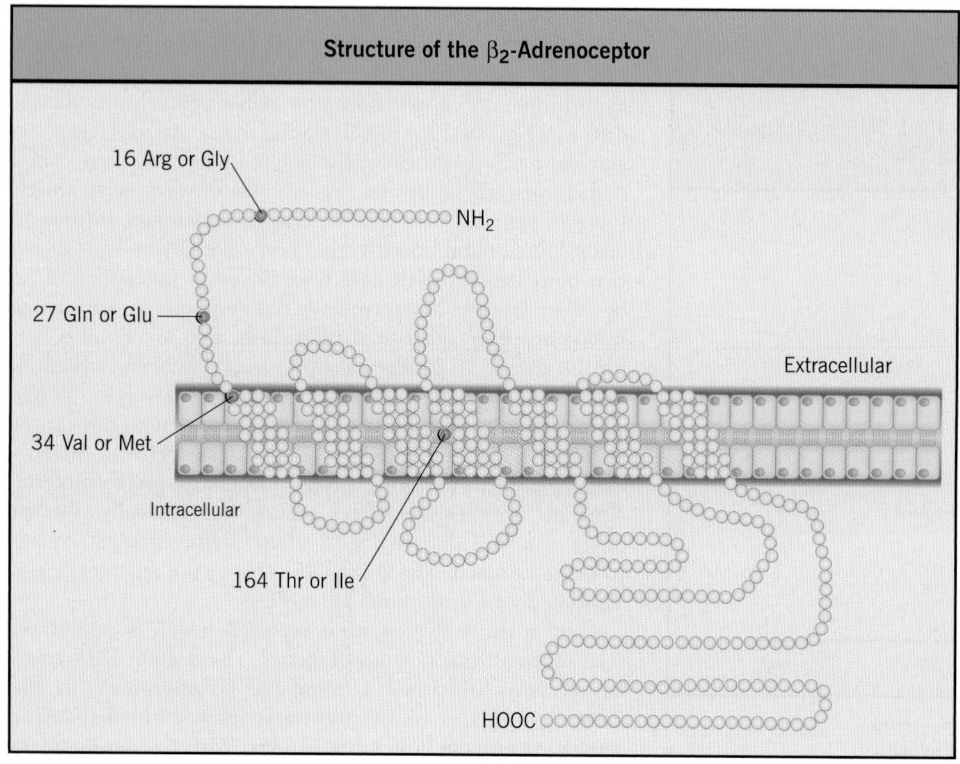

Fig. 14.29 Structure of the β_2-adrenoceptor showing the sites of polymorphisms at amino acids 16 and 27.

of 5-LO inhibitors and leukotriene receptor antagonists for the treatment of asthma, it will be important to determine whether polymorphisms affecting gene transcription will determine response to treatment. One recent example is the -444 A→C SNP of leukotriene C_4 synthase that not only predicts aspirin intolerant asthma but also is involved in generating reduced lung function in asthma and responsiveness to antileukotriene drugs since the polymorphic variant causes increased leukotriene C_4 production.

CONCLUSION

New techniques for scanning the human genome promise great advances in tracking the origins of disorders caused by multiple genes. However, it is clear from the studies presented in this overview that we are far from understanding the genetic basis of asthma and atopy and their interactions with the environment. It is also clear that agreement must be reached on definition of the phenotype and methods of ascertainment in order to carry out large, multicenter, collaborative studies. Positive findings need to be validated in different populations selected for the presence of the disease and then confirmed in a random population where the prevalence of asthma and atopy will also be expected to be significant.

A whole raft of genes is known to modify structural and functional changes of the airways, but their direct attribution to asthma has yet to be established. The concept that this is altered communication between the epithelium and underlying mesenchyme has created a new paradigm for chronic asthma that engages epithelial as well as mesenchymal genes (Fig. 14.29). What is proving a challenge, however, is to determine how, to what extent and at what times during human development environmental factors will influence the expression of susceptibility genes. The 'Hygiene Hypothesis' is a particularly good example of how, through environmental exposure, endotoxin present in bacteria could program the way the immune response develops and how polymorphic variation in these and related signaling molecules could influence this.

FURTHER READING

Allen M, Heinzmann A, Noguchi E, et al. Positional cloning of a novel gene influencing asthma from chromosome 2q14. Nat Genet. 2003; 35(3):258–263. Epub 2003 Oct.

Basehore MJ, Howard TD, Lange LA, et al. A comprehensive evaluation of IL4 variants in ethnically diverse populations: association of total serum IgE levels and asthma in white subjects. J Allergy Clin Immunol 2004; 114(1):80–87.

Blumenthal MN, Langerfeld CD, Beaty TH, et al. A genome-wide search for allergic response (atopy) genes in three ethnic groups: Collaborative study on the genetics of asthma. Hum Genet 2004; 114(2):157–164. Epub 2003 Oct.

Cakebreak JA, Haitchi HM, Holloway JW, et al. The role of ADAM33 in the pathogenesis of asthma. Springer Semin Immunopathol 2004; 25(3–4):361–375.

Cookson W. Genetics and genomics of asthma and allergic diseases. Immunol Rev 2002; 190:195–206.

Holloway JW, Holgate ST. Genetics. Chem Immunol Allergy 2004; 84:1–35.

Holloway JW, Keith TP, Davies DE, et al. The discovery and role of ADAM33, a new candidate gene for asthma. Expert Rev Mol Med 2004; 6(17):1–12.

Howard TD, Meyers DA, Bleecker ER. Mapping susceptibility genes for allergic diseases. Chest 2003; 123(suppl 3):363S–368S.

Knight DA, Holgate ST. The airway epithelium: structural and functional properties in health and disease. Respirology 2003; 8(4):432–446.

Kurz T, Altmueller J, Strauch K, et al. A genome-wide screen on the genetics of atopy in a multiethnic European population reveals a major atopy locus on chromosome 3q21.3. Allergy 2005; 60(2):192–199.

Chapter 15

Definition:

A term used for the hypothesis that asthma and allergy arise from influences present during fetal life and early childhood.

Early life origins of allergy and asthma

Patrick G Holt, Peter DL Sly, and Graham Devereux

INTRODUCTION

There is increasing evidence supporting the notion that the factors which determine susceptibility to persistent allergic disease and asthma exert their main influence(s) on disease pathogenesis early in life. Factors that are influential during fetal and early life have the potential to exert disproportionately potent effects because small perturbations in organogenesis can be exaggerated by rapid growth during fetal and early life. The activation of genes involved in organogenesis may enable gene–environment interactions to occur during fetal and early life that cannot occur when these genes are inactivated at later ages. Early life influences are also likely to be particularly relevant to immunologically mediated diseases such as allergy and asthma that are associated with the helper T cells type 2 (Th2) pattern of Th-cell differentiation in response to allergen stimulation. As will be described below, the immune system in the neonate is constitutively skewed towards the Th2 response phenotype, potentially biasing the long-term consequences of initial encounters between immature Th cells and allergen which occur in early life. This chapter will review recent developments in the understanding of early life influences on allergy and asthma, in particular on processes which impact on the innate and adaptive arms of immune function. The first part of the chapter focuses on antenatal factors, encompassing studies on cord blood mononuclear cells (CBMC), fetal allergen exposure, and antenatal factors that we have broadly grouped into the 'hygiene hypotheses', smoking, and maternal diet. The second half of the chapter focuses on early postnatal factors, in particular those associated with long-term 'programming' of immunologic and respiratory functions.

ANTENATAL ORIGINS OF ATOPY AND ASTHMA

Studies of cord blood mononuclear cells

The demonstration that CBMC can proliferate and secrete cytokines after in vitro stimulation with allergens has stimulated many areas of research investigating the immunologic mechanisms and associated antenatal influences that lead to the development of allergic disease and asthma. In particular, positive lymphoproliferation by CBMC in response to allergen has been widely interpreted as evidence that the immunologic changes leading to asthma and allergic disease start during fetal development. However, while some prospective studies have demonstrated that childhood asthma and allergic disease are associated with increased CBMC proliferative and cytokine responses, others have reported comparable associations with reduced CBMC responses. It is likely that differences in study size, study population, outcome definition and CBMC culture techniques have contributed to these inconsistencies,

Table 15.1 Reported associations with in vitro cord blood mononuclear cell responses

Parental atopic disease
Birth order
Race
Maternal allergen exposure
Maternal smoking
Maternal dietary vitamin E and fatty acid intake
Cord blood fatty acid composition
Childhood asthma
Childhood wheezing
Atopic dermatitis
Allergic rhinitis
Food allergy
Atopy

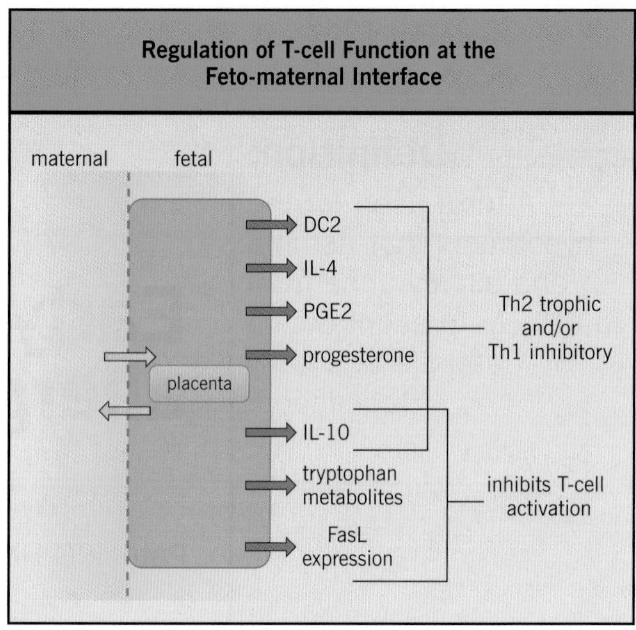

Fig. 15.1 Regulation of T-cell function at the fetomaternal interface. DC2, dendritic cells; FasL, Fas ligand; IL, interleukin; PGE_2, prostaglandin E_2; Th1, 2, helper T cells type 1, 2.

and hence the significance of these findings remains in contention. Very recent data also question the antigen specificity of these responses, and the issues arising from these findings are discussed in the following postnatal section.

Many antenatal factors have been reported to be associated with CBMC responses (Table 15. 1). In particular, qualitative and quantitative aspects of CBMC responses have been associated with parental history of atopic disease. While there are some conflicting reports, the majority of studies have reported that parental atopy is associated with reduced CBMC cytokine responses, principally interferon γ (IFNγ) but also interleukin-4 (IL-4). These reports are supported by more detailed studies on large panels of individual T-cell clones from infants at low versus high genetic risk of atopy, and more recently by data from the authors demonstrating that the 'low cytokine response' phenotype [reduced IFNγ and IL-4, and in this case tumor necrosis factor α (TNFα)] characteristic of high risk infants is mirrored by levels of circulating cytokines present in cord serum. The reported associations between parental atopy and CBMC responses are consistent with the suggestion that genetically determined mechanisms which are responsible for the enhanced risk of atopy and asthma in family history-positive children are already operative before birth. However, there may be additional non-genetic mechanisms whereby the immune system of the pregnant atopic mother can influence fetal immune development.

Fetal allergen exposure

The immunologic mechanisms preventing maternal rejection of her allogenic fetus are potentially relevant to the antenatal origins of allergic disease. Fetal and maternal placental tissues secrete a number of cytokines [IL-4, IL-10, IL-13, transforming growth factor β_2 (TGFβ_2)] that heavily bias the microenvironment of the fetomaternal interface against Th1 differentiation, such that Th1 biased sensitization and effector functions within the uterus are inhibited (Fig. 15.1). This has led to the suggestion that fetal allergen exposure and sensitization in this cytokine milieu increases the likelihood of Th2 biased responses and allergic disease.

Consistent with this latter suggestion, artificial placental perfusion has demonstrated the transplacental transfer of nutrient and inhalant allergens by passive diffusion and active transport pathways, some of which are IgG dependent. Fel d1 and Der p1 IgG immune complexes have been detected in cord blood. Der p1 has also been detected in low levels in amniotic fluid, suggesting minor amniochorionic transfer. It is thus theoretically possible that from at least 26 weeks' gestation the fetus is exposed to tiny amounts of ubiquitous nutrient allergens and, possibly, lower concentrations of perennial allergens such as house dust mite. However, the degree to which these ex vivo perfusion models reflect placental function in vivo remains to be established. Furthermore, a significant body of opinion questions the capacity of the (typically fluid phase) assay systems which have been utilized to detect aeroallergens in blood to accurately detect proteins at acceptable levels of specificity, over the very low concentration ranges claimed to exist in blood. The situation is less controversial in relation to dietary allergens, but further work is required to clarify the issues related to aeroallergen levels in blood, particularly in the fetal compartment.

Circulating fetal T cells can be detected from 15 weeks' gestation, and from 22 weeks' gestation they can proliferate after in vitro stimulation with allergens. Although fetal T cells have the capacity to respond by proliferation when stimulated by allergen, the literature on fetal T-cell allergen sensitization is contradictory and dependent on the premise that in vitro CBMC responses only occur if there has been fetal T-cell priming by maternally derived allergens. Several studies have positively associated maternal exposure to seasonal allergens during pregnancy to in vitro CBMC proliferative responses after stimulation with the seasonal allergens. These findings have been proposed as direct evidence that maternal allergen exposure leads to the in utero priming of fetal T cells. However, closer inspection of the data reveals that approximately 30–40% of CBMC samples proliferate in the absence of maternal exposure to the seasonal allergen. Furthermore, recent studies have failed to demonstrate associations between CBMC responses and maternal exposure to seasonal allergens and household house dust mite during pregnancy. These studies have concluded that in vitro CBMC responses cannot be used as evidence for in utero sensitization to inhalant allergens (further discussion below).

An alternative approach to the issue of whether genuine allergen-specific sensitization occurs before birth is to closely examine the effects of active allergen avoidance during pregnancy. Whilst several intervention studies have achieved successful reductions in maternal/fetal allergen exposure, interpretation of outcomes is complicated by the fact that most of the studies involve combined antenatal and postnatal allergen avoidance and additional environmental interventions. A systematic review of studies that have specifically reduced or totally avoided maternal dietary intake of nutrient allergens such as egg, peanuts, and dairy products has concluded that dietary allergen avoidance during pregnancy does not reduce the likelihood of atopic eczema or asthma during the first 12 to 18 months of life and may increase the severity of the disease when exposure ultimately occurs. It is difficult to specifically identify the consequences of reducing house dust mite exposure during pregnancy on childhood asthma and allergic disease because all of the reported studies include postnatal avoidance interventions. However recent data showing that postnatal avoidance of house dust mite allergen results in an *increased* rate of allergic sensitization argue strongly against this strategy.

Antenatal aspects of the 'hygiene hypothesis'

The 'hygiene hypothesis' was initially proposed as an explanation for the negative association between allergic disease and family size and number of older siblings. To date, numerous studies of postnatal microbial exposure have been unable to explain the birth order association. There is some evidence to suggest that the association between allergic disease and birth order is an antenatal phenomenon. Cord blood IgE is highest in first-born infants with sequential decrements with subsequent births; in vitro CBMC proliferative responses are claimed to be negatively associated with birth order and maternal IgE levels are related to the number of previous pregnancies.

Alterations in infant gut microflora have been implicated in the development of allergic disease. The fetal gut is sterile and exposure to maternal bacteria during delivery appears to be important in determining the gut microflora of an infant. It has been proposed that caesarean delivery may increase the risk of developing asthma and allergic disease because caesarean delivery delays and alters gut microbial colonization. To date, delivery by caesarean section has not been convincingly associated with an increased likelihood of allergic rhinitis, atopic eczema and atopy during childhood. Caesarean delivery has been positively associated with parentally reported food intolerance and atopy in children; however, these associations were not confirmed by objective food challenges and skin prick testing. Delivery by caesarean section has been inconsistently associated with CBMC responses; a very small study demonstrated a positive association between caesarean section and CBMC IFNγ and IL-12 responses; however, this was not confirmed by a larger study.

In contrast to allergic disease, some large studies have demonstrated that caesarean delivery is positively associated with the incidence of asthma up to the age of 28. Interpretation of these studies is complicated because factors associated with an increased likelihood of asthma, e.g. maternal asthma and increased fetal head circumference, are also associated with increased caesarean section rates. In the absence of an association between caesarean delivery and allergic disease, the adverse association with asthma may well be due to confounders rather than effects on immune maturation.

A number of obstetric complications during pregnancy and labor have been associated with an increased risk of asthma and allergic disease in children (Table 15.2). These complications may be a consequence of antenatal exposures, such as infections, that also increase the risk of asthma and allergic disease. Alternatively these complications may result from immunologic failure of the placenta resulting in progressive placental destruction by the maternal immune system. It is possible that immunologic failure and destruction of the placenta influences the fetal immune maturation and increases the risk of asthma and allergic disease.

Maternal infections during pregnancy, particularly during the first trimester, have been positively associated with asthma and allergic disease in children. The maternal use of antibiotics

Table 15.2 Summary of studies relating obstetric complications to the development of asthma and allergic disease

	Asthma	Allergic disease
Complicated but non-caesarean delivery: vacuum extraction, breech	–	–
Early, threatened labor	+	
Malpresentation, malposition: breech, transverse lie, face presentation	+	
Uterus-related complications: antepartum hemorrhage, preterm contractions, placental insufficiency, restricted uterine growth	+	+
Maternal infections during pregnancy: febrile episodes, vaginitis, bacterial, viral, yeast infections	+	+

during pregnancy has been inconsistently associated with asthma and allergic disease. Whilst maternal antibiotic use during pregnancy does not appear to increase the likelihood of parentally reported or confirmed food allergy, several studies have reported positive associations between maternal antibiotic use during pregnancy and childhood asthma, eczema and hayfever. It has been suggested that the adverse effects of antibiotics may be a consequence of antibiotic induced changes in maternal gut and possibly vaginal microflora. Maternal vaginal colonization during gestation with *Ureaplasma urealyticum* and *Staphylococcus aureus* has been positively associated with wheezing episodes and asthma during early childhood.

In utero exposure to maternal cigarette smoke

It is now clear that in utero exposure to maternal tobacco smoke is detrimental to infant and adult respiratory health. In 1986 cord blood IgE was reported to be elevated in neonates born to mothers who smoke during pregnancy. This paper has been widely cited as evidence that maternal smoking during pregnancy increases the likelihood of childhood allergic disease. However, this issue remains controversial, and a meta-analysis published in 1998 (Strachan and Cook) concluded that there is 'little or no effect of parental smoking on IgE concentrations in children in developed countries'. Since this review however, the German Multicenter Allergy Study has reported that fetal exposure to maternal smoke increases IgE sensitization to food allergens in children but not sensitization to inhalant allergens. More recent evidence (discussed below) also demonstrates that maternal smoking has significant effects on cytokine production in the fetus.

There is increasing evidence that in utero exposure to maternal tobacco smoke increases the likelihood of childhood asthma and respiratory symptoms. Several large epidemiologic studies have demonstrated that schoolchildren whose mothers smoked during pregnancy are more likely to have physician diagnosed asthma, asthma attacks, dry cough, episodes of wheezing and to use asthma treatment. The South Californian Child Health Study identified the 3% of children whose mothers stop smoking around the time of delivery. This prospective study has demonstrated that schoolchildren exposed in utero to maternal cigarette smoke are more likely to have physician diagnosed asthma, asthma with current symptoms, use asthma treatments, and to suffer wheezing symptoms during exercise, nocturnally and in the presence or absence of a cold.

A majority of studies have demonstrated that maternal smoking during pregnancy is independently associated with reduced ventilatory function in children. Studies of children in the first few days and weeks of life before any significant exposure to environmental tobacco smoke (ETS) have reported that ventilatory function is reduced in children whose mothers smoked during pregnancy and that this association is independent of lung size. Postnatal exposure to ETS further compromises lung function and the development of normal respiratory drive. Several epidemiologic studies of schoolchildren have demonstrated that maternal smoking during pregnancy is associated with reduced ventilatory function, particularly indices of small airway function, and that the associations with in utero maternal smoke exposure are greater in magnitude and independent of any associations with postnatal ETS exposure. As so few women actually alter their smoking habits during pregnancy, separating pre- and postnatal effects is extremely difficult.

The evidence to date suggests that in utero exposure to maternal cigarette smoke either damages or critically alters the developing fetal bronchial airways leading to reduced ventilatory function, increased bronchial hyperresponsiveness and a permanent predisposition to asthma and wheezing symptoms. Any adverse effect of maternal cigarette smoke is likely to permanently alter airway function for life because the bronchial airways are all present before the end of pregnancy. Susceptibility of fetal airways to the adverse effects of maternal cigarette smoke is, in part, genetically determined. The South Californian Child Health Study has demonstrated that the adverse effect of maternal smoking during pregnancy on childhood respiratory health is largely restricted to children with the null genotype for glutathione S-transferase M1 (GSTM1). It is possible that the absence of GSTM1 results in reduced metabolism of tobacco smoke-associated toxins and increased damage to the developing airways.

In addition to direct effects on the developing fetal airways maternal cigarette smoking may also influence the developing fetal immune system. Maternal cigarette smoking during pregnancy is associated with increased CBMC proliferative and secreted IL-13 responses. Moreover, a recent study from the authors on the large Raine birth cohort in Perth has demonstrated that the pattern of reduced IFNγ and IL-4 production which is characteristic of T cells from neonates at high risk of atopy, is mirrored by diminished levels of these cytokines in cord serum, and moreover that the latter deficit is markedly accentuated in the offspring of smoking mothers. This strongly suggests that at least part of the toxic effect of maternal smoking on disease development in their children may be mediated via tobacco smoke-mediated effects on immunologic processes in utero.

Aspects of fetal nutrition

Reports of associations between asthma/allergy and neonatal anthropometric measurements were amongst the first to highlight antenatal factors in the development of asthma and allergic disease. In 1994 Godfrey reported that elevated IgE levels in adults were associated with a larger head circumference at birth. Since this original study, increased head circumference at birth has been consistently associated with elevated IgE from birth to adulthood. Most studies indicate no association between birth head circumference and allergen specific IgE, positive skin prick tests (SPTs) or hayfever, although the largest study to date has demonstrated a positive association between head circumference and hayfever in adults. Increased head circumference at birth is a consequence of rapid fetal growth from early gestation; however, this rapid growth makes the fetus vulnerable to relative undernutrition during late gestation. If such relative undernutrition occurs, brain and head growth is maintained to the detriment of other organs, the limbs, the trunk and the thymus, possibly promoting Th2 biased immune responses. This hypothesis is not supported by reports of a positive association between birth head circumference and thymic size and that an increase in the ratio of head circumference to birth weight is associated with a reduction (and not the expected increase) in hayfever. The mechanism underlying the association between birth head circumference and serum IgE is not fully understood. It is known that birth head circumference is determined by the growth of the brain, which is influenced by numerous complex factors including fetal genetic growth potential, uterine and placental function and maternal nutrition, particularly lipids. The role of these factors has not been addressed in studies examining the associations between head circumference and IgE.

Many studies have demonstrated that reduced birth weight is associated with reduced ventilatory function, and increased risk of asthma. It is postulated that relative undernutrition during a critical period of fetal bronchial airway development leads to permanent airway changes predisposing the development of bronchial hyperreactivity, asthma and possibly chronic obstructive pulmonary disease (COPD). It is important to note that the association between asthma and reduced birth weight is not clear-cut; many studies have been unable to demonstrate such an association and some studies have demonstrated that reduced birth weight is associated with a reduced risk of asthma.

The studies relating birth measurements to asthma and allergy raise the issue of fetal nutrition. There is increasing interest in the role of maternal diet during pregnancy and the development of asthma and allergic disease; however, at present there are few studies directly investigating this. There is somewhat contradictory evidence consistent with the notion that maternal lipid intake may influence the development of childhood allergic disease. Elevated linoleic acid in cord blood lecithin has been associated with elevated cord blood IgE. The development of atopic disease has been associated with reduced cord blood arachidonic acid and dihomo-γ-linolenic acid levels. Elevated cord blood erythrocyte arachidonic acid has been associated with increased CBMC IFNγ responses, whilst elevated erythrocyte eicosapentaenoic acid (EPA) has been associated with reduced IFNγ and IL-10 responses. A maternal diet during pregnancy high in lipids has been associated with increased allergic disease in children. Dietary supplementation of atopic pregnant women with fish oil rich in EPA and docosahexaenoic acids is associated with a trend towards reduced in vitro CBMC cytokine responses.

In theory, oxidant stress during fetal airway development could potentially damage the airways and increase the likelihood of childhood asthma; these effects could potentially be ameliorated by dietary antioxidants. Maternal dietary antioxidant intake during pregnancy also has the potential to affect the fetal immune system. The potential effects of dietary antioxidants and oxidant stress during pregnancy on the development of childhood asthma and allergy have been highlighted by a number of recent studies. Paracetamol (acetaminophen) is a potential source of oxidative stress and its frequent use has been associated with an increase in childhood wheezing. There are very few studies relating maternal dietary antioxidant intake during pregnancy to the development of childhood asthma and allergic disease. A high maternal intake of vitamin E during pregnancy has been associated with reduced in vitro CBMC proliferative responses. During the second year of life a high maternal intake of vitamin E during pregnancy has been associated with reduced wheezing in the absence of a cold, and, in children born to atopic mothers, a reduced incidence of atopic eczema. A summary of possible antenatal influences on asthma and allergy is given in Table 15.3.

POSTNATAL EVENTS IN REGULATION OF ADAPTIVE IMMUNITY TO ALLERGENS

T-cell responses to inhalant allergens in early life: when does genuine T-cell 'memory' programming commence?

As noted above, a substantial literature exists which demonstrates T-cell responses to inhalant allergens in cord blood, and these findings have been widely interpreted as indicative of transplacental priming of the fetal immune system by allergens derived from the maternal circulation. However, earlier studies by some groups have pointed to the lack of correlation between levels of perennial allergen (such as house dust mite) in the maternal environment and ensuing T-cell responsiveness in their offspring. Moreover, T-cell epitope mapping studies in the authors' labs on neonatal T-cell responses to ovalbumin indicate recognition of large sections of the molecule, as opposed to a restricted range of 'immunodominant' regions as is seen in conventional T-memory responses, suggesting that mechanisms other than reactivation of T-memory cells should be considered to explain these responses.

In this context, a recent study from our group has demonstrated that the majority of $CD4^+$ Th-cell responses to allergens by CBMC are attributable to 'promiscuous' interactions between the allergens and T-cell receptors (TCRs) of functionally immature and immunologically naive recent thymic emigrants (RTE), which dominate the circulating $CD4^+$ Th-cell population in neonates. The promiscuity of the low affinity TCR/MHC II-peptide interactions in these responses may stem from structural differences relating to CDR3-region length between RTE and conventional functionally mature but immunologically naive T cells. During infancy the numbers of conventional naive

Table 15.3 Summary of possible antenatal influences on asthma and allergy

	Allergy	Asthma
Birth order	+	
Maternal allergen exposure	+/−	
Maternal cigarette smoking during pregnancy	+/−	++
Obstetric complications	+	+
Caesarean section	−	+
Maternal use of antibiotics during pregnancy	+/−	+/−
Maternal diet, polyunsaturated fatty acids, antioxidants	+/−	+/−

T cells increase progressively from very low frequencies at birth, to eventually dominate the circulating $CD4^+$ Th-cell pool. However, at birth and for a period yet to be defined during infancy, the circulating $CD4^+$ compartment predominantly comprises these RTE.

Our studies indicate that unlike the situation with $CD4^+$ $CD45RO^+$ T-memory cells responding to allergen, the response of $CD4^+$ $CD45RA^+$ RTE involves an initial burst of cytokine production, followed by death of the responding cells by apoptosis. Similar observations have been made in regards to neonatal $CD8^+$ T-cell responses in the mouse. Collectively, these data suggest the operation of a primitive mechanism in infancy for the provision of transient bursts of cytokines (i.e. 'cell mediated immunity') in tissue microenvironments at sites of antigen exposure, in advance of the development of conventional cognate Th-cell memory. This may provide a mechanism for inter alia local cytokine-induced activation of phagocytes at sites of microbial exposure during this life phase, when survival relies principally on a diminishing supply of maternal IgG. Intriguingly, our studies indicate that a further byproduct of these RTE responses to allergens is bystander activation/maturation of previously quiescent $CD4^+$ $CD25^+$ T-regulatory cells. It is not known whether these T-regulatory cells survive for long periods and hence play a role in subsequent regulation of allergic responses, but this possibility merits investigation.

If these early responses to allergy do not involve reactivation of conventional Th-memory cells, when is allergen-specific $CD4^+$ Th-memory primed? Our earlier studies on a small prospective birth cohort suggested upregulation of putative T-memory responses during the first 12 months of postnatal life (Prescott), but data were not available from that study on the 'stability' of this memory beyond the 12 month period. In a larger ongoing study on 240 infants at high risk of allergic disease (Rowe, Kusel, et al, in progress) we have recently observed the development of persistent allergen-specific IL-5 and IL-13 responses in infants between 6 and 12 months, in advance of the subsequent development of clinical sensitization (SPT reactivity) at age 2 years by the same infants, which suggests the development of genuine Th memory during this period. In contrast, the group who remain SPT-negative display progressively waning cytokine responses which decline over the same period, as non-specifically responding fetally-derived RTE die out and are replaced by fully functional naive T cells released from the thymus after birth. It remains to be determined whether postnatal Th memory generation in subsequently atopic children is influenced directly or indirectly by antenatal allergen exposure, either of the infant or the mother. In this context, we have recently shown that the Th1/Th2 balance in vaccine-specific responses in infants can be modulated by maternal-derived IgG-antivaccine antibody, present at the time of initial priming of the infant, and this provides a plausible precedent for the operation of similar mechanisms in relation to allergen-specific T-cell immunity.

Genetic risk for atopic sensitization: the role of developmental factors

Earlier studies from the authors and others indicate that genetic high risk (HR) for atopic sensitization during early childhood is associated with delayed postnatal maturation of Th-cell function, in particular with a slower-than-average rate of rebalancing the Th1/Th2 polarity of the adaptive immune system, which is strongly Th2 biased during fetal life. This results in prolonged persistence of relatively Th2-skewed immune function in HR infants, which increases the likelihood of allergen-specific Th-cell priming events leading to Th-memory cell differentiation down the Th2 pathway.

It is clear that the results of this genetically determined developmental deficiency go beyond risk for atopy, as HR children also display diminished capacity to mount stable Th1-polarized memory responses against vaccines such as BCG, pneumococcal polysaccharide, and diphtheria/pertussis/tetanus.

The mechanism(s) underlying this developmental deficiency, which is preferentially expressed in relation to Th1 immunity, are not fully understood. One possibility involves increased levels of methylation at/near transcription factor binding sites in the proximal promoter of the IFNγ gene, which we have demonstrated to be a major factor in the limitation of IFNγ gene expression in the neonatal/infant period. There is also accumulating evidence which suggests an important role for developmentally associated variations in the innate arm of the immune system, in particular in the antigen presenting cell (APC) compartment which controls the Th-cell priming process. In this regard, there is indirect evidence from our early studies, which suggest that the peripheral APC population which regulates T-cell responses to inhaled allergen, notably airway mucosal dendritic cells, are infrequent at birth, and develop into a dense network in airway tissues at a highly variable rate, between birth and weaning. It is likely that developmental changes within this network during this period are major determinants of both qualitative and quantitative aspects of the inhalant allergen-specific Th-cell priming process.

It has additionally become evident from recent studies that the developmental window within which Th1 function is reduced in the HR population, is restricted in many cases to infancy, and beyond infancy the maturation of Th1 competence rapidly accelerates in atopic children and overshoots the 'normal' range. Thus, while a deficiency in Th1 cytokine production in HR infants may contribute to the Th2 polarity of allergen-specific Th-memory responses which are primed in the early postnatal period, overcorrection of this developmental deficiency leading to hyperproduction of the same Th1 cytokines at later ages may potentially contribute towards atopy/asthma pathogenesis (Fig. 15.2).

Hygiene hypothesis

The identity of the gene(s) which contribute to these variations in the kinetics of postnatal maturation of immune function remains to be elucidated. One likely series of candidates are genes encoding pattern recognition receptors employed principally within the innate immune system. Two archetypal examples are CD14 and TLR2, both of which display polymorphisms associated with increased risk of allergy in childhood. It is likely that these genes (and other Toll receptor genes) are responsible for alerting the immune system to the change from a microbial-free to a microbial-infested outside environment following birth, and intracellular signaling from these receptor families is likely to play a central role in the differential upregulation of Th1 function in the infant immune system during early postnatal life. It is plausible to speculate that one aspect of the 'hygiene hypothesis' involves variations in the level of commensal and/or pathogen-mediated stimulation of this receptor system, i.e. reduced stimulation in a 'too clean' environment may reduce

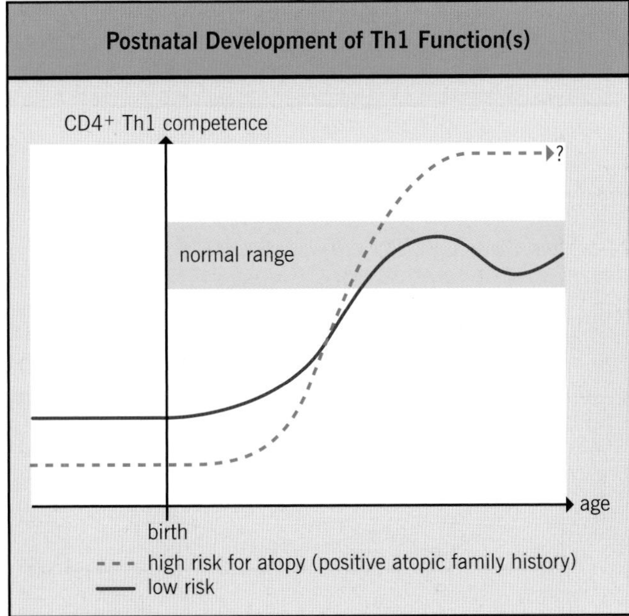

Fig. 15.2 Postnatal development of Th1 function(s).Th1, helper T cells type 1.

levels of signaling to below the critical threshold required to optimally drive this maturation process, particularly in individuals with genotype(s) associated with expression of pattern recognition receptors which are intrinsically less efficient than the population average.

CD4+ versus CD8+ Th-cell function

It is important to emphasize that the published data on the link between developmental deficiency in Th1 function and risk for atopy, are based primarily on studies on $CD4^+$ Th-cell responses. We have recently shown that developmental regulation of the expression of Th1 genes such as IFNγ in cell populations outside the $CD4^+$ Th-cell compartment differs qualitatively and quantitatively from that within $CD4^+$ Th cells. Notably, while levels of methylation in the proximal promoter of the IFNγ gene in $CD4^+$ Th cells are very high in infants relative to adults, corresponding age-related differences within $CD8^+$ T cells and natural killer (NK) populations are much less, to the extent that IFNγ production by these cells in neonates approaches that of adults. Additionally, we have recently shown that within a cohort of HR children, the expression of atopic disease at age 2 years is associated with *elevated* IFNγ responsiveness of $CD8^+$ T cells in cord blood, the opposite of what we and others have reported for $CD4^+$ T cells.

The resolution of this apparent paradox may lie in a clearer dissection of the precise contribution of each cell type to atopy pathogenesis. It is evident from the available literature that the primary role of $CD4^+$ Th-memory cells in atopy is at the level of atopic sensitization i.e. development of cytokine response patterns which drive the maturation of B cells to IgE class switching, and the parallel provision of effector T cells capable of secreting eosinophil-trophic IL-5 at allergen challenge sites. In contrast, while $CD8^+$ T cells are now recognized to also contribute towards Th2-cytokine secretion, their overall role appears to be more involved in driving disease pathogenesis at stages beyond the initial sensitization phase, in particular via Th1-like mechanisms. A compelling recent example is the demonstration of an association between numbers of activated IFNγ-producing $CD8^+$ T cells in peripheral blood and the expression of airway hyperresponsiveness in children. Consistent with the latter finding, the authors have also recently demonstrated an important role for IFNγ in synergizing with Th2 cytokines to drive asthma pathogenesis in 11 year olds. Thus the same gene operating in different cell populations may contribute to driving atopy via disparate mechanisms, acting at different stages of disease pathogenesis.

Risk for atopy versus risk for infection: double jeopardy?

As noted above, delayed postnatal maturation of Th1 function in HR children is associated not only with increased sensitization to inhalant allergens, but also with attenuated development of protective Th1-polarized immunity against microbial antigens in a variety of vaccines. A logical extension of these findings is the hypothesis that these same genetic mechanism(s) may contribute to increased risk for severe respiratory infections. Indirect evidence in support of this possibility comes from a variety of sources (review cited below). In particular, the expression of Th1 immunity appears impaired in infants and young children in whom respiratory infections attain a level of severity sufficient to trigger overt wheeze. Moreover, with viruses such as respiratory syncytial virus (RSV), it has been shown that the acquisition of RSV-specific cellular immune memory during infancy, a footprint of earlier severe infection, is most frequent in children displaying the slowest kinetics of postnatal upregulation of IFNγ response capacity. We have also shown in an ongoing study (Denburg, Holt, Sly, et al, to be published) that the development of wheeze during infancy in association with RSV infection is predicted by the number of IL-3 responsive eosinophil/basophil precursors present in cord blood. The latter represents an additional marker of overall 'Th2 polarity' of the immune system, in this case its innate component.

Synergistic interactions between infection and atopy in the pathogenesis of childhood asthma

It is clear from the results of large epidemiologic studies that while atopy is a major risk factor for asthma, it is usually not sufficient by itself to drive the disease process to chronicity, as less than 25% of atopics develop persistent asthma. The situation in childhood is further complicated by an additional series of development factors, related to postnatal maturation of respiratory function. Notably, a large proportion of children wheeze in infancy in response to airway infections, due principally to the small size of their airways. Most of these children grow through this phase and lose their tendency towards wheeze, simply as a result of airway growth (the so-called 'transient wheezers'). However, in a subset of these children, wheezing persists and may become more intense, in particular in children who develop sensitization to inhalants during infancy.

A series of large prospective birth cohort studies are progressively providing plausible mechanism(s) for the underlying processes and in doing so are supplying testable hypotheses for the etiology of persistent asthma in childhood. The key observations from these studies are:

- risk for asthma persisting beyond the preschool years is at least doubled if children become sensitized to inhalants;
- the degree of risk is inversely related to the age at which sensitization first occurs;
- risk for persistent asthma is also doubled if children contract a respiratory infection in infancy sufficiently serious to trigger wheeze;
- the risk is doubled again if more than one severe wheezing lower respiratory tract infection (wLRI) occurs during this period; and
- maximum risk, involving a further two-to-threefold increase in the odds ratios for persistent asthma, is encountered when both early sensitization to inhalant(s) and wLRI occurs in the same infant.

This suggests that inflammation due to airway allergy and airway infection can interact synergistically to drive asthma pathogenesis, presumably as a result of damage to local tissues during the critical stage of lung growth during early life. The implications are that when tissue damage attains supracritical threshold levels, irreversible changes occur to growth and differentiation programs, resulting in potentially permanent structure/function changes in lung and airway tissues, which are in turn responsible for the hyperresponsiveness to exogenous irritant stimuli characteristic of the asthmatic phenotype. This concept is supported by the results of prospective studies which indicate that analogous to long-term immunologic memory which is actively 'programmed' by experience of environmental (antigenic) stimuli (Fig. 15.3a), long- term respiratory function can similarly be shaped early in life by exogenous stimuli. Notably, infants who develop abnormal lung function tend to continue to track at the low end of the functional range as they grow into childhood, and are likely to track within this part of the range into adulthood, i.e. just as children's height tracks along centile lines as they grow, growth of lung function follows a similar process (Fig. 15.3b). This implies that insults that result in a relative loss of lung function in early life will have potentially permanent effects, and this possibility is supported by the results of recent studies.

Thus, the key to protection against asthma may lie in the early identification of children who are at HR of early lung and airway damage due to atopy and respiratory infection, with parallel development of more effective drugs for the amelioration of airway inflammation in this very young age group.

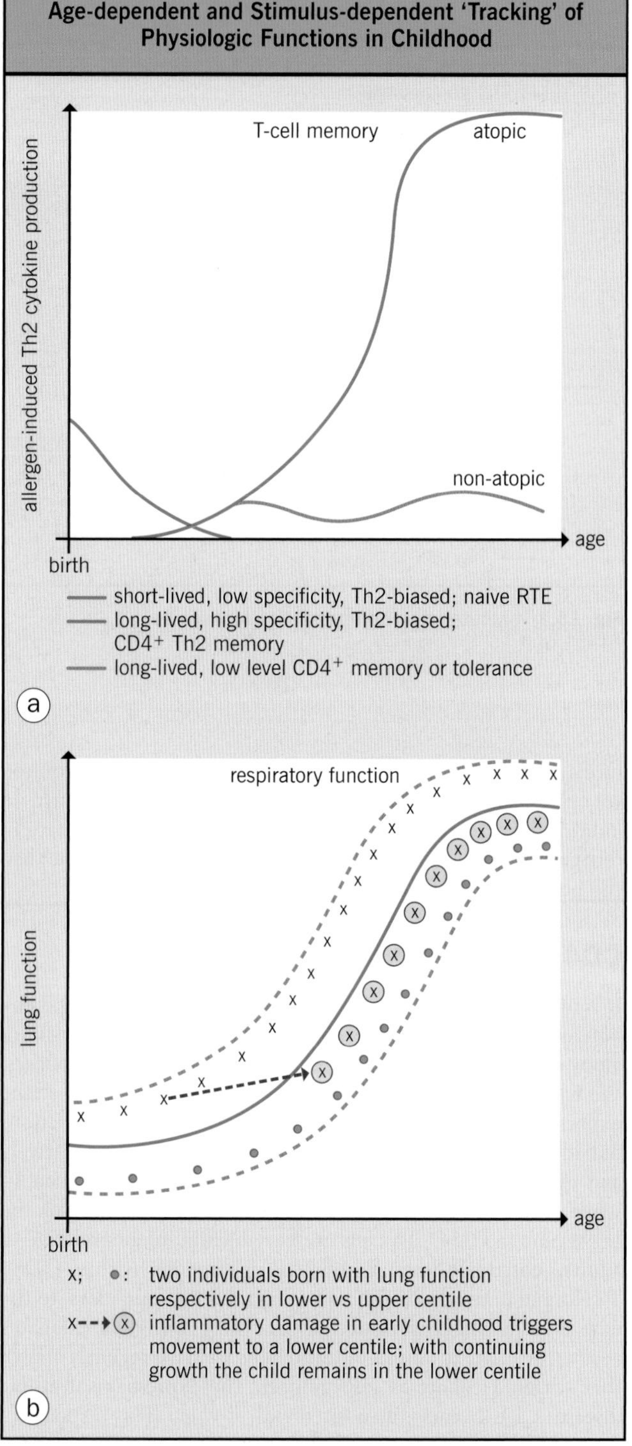

Fig. 15.3 Age-dependent and stimulus-dependent 'tracking' of physiologic functions in childhood (a) T-cell memory, (b) respiratory function. RTE, recent thymic emigrants; Th2, helper T cells type 2.

FURTHER READING

Gilliland FD, Li YF, Peters JM. Effects of maternal smoking during pregnancy and environmental tobacco smoke on asthma and wheezing in children. Am J Respir Crit Care Med 2001; 163:429–436.

Heaton T, Rowe J, Turner S, et al. An immunoepidemiological approach to asthma: identification of *in vitro* T-cell response patterns associated with different wheezing phenotypes amongst 11 year olds. Lancet 2005; 365:142–149.

Hibbert ME, Hudson IL, Lanigan A, et al. Tracking of lung function in healthy children and adolescents. Pediatr Pulmonol 1990; 8:172–177.

Holt, PG, Macaubas C. Development of long term tolerance versus sensitisation to environmental allergens during the perinatal period. Curr Opin Immunol 1997; 9:782–787.

Holt, PG, Sly PD. Interactions between respiratory tract infections and atopy in the aetiology of asthma. Eur Respir J 2002; 19:538–545.

Holt PG, Sly PD, Martinez FD, et al. Drug development strategies for asthma: in search of a new paradigm. Nature Immunol 2004; 5:695–698.

Katz KA, Pocock SJ, Strachan DP. Neonatal head circumference, neonatal weight, and risk of hayfever, asthma and eczema in a large cohort of adolescents from Sheffield, England. Clin Exp Allergy 2003; 33:737–745.

Kramer MS, Kakuma R. Maternal dietary antigen avoidance during pregnancy and/or lactation for preventing or treating atopic disease in the child. The Cochrane Database of Systemic Reviews 2003; volume 1.

Macaubas C, de Klerk NH, Holt BJ, et al. Association between antenatal cytokine production and the development of atopy and asthma at age 6 years. Lancet 2003; 362:1192–1197.

Prescott SL, Macaubas C, Smallacombe T, et al. Development of allergen-specific T-cell memory in atopic and normal children. Lancet 1999; 353:196–200.

Raghupathy R. Pregnancy: success and failure within the Th1/Th2/Th3 paradigm. Sem Immunol 2001; 13:219–227.

Strachan DP, Cook DG. Health effects of passive smoking 5. Parental smoking and allergic sensitisation in children. Thorax 1998; 53: 117–123.

Thornton CA, Vance GHS. The placenta: a portal of fetal allergen exposure. Clin Exp Allergy 2002; 32:1537–1539.

Thornton CA, Upham JW, Wikström ME, et al. Functional maturation of $CD4^+$ $CD25^+$ $CTLA4^+$ $CD45RA^+$ T-regulatory cells in human neonatal T-cell responses to environmental allergens. J Immunol 2004; 173:3084–3092.

Woodcock A, Lowe LA, Murray CS, et al. 2004. Early life environmental control: effect of symptoms, sensitization and lung function at age 3 years. Am J Respir Crit Care Med 2004; 170:433–439.

Chapter 16

Definition:

The epidemiology of allergic disease is concerned with the definitions, determinants and distribution of allergic disease and their prevention, management, morbidity and mortality.

Epidemiology of Allergic Disease

Julian Crane, Erika von Mutius, and Adnan Custovic

INTRODUCTION

Epidemiology is in part an extension of clinical practice to populations rather than individuals. It is thus concerned with the definition of disease, agents, or factors that might cause or predispose to disease, morbidity and mortality, and the effect of therapy and prevention, in populations rather than individuals. At the most straightforward level this involves defining a population and measuring disease frequency at a single point in time. Such population surveys may suggest factors that are associated with disease that can be quantified in terms of risk. A large number of such cross-sectional studies have been undertaken to measure the prevalence of allergic disease and explore risk factors. Where risk factors are thought to play an important role in early life, such as in the development of atopy, populations should be studied from birth and followed over time so that the temporal relationship between exposure and disease incidence can be established and problems of recall are minimized. Rather than examine a defined population for disease frequency, cases of a disease and suitable controls without disease may be compared for the frequency of known or suspected risk factors. Such an approach is particularly useful where the disease or an aspect of a disease is uncommon. Such a case control approach has been used for example to study asthma mortality, which is too uncommon to study prospectively.

This chapter will not attempt a complete review of the epidemiology of allergic disease. Rather, it will focus on asthma and follow a population 'clinical' approach, examining the definition and measurement of prevalence, changes in prevalence over time and by place; major risk factors, and in particular those associated with the hygiene hypothesis; and lastly discuss population 'treatment' or intervention studies of primary (preventing disease development) and secondary prevention (reducing morbidity or severity).

Population studies of asthma and rhinitis have been beset by three problems: the lack of agreed definitions; the need to distinguish the disease state from triggers of acute attacks; and the relationships between clinical disease and atopy. Epidemiologic studies rely heavily on reported symptoms of disease. For asthma, these include episodic wheezing, cough unassociated with upper respiratory tract infection, and shortness of breath. The frequency and severity of such symptoms are highly variable, ranging from occasional to persistent and from trivial to life threatening. The hallmark of descriptions of clinical asthma is that these symptoms are associated with episodes of airway obstruction that can be measured, and fall outside the range of normal variation. Such variability makes epidemiologic study difficult because serial measurement of lung function over time is usually impractical in population studies. One abnormality of the airway commonly associated with asthma that can be quantified is airway hyperresponsiveness (AHR). This refers to a heightened state of responsiveness of the airway to a wide variety of stimuli, including the increased ventilation with exercise, and a variety of non-specific bronchoconstrictor agonists, such as histamine and methacholine. Such agonists can be used to quantify an airway response in terms of the provocative dose causing a decrease in peak expiratory flow rate (PEFR), forced air expiratory volume in 1 second (FEV_1) or an increase in airways resistance. But airway hyperresponsiveness, while very common amongst those with asthma and often showing a relationship with asthma severity, is neither necessary nor sufficient. Studies that have examined seasonal asthma in relation to pollen exposure have shown that AHR increases and decreases in response to allergen exposure. In population studies, a proportion of subjects will demonstrate increased airway responsiveness without any clear history of asthma symptoms. A further practical difficulty is that AHR will reduce in the face of regular antiinflammatory treatment. Its value in the epidemiology of asthma has been the subject of considerable debate. Recently non-invasive methods of assessing airway inflammation such as exhaled nitric oxide have become available and reasonably standardized. Reliable portable methods of measurement may soon be available for epidemiologic studies.

Epidemiologic studies of rhinitis are arguably even more problematic than asthma and have been undertaken less frequently. Again, studies rely on reported symptoms of rhinitis that may be clearly seasonal (hayfever) and related to pollen exposure, or perennial. Symptoms include rhinorrhea, sneezing, nasal itching, and nasal blockage. Symptoms may include conjunctival irritation and lachrymation – rhinoconjunctivitis. Such symptoms are non-specific and in questionnaire surveys may be confused with viral upper respiratory tract infections. Allergic dermatitis presents similar problems. The peak incidence is in infancy when rashes are common. While the more severe cases of these diseases are clinically obvious, the less severe may be easily misinterpreted in questionnaire surveys. While atopy can be relatively easily assessed by skin prick tests or measurement of specific IgE, asthma, rhinitis, and dermatitis can all occur in the absence of atopy.

DEFINING ASTHMA

No agreed formal definition of asthma exists. There are no diagnostic tests or gold standards and thus what has been attempted are succinct descriptions. In recent years these have included statements noting airway inflammation and airway hyperresponsiveness. Almost all descriptions have included reference to the common symptoms of wheezing, coughing, and breathlessness and emphasized the importance of reversible airway obstruction. Measurable airway obstruction, usually with simple spirometry, remains the hallmark of clinical asthma. Symptoms, airflow obstruction and to a lesser extent AHR tend to be intermittent, and to improve with antiinflammatory treatment. It is thus possible in population surveys to find individuals with a history of asthma who have no symptoms, no evidence of airway obstruction, and no AHR at a single point in time. This has meant that definitions that include airway obstruction are not particularly useful for epidemiologic studies. Epidemiologic definitions have therefore tended to rely on self or a parental report of symptoms such as wheezing or attacks of asthma, usually confined to a short time period such as a year. A previous doctor's diagnosis of asthma or the use of asthma treatments, or a combination of symptom history and diagnosis and increased AHR have also been used in prevalence surveys. Such definitions, while useful in single reasonably uniform populations at one point in time, are likely to be less useful over time in the same population or between different populations with dissimilar community awareness or interpretation of symptoms, and with different management and treatment practices.

Having asthma versus having an attack of asthma

When considering the epidemiology of asthma and allergic disease it is useful to try and distinguish between attacks of asthma and their triggers and the underlying asthmatic state and factors that might predispose to it. 'Exercise induced asthma' for example is commonly referred to in asthma studies. Exercise induces bronchoconstriction in 70–80% of asthmatic children, but no amount of exercise will actually cause asthma. Inhaling allergen will also induce bronchoconstriction amongst asthmatics sensitized to that allergen. In contrast to exercise, allergen exposure leads to sensitization and to the development of the asthmatic state by inducing airway inflammation. Both are risk factors for an attack of asthma, but allergen exposure is also a risk factor for the development of the asthmatic state.

Allergic disease and atopy

The nomenclature for the three common allergic diseases has been problematic and has not kept pace with our understanding of them. Asthma is derived from the Greek meaning panting; eczema from the Greek meaning to boil out, used originally to describe any fiery pustules; hayfever, which describes neither the source of the allergenic material nor the clinical features is used to describe allergic seasonal rhinitis. Early qualifiers for asthma included bronchial or cardiac, the latter describing left ventricular failure. Later, extrinsic was used to describe asthma in which an obvious external cause was apparent, most commonly atopy, or intrinsic, where no obvious cause was apparent. These qualifiers have largely been dropped following studies in the early1990s that showed a linear relationship between total IgE and the risk of persistent asthma, independent of specific sensitization, suggesting that most asthma in childhood was related to allergy. Recently, these relationships have been questioned with evidence of recurrent wheezing in childhood where no obvious allergy is apparent; however no new nomenclature has been adopted. Various partial phenotypes have been described in childhood. For example, wheezing associated with respiratory infections is very common before 3 years of age. The majority of these children grow out of their wheezing by 6 years unless they become atopic. Nevertheless, persistent and severe wheezing in childhood is most commonly associated with atopy, with severity related to the degree of sensitization. Wheezy bronchitis, which was previously used to describe wheezing in early childhood associated with respiratory tract infections, was also dropped in the 1970s, and is discussed later in this chapter.

In this chapter the terms used will not follow a rigid nomenclature, given that the literature contains a variety of terms with varying definitions. In general, asthma will be used to describe recurrent episodic wheezing associated with airflow obstruction. Hayfever will be used interchangeably with allergic rhinitis, while acknowledging that hayfever usually denotes seasonal symptoms related to pollen exposure. Eczema will be used interchangeably with atopic dermatitis, while acknowledging that eczema occurs in the absence of atopy. Atopy is used to denote or describe individuals who produce specific IgE in response to an allergen, an allergen being anything that promotes the development of specific IgE.

ASTHMA PREVALENCE OVER TIME

The rise in the prevalence of asthma, allergic disease, and atopy is the most consistent epidemiologic observation about asthma and allergic disorders of the last 40 years. The evidence is based on a large number of repeat cross-sectional studies of the prevalence of asthma and allergic disease, predominantly in children and adolescents from many countries. The prevalence rates for asthma or wheezing reported in these studies vary from 2–3% to more than 40% and the annual rates of increase similarly show large variation. This is not surprising, given that there is wide variation in the definitions of asthma used in these studies. The majority of studies have relied on self-reported symptoms or a prior diagnosis of disease.

Interest in the rising prevalence of asthma and allergic disease especially in the last 30 years has not been confined to researchers but increasingly to healthcare funders, concerned with the management of asthma. Asthma tends to begin in childhood, often requires ongoing treatment with antiinflammatory therapy and intermittently with bronchodilators. For a very small minority with severe exacerbations, hospital treatment and intensive support in intensive care facilities may be required. For these reasons there has been considerable interest and concern over the rising prevalence and rising costs of asthma management.

Even when the definition is restricted, for example to a self-reported diagnosis in economically developed countries, there remains a wide variation in reported prevalence, and the rate of increase in prevalence (Fig. 16.1). Thus in the early 1990s the prevalence varied from 2.8% in Finland to over 10% in Scotland to 30% in Australia.

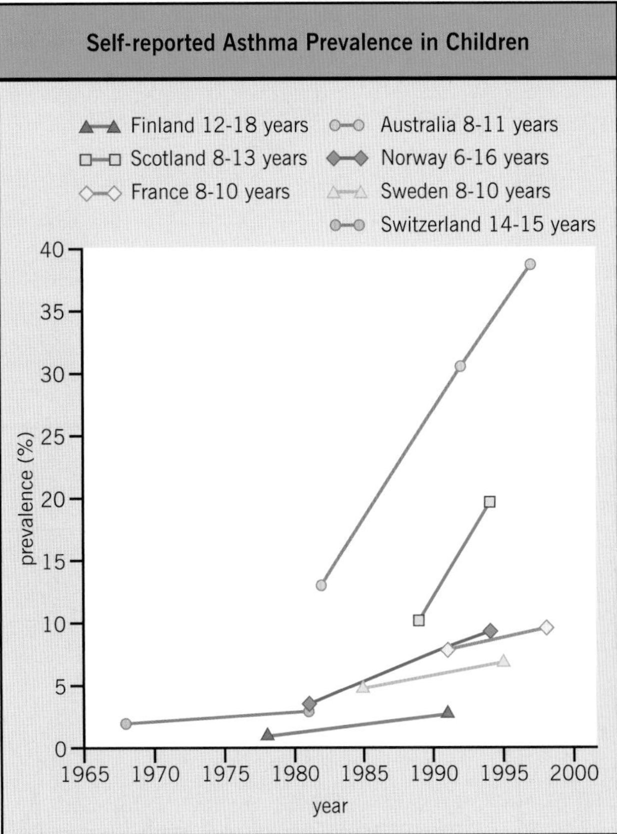

Fig. 16.1 Self-reported asthma prevalence in children.

It is of course impossible to study an identical population over time; either you must select similar subjects characterized by age and location or follow the same subjects through time, when age itself will affect the disease state. Repeat cross-sectional studies as in Figure 16.1 attempt the former approach. Populations of the same age are chosen in the same location, but geographic locations are also likely to change. In and out migration from cities or parts of cities may alter the distribution of ethnicity or socioeconomic status. Similarly programs of urban renewal and housing costs will alter the population mix. Diagnostic fashion will inevitably change over time. In turn this is likely to influence media awareness and, through the media, community awareness of disease and symptoms that are considered important. The rise of asthma societies and asthma campaigns will alter community and health professionals' perceptions of disease. Community perceptions are likely to be particularly important in cross-sectional studies where an increased emphasis on symptoms such as wheezing and their specific treatment is likely to significantly improve recall in questionnaire surveys.

Such a diagnostic shift occurred for asthma in the late 1960s and through the 1970s. Early surveys of asthma prevalence, particularly in the UK, collected information on asthma and wheezy bronchitis. The latter term was used to describe children who were wheezy only with respiratory tract infections. The term asthma was used to describe children who would wheeze with and without colds. In a national longitudinal birth cohort, the prevalence of a history of wheezing by the age of 7 years for children born in the UK in the 1950s was 18%. Of these, 3% were considered to have asthma and 15% wheezy bronchitis. The study also identified the poor recall of wheezing. Between the ages of 7 and 11 years, two-thirds of parents who had reported wheezy bronchitis before 7 years denied any history at 11 years amongst children who had not had recurring symptoms. The study illustrates how an increased awareness and medical emphasis on a symptom like wheezing could significantly increase recall. Just how prevalent wheezing is, has recently been shown in New Zealand. A longitudinal study from 3 years of age to early adulthood showed that 70% of the population reported wheezing on at least one occasion and 50% on at least two. Given that there will still be problems with recall of infrequent and mild symptoms, these results suggest that wheezing is a common, virtually universal phenomenon.

The change in labeling from wheezy bronchitis to asthma occurred in the late 1960s and early 1970s, particularly in English-speaking countries following recognition that apart from severity and frequency of symptoms, there was little difference in the natural history of asthma or wheezy bronchitis. In the 1980s, the therapeutic importance of this change was also emphasized. The majority of children with recurrent wheezing was not being labeled clinically as having asthma and consequently was rarely receiving bronchodilators. The majority was labeled as having wheezy bronchitis and received multiple courses of antibiotics. When a diagnosis of asthma was made, bronchodilators and inhaled corticosteroids were much more likely to

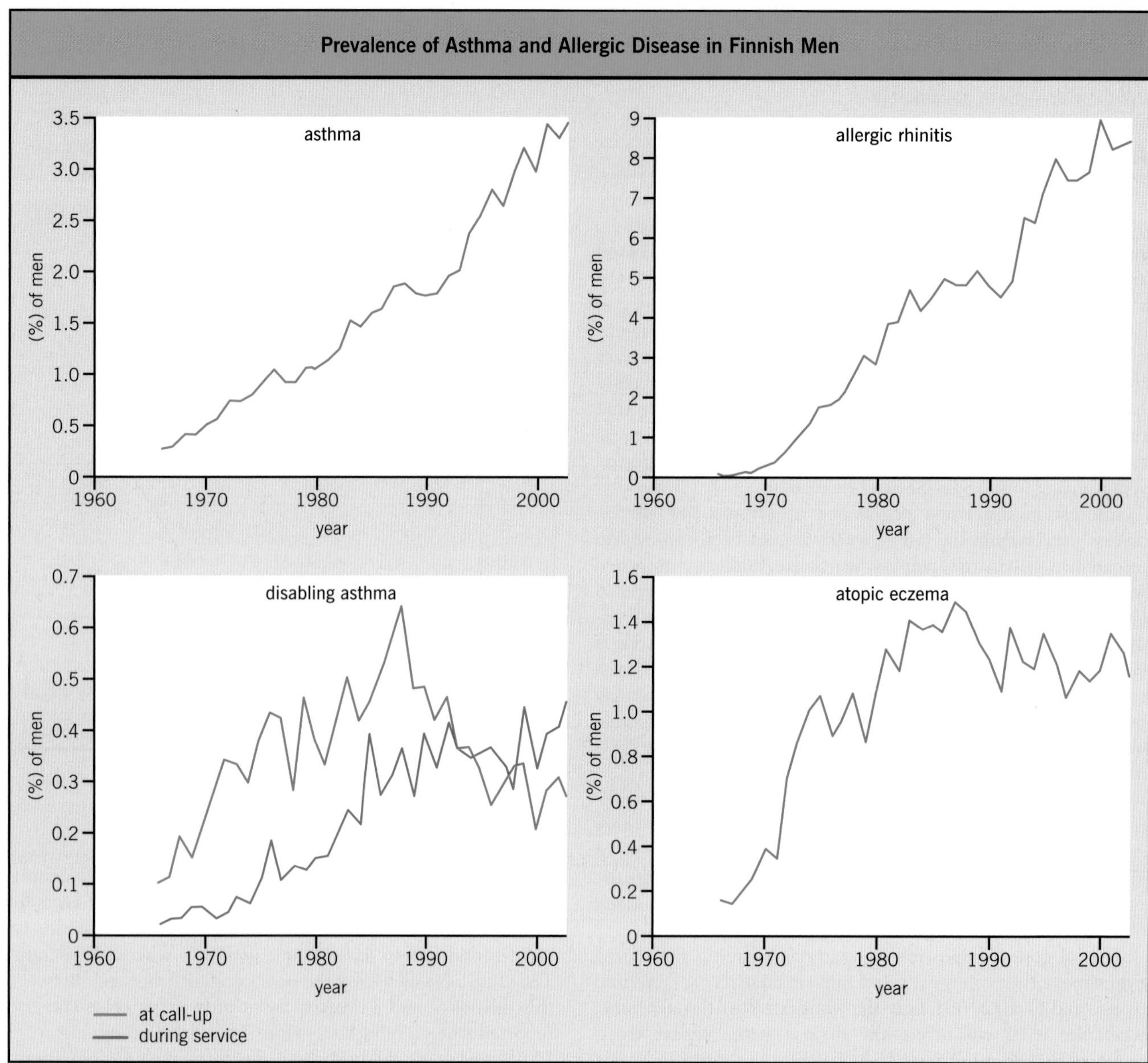

Fig. 16.2 Prevalence of asthma, allergic rhinitis and atopic eczema amongst Finnish conscripts and percentage of men discharged at call up or during service because of disabling asthma. Redrawn from Latvala J, Von Hertzen L, Lindholm H, et al. Trends in prevalence of asthma and allergy in Finnish young men: nationwide study 1966–2003. BMJ 2005; 330:1186–1187.

be prescribed. Treating these children with bronchodilators led to a marked improvement in their symptoms and absence from school. These studies had a marked influence on thinking about wheezing illness in childhood and the change in label led to a much greater use of asthma treatments. To what extent these factors are responsible for the increased prevalence of asthma and reported asthma symptoms is unknown and largely unknowable. They are, however, important to bear in mind when considering changes in asthma prevalence over time.

Despite these reservations, some studies do provide prevalence information that, while not entirely free of these issues, minimizes them. One such study from Finland initially reported data on a previous diagnosis of asthma from almost one million men called up for compulsory military service between 1960 and 1989, with some data from 1926 to 1938. The authors also reported data on subjects exempted from military service at call up because of disabling asthma and on subjects initially accepted but who were discharged early because of their asthma severity. The sample represented 98% of males in Finland aged 20 and issues of changes in economic status except at a national level are excluded. The data were not collected with any intention of looking at asthma prevalence but simply for the acceptability of recruits for military service. The data would be subject to the diagnostic fashion of medical practitioners between the 1960s and 1980s. However, the parallel increases in those declined entry and those discharged early because of asthma would not. Recently this study has been updated to 2003 (Fig. 16.2). The prevalence of reported asthma and allergic rhinitis only started to increase after 1960 and has continued to increase ever since. Reported atopic eczema appeared to plateau in the 1980s. Exemptions at call up for asthma have declined since the 1990s and during service have plateaued, suggesting that asthma management has improved.

Given the problems associated with collecting asthma prevalence data over time it is surprising that so few studies have included measurements of airway hyperresponsiveness as an objective marker associated with asthma. A study in Wales over 15 years amongst 11-year-old children showed an increase in reported symptoms but no rise in the prevalence of exercise induced bronchospasm. In Australia, a study in children showed an increased prevalence of symptoms and airway hyperresponsiveness over 10 years. The increase in AHR was predominantly amongst atopic individuals, although the prevalence of atopy was unchanged. A study amongst Belgian conscripts aged between 18 and 19 years that included measures of AHR showed an increase in the reported history of asthma and in AHR. The age adjusted proportion of asthmatics with AHR remained stable, suggesting that the increased reporting of asthma could not be wholly ascribed to changes in diagnostic labeling. Studies comparing prevalence over the last decade have suggested that the rise in prevalence, at least in economically developed countries, has reached a peak or may even have declined slightly.

The interpretation then, of trends in asthma and asthma symptom prevalence, is rather unsatisfactory. There is a serious dearth of studies with objective markers of asthma such as AHR, and in the few with such measures, conflicting evidence of an increased prevalence. There has undoubtedly been a large shift in ascribing wheezing illness to asthma rather than wheezy bronchitis; this must explain an indeterminate proportion of the increase in prevalence. Studies where these problems are minimized have also shown an increased prevalence, suggesting that the change in diagnostic labeling and the increased community awareness cannot explain all of the increase. Furthermore, despite large variation in studies repeated over a variable time period virtually all of them, whether in economically developed or less developed countries, show an increased prevalence, suggesting either multiple risk factors increasing simultaneously or a worldwide increase in one or more risk factors. The reasons for this worldwide rise in asthma prevalence and the recent plateau in developed countries are unknown. The evidence from Finland, and from other studies, particularly in the USA, suggests that the increased prevalence began in the early 1960s.

ATOPY PREVALENCE OVER TIME

In seeking a cause for the increased prevalence of asthma and allergic disease an increased sensitization to common environmental allergens is a prime candidate. In exploring allergen sensitivity the problems of diagnostic change are avoided. Changes to the materials or methods used for skin prick testing, for example, or analytical techniques for specific IgE remain a potential problem. Few repeat cross-sectional studies of sensitization in random populations have been undertaken. Where they have, they also tend to show significant increases in the prevalence of atopy. These studies in general populations show an increased prevalence of sensitization to local allergens rather than to any specific allergen.

ASTHMA AND ALLERGIC DISEASE PREVALENCE BY PLACE

Risk factors associated with disease can also be found by studying the variation in prevalence and risk factors between different communities. Only recently have such studies for allergic disease been undertaken using identical methods. Two such large initiatives have been developed, the European Community Respiratory Health Survey (ECRHS) in adults and the International Study of Asthma and Allergies in Childhood (ISAAC). The ECRHS study used validated questionnaires and measured airway responsiveness and atopy in 36 centers from 16 countries involving around 18 000 subjects in the early 1990s. The study was conducted in two phases, an initial one page questionnaire to 3000 20–44-year-old adults, followed by a random sample of phase 1 responders, and an enriched sample of positive wheezing responders, invited to undertake a methacholine challenge and an assessment of atopic status with skin prick tests and IgE. It was the first study to systematically explore asthma and allergic disease across a range of predominantly European countries. Many local center, country and combined analyses have been reported and were summarized in 2001. This study is by far the largest study in adults to determine prevalence of symptoms, AHR and atopy (Table 16.1). The study has also reported on many risk factors for asthma and allergic disease (Table 16.2). The database has been interrogated as new hypotheses are generated in smaller studies. Two key geographic findings were the high prevalence of asthma, AHR and atopy in English-speaking countries and the east–west gradient within Europe.

The ISAAC study is an even larger initiative in children that commenced at about the same time. This study took a slightly different approach by commencing with a simple written questionnaire to the parents of 5–6- year-old children and both written and video questionnaires to 13–14-year-olds. This approach was specifically adopted to allow many less economically developed countries to participate, many producing data on the prevalence of allergic disease for the first time. The prevalence of asthma symptoms from the written and video questionnaire, and allergic rhinoconjunctivitis and atopic eczema by country and center within countries is shown in Figure 16.3. A second phase of this study involving 30 centers in 20 countries measuring symptom prevalence, AHR and atopy, and a number of risk factors including allergen and endotoxin exposure has been completed but not yet reported. A repeat of the initial cross-sectional study has also just been completed and will provide information on changing asthma symptom prevalence internationally in more than 100 countries over a 5–10 year period.

A similar geographic pattern is seen in the ISAAC study as in the ECRHS, with a high prevalence of asthma and allergic disease in English-speaking countries, a clear east–west gradient within Europe and a lower reported prevalence in less economically developed countries. Some of the variation in ISAAC will be related to the translation of the term wheezing and the interpretation and importance attached to wheezing in the various communities. In an attempt to reduce this variation the video questionnaire sought information by showing wheezing and asking children if they recognized such symptoms in themselves. In general the prevalence of symptoms reported from the video questionnaire was lower than from the written one but the ranking of prevalence was highly correlated between the two questionnaires, suggesting that the differences in prevalence between countries were not related solely to interpretation.

The ECRHS study in adults and ISAAC in children are the first comprehensive international cross-sectional studies of

Table 16.1 Median prevalence percentage and ranges of various symptoms and exposures from the European Community Respiratory Health Survey (ECRHS)

	Centers	Median	Range
Symptoms			
Wheeze	48	20.7	41.1–32.0
Waking with breathlessness	47	7.3	1.5–11.4
Waking with cough	48	27.9	6.0–42.6
Asthma and rhinitis			
Current asthma (stage 1)	48	4.5	2.0–11.9
Current asthma (stage 2)	34	5.2	1.2–13.0
Nasal allergy and hayfever	45	20.9	9.5–40.9
Bronchial responsiveness			
$PD_{20} \geq 1$ mg	35	13.0	3.4–27.8
ECRHS slope (mean)	35	7.6	6.7–8.4
Allergic sensitization			
Mite	35	20.3	6.7–35.1
Cat	35	8.5	2.7–14.8
Timothy	35	18.0	8.1–34.6
Cladosporium	35	2.4	0.3–13.6
Any allergy	35	33.1	16.2–44.5
IgE (geometric mean) kU/L	35	35.9	13.2–62.2
Exposure			
Male smokers	34	38	17–65
Female smokers	34	33	14–52
Gas stoves	34	63.0	0–100
Cat ownership	35	20.1	3.7–68.6
Heredity			
Asthma prevalence in patients	30	5.8	3.4–10.6
Treatment			
Asthma medication (stage 1)	48	3.5	0.6–9.8
Inhaled bronchodilators	34	4.6	0.7–12.4
Inhaled antiinflammatory drugs	34	2.8	0.3–8.2
Oral antiasthmatics	34	1.4	0.2–6.5

The countries involved with the number of centers in parentheses are: Algeria (1), Australia (1), Austria (1), Belgium (2), Denmark (1), Estonia (1), France (5), Germany (2), Greece (1), Iceland (1), India (1), Ireland (2), Italy (3), Netherlands (3), New Zealand (4), Norway (1), Portugal (2), Spain (6), Sweden (3), Switzerland (1), UK (5), USA (1). PD_{20}, provocative dose that causes a 20% fall in forced expiratory volume in 1 second (FEV_1).

asthma and allergic disease to use the same validated instruments. They have confirmed, for the first time, large variations in the prevalence of allergic disease between and within countries. The ECRHS study has also provided evidence for both risk and protective factors that are associated with these diseases. Such large scale international studies have been commonplace in cardiovascular epidemiology for decades and have provided a wealth of data about risk and protective factors. Further collaborative studies to explore both the early development and prevention of allergic disease would seem likely and appropriate directions in the future.

RISK FACTORS FOR ASTHMA AND ATOPY

Studies of risk factors for atopy and allergic disease over the last decade have been dominated by the hygiene hypothesis. This hypothesis suggests that atopy is positively related to hygiene in its broadest sense. The mechanism postulated is that reduced infection and bacterial exposure in early life favors a helper T cell type 2 (Th2) phenotype that promotes the development of atopy. The concept of an inverse relationship between infectious and allergic disease was first suggested in the mid 1970s from studies of the Métis Indians in Saskatchewan who had shown very low levels of atopic disease associated with frequent bacterial, viral, and helminth infections. The associations were rediscovered in the late 1980s when a plausible immunologic mechanism was available. The hypothesis has many attractive features in terms of explaining some of the time trends for the rising prevalence of atopy and allergic disease and for the higher prevalence of allergic disease in wealthier countries and in the last decade has led to many avenues of enquiry.

The initial epidemiologic associations were from cohort studies in the UK where firstborn children had more hayfever than subsequent children. A greater exposure to infections from older siblings was suggested as the protective mechanism. Many studies have subsequently confirmed this sibling effect

Table 16.2 Variables explaining variation in the prevalence of wheeze, asthma, atopic sensitization and bronchial responsiveness in the European Community Respiratory Health Survey (ECRHS)

	Wheeze	Asthma	Bronchial responsiveness	Atopic sensitization
Age	(-)	(-)		-
Female sex		- (in childhood) + (in adulthood)	(+)	-
Rhinitis		+	+	+
Allergic sensitization	(+)	(+)	+	
Current smoking	(+)		(+)	+ (to mite) - (to grass and cat)
Indoor environment				
Gas cooking	+ (in women*)			
Cat ownership				+ (to cat in subjects without symptoms)
Damp dwelling	(+)	(+)	(+)	
Occupational exposure	+	+	+	
Genetic disposition				
Parental asthma		+	(+)	
Parental atopy				(+)
Childhood risk factors				
Number of siblings	(-)	(-)	(-)	-
Dog in childhood				-
Cat in childhood				- (to cat in subjects with atopic heredity)
Severe respiratory infections before the age of 5 years		(+)		

*, Heterogeneity between centers; +, positive association; -, negative association; parentheses indicate the association was shown in local analysis, as opposed to the whole data set. From Janson C, Anto J, Burney P, et al. European Community Respiratory Health S, II. The European Community Respiratory Health Survey: what are the main results so far? European Community Respiratory Health Survey II. Eur Respir J 2001; 18(3):598–611.

although the mechanism via infections remains to be proven. Further support comes from day care attendance in infancy and subsequent protection from allergic disease and atopy in later childhood. These children experience more wheezing in infancy (possibly related to increased viral respiratory infections) but less in later childhood (related to less atopic asthma). A variety of early life specific infections such as measles, hepatitis A, and a variety of orofecal and food-borne infections have been associated with reduced atopy and atopic disease in large population studies. Extensions of this hypothesis have explored antibiotic use and the gut microbiota.

Cross-sectional studies of antibiotic use particularly in the first year of life suggest an increased risk of allergic disease associated with early broad spectrum antibiotics. Causal hypotheses include early disturbance of the infant gut flora, thereby altering immune development. Reverse causation has been suggested as a non-causal explanation for these findings, and longitudinal studies have failed to confirm the relationship. Allied to these associations are studies of gut flora and their possible associations with the development of atopy. Infant gut flora has been shown to vary by atopy and in countries with high and low prevalence rates for atopy in small cross-sectional and prospective studies. Non-atopic children had higher counts of enterococci and bifidobacteria in the first year of life compared to atopic children, whereas atopic children were more likely to be colonized by staphylococci and clostridia. Probiotics in early infancy have been shown in one small randomized controlled trial to protect against the development of eczema at 2 years, but with no apparent effect on atopy. No obvious biological mechanism is apparent for why such differences in bowel flora might be immunologically important.

Amongst the most striking data supporting the hygiene hypothesis are those from studies of farming and non-farming rural children in central Europe. In a series of studies, 6–13-year-old children raised on farms in early life had significantly less atopy, asthma, and hayfever than children in the same rural environment but not raised on a farm. The protective effects were largely explained by contact with farm animals and unpasteurized milk in the first year of life. For children exposed to both in the first year compared to neither, the odds of having wheezing in the last year, atopy or hayfever were 0.17 (95%CI 0.07–0.45), 0.32 (95%CI 0.17–0.62), and 0.20 (95%CI 0.08–0.50) respectively. The authors then explored the relationships between mattress endotoxin and allergic outcomes in these children. The reduced prevalence was associated with higher mattress endotoxin exposure in the farming compared to the non-farming children. Polymorphisms for Toll-like receptors that increase receptor expression on antigen presenting cells appear to be associated with the apparent protective effect of farming and high endotoxin exposure but

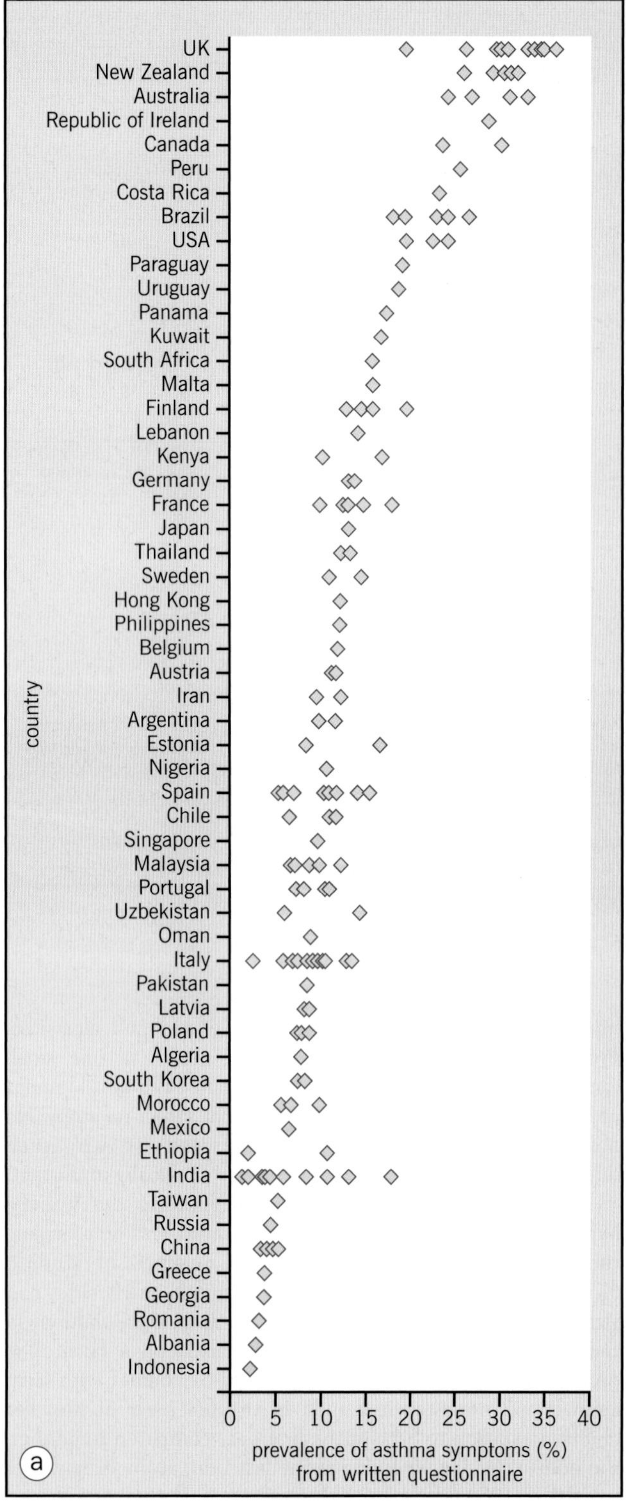

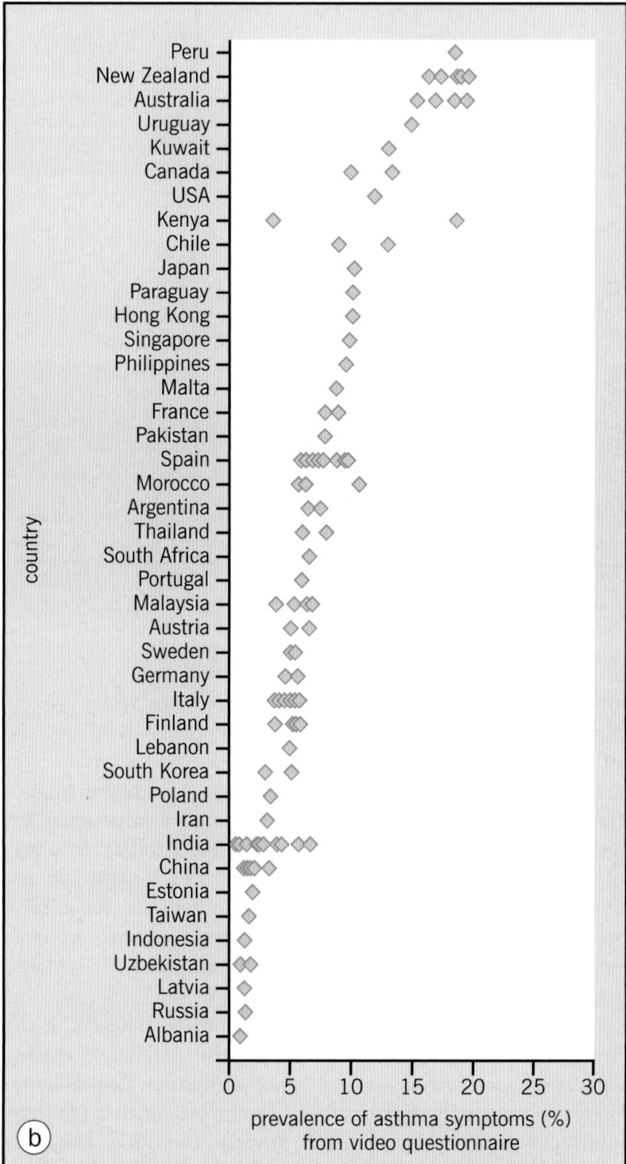

Fig. 16.3 (a) Prevalence of self-reported wheezing (%) in the last 12 months, from the written questionnaire, amongst 13–14-year-olds. [ISAAC Steering Committee. Worldwide variations in the prevalence of symptoms of asthma, allergic rhinoconjunctivitis and atopic eczema: The International Study of Asthma and Allergies in Childhood (ISAAC). Lancet 1998; 351:1225–1232)] (b) Prevalence of self-reported wheezing (%) in the last 12 months, from the video questionnaire, amongst 13–14-year-olds.

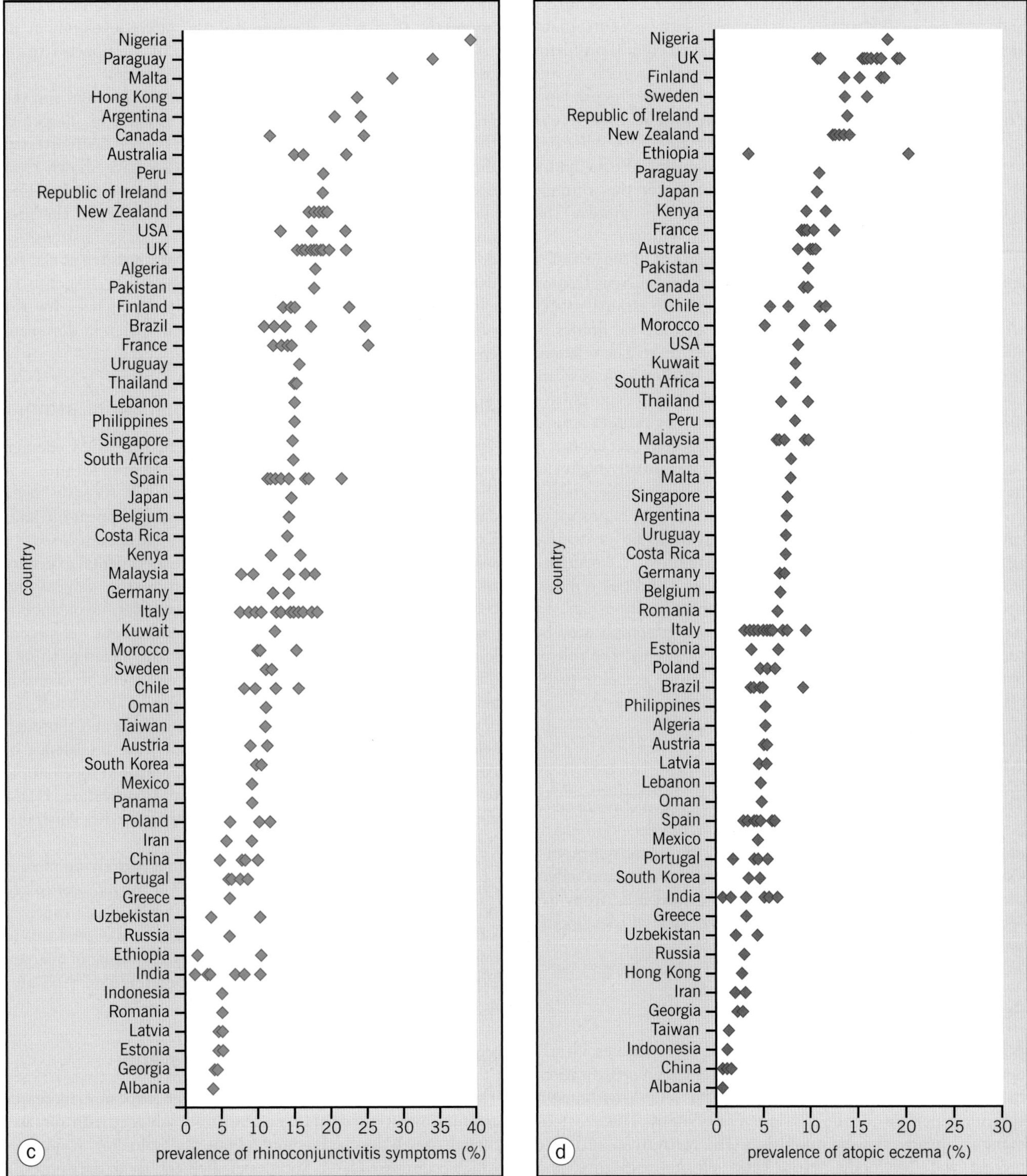

Fig. 16.3 cont'd (c) Prevalence of self-reported symptoms of rhinoconjunctivitis symptoms (%) in the last 12 months, amongst 13–14-year-olds. (d) Prevalence of self-reported atopic eczema (%) in the last 12 months amongst 13–14-year-olds.

have no effect in non-farming or low endotoxin environments. Endotoxin, which is the lipopolysaccharide component of Gram-negative bacteria (and fungal cell walls), is of particular interest. When inhaled it gives rise to wheezing in both asthmatic and non-asthmatic subjects, associated with a neutrophilic airway inflammation. It presents occupational clinical problems amongst those exposed to high concentrations such as pig farmers and sewage workers, and is thought to be the principal cause of byssinosis amongst cotton textile workers. Exposure in the domestic environment has been associated with wheezing in infancy. Paradoxically, it also has immunologic effects, and is an important bacterial recognition molecule for the immune system. In this way exposure in infancy may promote a Th1 phenotype and protect against Th2 mediated atopy.

The role of domestic pets in the development of sensitization and allergic disease is currently highly controversial. Sensitization to pet allergens is common and associations with asthma attacks well documented. Advice to remove pets from the homes of allergic children has been standard for many years. The relationships between pets and the development of allergic disease are complicated by three factors. Firstly, a number of reports have recently suggested that early dog exposure may protect against the development of allergic disease. A suggested mechanism is via increased exposure to endotoxin which is usually higher in homes with dogs. Some studies have suggested an independent protective effect unrelated to endotoxin. Secondly, exposure to cats and high cat allergen has been shown to be protective against sensitization to cat allergen, by a modified Th2 response associated with IgG4. Thirdly, pet avoidance and pet removal because of allergic disease will distort these relationships, by suggesting a spurious protective effect, further complicated by cat allergic families that choose dogs and vice versa. The role of pets in promoting or protecting against atopy remains to be resolved and will require longitudinal studies.

Allergen exposure

The relationships between allergens and allergic disease need to be considered in three stages: sensitization, the development of disease, and the maintenance and severity of disease symptoms. Only a proportion of the population acquires atopy, and only a proportion of those go on to develop allergic disease. Atopy has repeatedly been shown to increase the risk of developing asthma, hayfever and eczema.

Sensitization

Allergic disease clusters in families and twin studies clearly demonstrate an inherited component of allergen sensitization. In addition to genetic susceptibility, the fetal environment appears important for the development of atopy. This environment is already skewed towards a Th2 pattern in order to protect the developing fetus. Fetal allergen exposure first occurs in utero, with some evidence of a fetal response to this exposure. At a broader level, fetal growth and hence fetal nutrition may also be important in the late acquisition of atopy, as suggested by studies showing positive relationships between head circumference at birth and IgE.

Exposure to food and environmental allergens occurs immediately after birth. Exposure to food allergens both directly and via breast milk is associated with sensitization which is often transient during infancy and in turn sensitization is associated with the development of eczema in the first few years of life. Sensitization to indoor allergens, such as house dust mite (HDM), domestic pets and cockroach, appears more important than food allergens for the later development of asthma. Exposure in the first few years of life appears to be particularly important in relation to sensitization.

Exposure to an allergen is required for sensitization and the prevalence of sensitization varies by the amount of allergen in the environment. Cross-sectional studies have demonstrated these relationships and longitudinal studies have shown clear dose–response relationships between environmental HDM allergen concentrations in the infant environment and the later prevalence of sensitization. Such dose–response relationships do not appear to hold, however, for all allergens, such as cat, for example, discussed above. Such differences in response to allergen exposure may have important consequences for the prevalence of asthma in environments with different dominant environmental allergens.

Allergen exposure and the development of asthma

The view that allergen exposure, in particular HDM allergen exposure, is causally related to the development of asthma, was thought to be almost self-evident, but has recently been challenged. On the one hand, the relationships appear obvious. Exposure to HDM allergen in early childhood leads to sensitization in a dose–response manner, experimental exposure to HDM in an allergen challenge leads to the clinical and cellular manifestations of asthma, and complete avoidance is associated with a marked clinical improvement. A recent longitudinal birth cohort study from Germany failed to show a direct relationship between the early development of wheezing and infant HDM exposure. However, despite almost half the children being at high risk of developing asthma and thorough selection of children with a family history, the prevalence of current wheezing at age 7 was only 10%, compared for example to 30% in the general UK or New Zealand population. HDM allergen levels were also very low compared with Australia, New Zealand, or the UK.

That allergen exposure can cause asthma entirely de novo is evident from occupational exposures in many workplace settings; what is not clear is how important it is as a cause of asthma in populations exposed to much higher allergen loads in infancy. Intervention studies with effective lowering of allergen exposure from birth may shed more light on this issue (see later in this chapter).

Allergen exposure and asthma severity

There is general agreement that allergen exposure increases asthma severity and AHR in sensitized subjects with disease, though much less agreement about the value of avoidance, which is discussed later. Sources of allergen vary in the domestic environment. HDM tend to be concentrated on fabric surfaces in bedding, carpets, and furniture fabrics. They only become airborne following disturbance in a room or bed and the allergen tends to be found on larger particles. Exposure in the bedroom is thought to be the dominant source of HDM allergen. Cat and dog allergen is sticky, occurs on much smaller particles and tends to remain airborne continuously. They can be carried on clothing and while much higher levels are found in homes where pets regularly come indoors, significant allergen levels are found in homes with no history of pets coming inside.

Bedding is an important source of HDM and pet allergen. For example, infant sheepskins have been shown to have very high levels of HDM allergen and synthetic bedding materials (often recommended for allergic patients) contain much higher levels of HDM allergen than feather bedding. These differences are probably related to the much tighter weave on feather bedding encasement, compared to synthetic bedding, required to keep feathers in but also reducing ingress of mites. Synthetic bedding has been associated with an increased risk of severe asthma. These observations are supported by a number of studies showing less severe asthma amongst feather bedding users, after controlling for deliberate bedding modification because of asthma. Synthetic bedding in infancy has also been shown to be a risk factor for HDM sensitization and asthma in later childhood.

Non-allergic inhalant risk factors

Environmental tobacco smoke exposure has been consistently associated with asthma and a variety of respiratory symptoms in children. The relationships have recently been extensively reviewed, with strong evidence that parental smoking increases the prevalence and severity of asthma, that postnatal exposure was more important than prenatal and that the effect was greatest for wheezing in the first 2 years of life. A small effect of parental smoking on increasing AHR and decreasing FEV_1 was reported. In contrast parental smoking did not appear to be associated with atopy or allergic disease.

Indoor nitrogen dioxide, principally from gas cooking and unflued gas heating, has been associated with respiratory symptoms, though most studies have used gas appliance use rather than measures of direct exposure. Recently, upper respiratory tract viral infections in asthmatic children have shown a dose-related greater severity of lower respiratory tract symptoms for personal NO_2 exposure within current accepted air quality standards. A well blinded intervention study of replacing unflued gas heaters in schools was also associated with an improvement in asthma symptoms in the schools with replaced heaters. These studies suggest a role for NO_2 exposure in asthma severity.

Dampness and mold

A number of studies have reported positive relationships between asthma and damp homes. Most rely on self-reporting of symptoms and self-reporting of dampness or visible mold including mold odor, which has been shown to be a reasonable marker of active mold growth. Few studies have included independent housing surveys or independent markers of respiratory symptoms simultaneously to reduce the effects of over-reporting. Allergy to mold is uncommon in most studies and it is unclear to what extent associations between mold and asthma are mediated by specific mold IgE. Damp environments may also encourage HDM proliferation, although mites are able to grow and proliferate at humidity levels well below those that encourage fungal growth. Exposure to the cellular wall products from fungi and bacteria (which would also be likely to proliferate in damp conditions) may be responsible for increasing symptoms. An increased risk of viral upper respiratory tract infection in damp houses has been reported and could be a cause of increased asthma symptoms.

Viral respiratory tract infection

Viral respiratory infections have been implicated in the development of asthma, in the prevention of asthma and atopy, and as a frequent cause of exacerbations, especially amongst children. Respiratory syncytial virus (RSV) infection is very common in the first 3 years of life and is associated with bronchiolitis in infancy. In some studies RSV infection has been associated with the later development of asthma and AHR. It is unclear whether this association is directly causal or reflects susceptibility. Protection from the later development of atopy by early upper respiratory tract infection is postulated as part of the hygiene hypothesis (see above) to explain the protective effect of siblings and early daycare exposure on the development of allergic disease. Viral respiratory tract infection is the commonest cause of exacerbations in children, and a frequent cause in adults.

Outdoor Inhalant risk factors

Studies of outdoor air pollution and asthma are inherently difficult and exposures are invariably complex mixtures of chemicals such as oxides of sulfur and nitrogen, ozone, and particulates of varying size. Most studies have relied on comparing outdoor measurements with markers of asthma morbidity such as hospital admissions or emergency department visits. The results of these studies are inconsistent and where positive associations have been found they tend to be small. For the development of asthma in relation to air pollution the data support an inverse relationship (non-causal) as exemplified by the studies of asthma and atopy in East and West Germany prior to unification. Asthma and atopy were more prevalent in the less polluted West compared to the more polluted East, while symptoms of bronchitis showed the opposite and expected association. Such unexpected asthma pollution relationships led to examination of traffic air pollution and in particular diesel exhaust, both forms of pollution being more common in economically developed countries. A number of studies have shown increased asthma symptoms in association with traffic exposure, while others have failed to find an effect. Diesel exhaust has been shown to exert airway inflammatory effects in animal models and humans, and to have adjuvant effects on allergen sensitization in animal models.

Non-inhalant risk factors

Of recent interest have been the associations between obesity and asthma symptoms and AHR. The prevalence of both asthma and obesity has been increasing and obesity has been positively associated with asthma. In most cross-sectional studies the positive associations between obesity and asthma have been for symptoms rather than AHR and have been more apparent for females. In larger studies such as the ECRHS, in addition to the positive associations of obesity and asthma symptoms, a positive association with AHR to methacholine has also been found for both males and females. In some longitudinal studies in children there is evidence that the associations are recent although previously the lower prevalence of obesity would make such association less obvious. Intervention studies amongst morbidly obese patients with asthma have shown improvement in symptoms with weight loss but studies to date have been small and uncontrolled. A number of mechanisms have been suggested, both causal and non-causal. Non-causal mechanisms include reverse causation that asthma precedes obesity and results from it by lack of exercise. Obese asthmatics may perceive symptoms to a greater extent than non-obese and will have increased exercise breathlessness which may be confused with asthma. Causal associations include gastroesophageal reflux, hormonal effects to explain the predominance in women in some studies, or dietary factors that are associated with both obesity and asthma. Another explanation relates to airway mechanics. Deep inspiration both dilates the preconstricted airway and protects against constriction in the normal lung. Both these responses are impaired in asthma. Loss of elastic recoil and reduced tidal expansion associated with obesity could therefore increase bronchial responsiveness.

Diet has long been associated with allergic disease, most notably dietary proteins, especially cows' milk proteins associated with sensitization and eczema in infancy. The role of breastfeeding in the subsequent development of asthma and allergic disease has been controversial. Most longitudinal studies have shown reduced asthma and allergic disease associated with prolonged (> 4 months) exclusive breastfeeding. Some have shown no effect and others an increased risk. Exclusivity of breastfeeding is obviously important given that the introduction of foreign food proteins will increase the risk of sensitization. Maternal diet is also important as food allergens may be passed to the infant in breast milk. Sensitization to specific food proteins causing asthma on exposure is well documented but uncommon. Food dyes, such as tartrazine, and preservatives have also been associated with asthma attacks in a minority of asthmatics. More general dietary associations with the development of asthma have been suggested. Salt intake has been positively associated with asthma and AHR in some studies but not in others and reduction in salt in experimental studies has shown mixed results. More consistent have been the studies showing a positive association between salt intake and exercise-induced asthma. Regular consumption of oily fish containing n-3 polyunsaturated fatty acids has been shown to be associated with a reduced prevalence of asthma symptoms and AHR. This has recently been extended to maternal consumption during pregnancy and reduced asthma prevalence in children. Antioxidants have also been associated with asthma, with studies suggesting lower intakes amongst those with asthma and decreased AHR in those with higher intakes. Clinical studies of supplementation have proved disappointing though large well controlled trials have not been reported.

PREVENTION OF ASTHMA AND ALLERGIC DISEASE

Primary prevention

As discussed previously, sensitization to HDM allergen is related to exposure and sensitization is a risk factor for developing asthma. It makes sense then to try and reduce HDM exposure to reduce sensitization and in turn reduce prevalence. Table 16.3 summarizes data from six primary intervention studies, from Europe, Canada, and Australia. All have selected children at high risk of developing atopy by virtue of a family history of allergic disease. To date, these studies show variable results. They have all used slightly different interventions with variable reductions in HDM allergen in the home. All studies used some form of mattress encasement. It is important to recognize, however, that all but the Isle of Wight study can only be considered preliminary. Ascertainment of atopic status to environmental allergens at 2–3 years of age will be incomplete, and much of the wheezing will be unrelated to atopy. In the Isle of Wight study both wheezing and sensitization were reduced in the intervention group at 1 year but at 2 and 4 years there was no difference in respiratory symptoms. At age 8 however, the prevalence of current wheeze was halved and sensitization to HDM reduced to a third of the control group. After adjustment for potential confounders, intervention children were significantly less likely to report current wheeze, OR 0.26, (95% CI 0.07–0.96) or be atopic, OR 0.21, (95% CI 0.07–0.62). The Manchester study has by far the most stringent environmental intervention for HDM, including bedding interventions for the mother prior to birth, custom-made impermeable mattresses for the infant, and removal of bedroom carpets. At 3 years the intervention children were significantly *more* atopic, similarly wheezy but with better lung function as measured by specific airway resistance. It is tempting to speculate that this unexpected result is related to reduced exposure to endotoxin in the intervention group which improves lung function while predisposing to sensitization. For all of these studies, it will be the outcomes in later childhood and early adulthood that will determine the value of these primary interventions.

Secondary prevention

Most secondary prevention studies have explored HDM avoidance in asthma. These studies have proved both successful and unsuccessful depending on whether the patient or the mite is removed. Thus mite-sensitive asthmatic children taken to alpine sanatoria, where mites are unable to thrive due to the low humidity, have shown significant reductions in symptoms, and AHR and mite-specific IgE. Small studies using mechanical ventilation and heat recovery in homes have reduced mites and shown clinical benefit, but only in climates with dry cold winters. Most studies, however, using a variety of mite control procedures including barrier protection of bedding, acaricides, and hot washing of clothes and bedding, have been underpowered, of too short a duration, or have not demonstrated a sustained reduction in mite allergen. Not surprisingly, they have often failed to find any clinical benefit. Where these three conditions have been at least partially met, clinical improvements in asthma or a decrease in AHR have been observed with mite avoidance. Few studies consider concomitant asthma therapy, in particular the back titration of inhaled corticosteroids to ensure that a response to the intervention can be measured. A recent large intervention trial in adult asthmatics using impermeable bed covers alone failed to find any significant clinical benefit, but the intervention also failed to produce a sustained reduction in mite allergen levels. Recently, interventions targeted to an individual's atopic profile and including non specific irritants such as tobacco smoke avoidance have shown significant clinical benefit in children. Given the beneficial response when mite allergen is completely avoided as in an alpine environment, attempts to reduce allergen exposure should not be abandoned, particularly in patients whose asthma is poorly controlled despite adequate treatment and where multiple mite avoidance strategies can be employed.

Table 16.3 Summary of six current primary intervention studies

Study name (Year of last report)	Interventions	ATOPY	WHEEZE	OTHER
Isle of Wight Study (IoW) (8 years)	Food allergen avoidance mother + infant to 9 months. HDM mattress covers + acaricide	↓	↓	AHR ↓
Study of Prevention of Allergy in Children in Europe (SPACE) (1 year)	Hypoallergenic formula, food avoidance infant 12 months. HDM mattress encasement + advice	↓	↔	Eczema ↔
Childhood Asthma Prevention Study (CAPS) (Age 3 years)	Omega 3 FFA supplements. HDM bedding encasement + acaricidal wash	↓	↔	Eczema ↑
Prevention and Incidence of Asthma and Mite Allergy (PIAMA) (2 years)	HDM encasement mattress and pillows	↔	↔	
Canadian Asthma Primary Prevention Study (CAPPS) (2 years)	Maternal and infant food allergen avoidance, hydrolyzed infant formula. HDM bedding encasement and acaricide	↔	↓	
Manchester Asthma and Allergy Study (MAAS) (3 years)	Encasement parental and infant bedding, advice hot washing, acaricide, carpet removal infant bedroom + high filtration vacuum cleaner	↑	↓	Specific airway resistance ↓

AHR, airway hyperresponsiveness; FFA, free fatty acid, HDM, house dust mite

CONCLUSION

Epidemiologic study of asthma and allergic disease has provided significant insights into factors associated with increased and decreased risk of disease in the last two decades, despite the hindrance of poor definition and nomenclature. The etiology of airflow obstruction is clearly dominated by allergic inflammation but not confined to it and the nomenclature is in need of revision, in order to focus attention on very different risk factors for the different wheezing syndromes. While a substantial proportion of the increase in asthma prevalence is likely to be related to relabeling, this is unlikely to explain all of the change and the increases in atopy, allergic rhinitis, and eczema all support fundamental changes in population responses to allergens. The most likely explanation for these changes resides in the concepts suggested by the hygiene hypothesis, though at present the immunologic effects are only partially understood, and the environmental associations incomplete. There remains a need to continue to cast a wide net over factors that interact with the airway and its immune system. Increased understanding of the immunology and the way this is influenced by the environment, particularly coupled with genetic interactions, would seem to be the most likely route to eventually finding preventative solutions.

FURTHER READING

Arshad SH. Primary prevention of asthma and atopy during childhood by allergen avoidance in infancy: a randomised controlled study. Thorax 2003; 58:489–493.

Braun-Fahrlander C, Eder W, Schreuer M, et al. Exposure to farming environment during the first year of life protects against the development of asthma and allergy. Am J Respir Crit Care Med 2001; 163 (A157).

Braun-Fahrlander C, Riedler J, Herz U, et al. Environmental exposure to endotoxin and its relation to asthma in school-age children. N Engl J Med 2002; 347:869–877.

Chinn S. Obesity and asthma: evidence for and against a causal relation. J Asthma 2003; 40:1–16.

ISAAC Steering Committee. Worldwide variations in the prevalence of symptoms of asthma, allergic rhinoconjunctivitis and atopic eczema: The International Study of Asthma and Allergies in Childhood (ISAAC). Lancet 1998; 351:1225–1232.

Janson C, Anto J, Burney P, et al. The European Community Respiratory Health Survey: what are the main results so far? Env Respir J 2001; 18:598–611.

Latvala J, von Hertzen L, Lindholm H, et al. Trends in prevalence of asthma and allergy in Finnish young men: nationwide study, 1966–2003. BMJ 2005; 330:1186–1187.

Singh J, Schwartz DA. Endotoxin and the lung: Insight into the host-environment interaction. J Allergy Clin Immunol 2005; 115:330–333.

Strachan DP. Family size, infection and atopy: the first decade of the 'hygiene hypothesis'. Thorax 2000; 55 Suppl 1:S2–10.

Woodcock A, Lowe LA, Murray CS, et al. Early life environmental control: effect on symptoms, sensitization, and lung function at age 3 years. Am J Respir Crit Care Med 2004; 170:433–439.

Chapter 17

Allergens and Pollutants

Definition:
Allergens are antigens, usually proteinaceous in nature, that sensitize the host for allergic reactions. Their sources are diverse and include house dust mite products, pollens, fungal spores, animals, drugs, and foods.

Geoffrey A Stewart, Philip J Thompson, David Peden, and Neil Alexis

INTRODUCTION

Allergens and type 1 hypersensitivity

Humans are exposed to a variety of environmental, non-pathogen associated antigens which may induce the production of IgE, the antibody isotype associated with type I mediated diseases in about 10–20% of Western populations. These, supposedly innocuous, antigens are usually referred to as allergens to distinguish them from the myriad other substances that are routinely associated with the stimulation of IgA, IgG, and IgM production and referred to as antigens. The host may come into contact with such allergens via a number of routes but inhalation represents the most important. However, exposure by ingestion, injection, and passive absorption through the skin frequently occurs. The sequelae resulting from the interactions between allergens and IgE bound to cells such as the mast cell via these portals underlie diseases such as rhinitis, sinusitis, asthma, hypersensitivity pneumonitis, extrinsic allergic alveolitis, conjunctivitis, urticaria, eczema, atopic dermatitis, anaphylaxis and angioedema, allergic and migraine headache, and certain gastrointestinal disorders (Table 17.1). Type 1 mediated allergic diseases result from two temporally distinct stages. In the first, also known as the sensitization or antibody induction stage, inhaled, injected or ingested allergen is presented to the immune system by antigen presenting cells and this, in susceptible individuals, causes IgE antibody to be produced which then binds to mast cells and basophils via specific receptors including the high affinity FcεRI. In the second, effector phase, allergen interacts with receptor-bound IgE to cause cell degranulation within 5–15 minutes after the sensitized host is re-exposed. This process results in the release of inflammatory mediators which give rise to the characteristic features of type 1 mediated allergic disease. At both stages, it is assumed that allergens cross appropriate innate defense barriers such as skin, and mucous membranes to initiate disease.

Factors influencing allergenicity – intrinsic

Most allergens are proteins or glycoproteins with masses in the range 5000–100 000, although the glycan moiety of glycoprotein allergens does not usually stimulate specific IgE production. Allergens generally possess properties indistinguishable from those associated with conventional antigens which stimulate the production of the other immunoglobulin isotypes in a susceptible host, including biochemical and physicochemical properties (Table 17.2). However, some of the physicochemical and biochemical properties of allergens may influence the site of any resulting allergic

Table 17.1 Allergens and allergic disease

Allergens and Allergic Disease		
Asthma and/or rhinitis	**Anaphylaxis**	**Atopic Dermatitis**
Grass pollen	Insect venom	Dust mites
Tree pollen	Drugs	Food allergens
Weed pollen	Food allergens	Occupational allergens
Fungi		
Dust mites		
Animal dander		
Occupational allergens		
Food allergens		

Table 17.2 Factors that influence allergenicity

Factors Influencing Allergenicity	
Intrinsic	**Extrinsic**
Molecular complexity (size)	Pollutants
Concentration	Cigarette smoke
Solubility	Viral infection
Foreignness	Genetic predisposition and gender
Stability	Season of birth
Biochemical activity	Hygiene
Resistance to digestion (food allergens)	Birth weight
Resistance to cooking (food allergens)	

reaction. For example, it is possible that the resistance of some oral allergens to both heat and gut digestive enzymes may facilitate systemic responses whereas susceptibility to these processes may restrict responses to the oral cavity. A number of extrinsic factors, both endogenous and exogenous, may also contribute to their recognition by the immune system by altering normal homeostatic defense mechanisms, for example, genetic factors, industrial pollutants, cigarette smoke, or viral infections.

Factors influencing allergenicity – extrinsic

For initial sensitization to occur, the genetic characteristics of the host are important, not only in developing allergic disease per se but also in inducing allergic responses to specific allergens. Whilst the genes associated with allergic diseases such as those involved in IgE regulation, inflammation, and responsiveness to bronchodilator dilator therapy are currently being delineated, those associated with the production of allergen-specific IgE have been studied in some detail, particularly with regard to low-molecular-weight allergens (< 10 kDa). In this regard, genes involved in the induction of specific IgE responses to minor allergens from pollens such as *Ambrosia artemisiifolia* (ragweed) and *Lolium perenne* (rye grass) have been studied and found to code for proteins associated with major histocompatibility class I (HLA-A, -B, -C) and class II (HLA-DR, -DP, -DQ) genes. The latter cell membrane proteins, found on professional antigen presenting cells, are particularly important in presenting antigen and allergen fragments (peptides) known as epitopes to T helper cells for subsequent antibody production. As the size of an allergen increases and, therefore, the number of potential epitopes increases, it becomes increasingly difficult to delineate such associations. Information on regions of the allergen (agretope) which bind to the class II molecule and the region (epitope) which binds to the T-cell receptor or antibody combining site (paratope) is increasing rapidly due to their potential usefulness in the development of novel immunotherapeutic regimes.

Origins of allergens

Unless in the workplace, most individuals are exposed to mixtures of allergens rather than to single proteins. This is because many environmental allergens are important molecules playing major physiologic roles in the allergen source per se, and are associated with distinct, particulate structures. For example, allergens are to be found in pollen grains, fungal spores and arthropod feces, where they play roles in digestion (feces), somatic growth and fertilization (spores and pollen). Reflecting their role in their natural environment, allergens rapidly leach out of their particulate structures when they become hydrated on contact with mucosal surfaces. The most complex sources of allergens are fungi, pollen, and mites, with the least complex being animal dander and urine extracts (Table 17.3). Up to 60% of the proteins from a given source are allergenic and a sensitized patient may recognize more than one allergen. However, the precise number recognized reflects both the genetic capability of the host, the complexity of the source, and the assay used to determine allergenicity. The more frequently (> 50%) recognized proteins within a population exposed to a particular source are termed 'major allergens', in contrast to 'minor allergens'. However, these arbitrary divisions do not necessarily indicate that minor allergens will be clinically insignificant in certain individuals. Allergen exposure may occur in domestic and occupational settings and, in the former, they are sometimes referred to as indoor or outdoor allergens to reflect the origin of the allergen source. Typical outdoor allergens include pollens and fungi, whereas indoor allergens include animal dander, and mite and insect feces. In addition, the terms 'intrinsic' and 'extrinsic' are used to refer to allergens arising from sources within the host, e.g. fungi and helminthic parasites, and outside the host, respectively.

ALLERGEN SOURCES

Airborne allergens

Pollen allergens

Pollens represent some of the more clinically important allergen sources (10–20% of community allergic disease), and the most

Table 17.3 Common allergen sources

Allergen group	Examples	Seasonality
Common Allergen Sources		
Airborne		
Pollens		
Grasses	Rye, couch, wild oat, timothy, Bermuda, Kentucky blue, cocksfoot	Spring/early summer
Weeds	Ragweed, parietaria, plantain, mugwort	Summer/autumn
Trees	Alder, birch, hazel, beech, cupressae, oak, olive, cyprus	Winter/spring
Molds	*Aspergillus* spp., *Cladosporium* spp., *Alternaria* spp., *Candida* spp.	Perennial/variable
Cereal flours	Wheat, rye, oat	Perennial
Plant products	Latex, papain, bromelain	Perennial
Animal dander and urine	Cat, dog, horse, rabbit, guinea pig, hamster, mouse, rat, cow	Perennial
Bird feathers	Budgerigar, parrot, pigeon, duck, chicken	Perennial
House dust mite	*Dermatophagoides pteronyssinus, D. farinae, Euroglyphus maynei*	Perennial
Insects	Cockroach, fly, locust, midge	Seasonal
Oral		
Food	Seafood, legumes, peanuts, tree nuts, sesame, soya, cereals, dairy products, eggs, fruits, tomatoes, mushrooms, alcoholic beverages, coffee, chocolate	Non-seasonal
Drugs	Penicillins, sulfonamides and other antibiotics, sulfasalazine, carbamaepine	Non-seasonal
		Non-seasonal
Injected		
Insects	Bee and wasp stings, ant and mosquito bites	Summer
Drugs	Blood products, sera, vaccines, contrast media, drugs (including antiasthma drugs and antibiotics)	Non-seasonal

common disease presentation is rhinitis. The major allergenic pollens (grasses, weeds, and trees) are derived from wind-pollinated (anemophilous) rather than insect-pollinated (entomophilous) plants and, in this regard, the former possess a thin coat containing lipids and proteins, in contrast to the thick, sticky coats of insect-pollinated plants. The clinically important pollens will vary according to geographical location as well as season and microclimatic conditions (Fig. 17.1). Pollens from the anemophilous plants, in contrast to the entomophilous plants, are characterized by their buoyant density, ease of dispersion, and profusion, and grains from individual species may vary in size, ranging from 5 to over 200 μm. The pollen grain per se is the primary source of allergen but studies show that individuals may be exposed to submicronic particles derived from the grains themselves. Such particles are released from pollen in moist conditions that occur after rain and become airborne as the environment dries out. These particles such as starch grains (approx. 700/pollen) and wall precursor (P) particles are also released on contact with mucosal surfaces and are potent sources of allergen (Fig. 17.2). In addition to the submicronic particles, proteins and, therefore, allergens may be found within the pollen coat, as well as being secreted from within the pollen itself. A significant number of the released proteins will be involved in pollen tube growth as well as helping breach the stigma wall so that fertilization may occur. The constituent proteins from these various sources will vary between species as can be seen below. Pollens are absent from the atmosphere on wet days but frequently released when hot, dry conditions prevail. As a consequence, pollen release and atmospheric loading is usually seasonal, with late spring and summer representing the most important pollination seasons (Fig. 17.3). In this regard, the sequence of pollination is usually trees, grasses, and weeds. The number of pollen grains required to provoke disease is unclear although the amount of pollen required to initiate symptoms at the beginning of the hayfever season is greater than at the end. Approximately 20–100 grains/m^3 are considered to be a provoking dose. In addition to pollens, plants also produce pollen-related orbicules (0.2–1 μm) which contain allergens. These granules of sporopollenin accumulate proteins and carbohydrates during pollen formation, are released during pollination and outnumber pollen per se.

Fungal allergens

Fungi may be broadly divided into two groups based on their structure; namely, the yeasts which grow as single cells and fungi that produce hyphae and spores. Although allergen-producing yeasts have been identified, most of the clinically

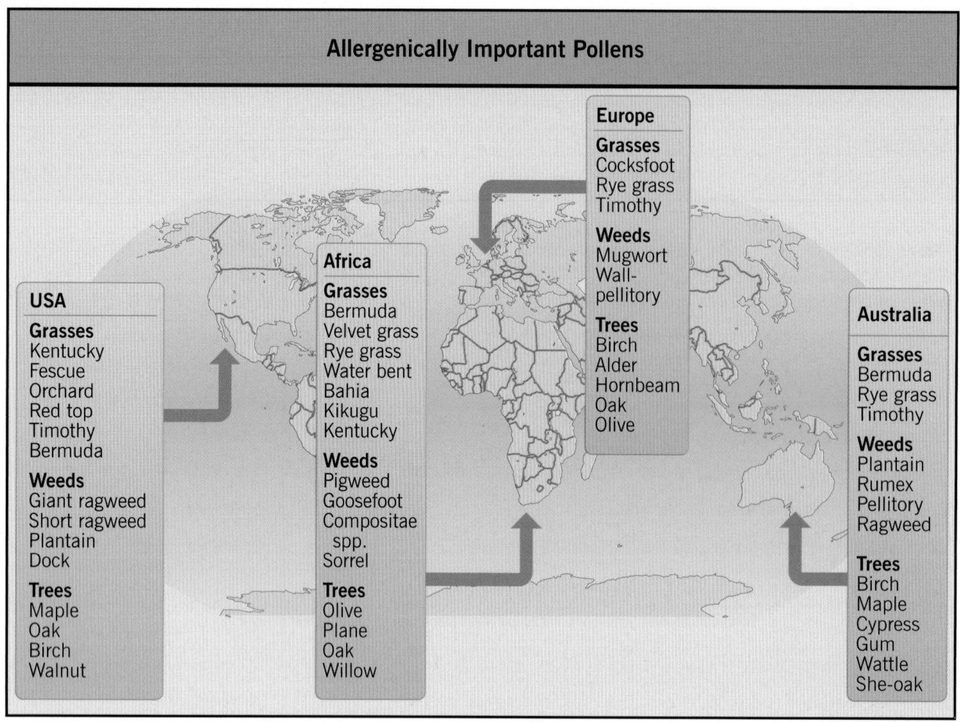

Fig. 17.1 Selected worldwide distribution of clinically important pollen allergens.

important allergen-producing species belong to the latter category, which may be further grouped according to their means of reproduction and morphology. The allergenicity (and pathogenicity) of several fungal species have been studied in detail, and those belonging to the Ascomycotina *(Aspergillus, Cladosporium, Penicillium* and *Alternaria* spp.) are important sources of allergen worldwide (Fig. 17.4). However, the Basidiomycotina spp. (mushrooms, puffballs, rusts, smuts and bracket fungi) are also thought to represent significant allergen sources in certain situations. Both produce spores which are often found in very large quantities in the air. The size of spores will vary between species, ranging from 1 to > 100 μm although in general most of the clinically important species produce spores in the range 7–12 μm. Theoretically, fungal allergens should be highly significant because spores containing them are the most abundant airborne particles (e.g. > 5000 spores/m^3) and small enough to penetrate deep into the respiratory tree, in contrast to pollen grains. Meteorological studies reveal that atmospheric conditions such as wind speed, temperature, and humidity influence the release of spores. For example, ascospores may be released after rainfall (*Didymella extalis*) or hot dry conditions (Cladosporium), and basidospores may be released due to humidity. *Aspergillus* and *Alternaria* spores appear to be particularly significant in asthma but those from *Cladosporium herbarium* and *Penicillium* species may also be important. Spore concentrations required to provoke symptoms will depend on the species (e.g. 50–100/m^3 for *Alternaria* and 3000/m^3 for *Cladosporium*). Fungal allergens are thought to be produced by both spores and/or hyphae as they develop, and then released into the environment. In addition to natural exposure, individual fungal allergens, often hydrolytic enzymes used in a variety of industries, have been shown to be allergenic.

Animal-derived allergens

Animal-derived allergens are also of major clinical significance, and the incidence of positive skin tests to such proteins in an unselected population is approximately 5%, which rises to over 30%. In domestic situations, allergy to cats and dogs is particularly common, whereas in occupational settings allergy to rats, horses, rabbits, mice, gerbils, and guinea pigs is common. In both settings, the allergens are derived from dander, epithelium, fur, urine, and saliva, although it is possible that the allergens originate from the same source, e.g. saliva or urine on the fur.

Arthropod allergens

The main arthropod allergen sources are to be found in the Classes Insecta and Arachnida, and include cockroaches, chironomid midges, moths, butterflies, locusts and mites (Fig. 17.5). Allergy to these insects may arise either through domestic contact or in scientific institutions where they are reared or studied. In such work-related situations, they may cause allergic disease in up to a third of workers. With regard to arachnids, house dust mites represent the most clinically important allergen sources worldwide (Fig. 17.6). Mite species are ubiquitous, but the most important are those in domestic dwellings and include the species *Dermatophagoides pteronyssinus, D. farinae, Blomia tropicalis* and *Euroglyphus maynei*. House dust mites live in carpets, soft furnishings and mattresses, and growth is dependent on microclimatic conditions; they proliferate best at 25°C and a relative humidity of 75%. It is because of their strong association with allergic rhinitis and asthma that mites and their allergens, and their global distribution, have been studied in considerable detail.

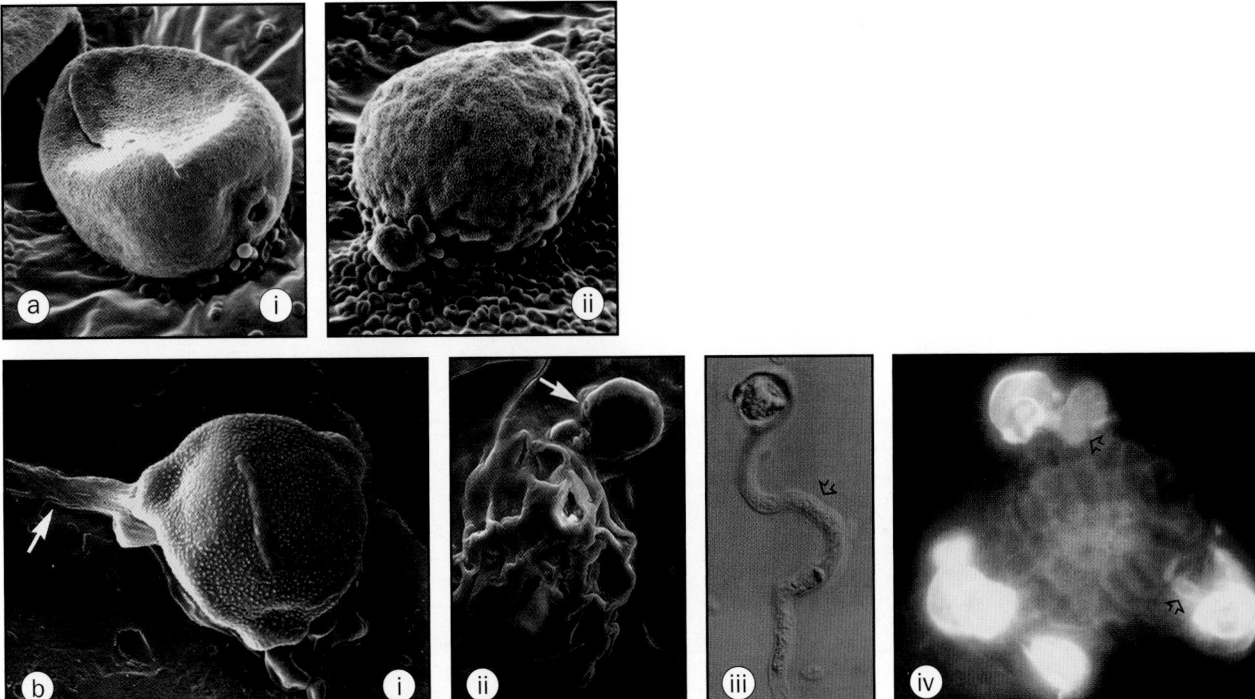

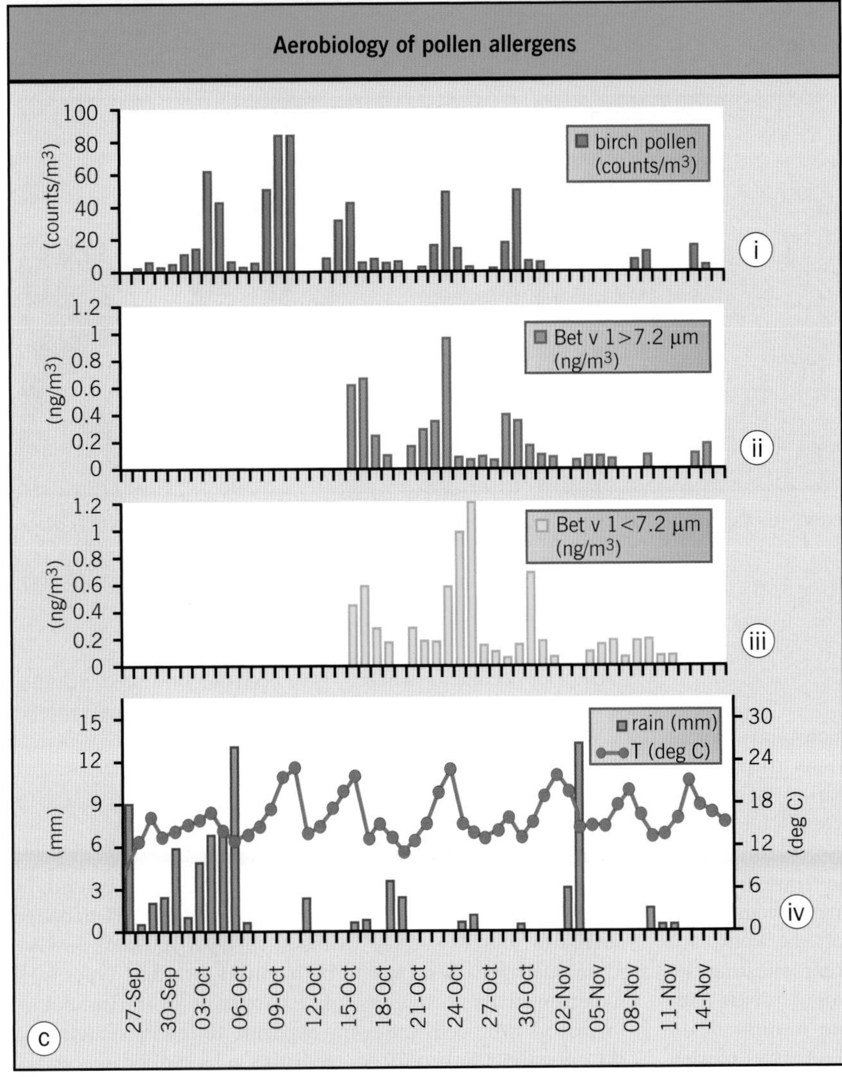

Fig. 17.2 (a) Scanning electron micrographs (SEM) of rye grass (*Lolium perenne*) pollen showing clearly the aperture through which pollen tube grows and starch granules are extended surrounded by starch granules. (b) Micrographs of germinating birch pollen and bursting pollen tubes. (i) SEM of a triporate birch (*Betula verrucosa*) pollen grain on a birch leaf. The pollen grain has germinated, producing a pollen tube (see arrow). (ii) SEM of birch leaf gland with one birch pollen grain nearby (see arrow). (iii) A germinated birch pollen grain with a pollen tube (see arrow) of about 90 µm showing dense cytoplasmic contents. This was viewed with Nomarski optics after being washed off a birch leaf. (iv) Germinating pollen accumulates around the birch leaf gland. Each grain produces a pollen tube (see arrows). Within hours of germinating, the pollen tube tips rupture releasing the cytoplasmic contents. Prominent amongst this discharged cytoplasm are numerous starch granules. (c) (i) Birch pollen counts (number/m^3); (ii) Bet v 1 concentrations (ng/m^3) in particles greater than 7.2 µm in diameter; (iii) Bet v 1 concentrations (ng/m^3) in inhalable particles less than 7.2 µm in diameter; (iv) rainfall (mm) and temperature (°C) in the atmosphere of Melbourne during the 1996 birch pollen season. Bet v 1 concentrations were determined from 16 October–15 November 1996. Bet v 1 data for 20 October and 3 November are not available.
[(a) Photographs courtesy of Professor Frank Murray, Murdoch University, Perth, Western Australia. (b) Photograph courtesy of Dr Cenk Suphioglu, Monash University, Melbourne, Australia and reproduced from Schäppi GF, Taylor PE, Staff IA, et al. Source of Bet v 1 loaded inhalable particles from birch revealed. Sex Plant Reprod 1997; 10:315–323, with permission of Springer Verlag. (c) Reproduced from Schäppi GF, Taylor PE, Staff IA, et al. Source of Bet v 1 loaded inhalable particles from birch revealed. Sex Plant Reprod 1997; 10:315–323, with permission from Springer Verlag.]

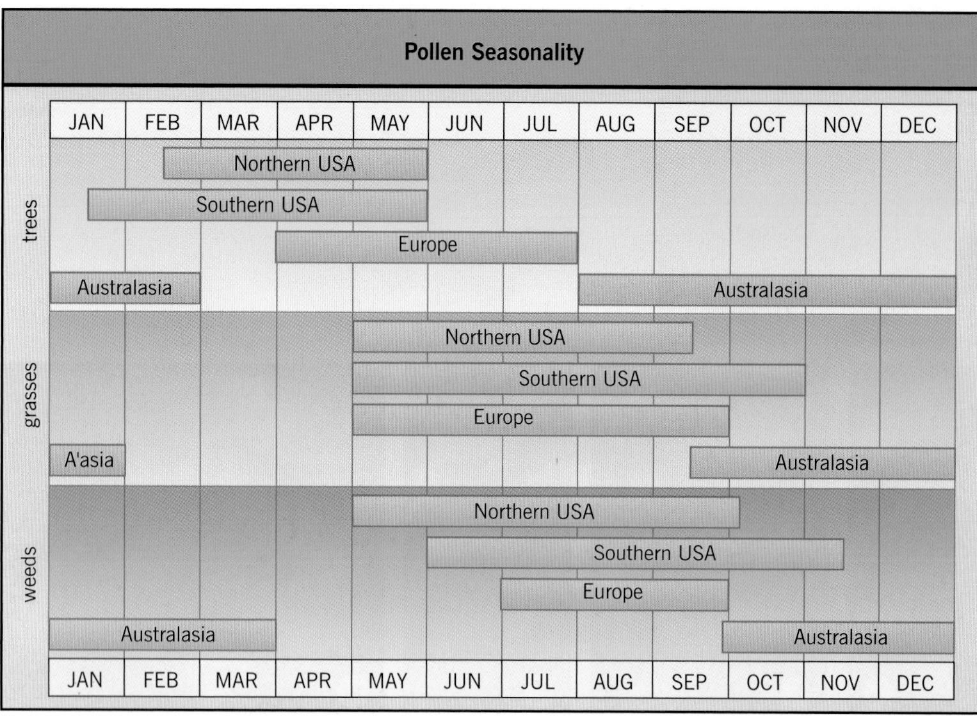

Fig. 17.3 Pollen seasons in USA, Australia and Europe. (Adapted from Sicherer SH, Eggleston PA. In: Lieberman P, Anderson J, eds. Environmental allergens in allergic diseases: diagnosis and treatment. Totowa: Humana Press Inc. 2000.)

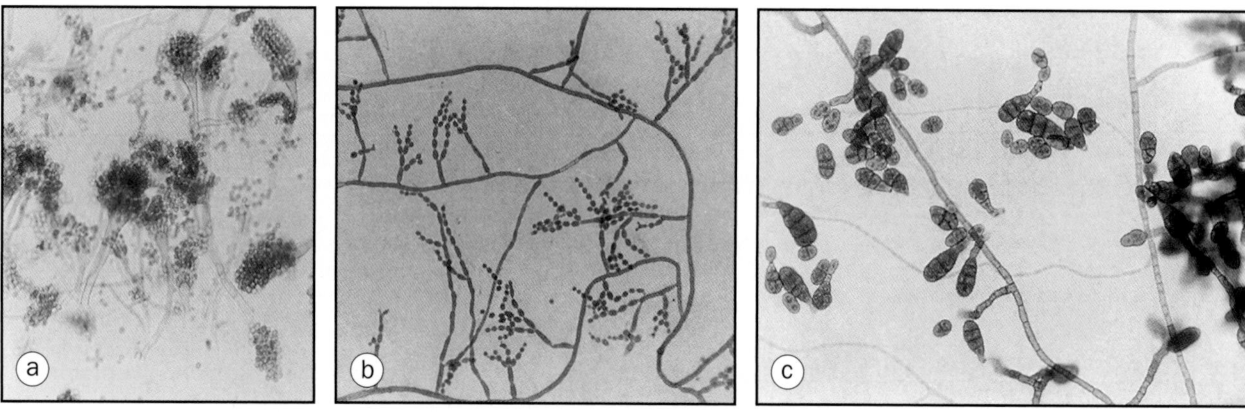

Fig. 17.4 Fungi commonly involved in allergic disease: (a) *Aspergillus fumigatus*, (b) *Cladosporium*, (c) *Alternaria*. (Photograph courtesy of Ms Rose McAleer, PathCentre, Western Australia.)

Occupational allergens

Occupational allergens range from low molecular weight chemicals of relatively simple structure through to complex proteins and glycoproteins derived from a variety of animal, arthropod, bacterial, fungal and plant sources (Table 17.4). Allergy may affect only a few individuals in the workforce or up to 30% of exposed workers. The response time between exposure and symptoms may be delayed by many hours, with the consequence that the subject may have left the workplace and be at home when symptoms occur, thus complicating the diagnosis. Recurrent exposure may lead to chronic disease with little variability being discernible, so making it difficult to associate disease with exposure. A number of predisposing factors for occupational allergy have been demonstrated including prior atopic status, duration of exposure and smoking history.

Oral and injected allergens

Food allergens

The frequency, severity, and variety of diseases caused by exposure to foods may be controversial although IgE-mediated allergy to sources such as peanuts, soybean and milk less so. Many mechanisms appear to be involved including types I–IV hypersensitivity responses, direct release of inflammatory mediators from cells following exposure to food products, and the presence of inflammatory mediators in food. Food intolerance

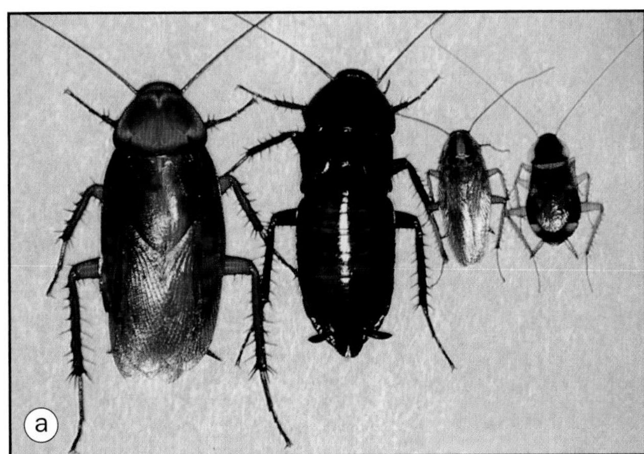

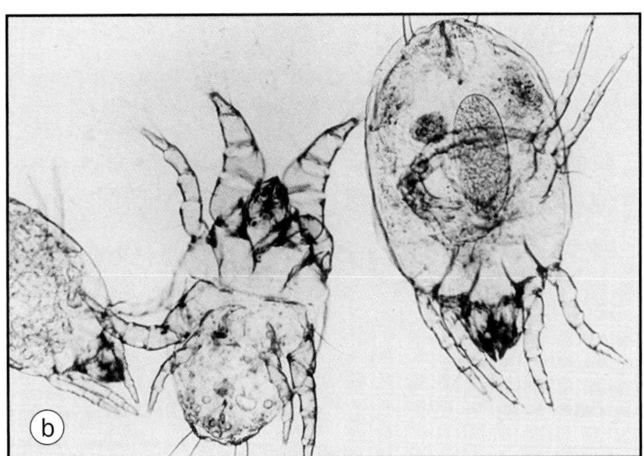

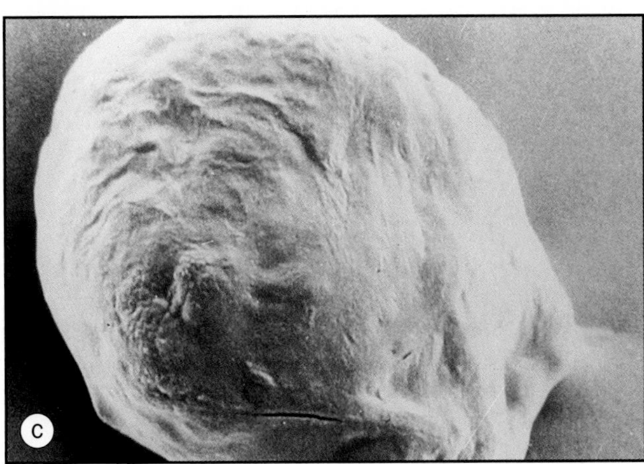

Fig. 17.5 Cockroaches (a) American, Oriental, German and Brown banded cockroaches from left to right), house dust mites (b) and house dust mite fecal pellet (c). (Photograph (a) courtesy of the Department of Entomology, University of Nebraska; photographs (b) and (c) courtesy of ALK-Abello, Horsholm, Denmark.)

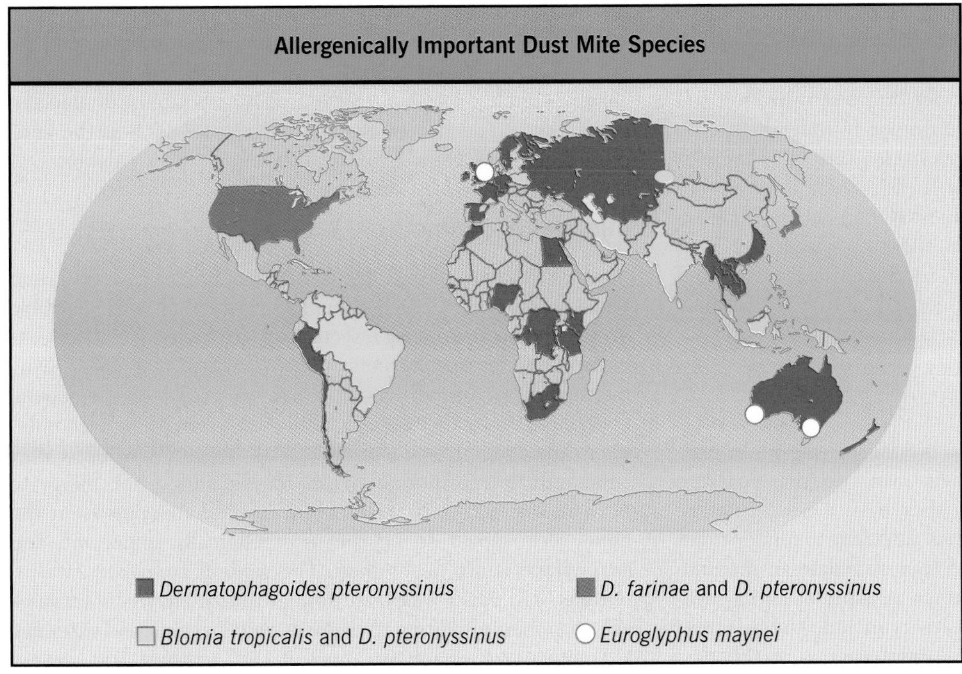

Fig. 17.6 Reported worldwide distribution of the major house dust mite species. [Modified from Colloff M, Stewart GA. In: Barnes PJ, Griretein MM, Leff AR, et al, eds. Asthma. Philadelphia: Lippencott-Raven; 1997 and van Bronswijk JEMH, Sinha RN. Pyroglyphid mites (Acari) and house dust allergy. J Allergy 1971; 47:31–52.]

Table 17.4 Common occupational allergens

Common Occupational Allergens		
Source	**Examples**	**Industry**
Low-molecular-weight		
Metals and their salts	Platinum, aluminum, vanadium, nickel and chromium salts	Metal-refining, plating, boiler-cleaning, welding
Chemicals	Chloramine T, colophony (pine resin), polyvinyl chloride, isocyanates, anhydrides, ethylenediamine, plicatic acid	Brewing, soldering, meat wrapping, plastics and chemical processing, wood processing
Drugs		
Antibiotics	Penicillin, tetracycline, cephalosporin	Manufacture, domestic use
Miscellaneous	Albuterol, methyldopa, opiates	Manufacture, domestic use
Animal proteins		
Miscellaneous–mammalian	Dander, urine, serum, feathers, droppings	Research, breeding
Miscellaneous – invertebrate	Scales, somatic debris, body fluids, fecal pellets	Research, breeding
Enzymes	Trypsin, pepsin, amylase, lysozyme, lipase	Manufacture, domestic use
Plants		
Vegetable dust	Wood, cereals, legumes	Carpentry, baking, milling, processing
Enzymes	Papain, bromelain, pectinase, cellulose, amylase	Pharmaceuticals, food-processing
Latex	Rubber	Healthcare workers, spina bifida patients
Bacterial		
Enzymes	Alcalase and esperase (serine proteases), amylase	Detergents

causes a variety of clinical entities, including anaphylaxis, and neurologic, gastrointestinal, cutaneous, and respiratory disorders. Diagnosis of food allergy may be difficult unless clear-cut evidence of food allergen-specific IgE can be detected. In addition to food allergens being responsible for direct sensitization and provocation, they may also initiate disease in individuals who are already sensitive to aeroallergens from a variety of sources, in particular from pollens (Table 17.5). Such diseases are referred to as 'oral allergy syndromes' (OAS) and result from allergenic cross-reactivity between allergens within the food and those in the aeroallergen source. OAS are usually associated with uncooked foods rather than cooked, and exposure may precipitate local (oral) or systemic reactions.

Drug allergens

Most drugs associated with allergic disease are low-molecular-weight substances which, on their own, do not sensitize susceptible individuals. However, they have a propensity to interact chemically with host proteins sufficient to render them foreign to the immune system and thus stimulate an immune response. Such compounds are known as haptens, and typical drugs involved in type 1 hypersensitivity include the β-lactam antibiotics such as the penicillins and cephalosporins, anesthetics, and muscle relaxants. With regard to the antibiotics, the β-lactam ring is central as it is chemically unstable and reacts with lysyl residues to form the penicilloyl epitope on cell membrane proteins. Allergic reactions may manifest as urticaria or anaphylaxis although the latter is usually associated with injected drugs. The frequency of sensitivity to drugs such as the antibiotics may vary from 1 to 10% of the general population.

Injected allergens

Allergen exposure via injection (natural or iatrogenic) is associated with certain insects which either sting or bite, or with injectable drugs. The major stinging insects associated with allergic disease include bees, wasps, hornets, and ants, which may inject many micrograms of venom at one time. About 3% of the general population may experience systemic reactions after envenomination, and about 15–30% of individuals become sensitized after being stung. Predisposing factors may include prior allergy to inhalant allergens. Of the stinging insects, allergens from the honey bee appear to be the most clinically important, and anaphylaxis is not uncommon. The venoms from bees, wasps, hornets, and paper wasps are similar in that they contain vasoactive amines in addition to peptides and enzymes, and extensive allergenic cross-reactivity may occur amongst the vespid

Table 17.5 Allergens involved in cross-reactivity syndromes

Sensitizing source	Provoking source	Cross-reacting allergen(s)
Plant-derived allergens		
Pollen–fruit		
Birch pollen	Apple, carrot, cherry, pear, peach, plum, fennel, walnut, potato, spinach, wheat, buckwheat, peanut, honey, celery, kiwi fruit, persimmon	Profilin, Bet v 1 and Bet v 6 analogs
Japanese cedar pollen	Melon, apple, peach, kiwi fruit	Pectate lyase
Mugwort pollen	Celery, carrot, spices, melon, watermelon, apple, camomile, hazelnut, chestnut	Lipid transfer proteins, profilins, 34 and 60 kDa allergens, Art v 1 analogs
Grass pollen	Melon, tomato, watermelon, orange, cherry, potato	Profilins
Ragweed pollen	Melon, camomile, honey, banana, sunflower seeds	Pectate lyase
Latex–fruit		
Latex	Avocado, potato, banana, tomato, chestnut, kiwi fruit, herbs, carrot	Patatin (e.g. Sol t 1), profilin, class I chitinases, Hev b 6, Pers a 1
Latex-mold		
Latex	*Aspergillus fumigatus*	Manganese superoxide dismutase
Animal-derived allergens		
Bird–egg		
Bird material	Egg yolk	Serum albumin (Gal d 5)
Egg–egg		
Egg white powder	Egg-containing foods	Lysozyme (Gal d 4)
Pork–cat		
Animal meat	Animal danders	Serum albumin
Arthropod–shellfish		
Mites	Shellfish, snails	Tropomysoin
Mites	*Anisakis simplex*	Tropomysoin
Cockroach	Shellfish, snails	Tropomysoin

species. With regard to the biting insects, the major allergenic species include ticks, ants, and mosquitos. Here, salivary proteins as well as venom proteins have been shown to be allergenic.

ALLERGEN NOMENCLATURE

The Allergen Nomenclature Subcommittee of the International Union of Immunological Societies (IUIS) (http://www.allergen.org) has introduced guidelines to facilitate the consistent naming of purified allergens from complex sources and in this regard data regarding novel allergens (as long as it is recognized by more than 5% of an allergic population) which have been isolated and sequenced should be submitted to this subcommittee for confirmation of its designation. For example, using the published guidelines, the designation for the cysteine protease allergen, Der p 1, from the house dust mite *Dermatophagoides pteronyssinus* is constructed by taking the first three letters of the genus (i.e. *Dermatophagoides*), together with the first letter of the species (i.e. *pteronyssinus*) and combining it with an arabic numeral which reflects the order in which the allergen was isolated or its clinical importance. In the case of Der p 1, this was the first mite allergen to be isolated and characterized, as well as cloned. If there is likely to be confusion with a previously named allergen, an additional letter may be used with either the genus or species name to avoid such a possibility. For example, the fungal alkaline serine protease allergen from *P. chrysogenum* is designated Pen ch 13 to distinguish it from the related allergen Pen c 13 from *P. citrinum*. Similarly, the allergen from *Candida albicans* is designated Cand a 1 to differentiate from the dog allergen, Can d 1. Allergens from different species within a genus or across genera will use the same numbering arrangement. For example, the related mite cysteine protease allergens from the species *D. farinae* and *Euroglyphus maynei* are referred to as Der f 1 and Eur m 1 respectively. Collectively, such related allergens are often referred to as belonging to a particular group, e.g. the 'group 1 mite allergens'. With the significant increase in the amount of sequence data generated due to the adoption of cloning technologies, it is apparent that a particular allergen source may contain a number of allergens with sequences that are very similar (> 67% sequence identity using the IUIS Allergen Nomenclature Subcommittee guidelines). In this case, such allergens are described as isoallergens and are given a suffix ranging from 00 to 99 (e.g. Amb a 1.01, Amb a 1.02). In situations where similar allergens are described that differ only in the occasional residue (polymorphism), these are described as variants, and an additional two digits are used in the description (e.g. Amb a 1.0101 – the first variant of the isoallergen Amb a 1.01).

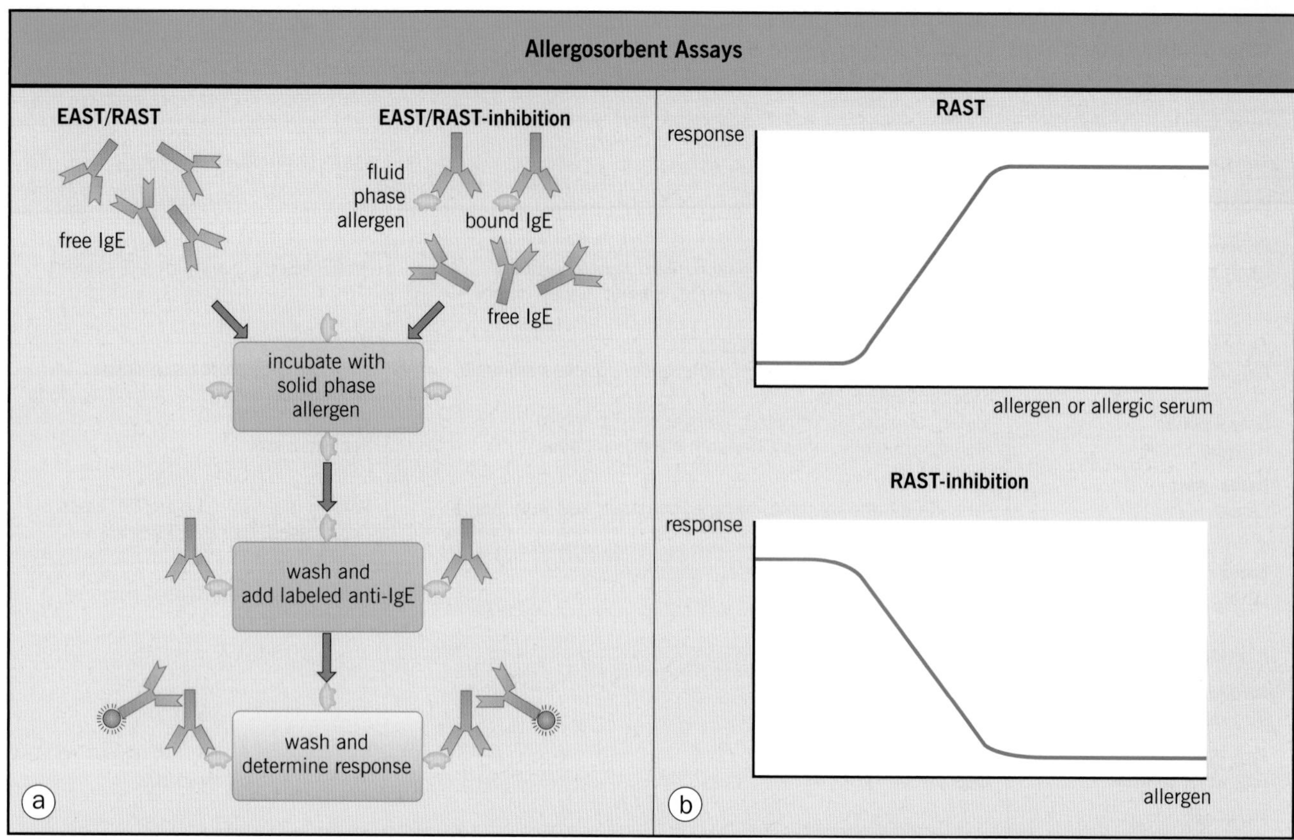

Fig. 17.7 Outline of the steps involved in allergosorbent and allergosorbent-inhibition assays. In enzyme-linked and radioallergosorbent assays (EAST/RAST) used for allergen characterization purposes, increasing concentrations of allergen are coupled to a solid phase and then incubated with a constant volume of serum from an allergic donor. For diagnostic purposes, a constant amount of allergen is coupled to the solid phase and varying dilutions of serum are then added. The amount of IgE bound is detected using a labeled anti-IgE. In each case, a positive dose response curve is obtained. In EAST/RAST inhibition, allergic serum is incubated with fluid phase allergen prior to incubation with solid phase allergen. The more potent the fluid phase allergen, the less free IgE is available to bind to the solid phase allergen. This gives rise to a negative dose response curve.

DETECTION OF ALLERGENS

Several techniques have been developed to determine whether an individual is allergic to a particular allergenic source or whether a protein isolated from a source is an allergen. Before the discovery of IgE and the development of serum-based immunochemical assays, the only methods available were biological, e.g. the skin prick test and the basophil degranulation assay. In the skin prick assay, the putative allergenic material is pricked into the epidermis of forearm skin of appropriately sensitized volunteers and the resulting wheal-and-flare reaction induced by sensitized mast cell degranulation recorded. In the basophil degranulation assay, sensitized (active or passive) basophils in whole blood are exposed to allergen and the resulting histamine release (or other mediators such as the leukotrienes) is measured. Despite their potential usefulness, the direct demonstration of IgE binding to a particular allergen or allergen source using serum-based methods has, in the main, supplanted the biological assays in monitoring allergenicity. However, in vivo or ex vivo assays may still be used in diagnostic situations (although they will not be described in this chapter) and may be used occasionally to confirm biological allergenic activity when characterizing novel allergens.

Allergosorbent tests

In allergosorbent tests (AST), allergen or allergen extract is immobilized onto an insoluble matrix such as plastic, cellulose nitrate, cellulose (paper) or agarose beads and incubated with sera from suspect patients. The IgE antibody binds to the immobilized allergen and is then detected by antibody specific for IgE. This antibody is conjugated with either radioisotope (radioallergosorbent test; RAST) or enzyme (enzyme allergosorbent test; EAST) (e.g. horseradish peroxidase) and the degree of IgE binding determined (Fig. 17.7) using appropriate detection systems. Variants of these methods include inhibition assays where varying concentrations of allergens are mixed with aliquots of the allergic serum before incubation with the matrix-bound allergen. If the soluble allergen has bound IgE in the serum, this is reflected in decreased IgE binding to the matrix. The results are expressed as the amount of allergen required to give 50% inhibition of maximum binding and, when comparing similar extracts, the lower the concentration required, the more potent. In addition, the slope of the inhibition curve obtained gives information regarding the range of allergens contained within an extract and this technique is regularly used in allergen standardization. More recently, our ability to produce recombinant

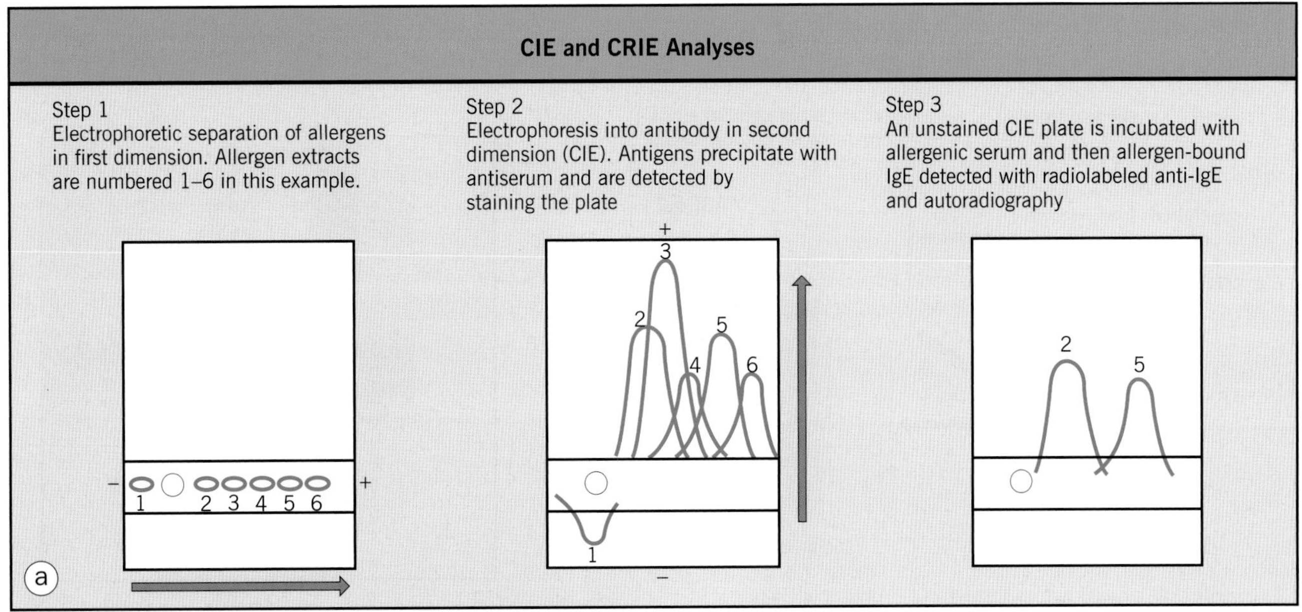
CIE and CRIE Analyses
Step 1
Electrophoretic separation of allergens in first dimension. Allergen extracts are numbered 1–6 in this example.
Step 2
Electrophoresis into antibody in second dimension (CIE). Antigens precipitate with antiserum and are detected by staining the plate
Step 3
An unstained CIE plate is incubated with allergenic serum and then allergen-bound IgE detected with radiolabeled anti-IgE and autoradiography
a

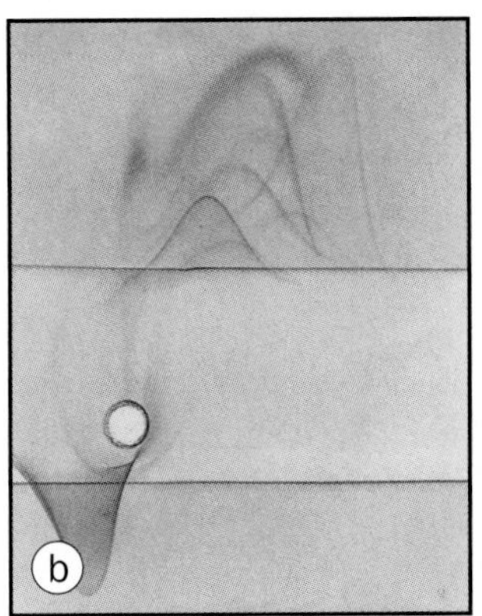
b

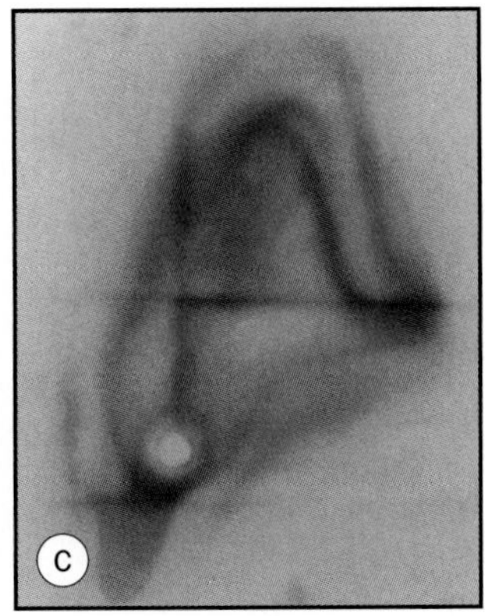
c

Fig. 17.8 Crossed immunoelectrophoresis (CIE) and crossed radioimmunoelectrophoresis (CRIE) analysis of allergen extracts, with CIE (b) and CRIE (c) analyses of *Lolium perenne* pollen extract.

allergens and the advances made in protein chip technology have given rise to the possibility of using this microarray technology to diagnose allergy. In this technique, small spots of allergen are bound to activated glass slides and then treated with serum as described above. The potential advantage of this technique lies in its ability to determine whether a patient is allergic to one or more of a large panel of allergens at once using minimal amounts of serum.

Crossed radioimmunoelectrophoresis

In crossed radioimmunoelectrophoresis (CRIE), allergen extracts are electrophoretically separated in an agarose gel, at the conclusion of which the gel is rotated 90 degrees and electrophoresis continued into agarose containing an antiserum raised against the whole allergen extract. The separated proteins migrate into the antibody-containing gel until they meet their homologous IgG antibodies which, because of their lack of charge in the chosen electrophoretic conditions, remain stationary. Once antibody and homologous antigen interact at optimal proportions, individual precipitates form, reflecting the number of antigens contained within the original mixture and the corresponding homologous antibodies in the polyclonal antiserum used. To determine which of the precipitated proteins are allergenic, the unstained crossed immunoelectrophoresis (CIE) gel is washed to remove non-precipitated proteins in both the antiserum and the allergen extract within the gel, and the washed gel is then incubated with allergic serum. Allergen-specific IgE binds to remaining epitopes on the precipitate which after washing is detected using radiolabeled anti-IgE (Fig. 17.8).

One- and two-dimensional SDS-PAGE gel electrophoresis and immunoblotting

In one-dimensional sodium dodecyl sulfate polyacrylamide electrophoresis (SDS-PAGE), individual protein components of an allergen extract are electrophoresed after denaturation and reduction of both intra- and interchain disulfide bonds with dithiothreitol. The proteins, which separate on the basis of their molecular weight in descending order, are then transferred electrophoretically or by capillary action to a cellulose nitrate or nylon membrane, during which time the proteins renature. After washing, the membranes are blocked with an extraneous, non-allergenic protein to reduce non-specific effects and then incubated with allergic serum. IgE binding to individual allergens is then visualized using a labeled anti-IgE reagent

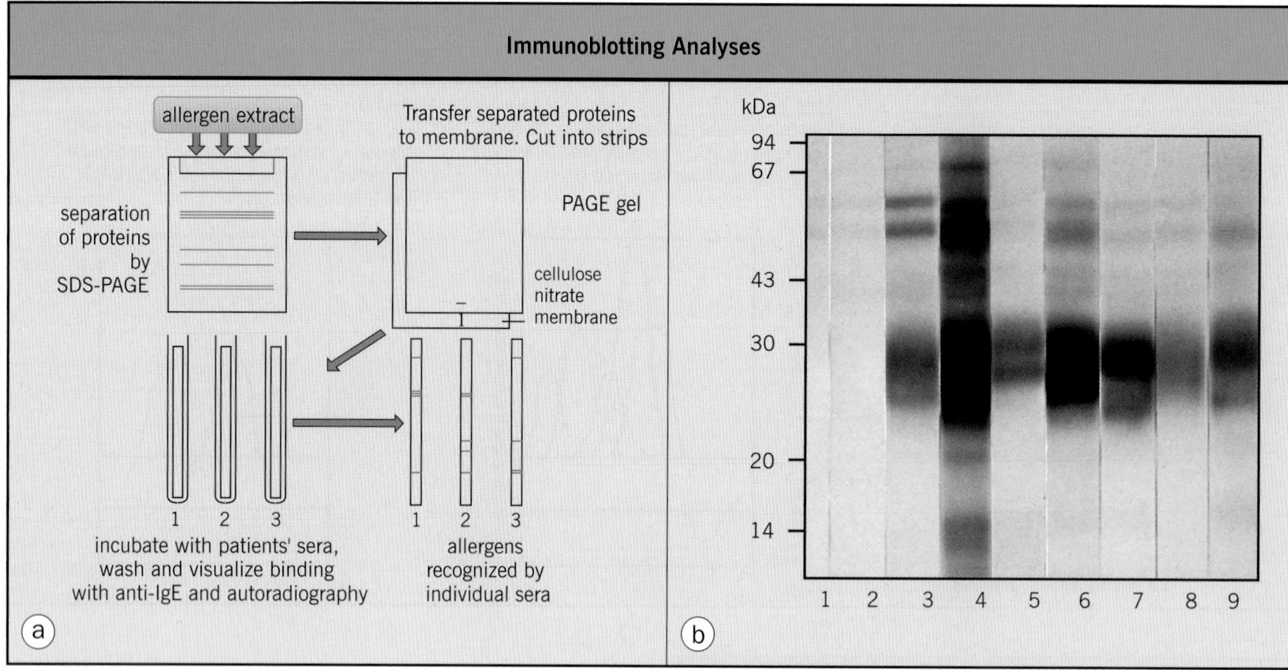

Fig. 17.9 Sodium dodecyl sulfate polyacrylamide electrophoresis (SDS-PAGE) and immunoblotting analysis of allergen extracts (left). SDS-PAGE-IgE immunoblot of *Lolium perenne* pollen extracts (right), demonstrating the responses obtained with sera from seven atopic individuals.

(Fig. 17.9). Immunoblotting provides information about the total number of allergens recognized by a sensitized individual as well as their apparent molecular weights. This technique is often used to determine the frequency of reactivities to allergenic components within an allergen extract. If this is the desired outcome, individual wells are filled with the same extract and the immunoblotted tracks are then incubated with individual sera in the study population. In two-dimensional electrophoresis, the allergen extract is first subjected to isoelectrophoresis in polyacrylamide gels containing ampholines which separate proteins on the basis of the isoelectric point (pI). The separated proteins within the gel are then subjected to SDS-PAGE at right angles to the isoelectrophoresis step. The resulting gels may then be immunoblotted as described above. This technique is superior to the one-dimensional approach in its resolving ability, and has been particularly useful in separating and characterizing allergens. Here, protein allergens may be digested in situ using proteolytic enzymes and the resulting peptides sequenced by Edman degradation or by mass spectroscopy.

ALLERGEN ISOLATION

Individual allergens are usually isolated from aqueous extracts prepared from the original allergenic source material. As most allergens are protein or glycoprotein, any of the physiochemical techniques available for isolating proteins in general (e.g. gel filtration, ion exchange, reverse phase chromatography) will suffice, including monoclonal antibody methodology, if purified allergens are available with which to immunize mice. More recently, recombinant DNA technology has become the method of choice for the characterization and production of recombinant allergens. In this regard, many of the clinically important allergens have now been cloned.

Cloning of allergens

In this technique, messenger (m)RNA is isolated from the allergen source, and complementary (c)DNA prepared by transcribing the RNA using the enzyme reverse transcriptase (Fig. 17.10). The single-stranded cDNA produced is then converted into double-stranded DNA with DNA polymerase and the resulting material inserted into appropriate vectors such as plasmids using restriction endonucleases, and cloned. The array of cDNA reflecting the starting mRNA represents the library which is then screened to isolate the cDNA coding for the allergens of interest. Screening may be accomplished by hybridization using oligonucleotide probes synthesized on the basis of amino acid sequences obtained by conventional protein sequencing of known allergens or, alternatively, using sera from allergic individuals. The latter technique is used when direct sequence information of the allergens is unavailable. Here, use is made of expression vectors which direct the synthesis of the recombinant allergen. Once cloned, the cDNA may be sequenced and the putative amino acid data checked to see if the allergen shows homology with any protein thus far sequenced. Such information may be useful in determining the role played by the allergen within the original source. These techniques may also be used to prepare allergen mutants where the allergenicity of specific recombinant allergens is reduced by substituting critical amino acid residues. This process has the potential to produce conformationally altered mutants that are unlikely to induce adverse reactions in sensitized individuals yet be capable of modulating specific T-cell responses during immunotherapy. The Allergen Nomenclature Subcommittee guidelines indicate that such recombinant allergens are identified by placing the letter 'r' in front of the allergen designation, e.g. rDer p 1 for the recombinant form of the mite cysteine protease allergen. If allergens are chemically synthesized, then the letter 's' must be used, e.g. sDer p 1.

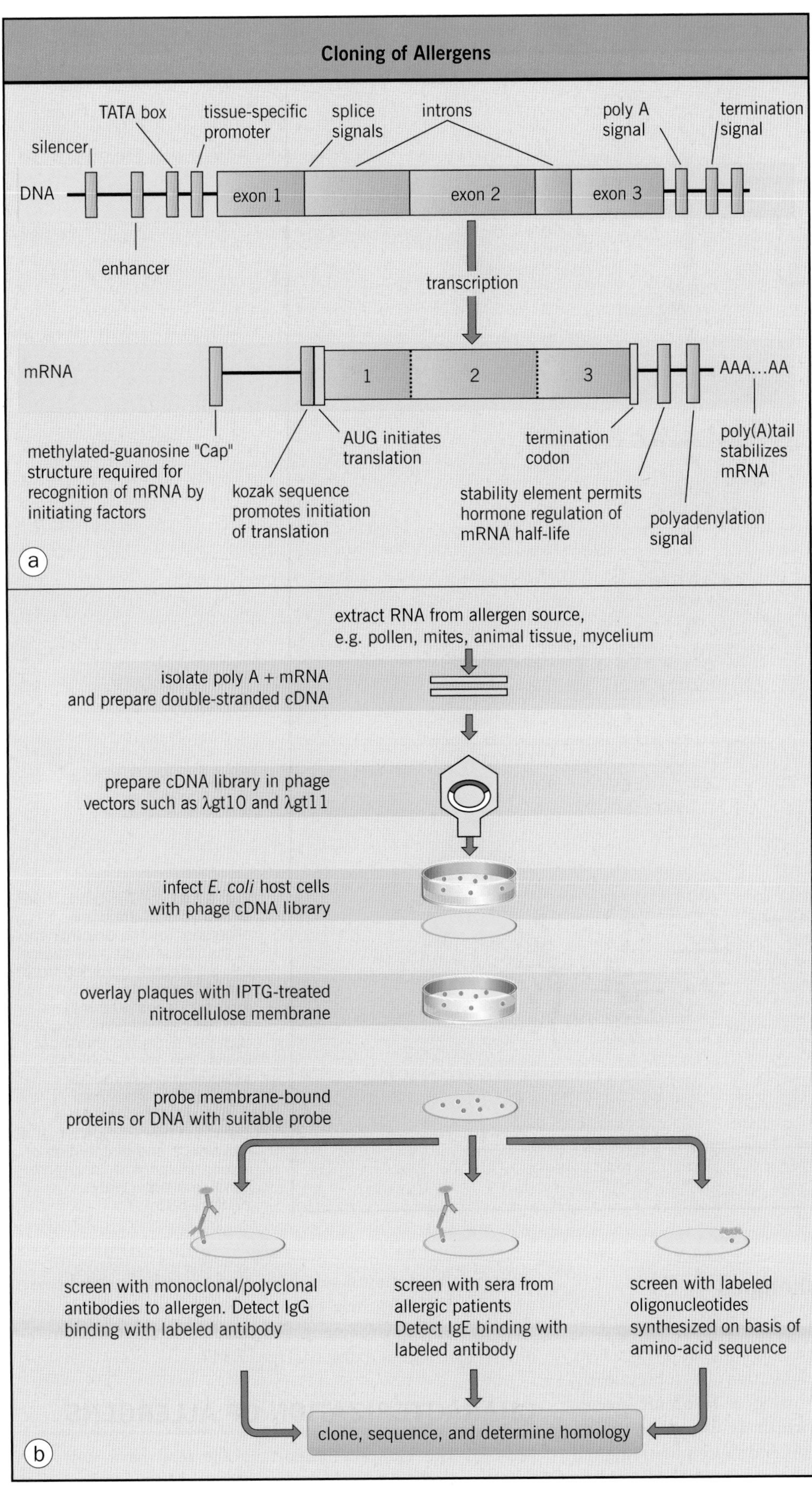

Fig. 17.10 (a) Schematic representation of (a) the structure of a typical eukaryotic gene coding for an allergen, (b) the steps involved in cloning allergen-specific cDNA into phage for subsequent expression as protein. (Modified from Stewart GA. Molecular biology of allergens. In: Busse WW, Holgate ST. Asthma and rhinitis. Oxford: Blackwell Scientific Publications; 1995.)

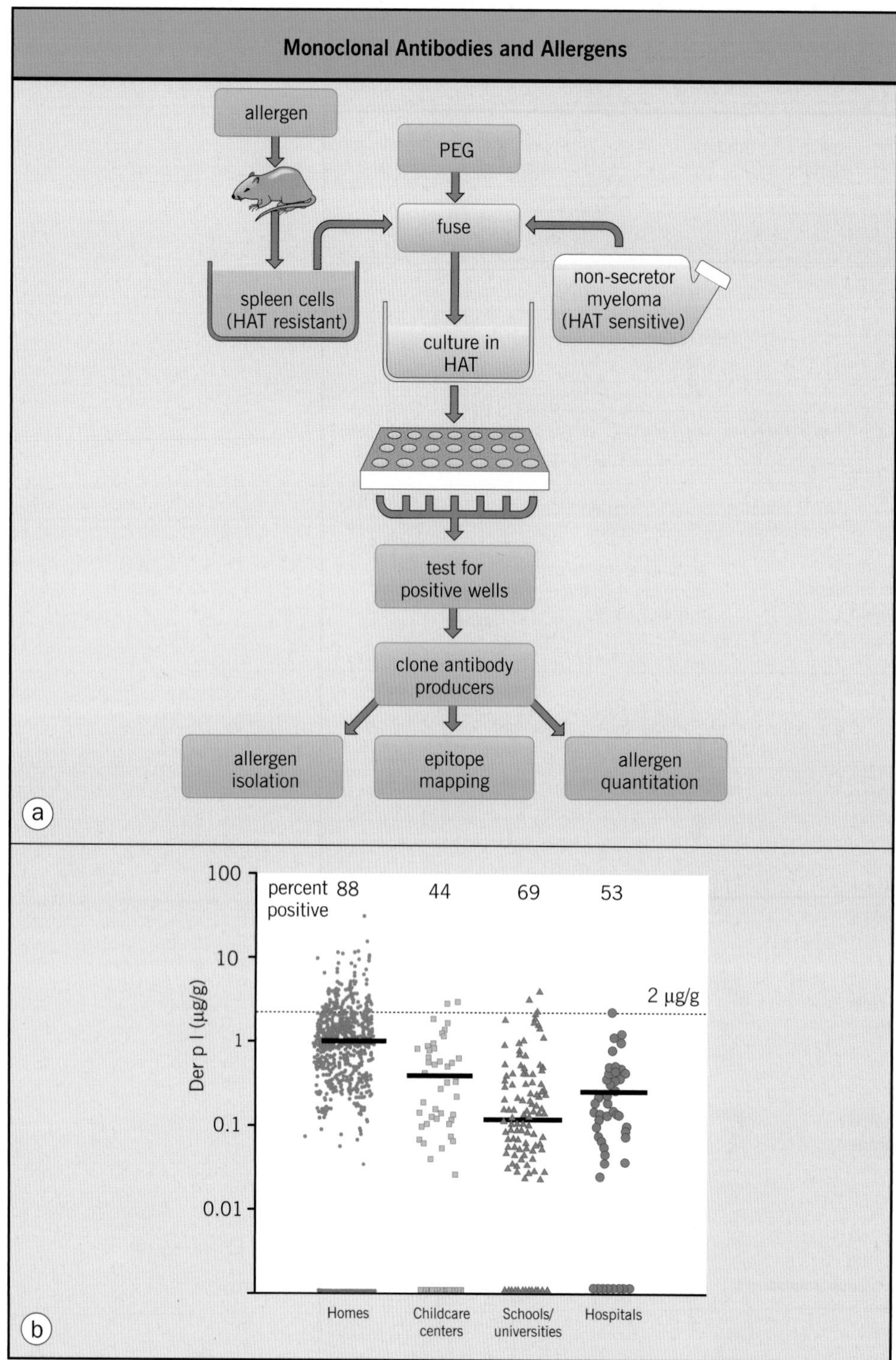

Fig. 17.11 (a) The production of monoclonal antibodies to allergens. (b) The determination of the house dust mite allergen Der p 1 in dust obtained from various locations. The bars represent geometric means and the dashed lines indicate currently accepted threshold levels. The mean levels of allergen in the home are significantly higher than elsewhere. (Modified from Zhang L, Chew FT, Soh SY, et al. Prevalence and distribution of indoor allergens in Singapore. Clin Exp Allergy 1997; 27:876–885.)

Monoclonal antibody techniques

In monoclonal antibody (mAb) techniques, mice are immunized with the purified allergen and spleen cells obtained a few weeks after primary and secondary immunization are subsequently fused with plasmacytoma cells using a fusogenic agent. Antibody-producing hybridomas which result are screened using appropriate selection chemicals and those possessing the appropriate specificity are isolated, cloned and then used to produce antibody in large quantities. Such hybridomas represent a potentially immortal supply of antibody which may be used to purify allergens, map epitopes, determine allergen concentrations in the environment, and standardize the concentration of allergens within extracts (Fig. 17.11).

CHARACTERIZATION OF ALLERGENS

Most of the clinically important allergens have now been cloned and their functions determined. Many are hydrolytic enzymes such as proteases, carbohydrases and ribonucleases

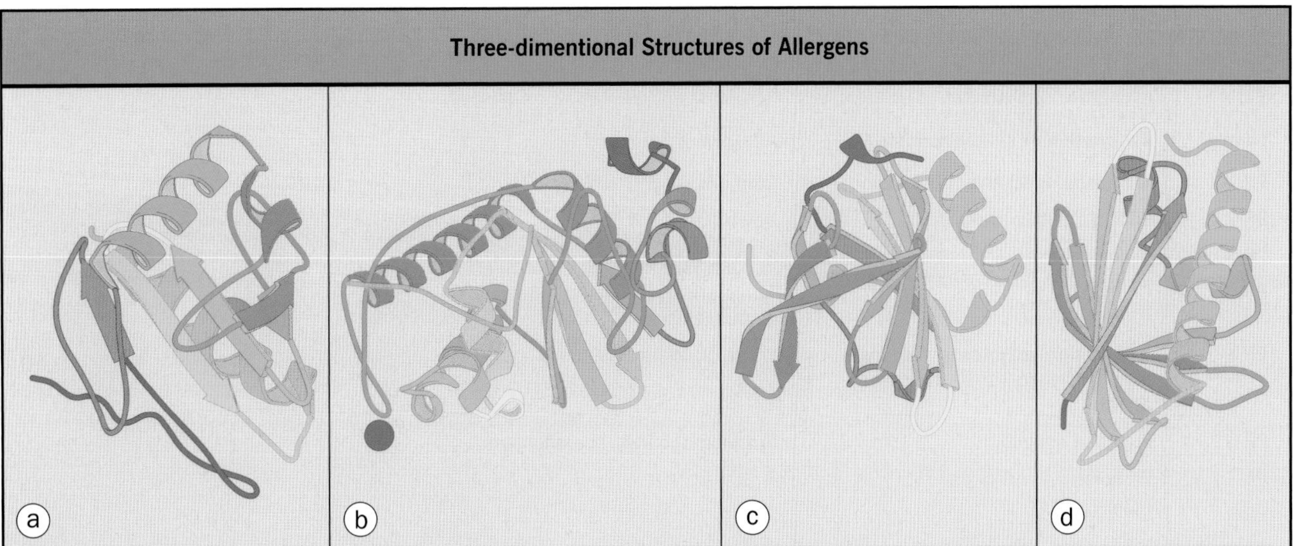

Fig. 17.12 Three-dimensional structures of allergens from (a) latex (Hev b v 8, profilin, 1G5U), (b) wasp venom (Ves v 5, 1QNX), (c) bovine dander (Bos d 2, 1BJ7) and (d) birch (Bet v 1, 1BV1). [The references for these structures are: Fedorov AA, Fedorov EV, Ganglberger E, et al. A comparative structural analysis of allergen profilins Hev b 8 and Bet v 2, to be published; Henriksen A, King TP, Mirza O, et al. Major venom allergen of yellow jackets, Ves v 5: structural characterization of a pathogenesis-related protein superfamily. Proteins 2001; 1; 45(4):438–448; Rouvinen J, Rautiainen J, Virtanen T, et al. Probing the molecular basis of allergy: three-dimensional structure of the bovine lipocalin allergen Bos d 2. J Biol Chem 1999; 274(4):2337–2343; Gajhede M, Osmark P, Poulsen FM, et al. X-ray and NMR structure of Bet v 1, the origin of birch pollen allergy. Nat Struct Biol 1996; 3(12):1040–1045; Berman HM, Westbrook J, Feng Z, et al. The protein data bank. Nucleic Acids Res 2000; 28(1):235–242.]

from mites, fungi, and pollens or non-hydrolytic enzymes such as pectin lyase from weed and tree pollen, the glycolytic enzymes from fungi such as enolase, alcohol dehydrogenase, aldolase and phosphoglycerate kinase, and glutathione transferases from cockroach and dust mites. Similarly, many show enzyme inhibitory activity or demonstrate marked sequence homology to known inhibitors, and are commonly found in seeds, potatoes, pollens, and hens' egg white. Many others are proteins involved in the transport of ligands such as lipids, pheromones, electrons, oxygen and iron, particularly the lipocalin allergens from animals such as rodents, dogs, cows, and horses. In addition, several pollen allergens have also been found to demonstrate homology with proteins known to transport a variety of ligands such as electrons, iron, oxygen, and lipid. Some allergens have been shown to be similar to a disparate but ubiquitous group of proteins known or considered to possess regulatory properties. These allergens are also encountered as antigens in parasite infection and autoimmunity and include profilins, the EF-hand calcium binding proteins, the cytoskeletal protein tropomyosin and heat shock proteins. Although their regulatory properties are varied, many appear to be associated with actin biology. The availability of cDNA coding of several of these allergens has now made it possible to determine the three-dimensional structures of some of the most important (Fig. 17.12).

Airborne allergens

Grass pollen aeroallergens

Allergens from a variety of grass pollens from species belonging to the clinically important subfamilies Pooideae (e.g. *Lolium* and *Phleum* spp., found in temperate climes), Chloridoideae (e.g. *Cynodon* spp., found in warmer climes) and Panicoideae (e.g. *Paspalum* spp., found in more tropical climes) have been described. The pollen allergens from the different grass species were originally divided into groups on the basis of marked physicochemical and immunochemical similarities, and this scheme has now been adopted for similar allergens derived from sources other than grass pollen. Grass pollen allergens may be divided into about 13 groups with varied functions associated with fertilization and pollen tube growth including expansins, extensins, ribonucleases, glucosidases, protease inhibitor-like proteins, calcium binding proteins and profilins (Appendix 17.1).

Weed pollen aeroallergens

The principal weed (referred to as such because they represent unwanted plants within a garden or field) pollen allergens associated with allergic disease are those belonging to the Asteraceae such as ragweed, mugwort, sunflower and feverfew, and wall-pellitory belonging to the Urticaceae. Several allergens from these species have been obtained but the most intensively studied source is ragweed. In this regard, the major allergens in this species are pectate lyases which are involved in the breakdown of pectin. A variety of other enzymes are necessary for pectin degradation such as polygalacturonase, polymethyl-galacturonase and pectin methylesterase, pectate lyase, pectin lyase and exopolygalacturonate lyase, all of which appear to be significant allergens in weed and tree pollens. Other common allergens include calcium binding proteins, profilins and lipid transfer proteins. The latter proteins are common allergens found in other sources such as seeds and belong to the prolamin superfamily (Appendix 17.2).

Table 17.6 The relationship between plant pathogenesis related proteins and allergens

Relationship Between Plant Pathogenesis Related Proteins and Allergens		
Family	**Description or characteristics**	**Allergen or source**
PR-1	Antifungal, mechanism unknown	Cum c 3
PR-2	Endo-β-1, 3-glucanase	Hev b 2, Ole e 4/9
PR-3	Endochitinase	Per s a 1, Hev b 11w
PR-4	Chitin binding proteins	Turnip prohevein, Hev b 6, wheat germ agglutinin
PR-5	Thaumatin-like proteins, antifungal, may have endo-β-1,3-glucanase activity	Pru av 2, Mal d 2, Jun a 3
PR-6	Protease inhibitor	Soy, wheat, barley, rice allergens
PR-7	Protease	?
PR-8	Chitinase	?
PR-9	Peroxidase	Wheat, barley allergens
PR-10	Plant steroid carrier	Bet v 1, Mal d 1, Pru av 1, Pyr c 1, Api g 1, Dau c 1 etc.
PR-11	Chitinase	Pru av 1, Pyr c 1, Api g 1
PR-12	Plant defensins	?
PR-13	Thionins	?
PR-14	Lipid transfer proteins	Pru p 3, Mal d 3, Gly m 1

PR-3 - type I (basic), II (acidic), IV, V, VI, VII chitinases; PR-4 - type I, II chitinases; PR-11 - type I chitinase; ?indicates that allergens belonging to a particular group have yet to be described.

Tree pollen aeroallergens

Several pollen allergens have been isolated from trees belonging to either the angiosperms (flowering trees) or the gymnosperms (conifers). It is clear that, in general, pollen allergens from species within the same family, for example, olive, lilac, ash and privet are related. Further, allergens from different families but within the same division are also similar, for example, the Fagales group (e.g. birch, alder, hornbeam) 1 and 2 allergens. However, there appears to be only limited similarity between orders. In this regard, the most potent allergens within the Order Fagales are the group 1 allergens which belong to or show homology with members of a diverse group of proteins known as pathogenesis-related proteins (Table 17.6). In contrast, in the Order Scrophalates (e.g. olive) they are proteins showing limited homology with known seed-derived protease inhibitors and in the division Pinopsida (gymnosperms) they are enzymes involved in pectin degradation. These differences are likely to reflect differences in pollen structure between angiosperms and gymnosperms (Appendices 17.3 and 17.4).

Non pollen-derived plant aeroallergens

A number of seed-derived allergens have been described both as aeroallergens and food allergens (Appendix 17.5). They are a significant source of allergens in occupational settings in industries such as baking and include flours prepared from wheat, barley, castor beans, mustard seed, green coffee beans, rice, cotton seed, Ispaghula and soy beans. The major seed-derived allergens usually belong to one of several types of storage proteins or proteins involved in protection against insects due to antimicrobial or enzyme inhibitory activites. These groupings include the cupin (vicilins and legumins) and prolamin (2S albumins, lipid transfer proteins) superfamilies and the pathogenesis-related proteins (PR). Some of the food allergens such as the lipid transport proteins appear to be highly resistant to digestion and heating, enabling them to cross epithelial barriers in a relatively intact form.

In addition to seeds, allergens may also be derived from other plant tissues including fruit, vegetables, and latex, which are generally important in occupational settings. Of importance are the latex allergens which may become absorbed into starch powder used as a lubricant in latex gloves which then becomes aerosolized. This results in a high prevalence of allergy in healthcare workers (20%) and patients with spina bifida (50%) who are exposed to latex products during surgical manipulations. Latex, a suspension of proteins in a water phase, is produced in response to deliberate cutting of the bark of the rubber tree and contains a variety of enzymes, proteins, and lectins for defensive purposes (c.f. the pathogenesis-related proteins. At least 13 allergens have now been described and include a rubber elongation factor, chitin-binding lectin, chitinase, profiling and endo-1,3-β glucosidase, as well as proteins of unknown function (Appendix 17.6).

Fungal aeroallergens

Several allergens from fungal species including *Alternaria alternata*, *Cladosporium herbarium*, *Aspergillus fumigatus*, *Penicillium* spp., and *Candida albicans* have been described because of their association with allergic disease as well as with aspergillosis and candidiasis. In addition, fungal enzymes used industrially have been shown to be allergenic. In this regard, enzymes such as amylase from *A. oryzae*, which is added to dough, have been shown to be potent allergens in the baking industry. The occupational fungal allergens are usually hydrolytic enzymes whereas the domestic fungal allergens are often enzymes associated with glycolysis or are of unknown function (Appendices 17.7 and 17.8).

Animal aeroallergens

A number of animal-derived aeroallergens have been described and are usually associated with dander, epithelium, fur, urine, or saliva. The major dander allergens, with the exception of the cat allergen Fel d 1, a psoriasin allergen and a mitochondrial allergen from the cow, belong to the lipocalin superfamily. Members of this family are involved in the transport of low molecular weight hydrophobic substances in hydrophilic environments. In addition to the lipocalins, serum proteins such as albumin and the immunoglobulins may also be allergenic (Appendix 17.9).

Insect aeroallergens

A number of insect-derived aeroallergens found in house dust or in occupational settings are clinically significant. Allergens from midges belonging to the Order Diptera such as the bloodworms (*Chironomus thummi thummi*), the green nimitti midge (*Cladotanytarsus lewisi*), and cockroach have been described. With regard to the two former insects, the hemoglobins have been shown to be major allergenic components whereas cockroach allergens comprise enzymes, lipocalins, and insect hemolymph-plated proteins (Appendix 17.10).

Arachnid allergens

Allergens from the house dust mites *Dermatophagoides pteronyssinus*, *D. farinae*, *D. microceras* and *Euroglyphus maynei*, the storage mites *Acarus siro* and *A. farris*, *Tyrophagus putrescentiae*, *T. longior*, *Glycyphagus domesticus* and *Lepidoglyphus destructor* and the tropical mite *Blomia tropicalis* have been characterized. They produce a variety of allergens, the majority of which are derived from fecal pellets. Many of the major allergens are hydrolytic enzymes involved in mite digestion, thus accounting for their presence in fecal pellets, whereas others remain biochemically undefined or are non-enzymatic proteins with diverse roles. The mite allergens include cysteine proteases, serine proteases, amylase, glutathione transferases, and tropomyosins. As with the grass pollens, the data indicate that each of the mite species within a family contains allergens which are biochemically and physicochemically similar but variations in the dominance of particular allergens between families may be observed (Appendix 17.11).

Occupational aeroallergens

The major occupational allergens are derived from various sources and most are hydrolytic enzymes, including the bacterial subtilisins (serine proteases) and amylases used in the detergent industry, fungal enzymes, and egg proteins used in the baking industry (Table 17.7).

Ingested food allergens

The important fish- bird- and mammal-derived allergens include the parvalbumins, tropomyosins, profilins, and lactalbumins, whereas in the plant-derived food allergens, they include the cupin, prolamin, and pathogenesis-related proteins. In OAS, many of the ingested allergens demonstrate significant sequences and therefore immunologic similarities with related proteins in pollens. Thus far, the major cross-reacting plant food allergens have been shown to correspond to the Fagales tree pollen group 1 and 2 allergens although other cross-reacting allergens such as the latex allergens chitinase, hevein, profilin and Hev b 5 also cross-react. The major invertebrate cross-reacting allergens are the tropomyosins (Appendices 17.12 and 17.13).

Injected insect allergens

The most important stinging insect allergens are those associated with the venom from bees (*Apis* spp.), wasps (yellow jackets; *Vespula* spp.), hornets (*Dolichovespula* spp.), paper wasps (*Polistes* spp.) and ants (*Solenopsis* spp.). They have been studied in detail given their importance in life-threatening anaphylaxis and the success of immunotherapy. The venoms contain a number of allergens which show homology with proteins associated with mammalian reproduction and it has been suggested that since the allergens are derived from stingers which represent modified ovipositors, it is feasible that the allergens may have played some ancestral role in insect reproduction. The allergens derived from stinging insects belonging to different families are structurally similar and include enzymes such as phospholipase, hyaluronidase and acid phosphatase as well as proteins of unknown function. Although the function of the vespid group 5 allergens is unclear, they demonstrate similarity with the plant pathogenesis-related proteins (Appendix 17.14).

Parasite allergens

Parasite allergens have been demonstrated in a variety of helminthic parasites. The major allergens include proteases and protease inhibitors as well as the lipid binding polyproteins (Appendix 17.15).

ALLERGEN USAGE AND STANDARDIZATION

Allergens, most usually in the form of aqueous extracts containing preservatives are used both diagnostically and to desensitize patients (termed allergen vaccines). Most of the available extracts used for these purposes are crude in that they contain not only allergens of interest but also irrelevant antigens. They have a finite shelf-life and there may be wide variation in potency between the same types of extract produced by different manufacturers. However, standardized allergen extracts are now becoming available which meet appropriate requirements of potency and reproducibility for both diagnostic and immunotherapeutic purposes and contain defined concentrations of specific allergens. With regard to using individual allergens for diagnostic and immunotherapeutic purposes, recombinant allergens as well as immunotherapeutic peptides are now being developed.

Monitoring allergen exposure

Monitoring the allergen source or individual allergen concentration can prove useful in several situations. For example, monitoring atmospheric pollen concentrations can warn people at risk of seasonal allergies. However, monitoring atmospheric concentrations of pollen and fungi should include a precise identification of the airborne particles and/or allergens so as to distinguish between allergenic and non-allergenic species. Specific allergen concentration monitoring may also be useful to determine whether atmospheric concentrations constitute a risk in the workplace or in the home. In the workplace it has proved relatively easy to monitor airborne allergen but in the home the allergen content of settled dust is usually sampled. Here, mAb assays have proved very useful and kits are available to measure allergen from mite, cockroach, and cat. These assays have helped in determining the concentrations of allergen associated with sensitization and provocation (Table 17.8). Such assays for measuring allergen concentrations are useful for assessing the effectiveness and timing of allergen avoidance measures.

Allergen avoidance and immunotherapy

One approach to reducing allergen-induced disease is to avoid the allergen source. This has had some success but, in many instances, total avoidance proves impossible. The simplest is to change jobs or move residence, but this is not often practical because of the social and financial circumstance involved and the possibility that other allergens in the new location may show cross-reactivity with the allergen being avoided. It is also possible to remove the source completely, e.g. by relinquishing the family pet, killing mites with acaracides, or installing high-efficiency filters to remove allergens from the atmosphere. A more recent approach is to attempt to modify the allergen itself so as to render it non-allergenic, e.g. by chemically modifying allergens such as those from the mite, with tannic acid. Allergens are also used in immunotherapy, particularly when patients are monosensitized. Despite our lack of understanding of the mechanisms underlying the clinical benefit observed, a number of novel methods for antigen delivery are currently under investigation. In this regard, 'naked' DNA vaccines comprising DNA coding for specific allergens rather than protein per se offers potential. For further details, the reader is directed to Chapter 12.

CONCLUSIONS

Over the last few years, progress in allergen research has been considerable and the majority of the clinically important allergens have now been characterized. All these developments should contribute significantly to our understanding of the nature of allergens and how they interact with the mechanisms involved in the disease process and, ultimately, result in better management of allergic conditions.

AIR POLLUTION

Definition: Pollutants are, in general, not allergens but they may exacerbate allergic diseases. Major pollutants, which may derive from both outdoor and indoor sources, include ozone, nitrogen dioxide, diesel fumes and cigarette smoke.

INTRODUCTION

The air that we breathe, whether indoors or outdoors, is universally contaminated by particles and gases emanating from both natural and artificial sources. These pollutants reach the eyes, the nose, the upper and lower airway, and the lung parenchyma (Fig. 17.13). Airborne allergens, of course, have a prominent role in causing and exacerbating allergic diseases, including hayfever and asthma. The effects of these non-allergenic substances are relevant to the allergist. Some of these pollutants augment responses to allergens, and people with allergic diseases tend to be more susceptible to a number of key indoor and outdoor pollutants. Symptoms caused by air pollutants, particularly at higher levels of exposure, may tend to mimic symptoms of allergic diseases. Patients with allergic diseases may turn to allergists for guidance concerning the self-management of their susceptibility to air pollution, particularly at a time when air pollution warnings are issued.

People with allergic diseases may be exposed to air pollutants in diverse indoor and outdoor environments (Fig. 17.14). The term microenvironment refers to locations that have unique air quality characteristics. For a typical adult, relevant microenvironments across the day might include the home, vehicles, the office, city streets, and various public places such as restaurants, bars, sports facilities, and shopping areas. For children, school and childcare facilities are relevant microenvironments in addition to the home and its environs. Exposures in any of the microenvironments may be clinically relevant, and a detailed and systematic history is needed to cover exposures in each microenvironment.

OUTDOOR AIR POLLUTION

Pollutants in outdoor air can come from natural sources, such as vegetation, the sea, and volcanoes; more relevant to health are the pollutants from artificial sources that contaminate not only urban areas but broader regions of entire countries, such as the central and eastern portion of the USA and many countries of the former Soviet Republic. These artificial sources can be broadly grouped as either stationary or mobile. The stationary sources include power-generating stations, which may burn coal, natural gas, or petroleum; fossil-fuel-burning industrial plants; and various additional manufacturing facilities. Mobile sources include gasoline- and diesel-fuelled vehicles.

The principal outdoor air pollutants relevant to persons with allergic diseases are typically present in complex mixtures, and the evidence for toxicity of the individual pollutants may not fully reflect the effect of the mixture. Fossil-fuel combustion typically generates primary particles in a size range that extends down to particles that are small enough to enter the lung. It also generates gases, including oxides of sulfur and nitrogen as well as carbon monoxide. The last of these impairs oxygen transport by binding to hemoglobin but it does not have toxicity that specifically affects people with allergic diseases. Sulfur oxides and nitrogen oxides undergo chemical transformation to form respirable secondary sulfate- and nitrate-containing particles, some of which are acidic. These small particles may also have heavy metals and organic chemicals on their surfaces, which can leach out in the airways to produce toxic effects. Sulfur dioxide, a highly soluble gas, is efficiently absorbed in the nose and upper airway whereas nitrogen dioxide, a less soluble gas, reaches the smaller airways of the lung.

In areas with both heavy vehicle traffic and high levels of sunlight, photochemical pollution or smog is generated. This type of pollution is a rich mixture of oxidative chemicals, generally indexed by the level of ozone (O_3). First identified in Los Angeles about 50 years ago, ozone pollution may become an increasingly widespread problem as urbanization has grown and cities have become progressively choked by vehicle traffic. In the USA, the problem of ozone pollution extends across the eastern portions of the country in the summer and affects many of the world's 'mega-cities'.

Various point sources of pollution may also affect persons with allergic diseases. Volatile organic compounds, which exist as gases at typical temperatures, and other respiratory irritants may contaminate air in communities and more specific sensitizing agents may also be released.

One of the best-known examples is the recent identification of the unloading of soybeans as the cause of sporadically occurring days of endemic asthma in Barcelona. Faulty equipment at a silo in the harbor resulted in the release of soy dust into the air; this dust contains an allergen now known to be a cause of asthma. Installation of filters ended the epidemic. Similar asthma episodes in New Orleans decades earlier have now also been linked to the unloading of soybeans. The Barcelona epidemic provides a reminder of the limits of our understanding of the environmental determinants of asthma.

INDOOR AIR POLLUTION

Indoor air pollutants are even more diverse than outdoor air pollutants, and many outdoor pollutants penetrate indoors. The indoor pollutants can be broadly grouped by source and type (Table 17.7). Indoor environments are, of course, principal microenvironments for exposure to allergens. Tobacco smoking releases fine particles and gases, including irritants such as acrolein and various aldehydes. The mixture of exhaled smoke and smoke released by the smoldering cigarette is referred to as environmental tobacco smoke. Nicotine is present as a gas in environmental tobacco smoke. Homes with smokers tend to have much higher levels of respirable particles than homes without smokers. Gas-fired ranges and ovens emit nitrogen dioxide, particularly if they have continuously burning pilot lights. Space heating devices also release nitrogen dioxide, and kerosene combustion may generate acids from sulfur that is present in the fuel. In the developing world, smoke from burning of biomass fuels is a dominant contributor to personal exposure. In developed countries, properly operated wood-stoves and fireplaces have little impact on indoor air quality.

Many different volatile organic compounds are found in indoor air; they come from building materials, furnishings, household products, office equipment, and other sources. Formaldehyde is the best known of this group of relatively low-molecular-weight chemicals that are in a gaseous form at room temperature. Concentrations are typically highest when a building is new and then decline as materials age. However, renovations and new processes and equipment, such as printers and copiers, may increase emissions of volatile organic compounds. Two other indoor pollutants – radon and asbestos – are carcinogens but are of no direct relevance to allergic diseases.

MECHANISMS OF TOXICITY

The toxicity of the various air pollutants depends on the site of deposition and the specific chemical properties of the pollutants (Table 17.9). The more water-soluble pollutants affect the mucous membranes of the eyes and upper airway and do not reach the lower airways and alveoli without the increased ventilation that results from exercise; less soluble gases, including nitrogen dioxide and ozone, can reach the lungs, where absorption from the airways is greatest. The site of particle deposition depends largely on the size of the particles, which is usually expressed as the aerodynamic diameter (Fig. 17.15). The larger airborne particles – those above approximately $10\,\mu m$ in aerodynamic diameter and referred to as PM10 – do not penetrate into the respiratory tract, and particles of size PM10 down to PM2.5 are filtered in the upper airway. Particles less than $2.5\,\mu m$ in diameter can enter the lower respiratory tract, whereas the smaller particles – those under $1\,\mu m$ in diameter – deposit in the small airways and alveoli.

Inflammation is central to the response of the respiratory tract, and probably also of the eye, to non-allergenic pollutants. Although specific mechanisms of action differ, all these pollutants initiate inflammation at the sites of deposition. In experimental studies, pollution exposure has been shown to provide cytokine release and neutrophil influx. The effects of prolonged exposures to most pollutants are not yet well characterized, although experimental and epidemiologic evidence indicates the possibility of airways fibrosis and narrowing and airspace enlargement, which leads to reduced ventilatory function. Increased frequency of respiratory symptoms is common.

This inflammation may be of consequence to the allergic disorders through several pathways. The presence of this non-specific inflammation may enhance responses to allergens – facilitation of allergen penetration as a result of increased permeability of the respiratory epithelium is a proposed mechanism. In experimental exposures of volunteers with asthma, exposures to ozone or nitrogen dioxide enhance the response to subsequent antigen challenge. There is also the possibility of synergism between inflammation caused by air pollution and that provoked by allergens. With regard to asthma, heightened airway responsiveness secondary to pollutant exposure might augment the response to allergens and make clinically relevant effects more frequent.

AIR POLLUTION AND ALLERGIC DISEASES

Allergic rhinitis

The nose acts as a filter, removing larger particles and soluble gases from inhaled air. Inflammatory responses of the nose following inhalation of various pollutants have been well described. Ozone characteristically causes burning and irritation of the eyes and upper airway, including the nose. Pollutant gases have been shown to induce inflammation in the nose and eyes. However, clinically relevant consequences of air pollution exposure for persons with allergic rhinitis have received little attention.

Table 17.7 Sources of common indoor contaminants

Sources of Common Indoor Contaminants	
Contaminant	**Source**
Asbestos	
Chrysotile, crocidolite, amosite, tremolite	Some wall and ceiling insulation installed between 1930 and 1950; old insulation on heating pipes and equipment; old woodstove door gaskets; some vinyl floor tiles; drywall joint finishing material and textures paint purchased before 1977; cement asbestos millboard and exterior wall shingles; some sprayed and troweled ceiling finish plaster installed between 1945 and 1973; fire retardant sprayed into some structural steal beams
Combustion by-products	
Carbon monoxide, nitrogen- and sulfur dioxide particulate soot, nitrogenated compounds	Gas ranges; wood and coal stoves; fireplaces; backdraft of exhaust flues; candles and incense
Tobacco smoke	
Carbon monoxide, nitrogen and carbon dioxide, hydrogen cyanide, nitrosamines, aromatic hydrocarbons, benzo[a]pyrene, particles, benzene, formaldehyde, nicotine	Cigarettes, pipes, cigars
Formaldehyde	
	Some particleboard, plywood, pressboard, paneling, some carpeting and carpet backing, some furniture and dyed materials, UFFI, some household cleaners and deodorizers, combustion gas, tobacco, wood, some glues and resins, tobacco smoke, cosmetics, permanent-press textiles
Microbiological organisms	
Fungal spores; bacteria; viruses; pollens; arthropods; protozoa	Mold, mildew, and other fungi, humidifiers with stagnant water, water-damaged surfaces and materials, condensing coils and drip pans in HVAC systems, refrigerator drainage pans, some thermophilics on dirty heating coils, animals, rodents, insects, humans
Radon	
Radon gas, ^{210}Bi, ^{218}Po, ^{210}Po, ^{210}Pb	Soil, rocks, water (gas diffuses through cracks and holes in the foundation and floor), well water, natural gas used near the source wells, some building material such as granite
Volatile organic compounds	
Alkanes, aromatic hydrocarbons, esters, alcohols, aldehydes, ketones	Solvents and cleaning compounds, paints, glue and resins, spray propellants, fabric softeners and deodorizers, combustion, dry-cleaning fluids, some fabrics and furnishings, store gasoline, out-gassing from water, some building materials, waxes and polishing compounds, pens and markers, binders and plasticizers

Modified from Samet JM et al. Indoor air pollution. In: Rom WN, ed. Environmental and occupational medicine. Philadelphia: Lippincott – Raven; 1998:1523–1537. HVAC, heating ventilation and air conditioning; UFFI, urea-formaldehyde foam insulation.

Asthma

The role of air pollution in causing and exacerbating asthma has been investigated extensively. Many of the relevant data come from epidemiologic studies that have been directed at either assessing risk factors for disease or determining if the status of people with asthma varies in relation to air pollution exposure. Additional data come from controlled air pollution exposures of volunteers with asthma, a research design often referred to as a clinical study. In clinical studies, exposures are of necessity brief and limited to lower levels of pollutants, and the protocols generally exclude people with more severe disease.

There is little indication that the general types of air pollution found in urban and industrialized areas contribute to the production of asthma. Some reports describe a higher prevalence of non-specific bronchial hyperresponsiveness in more polluted areas but definitive links to asthma have not been made. Some outbreaks of asthma have been linked to specific agents, such as the problem of soy bean asthma in Barcelona, but such episodes appear to be infrequent.

Table 17.8 Proposed allergen threshold concentrations

Proposed Allergen Threshold Concentrations		
Allergen source	**Specific allergen**	**Threshold concentration**
Dust		μg/g
House dust mite	Der p 1	< 2–10
Cow dander	Bos d 2	1-20
Cat dander	Fel d 1	8
Dog dander	Can f 1	10
Air		ng/m^3
Latex	–	0.6
Detergent enzymes	Subtilisin	15–60
Flour mixture	Asp o 2	0.25

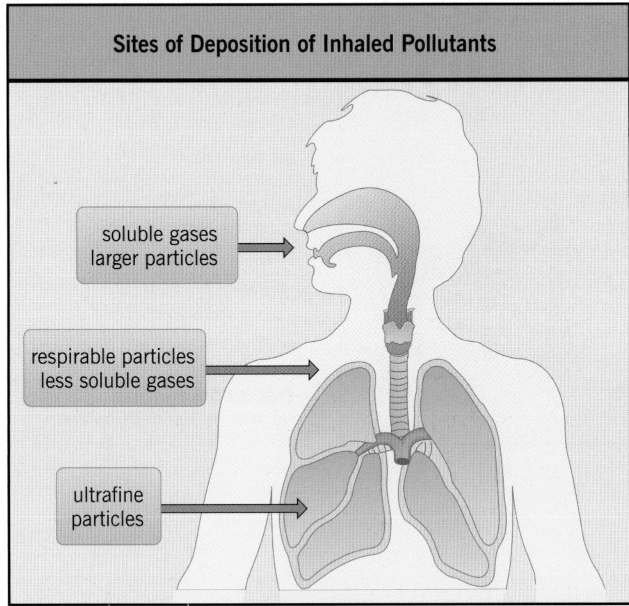

Fig. 17.13 Sites of absorption and deposition of inhaled particles and gases.

Indoor air pollutants have been identified as causes of asthma, although it is still not known whether onset of asthma is a reflection of environmental and genetic interaction, or if some patients develop asthma solely because of environmental factors. The level of house dust mite exposure predicts the age of initial wheezing in children at risk of asthma (Fig. 17.16). Of the many indoor air pollutants other than indoor allergens, passive exposure to tobacco smoke is most firmly established as a cause of asthma in young children (Fig. 17.17). Mounting evidence shows that children of mothers who smoke are at increased risk. The risk may partially reflect the consequences of in utero exposure to tobacco smoke components from maternal smoking during pregnancy. Physiologic testing shortly after birth shows that infants of smoking mothers have reduced airway function and a higher level of non-specific bronchial hyperresponsiveness compared to infants of non-smoking mothers (Fig. 17.18). Formaldehyde, a common indoor exposure, is infrequently found to be a cause of asthma.

Both indoor and outdoor air pollutants can adversely affect people with asthma. Indoor allergen exposure is, of course, tightly linked to the clinical status of asthmatics. For children, exposure to tobacco smoke increases the level of non-specific bronchial hyperresponsiveness and exposed children tend to use medical resources more often than non-exposed children. Some clinical studies indicate that nitrogen dioxide, another prevalent indoor gaseous agent, increases airway responsiveness and also the degree of response to inhaled allergens. Epidemiologic data on indoor nitrogen dioxide and exacerbation of asthma are limited.

Outdoor pollutants that may exacerbate asthma include particulate matter, sulfur dioxide, nitrogen dioxide, and ozone. Data on these pollutants have been gained from clinical studies, follow-up studies of people with asthma, and studies on rates of clinic and emergency room visits and hospitalization. Evidence from throughout the world indicates that these pollutants can exacerbate asthma. Particulate air pollution of diverse composition, including wood smoke particles and acidic particles, has been associated with measures of exacerbation (Fig. 17.19).

Clinical studies show that some asthmatics have exquisite sensitivity to sulfur dioxide, particularly when the dose delivered to the lungs is increased by exercise. The evidence from clinical studies that nitrogen dioxide can increase airway responsiveness is less clear. Extensive epidemiologic data show that ozone exposure can adversely affect people with asthma, although asthmatics are not more sensitive than non-asthmatics to the reduction of lung function that follows ozone exposure.

Clinical implications

The evidence for the link between indoor and outdoor air pollution and asthma has implications for the prevention of asthma and the management of patients with asthma. With regard to prevention, the damning evidence on maternal smoking during pregnancy and early childhood is sufficient to warrant educational intervention, particularly if parental history of allergic disease indicates that the child is at high risk of asthma. Reduction of allergen exposure would also be prudent for such children.

Exposures in both indoor and outdoor environments have been linked to exacerbation of asthma. For the indoor environment, source control can be recommended as a prudent strategy.

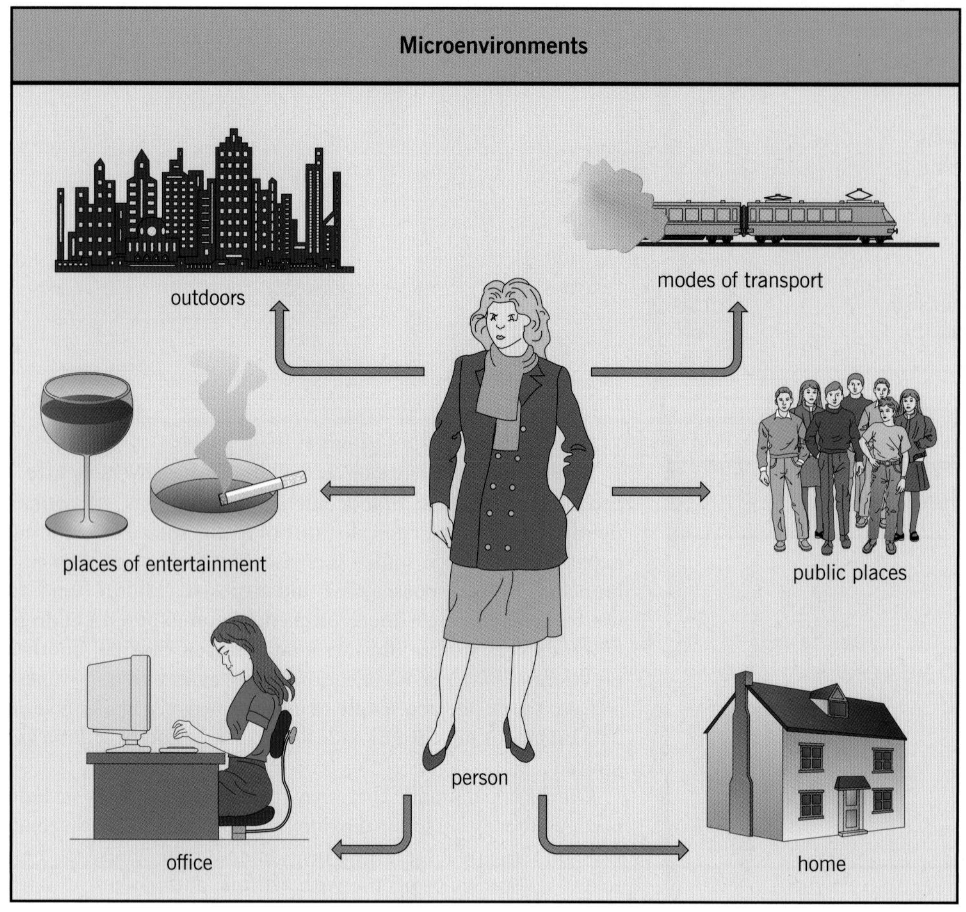

Fig. 17.14 Principal microenvironments for the average adult.

Table 17.9 Pathophysiologic responses of respiratory tract to environmental particles and gases

Pathophysiologic Responses of Respiratory Tract to Environmental Particles and Gases			
Site	**Agent**	**Response**	**Comments**
None	Pollen	Hayfever, rhinitis	Immunologic/non-immunologic mechanisms
Airways	Formaldehyde	Nasal cancer	Not conclusively established
	Sulfur dioxide, nitrogen dioxide	Bronchoconstriction	Reflex, irritant
	Aeroallergens	Asthma	Immunologic reaction
	Formaldehyde, wood smoke	Irritation, cough	Immunologic/non-immunologic mechanisms
	Radon asbestos	Cancer	Relations of environmental asbestos exposure and lung cancer uncertain
Parenchyma	Thermophilic actinomycetes, fungi	Hypersensitivity pneumoconiosis	Immunologic mechanisms
	Inorganic dust	Pneumoconiosis	Unrelated to environmental exposures

Modified from Utell MJ, Samet JM. Environmentally mediated disorders of the respiratory tract. Med Clin North Am 1990; 74:291–306.

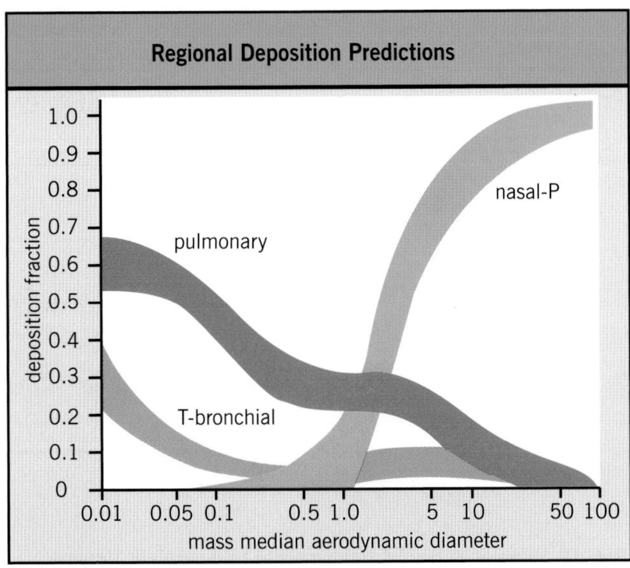

Fig. 17.15 Regional deposition predictions based on the model proposed by the International Commission on Radiological Protection Task Group on Lung Dynamics. (Modified from Wilson R, Spengler JD, eds. Particles in our air. Concentrations and health effects. Cambridge, MA: Harvard University Press; 1996.)

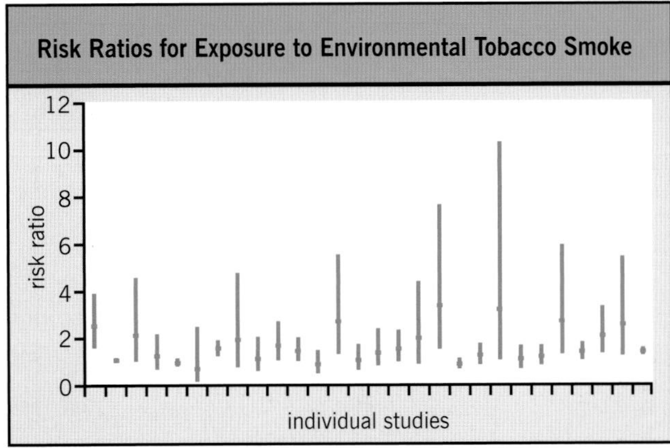

Fig. 17.17 Reported risk ratios (95% confidence intervals) in young children exposed to environmental tobacco smoke in studies that used clinically recognized asthma as an outcome. (From Office of Environmental Health Hazard Assessment, 1997.)

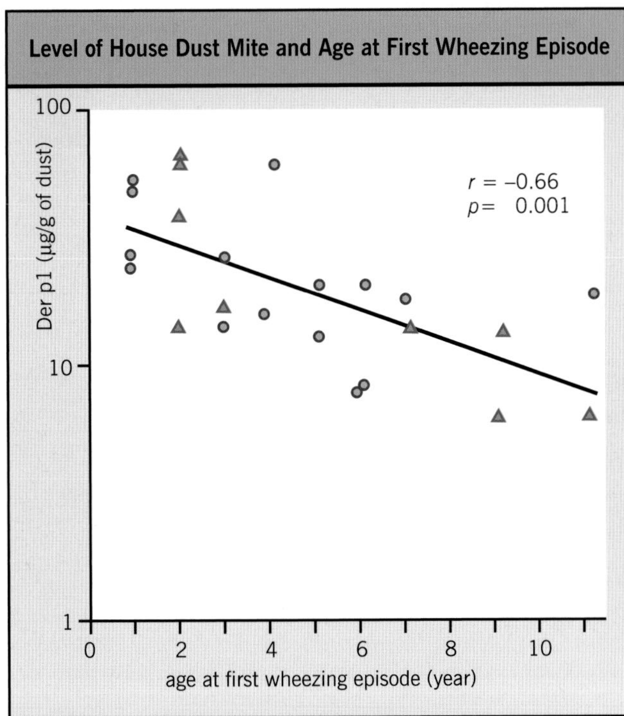

Fig. 17.16 Relation between the age at the onset of the first wheezing episode in 21 atopic children and the highest level of Der p 1 in house dust in 1979. (With permission from Sporik R, Holgate ST, Platts-Mills TAE, et al. Exposure to house-dust mite allergen (Der p 1) and the development of asthma in childhood. A prospective study. N Engl J Med 1990; 323:502–507, © Massachusetts Medical Society.)

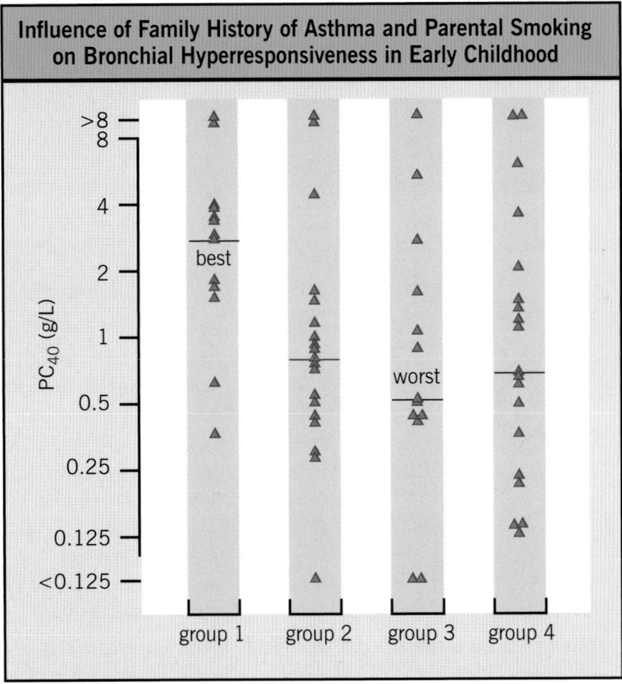

Fig. 17.18 Individual values for the histamine concentrations that provoked a decrease of 40% in maximal flow at functional residual capacity [V_{max}FRC (PC_{40})]. Group 1: no family history of asthma, both parents non-smokers; group 2: family history of asthma, both parents non-smokers; group 3: no family history of asthma, one or both parents smokers; group 4: family history of asthma, one or both parents smokers. The horizontal lines show the median PC_{40} for each group. Two infants in group 2 had baseline flow limitation and therefore could not be challenged with histamine. No PC_{40} value could be determined for one infant in group 4, in whom excessive upper-airway noise developed, necessitating discontinuation of the challenge. (With permission from Young S, Le Souf PN, Geelhoed GC, et al. The influence of a family history of asthma and parental smoking on airway responsiveness in early infancy. N Engl J Med 1991; 324:1168–1173, © Massachusetts Medical Society.)

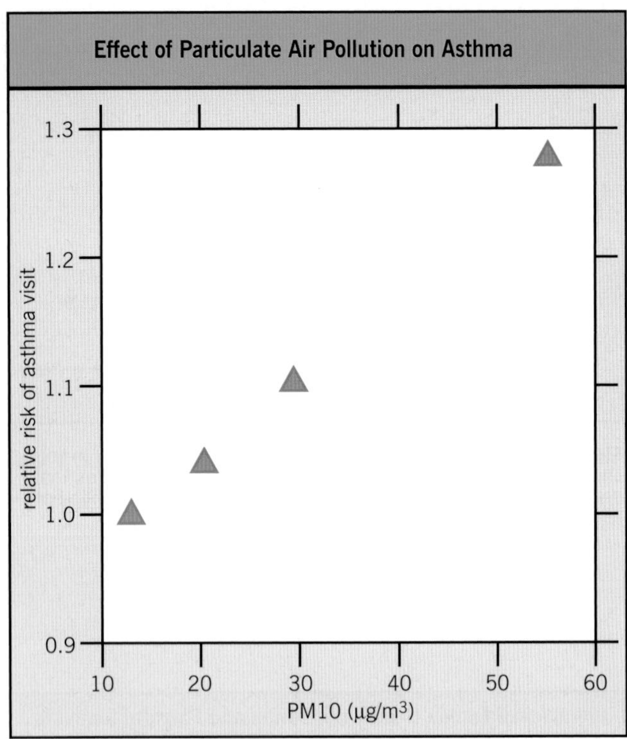

Fig. 17.19 Relative risk of asthma visits by quartile of airborne particles with aerodynamic diameter above approximately 10 μm (PM10) concentration, plotted against the mean PM10 concentration in the quartile. The relative risks are ajusted for temperature, season, day of week, hospital,time trends, age, and September peak. (With permission from Schwartz J, Slater D, Larson TV, et al. Particulate air pollution and hospital emergency room visits for asthma in Seattle. Am Rev Respir Dis 1993; 147:826–831, © American Lung Association.)

Table 17.10 Expected filter performance ratings for different filter types

Expected Filter Performance Ratings for Different Filter Types

Filter types	Filter media	Weight arrestance (%)	Atmospheric dust spot efficiency (%)	DOP efficiency (%)
Panel-type filter	Spun-glass, open cell foam, expanded metals and screen, synthetics, textile denier woven and non-woven, or animal hair	50–85		
Pleated panel-type filter	Fine denier nonwoven synthetic and synthetic-natural fiber blends, or all natural fiber	85–90	20–30	
Extended surface-type supported or non-supported	Fine glass fibers, fine electret synthetic fibers, or wet-laid paper of cellulose glass or all-glass fibers	95–99.7	30–98	0-90
Extended-area pleated HEPA-type filters	Wet-laid ultrafine glass fiber paper	99.99		99.7–99.99

From Am J Respir Crit Care Med 1997; 156:S31–S64, © American Thoracic Society. DOP, dioctyl phthalate; HEPA, high efficiency particulate air

Tobacco smoking in the home can be limited and many countries are implementing workplace regulations to prohibit or limit smoking. Increasingly, products are being manufactured with low emission rates of various volatile organic compounds. Proper venting of combustion appliances and use of gas cookers and ranges without pilot lights further reduce exposure to combustion gases.

Air cleaning devices can remove both particles and gases. The most up-to-date devices incorporate high-efficiency particulate air filters for particles and a sorbent for gases. Table 17.10 reviews the principal types of filters and their performances. These devices can clean pollutants from air but the volumes handled are limited in relation to room size. Clinically relevant effects have not been shown and most clinical trials on air cleaners have not had sufficiently large sample sizes.

Exposures to most outdoor pollutants can be reduced by staying indoors. The concentration of ozone, a reactive gas, is typically much lower indoors than outdoors. Small particles do penetrate indoors, but concentrations are generally lower than outdoors. At times when pollutant levels are high, people with asthma can be counseled to stay indoors and, in particular, to avoid vigorous exercise. The response to air pollutants may be blunted by inhaled sympathomimetics and cromolin sodium. Air pollution regulations in many countries have been devised to control adverse health effects for everyone, including those with asthma. However, protecting the most susceptible people may not be possible.

FURTHER READING

Aalberse RC. Structural biology of allergens. J Allergy Clin Immunol 2000; 106:228–238.

Alexis N, Barnes C, Bernstein I, et al. Rostrum article: Health effects of air pollution. What the allergist needs to know. J Allergy Clin Immunol 2004; 114 (5):1116–1123.

Alexis N, Lay JC, Almond M, et al. Inhalation of low dose endotoxin by human volunteers favors a local TH2 response profile and primes airway phagocytes in vivo, J Allergy Clin Immunol 2004; 114(6):1325–1331.

Arruda LK. Cockroach allergens. Curr Allergy Asthma Rep 2005; 5:411–416.

Breiteneder H, Mills EN. Molecular properties of food allergens. J Allergy Clin Immunol. 2005; 115:14–23.

Chen LL, Tager IB, Peden DB, et al. Effect of ozone exposure on airway responses to inhaled allergen in asthmatic subjects. Chest 2004; 125(6):2328–2335.

Douwes J, Le Gros G, Gibson P, et al. Can bacterial endotoxin exposure reverse atopy and atopic disease?, J Allergy Clin Immunol 2004; 114:1051–1054.

Eggleston PA. Improving indoor environments: reducing allergen exposures. J Allergy Clin Immunol 2005; 116:122–126.

Kurup VP. Fungal allergens. Curr Allergy Asthma Rep 2003; 3:416–423.

Peden DB. Effect of pollutants in rhinitis. Curr Allergy Asthma Rep 2001; 1(3):242–246.

Peden DB. Influences on the development of allergy and asthma. Toxicology 2002; 181–182, 323–328.

Stewart GA, Thompson PJ. The biochemistry of common aeroallergens. Clin Exp Allergy 1996; 26:1020–1044.

APPENDIX TO CHAPTER 17

Appendix 17.1 Physicochemical and biochemical characteristics of grass pollen aeroallergens

Allergen	[1]Frequency of reactivity	Mol. weight (K)	[2]CHO	Function
Group 1 (Lol p 1)	> 90	30	Yes	β-expansins involved in cell wall loosening; shows homology with groups 1–3 allergens
[3]Group 2 (Lol p 2)	> 60	11	No	Shows homology with groups 1–3 grass allergens
Group 3 (Lol p 3)	70	11	No	Shows homology with groups 1–3 grass allergens
Group 4 (Lol p 4)	50–88	57	Yes	Pectate lyase
[3]Group 5 (Lol p 5)	> 90	29–31	No	Ribonuclease
[3]Group 6 (Phl p 6)	76	12	Yes	Shows homology with group 5 allergens, associated with P particles
Group 7 (Cyn d 7)	10	9	No	Calcium binding protein, shows homology with Bet v 4
Group 10 (Lol p 10)	0–?	12	?	Cytochrome C
Group 11 (Lol p 11)	65	15	Yes	Function unknown; shows homology with tree allergen Ole e 1 and soybean trypsin inhibitor
Group 12 (Phl p 12)	20–35	12	No	Profilin, an actin binding protein
Group 13 (Phl p 13)	50	55–60		Polygalacturonase
Cyn d Bd46K	64	46		Shows homology with cytochrome c oxidase III from corn pollen
Cyn d BG60	?	60		Berberine bridge enzyme

[1]Frequency data presented in each of these tables have been derived from many sources and will be dependent on a variety of factors. In addition, the data presented may reflect immediate hypersensitivity diseases including atopic dermatitis and allergic bronchopulmonary aspergillosis (ABPA) as well as delayed type hypersensitivity disease. [2]Indicates presence of potential or demonstrated *N*- or *O*-glycosylation site. Specific examples of an allergen within the group are shown in parentheses. [3]Allergens in these groups do not appear to be present in pollens from grasses in the Chloridoideae [e.g. Bermuda grass (*Cynodon dactylon*)]. ? Indicates lack of data. Tables modified from Stewart GA, Robinson C. Allergen structure and function. In: Adkinson NFJ, Yunginger JW, Busse WW, et al, eds. Middleton's allergy: principles and practice. Philadelphia: Mosby; 2003:585–609.

Appendix 17.2 Physicochemical and biochemical characteristics of pollen-derived aeroallergens from weed and *Brassica* species

Allergen	Frequency of reactivity	Mol. weight (K)	CHO	Function
Asteraceae				
Short ragweed (*Ambrosia artemisiifolia*)				
Amb a 1	> 90	40	Yes	Pectate lyase
Amb a 2	> 90	41	Yes	Pectate lyase
Amb a 3	51	11	Yes	Shows homology with electron transport proteins
Amb a 5	17	5	No	Function unknown
Amb a 6	21	11	No	Lipid transfer protein
Amb a 7	20	12		Shows homology with electron transport proteins
Amb a 10	?	12		Cytochrome c
Profilin	?	14	No	Profilin, actin binding protein
Cystatin	30	10	No	Cysteine protease inhibitor
Mugwort (*Artemisia vulgaris*)				
Art v 1*	> 90	11	Yes	Function unknown; contains antifungal plant defensin-like domain and a hydroxyproline/ praline rich domain
Art v 2	33	20	Yes	Function unknown
Art v 3	?	10		Lipid transfer protein
Profilin	?	14	No	Profilin
Feverfew (*Parthenium hysterophorus*)				
Par h 1	> 90	31	Yes	Extensin
Sunflower (*Helianthus annus*)				
Hel a 2	31	14	No	Profilin
Hel a 5	?	?		Expansins

Appendix 17.2 Physicochemical and biochemical characteristics of pollen-derived aeroallergens from weed and *Brassica* species—cont'd

Allergen	Frequency of reactivity	Mol. weight (K)	CHO	Function
Urticaceae				
Wall-pellitory (*Parietaria* spp.)				
Group 1 (Par o 1)	100	14	Yes	Lipid transfer protein
Group 2 (Par o 2)	82	11	Yes	Lipid transfer protein
Group 3 (Par j 3)	?	14	No	Profilin
Brassicaceae				
Oilseed rape (*Brassica napus*)				
Bra n 1	?	9		Calcium binding protein, shows homology with grass Cyn d 7 allergen
Bra n 2	?	9		Calcium binding protein
6/8 kDa protein	50	6/8		Calcium binding protein
14 kDa protein	34	14		Profilin
27–69 kDa cluster	80	27–69		Shows homology with grass pollen group 4 allergens, pectate lyase?
40 kDa protein	?	40		Receptor-like protein kinase
43 kDa protein	28–56	43	Yes	Polygalacturonase
70 kDa protein	?	70		Berberine bridge protein
80 kDa protein	?	80		Cobalamin-independent methionine synthetase
TRX-H-1	?	14		Thioredoxin
PCP-1	?	9		Pollen coat protein
Turnip (*Brassica rapa*)				
Bra r 1	?	9		Calcium binding protein, shows homology with grass Cyn d 7 allergen
Bra r 2	?	9		Calcium binding protein
PEC-1	> 30	13		Lipid transfer protein
PEC-2	?	14		Thioredoxin
PCP-1	?	9		Pollen coat protein
Euphorbiaceae				
Mercurialis annua				
Mer a 1	> 59	14		Profilin, an actin binding protein
Chenopodiaceae				
Chenopodium album				
Che a 1	77	17	Yes	Shows homology with Ole e 1

*Art v 1 was previously described as a 47–60 kDa allergen. In the absence of sequence data, it has now been replaced by the 11 kDa allergen.

Appendix 17.3 Physicochemical and biochemical characteristics of angiosperm tree pollen aeroallergens

Allergen	Frequency of reactivity	Mol. weight (K)	CHO	Function
Fagales (Birch, Alder, Hornbeam, Oak, Chestnut, Hazel)				
Group 1 (Bet v1)	> 95	17	Yes	Plant steroid carrier; shows homology with pathogenesis-related proteins (PR-10)
Group 2 (Bet v 2)	20	14	No	Profilin, an actin binding protein
Group 3 (Bet v 3)	< 10	23	No	Calcium binding protein
Group 4 (Bet v 4)	20	9	No	EF hand calcium binding protein, a polycalcin; shows homology with Aln g 4, Ole e 3, Syr v 3
Group 5 (Bet v 5)	32	35	Yes	Isoflavone reductase
Group 7 (Bet v 7)	21	18		Peptidyl-prolyl isomerase (cyclophilin)
Pectin methylesterase	66	65		Pectin methylesterase

Appendix 17.3 Physicochemical and biochemical characteristics of angiosperm tree pollen aeroallergens—cont'd

Allergen	Frequency of reactivity	Mol. weight (K)	CHO	Function
Lamiales (Olive, Lilac, Privet, Ash, English plantain)				
Group 1(Ole e 1)	> 90	16	Yes	Shows limited homology with soybean trypsin inhibitor and Lol p 11
Group 2 (Ole e 2)	> 40	14	No	Profilin
Group 3 (Ole e 3)	20–>50	9	No	Calcium binding protein
Group 4 (Ole e 4/9)	65–80	32–46	Yes	1,3-β-glucanase
Group 5 (Ole e 5)	35	16	No	Superoxide dismutase
Group 6 (Ole e 6)	5–20	6		Cysteine rich protein
Group 7 (Ole e 7)	>60	10		Lipid transfer protein
Group 8 (Ole e 8)	3–4	19	No	Calcium binding protein
Group 10 (ole e 10)	55–70	11	Yes	1,3-β -glucosidase; shows homology with Ole e 9

Appendix 17.4 Physicochemical and biochemical characteristics of gymnosperm tree pollen aeroallergens

Allergen	Frequency of reactivity	Mol. weight (K)	CHO	Function
Taxoidiaceae				
Japanese cedar (*Cryptomeria japonica*)				
Cry j 1	> 85	39	Yes	Pectate lyase; shows homology with bacterial pectate lyase and Amb a 1 and 2
Cry j 2	76	37	Yes	Polymethylgalacturonase
Cupressaceae				
Japanese juniper (*Juniperus rigida*)				
70 kDa allergen	100	70	Yes	Function unknown
Mountain cedar (*Juniperus ashei*)				
Jun a 1	71	40	Yes	Pectate lyase
Jun a 2	100	43	Yes	Polymethylgalacturonase
Jun a 3	43	30	Yes	Shows homology with thaumatin, osmotin and amylase/trypsin inhibitor
Eastern red cedar (*Juniperus virginiana*)				
Jun v 1	46-92	43	Yes	Pectate lyase
Jun v 3	?	10	No	Shows homology with thaumatin, osmotin and amylase/trypsin inhibitor
Jun v 4	85	145		Function unknown
Prickly juniper (*Juniperus oxycedrus*)				
Jun o 1	?	40	Yes	Pectate lyase
Jun o 4	?	18	Yes	Calcium binding protein
Cypress (*Cupressus sempervirens*)				
Cup s 1	81	42	Yes	Pectate lyase
Cypress (*Cupressus arizonica*)				
Cup a 1	57	43	Yes	Pectate lyase
Cup a 3	?	?	No	Shows homology with thaumatin, osmotin and amylase/trypsin inhibitor
Japanese cypress (*Chamaecyparis obtusa*)				
Cha o 1	> 50	38	Yes	Pectate lyase
Cha o 2	83	46	Yes	Polymethylgalacturonase

Appendix 17.5 Physicochemical and biochemical characteristics of non-pollen, plant aeroallergens

Allergen	Frequency of reactivity	Mol. weight (K)	CHO	Function
Brassicaceae				
Yellow mustard seed (*Sinapis alba* L.)				
Sin a 1	?			2S albumin
Short chain		4	No	
Long chain		10	No	
Oriental mustard seed (*Brassica juncea*)				
Bra j 1	?			2S albumin
Short chain		4	No	
Long chain		10	No	
Oilseed rape (*Brassica napus*)				
BnIII (Bra r 1)	?			2S albumin
Short chain		4	No	
Long chain		10	No	
Euphorbiaceae				
Castor bean (Ricinus communis)				
Ric c 1	96			2S albumin
Short chain		4	No	
Long chain		7	No	
Ric c 2	?	47		11 S crystalloid protein
Ric c 3	?	47–51		Function unknown
Leguminosae				
Seed husk allergens				
Soybean (*Glycine max*)				
Gly m 1	95	8		Cysteine rich, hydrophobic seed protein, member of lipid transfer protein family
Gly m 2	95	8		Function unknown
Flour				
*Soybean (*Glycine max*)				
Trypsin inhibitor (B)	86	20	No	Kunitz protease inhibitor
Lipoxygenase	?	94	Yes	Lipoxygenase
Poaceae				
Barley (*Hordeum vulgare*)				
Hor v 15	?	14		α-Amylase/trypsin inhibitor; shows homology with wheat allergens and 2S albumin allergens (BMAI-1)
Hor v 16	> 96	64		α-Amylase (1,4,-α-D-glucan glucanohydrolase)
Hor v 17	> 96	60		β-Amylase (1,4-α-D-glucan maltohydrolase)
Hor v 21	[a]91	34		Hordein, shows homology with rye secalins and wheat gliadins
Rice (*Oryza sativa*)				
Ory s 1	> 90	15		α-Amylase inhibitor; shows homology with wheat and barley α-amylase/trypsin inhibitor allergens
33 kDa protein	?	33		Glyoxalase I
Wheat (*Triticum* spp.)				
Tr i a 3				Function unknown; found in wheat ovaries; shows homology with pollen allergens
Tri a 18	?	17		Lectin
Tri a 19	100	65		α-Gliadin, shows homology with rye secalins and barley hordein
CM16	> 50	13	Yes	Wheat α-amylase/trypsin inhibitor; shows homology with barley allergens and 2S albumin allergens

Appendix 17.5 Physicochemical and biochemical characteristics of non-pollen, plant aeroallergens—cont'd

Allergen	Frequency of reactivity	Mol. weight (K)	CHO	Function
WMAI-1	?	13	Yes	Wheat α-amylase/trypsin inhibitor; shows homology with barley allergens and 2S albumin allergens
27 kDa allergen	?	27		Shows homology with acyl-CoA oxidase from barley and rice
Tri a Bd36K	60	36	Yes	Peroxidase
Gliadin	72	40		α-Gliadin
37 kDa allergen	?	37		Fructose biphosphate-aldolase
Rye (*Secale cereale*)				
Sec c 1	> 50	14	No	α-Amylase/trypsin inhibitor; shows homology with wheat allergens and 2S albumin allergens
Sec c 20	?	?		Secalin
34 kDa protein	[a]83	34		Rye γ-35 secalin, shows homology with wheat gliadins and barley hordeins
70 kDa protein	[a]91	70		Rye γ-70 secalin, shows homology with wheat gliadins and barley hordeins

*See Appendix 17.13 for ingested allergens from these sources.

[a]Frequency based on patients with wheat-dependent, exercise-induced anaphylaxis.

Appendix 17.6 Physicochemical and biochemical characteristics of latex allergens

Allergen	Frequency of reactivity	Mol. weight (K)	CHO	Function
Euphorbiaceae				
Rubber tree (latex; *Hevea brasiliensis*)				
Hev b 1	50–82	15		Rubber elongation factor, exists as homotetramer with mol. wt of 58 kDa and pI of 8.5
Hev b 2	20–61	30		Endo-1, 3-β-glucosidase
Hev b 3	79	24	No	Shows some homology with rubber elongation factor, Hev b 1
Hev b 4	65–77	50–57		Microhelix component
Hev b 5	56–92	*16		Shows homology with an acidic protein from kiwifruit and potato
Hev b 6	83	20		Prohevein; chitin binding lectin, causes latex agglutination; native hevein exists as 5 kDa protein
Hev b 7	8–49	44		A patatin-like protein with lipid acyl-hydrolase and PLA_2 activity, shows cross-reactivity with Sol t 1
Hev b 8	24	14		Profilin, plays role in actin polymerization
Hev b 9	15	51		Enolase
Hev b 10	4	26	Yes	Manganese superoxide dismutase, shows homology with Asp f 6
Hev b 11	3	30		Class I chitinase
Hev b 12		9		Lipid transfer protein
Hev b 13	78	42–46	Yes	Esterase; shows homology with early nodule-specific protein from legumes

*Hevein is a 4.7 K chitin binding domain from this precursor.

Appendix 17.7 Physicochemical and biochemical characteristics of domestic fungal aeroallergens

Allergen	Frequency of reactivity	Mol. weight (K)	CHO	Function
Ascomycota				
Alternaria alternata				
Alt a 1	> 80	14	Yes	Function unknown
Alt a 2	61	20		EIF-2 α kinase
Alt a 3	?	70	Yes	Heat shock protein 70
Alt a 4	?	57		Protein disulfide isomerase
Alt a 6	8	11	Yes	Ribosomal P2 protein, shows homology with Cla h 4
Alt a 7	7	22	No	1,4-benzoquinone reductase, shows homology with Cla h 5
Alt a 10	2	54	Yes	Aldehyde dehydrogenase, shows homology with Cla h 3
Alt a 11	50	46	Yes	Enolase
Alt a 12	?	12		Ribosomal P1 protein
22 kDa allergen	< 50	22	No	trp repressor-binding protein; shows homology with flavodoxins
Aspergillus fumigatus				
Asp f 1	85	17	No	Ribonuclease; shows homology with mitocillin
Asp f 2	96	36	Yes	Shows homology with *Candida albicans* fibrinogen binding protein
Asp f 3	84	19	Yes	Peroxisomal membrane protein, belongs to the peroxiredoxin family, thiol-dependent peroxidase
Asp f 4	*78–83	40	No	Shows homology with bacterial ABC transporter binding protein, associated with peroxisome
Asp f 5	74	40		Metalloprotease
Asp f 6	*42–56	27	No	Manganese superoxide dismutase, shows homology with Hev b 10
Asp f 7	29	12	No	Shows homology with fungal riboflavin, aldehyde-forming enzyme
Asp f 8	8–15	11	No	Ribosomal P2 protein
Asp f 9	31	34		Shows homology with plant and bacterial endo-β-1,3-1,4 glucanases
Asp f 10	3	34		Aspartic protease
Asp f 11	?	24		Peptidyl-prolyl isomerase (cyclophilin)
Asp f 12	?	90	Yes	Heat shock protein 90
Asp f 13	> 60	34	Yes	Alkaline serine protease
Asp f 15	?	16	Yes	Shows homology with a serine protease antigen from *Coccidioides immitis*, also designated Asp f 13
Asp f 16	70	43		Shows homology with Asp f 9
Asp f 18	79	34		Vacuolar serine protease
Asp f 22	30	47	Yes	Enolase, shows homology with Pen c 22
Cladosporium herbarium				
Cla h 1	> 60	13		Function unknown
Cla h 2	43	19	Yes	Function unknown
Cla h 3	36	53	Yes	Aldehyde dehydrogenase
Cla h 4	22	11	Yes	Ribosomal P2 protein
Cla h 5	22	22	No	1,4-benzoquinone reductase, shows homology Cla h 5
Cla h 6	20	48		Enolase
Cla h 12	?	11		Ribosomal P1 protein
HSP 70	?	70	Yes	Heat shock protein, also denominated Cla h 4
Penicillium chrysogenum/notatum				
Pen ch 13	> 80	34	Yes	Alkaline serine protease
Pen ch 18	> 80	28–34		Vacuolar serine protease
Pen ch 20	56	62	Yes	Shows homology with β-*N*-acetylglucosaminidase from *Candida albicans*
Penicillium citrinum				
Pen c 3	46	18		Peroxisomal membrane protein, belongs to the peroxiredoxin family, thiol-dependent peroxidase
Pen c 13	100	33	Yes	Alkaline serine protease

Appendix 17.7 Physicochemical and biochemical characteristics of domestic fungal aeroallergens—cont'd

Allergen	Frequency of reactivity	Mol. weight (K)	CHO	Function
Pen c 19	41	70		Show homology with hsp 70 heat shock protein
Pen c 22	?	46		Enolase
Candida albicans				
Cand a 1	?	40	Yes	Alcohol dehydrogenase
Cand a 3		29		Peroxisomal protein
37 kDa allergen	?	37		Aldolase
43 kDa allergen	?	43		Phosphoglycerate kinase
48 kDa allergen	50	46	Yes	Enolase
Acid protease	75	35	No	Aspartate protease
Trichophyton tonsurans				
Tri t 1	54	30		Function unknown; possible
Tri t 2	42	30		Subtilisin-like protease, shows homology with Pen ch 13, Pen c 13
Tri t 4	61	83		Dipeptidyl peptidase
Trichophyton rubrum				
Tri r 1/2	?	30		Subtilisin-like protease, shows homology with Pen ch 13, Pen c 13
Tri r 4	?	83		Dipeptidyl peptidase
Basidiomycota				
Malassezia furfur				
Mala f 1	61	36	Yes	Function unknown; cell wall protein
Mala f 2	72	21	Yes	Peroxisomal membrane protein, belongs to the peroxiredoxin family, thiol-dependent peroxidase, shows homology with Asp f 3
Mala f 3	70	20	Yes	Peroxisomal membrane protein, belongs to the peroxiredoxin family, thiol-dependent peroxidase, shows homology with Asp f 3 and Mala f 2
Mala f 4	?	36		Mitochondrial malate dehydrogenase
Mala f 5	?	18		Peroxisomal membrane protein, belongs to the peroxiredoxin family, thiol-dependent peroxidase, shows homology with Mala f 2/3 and Asp f 3
Mala f 6	?	17		Peptidyl-prolyl isomerase (cyclophilin)
Mala f 7	89	16		Function unknown
Mal f 8	?	19		Shows homology with immunoreactive mannoprotein from *Cryptococcus neoformans*
Mala f 9	44	14		Function unknown
Coprinus comatus				
Cop c 1	25	9		Leucine zipper protein
Cop c 2	19	12		Thioredoxin
Cop c 3	?	37		Function unknown
Cop c 5	?	16		Function unknown
Cop c 7	?	16		Function unknown
Psilocybe cubensis				
Psi c 1	> 50	46		Function unknown
Psi c 2	> 50	16		Peptidyl-prolyl isomerase (cyclophilin)
Rhodotorula mucilaginosa				
Rho m 1	21	47		Enolase
Rho m 2	?	31		Vacuolar serine protease

*Frequency determined in ABPA patients

Appendix 17.8 Physicochemical and biochemical characteristics of occupational aeroallergens

Allergen	Frequency of reactivity	Mol. weight (K)	CHO	Function
Fungal allergens				
Aspergillus niger				
Asp n 14	14	105		β-Xylosidase
Asp n 18	?	?		Vacuolar serine protease
Asp n 25	> 50	50	Yes	Histidine acid phosphatase (phytase)
Pectinase	?	35	Yes	Poly(1,4)-α-D-galacturonidase
Cellulase	8	26		1,4-(1,3;1,4)-β-D-glucan glucanhydrolase
Glucoamylase	5	66	Yes	1,4-α-D-glucan glucanhydrolase
Aspergillus oryzae				
Asp o 13	?	34	Yes	Alkaline serine protease; belongs to subtilase family
Asp o 21	56	52	Yes	α-Amylase
Lactase	?	?		1,4-β-D-Galactoside galactohydrolase
Cryphonectira parasitica				
Renin	?	34	No	Aspartate protease; shows homology with mammalian and cockroach pepsins
Bacterial proteases				
Bacillus subtilis				
Alcalase	> 50	28	Yes	Subtilisin serine protease
Bacillus licheniformis				
Esperase	> 50	28	Yes	Subtilisin serine protease
Clostridium histolyticum				
**Collagenase	> 50	68–125		Metalloprotease
Caricaceae				
Pawpaw (*Carica papaya*)				
Car p 1	?	23	No	Papain, cysteine protease
Kiwi fruit (*Actinidia chinensis*)				
Act c 1	100	30	No	Actinidin, cysteine protease
Act c 2	100	24	Yes	Thaumatin-like protein, possesses antifungal activity
Bromelaceae				
Pineapple (*Ananas comosus*)				
Ana c 1	?	23	Yes	Bromelain, cysteine protease
Mammalian proteases				
Trypsin (porcine)	?	24		Serine protease; shows homology with mite groups 3, 6 and 9 allergens
Chymotrypsin (bovine)	?	25		Serine protease; shows homology with mite groups 3, 6, and 9 allergens
Pepsin (porcine)	?	35		Aspartate protease; shows homology with Bla g 2 and renin
Chicken egg allergens				
Chicken (*Gallus domesticus*)				
Egg white				
Gal d 1	34–38	20	Yes	Ovomucoid, protease inhibitor
Gal d 2	32	43	Yes	Ovalbumin, function unknown but protein shows homology with serine protease inhibitors
Gal d 3	47–53	76	Yes	Conalbumin (ovotransferrin), iron transport protein
Gal d 4	15	14	No	1, 4-β-*N*-acetylmuramidase (lysozyme)

Appendix 17.8 Physicochemical and biochemical characteristics of occupational aeroallergens—cont'd

Allergen	Frequency of reactivity	Mol. weight (K)	CHO	Function
Egg yolk				
Gal d 5	> 50	65–70		Serum albumin (α-livetin)
Brassicaceae				
Yellow mustard seed (*Sinapis alba* L.)				
Sin a 1	?			2S albumin
Short chain		4	No	
Long chain		10	No	
Oriental mustard seed (*Brassica juncea*)				
Bra j 1	?			2S albumin
Short chain		4	No	
Long chain		10	No	
Oilseed rape (*Brassica napus*)				
BnIII (Bra r 1)	?			2S albumin
Short chain		4	No	
Long chain		10	No	
Euphorbiaceae				
Castor bean (*Ricinus communis*)				
Ric c 1	96			2S albumin
Short chain		4	No	
Long chain		7	No	
Ric c 2	?	47		11 S crystalloid protein
Ric c 3	?	47–51		Function unknown
Leguminosae				
Seed husk allergens				
Soybean				
(*Glycine max*)				
+Gly m 1	95	8		Cysteine rich, hydrophobic seed protein, member of lipid transfer protein family
Gly m 2	95	8		Function unknown
Flour				
*Soybean (*Glycine max*)				
Trypsin-inhibitor (B)	86	20	No	Kunitz protease inhibitor
Lipoxygenase	?	94	Yes	Lipoxygenase
Poaceae				
Barley (*Hordeum vulgare*)				
Hor v 15	?	14		α-Amylase/trypsin inhibitor; shows homology with wheat allergens and 2S albumin allergens (BMAI-1)
Hor v 16	> 96	64		α-Amylase (1,4,-α-D-glucan glucanohydrolase)
Hor v 17	> 96	60		β-Amylase (1,4-α-D-glucan maltohydrolase)
Hor v 21	[a]91	34		Hordein, shows homology with rye secalins and wheat gliadins
Rice (*Ores sativa*)				
Ory s 1	> 90	15		α-Amylase inhibitor; shows homology with wheat and barley α-amylase/trypsin inhibitor allergens
33 kDa protein	?	33		Glyoxalase I
Wheat (*Triticum* spp.)				
Tr i a 3				Function unknown; found in wheat ovaries; shows homology with pollen allergens
Tri a 18	?	17		Lectin

Appendix 17.8 Physicochemical and biochemical characteristics of occupational aeroallergens—cont'd

Allergen	Frequency of reactivity	Mol. weight (K)	CHO	Function
Tri a 19	100	65		ω-Gliadin, shows homology with rye secalins and barley hordein
CM16	> 50	13	Yes	Wheat a-amylase/trypsin inhibitor; shows homology with barley allergens and 2S albumin allergens
WMAI-1	?	13	Yes	Wheat α-amylase/trypsin inhibitor; shows homology with barley allergens and 2S albumin allergens
27 kDa allergen	?	27		Shows homology with acyl-CoA oxidase from barley and rice
Tri a Bd36K	60	36	Yes	Peroxidase
Gliadin	72	40		α-Gliadin
37 kDa Allergen	?	37		Fructose biphosphate-aldolase
Rye (*Secale cereale*)				
Sec c 1	> 50	14	No	α-Amylase/trypsin inhibitor; shows homology with wheat allergens and 2S albumin allergens
Sec c 20	?	?		Secalin
34 kDa protein	[a]83	34		Rye γ-35 secalin, shows homology with wheat gliadins and barley hordeins
70 kDa protein	[a]91	70		Rye γ-70 secalin, shows homology with wheat gliadins and barley hordeins

*See Appendix 13 for ingested allergens from this source.
**Represents a mixture of proteases.
[a]Frequency based on patients with wheat-dependent, exercise-induced anaphylaxis.

Appendix 17.9 Physicochemical and biochemical characterization of animal and dander allergens

Allergen	Frequency of reactivity	Mol. weight (K)	CHO	Function
Cat (*Felix domesticus*)				
Fel d 1	> 80	33–39*	β Chain	Heterodimer (α & β chains), function unknown; a chain shows homology with 10 kDa secretory protein from human Clara cells, mouse salivary androgen binding protein subunit; rabbit uteroglobin and a Syrian hamster protein
Fel d 2	15–22	69	Yes	Serum albumin
Fel d 3	60–90	11		Cystatin
Fel d 4	63	20		Lipocalin
Dog (*Canis familiaris*)				
Can f 1	> 70	19–25		Lipocalin; shows homology with Von Ebner's gland protein which has cysteine protease inhibitory activity
Can f 2	70	27		Lipocalin; shows homology with other lipocalin allergens
Can f 3	35–77	69		Serum albumin
IgG	88	150	Yes	Immunoglobulin G
Horse (*Equus caballus*)				
Equ c 1	100	22	Yes	Lipocalin; shows homology with rodent urinary proteins
Equ c 2	100	16		Lipocalin; shows homology with rodent urinary proteins
Equ c 3	?	67		Serum albumin
Equ c 4	?	19		Shows homology with rat mandibular gland protein A
Equ c 5	?	17		Function unknown
Cow (*Bos domesticus*)				
Bos d 2	97	18	No	Function unknown; shows homology to the rodent lipocalin allergens
AS1	31	21		Oligomycin sensitivity-conferring protein of the mitochondrial adenosine triphosphate synthase complex

Appendix 17.9 Physicochemical and biochemical characterization of animal and dander allergens—cont'd

Allergen	Frequency of reactivity	Mol. weight (K)	CHO	Function
BDA 11	?	12	Yes	Shows homology with human calcium binding psoriasin protein
Guinea pig (*Cavia porcellus*)				
Cav p 1	70	20	No	Lipocalin, shows homology with Cav p 2
Cav p 2	55	17	No	Lipocalin, shows homology with Bos d 2
Mouse (*Mus musculus*)				
Mus m 1	> 80	19	No	Major urinary protein; shows homology with lipocalins such as β-lactoglobulin, odorant binding proteins, Rat n 2 Rat (*Rattus novegicus*)
Rat (*Rattus norvegicus*)				
Rat n 1	> 80	21	Yes	Lipocalin; shows homology with lipocalins such as β-lactoglobulin, odorant binding proteins, Mus m 1
Albumin	24	69		Serum albumin
Check transferrin				
Rabbit (*Oryctolagus cuniculi*)				
Ory c 1	?	18		Odorant binding protein, lipocalin, shows homology with Ory c 2
Ory c 2	?	21		Odorant binding protein
8 kDa allergen	?	8		Shows homology with rabbit uteroglobin
Albumin	< 50	69		Serum albumin

*Truncated variants of β chain present in extracts. Mol. wt given represents dimer; each chain approx. 18 K.

Appendix 17.10 Physicochemical and biochemical characteristics of insect aeroallergens

Allergen	Frequency of reactivity	Mol. weight (K)	CHO	Function
Chironomidae				
Blood worm (*Chironomus thummi thummi*)				
Chi t I to 9	> 50	15	No	Hemoglobin
Midges				
Cladotanytarsus lewisi				
Cla l 1	> 50	17		Hemoglobin
Polypedium nubifer				
Pol n 1	> 50	17		Hemoglobin
Chironomus kiiensis				
Chi k 10	?	33		Tropomyosin
Blattidae				
German cockroach (*Blattella germanica*)				
Bla g 1	50	25		Shows homology with Per a 1 allergen, Cr PII, and with ANG12 secretory mosquito protein
Bla g 2	58	36	Yes	Aspartate protease (inactive)
Bla g 4	40–60	21		Lipocalin
Bla g 5	70	23	No	Glutathione transferase
Bla g 6	50	27		Troponin C
American cockroach (*Periplaneta americana*)				
Per a 1	50	24		Shows homology with Bla g 1 allergen, Cr-PII and ANG12 secretory mosquito protein
Per a 3	83	78	Yes	Hexamerin, subunit protein showing homology with larval insect storage proteins
Per a 7	50	72		Tropomyosin
Indian meal moth (*Plodia interpunctella*)				
Plo i 1	25	40	Yes	Arginine kinase

Appendix 17.11 Physicochemical and biochemical characteristics of mite aeroallergens

Allergen	Frequency of reactivity	Mol. weight (K)	CHO	Function
Pyroglyphidae/Glycyphagidae/Acaridae/Echimyopodidae				
Group 1 (Der p 1)	> 90	25	Yes	Cysteine protease
Group 2 (Der p 2)	> 90	14	No	Shows homology with putative human epididymal protein, possible cholesterol binding protein
Group 3 (Der p 3)	90	25	No	Trypsin
Group 4 (Der p 4)	25–46	56		Amylase
Group 5 (Der p 5)	9-70	13		Function unknown
Group 6 (Der p 6)	39	25	No	Chymotrypsin
Group 7 (Der p 7)	53–62	11–29	Yes	Function unknown
Group 8 (Der p 8)	40	26	Yes	Glutathione transferase
Group 9 (Der p 9)	> 90	28	No	Collagenase-like serine protease
Group 10 (Der p 10)	81	33	No	Tropomyosin
Group 11 (Der f 11)	82	98		Paramyosin
Group 12 (Blo t 12)	50	16		May be a chitinase, shows homology with Der f 15
Group 13 (Lep d 13)	11-23	15		Fatty acid binding protein
Group 14 (Der f 14)	84	190		Vitellogenin or lipophorin
Group 15 (Der f 15)	95	*63/98		Chitinase, shows homology with Blot 12 allergen
Group 16w (Der f 16)	35	53		Gelsolin
Group 17w (Der f 17)	35	30		Calcium binding protein
Group 18w (Der f 18)	?	60		Chitinase
Mag29	?	67		Heat shock protein

*Glycosylated and non-glycosylated form. Frequency determined in dogs with atopic dermatitis.

Appendix 17.12 Physicochemical and biochemical characteristics of ingested, animal-derived food allergens

Allergen	Frequency of reactivity	Mol. weight (K)	CHO	Function
Mammalian-derived				
Cow (*Bos domesticus*)				
Bos d 4	6	14	Yes	a-Lactalbumin, lactose synthase
Bos d 5	13	18	No	β-Lactoglobulin, lipocalin
Bos d 6	29	67	No	Serum albumin
Bos d 7	83	160	Yes	Immunoglobulin
Bos d 8	100	20–30		Caseins
75 kDa allergen	16	75		Transferrin
Fish/shellfish/amphibian-derived				
Atlantic salmon (*Salmo salar*), Cod (*Gadus callarias*)				
Group 1	100	12	No	Parvalbumin, calcium binding protein
Shrimp (*Metapenaeus* spp., *Penaeus* spp.)				
Group 1 (Met p 1)	> 50	34–36		Tropomyosin
Group 2 (Pen m 2)	70	39		Arginine kinase

Appendix 17.12 Physicochemical and biochemical characteristics of ingested, animal-derived food allergens—cont'd

Allergen	Frequency of reactivity	Mol. weight (K)	CHO	Function
Crab (*Charybdis feriatus*)				
Group 1 (Cha f 1)	> 50	34		Tropomyosin
Squid (*Todarodes pacificus*)				
Group 1 (Tod p 1)	> 50	38		Tropomyosin
Edible frog (*Rana esculenta*)				
Rana e 1		12		Parvalbumin α
Rana e 2		12		Parvalbumin β

Appendix 17.13 Physicochemical and biochemical characteristics of ingested seed and fruit allergens

Allergen	Frequency of reactivity	Mol. weight (K)	CHO	Function
Leguminosae				
Peanut (*Arachis hypogaea*)				
Ara h 1	> 90	63	Yes	Vicilin, seed storage protein
Ara h 2	> 90	17		Conglutin, seed storage protein
Ara h 3/4	35–53	14–60		Glycinin, seed storage protein
Ara h 4	43	36		Glycinin, seed storage protein
Ara h 5	16	14		Profilin, an actin binding protein
Ara h 6	38	16		Similar to conglutin
Ara h 7	43	15		Similar to conglutin
Ara h 8	85	17		Shows homology with Bet v1
Peanut agglutinin	50	*27		Lectin
**Soybean (*Glycine max*)				
Gly m 3	69	14	No	Profilin, an actin binding protein
Gly m Bd 30K/P34	90	34	Yes	Syringolide receptor, seed vacuolar protein; shows homology with mite group 1 allergen, papain and bromelain but not active
Gly m Bd 28K	> 50	22	Yes	Vicilin-like glycoprotein, shows homology with Ara h 1
21 kDa allergen	?	22		A member of the G2 glycinin family
G1 glycinin	?	40		A member of the G1 glycinin family, shows homology with Ara h 3
Gly m Bd 60K	25	60		β-Conglycinin seed storage protein
Juglandaceae				
Brazil nut (*Bertholletia excelsa*)				
Ber e 1	100	9		2S albumin
Lecythidaceae				
English walnut (*Juglans regia*)				
Jug r 1	?	?		2S albumin
Jug r 2	60	47		Vicilin-like glycoprotein
Polygonaceae				
Buckwheat (*Fagopyrum esculentum* Moench)				
Fag e 1	> 50	26		β chain of 11S globulin
18 kDa protein	78	18		2S albumin, shows homology with BW10KD
16 kDa protein	< 50	16		2S albumin, shows homology with BW10KD
9 kDa protein	50	9		Trypsin inhibitor
BW10KD	57	10		2S albumin
BW24KD	> 50	24		Legumin-like storage protein

Appendix 17.13 Physicochemical and biochemical characteristics of ingested seed and fruit allergens—cont'd

Allergen	Frequency of reactivity	Mol. weight (K)	CHO	Function
Heliantheae				
Sunflower (*Helianthus annus*)				
16 kDa allergen	66	16/17		2S albumin
Apiaceae				
Celery (*Apium graveolous*)				
Api g 1	100	16		Pathogenesis-related protein; homolog ; shows homology with Bet v 1
Api g 4	?	14	No	Profilin
Api g 5	?	?		Flavin adenine dinucleotide-dependent oxidase
Rosaceae				
Apple (*Malus domestica*)				
Mal d 1	?	18		Pathogenesis related protein; shows homology with Bet v 1
Mal d 2	?	?		Thaumatin-like protein
Mal d 3		11	No	Non-specific lipid transfer protein
Mal d 4	?	14	No	Profilin
60 kDa allergen	?	60		Phosphoglyceromutase
Prunoideae				
Cherry (*Prunus avium*)				
Pru av 1	89	18		Pathogenesis related protein; shows homology with Bet v 1
Pru av 2?	100	23		Thaumatin-like protein
Pru av 3	?	10	No	Non-specific lipid transfer protein
Pru av 4	?	14	No	Profilin
Peach (*Prunus persica*)				
Pru p 1	?	9	No	Non-specific lipid transfer protein
Solanaceae				
Potato (*Solanum tuberosum*)				
Sol t 1	74	43		Patatin, defense related storage protein, has PLA_2 activity
Sol t 2	51	20		Cathepsin D protease inhibitor, kunitz type protease inhibitor
Sol t 3	43	20		Cysteine protease inhibitor
Sol t 4	58	20		Aspartate protease inhibitor
Cucurbitaceae				
Melon (*Cucumis melo*)				
Cuc m 1	100	54	Yes	Cucmisin; subtilisin serine protease
Cuc m 2		14	No	Profilin, an actin binding protein
Cuc m 3	71	16		Pathogenesis related protein; shows homology with the vespid group 5 allergens

**See also Appendix 17.8

Appendix 17.14 Physicochemical and biochemical characteristics of stinging and biting insect allergens

Allergen	Frequency of reactivity	Mol. weight (K)	CHO	Function
VENOM ALLERGENS				
Aidae				
Honey bee (*Apis mellifera*)				
Api m 1	> 90	15	Yes	Phospholipase A_2
Api m 2	95	41	Yes	Hyaluronidase
Api m 3	> 50	49	No	Acid phosphatase prostatic
Api m 4	< 50	3		Melittin
Api m 6	> 42	8		Function unknown
Api m 7	?	?		CUB serine protease
Bumble bee (*Bombus pennsylvanicus/ terrestris*)				
Bom p 1	?	?		Phospholipase A_2
Bom p 4	?	?		Protease
Bom t 1	?	49		Acid phosphatase
Vespidae				
White faced and yellow hornets (*Dolichovespula* spp.), paper wasps (*Polistes* spp.) and yellow jackets (*Vespula* spp.)				
Group 1 (Pol a 1)	46	34	Yes	Phospholipase A_1
Group 2 (Pol a 2)	26	39	Yes	Hyaluronidase
Group 3	?	49		Acid phosphatase
Group 4 (Pol d 4)		32–34		Serine protease
Group 5 (Pol a 5)	8	26	Yes	Shows homology with cysteine rich secretory protein found in epididymis, testis and salivary gland, and pathogenesis related proteins
Formicidae				
Fire ant (*Solenopsis invicta*)				
Sola i 1	26	37		Phospholipase A_1
Sola i 2	87	13	No	Function unknown
Sola i 3	17	24	Yes	Shows homology with the vespid group 5 allergens
Sola i 4	26	13	No	Shows homology with Sol i 2
Australian jumper ant (*Myrmecia pilosula*)				
Myr p 1	> 50	9	No	Pilosulin 1, function unknown
Myr p 2	35	5	No	Function unknown
SALIVARY ALLERGENS				
Culicidae				
Mosquito (*Aedes aegyptii*)				
Aed a 1	29–43	68		Apyrase
Aed a 2	11	37		Function unknown
Aed a 3	32	30		Function unknown
Pulicidae				
Flea (*Ctenocephalides felis*)				
Cte f 1	80	20		Function unknown
Cte f 2	?	30		Salivary protein, shows homology with ant Sol i 3 allergen, and vespid group 5 allergens
Reduviidae				
Kissing bug (*Triatoma protracta*)				
Tria p 1	89	19	No	Procalin, a member of the lipocalin family; shows homology with triabin, a thrombin inhibitor

Appendix 17.15 Physicochemical and biochemical characteristics of parasite allergens

Allergen	Frequency of reactivity	Mol. weight (K)	CHO	Function
Ascaridida				
Anisakis simplex				
Ani s 1	?	24		Function unknown
Ani s 2	?	97		Paramyosin
Ani s 3	?	41		Tropomyosin
Ani s 4	75	9		Function unknown
Ascaris suum				
ABA-1	> 80	14	Yes	Polyprotein, lipid binding protein
Cyclophyllidae				
Echinococcus granulosus				
EA21	80	17	Yes	Peptidyl-prolyl isomerase (cyclophilin) shows homology with Mal f 6 and Asp f 11
EgEF-1 β/λ	56–90	14		Elongation factor
EgHSP70	57	70		Heat shock protein
AgB	?	12		Protease inhibitor
Antigen 5	?	67		Dimer, 22 kDa chain and 38 kDa chain with tryspin-like similarity although not active
Spirurida				
Brugia malayi				
58 kDa allergen	100	58		γ-Glutamyl transpeptidase
Bm 23–25	?	23–25		Function unknown
Dirofilaria immitis				
DiAg	?	?		Polyprotein, function unknown
Trichurida				
Trichinella spiralis				
Serine proteases	?	18, 40, 50		Serine proteases
Strongylida				
Trichostrongylus c oubriformis (Sheep parasite)				
31 kDa allergen	?	31	No	Aspartyl protease inhibitor homolog (Aspin)
Necator americanus				
60 kDa protein	?	60		Calreticulin
Strigeatida				
Schistosoma japonicum				
23 kDa protein	> 50	23	Yes	Function unknown
Schistosoma haematobium				
90 kDa protein	?	90	?	Serine protease inhibitor

Chapter 18

IgE Structure, Receptors, and Signaling

Rebecca L Beavil, Andrew J Beavil, and Ilona G Reischl

Definition:

To the layman the word allergy brings to mind the symptoms of hayfever, asthma, eczema, and reactions to particular foods and bee stings, or the substance (allergen) that induces these explosive and occasionally fatal reactions in sensitive individuals. Atopic allergy refers to the common mechanism underlying these responses. Immunoglobulin E (IgE) antibodies and IgE receptors, FcεRI and CD23, essential proteins in this mechanism, are the subjects of this chapter.

IGE STRUCTURE AND RECEPTORS

The allergic response differs from other immune responses in its dependence on immunoglobulin E (IgE), its high-affinity receptor FcεRI, and the nature of the primary effector cell – the tissue mast cell. IgE binds to cells that express FcεRI with such a high affinity that they are permanently coated with IgE, and thus sensitized for rapid activation when challenged with allergen. This activation, triggered by aggregation of a few hundred receptor molecules by multivalent allergen, leads to the release of molecules that provoke the symptoms of immediate hypersensitivity (Fig. 18.1). The high affinity of the IgE–receptor complex is mainly due to its extremely slow rate of dissociation: the half-life of the IgE–FcεRI complex in solution is around 20 hours (versus seconds for IgG), but over 2 weeks in body tissues such as the skin, where diffusion is restricted and reassociation is favored. The stability of the IgE–FcεRI complex, relative to that of IgG–receptor complexes [association constant (K_a) ~ 10^{10} M^{-1} for IgE, as against maximum $K_a < 10^8$ M^{-1} for IgG], is one of the major reasons for the greater sensitivity and duration, which is so characteristic of the IgE response in contrast to that of IgG. Another essential difference is the localized nature of allergic reactions, which can be attributed to the fact that IgE is produced locally in tissue by B cells, and FcεRI is expressed only on tissue mast cells, effector cells and antigen-presenting cells (APCs), and not on their precursors in the circulation.

The IgE–receptor complexes on other cell types are also important in the stages that precede and follow the immediate reaction to an allergen. During the first few hours after the immediate response, cytokines and other mediators, released by the activated mast cell, act on the local endothelium to attract T cells and inflammatory cells, especially eosinophils, into the tissue. IgE secreted by B cells in allergic tissue binds to FcεRI on the inflammatory cells, which can then contribute to the late response in both IgE-antibody-dependent and -independent modes.

When allergen binds to IgE–FcεRI complexes in effector cells, the ternary complex is internalized and digested by proteolytic enzymes. Although IgE and receptors are consumed in these reactions, they are soon replaced. Dendritic cells, 'professional' APCs in the tissue, also bear IgE–FcεRI complexes, which bind allergen to initiate the sequence of events culminating in the *de novo* synthesis of specific antibodies against the allergen. This process involves the activation and differentiation of T cells, which in turn activate cognate B cells. In allergic tissue, the activated B cells undergo heavy-chain class switching to IgE and secrete IgE antibodies. These then bind to mast cells to complete the cycle (see Fig. 18.1).

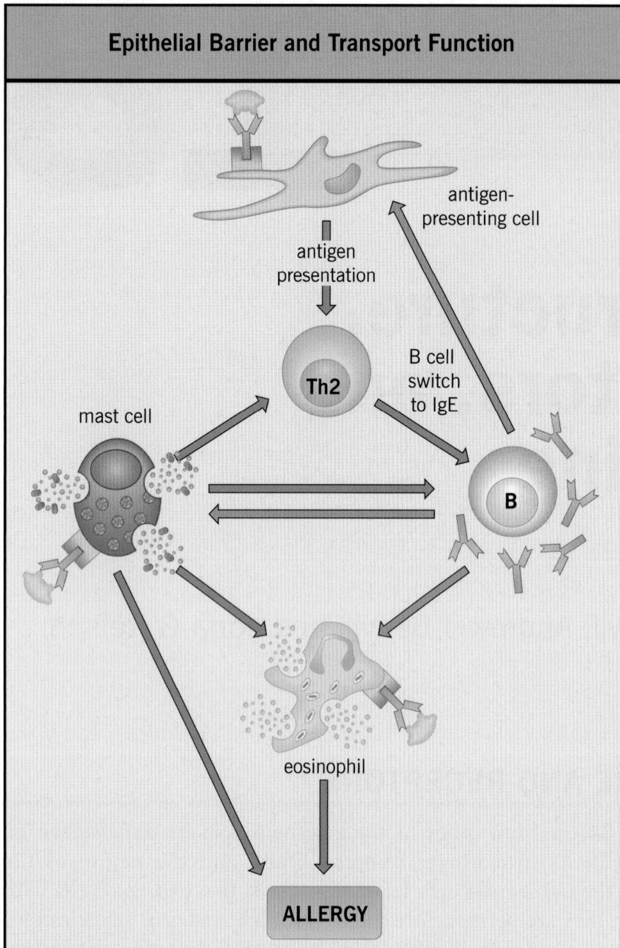

Fig. 18.1 The positive feedback mechanism in IgE synthesis. Shown here are the important functions of interleukin-4 (IL-4, blue arrows) and IgE (green arrows) in the allergic response, and the involvement of several types of cells, which either mediate the allergic reaction (mast cells and eosinophils) or maintain the hypersensitive state of allergic individuals (antigen-presenting cells, T cells, and B cells). This is a positive feedback mechanism, since IgE sensitizes the mast cell, and the allergen-activated mast cell initiates the series of events leading to *de novo* IgE synthesis.

Table 18.1 The essential characteristics of human IgE

Essential Characteristics of Human IgE	
Cell distribution	Committed B cells
Subunit structure	Two (κ or γ) light chains and two ε heavy chains
No. of amino acids	556 for IgE ND
Molecular weight	170 kDa protein + 20 kDa carbohydrate
Post-translational modifications	Six N-glycosylation sites
Isoforms (Fig. 18.3)	Secreted IgE (IgE) Membrane-bound (mIgE)
Regulation	IL-4: commitment (switching) CD23: rescue of cells from apoptosis Unknown factors: splicing to general IgE or mIgE

The low-affinity IgE receptor CD23 (or FcεRII) exerts feedback control of IgE synthesis (see below). This ensures that this highly amplified and potentially harmful immune response (the allergic reaction) does not get out of control. Indeed, IgE concentrations in serum are the lowest of any Ig class: 50–200 ng/mL as compared to 10 mg/mL for IgG in the serum of normal subjects. The various functions of IgE and its receptors in the allergic response are illustrated in Figure 18.1, and Tables 18.1 and 18.2. In this chapter we consider the structures and interactions of IgE and its receptors, and examine the process of signal transduction through FcεRI in mast cells.

The structure of IgE and the location of receptor-binding sites

Like all other antibody classes (IgM, IgD, IgG, and IgA) IgE comprises two identical light (L) and two identical heavy (H) chains; each chain is made up of structural units of about 110 amino acids, called immunoglobulin (Ig) domains, covalently linked by disulfide bonds, as shown in Figure 18.2. The L-chain has one N-terminal variable (V_L) domain, and one constant (C_L) domain and the H-chain one N-terminal V (V_H) and four C (C_H) domains. The antibody class is determined by the C_H sequence, designated $C\mu$, $C\delta$, $C\gamma$, $C\alpha$, and $C\varepsilon$, respectively, in IgM, IgD, IgG, IgA, and IgE, and the sequence of Cε is shown in Figure 18.3.

A given B cell produces an antibody with just one specificity, defined by the V_L and V_H combination, but during the antibody response it can 'switch' classes. What is involved in this switch is genetic recombination, which shifts the V_H, initially linked to $C\mu$, to one of the downstream C genes in a tandem array on chromosome 14, in this case the Cε gene (see also Ch. 19). Heavy-chain switching allows the antibody to exert a new range of effector functions in the immune response, and IgE is the effector of the allergic response. The only known benefit of this response is the resistance to infection by certain parasites.

Immunoglobulin domains are formed from two β sheets, referred to as a β-sheet sandwich. Each β sheet is made up of three to six strands, named in alphabetical order from the N terminus. The sandwich is opened out in Figure 18.4 to reveal how the strands are interwoven between the two sheets in V- and C-type immunoglobulin domains. In C domains ABDE and CGF strands form the opposing sides of the domain. Alternating residues in the amino acid sequence point inwards towards the hydrophobic interface between the two β sheets and outwards to make up the two exposed surfaces on opposite sides of the domain. In the domains that dimerize (e.g. Cε4 in IgE and Cγ3 in IgG), the exposed surfaces that interact with each other are also predominantly hydrophobic. The hydrophobicity favors interaction between protein surfaces over exposure to water.

Structurally, the ε heavy chain is most similar to the μ chain of IgM, in that it has four constant region domains (Cε1–Cε4), as compared to three in IgD, IgG, and IgA (C_H1–C_H3; see Fig. 18.2). Cε3 is homologous to Cγ2 and Cε4 to Cγ3 in IgG, while Cε2 takes the place of the hinge in IgG. IgG and IgE each contain a papain-sensitive site, located in the hinge region of

Table 18.2 The essential properties of receptors for human IgE

Essential Properties of Receptors for Human IgE

	FcεRI	**CD23**
Other names	High-affinity receptor	FcεRII; Low-affinity receptor
Affinity for monomeric IgE	$K_a = 10^{10}\ M^{-1}$	$K_a = 10^7\ M^{-1}$ for trimer $K_a = 10^6\ M^{-1}$ for monomer
Cell distribution	Mast cells, basophils, Langerhans' cells, platelets, eosinophils, macrophages	B cells, T cells, eosinophils, platelets, follicular dendritic cells
Subunit composition (number of amino acids)	α chain (260); β chain (263); two γ chains (86)	Trimer (321)
Orientation of polypeptide	Intracellular C terminus	Intracellular N terminus
Ligands	IgE	IgE, CR2(CD21), CR3(CD11b, CD18), CR4(CD11c, CD18), other integrins
Structural motifs	Two Ig domains per α chain	Animal C-type lectin, α-helical coiled-coil stalk; RGD adhesion, YSEI trafficking signal
Post-translational modifications	Serine, threonine, and tyrosine phosphorylation sites in β and γ chain Seven carbohydrates sites in α chain	One N-glycosylation site per chain Three protease processing sites per chains
Isoforms	One known	CD23a and CD23b
Binding site on IgE	Cε3	Cε3
Function	Mast cell activation and degranulation Antigen presentation IgE ADCC	Growth and/or differentiation factor for hematopoetic cells, anti-apoptosis, antigen presentation, IgE expression, IgE ADCC
Associated disease states	Immediate hypersensitivity	Inflammation, EBV transformation of cells

ADCC, antibody-dependent cell-mediated cytotoxicity; EBV, Epstein–Barr virus; K_a, association constant.

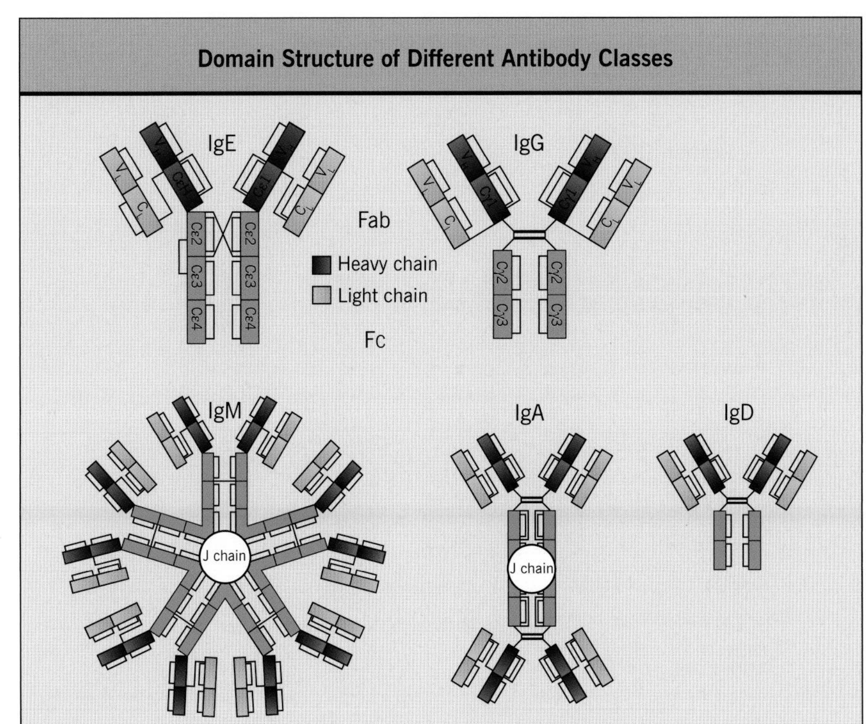

Fig. 18.2 The domain structure of different antibody classes. IgE is shown on the same scale as IgG for comparison, and IgM, IgA, and IgD are shown on a smaller scale to give an impression of their relationship to each other. Antigen-binding (Fab) regions are shown, with light blue representing the light chain and red the heavy chain; the receptor binding (Fc) regions are shown in green. Intra- and interchain disulfide bonds are in black.

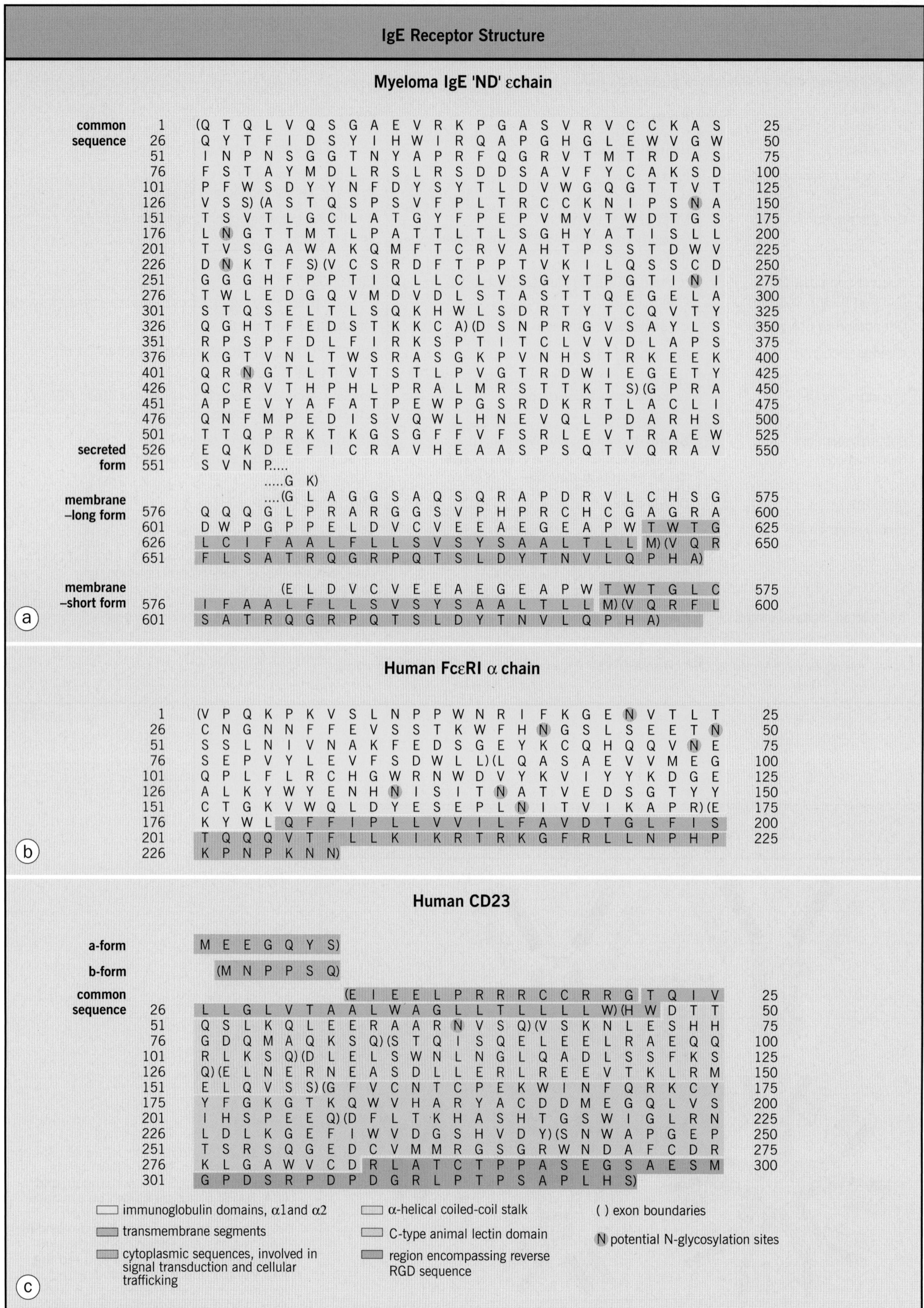

Fig. 18.3 The primary structure of a human myeloma ε chain, the α chain of FcεRI and CD23. (a) The common sequence (at the top) and the extra additional acid sequences at the C-terminal end of the secretory form, and the long and short membrane-bound forms (in that order from the top) of the myeloma ND ε sequence are shown. (b) A sequence of the human FcεRIα. (c) A sequence of human CD23.

IgG, giving rise on cleavage to the Fab and Fc fragments. In IgE, papain cleaves between Cε1 and Cε2 to produce the Fab fragment and an 'Fc' fragment, containing Cε2–Cε4. The terms Fab and Fc are historical, and derive from the presence of the antigen-binding site in the former, while the latter was termed the 'crystallizable' fragment from IgG.

As with other antibodies, the two antigen-combining sites in IgE are formed by the pairing of V_L and V_H domains, while the cell-receptor (FcεRI and CD23)-binding sites are formed by the dimerized region of the ε chains (the 'Fc'). From studies with recombinant peptides and chimeric antibodies, in conjunction with various binding and functional assays, the receptor-binding sites in IgE have been mapped to the Cε3 domain of IgE. The details of the interaction with FcεRI are further revealed by the X-ray structure of the complex between a fragment of IgE–Fc (Fcε3–4) and a soluble form of the receptor. Also, as with other antibodies, IgE is expressed in membrane-bound form(s) prior to antigen activation and in the secreted form following antigen activation and induction of B-cell differentiation. The primary structures of the secreted and membrane-bound forms of the ε-chain constant region secreted by myeloma ND are shown in Figure 18.3a. Membrane and secreted forms result from differential splicing of the mRNA precursor, which makes use of one terminal exon to encode the secreted form of the ε chain or an internal splice site in this exon to join the mRNA to a separate membrane exon.

There are a number of atomic structures of IgE–Fc and fragments. The whole Fc portion (Cε2–Cε4) has been studied by X-ray crystallography and the structure is shown in Figure 18.5. The Cε4 and Cε3 domains adopt a configuration more compact than that seen for Cγ3 and Cγ2 respectively in IgG–Fc, with the Cε4 domains dimerizing and the Cε3 domains positioned asymmetrically and making no contact with one another. The two Cε2 domains also form a dimer with two interchain disulfide bonds linked in a crossed arrangement, with Cys249 of one chain linked to Cys337 on the other and vice versa. The Cε2 pair exhibits a distinctive mode of Ig domain association; both less extensive and more hydrophilic than other Ig domains in Fab (C_H1:C_L) or Fc (Cγ3–Cγ3 or Cε4–Cε4). The overall

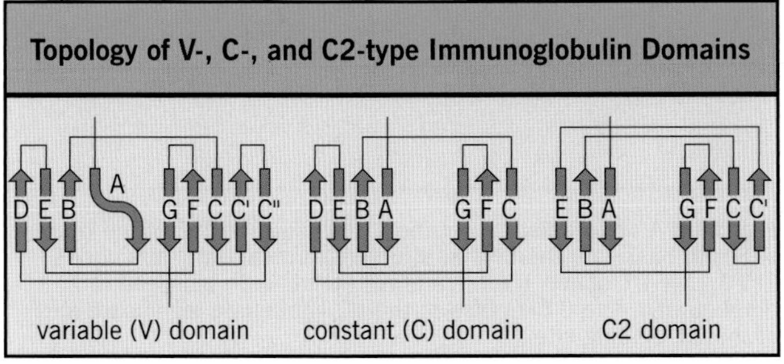

Fig. 18.4 The topology of variable (V)-, constant (C)-, and C2-type immunoglobulin (Ig) domains. The interconnection between strands in the two sheets comprising Ig or Ig-like domain for antibody V- and C-type Ig domains and the C2-type Ig-like domains in the α chains of FcεRI and IgG receptors is illustrated by opening out the β-sheet sandwich. Strands are designated in alphabetical order from the N terminus but are interwoven between the two sheets in a characteristic manner for each of the three topologies.

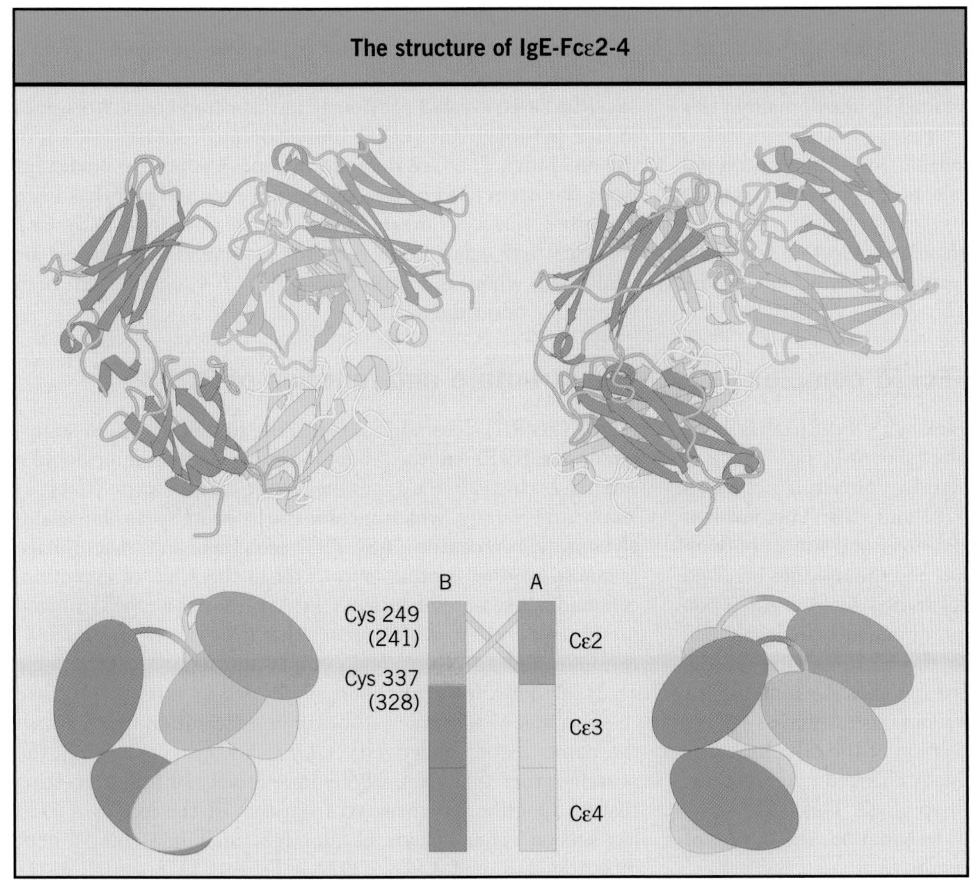

Fig. 18.5 Two orthogonal views of the X-ray crystal structure of IgE–Fcε2–4 (protein databank code 1LS0). The two Cε2 domains (red and orange) bend across and touch the Cε3 of one chain (yellow). The schematic diagram below indicates the color scheme used. The crossed disulfide bonds between Cys249 in one chain and Cys337 are shown in yellow (numbering in brackets denotes the alternative Bennich numbering commonly used).

structure is acutely and asymmetrically bent at the Cε2–3 linker region with the two Cε2 domains folded back onto the rest of the structure so that one of them makes extensive contacts with Cε3 of the opposite chain, and even touches Cε4. In contrast, the other Cε2 domain makes very few contacts with Cε3 and none with Cε4.

There are also X-ray structures of a truncated fragment of the Fc containing domains Cε3 and Cε4 (termed Fcε3–4), both alone and in complex with FcεRIα, and a nuclear magnetic resonance (NMR) structure of a monomeric Cε2 domain: these will be discussed in the context of the Fc receptor complex.

The structure of FcεRI

The high-affinity receptor FcεRI is composed of four polypeptide chains, an α chain, a β chain, and two γ chains. The α chain has an appreciable length of extracellular sequence but only a short cytoplasmic sequence. A soluble fragment of the α chain binds to IgE with full affinity and so the other subunits do not participate in binding. The predominantly cytoplasmic β and γ chains are responsible for signal transduction, as described in the last part of this chapter. Here we focus on the structure of the α chain, and more particularly its extracellular sequence.

For the primary structure of the FcεRI α chain see Figure 18.3b. The extracellular sequence is organized into immunoglobulin-like domains, resembling the α chains of all three IgG receptors (FcγRI, FcγRII, and FcγRIII) and the IgA receptor (FcαR). These are designated as C2-type immunoglobulin domains to distinguish them from the V- and C-type domains of antibodies. They are somewhat smaller (approx. 80 as against 110 amino acids) and they have a different arrangement of strands compared to V and C domains (see Fig. 18.4). The two Ig domains in the FcεRI α chain are designated α1 and α2, reading from the N terminus; thus α1 is the membrane-distal- and α2 is the membrane-proximal Ig-like domain in this type-I integral membrane protein.

Several structures are now available for different crystal forms of the solubilized ectodomain of the receptor FcεRIα (sFcεRIα) (Protein databank codes 1F2Q;1J86-9). All these structures show the two C2 domains anticipated from the primary sequence (Fig. 18.6), and essentially differ only in the conformation of the CC′ loop of α2.

The Tertiary Structure of IgE and FcεRI

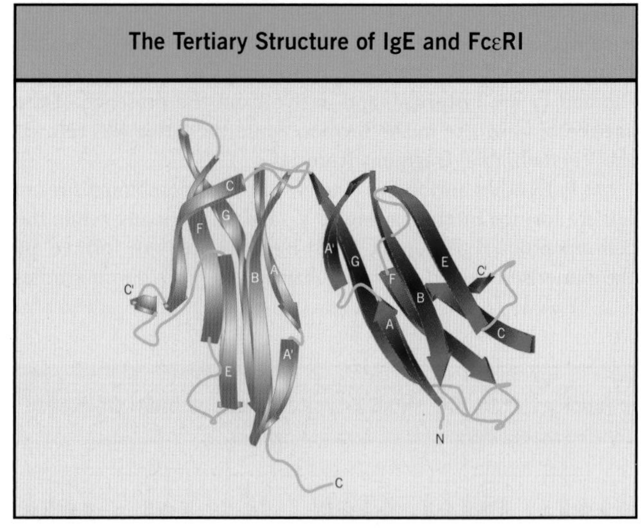

Fig. 18.6 A ribbon diagram of the extracellular region of the α chain of FcεRI, based on the crystal structure (protein databank codes 1F2Q;1J86-9), shows the α1 and α2 domains (in blue and red, respectively). The C′CFG face of the α2 contains a significant part of the IgE-binding site.

Comparison of the structures of Fcε3–4 in the presence and absence of the receptor reveals that the Cε3 domains are positioned differently. In the bound state, the two domains are further apart (termed the 'open'' conformation) allowing the receptor access to both sites 1 and 2. In the absence of receptor the Cε3 domains appear 'closed' with the receptor site partially occluded. The structure of the uncomplexed Fcε2–4 is intermediate between the two with one Cε3 domain in the open position and one in the closed position.

Additionally, the structure of a monomeric fragment of Cε2 has been solved by NMR spectroscopy, and titrations with sFcεRIα have revealed previously unsuspected contact residues in Cε2 (although not yet the corresponding contact residues in the receptor). The Cε2 domains in Fcε2–4 appear to be distant from the expected position of the receptor and so it has been suggested that a conformational change involving both Cε2 and Cε3 may occur upon receptor binding. This will only be confirmed when the structure of Fcε2–4 complexed with receptor is determined.

The structure of the IgE–FcεRI complex

The structure of Fcε3–4 in complex with FcεRIα has been determined by X-ray crystallography (shown in Fig. 18.7). A single receptor molecule binds to IgE by contacting both Cε3 domains at the junction between Cε2 and Cε3. This involves two distinctly different sites (termed site 1 and site 2) both on the receptor and on the Cε3 domains, and the residues involved are shown in Figure 18.7. The total buried surface area upon binding is extensive (1850Å^2) and predominantly hydrophobic, which undoubtedly contributes to the high stability of the complex. Binding across the two Cε3 domains explains the 1:1 stoichiometry which is required to avoid receptor cross-linking which would otherwise lead to activation of the effector cell.

The structure of FcεRIα is minimally changed upon binding, except for the region of the C–C′ loop of α2. This is the same loop that showed conformational freedom in the range of structures of the uncomplexed receptor.

The structure and function of CD23

CD23 (FcεRII) does not belong to the immunoglobulin superfamily like FcεRI and the receptors of the other immunoglobulin subclasses. Instead it is a member of the calcium-type (C-type) lectin superfamily, which includes such proteins as the asialoglycoprotein receptor (ASGPR), selectins, and macrophage mannose-binding protein, and lower in the scale of evolution, echinoidin, a sea-urchin lectin. Like ASGPR it is a type II integral membrane protein, which means that it has an extracellular C terminus and an N-terminal cytoplasmic sequence (see Table 18.2). Other known members of the lectin superfamily have the function of selective carbohydrate recognition (from which the name 'lectin' is derived). CD23, however, recognizes the protein rather than the carbohydrate moiety of IgE, suggesting that its function has diverged from that of the lectins. CD23 has several other ligands besides IgE, including complement receptors 2, 3, and 4 (i.e. CD21, CD11b/CD18, and CD11c/

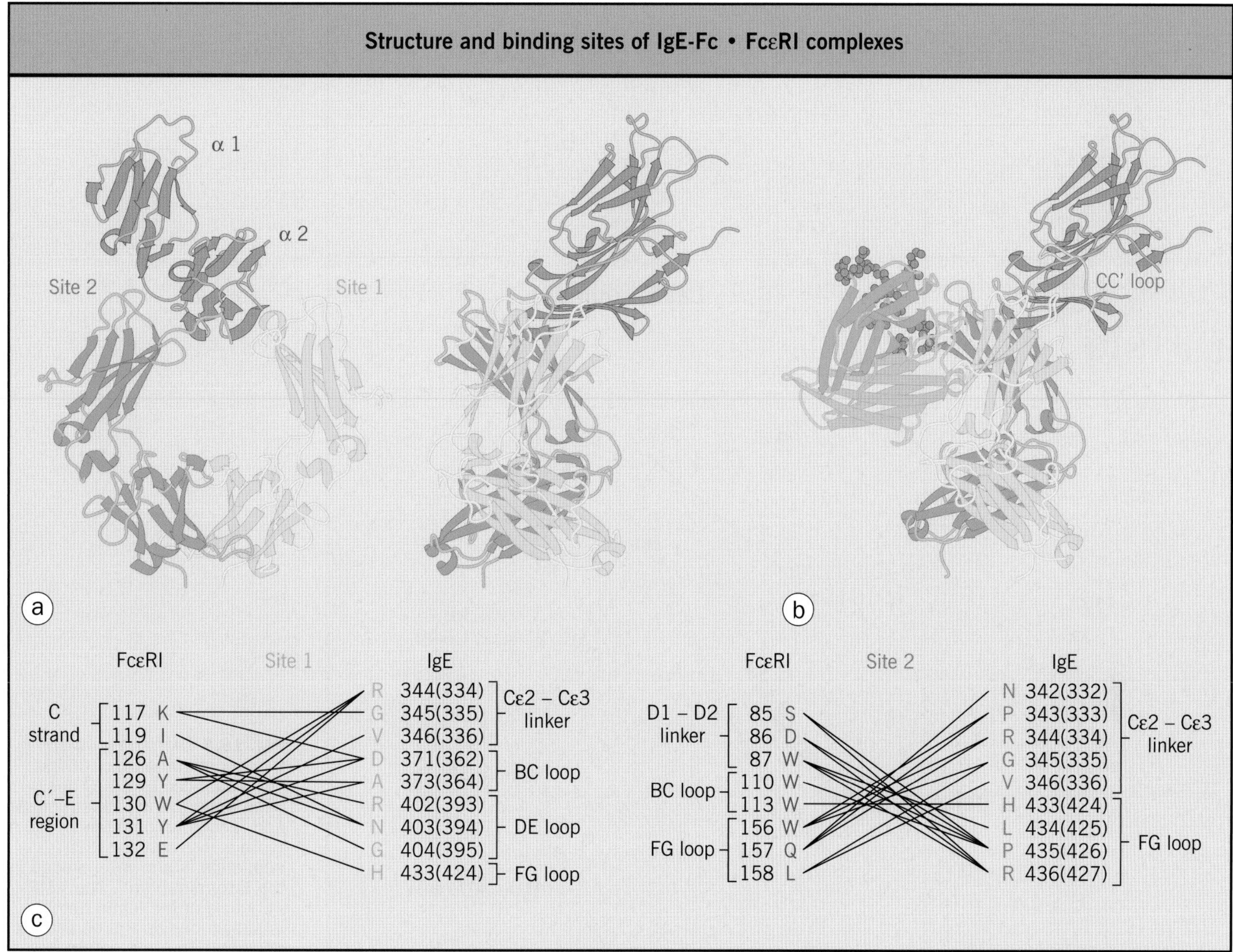

Fig. 18.7 (a) A ribbon representation of two orthogonal views of the X-ray crystal structure of Fcε3–4 (yellow and red) complexed with FcεRIα (blue) (protein databank code 1F6A). The α2 domain of the receptor binds both Cε3 domains (termed site 1 and site 2). (b) A model of the possible mode of interaction between Fcε2–4 and FcεRIα. The receptor is docked onto the Cε3 domains as in (a). The residues identified as contact residues in Cε2 are shown space-filled in blue. (c) Tables showing the residues in Fcε3–4 and FcεRIα that make contact in the complex. The residues in IgE are numbered according to the ND sequence in Fig.18.3 (with alternative numbering according to Bennich in brackets).

CD18), which are heavily glycosylated. There is evidence that the carbohydrate may be important in the recognition of these ligands.

The primary sequence of CD23, a 45 kDa polypeptide chain, is shown in Figure 18.3c. CD23 contains a variety of structural motifs, each corresponding to a different function in the protein (Fig. 18.8). Starting at the C terminus is a sequence of unknown structure, which contains a reverse RGD motif; it is conjectured that this may have an integrin-binding function. Adjoining this sequence is the lectin domain itself. It has conserved features found in all members of the family, such as the pattern of disulfide bonds and calcium-binding sites. The 3D structure of the lectin domain of CD23 has been determined by NMR (protein data bank code 1T8D) (see Fig. 18.8). The domain unfolds and ligand binding is lost if calcium is removed by the calcium chelating agents, ethylene glycol bis (2-aminoethyl ether) tetraacetic acid (EGTA) or ethylenediaminetetraacetic acid (EDTA). The lectin domain has been expressed as a recombinant fragment and binds to both IgE and CD21. The affinity of the monomeric lectin domain for IgE is an order of magnitude lower than that of native CD23, i.e. $K_a = 10^6 M^{-1}$ as against $10^7 M^{-1}$.

The lectin domain is connected to the transmembrane sequence by three imperfectly repeated 21 amino acid motifs. These, and the immediate flanking sequences, contain heptad hydrophobic repeats, the signature of sequences that form α-helical coiled coils; this domain is responsible for the association of CD23 into a homotrimer. The coiled coil is a very rigid structure constituting a 15 nm 'stalk', at the end of which the three lectin domains are placed to interact with soluble ligands and the counter-receptors on other cells, e.g. membrane IgE, CD21 (CR2), CR3, and CR4.

Next in the sequence is the hydrophobic transmembrane domain, followed by the cytoplasmic 'tail'. The cytoplasmic sequence can be either of two forms, CD23a or CD23b, which differ by seven and six amino acids at the N terminus respectively. CD23a is constitutively expressed on activated B cells and contains the YSEI motif, which serves as a targeting signal for coated pits. This is the form that is active in antigen presentation by B cells, a process not unlike the endocytosis

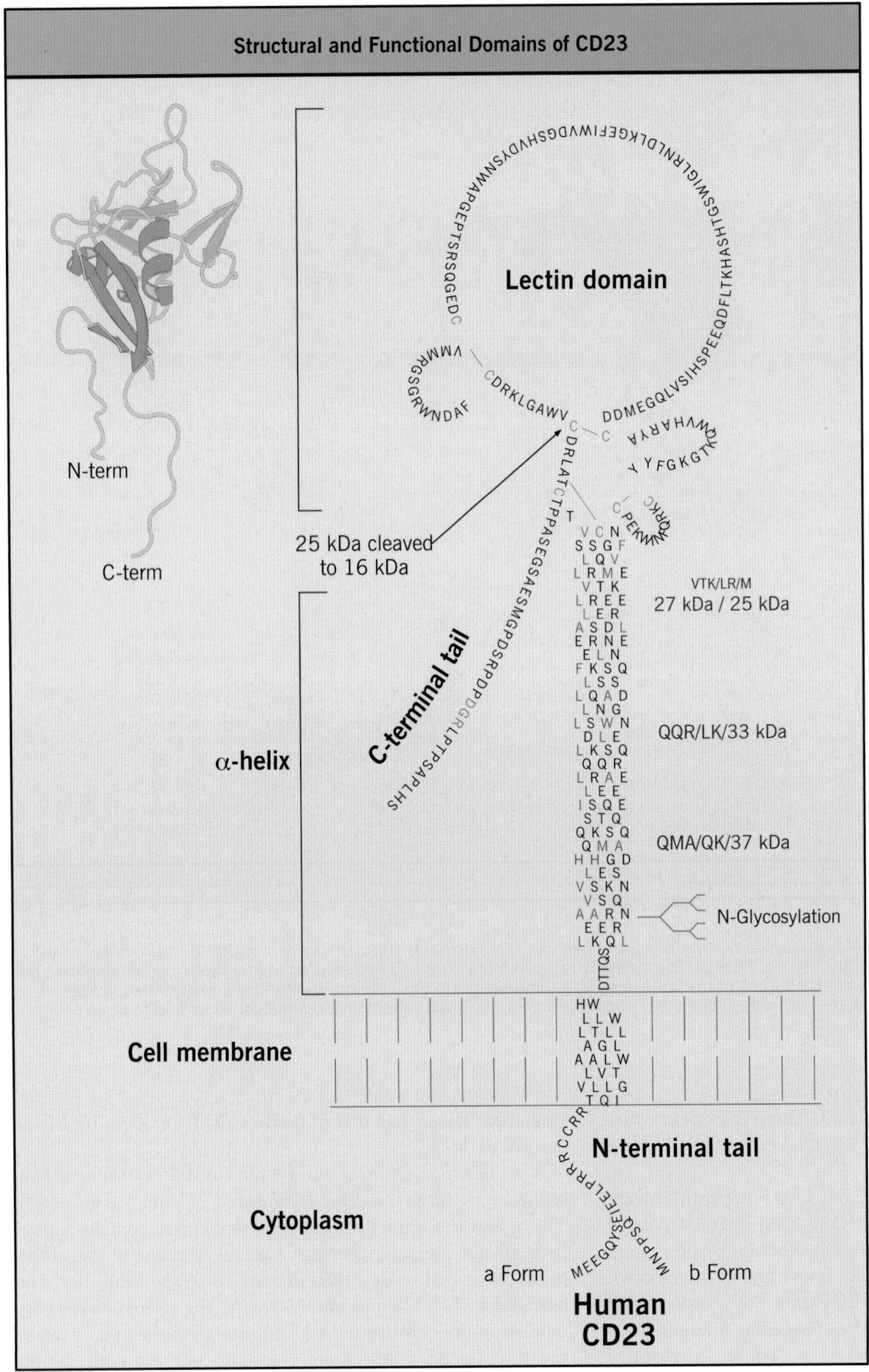

Fig. 18.8 The structural and functional domains of CD23. The sequence of CD23 has been used to indicate structural and functional domains of the protein. The reverse RGD sequence is shown in orange in the C-terminal 'tail'. The NMR structure of the lectin domain is shown beside the equivalent sequence (protein databank code 1T8D). Disulfide bonds are indicated in magenta. The α-helical sequence is laid out in a 4–3 repeating pattern to simulate the relative positions of the residues around the α-helix. Hydrophobic residues are colored cyan, and these clearly lie along one side of the helix, which forms the trimerization interface. Proteolytic cleavage sites, and the sizes of the fragments released, are shown in blue and the single N-glycosylation site in green. The transmembrane sequence is also laid out as an α-helix and this is followed by a representation of alternative forms of the N-terminal 'tail', which give rise to CD23a (containing the YSEI motif for targeting to coated pits) and CD23b.

and catabolism of glycoproteins by the homologous protein ASGPR. After limited proteolysis of the antigen within the cell, antigenic peptides are picked up by major histocompatibility complex (MHC) II molecules and returned to the surface for presentation to T cells.

CD23b lacks the YSEI signal sequence, because its N-terminal domain is encoded by a separate exon, situated between the first exon for CD23a and a common second exon. CD23b then has a different promoter sequence, and this contains a response element for interleukin-4 (IL-4). CD23b is thus upregulated by IL-4 in a wide range of hematopoietic cells and in epithelial cells. CD23b mediates IgE antibody-dependent phagocytosis by macrophages. Both CD23a and CD23b may function as adhesion molecules in cell trafficking.

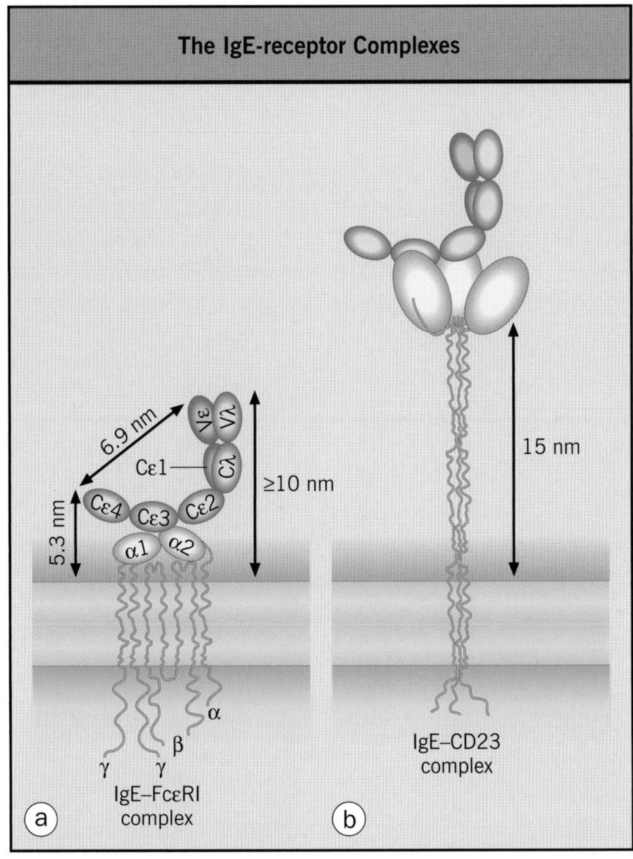

Fig. 18.9 The IgE-receptor complexes. (a) The IgE–FcεRI complex; the following features are shown: (1) The 1:1 stoichiometry of the complex. (2) The binding sites in Cε3 and α2. (3) The bent structures of IgE and FcεRIα. (4) Measured distances between IgE and the cell membrane (requiring the flattening of the α chain along the surface of the cell. (b) The IgE–CD23 complex, which incorporates the trimeric nature of the CD23, is illustrated, along with the association between IgE and the lectin domain.

For a model of the binding of IgE to trimeric CD23, see Figure 18.9. The higher affinity of the native trimer compared to the recombinant monomeric lectin domain of CD23 for IgE could result merely from the greater avidity of a protein containing three identical binding sites for IgE. However, CD23 monomers form a 2:1 complex with IgE in solution, so it appears that there are two binding sites in IgE. According to the model of the trimeric CD23, two lectin domains could only make contact with IgE if they bind to different sites. Correspondingly, there must be two different IgE binding sites in CD23 (see Fig. 18.9b).

The coiled-coil stalk of CD23 contains several sites that are cleaved by endogenous proteases (such as the metalloprotease ADAM 8) to release fragments containing the lectin domain and different lengths of stalk (see Fig. 18.8). These fragments are found at a concentration of about 2 ng/mL (10 nM) in the serum of normal individuals and at higher concentrations in those with inflammatory diseases, e.g. allergy and autoimmune diseases. The first cleavage occurs at the site nearest the membrane to yield a large (37 kDa) extracellular fragment. This fragment should be released as a trimer, although it is possible that the coiled-coil stalk may unravel from the N-terminal ends when it is liberated from the cell membrane. Subsequent digestion produces fragments with progressively shorter remnants of the stalk until only the lectin domain remains (25 and 16 kDa fragments). IgE binding to membrane-bound CD23 protects the protein from proteolysis, even though the binding site (in the lectin domain) is remote from the site of proteolytic cleavage (in the stalk).

The larger fragments of CD23 have been shown to upregulate IgE synthesis in cell culture by binding to CD21 on B cells, and the smaller ones antagonize this activity. CD21 is the complement receptor for the iC3b and C3dg fragments of the C3 component of complement and the receptor for the Epstein–Barr virus (EBV in Table 18.2). The complement fragments covalently attach to antigen and then co-ligate CD21 and antigen receptor (the membrane-bound antibody, specific for the antigen) in the B-cell membrane. This interaction gives rise to synergistic signaling, which empowers the B cell to respond to antigen concentrations several orders of magnitude lower than required for signaling by the antigen receptor alone. These signals stimulate B-cell proliferation and clonal expansion and account for the antigen specificity of the immune response.

CD23 gene knock-out and overexpression in mice reveals that the dominant effect of CD23 in this species is the downregulation of IgE synthesis. Paradoxically, CD23 appears to act in both the upregulation and downregulation of IgE synthesis (Fig. 18.10). The above information concerning the interacting proteins (IgE, CD23, and CD21), however, suggests a resolution of this paradox. CD23a is expressed on antigen-activated B cells and CD23b on IL-4-stimulated B cells and inflammatory cells. In the absence of IgE, which inhibits the proteolysis of CD23, fragments are released from these cells. By analogy to the mechanism of action of the C3-antigen complex in stimulating B-cell proliferation, trimeric CD23 fragments may co-ligate membrane IgE and CD21 on cells committed to IgE synthesis, binding IgE by two of its lectin domains and CD21 by the third (right hand side, Fig. 18.10). This could account for the selective expansion of the population of B cells committed to IgE synthesis and expressing the membrane form of IgE.

IgE concentrations in tissues would then rise from an initial level of 50–200 ng/mL (which is $0.3–1.2 \times 10^{-11}$ M) in the tissue to approach the dissociation constant (K_d) of the IgE–CD23 complex (10^7 M^{-1}). Above this IgE concentration, further release of CD23 fragments would be inhibited by binding of the excess IgE to CD23, and stimulation of IgE synthesis would therefore cease. Co-ligation of membrane IgE and CD23 by allergen–IgE complexes may also directly downregulate IgE synthesis in B cells (Fig. 18.10, left hand side), resembling the mechanism of the feedback regulation of IgG synthesis by the low-affinity IgG receptor (FcγRIIβ/CD32). These two inhibitory mechanisms may both operate to provide a concerted mechanism in the case of IgE. These activities would be negligible at IgE concentrations below 10^{-7} M. However, local concentrations in allergic tissues are likely to exceed this level.

Positive feedback may be an important feature of the mechanism that operates to upregulate IgE. Activated mast cells and T cells release IL-4, which upregulates IgE synthesis, and the resulting IgE binds to mast cells, and so on ad infinitum (see Fig. 18.1). CD23 provides a counterbalancing negative feedback mechanism, which, in the mouse, is important in the homeostasis of IgE. (Mouse and human CD23 differ, in that murine CD23 does not bind to CD21. This may account for the dominance of IgE suppression in this species.) The positive and negative effects of CD23 on IgE synthesis are represented

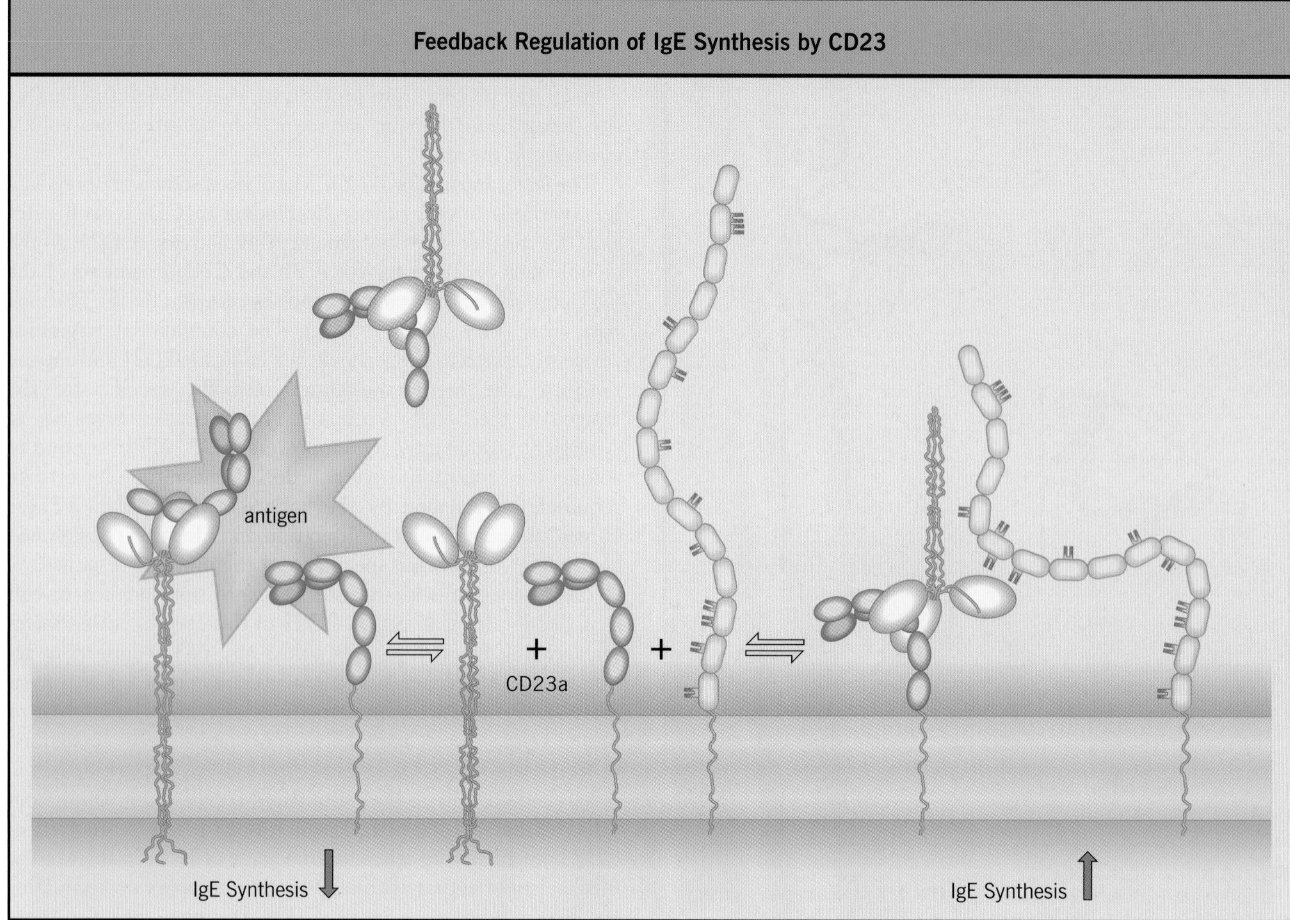

Fig. 18.10 The feedback regulation of IgE synthesis by CD23. In the window of opportunity (between 10^{-10} and 10^{-7} M IgE, which are the K_d values of IgE–FcεRI and IgE–CD23 complexes respectively) the upregulation of CD23a by antigen activation of B cells and IL-4 activation of CD23b on various cells is expected to stimulate IgE synthesis (on the right). But as IgE concentrations in the tissue – due to this stimulation – approach and then exceed the upper limit, there are two possible mechanisms by which further IgE synthesis may be suppressed by the product (on the left): (1) Binding of secreted IgE to soluble CD23 fragments – this inhibits IgE synthesis by competing with CD23 binding to membrane IgE. (2) Negative signaling induced by the co-ligation of IgE and CD23 in the B-cell membrane. IgE regulation by CD23 is represented here as a competition between CD21 and CD23 in the cell membrane. Note that IL-4, released by both mast cells and T cells in the allergic response, simultaneously induces IgE synthesis in B cells and upregulates CD23b on nearly all the cells that populate the tissue; the dual action of IL-4 may thus ultimately determine the physiologic concentrations of IgE. K_d, dissociation constant. IL-4 interleukin-4.

in Figure 18.10 as a competition between CD21 and CD23 for IgE in the B-cell membrane. Thus, IgE concentrations regulate the switch between upregulation of IgE (at low IgE concentrations) and downregulation of IgE (at high IgE concentrations) mediated by CD23.

CD23 is highly expressed on the follicular dendritic cells (FDC) of the lymphoid node germinal centers and appears to play a role in the differentiation of B cells into plasmacytes. No selectivity for IgE-committed cells is apparent in this process, probably because the FDC express CD21 and IgG receptors. Co-ligation of antigen receptors and CD21 on the B-cell membrane does not then require an antigen receptor of the IgE class. For example, a membrane IgM or IgG antibody on the B cell could be linked to the FDC through a soluble antigen-IgG antibody or an antigen–C3 complex, linked in turn to the FDC through an IgG receptor or CD21, respectively. CD23 on the FDC would then provide the second signal through CD21 on the B cell.

The little that is known about signaling pathways through CD23, whether as a membrane receptor for IgE or the ligand for CD21 and membrane IgE on B cells is described at the end of this chapter. It is known that CD21 signaling leads to the upregulation of bcl-2 gene expression in the nucleus; bcl-2 protein rescues B cells from apoptosis, and thus contributes to cell survival and proliferation. The same signaling pathway probably participates in the selective upregulation of IgE by fragments of CD23 (see Fig. 18.10, right hand side).

CELLULAR SIGNALING – GENERAL INTRODUCTION

Cellular signaling is a tightly controlled and complex multistep process that coordinates cellular responses to external or metabolic stimuli. The interplay of multiple regulatory loops ensures adequate responses and the prevention of aberrant or excessive activation. Although presented here in the context of

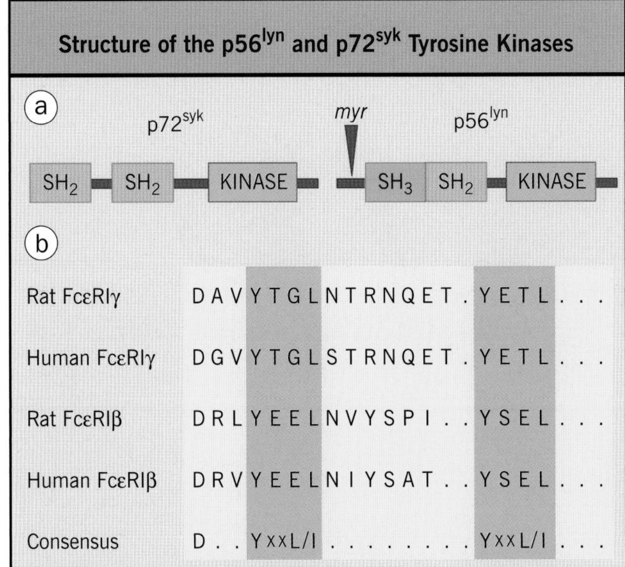

Fig. 18.11 (a) The structure of the Syk and Lyn tyrosine kinases – myr represents the N-terminal myristoylation site. (b) The sequences of the ITAMs contained within the rat and human FcεRIβ and γ subunits. The illustration shows the consensus sequence, which is also found in the ITAMs contained within the T-cell receptor ζ chain and the B-cell receptor IgA and IgB chains. The SH_2-binding tyrosine motifs are indicated by the darker shading. ITAMS, immunoreceptor tyrosine activation motifs; SH_2, src homology 2.

FcεRI, signaling cascades share basic concepts, some of which are presented in the following:

- Signaling in general and protein interaction in particular are not random processes. Proteins can be subdivided into functional modules (domains), and families of proteins are defined based on similar domain combinations. Domains were identified as stretches of similar amino acid sequence with defined function and shared binding partners. A central recognition motif tends to be flanked by amino acids that convey specificity of interaction. Classic examples are the interactions of the src homology 2 (SH_2) domains with phospho-tyrosine residues, or SH_3 domains with proline-rich regions (Fig. 18.11). With the increasing number of well-characterized domains, it has become possible to predict the function of many proteins by their amino acid sequence.
- Many protein interactions only occur after activation-induced modifications, such as the above-mentioned phosphorylation of tyrosine residues. Similarly, catalytic activity of signaling proteins can be modulated by phosphorylation of critical tyrosines. Other signaling-induced modifications that influence protein interactions are serine/threonine phosphorylation, methylation, ubiquitination, etc.
- Location plays an important role in signal propagation: components of signaling cascades are frequently spatially restricted within the cell and associate only upon activation-induced movement. As an example, translocation may occur from the cytoplasm to the membrane, as is the case for phospholipase Cγ1, which requires activation for transport to its membrane associated substrate phosphatidylinositol 4,5-bisphosphate (PIP_2). Activation may also alter the position of proteins within the membrane. Although their exact nature is still under investigation, cellular subdomains were identified based on their differential solubility in detergents and were alternatively termed glycolipid-enriched membranes (GEMs), detergent insoluble glycolipid-enriched membranes (DIGs) or lipid rafts. Proteins can be targeted to rafts based on lipid modifications (myristoylation and palmitoylation) or hydrophobicity. An aggregation-induced change in the latter is thought responsible for the observed movement of activated FcεRI complexes into lipid rafts.
- Since virtually every cellular activation process simultaneously activates inhibitory mechanisms, signaling is best viewed as a series of dynamic equilibria, rather than an 'on–off' phenomenon.
- Finally, multistep signaling cascades can incorporate receptor-interaction time as a regulatory factor. Simplified, the concept of 'kinetic proofreading' is based on the premises that the duration of ligand/receptor interaction is determined by affinity, and that progression through signaling steps takes time. It predicts that the ligand needs to bind to its receptor sufficiently long for the signal to proceed to a given threshold step, whereas the cascade would not be completed in case of shorter, low affinity interaction. While this concept does not apply to all aspects of signaling, it provides an outline of how cells could quantitatively and qualitatively fine-tune their responses according to ligand affinity.

FCεRI SIGNALING

In its 'classical' form, FcεRI is expressed as the above-described heterotetramer comprising α, β, and two γ chains. However, in human cells, FcεRI can also reach the cell membrane as an $\alpha\gamma_2$ complex. The complete $\alpha\beta\gamma_2$ complex is expressed on cell types primarily responsible for effector functions, e.g. mast cells and basophils, while the $\alpha\gamma_2$ heterotrimer is found on human APCs, including dermal and blood dendritic cells, epidermal Langerhans' cells and monocytes/macrophages. The α chain confers ligand recognition and carries seven N-linked glycosylation sites, which are essential for proper folding in the endoplasmic reticulum. It also carries a retention motif, which needs to be masked through γ-chain association for transport of FcεRI to the cell surface. The FcεRI β chain has been ascribed a receptor-stabilizing and signal-amplifying role which appears in line with more robust FcεRI signals on effector cells, compared with a more mobile FcεRI on APCs, that facilitates antigen uptake and processing. Additionally a truncated version of the FcεRI β chain has been described as a negative regulator of receptor expression. Finally the γ dimer is essentially for signaling, but not unique to FcεRI, since it is also found in other Fc receptor complexes.

The network of FcεRI signaling has mostly been explored in rodent mast cell models, such as rat peritoneal and murine mast cells and the rat basophil leukemia (RBL) cell line, all of which carry the $\alpha\beta\gamma_2$ complex. In comparison to human primary cells, these systems have the advantage of abundant cell availability, ease of manipulation and reproducibility. Available results indicate that principal signaling events are similar but not identical between these models and primary cells. Restriction to human cells, limited cell numbers, low intensity of receptor expression and weaker signals are challenges for the exploration of signaling via the $\alpha\gamma_2$ complex on APCs.

Aggregation of FcεRI by IgE–allergen complexes or antibodies in experimental systems, initiates the events that lead to mast cell degranulation, the de novo synthesis and release of preformed mediators, and the induction of cytokines. While the early events and their outcome are reasonably well known, much remains to be learned about the intermediate steps and the interaction and regulation of signaling proteins involved.

Receptor aggregation (Fig. 18.12)

The FcεRI complex by itself does not have kinase activity, therefore signaling is initiated through the aggregation of two or more receptors by IgE bound to multivalent antigen. A proportion of the FcεRI β chain is constitutively associated with a small amount of the protein tyrosine kinase $p56^{lyn}$ (Lyn), which after aggregation, also termed cross-linking, transphosphorylates approximated immunoreceptor tyrosine activation motifs (ITAMs) on the β- and γ-receptor subunits. These ITAMs are stretches of approximately 20 amino acids, which possess two tyrosine-containing motifs (YXXL/I) separated by six to eight amino acids (Fig. 18.11). Their phosphorylation results in an increased association of Lyn with FcεRIβ and binding of $p72^{syk}$ (Syk) to FcεRIγ. The interaction of Syk with the γ chain facilitates the phosphorylation of Syk by Lyn, increasing the catalytic activity of Syk. Accompanying these early events is the translocation of aggregated FcεRI into lipid rafts and the phosphorylation of scaffolding proteins, such as the transmembrane adaptor LAT. These docking molecules are the backbones for the assembly of signaling complexes, also termed 'signalosomes'.

In a Lyn independent, parallel pathway, receptor aggregation also activates the Src-kinase Fyn.

As discussed in the introduction, cellular signaling is a dynamic balance of activation and inhibition and the phosphorylation of β- and γ-chain ITAMs by Lyn is reversed by the two phosphatases (PTPs) SHP1 and SHP2, which associate with the FcεRI subunits. Mast cells express a number of PTPs including CD45, PTP1C, PTP1D, and HePTP, which regulate multiple inhibitory and stimulatory signaling pathways.

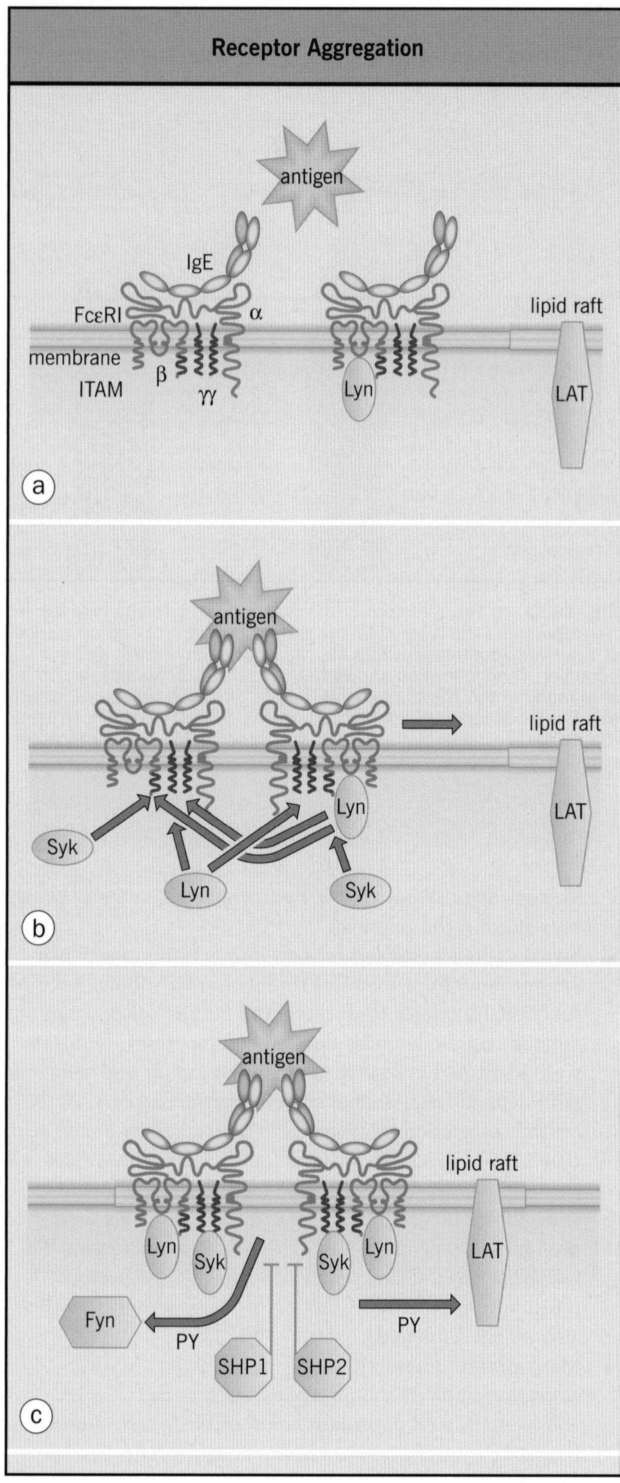

Fig. 18.12 Early events following FcεRI aggregation. Turquoise regions on the receptor subunits represent the ITAMs. (a) In the resting cell, Lyn, but not Syk, is associated with FcεRI. (b) Following antigen-dependent FcεRI aggregation, Lyn is activated and phosphorylates the FcεRIβ and FcεRIγ ITAMs. (c) Following binding of Lyn and Syk SH_2 domains to the FcεRIβ and FcεRIγ ITAMs respectively, Syk is phosphorylated thereby increasing its catalytic activity. Receptor aggregation also leads to the phosphorylation of the tyrosine kinase Fyn and the adaptor protein LAT. The phosphatases SHP1 and SHP2 dephosphorylate FcεRI subunits. ITAMS, immunoreceptor tyrosine activation motifs; SH_2, src homology 2.

Downstream signals

Subsequent to receptor aggregation, several signaling branches are initiated with a large number of proteins involved. These branches intersect at multiple stages and are linked through feedback loops, but will be discussed separately for the sake of simplicity. In the following, proteins are grouped according to essential signaling events: calcium signals, the activation of Ras/Raf or phosphatidylinositol-3 kinase (PI3 kinase), sphingosine metabolism, cyclic adenosine monophosphate (cAMP) and ubiquitination. Together they coordinate the release of preformed mediators (histamine, serotonin, and proteases), the de novo synthesis of prostaglandins, leukotrienes and cytokines, and other cell responses, such as migration.

Phospholipase C, calcium mobilization and protein kinase C activation (Fig. 18.13)

Similar to many receptors, the stimulation of FcεRI triggers calcium fluxes through activation of phospholipases (PLCs). These fall into three major classes, PLCβ, PLCδ, and PLCγ of which the β_1, β_2, β_3, γ_1 and γ_2 isoforms are expressed in mast

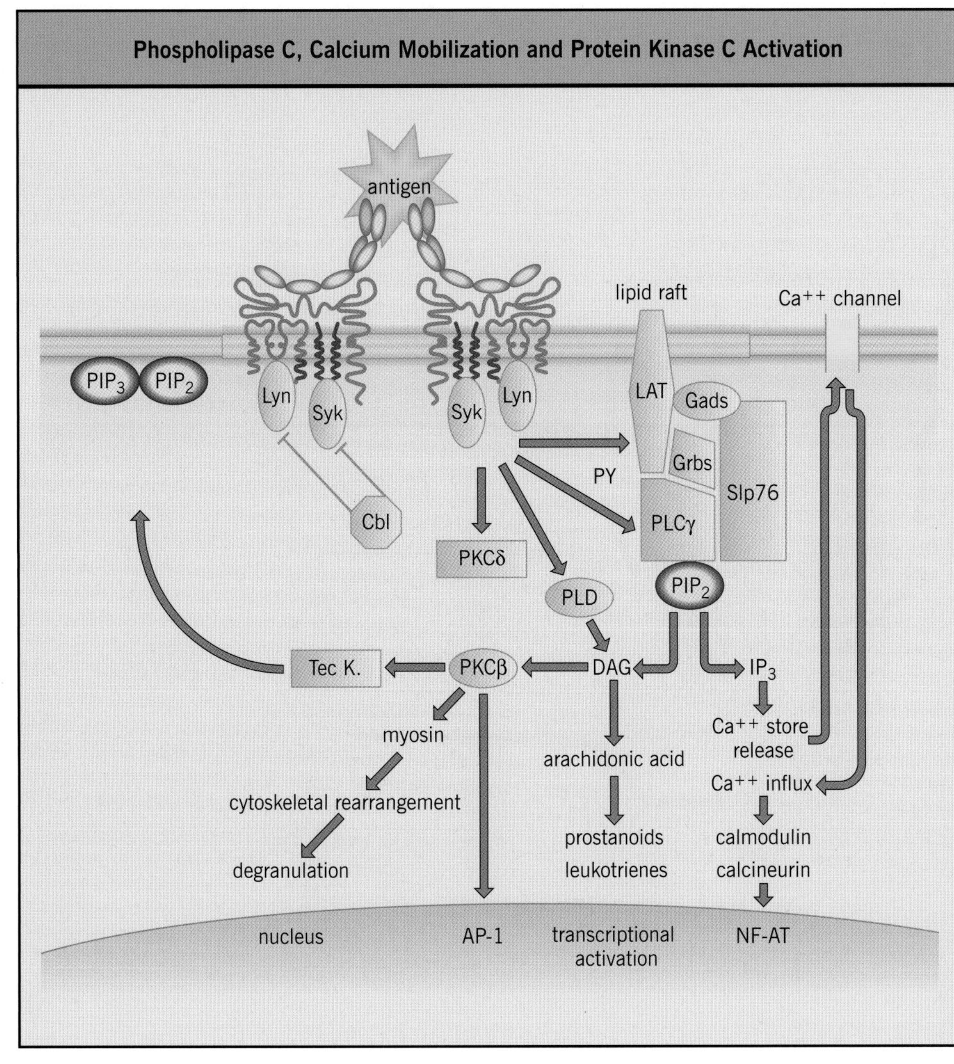

Fig. 18.13 Phospholipase C, calcium mobilization and protein kinase C activation. The phosphorylation of LAT nucleates a signaling complex of PLCγ, Slp-76, Grb2 and Gads. Subsequently PLCγ hydrolyses PIP_2 to IP_3 and DAG. The latter is also produced through the activation of PLD, activates PKCβ and stimulates the production of arachidonic acid, leukotrienes and prostaglandins. IP_3 mediates the initial release of calcium from intracellular stores, which is followed by calcium influx, calcineurin activation and the initiation of transcription. PKCβ mediates cytoskeletal rearrangement and phosphorylates Tec kinases, which require phosphorylation and membrane recruitment for their full activity. Cbl inhibits signaling by catalyzing the transfer of polyubiquitin chains to target proteins, such as Lyn and Syk, a mark for degradation by the proteasome. AP-1, activated protein-1; DAG, 1,2-diacylglycerol; IP_3, inositol trisphosphate; NF-AT, nuclear factor of activated T cells; PIP_2, phosphatidylinositol 4,5-bisphosphate; PIP_3 phosphatidylinositol-3,4, 5-trisphosphate; PKC, protein kinase C. PLC, PLD, phospholipases.

cells. As a consequence of Syk kinase activation, the raft localized adaptor LAT and cytosolic PLCγ are phosphorylated. Reports indicate that $PLC\gamma_1$ is dominantly expressed and activated in human mast cells, whereas rodent mast cells utilize both $PLC\gamma_1$ and $PLC\gamma_2$. The phosphorylation of LAT creates docking sites for PLCγ, which translocates to the membrane, where it hydrolyzes its substrate PIP_2 to inositol 1,4,5-trisphosphate (IP_3) and 1,2-diacylglycerol (DAG) (Fig. 18.14). A LAT-related protein was identified recently and named NTAL (non-T-cell activation linker). It has similar, but non-overlapping adapter functions, and appears not to couple to $PLC\gamma_1$. Proteins that form a complex with PLCγ are Grb2, which binds to LAT, and Slp-76, which in turn binds PLCγ. Gads (Grb2-related adaptor downstream of Shc), another bridging protein, binds to Slp-76 and LAT.

IP_3 production causes the release of calcium ions from intracellular stores in the endoplasmic reticulum. The initial calcium spike triggers the opening of membrane calcium channels and is followed by a more substantial second wave of calcium influx from the extracellular space, in a process termed capacitive entry. Free calcium binds to calmodulin, and activates the calcium- or calmodulin-dependent serine/threonine phosphatase, calcineurin, which dephosphorylates the NF-AT family of transcription factors (*n*uclear *f*actor of *a*ctivated *T* cells) and causes their translocation to the nucleus. Calcineurin is the target of the immunosuppressive drug ciclosporin and the novel non-steroidal therapeutic agents for atopic dermatitis, tacrolimus and pimecrolimus.

Transcription factors are also activated through calcium dependent isoforms of protein kinase C (PKC), which is downstream of DAG and translocates to the membrane upon activation. The PKC family comprises at least 11 isoforms grouped into conventional (α, β, γ), novel (δ, ε, θ) and atypical (ζ, λ) PKCs. Conventional and novel PKCs require DAG for activation, but only conventional PKCs also depend on calcium. The atypical PKCs are independent of both. Mast cells express the calcium-dependent isoforms α, β_1, β_2 and δ and the calcium-independent isoforms ε, θ and ζ.

PKCβ connects to mitogen activated protein (MAP) kinase activation via Ras and mobilizes transcription factors, such as activated protein-1 (AP-1) for the initiation of cytokine production. Further targets of this pathway are the light and heavy chains of myosin, whose activation promotes the reorganization of myosin filaments and their association with actin. These contractile elements aid in the movement of secretory granules to the apical membrane and granule release,

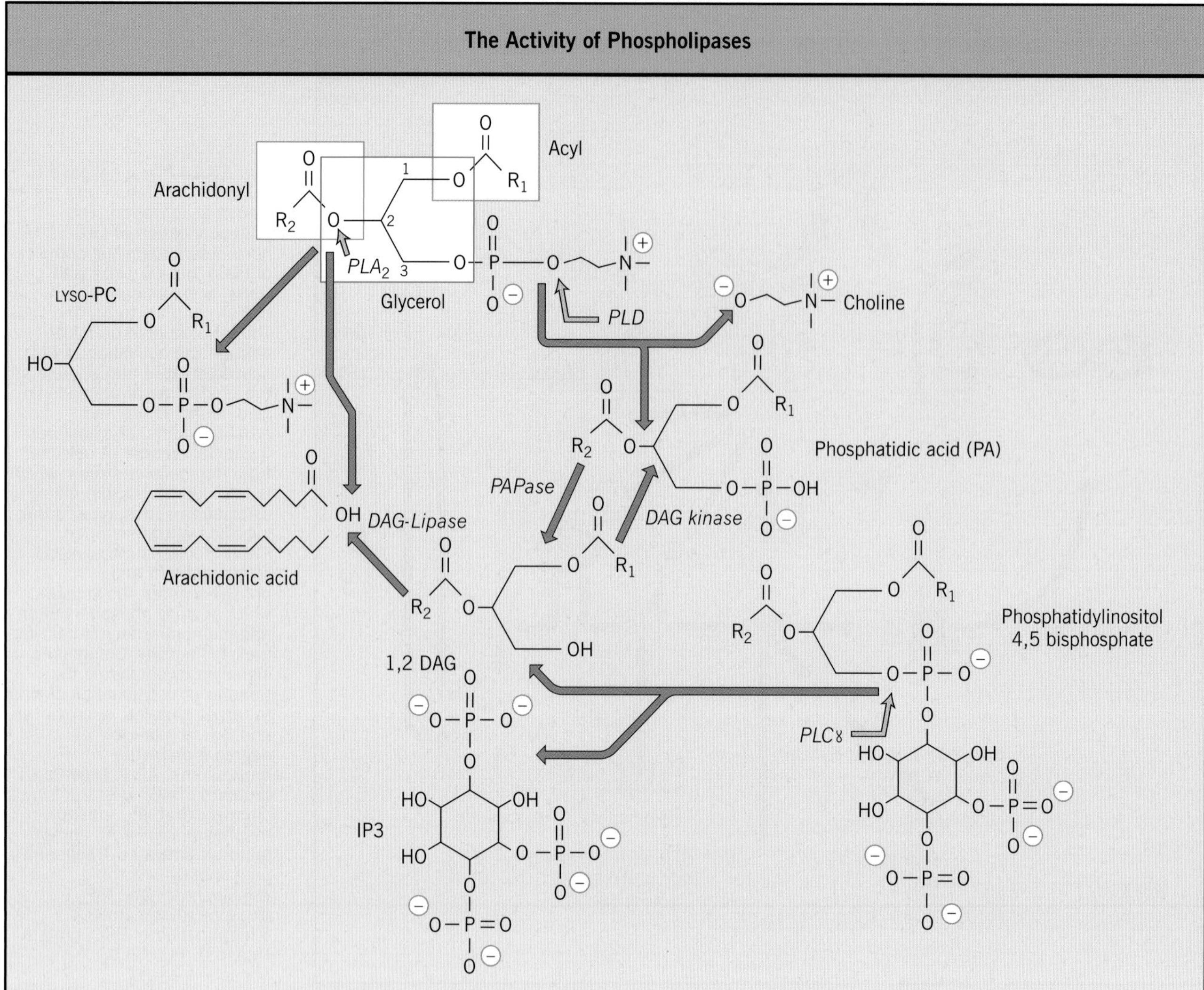

Fig. 18.14 Phospholipases are classified according to their cleavage site on phospholipids. Phospholipase A1 (PLA1) catalyses the hydrolysis of the fatty acid on C1 from the glycerol backbone of phospholipids. PLA2 cleaves on position C2 releasing lysophosphatidylcholine (lyso-PC) plus free fatty acid, most commonly arachidonic acid. PLCγ hydrolyzes between glycerol and the phosphate group, releasing 1,2-diacylglycerol (DAG) and inositol-1,4,5-trisphosphate (IP3) from phosphatidylinositol 4,5 bisphosphate. PLD cleaves the headgroup to yield choline plus phosphatidic acid (PA), which is further cleaved by phosphatidic acid phosphatase (PAPase) to DAG. DAG lipase hydrolyses the C2 arachidonic acid, while DAG lipase converts DAG to PA.

supported by the FcεRI-induced activation of myosin light chain kinase, which phosphorylates specific serine residues on the myosin light chain. Mast cells from PKCβ-deficient mice demonstrate defective degranulation; in contrast, elimination of PKCδ results in increased secretory responses in a mechanism that is currently unclear. PKCδ associates directly with the FcεRI γ chain and promotes the hydrolysis of inositolphosphate. PKCθ has recently received attention in the context of T-cell stimulation and its recruitment to the immunologic synapse; in mast cells its activation is linked to the transcription factors AP-1 and NF-κB via intermediates that are currently not characterized.

Finally, PKC also regulates the activity of the Tec family kinases, which integrate calcium mobilization and PI3 kinase signaling. Their serine phosphorylation by PKC generates a binding site for the Grb2/Sos complex, which contributes to the full activation of the Ras/Raf pathway.

Although specific DAG production by $PLC\gamma_1$ results in the activation of PKC, most DAG formed upon mast cell activation is dependent upon the phospholipase D (PLD)-catalyzed hydrolysis of phosphatidylcholine (Fig. 18.14). In addition to DAG, PLD releases phosphatidic acid, which can trigger mitogenesis, and free arachidonic acid, which contributes to the pool of arachidonic acid used for the synthesis of prostanoids and leukotrienes. FcεRI-dependent activation of PLD requires calcium, and the phospholipase can also be activated by PIP_2, phosphatidylinositol-3,4,5-trisphosphate (PIP_3) and G proteins (Arf1, RhoA, and Rac1).

GTPase pathway (Fig. 18.15)

Small monomeric guanosine triphosphate (GTP) binding proteins (G proteins) orchestrate cytoskeletal changes, lipid and protein kinase cascades, and the induction of gene transcription in mast cells. In contrast, members of the heterotrimeric class of G proteins including Gi and Gs are expressed by mast cells, but do not appear to couple to FcεRI signaling. Small GTPases alternate between an inactive guanosine diphosphate (GDP)- and the active GTP-bound state, in which they interact with target proteins. This exchange is controlled by two opposing groups of proteins; the guanosine nucleotide exchange factors

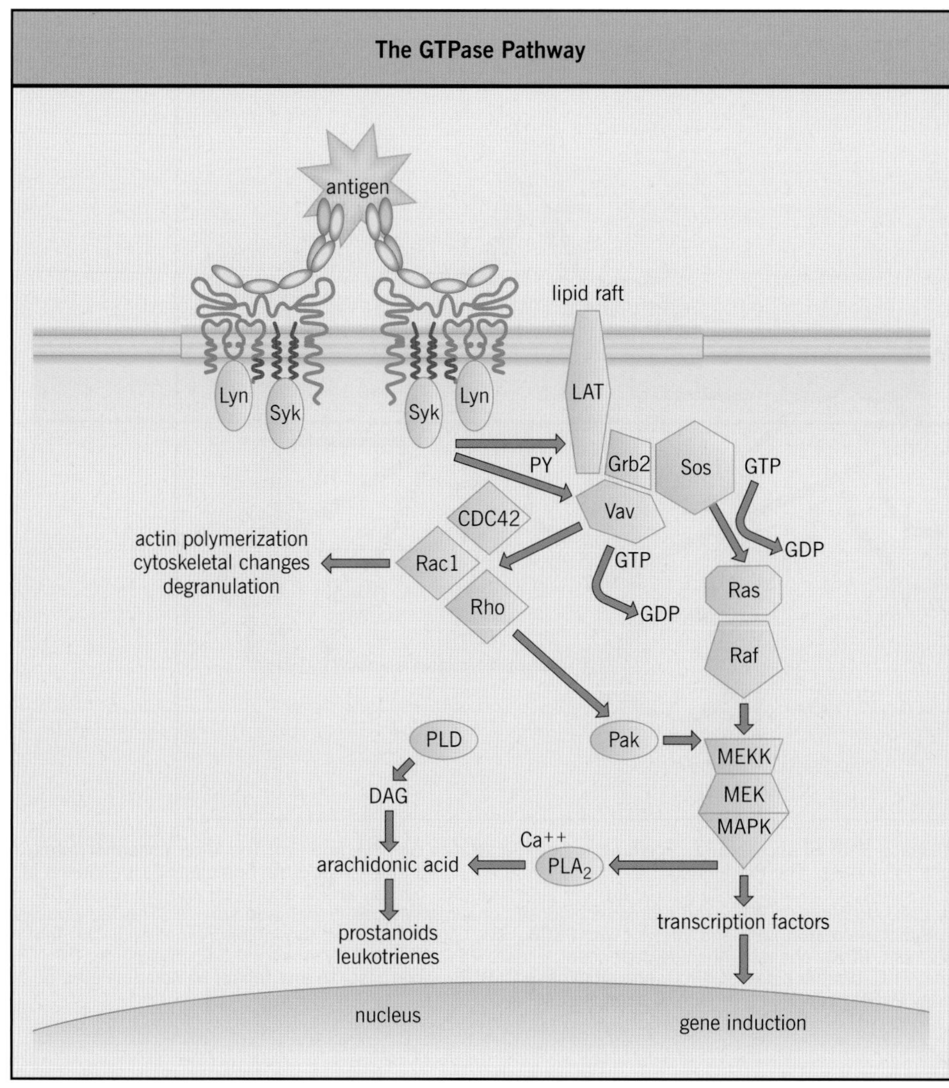

Fig. 18.15 The activation of the GTPase pathway. Small GTPases are activated through the exchange of GDP for GTP by GEFs (guanosine nucleotide exchange factors). At the membrane, Vav, Grb2 and Sos are part of the signaling complex linked to LAT. Vav functions as GEF for the Rho-family of GTPases (Rac, CDC42, Rho) which bind to cytoskeletal components. Sos is the GEF for Ras, which activates the serine/threonine kinase Raf and the MAP kinase complex, consisting of a MAP kinase kinase kinase (MAPKKK), MAP kinase kinase (MAPKK), and MAP kinase (MAPK). Downstream of MAPK is the phosphorylation of transcription factors, and activation of PLA_2. DAG, 1,2-diacylglycerol; GDP, guanosine diphosphate; GTP guanosine triphosphate; IP_3, inositol trisphosphate; MAP, mitogen activated protein; PLA, PLD, phospholipases.

(GEFs), which promote activation, and GTPase activating proteins (GAPs) that promote their deactivation. Small GTPases are usually grouped into the Ras family, activated through the GEF Sos, and Rho family, activated through Vav. Ras couples to the downstream activation of cytokine genes in conjunction with calcium signals, while the small GTPases (Rho, CDC42, and Rac1) control cytoskeletal responses that are crucial for secretion, migration and cell–cell contact. The two cascades are linked through feedback-loops, and proteins such as the serine/threonine kinase PAK (p21 activated kinase), which is activated by Rac/CDC42 and supports MAP kinase activation by Ras/Raf.

The hematopoietic-specific GEF Vav is activated and phosphorylated by Syk and mediates GDP–GTP exchange on Rac1. Rac1 binds to tubulin, regulates the formation of membrane ruffles, and contributes to the activation of the transcription factor NF-AT, while CDC42 controls cell adhesion and actin plaque assembly. Genetic defects in this pathway characterize hereditary human diseases such as Wiscott–Aldrich syndrome.

After FcεRI aggregation, Vav forms a multimeric membrane-signaling complex with Shc, Grb2 and Sos, and Slp-76. This interaction mediates the downstream activation of the MAP kinase cascade via Ras and Raf. Both Ras and Raf translocate to the membrane upon activation. They subsequently activate the MAP kinase complex, which is a three-component module of a MAP kinase that is activated by a MAP kinase kinase (MAPKK), which in turn is activated by a MAP kinase kinase kinase (MAPKKK). The three major families of MAP kinases are the extracellular-signal related kinases (ERKs), the Jun-amino-terminal kinases and the p38 family of proteins. They couple to specific MAPKKs, but may be activated through various MAPKKKs. Activated MAP kinases either modulate gene expression through cytoplasmic targets and post-transcriptional mechanisms, or they may translocate to the nucleus, where they activate transcription factors such as the AP-1 complex.

One function of MAP kinases is to regulate phospholipase A_2 (PLA_2), via serine phosphorylation, which increases its catalytic activity. PLA_2 finds access to its major substrates, phosphatidylcholine (PC) and phosphatidylethanolamine (PE) after calcium-dependent translocation from the cytosol to the nuclear membrane (Fig. 18.14). Phospholipid hydrolysis by PLA_2 yields lyso-PAF (platelet activating factor), which on acylation produces PAF and lysophospholipid, a potent membrane detergent capable of causing cell lysis. PLA_2 is also primarily responsible for the release of arachidonic acid, which

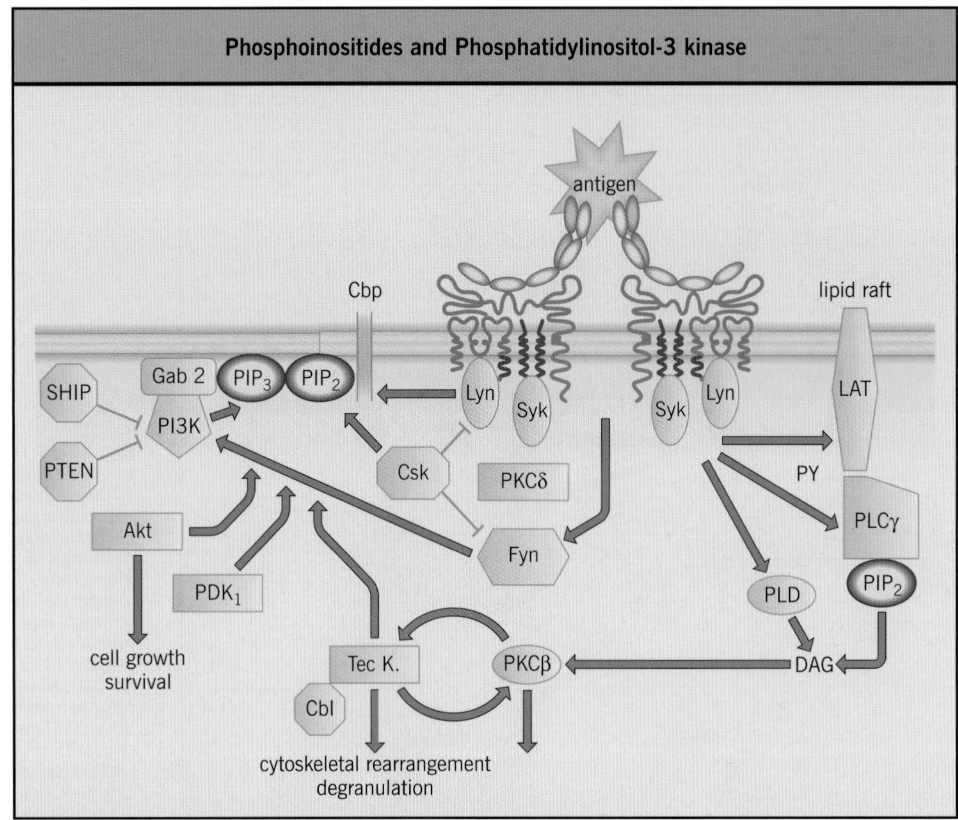

Fig. 18.16 The phosphatidylinositol-3 kinase (PI3) kinase pathway. FcεRI aggregation activates Lyn, Syk and Fyn. The latter phosphorylates the adaptor protein Gab2, which recruits PI3 kinase. The PI3 kinase products PIP_2 and PIP_3 bind to the Pleckstrin homology (PH) domains of Vav, Rac, Tec kinases, Akt and PLCγ. Physiologic inhibitors of PI3 kinase are the phosphatases SHIP1, SHIP2 and PTEN and the kinase Csk, which is recruited to the membrane by Cbp. Akt binds to PDK_1 and promotes glucose consumption, cell growth and survival. The Tec kinases are activated by phosphorylation and membrane recruitment and interact with $PKC\beta_1$, Syk, Slp-76, Vav, and the inhibitory molecule Cbl. Tec kinases promote cytoskeletal rearrangement. PDK_1, phosphoinositide-dependent kinase; PIP_2, phosphatidylinositol 4,5-bisphosphate; PIP_3 phosphatidylinositol-3,4,5-trisphosphate; PKC, protein kinase C; PLC, phospholipase C; PTEN, phosphatase and tensin homolog deleted on chromosome 10; SHIP1, 2, src homology 2 (SH_2)-containing inositol 5-phosphatases.

is metabolized by cyclooxygenases and lipoxygenases into eicosanoids. Their primary products in mast cells are prostaglandin D_2 and leukotriene C_4 respectively.

Phosphoinositides and phosphatidylinositol-3 kinase (Fig. 18.16)

PI3 kinases are both serine/threonine kinases and lipid kinases, and mediate the phosphorylation of phosphoinositides at the D-3 position of the inositol ring. PI3 kinases are heterodimers of a regulatory and a catalytic subunit and convert PIP_2 to PIP_3. FcεRI-mediated PI3 kinase activation is thought of as Lyn independent and instead links the kinase activity of Fyn, another Src-family kinase. Fyn phosphorylates the adaptor protein Gab2, which is essential for PI3 kinase recruitment to the membrane and activation in mast cells. The local production of 3-phosphoinositides creates binding sites for proteins that carry Pleckstrin homology (PH) domains, such as Vav, Rac, Tec kinases, the serine/threonine kinase Akt (or protein kinase B/PKB) and PLCγ, and thus modulates their activity. It is therefore not surprising that chemical inhibitors of PI3 kinase abrogate mast cell calcium responses, e.g. wortmannin, LY29002. Physiologically, PI3 kinase products are inactivated by lipid phosphatases, such as the SH_2-containing inositol 5-phosphatases (SHIP1 and SHIP2), which dephosphorylate position D-5 on the inositol ring, and PTEN (phosphatase and tensin homolog deleted on chromosome 10), which dephosphorylates position D-3. Inhibition of this pathway is further possible through a feedback-loop of Csk (C-terminal Src-kinase) association with the raft-localized adaptor Cbp (Csk binding protein). Csk phosphorylates inhibitory regulatory tyrosines on Src kinases (Lyn, Fyn) when targeted to the membrane by phosphorylated Cbp.

The serine/threonine kinase Akt is recruited to the membrane by PIP_2 and PIP_3, as is PDK_1 (phosphoinositide-dependent kinase), which activates Akt by serine phosphorylation. Akt then associates with and phosphorylates proteins that promote glucose consumption, cell growth and survival.

The Tec kinase family of protein tyrosine kinases integrates a number of signaling pathways through their protein interactions. They are activated by translocation to the membrane and phosphorylation by Src kinases, bind to the products of PI3 kinase activation and interact with $PKC\beta_1$, Syk, Slp-76, Vav, the inhibitory molecule Cbl (discussed below) and F-actin. The symptoms of human gene defects in Tec kinases reflect the multifaceted action of these proteins. The defects range from cytoskeletal abnormalities to defective calcium responses, cellular development and function; an example is X-linked agammaglobulinemia, with reduced mature B cells and immunoglobulin production. Tec kinases promote the formation

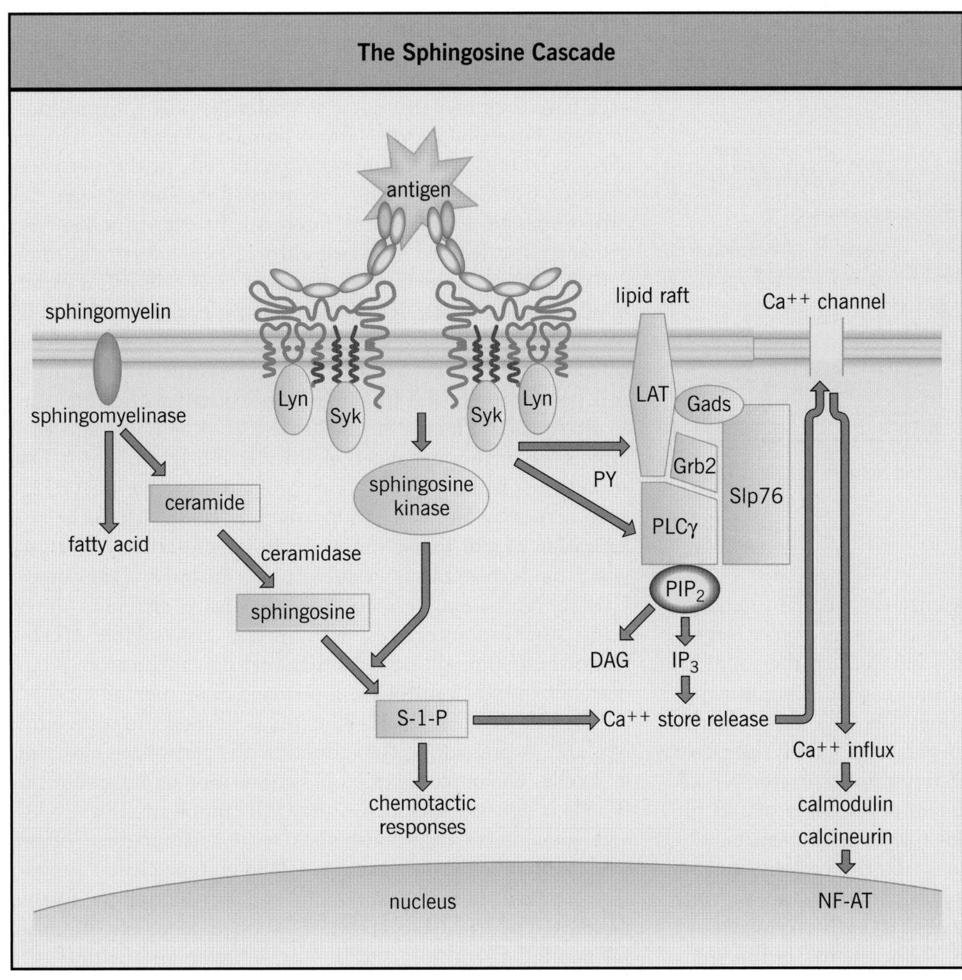

Fig. 18.17 The sphingosine pathway. A variety of inflammatory and stress signals activate sphingomyelinase in the membrane to metabolize sphingomyelins into fatty acid and ceramide. Ceramidase then acts on ceramide to produce sphingosine, the substrate for sphingosine kinase. FcεRI activation increases the activity of sphingosine kinase and results in the production of sphingosine-1-phosphate (S-1-P), which liberates intracellular calcium independently of IP_3 produced by PLCγ. DAG, 1,2-diacylglycerol; IP_3, inositol trisphosphate; NF-AT, nuclear factor of activated T cells; PIP_2, phosphatidylinositol 4,5-bisphosphate; PLC, phospholipase C.

of actin filament bundles and co-localize with focal adhesion kinase (FAK, pp125FAK) at membrane ruffles. FAK depends on calcium flux for activation and in turn phosphorylates FAP (FAK *a*ssociated *p*rotein) and paxillin, which may play a role in cell secretion, and Pyk2 (proline rich tyrosine kinase 2, RAFTK), a member of the FAK family, which phosphorylates potassium channels and acts as a transcriptional regulator.

The sphingosine cascade (Fig. 18.17)

FcεRI signaling also couples to the ceramide–sphingosine pathway, which previously has been linked to growth factor signaling and cell differentiation. Antigen challenge of mast cells increases cellular sphingosine-1-phosphate (S-1-P) as a direct consequence of sphingosine kinase activation by FcεRI. Sphingosine, the substrate for sphingosine kinase, is generated through the sphingomyelinase-mediated hydrolysis of sphingomyelin to ceramide plus fatty acid and sphingosine. A number of sphingomyelinases have been characterized that operate at different enzymatic pH optima and can be activated by a variety of inflammatory and stress stimuli. Sphingosine opposes calcium responses through inhibition of PKC and PLCγ, whereas S-1-P promotes them. The release of calcium ions from intracellular stores can therefore be initiated through the presumed independent pathways of IP_3 or S-1-P production. In addition, S-1-P is a potent chemotactic agent that is secreted upon cell stimulation, binds to specific membrane receptors and promotes mast cell migratory responses.

Cyclic adenosine monophosphate and protein kinase

FcεRI aggregation leads to an activation of adenylyl cyclase and a consequential increase in intracellular cAMP. This leads to the activation of cAMP-dependent protein kinase (PKA). PKA appears to regulate inhibitory pathways for degranulation, arachidonic acid metabolite synthesis, and cytokine generation. Although the precise mechanism by which the cAMP–PKA axis modulates mast cell function is far from clear, effects at the level of phospholipases or calcium flux have been suggested. The ability of β-adrenoceptor and cAMP phosphodiesterase inhibitors to elevate intracellular cAMP levels and inhibit mast cell function may contribute to the efficacy of this class of drugs in allergic disease.

Ubiquitination

A general mechanism of signal modulation is the covalent transfer of ubiquitin, a small (8.5 kDa) evolutionary conserved protein, to the amino group of a lysine on the target protein. The process requires ATP and is catalyzed by enzymes that are grouped according to function into E1 (ubiquitin activating

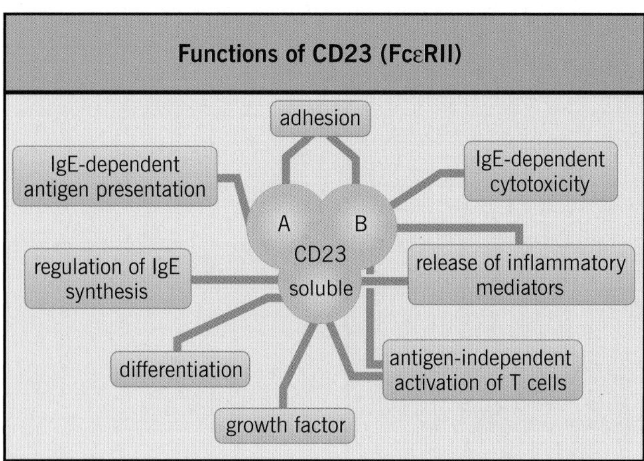

Fig. 18.18 The roles of CD23a, CD23b, and soluble CD23 in the immune response.

enzymes), E2 (ubiquitin conjugating enzymes) and E3 (ubiquitin protein ligases). The attachment of ubiquitin chains targets proteins for proteasomal degradation and thus has the ability to terminate signaling. FcεRI itself is internalized, ubiquitinated and degraded following aggregation. On the other hand, ubiquitination should not be viewed as a purely negative mechanism of regulation, since the transcription factor NF-κB requires ubiquitination and subsequent degradation of IκB for its activation and plays an important role in inflammation.

A well-characterized E3 enzyme is Cbl, the protein product of the c-cbl protooncogene. Cbl is phosphorylated upon FcεRI engagement by Lyn and Syk and exerts its negative regulatory function through ubiquitin transfer. Additionally Cbl functions as adaptor protein, and interacts with Vav, PI3 kinase, and Grb2.

In summary, FcεRI aggregation triggers a plethora of signaling events and much remains to be learned about the molecular interactions and their regulation, particularly in view of the development of potential therapeutics that interfere with signaling.

One approach to better understand and predict these complex processes is the development of computer-based mathematical models. To generate these models, hypotheses are extrapolated from experimental data and translated into equations, which allow the prediction of measurable outcomes of signaling. If the predicted outcome, such as the kinetics of phosphorylation of a particular protein, matches the prediction, the hypotheses can be accepted, if not, rejected. These models will become increasingly important in studies with an integrated view of multiple signaling events.

FCεRII SIGNALING

FcεRII (CD23), which exists in membrane-associated and soluble forms (Fig. 18.8), has three major biological functions. First, as a receptor for IgE it mediates enhanced antigen presentation of IgE complexes by B cells to T cells and thus plays a prominent role in the allergic immune response (see Ch. 19). Secondly, CD23 acts as an adhesion molecule, interacting with CD21, CD11b, CD11c, galactose- or L-fucose-containing glycoproteins, and extracellular matrix to enhance homo- and heterotypic cell adhesion. Thirdly, soluble CD23 fragments mediate pleiotropic cytokine-like effects (Fig. 18.18).

CD23 expression

As outlined at the beginning of this chapter, CD23a and CD23b each have their own promoter and differ by only a few residues in their N-terminal cytoplasmic domain (Fig. 18.8). Human surface IgD+/IgM+ double-positive B cells in the periphery express CD23a prior to isotype switch and plasma cell differentiation. Of diagnostic interest is its overexpression as a characteristic feature of B-cell chronic lymphocytic leukemia cells. CD23b is inducible by cytokines on B cells and a variety of other cell types, e.g. lymphoid, monocytic, and dendritic cells.

On human B cells, membrane CD23 is involved in cell activation, antigen presentation, and IgE synthesis (see Ch.19). It is both spatially and functionally associated with MHC class II molecules. Inducers of CD23b are IL-4 or IL-13 and their effects are further enhanced in vitro by anti-IgM or anti-CD40 stimulation, leukotriene B_4, IL-5, or lipopolysaccharide. CD23b gene activation by IL-4 is mediated by the post-translational activation of the transcription nuclear factor IL-4 (NF-IL-4), which binds, possibly as a dimer, to specific binding sites on the CD23b promoters, termed IL-4 responsive elements. Interferon γ (IFNγ) interferes with surface and soluble CD23b biosynthesis through post-translational downregulation, which destabilizes CD23 mRNA and cleavage of membrane CD23.

The role of IL-4 and IL-13 extends beyond the stimulation of CD23 expression to the induction of ε germ-line transcripts in B cells. The outcome of CD23 stimulation on IgE-producing B cells is epitope specific, in that IgE complexes (Fig. 18.10) and some anti-CD23 antibodies have a suppressive effect, while antibodies against another CD23 epitope cluster support IL-4-induced B-cell stimulation. IgE production is further modulated by IL-2, IL-6, and IL-9, which preferentially stimulate IgE and IgG4 synthesis, and IL-7, which synergizes with IL-4 in a T-cell-dependent manner via soluble CD23 and IL-9. In contrast, IFNα, IFNγ, transforming growth factor β (TGFβ), IL-10, IL-12, and prostaglandin E_2 counteract the effect of IL-4.

As described earlier, metalloproteinases or the major house dust mite allergen, Der p 1, can cleave the 45 kDa membrane into 37, 33, 29, 25, and 16 kDa fragments (Fig. 18.8). The fragments all retain IgE-binding capacity in the presence of calcium and mediate their cytokine effects via epitopes overlapping with, but distinct from, the IgE-binding site. The unstable 37 and 33 kDa fragments degrade to a stable 25 kDa form. The 16 kDa fragment is both deleted at the COOH terminus and cleaved from the membrane. Soluble CD23 fragments have been reported as promoting the cell growth of myeloid precursors, supporting the differentiation of pro-thymocytes in synergy with IL-1, preventing germinal center B-cell apoptosis and increasing histamine release by basophils. IgE production by B cells is supported by the 37 kDa fragment, but suppressed by 16 kDa sCD23. The 25 kDa sCD23 is detectable in the serum of healthy individuals but does not correlate with IgE levels.

CD23 signals

The intracellular signals elicited upon CD23 activation remain poorly understood. Although the two CD23 isoforms differ only by a short stretch of amino acids, this variation accounts for considerable differences in signal transduction, illustrated for example by the prediction that tyrosine 6 and serine 7, unique to CD23a, are sites for sulfation and casein kinase II phosphorylation. The B-cell-specific CD23a mediates endocytosis,

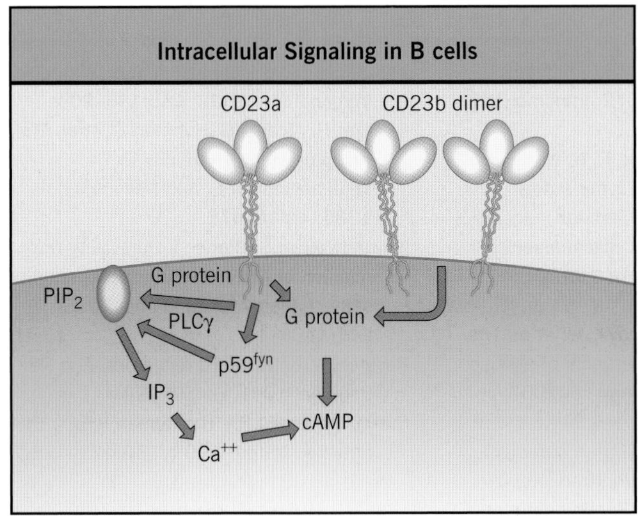

Fig. 18.19 Intracellular signaling events in B cells. Ligation of CD23a or b increases intracellular cyclic adenosine monophosphate (cAMP) levels, possibly via GTP-binding proteins. G proteins and/or Fyn activate PLCγ resulting in calcium signals through the hydrolysis of PIP_2 to IP_3 and DAG. Elevated intracellular calcium then promotes a further rise of cAMP. DAG, 1,2-diacylglycerol; IP_3, inositol trisphosphate; GTP guanosine triphosphate; PIP_2, phosphatidylinositol 4,5-bisphosphate; PLC, phospholipase C.

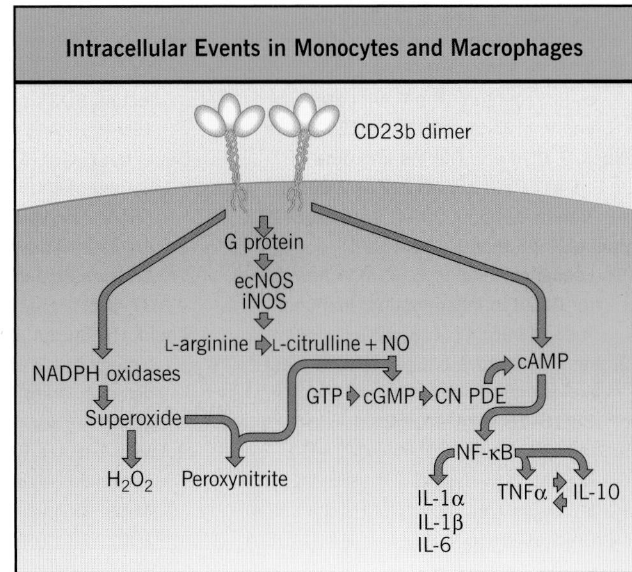

Fig. 18.20 Intracellular signaling events in monocytes and macrophages. Monocyte nitric oxide (NO) production is activated via CD23b through G-protein-mediated activation of the nitric oxide synthases (NOS) ecNOS and iNOS. They catalyze the conversion of L-arginine into L-citrulline and NO, and the latter acts on soluble guanylate cyclase (sGC) to generate cyclic GMP from GTP. Cyclic GMP regulates the activity of cyclic nucleotide phosphodiesterase (CN PDE), which induces the delayed accumulation of cAMP, and the activation of the NFκB and gene transcription. Increased cAMP activates NADPH (reduced form of nicotinamide adenine dinucleotide phosphate) oxidase which produces cytotoxic superoxide. NO reacts with superoxide to form peroxynitrite, another reactive oxygen species. cAMP, cyclic adenosine monophosphate; GMP, guanosine monophosphate; GTP, guanosine triphosphate.

which is consistent with the role of the B cell in IgE-dependent antigen presentation (see Ch.19). CD23b promotes the phagocytosis of IgE-coated particles, which has been related to the role of macrophages and eosinophils in defense against parasites.

Triggering CD23 on B cells promotes their progression into the G1 phase of the cell cycle and increases DNA synthesis stimulated via IL-4 and CD40. CD23a, but not b, is coupled to the PLCγ/calcium pathway (Figs 18.19 and 18.20). It is currently hypothesized that the tyrosine kinase Fyn alone or in concert with GTP-binding proteins activates PLCγ, and causes a rise in intracellular calcium levels through the hydrolysis of PIP_2 to IP_3 and DAG (as described above). CD23a stimulation also directly stimulates the production of cAMP and indirectly via calcium mobilization. The detailed mechanism is unknown and the downstream targets uncharacterized. Other cellular systems however suggest PKA as the most likely target.

In analogy to CD23a, stimulation of CD23b leads to increased cAMP production (Fig. 18.20). Further, stimulation of this isoform activates the generation of reactive oxygen species and nitric oxide (NO), which have been linked to the release of proinflammatory mediators, cell differentiation, and apoptotic cell death. Monocytes and macrophages contain two of the three isozymes that convert the substrate L-arginine into L-citrulline; the constitutive endothelial nitric oxide synthase, ecNOS, or type III, and the inducible NOS (iNOS, type II). Both proteins require calcium/calmodulin binding for their activity. EcNOS is also present in B and T cells and synthesizes low amounts of NO for a short amount of time. In contrast, inflammatory cytokines (IFNγ, TNFα, IL-1β) stimulate the expression of iNOS, which produces large amounts of NO over extended time periods. Full activation of iNOS requires (IFNγ-induced) monocyte maturation into macrophages, the induction and ligation of CD23, and the production of TNFα, which contributes to iNOS mRNA and protein synthesis in an autocrine loop. NO generates most of its effects through the activation of soluble guanylate cyclase, which catalyzes the conversion of GTP to cyclic guanosine monophosphate (GMP) (cGMP). This stimulates the cyclic nucleotide phosphodiesterase and leads to the delayed accumulation of cAMP, similarly to the B cell.

In a parallel pathway, CD23 stimulates the formation and release of reactive oxygen species, a hallmark of inflammatory reactions. These oxidants are now considered as second messengers in signaling and mediate effects beyond their cytotoxic activity. The first step in the generation of reactive oxygen species is catalyzed by NADPH (reduced form of nicotinamide adenine dinucleotide phosphate) oxidase, a pentameric enzyme that gains full functional activity only after the recruitment of all its subunits to the membrane, and produces superoxide anions. This highly reactive species is converted to hydrogen peroxide by superoxide dismutases, but can also react with NO to form peroxynitrite, another strong oxidant that targets proteins as well as DNA. Peroxide can inactivate protein tyrosine phosphatases by oxidizing a redox-sensitive cysteine and has also been demonstrated to activate the transcription factor NF-κB.

Soluble CD23 activates ecNOS in resting monocytes via a transient calcium flux, and it is hypothesized that the synthase promotes cell differentiation and the late onset of iNOS activity.

Cytokines reportedly activated by CD23 are TNFα, IL-1α, IL-1β, IL-6, and IL-10. These factors either have a potentiating (TNFα) or a downregulatory effect on CD23 signaling. IL-10, the endogenous inhibitor of NO production, and TNFα are linked through feedback control. Both NO and TNFα production have also been demonstrated in human keratinocytes and eosinophils and are elicited by either membrane or soluble CD23.

FURTHER READING

Beaven MA, Metzger H. Signal transduction by Fc receptors: the FcεRI case. Immunol Today 1993; 14:222–226.

Blank U, Rivera J. The ins and outs of IgE-dependent mast-cell exocytosis. Trends Immunol 2004; 25(5):266–273.

Bonnefoy J-Y, Plater-Zyberk C, Lecoanet-Henchoz S, et al. A new role for CD23 in inflammation. Immunol Today 1996; 17:418–420.

Draber P, Draberova L. Lipid rafts in mast cell signaling. Mol Immunol 2002; 38(16–18):1247–1252.

Durham SR, Gould H, Hamid QA. IgE regulation in tissues. In: Vercelli D, ed. IgE regulation: molecular mechanisms. Chichester: John Wiley; 1997:21–36.

Gordon J. B-cell signaling via the C-type lectins CD23 and CD72. Immunol Today 1994; 15:411–417.

Gould HJ, Beavil RL, Reljic R, et al. IgE homeostasis: Is CD23 the safety switch? In: Vercelli D, ed. IgE regulation: molecular mechanisms. Chichester: John Wiley; 1997: 37–59.

Gould, HJ, Sutton, BJ, Beavil, AJ, et al. The biology of IgE and the basis of allergic disease. Annu Rev Immunol 2003; 21:579–628.

Holowka D, Baird B. FcεRI as a paradigm for a lipid raft-dependent receptor in hematopoietic cells. Semin Immunol 2001; 13 (2):99–105.

Metzger H. Molecular versatility of antibodies. Immunol Rev 2002; 185:186–205.

Metzger H, Alcaraz G, Hohman R, et al. The receptor with high affinity for immunoglobulin E. Ann Rev Immunol 1986; 4:419–470.

Novak N, Kraft S, Bieber T. Unraveling the mission of FcεRI on antigen-presenting cells. J Allergy Clin Immunol 2003; 111(1):38–44.

Ravetch JV, Kinet J-P. Fc receptors. Ann Rev Immunol 1991; 9:457–492.

Sutton BJ, Gould HJ. The human IgE network. Nature 1993; 366:421–428.

Chapter 19

Definition:

The production of allergen-specific IgE underpins all allergic diseases. IgE synthesis is stimulated when antigen-presenting cells present allergen to T lymphocytes which in turn stimulate B lymphocytes to initiate antibody production.

Antigen Presentation and IgE Synthesis

Natalija Novak, Hans Oettgen, Thomas Bieber, and Patrick G Holt

CELLS INVOLVED IN ANTIGEN PRESENTATION AND IgE SYNTHESIS

Introduction

In health and disease, antigen-presenting cells (APCs) perform a central role in directing immune responses. Several different APC/accessory cells are known; among them are dendritic cells (DCs), monocytes/macrophages, B cells, and non-bone-marrow-derived follicular dendritic cells (FDCs). Antigen presentation principally involves interactions between the APCs and helper T cells (Th) cells, in which the APCs initially internalize antigen and degrade it in their lysosomal compartments, after which short peptides (of 15–20 amino acids) of the original antigen appear in the major histocompatibility complex (MHC) class II molecules of the APCs. T cells recognizing these peptides presented in the class II molecules present on the APCs will become activated.

The one exception to this rule is antigen presentation to B cells by FDCs in germinal centers, which will be discussed in the section on class switching and affinity maturation later in this chapter.

Dendritic cells

Together with skin, the mucosal surfaces of the gastrointestinal and respiratory tracts provide the principal interface between the immune system and the outside environment. These areas are under continuous challenge from a wide variety of both pathogenic and trivial antigens. Accordingly, highly efficient antigen surveillance mechanisms are required at these sites in order to maintain local homeostasis. It is clear from independent evidence derived in a range of laboratories that the key cell populations involved in this process are DCs, which are found in high density in these tissues. The development of specialized tangential sectioning techniques, which permit the visualization of the facing intraepithelial DCs, has simplified the accurate quantification of population size, i.e. 500–700 cells/mm^2 of the epithelial surface of the airway mucosa, comparable to the Langerhans' cell (LC) compartment in the epidermis.

Together with monocytic (phagocytic) cells the dendritic cells are the most well known APCs (Fig. 19.1). At present it is still not clear whether monocytes and dendritic cells (apart from the non-bone-marrow-derived FDCs) belong to the same lineage or whether they have different precursor stem cells. However, accumulating evidence points in the direction of a common stem cell for monocytic and dendritic

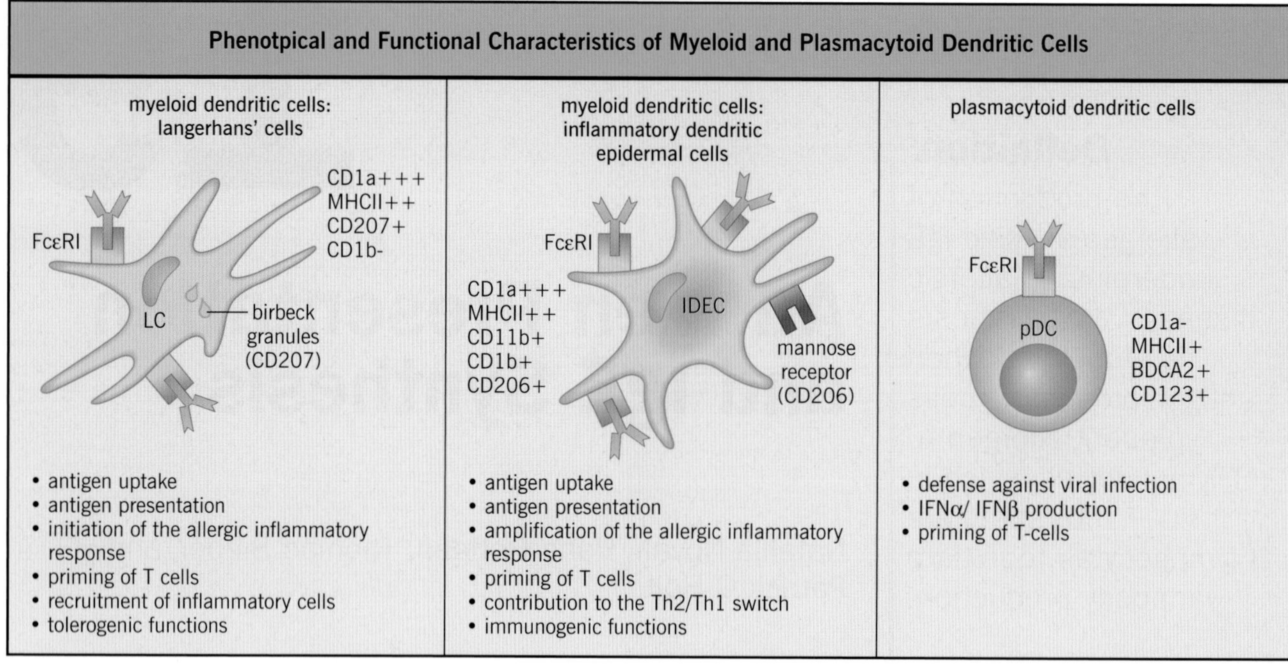

Fig. 19.1 Dendritic cells (DC), such as the Langerhans' cells (LC), inflammatory dendritic epidermal cells (IDEC) and plasmacytoid DCs (pDC) are morphologically distinct and play a key role in enhancing immunogenicity. Th, helper T cells.

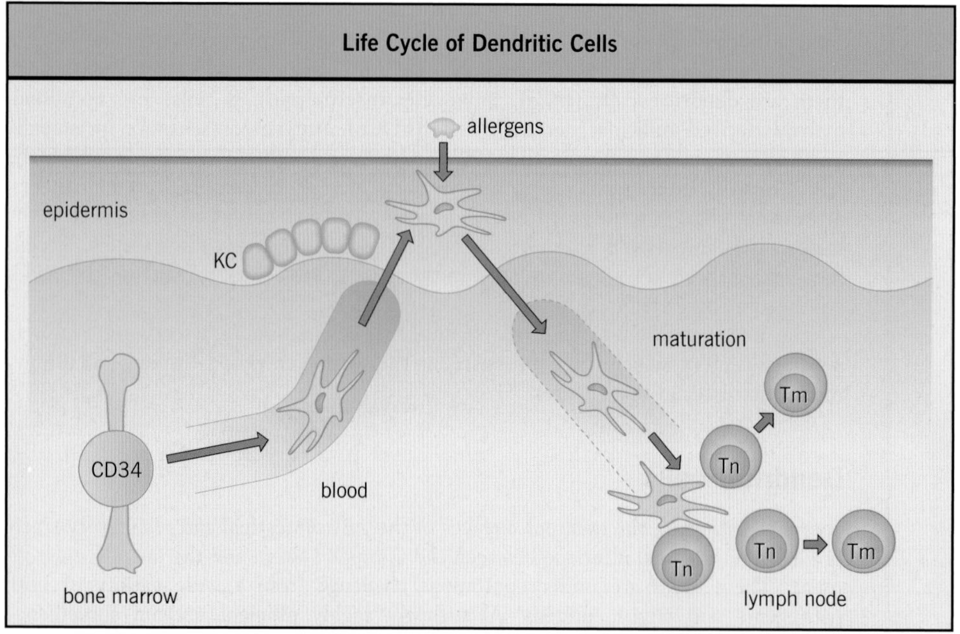

Fig. 19.2 Schematic representation of suggested migration patterns and the relationship between the various subsets of dendritic cells normally present in healthy skin and draining lymph system. Monocytes from the bone marrow migrate through the circulation and mature into dendritic cells in the skin. KC, keratinocyte; Tn, naïve T-cells; Tm, memory T-cells.

cells. Based on cell surface marker expression and indirect evidence obtained from antigen challenge experiments in vivo, it is generally accepted that dermal DCs, LCs, veiled cells, and interdigitating cells are different maturation stages of one single cell type (Fig. 19.2). Phagocytic cells, although excellent in antigen trapping, are not the most efficient professional APCs. This title is definitely reserved for the DCs.

The role and function of macrophages is detailed in Chapter 21.

LANGERHANS' CELLS

LCs are highly specialized professional APCs usually located at surveillance interfaces of the human body such as the skin or mucosa, and they are thought to play an important role in the generation and regulation of immune responses. Compelling evidence suggests that LCs and another DC subtype, the so-called inflammatory dendritic epidermal cells (IDECs), are instrumental in the pathophysiology of IgE-mediated diseases such as atopic eczema (AE).

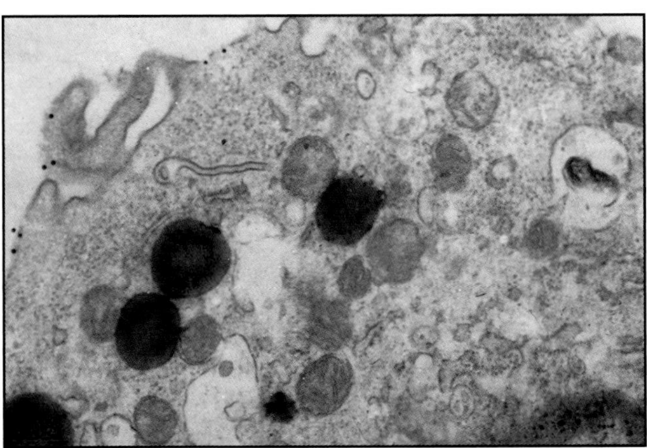

Fig. 19.3 Electron microscopy of a Langerhans' cell showing the characteristic Birbeck granule shaped like a tennis racket.

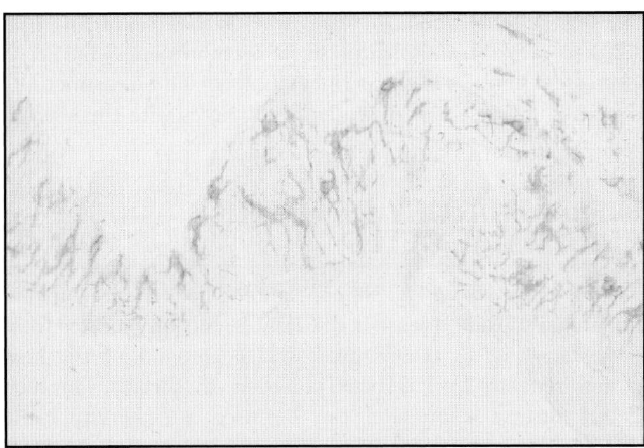

Fig. 19.4 Pattern of CD1a+ cells in the epidermis.

LCs have been identified by the medical student Paul Langerhans and act as resident APCs in the skin. LCs can be detected even in healthy, non-inflammatory skin. LCs are characterized by their distinctive morphology and their primary marker, the tennis-racket shaped Birbeck granules in their cytoplasm, which are composed by the newly characterized protein langerin (Fig. 19.3), and the surface expression of the cluster of differentiation 1a marker (CD1a) (Fig. 19.4). LCs are immature DCs, indicated by the low expression of B7.2 (CD86) and no expression of B7.1 (CD80). Both receptors, however, are instantly upregulated when the LCs are stimulated by granulocyte–macrophage colony-stimulating factor (GM-CSF), which induces maturation of these cells. LC represent the oldest member of the DC system and reside at sites of maximum antigen encounter in the basal and suprabasal layers of the epidermis. LCs are non-phagocytic and express MHC class II molecules on their cell surface for professional antigen presentation (Fig. 19.1). Their primary function in uninflamed skin is to maintain a state of tolerance against invading antigens and allergens under immunologic steady state condition. By contrast, in response to arriving danger signals such as inflammation, multiple changes occur. Among these is the release of monocyte-chemoattractant protein (MCP) chemokines by skin cells which induce the recruitment of LC progenitors from the bone marrow (Fig. 19.2). Other factors initiate LC migration to the peripheral lymph node. Altogether, this leads to the breakdown of tolerance and the rapid induction of an immune response at this site. In this manner, in the acute phase of allergic and inflammatory diseases, LC precursors and other DC subtypes are immediately recruited by chemotactic signals to the site of inflammation.

In the mid-1980s, the presence of IgE molecules on the surface of LCs from patients presenting with AE was first reported. Later on, a new pathophysiologic concept was proposed whereby LCs armed with allergen-specific IgE trigger eczematous inflammation. One key element of this concept is the expression of the high affinity receptor for IgE, namely FcεRI, on these APCs.

LCs exist in the skin in an immature state dedicated to capturing antigens, and in the subcutaneous lymph nodes in a mature state to present those antigens to T cells. The phenotypic changes undergone by LCs during maturation, and the correlation of these changes with tissue localization, have been generally considered as a paradigm for all DCs. Classical LCs are characterized ultrastructurally by a clear cytoplasm, a lobulated nucleus, the lack of desmosomes, melanosomes or Merkel cell granules and most importantly, by the presence of highly specific tennis racket shaped, cytoplasmic Birbeck granules. They show a relatively invariable CD1a+++, FcεRII++, HLA-DR+++, CD1b immunophenotype (Fig. 19.1).

STRUCTURE OF THE HIGH AFFINITY RECEPTOR FOR IgE (FcεRI) ON DENDRITIC CELLS

Initially it has been assumed that FcεRI is exclusively expressed on mast cells and basophils involved in cell activation of immediated-type hypersensitivity reactions. In 1992, two different research groups reported the presence of specific transcripts for FcεRI chains as well as surface protein expression of the FcεRI complex in DCs in the epidermis of atopic skin lesions, which resulted in a new view of the cellular distribution and functionality of this structure. The classical, tetrameric FcεRI expressed on effector cells of anaphylaxis consists of three distinct protein species ($\alpha\beta\gamma_2$). The heavily N-glycosylated α chain exhibits two Ig-like domains that mediate binding to the Fc portion of IgE. The β chain acts as an amplifier of signaling downstream of the receptor. In addition, the β chain augments the maturation of the α chain and its intracellular trafficking to the cell surface, thus leading to increased surface expression. The γ chain dimer, which is shared by other Fc-receptor complexes, carries two immunoreceptor tyrosine-based activation motifs in its cytoplasmic tail for downstream signal propagation. In DCs only specific transcripts for the α and γ chain are present, whereas the putative β subunit is completely lacking. This shows that FcεRI has a modular structure in the human system: the tetrameric form ($\alpha\beta\gamma_2$) on effector cells and the trimeric variant ($\alpha\gamma_2$) on APCs.

In addition FcεRI is differentially regulated in atopic and non-atopic individuals. The FcεRI γ chain, which stabilizes surface expression of the FcεRI complex, is present in low amounts in professional APCs from non-atopic individuals, limiting the surface expression of the FcεRI complex and their IgE binding capacity. In contrast, DCs of atopic individuals express substantial amounts of FcεRI, and the IgE/FcεRI binding stabilizes and increases the surface expression of this receptor. This explains also, at least in part, why FcεRI expression on DCs in the peripheral blood and on distinct DC subtypes in the skin of AE patients correlates with their serum IgE level.

INFLAMMATORY DENDRITIC EPIDERMAL CELLS

The second myeloid DC subpopulation which is detectable in inflammatory skin disease is the IDECs. In skin biopsies from patients with AE, IDECs express high amounts of the high affinity receptor for IgE (FcεRI) on their cell surface. This high FcεRI surface expression can be used to phenotypically differentiate eczematous skin lesions of patients with AE from other inflammatory skin diseases such as psoriasis, contact dermatitis, or cutaneous T-cell lymphoma. The ultrastructure of IDECs resembles that of LCs because of their clear cytoplasm, lobulated nucleus and lack of desmosomes, melanosomes and Merkel cell granules, but IDECs do not contain any Birbeck granules. Although it has been claimed by a number of authors that they had identified LCs as the IgE-binding and FcεRI-expressing epidermal cell population in AE lesions, it is now clear that IDECs and LCs are the relevant IgE-binding and FcεRI-expressing cells. In addition, IDECs are expressing CD1b, CD11a, CD11b and CD11c, the thrombospondin receptor CD36 and the mannose receptor (CD206), which is known to be involved in the uptake of bacterial components by endocytotic processes (Fig. 19.1). Both cell types, i.e. LCs and IDECs, express the co-stimulatory molecules CD80 (B7.1) and CD86 (B7.2) on their cell surface. In contrast to LCs, the expression of some surface markers on IDECs is highly variable and seems to be influenced by the state and type of the underlying skin disease. The high expression of FcεRI on IDECs in AE could be detected with a high sensitivity and specificity compared to other inflammatory skin diseases and provides a diagnostic application of a standardized phenotyping procedure, in which the expression of the FcεRI/FcγRII ratio is used to distinguish between extrinsic and intrinsic AE and other inflammatory skin diseases.

Recent concepts support the hypothesis that IDECs, which are assumed to be of a rather monocytic origin, are recruited in the acute phase of AE into the epidermis by signals mediated from cells of the inflammatory micromilieu. Interestingly, after successful topical treatment of the AE lesions, the number of IDECs in the epidermis decreases below the detectable level, indicating that this cell type is strongly related to the state of inflammation of the skin.

PLASMACYTOID DENDRITIC CELLS

In addition to myeloid DCs, such as LCs and IDECs, a second DC subtype, the so-called plasmacytoid DC (pDC) has been identified. pDCs consist of two subpopulations, $CD123^{dim}$ and $CD11c^{bright}$ DCs which have monocytic features and $CD123^{bright}$ CD11c- blood DCs which display plasmacytoid features. pDCs can be distinguished from myeloid DCs by the surface expression of CD123, blood dendritic cells antigen (BDCA)4+ and MHC class II molecules and the absence of CD11c expression. pDCs are important in protecting from viral infections via the production, in large amounts, of type I interferons such as IFNα and IFNβ (Fig. 19.1).

pDCs express Fc receptors including the high affinity receptor for IgE. Further on in patients with AD, the amount of IgE bound to FcεRI on the surface of pDCs is related to the disease state and the serum IgE levels. It has been shown very recently that pDCs are capable of processing allergens via FcεRI–IgE, thereby promoting Th2 type immune responses.

Although the number of pDCs is increased in the peripheral blood of AD patients, only a limited number of pDCs are detectable in the epidermal skin lesions of AD patients in contrast to patients with other inflammatory skin diseases such as psoriasis or allergic contact dermatitis. Several mechanisms have been proposed to explain the deficiency of pDCs in the skin of AD patients, including impairment in pDC recruitment from the blood into the skin or a higher sensitivity of these cells to pro-apoptotic signals within AD skin. Recently it has been shown that pDCs, which have been stimulated via FcεRI by allergen challenge, display a reduced capacity to produce IFNα and IFNβ as a consequence of stimulation with viral components. Therefore the relatively lower amount of IFNα and β-producing pDCs in the skin of patients with AD might account for the higher susceptibility of these patients to viral infections.

ROLE OF LANGERHANS' CELLS AND INFLAMMATORY DENDRITIC EPIDERMAL CELLS IN ANTIGEN PRESENTATION

Sequential skin biopsies from patients with AE subjected to allergen-induced lesions are characterized by a biphasic cytokine profile. While early lesions are characterized by the expression of a Th2-predominant pattern, a Th1/Th0 dominant pattern emerges during the subacute and chronic phase. This observation challenges the current belief that AE is a typical Th2 disease.

Studies with LCs and IDECs isolated ex vivo and in vitro-generated LCs and IDECs provide evidence that they contribute distinctly to the biphasic nature of the disease.

After IgE-mediated binding and internalization, the antigen-bearing LCs migrate to the peripheral lymph nodes and present the processed allergens efficiently to T cells (Fig. 19.5). Antigen presentation following FcεRI binding is associated with Th2-type immune responses characterized by interleukin-4 (IL-4), IL-5 and IL-13-producing T cells. The activated LCs present allergen-derived peptides locally to transiting antigen-specific T cells and thereby induce a classical T-cell mediated secondary immune response. Concomitantly, aggregation of FcεRI on the surface of LCs induces the release of chemotactic factors such as IL-16, macrophage-derived chemokine (MDC), thymus- and activation-regulated chemokine (TARC) and most importantly, monocyte chemoattractant protein-1 (MCP-1). These cytokines and chemokines are hypothesized to recruit IDECs into the skin. In contrast to LCs, IDECs are only present at inflammatory sites and do not bear any Birbeck granules but display a high surface expression of FcεRI. IDECs can be found exclusively at inflammatory skin sites and have been shown to produce high amounts of proinflammatory cytokines and chemokines following FcεRI cross-linking. IDECs display a high stimulatory capacity toward T cells and serve as amplifiers of the allergic-inflammatory immune response. In contrast to LCs, stimulation of FcεRI on the surface of IDEC with allergen/IgE complexes induces the release of IL-12 and IL-18 in high amounts and enhances the priming of T cells of the Th1 type, characterized by increased IFNγ production (Fig. 19.6). These mechanisms

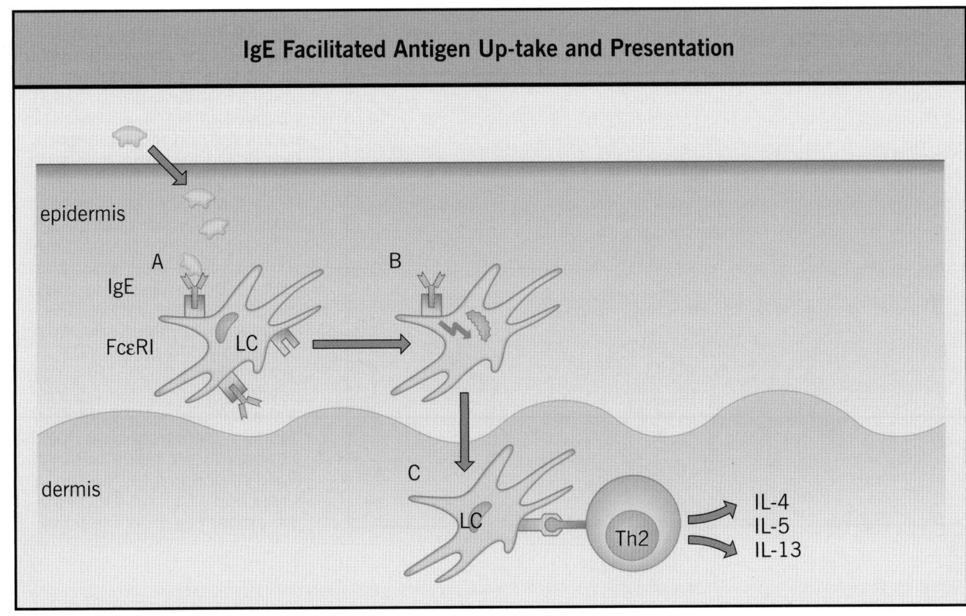

Fig. 19.5 Langerhans' cells take up allergens which penetrate the epidermis, internalize them and present the processed antigen to allergen-specific T cells.

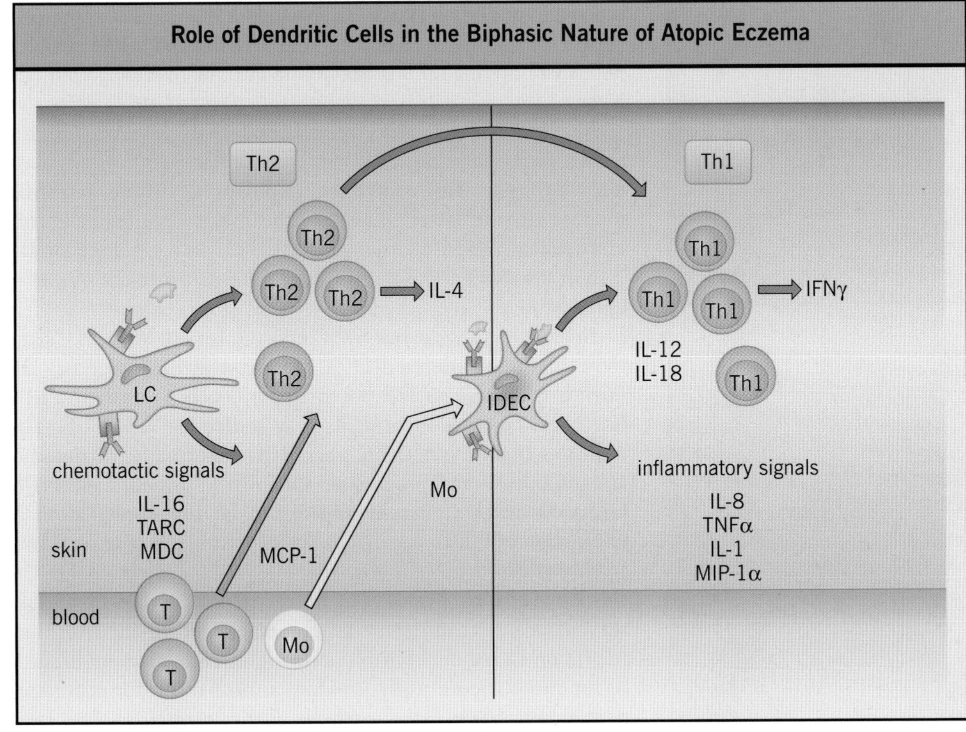

Fig. 19.6 Distinctive contribution of Langerhans' cells (LCs) and inflammatory dendritic epidermal cells (IDECs) to the biphasic nature of atopic eczema. LCs take up allergens invading the epidermis and release chemotactic signals. IDECs invade into the epidermis and contribute to the amplification of the inflammatory reaction and to the switch of the initial immune response of the Th2 type into a Th1 immune response. IFNγ, interferon γ; IL-1, interleukin-1; MDC, macrophage-derived chemokine; MIP-1α, macrophage inflammatory protein-1α; Mo, monocyte; TARC, thymus- and activation-regulated chemokine; Th, helper T cell; TNFα, tumor necrosis factor α.

may lead to the switch from the initial Th2 immune response associated with acute AE to the Th1 phenotype associated with the chronic phase of this disease.

The atopy patch test (APT) represents a novel diagnostic tool which can be used as an experimental model for AE. In this test, aeroallergens and food allergens are applied epicutaneously to a patient's back and in the majority of cases this results in an eczematous skin lesion in sensitized patients. Skin biopsies from APT lesions have demonstrated the kinetic interplay of DC subtypes and skin migration. Seventy-two hours after allergen challenge, high numbers of IDECs invade the epidermis (Fig. 19.7). Later on, alterations of the phenotype of LCs and IDECs occur, including the upregulation of the high affinity receptor for IgE. These observations support the hypothesis that the interplay of FcεRI-bearing DC subtypes is crucial for the development of the skin lesions in AE. In contrast, after successful topical treatment the FcεRI surface expression of LCs in the epidermis is reduced and the number of IDECs in the epidermal skin lesions decreases below the detectable level.

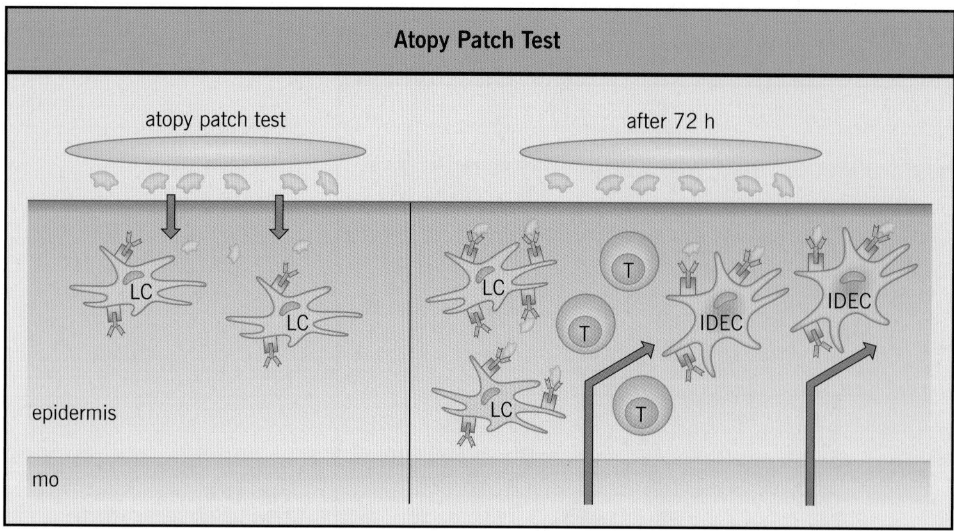

Fig. 19.7 In an atopy patch test (APT) the antigen is applied to the skin in an aqueous solution under a patch, which is removed after 24–48 hours, in contrast to an intracutaneous test (ICT) where the antigen is injected into the dermis. The APT induces a positive reaction when sufficient amounts of antigen penetrate the epidermis, where Langerhans' cells (LCs) capture the antigen and finally present it to the T cells. The presence of antigen-specific IgE bound to FcεRI on the LCs reduces the amounts of antigen needed for a positive reaction. Within 72 hours inflammatory dendritic epidermal cells (IDECs) invade into the epidermis and FcεRI is upregulated on the surface of LCs and IDECs in the epidermis of APT lesions.

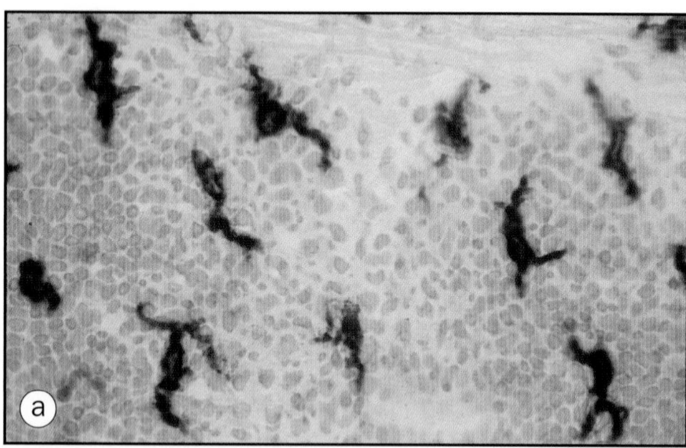

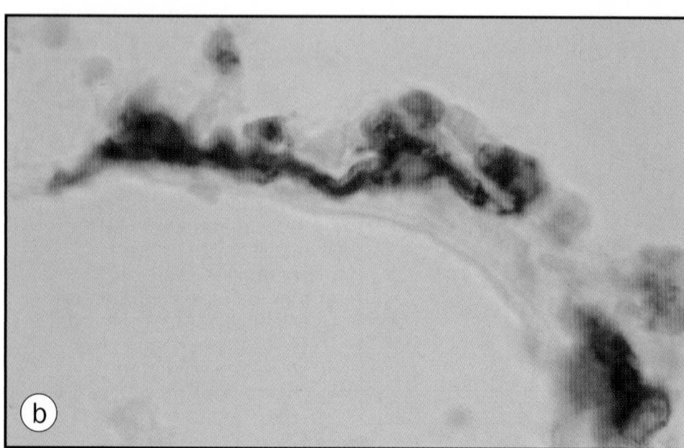

Fig. 19.8 Dendritic cell networks in the respiratory tract. (a) Airway dendritic cells (rat) stained for major histocompatibility complex (MHC) II (normal healthy airway epithelium, tangential section; (b) MHC II+ dendritic cells in rat alveolar septal wall.

Dendritic cells at mucosal surfaces

Distinct populations of DCs are localized within the airway epithelium, the underlying airway mucosa, the lung parenchyma (notably within the interstitium at alveolar interseptal junctions) (Fig. 19.8), and the pleura. Also, in small numbers, they occur on the alveolar surface as part of the bronchoalveolar lavage population. Within the airway mucosa a large subset of these DCs is found in association with the epithelial basement membrane and underlying basal lamina and, in many cases, these cells appear physically attached to the basal lamina while simultaneously ramifying their processes up into the overlying epithelial layer.

Respiratory tract DCs commonly occur in close proximity to local macrophage populations, and similar relationships have been reported for equivalent populations in the intestinal mucosa. In the latter, however, the major population is subepithelial as opposed to intraepithelial, and a subset of the former also appears to ramify their processes into the overlying epithelium.

Analogous to what has been reported for epidermal LCs and most of the gut-derived DCs, this type of lung mucosal DC does not express its full potential for T-cell activation until it has been cultured overnight in a source of GM-CSF. This indicates that its functional phenotype is normally restricted to antigen uptake and processing. One of the principal effects of GM-CSF in this context appears to be the upregulation of expression of CD1a and B7, B7 being expressed only weakly in freshly isolated cells. Thus, the role of lung mucosal DCs in the steady state is likely to be restricted to that of antigen surveillance, with antigen presentation only occurring after their migration to regional lymph nodes. This compartmentalization of functions theoretically provides a mechanism for protection of the delicate epithelial surfaces of the respiratory tract from the consequences of repeated local T-cell activation and ensuing cytokine release.

It has also been demonstrated that while resident within lung tissue, the capacity of DCs to mature into active APCs is inhibited by signals from resident tissue macrophages, in particular nitric oxide (NO), which blocks their capacity to respond to GM-CSF. The potency of this mechanism in vivo has been clearly demonstrated in studies showing that selective in situ depletion of pulmonary alveolar macrophages by the intratracheal administration of liposomes containing dichloromethylene diphosphonate renders mice and rats hyperresponsive to recall antigens administered by aerosol or intratracheal inoculation. Interestingly, the ensuing responses display a bias towards the

Table 19.1 Dendritic cell turnover times in different tissues

Dendritic Cell Turnover Times in Different Tissues	
Tissue	**Turnover time**
Spleen	10 days to 2 weeks
Peripheral LN	3–10 days
Heart	2–4 weeks
Kidney	2–4 weeks
Skin	> 21 days
Intestinal wall	3 days
Airway epithelium	3 days
Lung parenchyma	7–10 days

LN, lymph node.

production of Th2-dependent antibody isotypes (notably IgE), suggesting that such a mechanism may be important in limiting allergic responses to inhaled allergen.

The NO production by airway epithelial cells, which is a distinguishing feature of atopic asthma, may therefore be part of a feedback loop contributing towards the damping down of local T-cell activation via the inhibition of the APC functions of intraepithelial DCs in the airway mucosa. However, it may have the deleterious side-effect of further distortion of the equilibrium between Th1 and Th2 cells in underlying allergen-specific immune responses.

The DC turnover in gut mucosa and resting respiratory tract tissues is much higher than in skin, reflecting its important role in antigen surveillance at those sites of continuous antigen exposure (Table 19.1).

It is also evident that this rapid turnover at mucosal sites can be further upregulated by local exposure to bacterial (Fig. 19.9),

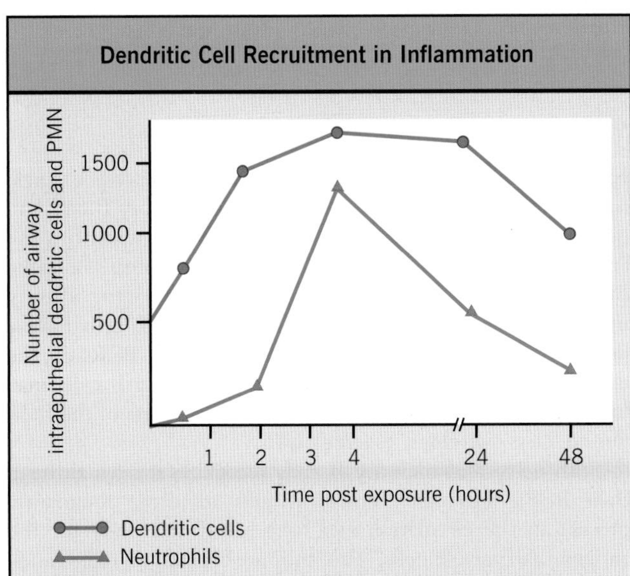

Fig. 19.9 Rapid dendritic cell recruitment into the airway epithelium is a hallmark of the acute inflammatory response. The number of dendritic cells and PMN is shown following 30 minutes' exposure to aerosolized *Moraxella catarrhalis*. PMN, polymorphonuclear cell.

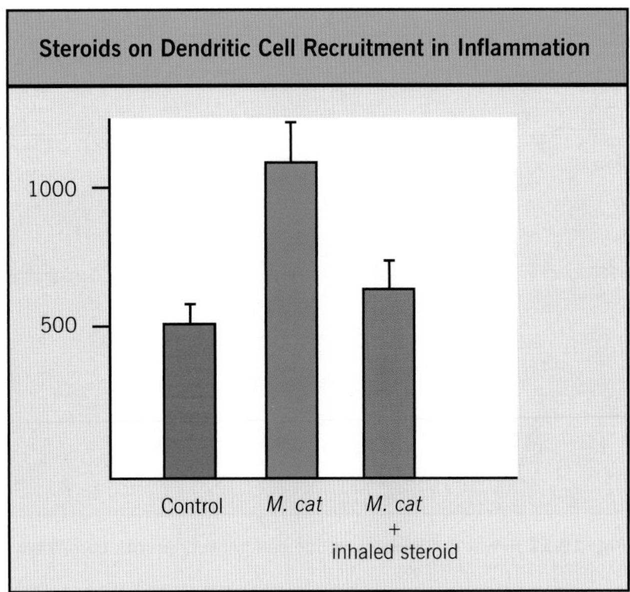

Fig. 19.10 Recruitment of dendritic cells into the airway epithelium (rat) during acute inflammation is efficiently blocked by inhaled steroids (equivalent blocking obtained with budesonide and fluticasone propionate). *M. cat, Moraxella catarrhalis.*

viral, or (recall) antigenic stimuli, which elicit the rapid influx of immature DCs into the airway mucosa. DC recruitment is, therefore, an integral component of the acute host response to the challenge of mucosal surfaces, and these cells may provide the essential link between the innate and adaptive arms of the host defense system.

Situations of chronic stimulation of the respiratory tract lead to the expansion of local mucosal DC populations (Fig. 19.10), in particular in atopics exposed to inhalant allergens. In addition, several function-associated surface molecules become upregulated as has been shown for LCs in the epidermis, indicating the in situ maturation or activation of immature dendritic cells. It is possible that the precocious expression of APC activity by these resident DCs [from patients with atopic asthma and those with atopic dermatitis (AD)] may underlie the excessive local T-cell activation which is the hallmark of these diseases.

Note that while inhaled steroids inhibit airway DC recruitment during acute inflammation (Fig. 19.11), the APC activity of these cells is only partially blocked.

Lymphocytes

B cells are derived from bone marrow and their main function is antigen recognition, through specific antigen receptors [B-cell receptors, (BCRs)], and subsequent differentiation to antibody-producing plasma cells (Fig. 19.12).

B cells can also present antigens to T cells but only after recognition of the antigen by their BCRs. The antigen–BCR complex is then internalized, and as occurs in monocytes and DCs the antigen is degraded in the lysosomal compartment of the B cell. Peptides derived from the antigen are subsequently presented by the class II MHC molecules of the B cell. T cells recognizing the peptide–class II complex will become activated and in return produce cytokines and express cell surface CD40L

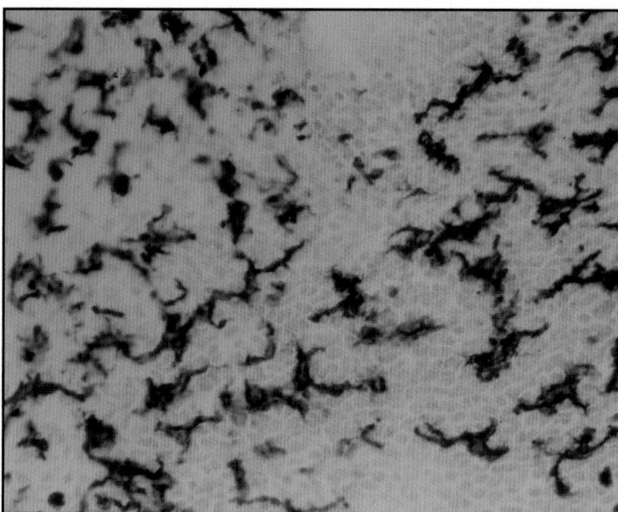

Fig. 19.11 Airway epithelial dendritic cell network in rats chronically exposed to pine shavings.

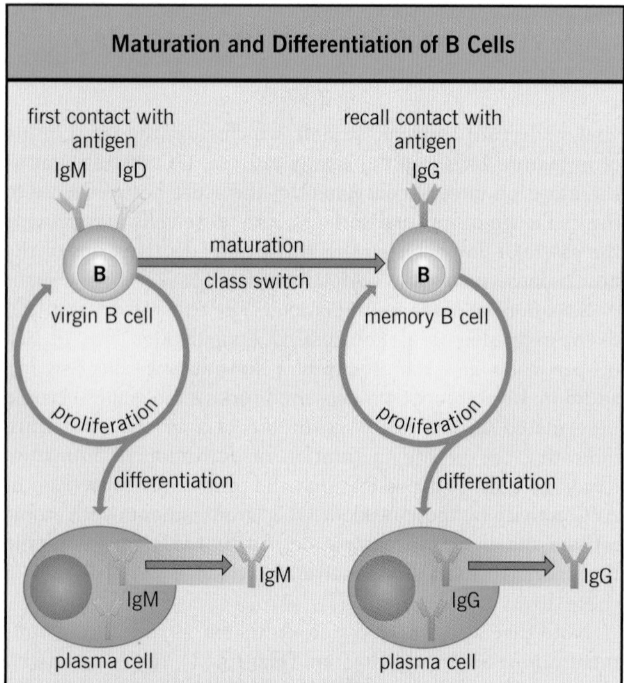

Fig. 19.12 Virgin B cells recognize antigen through their B-cell receptors (BCRs), typically of IgM and IgD isotypes. The cells proliferate heavily in the germinal centers, and part of the cells differentiate into plasma cells producing IgM antibodies whereas others undergo class switching and mature into memory B cells expressing a BCR of a different isotype (e.g. IgG) and higher affinity for the antigen that induced the process. When B cells differentiate into plasma cells their function changes from antigen capture/recognition (through the BCR) to the production of antibodies.

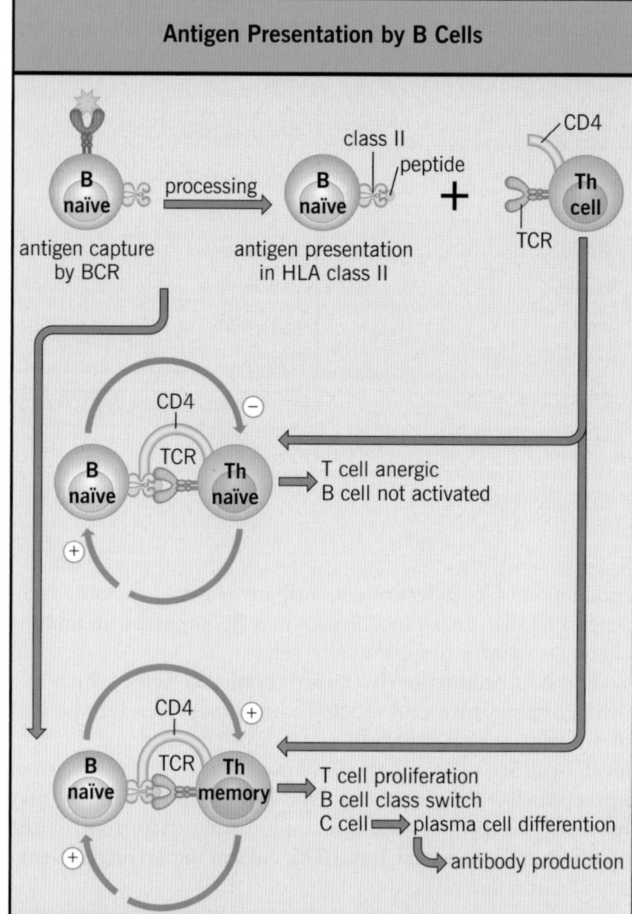

Fig. 19.13 B cells recognize antigen through the B-cell receptors (BCRs). The antigen/BCR complex is internalized and the antigen is processed. Small peptides of the original protein antigen appear in the class II molecules of the B cells and are 'presented' to helper T (Th) cells, which recognize the complex of peptide/class II molecules. The CD4 molecule on the T cell interacts with the class II molecule. When virgin/naïve B cells present antigen to naïve T cells, the end result is T-cell anergy and the B cells do not class switch and do not differentiate into plasma cells. However, naïve B cells are able to stimulate memory T cells, which in return will induce a class switch and/or plasma cell differentiation in the antigen-presenting B cell. TCR, T-cell receptor.

which act in concert to control antibody affinity maturation and immunoglobulin isotype switching in the activated B cell (see later in this chapter).

Two types of B cell can be recognized on the basis of BCR expression: naïve B cells (which co-express BCRs of IgM and IgD isotypes) and memory B cells (which express a single isotype BCR, i.e. IgM, IgG, IgA, or IgE). Memory B cells are derived directly from naïve B cells after first contact with the antigen. As a consequence, they essentially express the same BCR (or antigen specificity). However, due to 'affinity maturation' (see below) the BCRs of memory B cells have a higher affinity for the antigen than the original BCRs on the naïve B cells. In addition, the BCRs of memory B cells may have a different Fc part as indicated by the isotype of the BCR due to 'class switching' (see below).

Both naïve and memory B cells recognize antigen through their BCRs, although memory B cells are more abundantly present in the circulation and have a higher affinity for the antigen than naïve B cells. Also, they are considered to be much more efficient in plasma cell differentiation and antigen presentation. Antigen presentation by naïve B cells may induce anergy in naïve T cells (Fig. 19.13). Both naïve and memory B cells can efficiently present antigen to memory T cells.

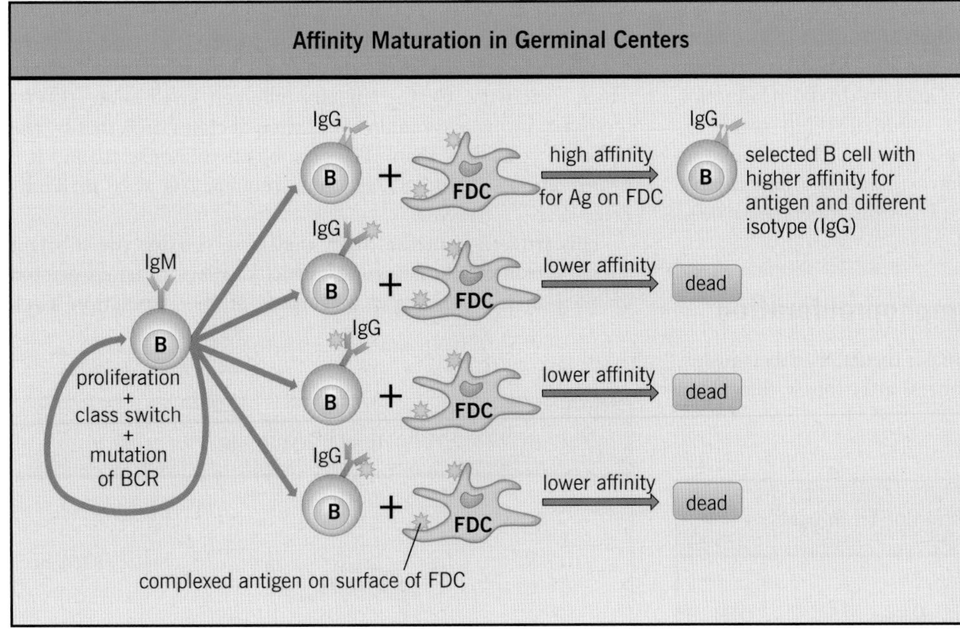

Fig. 19.14 In the process of proliferation, after antigen contact, B cells switch the isotype of their B-cell receptors (BCRs); also, mutations in the antigen-binding part of the BCR take place. BCR, with higher affinity for the antigen, will be positively selected through recognition of the antigen complexed on the FDC, which expresses the CD40 ligand; the ligand is necessary to prevent apoptosis of the B cells. Those B cells with a lower affinity for the antigen will not be rescued and so will eventually die. FDC, follicular dendritic cell.

Affinity maturation and isotype switching

Recognition of antigen is the first step in the maturation from naïve B cell into memory B cell. The second step is internalization and processing of the (protein) antigen, after which antigen presentation to T cells takes place. T cells, in contrast to B cells, only recognize processed antigens which are presented in the MHC class II molecules of APCs. As described in more detail in the next section, the interaction between the APC and the (naïve) T cell may dictate the phenotype of the T cell with respect to the constellation of cytokines produced by the T cell upon activation.

The last step in the maturation to memory B cell is driven by antigen presentation by FDCs in the germinal centers of secondary lymphoid tissue. Upon activation by antigen 'cognate' interaction with T cells (e.g. interaction with T cells recognizing the same antigen in processed form), B cells enter the cell cycle. Th cytokines, along with CD40L, drive B cell proliferation, immunoglobulin isotype switching, and the generation of mutations in the hypervariable regions of their BCR genes encoding both the heavy and light chains. This process of hypermutation alters the primary structure of the antigen-binding complementarity determining regions of antibodies and is responsible for affinity maturation in which B cell clones arise which express BCRs with a higher affinity for the original antigen. These high-affinity B cells are then preferentially further expanded by ongoing antigenic stimulation leading to the production of increasingly high-affinity antibodies (Fig. 19.14).

In addition to memory formation, part of the B-cell population will differentiate into antibody-producing plasma cells. The antibodies produced are identical to the BCR of the B cell that was induced to differentiate. Class switching and affinity maturation do not continue after the B cell becomes a plasma cell.

T cells

T cells are derived from bone marrow progenitors which migrate into the thymus to be either 'educated' into mature T cells selected for their ability to recognize antigenic peptides in the presence of self-MHC ('positive selection') or eliminated if they have high-affinity interactions with self-MHC or processed autologous antigens. T cells express an antigen-specific T cell receptor (TCR), which responds to antigenic peptides presented in the class I or II molecules of APCs. In general, Th cells, which are important for supporting antibody production by B cells, and some regulatory T cells express the CD4 marker and recognize antigen presented by class II molecules. In contrast, cytotoxic T cells and suppressor T cells as well as some Th cells express CD8 and recognize peptides presented in class I molecules. A further functional subdivision of CD4+ Th cell populations can be made on the basis of their pattern of cytokine production profiles after antigenic stimulation (Fig. 19.15).

Th cells have been divided into Th0, Th1, and Th2 according to cytokine secretion profiles. Th0 cells produce IL-2, IL-4, IL-5 and IFNγ; Th1 cells produce IL-2 and IFNγ; and Th2 cells produce IL-4 and IL-5.

Comparative studies of atopic and non-atopic adults show that active T-cell immunity against inhalant allergens is universal. However, the cytokine phenotypes of the dominant T-memory cell populations differ markedly between these groups, with a Th2 or sometimes Th0 pattern in atopic subjects, versus the Th1 pattern in normal subjects.

DEVELOPMENT OF LONG-TERM T-CELL MEMORY

Several laboratories have reported the presence of food and aeroallergen-specific T cells in umbilical cord blood (CB). This has prompted the theory that T cell priming occurs during fetal life, via transplacental transfer of a allergens (Fig. 19.16). CB lymphocytes of neonates with or without an atopic family history almost universally display allergen-specific Th2-like cytokine mRNA responses, characterized by antigen-driven production of IL-4 and IL-5 with relatively minimal IFNγ responses (Table 19.2). However, recent findings that the responding T cells express the CD45RA+ naive phenotype and rapidly apoptose after stimulation, indicate that this theory may need revision.

Postnatal regulation – lymphoproliferation

Initial insight into the nature of the major regulatory mechanisms, which reshape these T-cell responses after birth, has been obtained in cross-sectional studies of lymphoproliferative responses. These studies indicate a marked divergence postnatally between responses to dietary and inhalant allergens. Thus, reactivity to the dietary allergen ovalbumin (OVA) increases during early infancy but then declines such that by the age of 5 years less than 10% of subjects demonstrate in vitro proliferation. A similar response frequency is seen in adults (Fig. 19.17).

This pattern contrasts with that observed for the inhalant allergens from house dust mites, which displays an age-associated increase in frequency and magnitude at the population level,

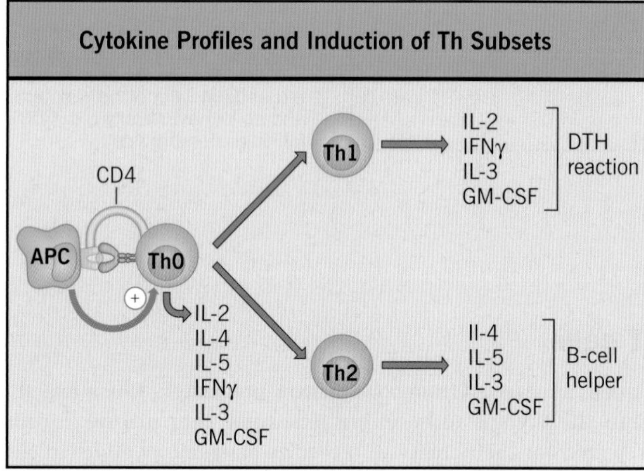

Fig. 19.15 Naïve Th0 cells can be induced to differentiate into Th1 or Th2 cells by the antigen-presenting cell (APC). In the presence of IL-12/IFN, the Th0 cells develop into Th1 cells, whereas the presence of IL-4 induces Th2 cells. DTH, delayed-type hypersensitivity; GM-CSF, granulocyte–macrophage colony-stimulating factor; IFN, interferon; IL, interleukin; Th, helper T cell.

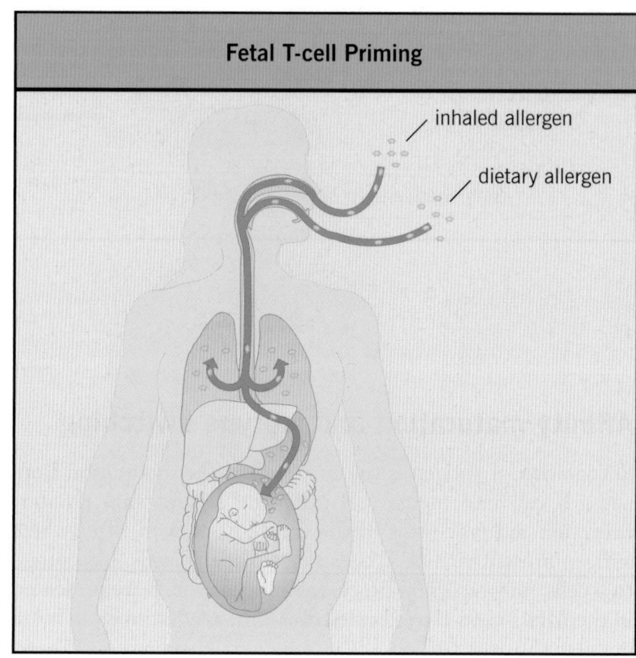

Fig. 19.16 Fetal T-cell priming against allergens encountered by the mother during pregnancy, i.e. transplacental leakage theory.

Table 19.2 Case control study of allergen-specific responses to OVA/HDM in atopic/non-atopic 5-year-olds selected from an ongoing prospective cohort. Five-year-old atopics were SPT-reactive to HDM and at least two other inhalant allergens; the population was OVA-SPT–. The data shown are relative levels of allergen-specific mRNA production post-24-hour in vitro stimulation of PBMC, as determined by sqRT-PCR. Atopic subjects comprised 35% of the overall study population

Monocyte Cytokine Production in Children							
	IL-4	IL-5	IL-6	IL-9	IL-10	IL-13	IFNγ
Cord blood (all):							
HDM	±	+	+	+	+++	+	±
OVA	+	+	+	+	++++	+	±
5-year-olds (non-atopic):							
HDM	–	–	+	–	–	–	±
OVA	–	–	++	–	±	±	–
5-year-olds (atopic):							
HDM	++	+	+	+++	+	++	–
OVA	–	–	++	–	–	±	–

HDM, house dust mite; IFN, interferon; IL, interleukin; OVA, ovalbumin; PBMC, peripheral blood mononuclear cells; SPT, skin prick test; sqRT-PCR, semi-quantitative reverse transcription-polymerase chain reaction

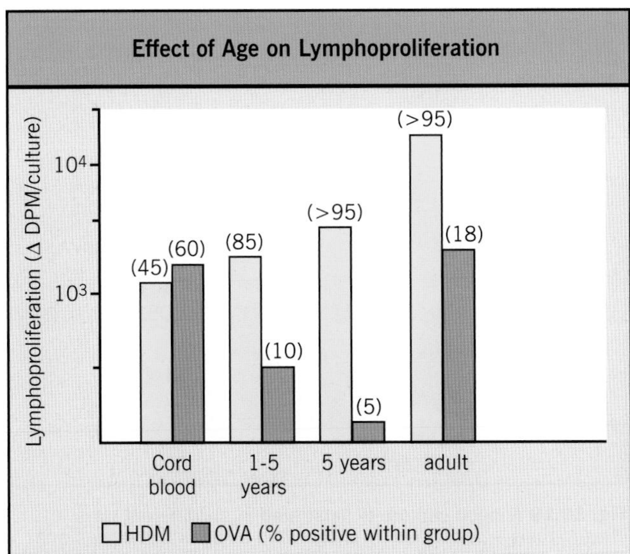

Fig. 19.17 Age-dependent changes in lymphoproliferative responses to dietary (OVA) against inhaled (HDM) allergens. Bars are the group medians and the numbers in parentheses are the positive percentages in each group. HDM, house dust mite; OVA, ovalbumin.

such that over 95% of adults manifest high-level lymphoproliferative responses (see Fig. 19.17).

These findings give rise to the hypothesis that repeated postnatal exposure of the immature T-cell system to inhalant allergens leads ultimately to the selection of either Th1-polarized or Th2-polarized memory i.e. either boosting of immature Th2-like responses or their deviation towards the Th1 phenotype. This contrasts with the progressive silencing of responses to the dietary allergens via T cell deletion or anergy. The issue of precisely when priming occurs remains to be resolved.

As mentioned above, the operation of these distinct regulatory pathways for the two classes of allergen may be simply a function of antigen dosage, i.e. low-zone tolerance (immune deviation) driven by nanogram or microgram exposure to the inhalant as opposed to high-zone tolerance (deletion or anergy) driven by milligram or gram levels of the dietary allergen.

Postnatal regulation – cytokine production

The recent analysis of allergen-specific cytokine responses in samples from preschool children has further clarified the nature of these regulatory processes. With respect to OVA-specific responses, by 18 months of age the Th2-like CB pattern of allergen-specific cytokine production wanes in the atopic family history negative population (FH-) to virtual unresponsiveness whereas FH+ infants display weak Th0-like reactivity. However, by the age of 5 years, the only consistent OVA-specific cytokine response detectable in either population is IL-6, the greater part of which is attributable to monocytes (see Table 19.2).

In contrast, consistent with the above predictions based on lymphoproliferation data, cytokine responses to house dust mites become consolidated into unequivocal Th1-like or Th2-like patterns, which manifest by the age of 5 years. Thus the population who are skin prick test positive (SPT+) to house dust mites display in vitro house dust mite-induced cytokine responses characterized by IL-4, IL-5, IL-9, and IL-13, whereas the responses of the house dust mite-SPT- population are restricted to low-level IFNγ. These findings suggest that important aspects of the programming of the T-cell system (for subsequent clinical responsiveness versus unresponsiveness to environmental allergens) occur within a relatively short 'window' during early life.

Th1 versus Th2 polarization

Why do allergies to inhalant and food allergens follow a different course? Is the polarization of Th1 versus Th2 responses different in atopic subjects when compared with normal subjects? The answers to these questions are of primary importance in understanding the development of allergy.

Recent developments in understanding the immunology of pregnancy provide a plausible explanation for the generalized Th2 polarity of fetal allergen responses. Thus it is clear that pregnancy is a Th2 state in which the production of high levels of IL-4, IL-10, prostaglandin E_2 (PGE_2), and progesterone, inter alia via the placenta, maintain a strong barrier against the induction of Th1 immunity at the fetomaternal interface.

During postnatal life the capacity to generate Th1 immunity increases progressively with age but remains 'deficient' relative to adulthood for various periods during early life. This conclusion is based primarily on animal studies during infancy, particularly in relation to the Th1–Th2 imbalance responsible for the phenomenon of neonatal tolerance. However, it is clearly of equivalent relevance to humans, reflected particularly by the low capacity for production by peripheral blood mononuclear cells (PBMC) of key Th1 cytokines such as IFNγ during infancy and early childhood.

In mice, the Th1 'deficit' in neonatal life can be attributed principally to a failure on the part of APCs, in particular DCs, to provide appropriate immune-deviating signals during T-cell activation. A similar situation is likely to pertain in humans, given that the failure of infant PBMC to produce high levels of IFNγ during in vitro stimulation can be markedly improved by the supplementation of cultures with maternal APCs.

Several independent lines of evidence suggest that this developmental 'deficit' in Th1 function, which is clearly left over from fetal life, is more pronounced in subjects with the atopic genotype.

The possible role of dendritic cells

Airway intraepithelial DC populations mature extremely slowly during early postnatal life and (at least in rodents) do not appear to obtain adult equivalence until a significant period after weaning (Fig. 19.18). The functions which are defective during this period include MHC II expression and responsiveness to cytokines such as GM-CSF and IFNγ, all of which are central to airway intraepithelial cell activity as APCs.

Given earlier studies indicating that, in resting airway and lung tissue, DCs represent the major (often sole) resident APC population, it is axiomatic that they must play a central role in responses to inhaled allergens. It is feasible that the kinetics of postnatal maturation of these DC populations may be one of the major determinants of the efficiency of the immune deviation process, which ultimately protects against the development of inhalant allergy.

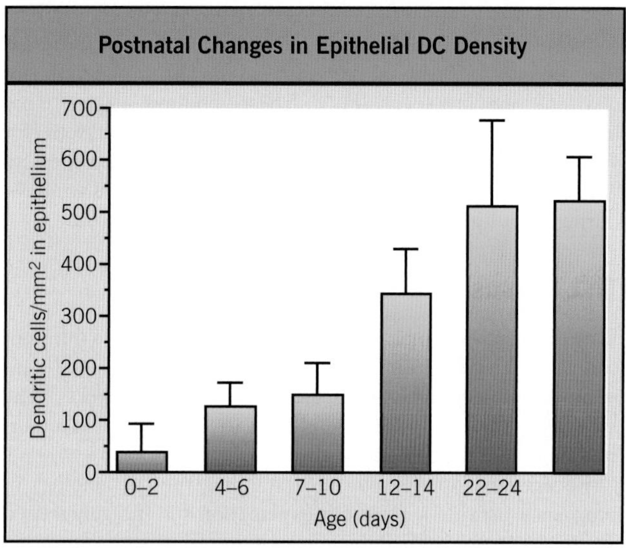

Fig. 19.18 Postnatal maturation of airway epithelial dendritic cell network in a rat (22–24 days of weaning).

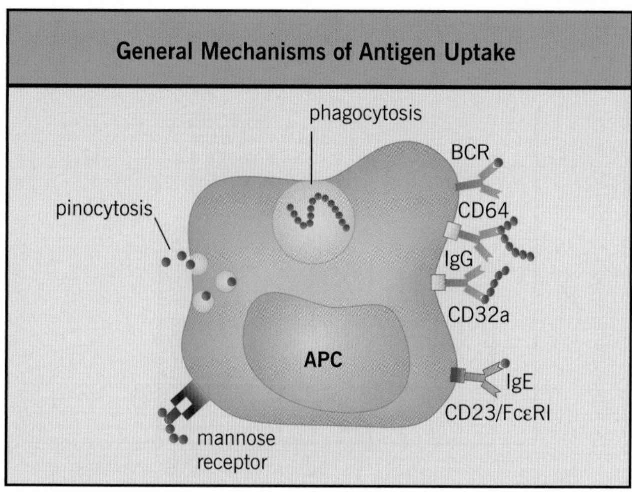

Fig. 19.19 Antigen capture is illustrated in six different ways. (i) Phagocytosis – performed by phagocytes such as monocytes and macrophages, (ii) B-cell receptor (BCR) – very efficient, performed by antigen-specific B cells only, (iii) Fcγ receptors – CD64 is expressed by monocytes and macrophages; CD32a is expressed by many different antigen-presenting cells (APCs) dependent on the number of IgG molecules or antigens for a stable interaction with the low-affinity receptors, (iv) Fcε receptors – very efficient, performed by dendritic cells (FcεRI), monocytes (FcεRI) and B cells (CD23); especially important in allergy; CD23 can be induced on dendritic cells and monocytes by IL-4, (v) mannose receptors – very efficient and allow APCs (mostly dendritic cells) to bind sugar (mannose) residues of glycosylated proteins, (vi) pinocytosis – not efficient as large quantities of antigen are needed; theoretically performed by all types of APC.

PRESENTATION OF ANTIGEN AND STIMULATION OF IgE SYNTHESIS

General mechanisms of antigen presentation

The immune response to foreign proteins is strongly dependent on the efficiency and selectivity of antigen uptake by APCs. Internalized antigen is then processed and presented to the T cells in an HLA class II-restricted way. Until now six mechanisms of antigen trapping by APCs have been generally accepted (Fig. 19.19).

Phagocytosis of particles is the means by which cells of the mononuclear phagocyte system take up antigens, allowing both primary and recall antigens to be internalized and processed. Phagocytosis is enhanced by the opsonization of particles with IgG, which interacts with IgG Fc receptors (FcγR) or with complement receptors on these mononuclear cells. Dendritic cells and B cells are not able to use phagocytosis but they may utilize the more general process of pinocytosis. B cells may also use antigen-specific surface immunoglobulin for antigen capture. This process is the more efficient, since the required antigen concentrations are 1000 times less than for pinocytosis. However, despite the efficient binding by B cells, this process may be limited by the relatively small number of specific B cells, and those B cells which produce rheumatoid factor. DCs have recently been shown to have an additional means of capturing glycosylated protein antigens through the so-called mannose receptor.

Recently, several groups have reported a sixth possible mechanism for antigen trapping, both in vivo and in vitro. The APC may, by means of an FcεR, bind monomeric antigen-specific IgE, which will then capture the antigen and increase the efficiency of antigen presentation (Fig. 19.20). Furthermore, IgE–antigen complexes may be used by the APC for antigen focusing. This mechanism, which is comparable to antigen-specific binding by B cells, is especially of importance in allergy where high levels of IgE antibodies are found in the serum of the patients.

IgE-mediated antigen presentation via FcεRI

The concept of IgE as an antigen-capturing antibody was first described for mast cells. Allergen may bind to 'empty' IgE bound to the FcεRI on the surface of the mast cell (see Ch. 18). Cross-linking of the receptors will then cause the release of inflammatory mediators, which are involved in immediate-type hypersensitivity reactions. In order to cause cross-linking, the IgE on the surface of the mast cell must be relatively monoclonal.

The first evidence that IgE may play a role in antigen capture by APCs was found in patients with AD (see Ch. 7). In AD IgE may be found on epidermal LCs (which has been confirmed) while in allergic rhinoconjunctivitis it is found on the nasal and conjunctival DCs. The Fc receptor for binding the IgE on these cells has been identified as the high-affinity receptor for IgE (FcεRI).

Aggregation of tetrameric FcεRI on effector cells of anaphylaxis is involved in immediate-type hypersensitivity reactions by the release of preformed mediators stored in granules such as the amines histamine or heparin, and the rapid synthesis of prostaglandins and leukotrienes. In contrast, the key role of the trimeric variant of FcεRI on APCs is believed to be antigen focusing (Fig. 19.21).

Early observations on LCs suggested that allergen presentation by these cells is mediated by IgE. Detailed studies using pollen allergen, which were recognized by antigen-specific IgE bound to APCs via FcεRI, showed that FcεRI represents the most important IgE-binding structure which mediates IgE-dependent antigen presentation to T cells. This process is about 100–1000-fold more efficient than non-specific uptake of allergens. After polyvalent ligation, FcεRI-bound IgE is internalized into acidic,

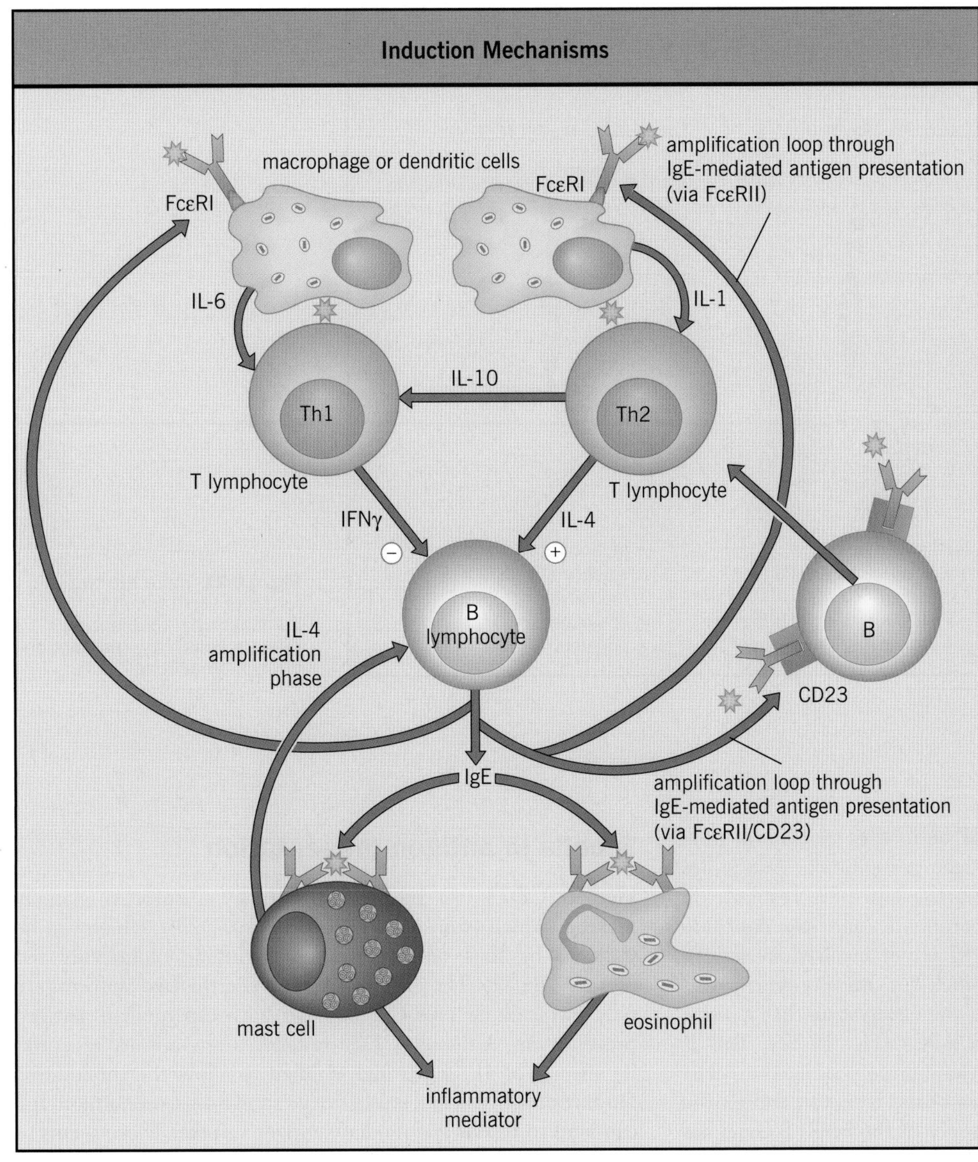

Fig. 19.20 Interrelationship between inducer and effector mechanisms of allergic inflammation.

proteolytic compartments, degraded and delivered into organelles containing MHC class II, HLA-DM and lysosomal proteins. Thus, multimeric ligands captured by FcεRI and IgE are channeled efficiently into MIIC (MHC class II compartment)-like organelles of DCs, instead of being delivered into a recycling MHC class II pathway. In MIIC, cathepsin S-dependent ligand peptide loading of newly synthesized MHC class II molecules occurs. The decision to take up and to present Ag in an IgE-dependent manner is made on the basis of whether Ag or pathogens carry repetitive or multiple distinct IgE epitopes. Together, these observations led to the development of the concept of an 'IgE-mediated delayed-type hypersensitivity reaction' by which FcεRI-bearing APCs play a role in the pathophysiology of atopic diseases. Further on, there is some evidence that the quality of the signal transduction events triggered after FcεRI aggregation differs profoundly in atopic and non-atopic individuals. It leads to the rapid tyrosine phosphorylation of proteins. However, calcium mobilization, which is dependent on tyrosine phosphorylation and the activation of phospholipase Cγ, occurs exclusively in dendritic cells of atopic donors in consequence of FcεRI aggregation. Together, this implies that some key steps in the signal transduction pathway are upregulated in DCs of atopic individuals, in which FcεRI ligation on DCs is capable of inducing NF-κB activation and is thereby able to regulate genes involved in inflammatory immune responses.

On the other hand, CD23 – which is the low-affinity receptor for IgE [10^{-8} dissociation rate constant (K_d)] (see Ch. 18) – is also able to mediate antigen uptake. CD23 is constitutively expressed by naïve B cells and can be induced on most APCs by means of IL-4, a cytokine upregulated in allergic disease.

In vivo IgE-mediated antigen presentation

IgE-mediated antigen presentation by CD23 in vivo has been demonstrated by the observation that 2,4,6-trinitrophenyl (TNP)-specific IgE – injected intravenously before bovine serum albumin (BSA)-TNP – enhances antigen capture and presentation, and leads to strong IgG anti-BSA production in the absence of adjuvants. Not only are IgG antibodies induced

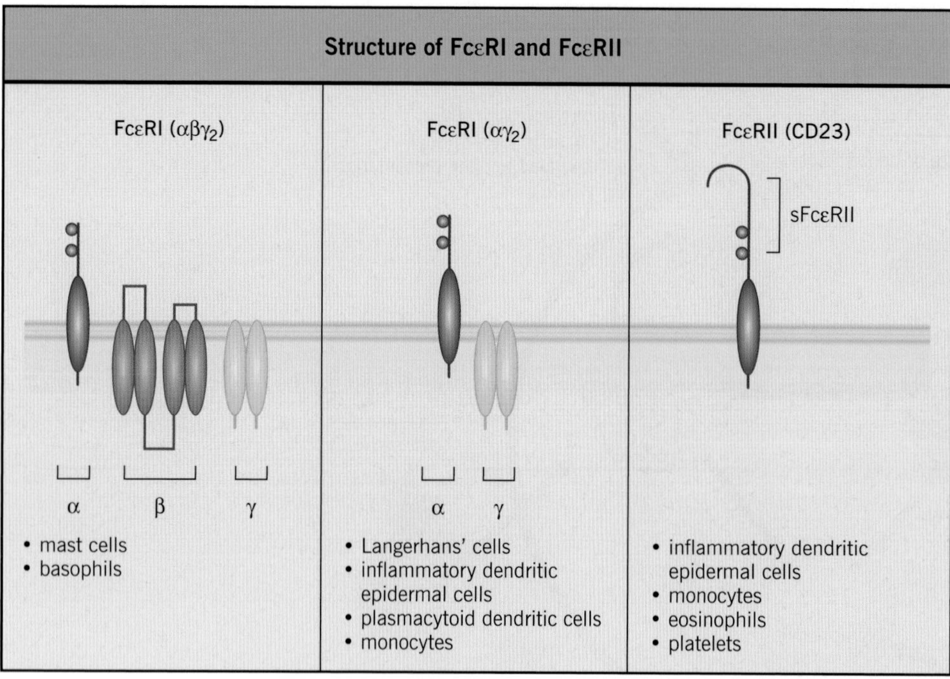

Fig. 19.21 There are two forms of FcεRI found in humans: $\alpha\beta\gamma_2$ (present on effector cells); $\alpha\gamma_2$ (present on antigen-presenting cells).

but also IgM and, importantly, IgE antibodies specific for BSA are found after IgE-mediated antigen presentation. Antibodies against CD23 completely inhibit the anti-BSA response in these animals. From these experiments, one can conclude that, in the mouse at least, FcεRI is not involved in antigen presentation. Indeed, CD23 knock-out mice confirm this conclusion, and this also fits with the observation that in mice no FcεRI has been detected on APCs (Fig. 19.22). This is probably due to the fact that in the murine system, the FcεRI β chain is necessary for expression of the receptor, and on the APC, at least in humans, the presence of the FcεRI β chain has not been demonstrated (Fig. 19.21).

In mice, only two cell types express CD23 constitutively: FDCs and naïve B cells. It was found that in IL-4 knock-out mice, IgE-mediated antigen presentation induced comparable levels of IgG anti-BSA. As in wild type mice, the involvement of other APCs, on which IL-4 may have induced the expression of CD23, was excluded.

Using irradiated CD23 knock-out mice, reconstituted with the blood of CD23+ donor cells, and irradiated wild type mice, reconstituted with blood from CD23 knock-out mice, Heyman's group (see Further Reading) showed that it is most likely that the naïve B cells, and not the FDCs, are responsible for the APC function. Importantly, they never found any upregulation of 'bystander' antigen presentation, indicating that in their in vivo model with naïve animals, IgE-mediated antigen presentation only occurs by antigen-specific B cells, which in addition are CD23+. This implies that, in contrast to dogma, naïve B cells can present antigen to naïve T cells, when the antigen is captured though BCRs and CD23 at the same time. Clearly, these elegant studies need confirmation by different groups and in different systems, but they also indicate the potency of IgE in antigen uptake and antigen presentation.

B cells in antigen presentation

Human CD23 can be expressed in two isoforms, namely CD23a, which is on naïve B cells, and CD23b, which can be induced by IL-4 on many APCs including monocytes and memory B cells. The differences between the two isoforms are only intracellular (see Ch. 18) and both can mediate antigen presentation. Although CD23 is called a low-affinity receptor, its affinity of 10^{-8} K_d is high enough to allow the monomeric binding of IgE. Several studies have shown that monomeric IgE can bind to B cells and mediate antigen uptake. There seems to be no advantage in cross-linking the receptor, which is in contrast to FcεRI, which needs cross-linking for activation. The potency of IgE on B cells for antigen uptake is overwhelming. B cells preincubated with 10 ng/mL monomeric-specific IgE, induced a strong antigen-specific T-cell response (Fig. 19.23). This amount of IgE is not detectable on the surface of the B cells using a fluorescence-activated cell sorter. Furthermore, less than 10^{-12} M of antigen is sufficient to mount a specific T cell response in vitro, even when the IgE-preincubated B cells are allowed to catch the antigen for 1 hour only.

Similar data have been described for DCs incubated with IgG–antigen complexes. However, in that study the DCs were allowed to interact with the antigen for the whole culture period.

In conclusion, IgE-mediated antigen presentation by B cells is the most efficient antigen-presenting system described to date.

IgG-mediated antigen presentation

As described above, not just IgE but also IgG antibodies can be used by APCs for antigen presentation. For this, two FcγRs have been implicated: CD64 (also called FcγRI) and CD32 (FcγRII). On B cells and DCs only CD32 is expressed whereas monocytic cells express both CD32 and CD64. CD64 has an

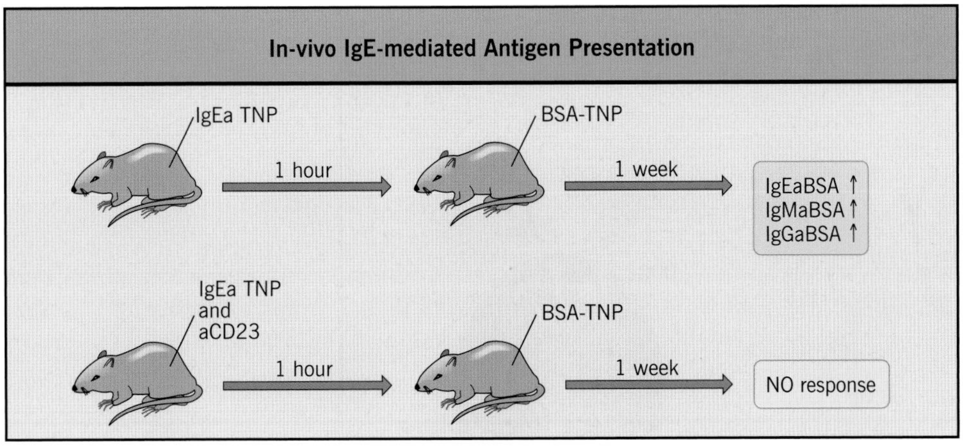

In-vivo IgE-mediated Antigen Presentation

IgEa TNP
1 hour
BSA-TNP
1 week
IgEaBSA ↑
IgMaBSA ↑
IgGaBSA ↑
IgEa TNP and aCD23
1 hour
BSA-TNP
1 week
NO response

Fig. 19.22 Naïve mice are injected with TNP-specific IgE antibodies and subsequently OVA-TNP in a single injection. After 1 week, OVA-specific IgE, IgM and IgG can be measured in the serum of the mice. Co-injection of neutralizing CD23a antibodies completely abrogates this reaction. BSA, bovine serum albumin; OVA, ovalbumin; TNP, trinitrophenol.

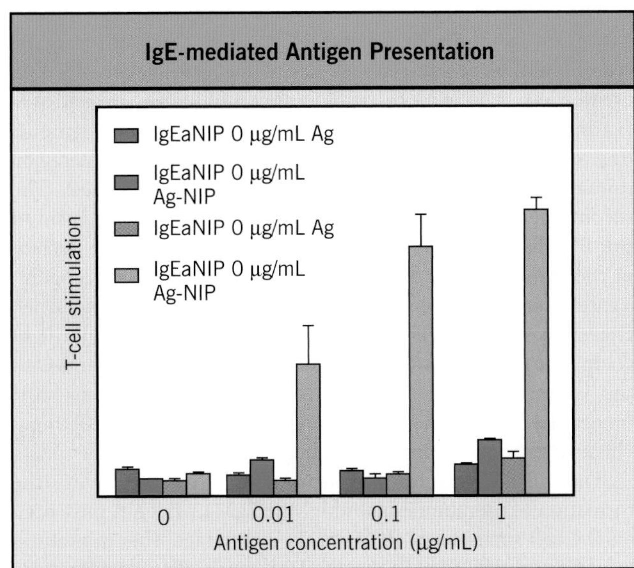

Fig. 19.23 Only when IgE recognizes the antigen (NIP) is there stimulation of the T cells. (Data from Santamaria LF, Bheekha R, Van Reijsen FC, et al. Antigen focusing by specific monomeric immunoglobulin E bound to C23 on Epstein–Barr virus-transformed B cells. Hum Immunol 1993; 37:23–30, American Society of Histocompatibility & Immunogenetics.)

affinity of 10^{-8} K_d and can bind monomeric IgG, but CD32 only binds IgG in complexed form due to a low affinity of 10^{-6} K_d. It has been calculated that antigens need more than 10 epitopes for IgG molecules to allow complex formation, which is sufficiently large for a stable binding to CD32. This implies that CD32, although able to mediate antigen presentation, will only be involved in antigen capture when the complexes are around for a relatively long time, such as in the experiment described above. Preincubated allergen–IgG complexes will not bind to the cells with any stability unless CD64 is present, although allergen complexes in vivo most likely consist of IgE and IgG molecules, in which case both the FcεR and the FcγR are involved in binding the complex. For monocytic cells this does not appear to have any consequences but for B cells the impact may be more dramatic.

B cells (in contrast to DCs and monocytic cells) express the CD32b isoform, of which two subtypes exist; CD32bI and CD32bII are both expressed on resting B cells. The other APCs express the CD32a form. Importantly, these three different isoforms have different functions:

- CD32a is involved in antigen uptake when complexed IgG interacts.
- CD32bII can also be internalized but is not as efficient as CD32a.

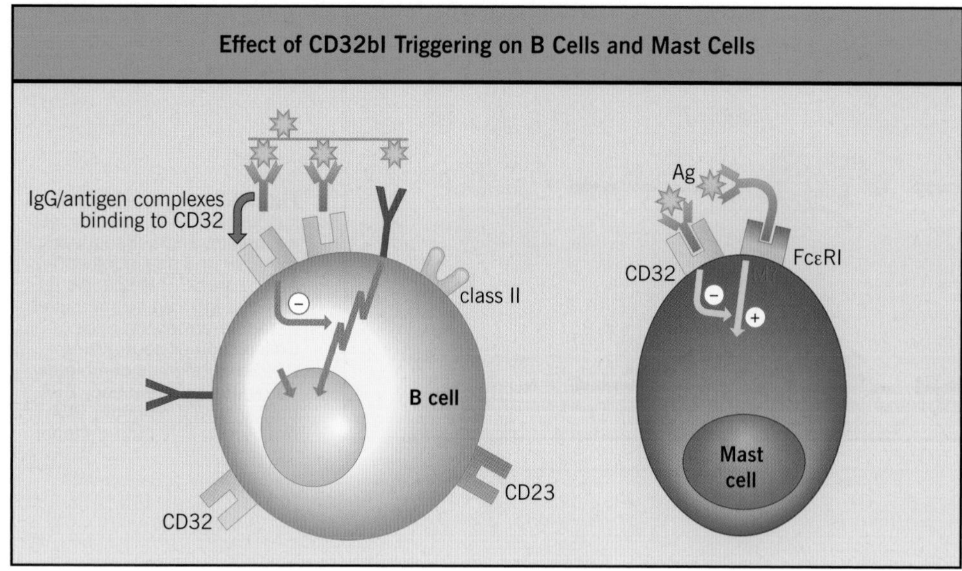

Fig. 19.24 Co-cross-linking of CD32bI with B-cell receptors blocks B9cell activation; co-cross-linking of CD32bI with FcεRI blocks mast-cell activation through FcεRI.

- The CD32bI isoform cannot mediate receptor endocytosis – this receptor is involved in 'negative signaling'.

Co-cross-linking of BCRs and CD32bI completely blocks B-cell activation. Interestingly, the mast cell CD32bI is also found, and co-cross-linking this receptor with the FcεRI blocks antigen-induced mast cell degranulation (Fig. 19.24).

Consequences of CD23- and IgE-mediated antigen presentation

As shown above, CD23- and IgE-mediated antigen presentation is a potent system for antigen uptake. The danger of this mechanism may be in the constitutive expression of CD23 on naïve B cells, to which cells are able to switch their isotype after antigen contact and interaction with antigen-specific T cells (as above). When naïve B cells interact with Th2 cells (see below) they will receive IL-4, which induces a class switch to IgE in these B cells.

It has therefore been speculated that in allergy, where high IgE titers and large numbers of allergen-specific Th2 cells are found, the chance that naïve B cells pick up the allergen through IgE or CD23 is relatively high. When these naïve B cells simultaneously become activated by their natural antigen (call it Ag-X) through binding to their BCRs, as well as through CD23 and IgE–Al-Y, these B cells present two antigens at the same time (Ag-X and Al-Y) (Fig. 19.25).

The type of responding T cells for the Al-Y is most likely to be a Th2 cell, which leads to IL-4 production and a subsequent class switch to IgE. Since the B cells only produce BCRs with specificity for Ag-X, the antibodies against Ag-X will be of the IgE type and the patient, who originally was only allergic to Al-Y will now also become allergic to Ag-X.

IgE synthesis

The production of allergen-specific IgE by B cells is a tightly regulated process that requires an orchestrated series of molecular genetic rearrangements. The first step in this process is the production a complete immunoglobulin molecule, expressed at the cell surface as a BCR. Random somatic recombination of cassettes of germ line gene fragments first creates a μ chain gene by recombination of an assortment of V (variable), D (diversity), and J (joining) gene segments upstream of the gene exons encoding the Cμ, constant region domains of the μ heavy chain of IgM antibodies. The recombined VDJCμ gene product appears in the cytoplasm of pre-B cells as μ chain and is then assembled at the surface of the pre-B cell in a complex with the 'surrogate light chains', V-pre B and λ-5. Expression of this pre-B cell receptor then triggers a similar series of events at the immunoglobulin light chain loci (κ or λ) in which V and J segments recombine with the Cκ or Cλ gene segments to construct a gene encoding functional Ig light chain that can assemble with the existing μ chain to produce an immunoglobulin molecule.

The mRNA splicing mechanism at this stage favors the formation of membrane-bound IgM (mIgM), which is presented on the cell surface as a BCR. In the next stage, the 'immature' mIgM-expressing B cells mature into 'virgin' B cells expressing both mIgM and mIgD (Fig. 19.26). The co-expression of mIgM and mIgD is possible on a single B cell because the proximity of the Cμ and Cδ loci permits the formation of a single large RNA consisting of VDJCμCδ, which is subsequently differentially spliced into VDJCμ mRNA and VDJCδ mRNA. Although B cells at this stage produce fully functional antibodies of a broad range of specificities (generated by the huge number of potential permutations of recombined V, D, and J segments encoding the complementarity determining regions of the antibodies), their affinity for specific antigens is still generally low and the biological activities of the antibodies restricted to those mediated by the Fc portions of IgM and IgD. Additional steps are required to generate high-affinity antibodies and to produce isotypes, such as IgE, with specific effector functions.

In order to enhance antigen specificity and to produce specific immunoglobulin isotypes, naïve antigen-specific B cells undergo processes known as affinity maturation and isotype

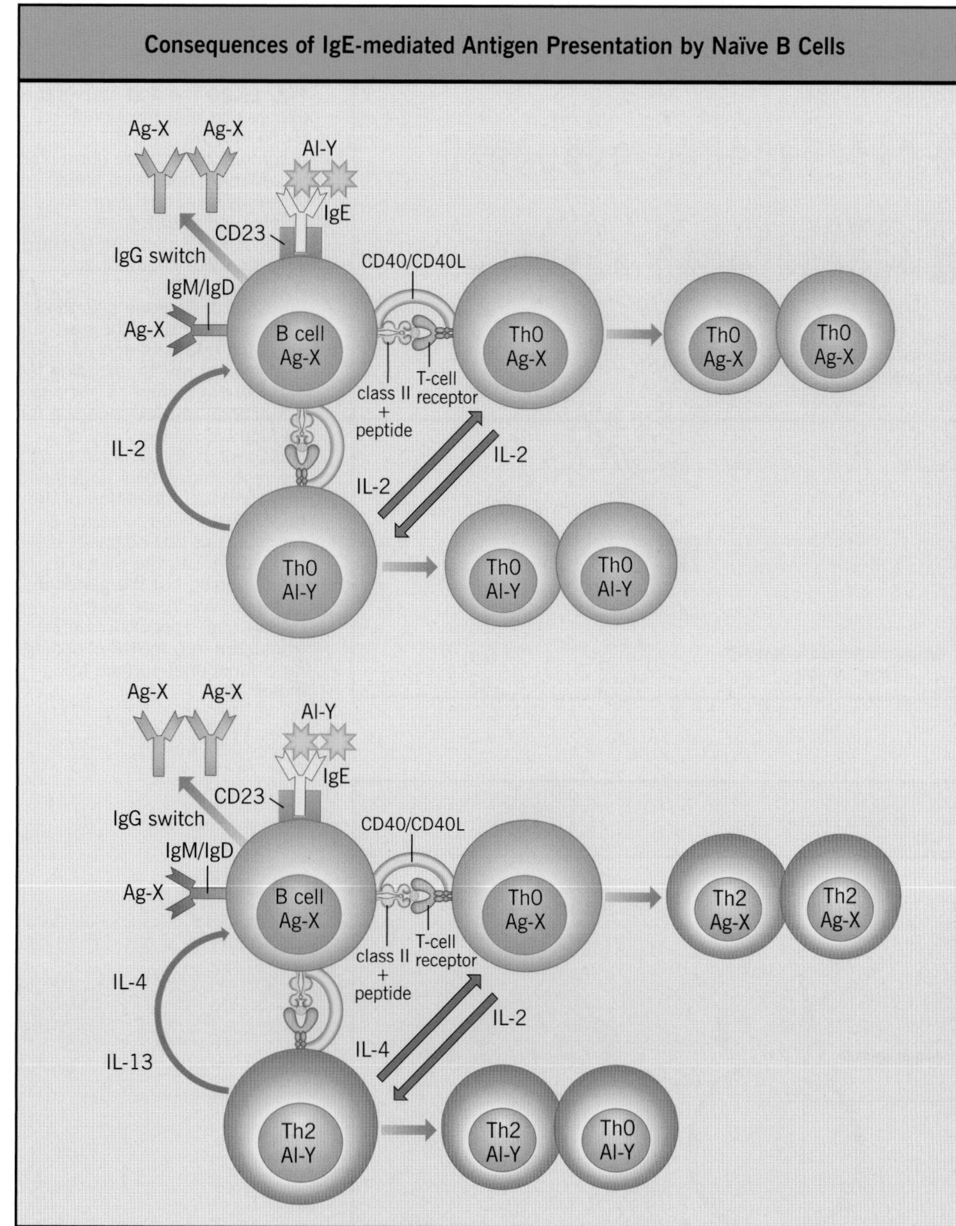

Fig. 19.25 Naïve B cells can use their B-cell receptors (IgM or IgD) to capture antigen (Ag-X). Also, through CD23 expression, naïve B cells can bind IgE, which recognizes an allergen (Al-Y). Both antigens will be presented to specific T cells. When the Al-Y-specific T cell is of the Th0 phenotype (upper part) a normal secondary immune response will be initiated leading to IgG memory B cells and finally Ag-X-specific IgG antibody production. When the responding allergen-specific T cell is of the Th2 phenotype (lower part) the B cell may switch to IgE as a result of the IL-4 production by the Th2 cell, leading to formation of new IgE antibodies with specificity for Ag-X. Also, the IL-4 produced by the Al-Y-specific Th2 cells may influence the phenotype of naïve Ag-X-specific T cells by changing these T cells into Th2 cells. Similarly, the IL-2 produced by the Ag-X-specific Th0 cell will lead to the proliferation of the Al-Y-specific Th2 cell. IL, interleukin; Th, helper T cell.

class switching (Fig. 19.27). Affinity maturation occurs in germinal centers, specialized regions of lymph nodes draining antigen-exposed sites. In the germinal center the gene sequences encoding immunoglobulin complementarity determining regions are subjected to a process of 'hypermutation' leading to the production of antibodies with altered antigen-binding capacity. B cells expressing high-affinity antibodies are selected, and others are eliminated by apoptosis, within a few days. The mechanism of somatic hypermutation involves the introduction of double-strand DNA breaks and is initiated by the process of RNA transcription. The enzyme activation-induced adenosine deaminase, which is also involved in isotype switching (another transcription-dependent process, see below) participates in this process of hypermutation and individuals with mutations in the AID gene have defects both in the production of high-affinity antibodies and in the production of immunoglobulin isotypes other than IgM.

In the process of isotype switching, B cells undergo rearrangements which result in the production of antibodies which retain their antigen specificity but change the structure of the heavy chain constant region domains to facilitate the production of antibodies with distinct effector functions (including IgG1–4, IgA1, IgA2, or IgE). This heavy chain switch diversifies the effector function of antibodies by enabling the production of antibodies which retain their original antigenic specificity but bind to specific receptors, which are differentially expressed on different types of cells, e.g. FcεRI is found on mast cells and basophils as well as on APCs.

Like affinity maturation, isotype switching takes place in germinal centers. The direction of switching is determined by the cytokine milieu of the B cell (Fig. 19.28). Specific patterns of cytokine signaling result in the activation of distinct gene promoters located upstream of each heavy chain gene segment. IL-4 and IL-13 activate transcription at the Iε promoter

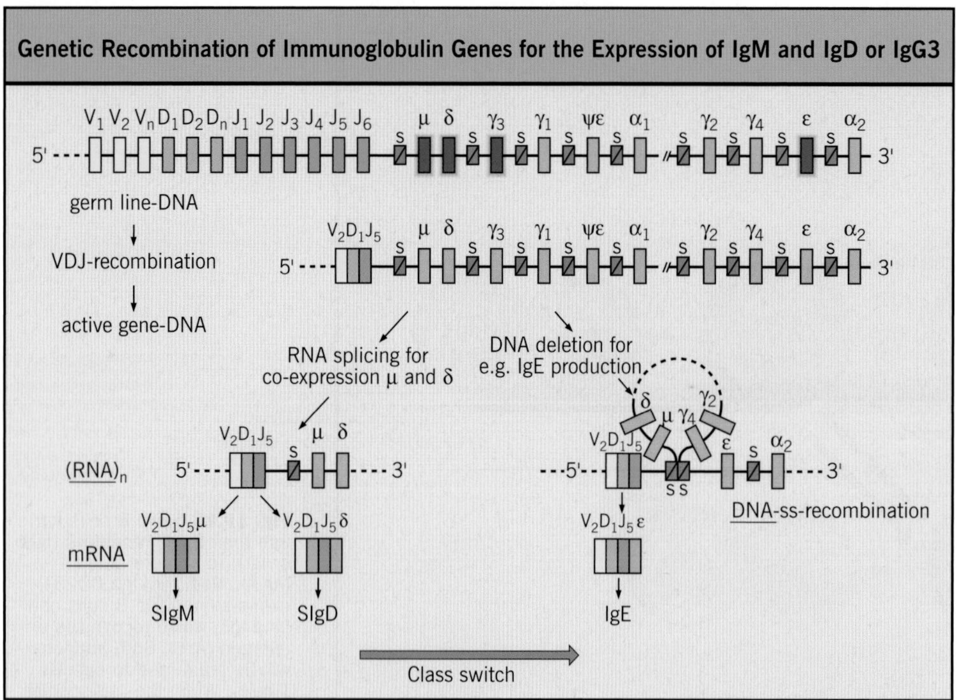

Fig. 19.26 The first step in the expression of a functional B-cell receptor is DNA recombination of one germ line V (variable), one germ line D (diversity) and one germ line J (joining) gene to form a particular VDJ gene. In the next step this VDJ segment is translated into mRNA including the Cμ and Cδ gene segments (C for constant). In the next step this mRNA is spliced into a functional mRNA encoding for surface expression of IgM and a functional mRNA encoding for surface IgD. In the case of a class switch (for example to IgE) the recombined DNA undergoes a second recombination of the heavy chain genes in such a way that the VDJ segment is connected with the Cε gene while looping out the genes in between, which are lost for further use. This DNA is then translated into mRNA encoding for a functional surface IgE molecule.

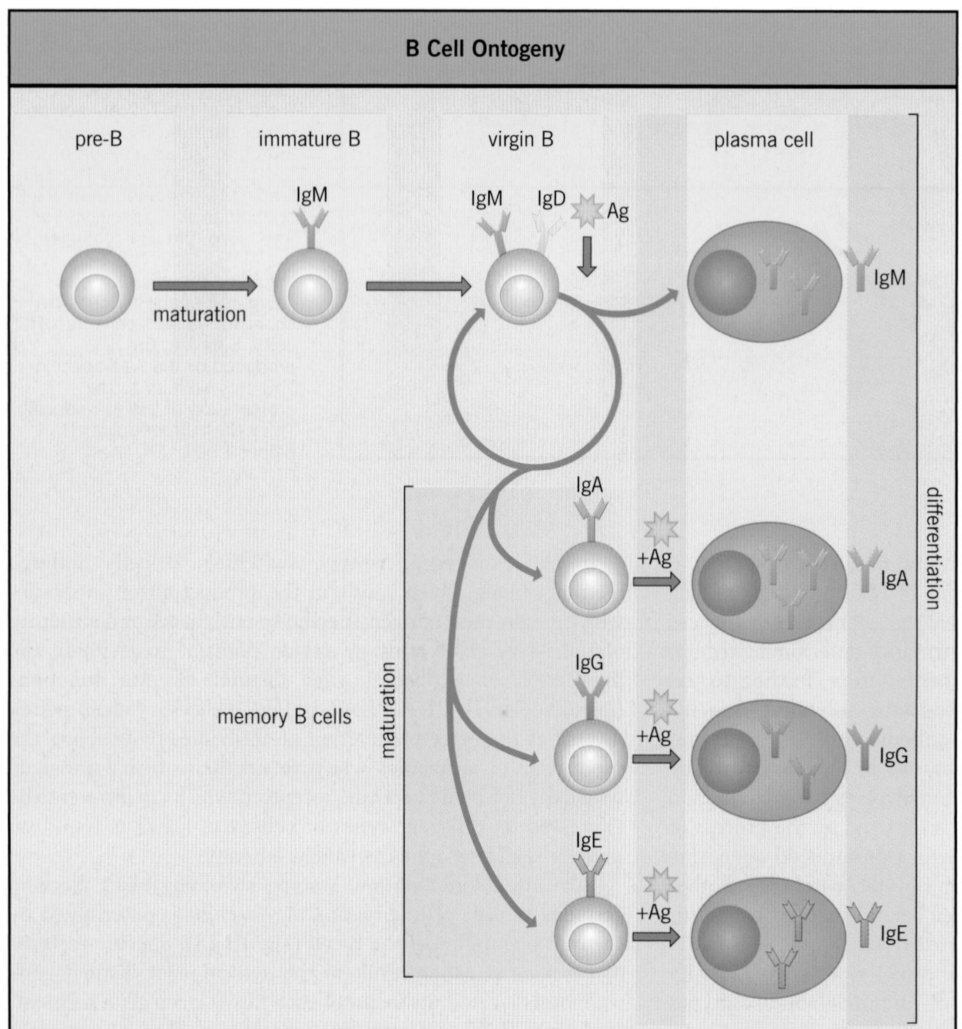

Fig. 19.27 Pre-B cells, characterized by intracellular μ heavy chains in the absence of light chains, are found in the bone marrow. They mature via an IgM-expressing immature B-cell stage (mostly in the bone marrow) into mature, virgin B cells, which co-express IgM and IgD and can be found in the blood. The virgin B cells, upon antigen contact, differentiate into IgM-producing plasma cells or further mature into memory B cells that have undergone class switch and affinity maturation.

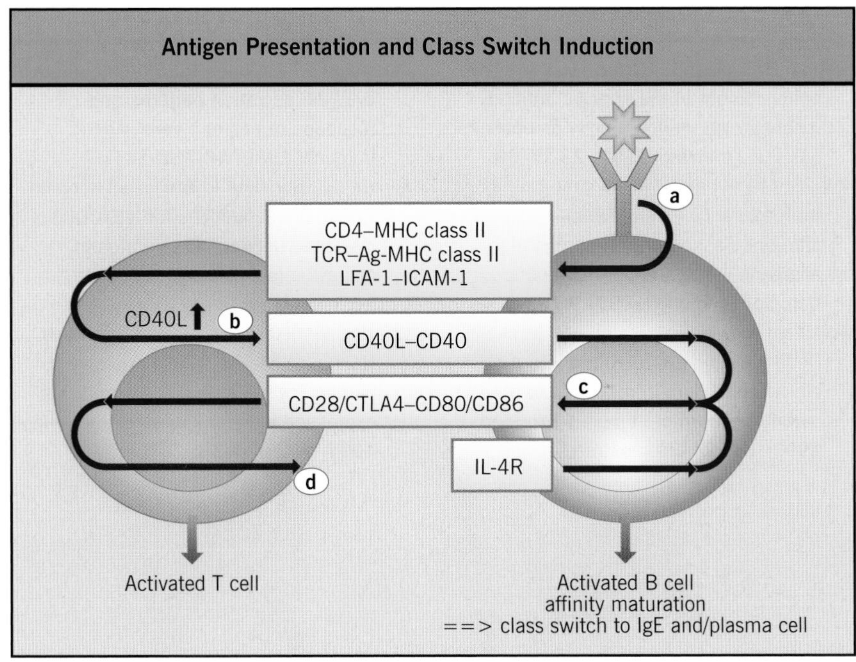

Fig. 19.28 (a) Antigen capture by B-cell receptor internalization and antigen processing of TCR-Ag recognition, CDR-class II, LFA-1–ICAM-1. (b) T cell upregulates the CD40 ligand, which binds to CD40 on the B cell. (c) B cell upregulates CD80 and CD86 binds to CD28 on the T cell. (d) T cell produces IL-4, which binds the IL-4 receptor on the B cell. LFA, lymphocyte function-associated; MHC, major histocompatibility complex; TCR, T-cell receptor.

upstream of the Cε locus. IL-4 and IL-13 signaling leads to the nuclear translocation of the DNA binding protein STAT6. STAT6 is the critical regulator of activation of the Iε promoter of the Cε gene. In rodents, IgE is co-regulated with IgG1, whereas in humans IgE and IgG4 occur together. The RNAs which are transcribed at this stage do not encode functional proteins and are hence referred to as 'germ line' or 'sterile' transcripts. However, the process of cytokine-driven germ line RNA transcription is critical to regulation of isotype switching. Completion of the isotype switch requires a second signal in addition to cytokines. This signal is provided by the interaction of CD40L on activated T cells with CD40 on the B cell. CD40 signaling induces the expression of activation-induced cytidine deaminase (AID). AID serves to recruit enzymes involved in DNA repair to sites of immunoglobulin germ line transcription. Double strand DNA breaks are subsequently introduced upstream of Cμ and upstream of the cytokine-activated, transcriptionally-activated CH locus targeted for switching. Intervening DNA is excised as a large loop and the remaining VDJ and CH segments annealed, resulting in the assembly of a new immunoglobulin heavy chain gene.

Overproduction of IgE leads to allergy. Effector cells such as mast cells, basophils and eosinophils are all triggered by IgE to release pathologic mediators. In addition, APCs use IgE to lower the threshold for antigen presentation, and B cells may use CD23/IgE-mediated antigen presentation to further drive immune responses to allergens. Therefore the production of IgE needs to be tightly controlled. In general, IgE synthesis is influenced primarily by the balance of positive (IL-4, IL-13) and negative (IL-12, IFNγ) influences of specific cytokines produced by T cells on Cε-directed isotype switching. Myriad host and environmental factors interact to define the cytokine profile of antigen-specific T cells. These include the nature of the antigen, exposure adjuvants (as when animals are artificially immunized), the route of entry of antigen, and the histocompatibility type of the individual.

Genetic predispositions towards allergy on the basis of enhanced production of IL-4 and/or IL-13 or impaired production of IFNγ are thought to account in part for the linkage of the allergic phenotype to the genetic loci encoding these cytokines. The induction of Th2 cells appears to be partly controlled at the level of DCs and there is functional heterogeneity among DCs with respect to the ability to induce Th1 versus Th2 T-helper responses. 'DC1s', which produce IL-12, favor the induction of Th1 responses whereas 'DC2s' preferentially stimulate Th2 responses. Microbial products may affect DC phenotype. Conserved microbial structures, which signal via the Toll-like receptor (TLR) family of receptors, can shift DC polarity. These receptors, which bind microbial lipid and polysaccharide structures, are conserved from *Drosophila* to humans, and are critical in the early 'innate' response to pathogens. DCs express a range of TLR family receptors and the specific effects of ligand binding by each of these receptors on DC phenotype remain to be worked out.

Although allergen-specific Th2 cells are a major source of IL-4 in allergic tissues, several other cell types can provide IL-4 and IL-13. Mast cells, which are abundant in the respiratory and gastrointestinal mucosa, are excellent producers of both IL-4 and IL-13. Natural killer (NK)1.1+ CD4+ T cells are another IL-4 source. These NK1.1+ cells express a very restricted repertoire of αβ T cell receptors and interact with the non-classical MHC class I molecule, CD1. NK cells may also provide IL-4 early in immune responses to allergens. Both cultured and freshly-isolated human NK cells have been shown to be differentiated to produce either IL-10 and IFNγ (NK1) or IL-5 and IL-13 (NK2), a polarity analogous to that observed in Th1 versus Th2 T-helper cells. In light of the strong association between asthma flares and viral respiratory infections, particularly early in life, the NK contribution to tissue cytokine levels may be important in regulating IgE responses.

FURTHER READING

Banchereau J, Bazan F, Blanchard D, et al. The CD40 antigen and its ligand. Annu Rev Immunol 1994; 12:881–922.

Bruijnzeel-Koomen CAFM, van Wichen DF, Toonstra J, et al. The presence of IgE molecules on epidermal Langerhans cells from patients with atopic dermatitis. Arch Dermatol Res 1986; 278:199–205.

Daëron M, Malbec O, Latour S, et al. Regulation of tyrosine-containing activation motif-dependent cell signalling by FcgammaRII. Immunol Lett 1995; 44:119–123.

Heyman B, Tianmin L, Gustavsson S. In-vivo enhancement of the specific antibody response via the low-affinity receptor for IgE. Eur J Immunol 1993; 23:17–39.

Holt PG, Macaubas C. Development of long term tolerance versus sensitisation to different classes of environmental allergens during the perinatal period. Curr Opin Immunol 1997; 9:782–787.

McWilliam A, Napoli S, Marsh AM, et al. Dendritic cells are recruited into the airway epithelium in response to a broad spectrum of stimuli. J Exp Med 1996; 184:24–29 (abstract).

Mosmann TR, Coffman RL. Heterogeneity of cytokine secretion patterns and functions of helper T cells. Adv Immunol 1989; 46:111–147.

Mudde GC, Bheekha R, Bruijnzeel-Koomen CAFM. Consequences for IgE/CD23 mediated antigen presentation in allergy. Immunol Today 199; 16:380–383.

Van den Herik-Oudijk IE, Westerdaal NAAC, Henriquez NV. Functional analysis of human FcgammaRII (CD32) isoforms expressed in B lymphocytes. J Immunol 1994; 152:574–585.

Chapter 20

Definition:

Cytokines are low-molecular-weight glycoprotein-signaling molecules, produced and released by a wide variety of cells, that mediate and regulate cell-to-cell communication, and are involved in cell growth and differentiation, inflammation, immunity and tissue repair.

Cytokines, Chemokines, and Adhesion Proteins

David H Broide

CYTOKINES

Introduction

Cytokines are extracellular signaling molecules which bind to specific cell surface cytokine receptors to regulate the immune and inflammatory response. They predominantly act on closely adjacent cells (the paracrine effect), but can also act on the cells of their origin (the autocrine effect), and occasionally on distant cells in another organ (the endocrine effect). Cytokines are involved in orchestrating the initiation and maintenance of the allergic inflammatory response. In allergic inflammation, cytokines are both active in the bone marrow where they regulate the development and differentiation of inflammatory cells [e.g. interleukin-5 (IL-5) induces eosinophilopoesis], and are also expressed at tissue sites of allergic inflammation (e.g. lower airway in asthma) where they regulate the immune and inflammatory response. Cytokines function through complex cytokine networks to promote or inhibit inflammation. During an inflammatory response the profile of cytokines expressed, as well as the profile of cytokine receptors expressed on responding cell types, will determine whether the response is predominantly pro- or anti-inflammatory. Activation of high-affinity cytokine receptors on target cells induces a cascade of intracellular signaling pathways which regulate the transcription of specific genes and the ultimate cellular inflammatory response. Considerable progress has been made in characterizing the cellular sources and actions of the numerous cytokines involved in allergic inflammation (Table 20.1). Overall, these studies suggest that cytokines exhibit redundancy (i.e. several cytokines can often subserve the same function), and that several cell types can generate or respond to the same cytokine. Thus, therapeutic strategies in allergic inflammation aimed at neutralizing a single cytokine may not always be successful if an alternate cytokine can subserve the same function. However, in rheumatoid arthritis, a disease associated with expression of multiple cytokines, neutralizing a single cytokine [e.g. tumor necrosis factor (TNF)] has resulted in a significant therapeutic benefit. Thus, in allergic inflammation an improved understanding of the mechanism through which cytokines promote allergic inflammation may identify key cytokine targets for therapeutic intervention.

Role of cytokines in the early life origins of allergy

Cytokines have an important role in controlling the functional maturation of the developing fetal immune system, conditioning it for participation in the postnatal

Table 20.1 Cytokines in allergic inflammation

Cytokine	Cell source	Gene	Actions
IL-1(IL-1α, IL-β)	Predominately monocytes, macrophages. Also smooth muscle, endothelium, epithelium	2q13-21	Activation of T cells and endothelial cells. Promotes B-cell proliferation
IL-2	Predominantly T cells. Also NK cells	4q26-27	Promotes T-cell proliferation and clonal expansion
IL-3	T cells, mast cells, eosinophils	5q23-31	Stimulates development of mast cells and basophils. Promotes eosinophil survival
IL-4	Predominantly T cells, and basophils	5q23-31	Promotes T-cell differentiation to Th2 phenotype. Promotes B-cell growth, differentiation, and class switching to IgE production. Promotes eosinophil recruitment by upregulation of VCAM-1 on endothelial cells
IL-5	T cells, eosinophils, mast cells	5q23-31	Promotes eosinophil growth, differentiation and survival
IL-6	Predominantly monocytes, macrophages. Also eosinophils, mast cells, fibroblasts	7p21	Differentiation of T cells into cytotoxic cells and B cells into plasma cells
IL-8	Predominantly macrophages. Also T cells, mast cells, endothelial cells, fibroblasts, neutrophils	4q12-13	Neutrophil activation and differentiation. Chemotactic factor for neutrophils
IL-9	T cells	5q31	Enhances mast-cell growth. Increases mucus expression
IL-10	T cells, B cells, macrophages, monocytes	1q31-32	Inhibits T-cell proliferation and downregulates pro-inflammatory cytokine production by Th1 and Th2 cells
IL-12	Predominantly monocytes, macrophages, dendritic cells	5q31	Inhibits Th2 development and cytokine expression. Suppresses IgE production. Promotes Th1 phenotype and IFNγ production
IL-13	Predominantly T cells Also mast cells, basophils, eosinophils	5q31	Promotes B-cell differentiation, proliferation, and class switching to IgE production. Promotes eosinophil accumulation by increased expression of VCAM-1 on endothelial cells
IL-16	Predominantly CD8 + T cells. Also mast cells, airway epithelium	15q26.1	Recruitment of CD4 + T cells and eosinophils
IL-18	Predominantly macrophages. Also airway epithelial cells	Not known	Activates B cells. Induces IFNγ, promoting Th1 phenotype
IL-25	Predominantly Th2 lymphocytes	–	Stimulates IL-4, IL-5 and IL-13 release from non-lymphoid accessory cell
GM-CSF	Macrophages, eosinophils, neutrophils, T cells, mast cells, airway epithelial cells	5q23-31	Priming of neutrophils and eosinophils. Prolongs survival of eosinophils
TNFα	Mast cells, macrophages, monocytes, epithelial cells	6	Upregulates endothelial adhesion molecule expression. Chemoattractant for neutrophils and monocytes
TGFβ_1	Eosinophils, macrophage, epithelium	–	Profibrotic effects, involved in airway remodeling. Chemotactic for monocytes, fibroblasts, and mast cells.
IFNγ	T cells, NK cells	12q	Suppression of Th2 cells. Inhibits B-cell switching to IgE. Increases ICAM-1 expression on endothelial and epithelial cells

GM-CSF, granulocyte–macrophage colony-stimulating factor; ICAM-1, intercellular adhesion molecule-1; IFNγ, interferon-γ; NK cells, natural killer cells; TGFβ_1, transforming growth factor β_1; TNFα, tumor necrosis factor α; VCAM-1, vascular cell adhesion molecule-1.

immune response to environmental allergens and pathogens. Thus, even in pregnancy, infancy, and early life, cytokines are considered to play an important role in determining the subsequent development of the atopic phenotype. During normal pregnancy the immune response deviates away from a helper T cell type 1 (Th1)-type cell-mediated immune response towards a Th2-type humoral-immune response to prevent rejection of the immunologically distinct fetal allograft. As a consequence of the enhanced Th2 cytokine milieu at the placental maternofetal interface, the fetal immune system in genetically predisposed atopic individuals may deviate towards a sustained Th2 response, predisposing to the later development of atopy.

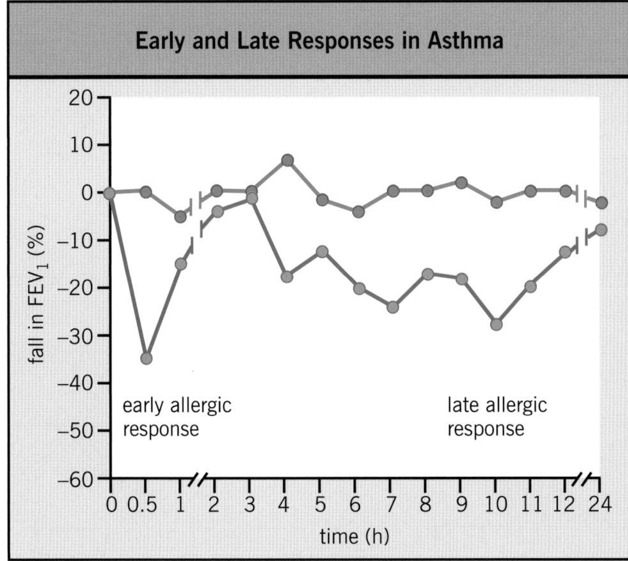

Fig. 20.1 Early and late phase responses in asthma. The asthmatic response to allergen inhalation challenge with house dust mite allergen (green line) and diluent control (red line), demonstrating both an early and a late phase allergic response. FEV_1, forced expiratory volume in 1 second.

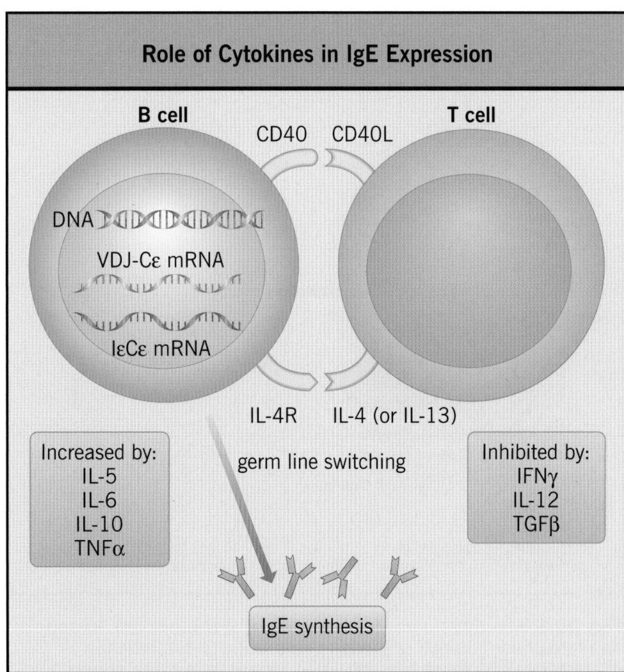

Fig. 20.2 Role of cytokines in IgE production. IεCε mRNA, germ line mRNA; VDJ-Cε mRNA, IgE mRNA. Following appropriate stimulation of the B cell with two signals (cytokine and co-stimulation), B cells can alter the isotype of the antibodies they produce to IgE. The first signal is provided by cytokines (IL-4 or IL-13); the second signal is provided by activation of CD40 on B cells. In this process, genomic DNA in the B cell is spliced and rejoined to juxtapose the VDJ elements of the antibody (which defines the antigenic specificity of the antibody) to the constant (C) region exons that encode the ε chain of IgE. As the intervening DNA between the VDJ region and the downstream C region exons is excised when they are joined, the mechanism is referred to as deletional switch recombination.

Environmental exposures in genetically predisposed individuals in early life (which predispose to Th1 or Th2 immune responses) may also determine the likelihood of the subsequent development of the atopic Th2 phenotype. These environmental immune modulating exposures include childhood infections, in utero and postnatal allergen exposure, pets, and exposure to indoor and outdoor pollution.

Cytokine regulation of IgE synthesis

The hallmark of the allergic response is the presence of increased levels of circulating allergen-specific IgE in atopic subjects. The triggering of high-affinity IgE receptors on the surface of mast cells results not only in the immediate release of histamine, tryptase, leukotrienes, and prostanoids manifesting as the early phase response (Fig. 20.1), but also triggers transcription and release of cytokines from mast cells. Mast cells also store cytokines such as TNF-α preformed in mast cell cytoplasmic granules. Triggering of mast cell IgE receptors rapidly releases this preformed TNF-α which is able to induce upregulation of adhesion molecules on endothelium and consequently contributes to recruitment of circulating leukocytes including eosinophils in the late phase reaction (LPR).

Cytokines such as IL-4 and IL-13 control IgE synthesis by regulating isotype class switching in B cells in the lymph nodes and spleen. Initially, all B cells produce IgM antibodies. Following appropriate stimulation of the B cell with two signals (cytokine and co-stimulation), B cells can alter the isotype of the antibodies they produce from IgM to IgE while retaining the antigenic specificity of the antibody. In the case of IgE, two types of signals induce this process in B cells: the first signal is provided by cytokines (IL-4 or IL-13); the second signal is provided by activation of CD40 on B cells. In this process, genomic DNA in the B cell is spliced and rejoined to juxtapose the VDJ elements of the antibody (which defines the antigenic specificity of the antibody) to the constant (C) region exons that encode the ε chain of IgE. As the intervening DNA between the VDJ region and the downstream C region exons is excised when they are joined, the mechanism is referred to as deletional switch recombination (Fig. 20.2).

While Th2 lymphocytes support B cell synthesis of IgE, other cells in addition to Th2 cells (e.g. basophils, mast cells, eosinophils) present at sites of allergic inflammation in vivo may also be involved in inducing B-cell synthesis of IgE. For example, basophils, mast cells, and eosinophils all express the molecules needed for inducing B cells to express IgE, namely IL-4 and CD40L. The presence in asthmatic airways of Th2 cells, B cells, and non-T cell populations capable of expressing IL-4 and CD40L suggests that this mechanism of IgE synthesis may also contribute to local mucosal IgE production.

The role of cytokines in the late phase allergic response

In allergic asthmatics the response to allergen inhalation is characterized by an immediate or early phase response (EPR) which is followed in approximately 50% of adults and 70% of children by a late phase response (LPR). The EPR is characterized by a fall in FEV_1 (forced expiratory volume in 1 second) which develops within approximately 10 minutes of allergen exposure, reaching a maximum at 30 minutes, and resolving within 1–2 hours. In the absence of further allergen inhalation, a LPR (characterized by a fall in $FEV_1 > 12\%$) may also occur, reaching a maximum at 6–12 hours and resolving by 24 hours

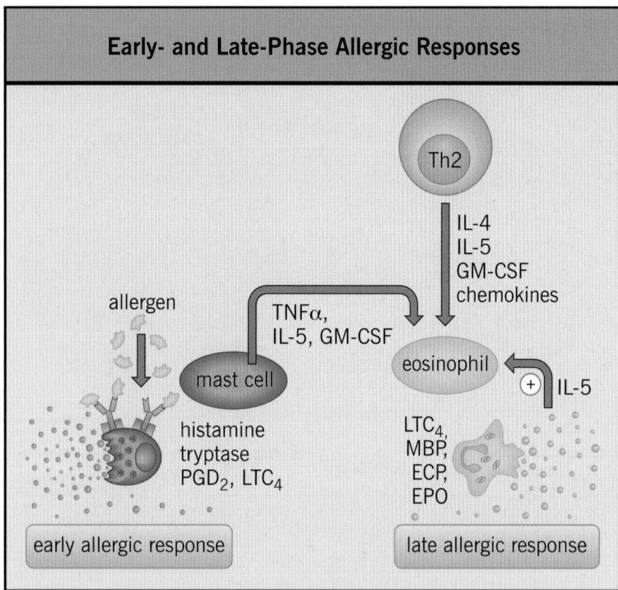

Fig. 20.3 Inflammatory cells, cytokines, and chemokines in early and late-phase allergic responses. The early phase reaction is characterized by mast cell activation, whereas the late phase reaction is characterized by activation of Th2 cells and eosinophils.

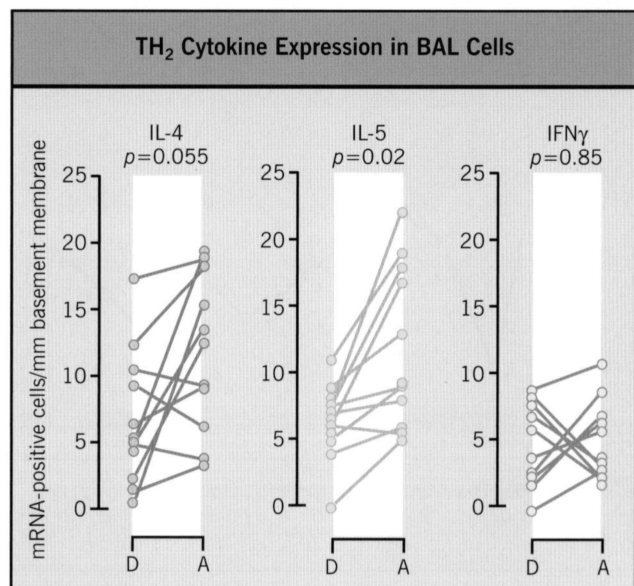

Fig. 20.4 Cytokine mRNA expression in bronchoalveolar lavage (BAL) cells. The BAL cells, were obtained from atopic asthmatic subjects, who had been either challenged with allergen (A) or with diluent (D) (control). (Modified from Bentley AM, Kay AB, Durham SR. Human late asthmatic reactions. Clin Exp Allergy 1997; 27(suppl 1):71–86, Blackwell Science Ltd.)

(Fig. 20.1). The EPR results from IgE-dependent activation of mast cells which release preformed mediators including histamine, as well as newly generated lipid mediators including leukotrienes (LTC_4, LTD_4, and LTE_4), and prostanoids [prostaglandins D_2, $F_{2\alpha}$ (PGD_2, $PGF_{2\alpha}$) and thromboxane A_2 (TXA_2)] (Fig. 20.3). A characteristic feature of the LPR in asthma is the infiltration of the airways with inflammatory cells, particularly eosinophils, as well as CD4+ Th2 cells, mononuclear cells, and basophils. These inflammatory cells recruited from the circulation release cytokines and proinflammatory mediators in the airway which contribute to mucus expression, epithelial damage, and associated bronchial hyperresponsiveness (BHR). Studies using allergen inhalation challenge in asthmatics have shown an increased number of activated CD4+ Th2 cells and eosinophils in bronchial biopsies after allergen challenge (Fig. 20.4). The profile of cytokines released during the LPR is characterized by the expression of Th2 cytokines (IL-4, IL-5, IL-9, IL-13) rather than Th1 cytokines [interferon γ (IFN-γ), IL-12]. Several cells contribute to IL-5 expression in the airway in asthma including T cells and eosinophils. Corticosteroids have an inhibitory effect on the LPR and also reduce the number of cells expressing IL-4 mRNA and IL-5 mRNA, and the number of eosinophils in BAL and bronchial biopsies.

Cytokines play a key role in the recruitment of inflammatory cells involved in the LPR by upregulating adhesion molecule expression on the surface of endothelial cells. Endothelial cells in blood vessels in the lung do not constitutively express adhesion molecules, and thus under normal conditions of blood flow circulating leukocytes do not adhere to the lumenal surface of the blood vessel. However, within minutes to one hour following allergen inhalation preformed cytokines (e.g. TNF-α) and histamine stored in mast cell granules are released and promote lung vascular endothelial adhesion molecule expression [P-, and E-selectin, vascular cell adhesion molecule-1 (VCAM-1), and intercellular adhesion molecule-1 (ICAM-1)]. Subsequent expression of cytokine transcripts (IL-4, IL-13, TNF-α) by resident lung cells (mast cells, macrophages) as well as by recruited leukocytes (T cells, eosinophils, basophils) also contributes to continued expression of cytokines which further upregulate adhesion molecule expression by endothelium. While TNF-α upregulates expression of several endothelial expressed adhesion molecules (P-, and E-selectin, VCAM-1, and ICAM-1), IL-4 and IL-13 have a more restricted effect on endothelial adhesion molecule expression, upregulating only VCAM-1 expression.

The Th1–Th2 cytokine paradigm and allergic inflammation

CD4+ T cells have been classified in the mouse into functionally distinct Th1 or Th2 subsets on the basis of distinct cytokine profiles expressed by each subset (Table 20.2). Th1 cells play a prominent role in cellular immunity by expressing cytokines which promote the development of cytotoxic T cells and macrophages (e.g. IFN-γ, IL-2, and TNF-β), while Th2 cells promote humoral immune responses. Th2 cells express cytokines which regulate IgE synthesis (IL-4), eosinophil proliferation (IL-5), mast cell proliferation (IL-9), and airway hyperreactivity (IL-13). A Th2 pattern of cytokine expression is noted in allergic inflammation and in parasitic infections, conditions both associated with IgE production and eosinophilia. While Th1/Th2 polarization is clear-cut in murine models, the situation is not so clear-cut for human T-cell subsets, which can secrete a mixed pattern of cytokines (Table 20.2). Thus, Th1 and Th2 cells are not two distinct CD4+ T-cell subsets, but rather represent polarized forms of the highly heterogenous CD4+ Th cell-mediated immune response.

The cytokine environment encountered by a naïve T cell plays a prominent role in determining whether that naïve T cell develops into a Th1 or Th2 cell. Thus, the same naïve Th cell

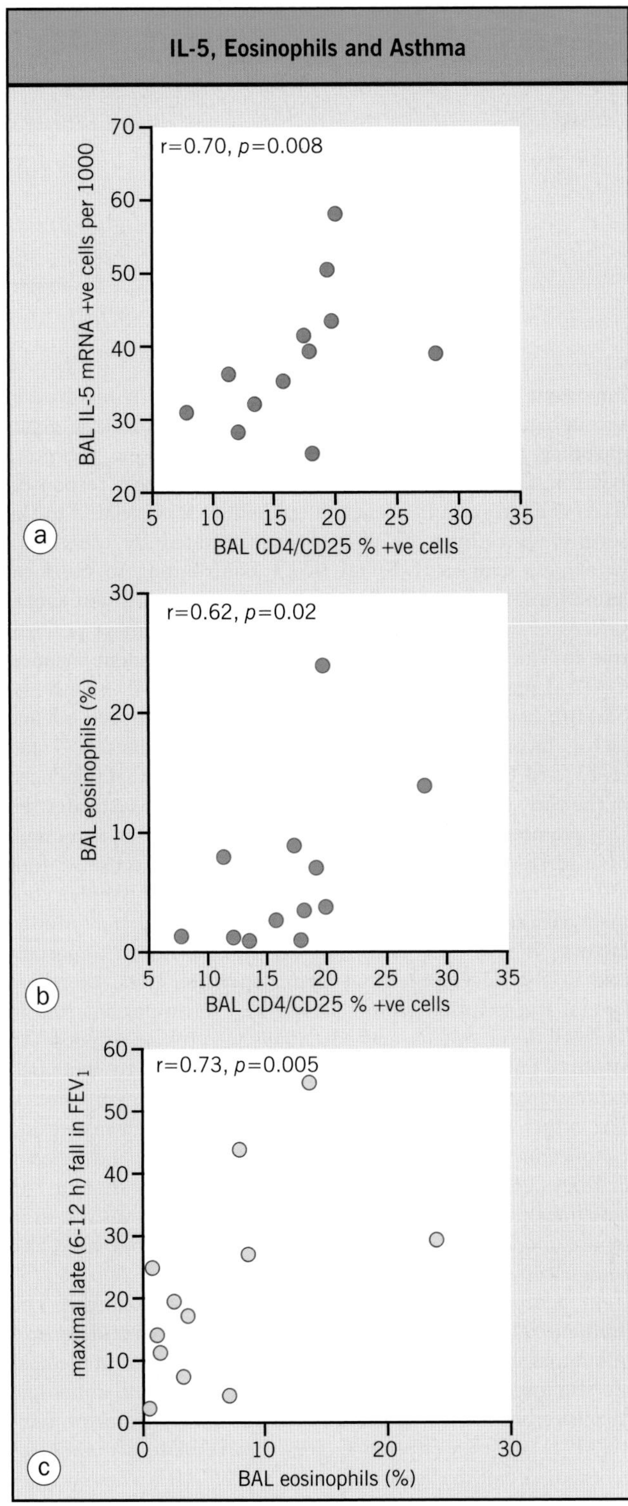

Fig. 20.5 Interleukin-5 (IL-5), eosinophils and asthma. Significant relationships are shown between numbers of BAL-fluid-activated (a) CD4+ cells and IL-5 mRNA +ve cells, as well as between (b) CD4+ cells and BAL eosinophils. The percentage of BAL eosinophils also correlated with the late phase fall in FEV_1 24 hours after allergen challenge in sensitized asthmatics (c). BAL, bronchoalveolar lavage; FEV_1, forced expiratory volume in 1 second. (Modified from Robinson DS, Hamid Q, Bentley A, et al. Activation of CD4+ T cells increased TH2-type cytokine mRNA expression, and eosinophil recruitment in bronchoalveolar lavage after allergen inhalation challenge in patients with atopic asthma. J Allergy Clin Immunol 1993; 92:313–324.)

Table 20.2 Cytokine production by murine and human T cell clones of Th1 and Th2 types

Cytokine Production by Murine and Human T-cell Clones			
	Th1 type	**Th2 type**	**Th1 and Th2 types**
Murine	IFNγ IL-2 TNFβ	IL-4 IL-5 IL-9	IL-3 IL-13 GM-CSF TNFα
Human	IFNγ IL-2 TNFβ	IL-4 IL-5 IL-9	IL-3 IL-6 IL-10 IL-13 GM-CSF TNFα

GM-CSF, granulocyte–macrophage colony-stimulating factor; IFN, interferon; IL, interleukin; TNF, tumor necrosis factor.

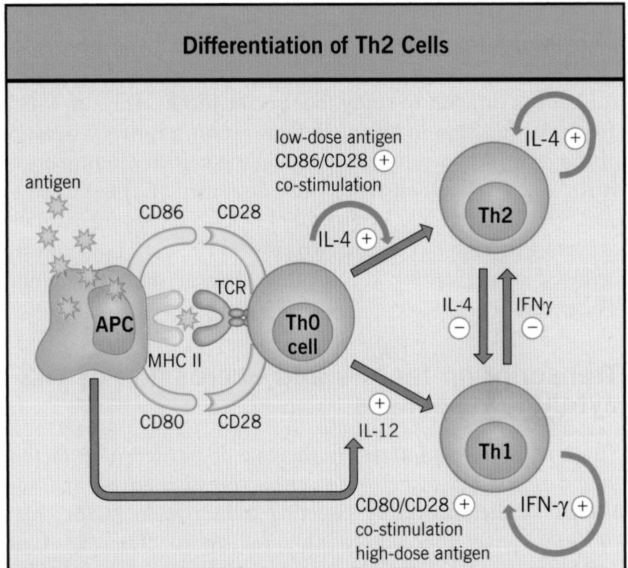

Fig. 20.6 Factors involved in the differentiation of Th2-type CD4+ cells. The cytokine mileu (IL-4 vs IFN-γ), as well as the dose of antigen (high vs low), influence differentiation of Th0 cells to Th1 vs Th2 cells.

can give rise to either Th1 or Th2 cells under the influence of both environmental (e.g. cytokine) and genetic factors acting at the level of antigen presentation. In particular cytokines such as IL-4 play a prominent role in deviating naïve T cells to develop into Th2 cells, whereas IFN-γ and IL-12 are important in the development of Th1 cells. In addition to the local cytokine environment, the level of antigen-induced activation of the T-cell receptor (high versus low dose antigen), the delivery of co-stimulatory signals from the antigen-presenting cell (APC), and the number of post-activation cell divisions influence the development of Th1 versus Th2 cells (Fig. 20.6). While the source of IL-4 that is likely to be responsible for deviating naïve T cells to Th2 cells at the beginning of the allergic immune response is not completely understood, several cell types are candidates for being the source of IL-4 including naïve Th cells themselves, mast cells, basophils, eosinophils, and natural killer (NK)1.1+ T cells.

A large number of studies have supported the hypothesis that Th2-type responses are involved in the pathogenesis of several allergic diseases including atopic asthma, allergic rhinitis, and atopic dermatitis. However, there are still aspects of this paradigm that require further investigation. For example, in mouse models of asthma, adoptive transfer of antigen specific Th1 cells aggravates airway inflammation and airway responsiveness, while in humans with asthma, administration of Th1 cytokines (IFN-γ or IL-12) does not reduce airway responsiveness.

T regulatory cytokines and allergy

The term regulatory T cell (Treg) refers to cells that actively control or suppress the function of other cells, generally in an inhibitory fashion. Thus in allergic inflammation Treg cells which suppress the function of Th2 cells may have an important role in limiting allergic responses. For example, allergen immunotherapy induces Treg cells which express cytokines [IL-10, transforming growth factor β (TGFβ)] that can downregulate the allergic inflammatory response. Thus, one potential mechanism through which immunotherapy is hypothesized to be effective in allergic rhinitis is through induction of Treg cells. It has been difficult to study the specific mechanisms by which Treg cells function in allergic inflammation, primarily because of the difficulty in culturing these cells in sufficient numbers in vitro. Several Treg cells have been described (CD4+CD25+, Th3, TR1, TR, and NK T cells). CD4+CD25+ cells are naturally occurring regulatory cells that express IL-10, and TGFβ and are involved in preventing autoimmune disease, and also inhibit Th2 responses.

Transcription factors and expression of Th2 cytokine responses

There is increasing interest in the role of transcription factors in the regulation of cytokine gene expression in asthma and allergy, as therapeutically targeting transcription factors may provide a novel approach to inhibiting the function of several cytokines important to the genesis of allergic inflammation. Transcription factors are intracellular signaling proteins that bind to regulatory sequences of target genes, resulting in the promotion (transactivation) or suppression (transrepression) of gene transcription, with resultant effects on subsequent cytokine mRNA and protein production. Transcriptional control of genes involved in allergic inflammatory responses is mediated by several classes of signal-dependent transcription factors which can be categorized according to their structure. Several transcription factors are important in mediating Th2 immune responses [STAT-6, GATA-3, c-MAF, nuclear factor of activated T cells (NF-ATc)], while additional transcription factors are important in mediating Th1 immune responses (STAT-4, T-bet) (Table 20.3). The importance of these transcription factors to Th2 immune responses has been demonstrated in vitro in investigations of Th2 cell development, and in vivo assessing Th2 responses using mice deficient in these transcription factors. In addition, immunohistochemical studies have demonstrated expression of these Th2 promoting transcription factors in the airway in asthma. How might these individual transcription factors be important to Th2 responses in asthma? STAT-6 is involved in the upregulation of IL-4-dependent genes, such as the genes encoding the IL-4 receptor, IgE, and chemokine receptors (CCR4, CCR8), which play key roles in allergic responses. STAT-6 expression in bronchial epithelium is correlated to the severity of asthma. STAT-6 is also activated by other Th2 cytokines, such as IL-5 and IL-13, contributing to the local amplification of the Th2 response. The transcription factor GATA-3 is selectively expressed in Th2 cells and plays a critical role in Th2 differentiation in a STAT-6-independent manner. GATA-3 regulates the transcription of IL-4 and IL-5, and like STAT-6, has been suggested to act as a chromatin-remodeling factor, favoring the transcription of Th2 cytokines IL-4 and IL-13. c-MAF is a Th2-specific transcription factor that is induced in the early events of Th2 differentiation and transactivates the IL-4 promoter. Asthmatic patients display an increased expression of c-MAF. The NF-AT transcription factors comprise four different members which are expressed in T and B lymphocytes, mast cells, and natural killer cells. One of the NF-AT transcription factors NF-ATc (also known as NF-AT2) plays an important role in the development of Th2 responses. Thus, there are several transcription factors which play an important role in Th2 cell development, and potentially in cytokine responses in asthma. Enhanced Th2 responses can be due to increased expression of transcription factors which regulate expression of Th2 cytokines, or alternately due to deficiencies in transcription factors which regulate Th1 responses. For example, a deficiency in T-bet (a transcription factor that regulates expression of Th1 cytokines) is associated with increased airway responsiveness in mouse models of asthma. Reduced levels of T-bet have also been noted in the airway of human asthmatics.

Table 20.3 Transcription factors involved in the regulation of Th1 and Th2 responses

Th1	Th2
STAT-4	STAT-6
T-bet	c-MAF
	GATA-3
	NF-ATc

In addition to transcription factors which regulate Th2 immune responses, transcription factors which regulate pro-inflammatory cytokines, chemokines, and adhesion molecules are also important potential regulators of allergic inflammation. In this regard nuclear factor κB (NF-κB) and activator protein-1 (AP-1) are transcription factors that regulate a number of genes important to allergic inflammation. NF-κB is a heterodimer consisting of two subunits (usually p65 and p50), although other dimer forms exist. In resting cells NF-κB is in an inactive form in the cytoplasm bound to the regulatory subunit inhibitory κB protein (IκB), which covers its nuclear localization signals. Upon cell activation, the inhibitory protein I-κB is phosphorylated and degraded, a process that allows freed NF-κB to rapidly enter the nucleus, where its subunits can bind to κB motifs located on promoters of specific genes (Fig. 20.7). NF-κB plays an important role in the regulation of genes involved in allergic inflammation, such as those encoding inflammatory cytokines, chemokines, adhesion receptors, enzymes, and inducible nitric

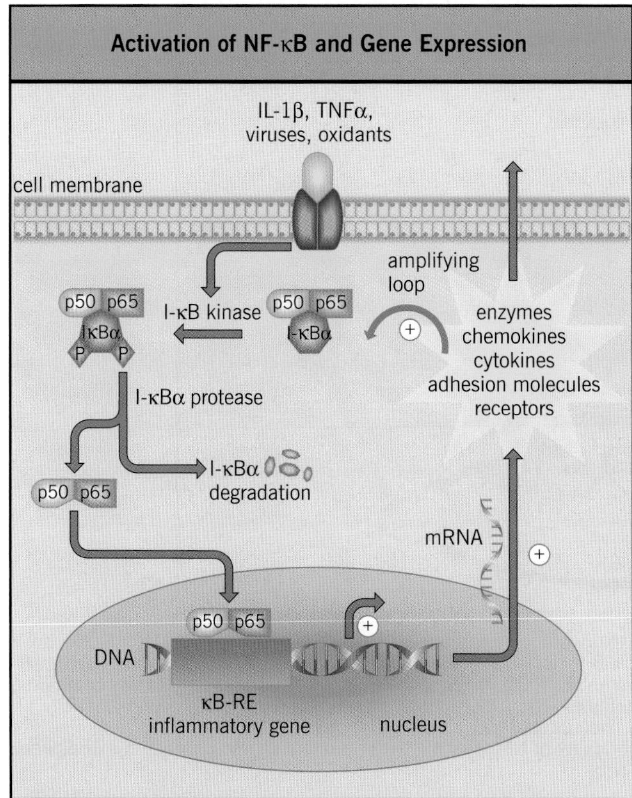

Fig. 20.7 Activation of nuclear factor κB. NF-κB is a heterodimer consisting of two subunits (usually p65 and p50). In resting cells NF-κB is in an inactive form in the cytoplasm bound to the regulatory subunit inhibitory κB protein (IκB), which covers its nuclear localization signals. Upon cell activation (e.g. TNF-α, viruses, etc) the inhibitory protein IκB is phosphorylated by IκB kinase and degraded, a process that allows freed NF-κB to rapidly enter the nucleus, where its subunits can bind to κB motifs located on promoters of specific genes.

Table 20.4 Nuclear factor κB (NF-κB) regulation of gene expression

NF-κB Regulation of Gene Expression	
Pro-inflammatory cytokines	TNFα IL-1β IL-2 IL-6 GM-CSF G-CSF M-CSF
Chemokines	IL-8 MIP-1α MCP-1 Gro-α, -β, -γ Eotaxin RANTES
Adhesion molecules	ICAM-1 VCAM -1 E-selectin
Receptors	IL-2R (α chain) T-cell receptor (β chain)
Inflammatory enzymes	Inducible nitric oxide synthase (iNOS) 5-lipoxygenase Inducible cyclooxygenase-2 (COX-2) Cytosolic phospholipase-A_2

G-CSF granulocyte colony-stimulating factor; GM-CSF, granulocyte–macrophage colony-stimulating factor; ICAM-1, intercellular adhesion molecule-1; IL, interleukin; MCP, monocyte chemotactic protein; M-CSF, macrophage colony-stimulating factor; MIP, macrophage inflammatory protein. TNF, tumor necrosis factor; VCAM-1, vascular cell adhesion molecule-1.

oxide synthase (Table 20.4). Many stimuli encountered in the airway in asthma, including cytokines (IL-1β, TNFα), viruses, and oxidants can activate transcription factors such as NF-κB.

Corticosteroids and cytokine expression

Corticosteroids are our most effective therapy in allergic inflammation and asthma. Therefore an improved understanding of the mechanism of action of corticosteroids may provide important insight into how they regulate cytokine production and inhibit allergic inflammation. Glucocorticoids act by binding to a glucocorticoid receptor (GR) in the cytoplasm which then rapidly translocates into the nucleus (Fig. 20.8). Within the nucleus, the glucocorticoid and GR complex bind as a dimer to specific glucocorticoid response elements present in DNA within the promoter region of glucocorticoid-responsive genes. The binding of the glucocorticoid and GR complex to negative glucocorticoid response elements (nGREs) or positive ones (pGREs) in the nucleus inhibits or promotes gene transcription (Fig. 20.8). Corticosteroids may also inhibit the activation of NF-κB via a direct interaction between the activated GR and the p65 subunit of NF-κB. In T cells and monocytes, glucocorticoids have also been shown to increase gene transcription for I-κB, which binds to activated NF-κB in the nucleus and induces the dissociation of NF-κB from κB binding sites on target genes.

Corticosteroid regulation of histone acetylation may also be a key mechanism of action of corticosteroids in regulating gene expression. Acetylation of core histones around which DNA is wound in the nucleus of cells opens up the chromatin structure allowing gene transcription and synthesis of genes, including cytokine genes, to proceed. Glucocorticoids inhibit transcription factors, such as AP-1 as well as NF-κB, from activating their target genes by inhibition of acetylation of specific lysine residues in histone H4 in the nucleus, which keeps the chromatin structure closed and prevents gene transcription. As increased gene transcription is associated with an increase in histone acetylation, whereas hypoacetylation is correlated with reduced transcription or gene silencing, corticosteroid regulation of histone acetylation may be a key mechanism of action of corticosteroids in regulating gene expression. An improved understanding of the mechanisms of action of corticosteroids may lead to the development of novel therapeutic agents in allergic inflammation.

Cytokine modulation as a therapeutic strategy in allergic inflammation

Corticosteroids are effective therapeutic agents for allergic inflammatory diseases. They exert several anti-inflammatory effects which may account for their beneficial effect in allergic

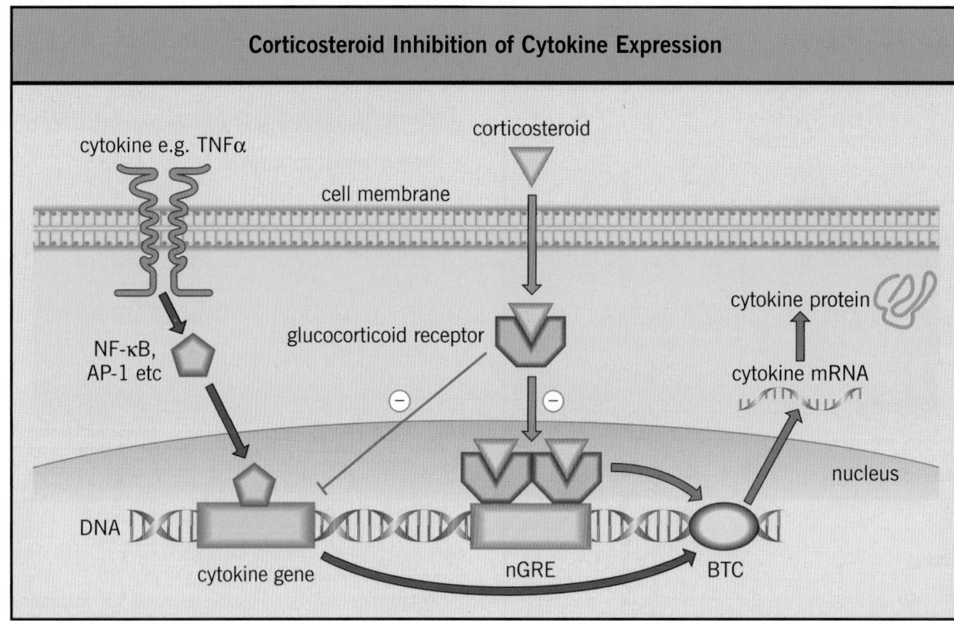

Fig. 20.8 Mechanisms by which corticosteroids inhibit cytokine action. Cytokines such as tumor necrosis factor (TNF-α) bind to specific cell surface cytokine receptors which activate transcription factors such as nuclear factor κB (NF-κB) or activator protein-1 (AP-1). The transcription factor translocates from the cytoplasm to the nucleus and binds to the promoter region of responsive genes. This stimulates transcription of cytokines or other genes following recruitment of the basal transcription complex (BTC). Corticosteroids inhibit gene expression by initially binding to a cytoplasmic glucocorticoid receptor which translocates to the nucleus and binds either to a negative glucocorticoid response element (nGRE) in the promoter of the cytokine gene, or directly blocks the ability of NF-κB or AP-1 from enhancing cytokine gene expression. GR, glucocorticoid receptor; nGRE, negative glucocorticoid response element.

inflammation, including downregulating the expression of transcription factors (e.g. NF-κB), and Th2 cytokines (IL-4, IL-5, and IL-13) important to allergic inflammation. However, a proportion of asthmatics are not well controlled on corticosteroid treatment, or develop significant side-effects, prompting a search for more selective therapies, including therapies that modulate cytokine expression. Therapeutic options to inhibit cytokines include drugs that inhibit cytokine synthesis (e.g. ciclosporin or tacrolimus); blocking antibodies to cytokines or their receptors; soluble cytokine receptors; cytokine receptor antagonists; inhibitors of cytokine signal transduction; inhibitors of transcription pathways used by cytokines; and treatment with anti-inflammatory cytokines (Fig. 20.9). Many of these approaches have been tested in animal models of asthma and several have started to be tested in humans with asthma.

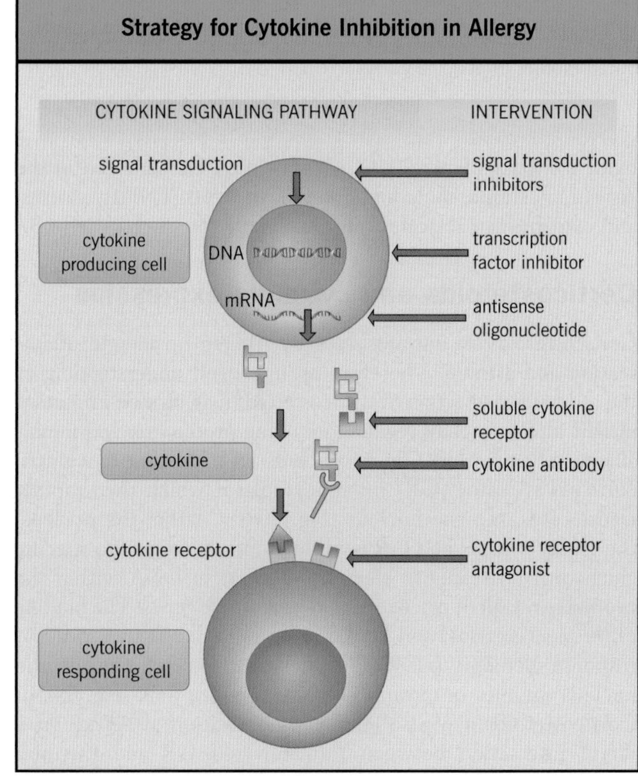

Fig. 20.9 A strategy for cytokine inhibition in allergy. Inhibition of cytokines can either be accomplished by targeting the cytokine producing cell, the extracellulary released cytokine, or the target cell responding to the cytokine.

Cytokine IL-1

Increased levels of IL-1 are detected in the airway of symptomatic asthmatics. IL-1 upregulates adhesion molecule expression on endothelium and thus indirectly promotes circulating leukocyte recruitment to tissues. The IL-1 receptor antagonist (IL-1ra) binds to IL-1 receptors and inhibits the action of IL-1. IL-1ra has been shown to reduce BHR in animal models of asthma, but clinical trials of a humanized IL-1ra have thus far proved disappointing.

Cytokine IL-4

IL-4 plays a central role in regulating IgE production, adhesion molecule expression, and development of Th2-cells. IL-4 receptor blockade has been shown to inhibit IgE production, BHR, and airway eosinophilia in mouse models of asthma, prompting the development of anti-IL-4 receptor antagonists. While initial small-scale studies of a soluble IL-4 receptor antagonist showed promise in the treatment of asthma, subsequent large-scale studies did not demonstrate a clinical benefit in asthmatics of moderate severity.

Cytokine IL-5

IL-5 is an important lineage specific eosinophil growth factor which is expressed at increased levels in the airways of asthmatics. In asthmatics an anti-IL-5 antibody significantly inhibits blood and sputum eosinophilia by over 90%, but only reduces airway eosinophils by approximately 55%. In mild asthmatics anti-IL-5 did not reduce the LPR or airway responsiveness to methacholine. Subsequent studies have demonstrated that anti-IL-5 reduces levels of airway remodeling in asthmatics. Treating asthmatics with an anti-IL-5 antibody significantly reduced the expression of extracellular matrix proteins (tenascin, lumican), and procollagen III in the bronchial mucosal reticular basement membrane. In addition, anti-IL-5 treatment was associated with a significant reduction in the number of airway eosinophils expressing mRNA for TGF-β_1 and the concentration of TGF-β_1 in bronchoalveolar lavage fluid. Thus, further studies will help to define whether anti-IL-5 alone and/or in combination with another eosinophil depleting agent (e.g. anti-CCR-3) will have any role in the treatment of asthma.

Cytokine IL-9

In animal models of asthma IL-9 appears to be important in mediating mucus secretion. Increased levels of mucus and IL-9 are noted in bronchial biopsies in asthma. At present there are no published studies of IL-9 inhibitors in human asthma.

Cytokine IL-10

IL-10 is an anti-inflammatory cytokine for both Th1- and Th2-type immune responses and inhibits the synthesis of many inflammatory proteins, including cytokines [TNF, granulocyte–macrophage colony-stimulating factor (GM-CSF), IL-5, chemokines] and inflammatory enzymes [inducible nitric oxide synthase (iNOS)] that are overexpressed in asthma. Recombinant human IL-10 has proved to be effective in controlling inflammatory bowel disease and psoriasis, and may be given as a weekly injection. Although IL-10 is reasonably well tolerated, there are potential hematologic side-effects. Results of IL-10 therapy in asthma are not currently available.

Cytokine IL-12

IL-12 has important functions in promoting Th1 immune responses. IL-12 inhibits allergen-induced IgE production, BHR, airway eosinophilia, and Th2 expression (IL-4, IL-5) in mouse models of asthma. In patients with mild asthma, weekly infusions of human recombinant IL-12 for 1 month caused a progressive fall in blood eosinophils (approx. 85% decrease), and blunted the normal rise in circulating eosinophils after allergen challenge. There was a concomitant reduction in eosinophils in induced sputum (approx. 55%). However, there was no reduction in either EPR or LPR to inhaled allergen challenge or any reduction in BHR. Furthermore, most of the patients suffered from malaise and one out of the 12 subjects had an episode of cardiac arrhythmia. This suggests that IL-12 may not be a suitable treatment for asthma.

Cytokine IL-13

Studies in animal models of asthma suggest an important role for IL-13 in mediating airway hyperresponsiveness (AHR). Clinical trials in human asthma are currently evaluating whether inhibiting IL-13 will be of clinical utility.

Cytokine TNF-α

Increased levels of TNF-α are detected in the airway of symptomatic asthmatics. As patients with rheumatoid arthritis have shown a dramatic clinical response when treated with either soluble TNF receptor antagonists or with anti-TNF antibodies, studies are currently evaluating their potential role in the treatment of asthma.

Cytokine IFN-γ

IFN-γ has been shown to have an inhibitory activity on Th2 responses. Exogenous IFN-γ administration prevents allergen-induced airway eosinophil infiltration in mice. However, administration of IFN-γ to asthmatics or patients with allergic rhinitis has resulted in no significant clinical improvement.

CHEMOKINES

Definition: Chemokines are a group of structurally related cytokine proteins of low molecular weight (8–10 kDa), expressed by a wide variety of cell types and tissues, that induce activation and the directed migration of specific leukocyte subsets to sites of inflammation.

Introduction

The chemokines are a large family of chemotactic cytokines that have been divided into four groups, designated CXC, CC, C, and CXXXC (or CX3C), depending on the spacing of conserved cysteines (C is cysteine; X is any amino acid). Over 50 different chemokines are now recognized and many of these chemokines are involved in the recruitment of inflammatory cells from the circulation in asthma. The CC chemokines (Table 20.5) target a variety of cell types important to allergic inflammation including eosinophils, basophils, lymphocytes, macrophages, and dendritic cells, whereas the CXC chemokines mainly target neutrophils and mononuclear cells.

Many of the stimuli for secretion of chemokines are the early signals elicited during innate immune responses. For example, bacterial products [such as lipopolysaccharide (LPS)], viral infection, and pro-inflammatory cytokines (such as IL-1 and TNFα) induce expression of a variety of chemokines. Chemokines are induced rapidly (i.e. within 1 hour) by these triggers and provide an important link between early innate immune responses and adaptive immunity (by recruiting and activating T cells) (Table 20.6). Chemokines are produced by a variety of cells in the lung in asthma especially structural cells such as epithelium, as well as recruited inflammatory cells (monocytes, lymphocytes) (Table 20.6). The chemokine gradient

Table 20.5 CC chemokines and CC receptors to which they bind

CC Chemokine (CCL 1-27)	Corresponding Chemokine Receptors (CCR 1-10)
CCL1 (or I-309)	CCR 8
CCL2 (MCP-1)	CCR 2
CCL3 (MIP-1α)	CCR 1, 5
CCL4 (MIP-1β)	CCR 5
CCL5 (RANTES)	CCR 1, 3, 5
CCL6 (Unknown)	Unknown
CCL7(MCP-3)	CCR 1, 2, 3
CCL8(MCP-2)	CCR 3
CCL9 (Unknown)	Unknown
CCL10 (Unknown)	Unknown
CCL11 (Eotaxin-1)	CCR 3
CCL12 (Unknown)	CCR 2
CCL13 (MCP-4)	CCR 2, 4
CCL14 (HCC-1)	CCR 1
CCL15 (HCC-2)	CCR 1, 3
CCL16 (HCC-4)	CCR 1
CCL17 (TARC)	CCR 4
CCL18 (PARC)	Unknown
CCL19 (ELC)	CCR 7
CCL20 (LARC)	CCR 6
CCL21 (SLC)	CCR 7
CCL22 (MDC)	CCR 4
CCL23 (MPIF 1)	CCR 1
CCL24 (eotaxin-2)	CCR 3
CCL25 (TECK)	CCR 9
CCL26 (eotaxin-3)	CCR 3
CCL27 (CTAP)	CCR 10

CCL, CC chemokine ligand; CCR, CC chemokine receptor; MCP, monocyte chemotactic protein; MIP, macrophage inflammatory protein; HCC, hemofiltrate derived CC chemokine; RANTES, regulated on activation normal T cell expressed and secreted.

from the airway epithelium (high concentration of chemokine) to the blood vessel (lower concentration of chemokine) assists in directing the migration of extravascular leukocytes to the epithelium (Fig. 20.10). Chemokines also play a role in activation-dependent adhesion of circulating leukocytes to endothelium. In the vascular lumen, chemokines presented by endothelial cells bind to chemokine receptors on circulating leukocytes when the leukocytes are tethering to the endothelium. This binding of chemokines to chemokine receptors on the tethering leukocyte induces a rapid change in affinity of integrin adhesion receptors on the circulating leukocyte. This change in leukocyte integrin affinity from a low affinity to a high-affinity integrin binding state leads to tight adherence of the leukocyte to endothelium and subsequent leukocyte extravasation. Once the leukocyte extravasates between endothelial cells into the extracellular space, the chemokine concentration gradient promotes directed cell migration to the site of inflammation.

While chemokines play a primary role in mediating leukocyte chemotaxis in tissues, several chemokines also have a number of other functions including antiviral activity, as well as modulating effects on the control of hematopoiesis, angiogenesis, cell growth, and metabolism. Chemokines including eotaxin, monocyte chemotactic protein (MCP-1, -2, and -3), macrophage inflammatory protein-1α (MIP-1α) and RANTES can promote histamine release by an IgE-independent mechanism. RANTES also promotes eosinophil activation for mediator release.

Chemokine receptors

Chemokine receptors (currently 20 known) belong to the seven transmembrane receptor superfamily of G-protein-coupled receptors. Ten human CC chemokine receptor genes (they are known as CCR1 through CCR10) (Table 20.5), and six CXCR receptors have been identified (they are referred to as CXCR1 through CXCR6). The CCR are expressed on macrophages, eosinophils, basophils, and dendritic cells, whereas the CXCR are expressed mainly on neutrophils and lymphocytes. Chemokine receptors are for the most part inhibited by pertussis toxin, which indicates that they are primarily coupled to Gi proteins. Activation of chemokine cell surface receptors by specific chemokines results in activation of a cascade of intracellular signaling pathways, including guanosine triphosphate-binding proteins of the Ras and Rho families, leading ultimately to the formation of cell surface protrusions termed uropods and lamellipods, which are required for cellular locomotion. Some chemokine receptors are expressed only on certain cell types, whereas other chemokine receptors are more widely expressed. In addition, some chemokine receptors are expressed constitutively while others are expressed only after cell activation. For example, CCR1 and CCR2 are constitutively expressed on monocytes but are expressed on lymphocytes only after IL-2 stimulation. A given leukocyte often expresses multiple chemokine receptors, and more than one chemokine typically binds to the same receptor. Examples of chemokine receptor expression by circulating cells important to allergic inflammation include: eosinophils which express the CC chemokine receptors CCR1 and CCR3; basophils which express CCR1, CCR2, and CCR3; and monocytes which express CCR1, CCR2, CCR5, and CCR8 (Fig. 20.11). In addition to expression of CC chemokine receptors, eosinophils, basophils, and mononuclear cells express the CXC chemokine receptor CXCR4 which is also expressed on neutrophils. The ligand for CXCR4 is the CXC chemokine SDF-1 (stromal cell derived factor-1). In the tissues eosinophils express additional CC receptors (CCR2, CCR4, CCR5) which are not expressed on circulating eosinophils (Fig. 20.11). Subsets of T cells can also be distinguished based on their profile of expression of CCR and CXCR. For example, Th1 cells express CCR5, CXCR3, and CXCR6, whereas Th2 cells express CCR3, CCR4, and CCR8 (Fig. 20.12).

CC chemokines and allergic inflammation

As CC chemokines are expressed at sites of allergic inflammation and attract cells important to the perpetuation of the allergic inflammatory response (e.g. eosinophils, basophils, monocytes, and lymphocytes), they have received increasing

Table 20.6 Cell sources of chemokines

Cell Sources of Chemokines	
Cells of origin	**Chemokine**
Monocytes	IL-8, Gro-α, -β, -γ, MCP-1, MCP-2, MIP-1α
Lymphocytes	RANTES; I-309; MIP-1α, -1β
Neutrophils	IL-8, Gro-α, -β, MIP-1α
Eosinophils	IL-8
Epithelial cells	IL-8, Gro-α, -β, -γ, MIP-1α, ENA-78, MCP-1, RANTES, eotaxin, TARC
Airway smooth muscle cells	RANTES, IL-8, MIP-1α, eotaxin
Vascular endothelial cells	RANTES

*After priming with GM-CSF. GM-CSF, granulocyte–macrophage colony-stimulating factor; IL, interleukin; MCP, monocyte chemotactic protein; MIP, macrophage inflammatory protein.

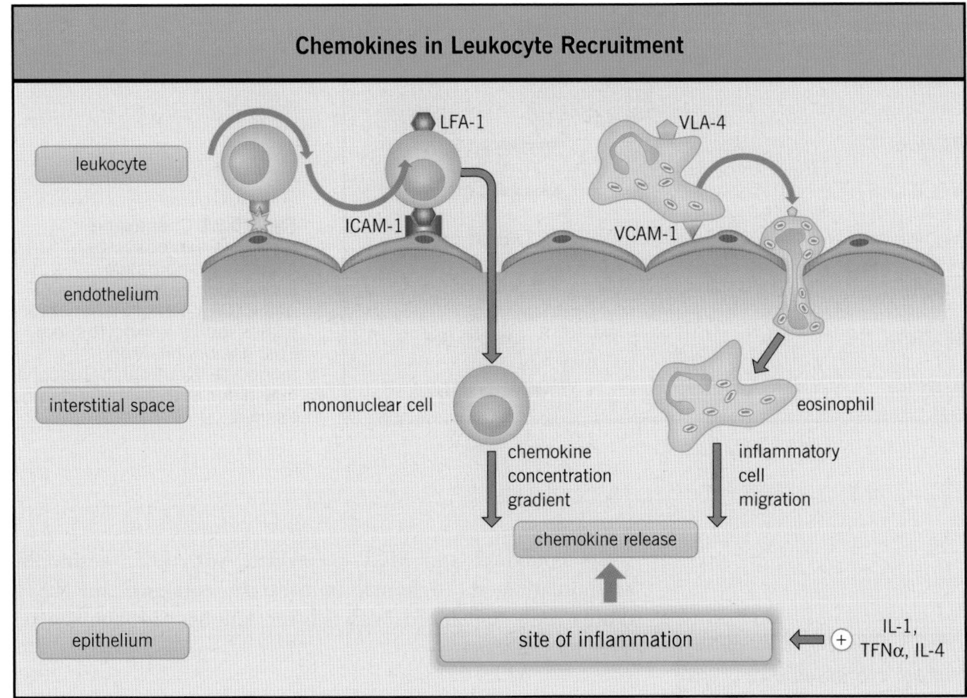

Fig. 20.10 Chemokines in leukocyte recruitment. Circulating leukocytes (e.g. eosinophil) adhere to endothelial adhesion molecules, diapedese between endothelial cells, and migrate along the chemokine gradient towards the site of inflammation. Chemokines upregulate the affinity of integrins on leukocytes [e.g. VLA-4, or lymphocyte function-associated antigen (LFA-1)] promoting tight adhesion of leukocytes to corresponding counter-receptor molecules expressed by vascular endothelium [e.g. vascular cell adhesion molecule-1 (VCAM-1) or intercellular adhesion molecule-1 (ICAM-1)]. In addition, chemokines play a primary role in promoting chemotaxis of leukocytes into inflamed tissues.

attention as a target to modulate the allergic inflammatory response. Studies in mouse models of asthma have demonstrated an important role for several CC chemokines in leukocyte recruitment to the airway. Studies in humans with asthma have established that CC chemokines are expressed by airway epithelial cells, and that allergen challenge can upregulate expression of chemokines in the airway. The levels of chemokines expressed during allergen-induced late phase responses demonstrate correlations between individual chemokines and subsets of leukocytes which respond to these chemokines. During inflammatory responses epithelial cells, macrophages and, to a lesser extent, eosinophils and lymphocytes localized to the subepithelial layer are significant sources of chemokines. Chemokines detected in asthma include CC chemokines (eotaxin or CCL11, RANTES or CCL5, MCP-1 or CCL2, MCP-4 or CCL13, MIP-1 or CCL3, thymus and activation-regulated chemokine or CCL17) (Table 20.5) and CXC chemokines (IL-8). Eotaxin has three isoforms (eotaxin -1, -2, -3; or CCL11, CCL24, CL26, respectively) which are induced with different kinetics following allergen challenge. In humans following allergen challenge, eotaxin-1 is induced early (at 6 hours) and correlates with early eosinophil recruitment,

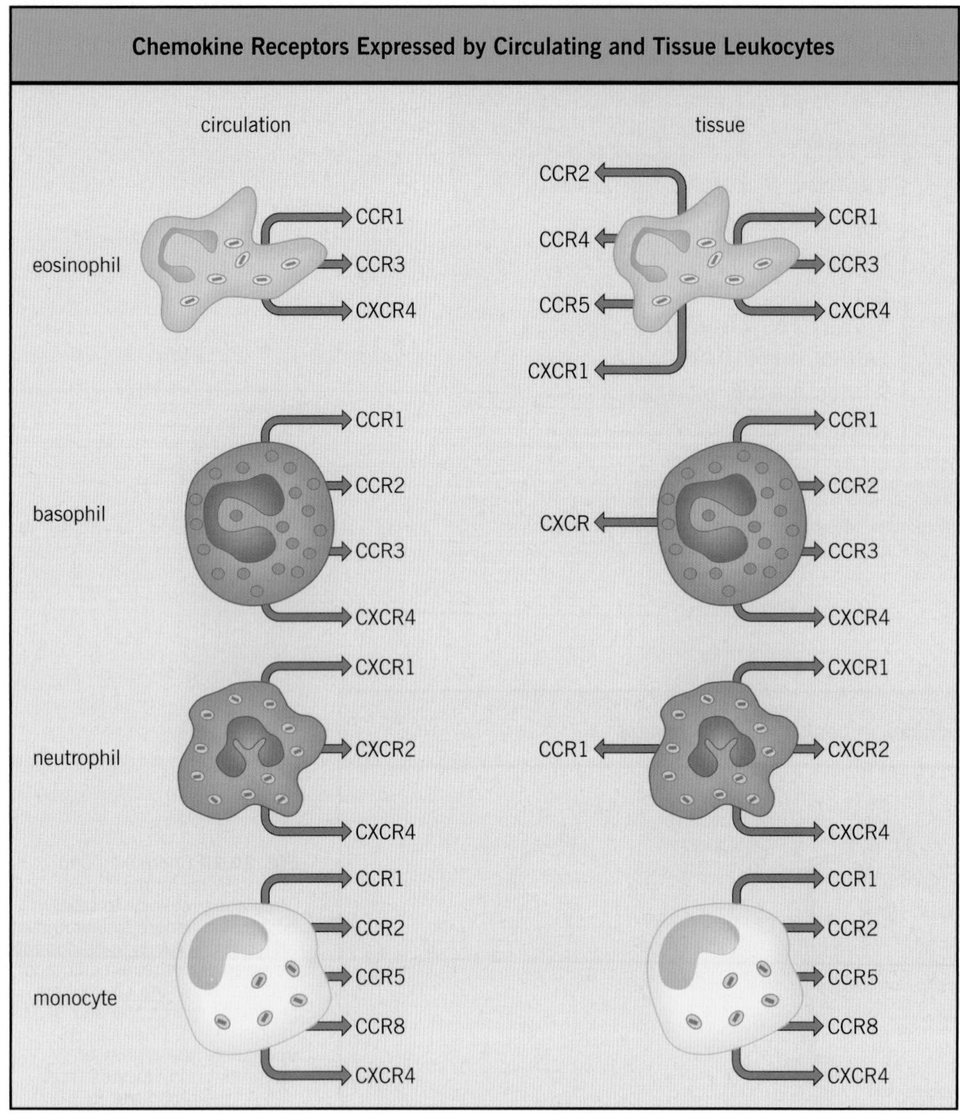

Fig. 20.11 Chemokine receptors expressed by circulating and tissue leukocytes. The profile of CCR and CXCR chemokine receptors expressed by leukocytes (e.g. Eos, eosinophil, Mono, monocyte, Neutrophil, Basophil) may differ in the circulation and tissues.

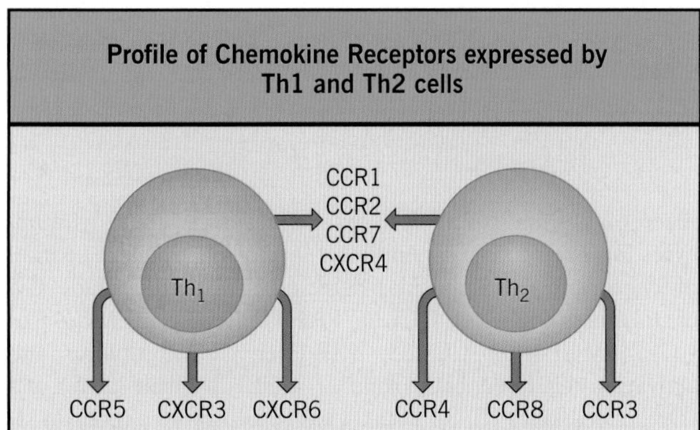

Fig. 20.12 Profile of chemokine receptors expressed by Th1 vs Th2 lymphocytes. Th1 and Th2 cells both express CCR1, CCR2, CCR7, and CXCR4. In addition, Th1 cells express CCR5, CXCR3, and CXCR6, while Th2 cells express CCR4, CCR8, and CCR3.

while eotaxin-2 and MCP-4 correlate with later eosinophil accumulation at 24 hours. In contrast, eotaxin-3 mRNA is dramatically enhanced with slower kinetics 24 hours after allergen challenge.

CCR3 antagonists and asthma

The CC chemokine receptor CCR3 is expressed on multiple cells important to the allergic inflammatory response including eosinophils, basophils, and activated Th2-type lymphocytes. As several CC chemokines (eotaxin-1, eotaxin-2, eotaxin-3, RANTES, MIP-1, macrophage chemoattractant protein-2, -3, -4 or MCP-2, -3, -4) activate a common CCR-3 receptor on eosinophils, there has been particular interest in the therapeutic potential of using chemokine-receptor antagonists such as anti-CCR3 to inhibit the actions of multiple CC chemokines on eosinophils and to prevent the subsequent airway infiltration with eosinophils typically noted in asthma. In asthmatics there is increased expression of both CC chemokines which bind to CCR3 (e.g. eotaxin, eotaxin-2, MCP-3, MCP-4) and CCR3 in the airways, which correlates with increased AHR. Several small molecule inhibitors of CCR3 are effective in inhibiting eosinophil recruitment in allergen challenge animal models of asthma and are currently undergoing clinical trials in asthma.

ADHESION MOLECULES

Definition: Adhesion molecules are glycoproteins expressed on the surface of cells that mediate cell-to-cell, as well as cell-to-extracellular matrix, contact and communication.

Introduction

The role of adhesion molecules expressed by circulating leukocytes and adhesion counter-receptors expressed by endothelial cells has been extensively investigated to determine pathways for general tissue recruitment of leukocytes, as well as to identify mechanisms that mediate selective tissue recruitment of leukocyte subpopulations (e.g. eosinophils at sites of allergic inflammation). In order to accumulate in the airway in diseases such as asthma, circulating leukocytes must adhere to the endothelium lining the blood vessels of the bronchial microcirculation, penetrate the vessel wall, and migrate to the airway lumen. Cell adhesion molecules are involved in all stages of this process. In addition, adhesion molecules present on mast cells, dendritic cells, macrophages, and nerve cells also contribute to the localization and activation of the inflammatory response.

Cell adhesion molecules and leukocyte adhesion to endothelium

Adhesion molecules involved in leukocyte trafficking are grouped into three families based on structural features: the selectins, the integrins, and the immunoglobulin (Ig) gene superfamily (Table 20.7). Studies of leukocyte adhesion to endothelium in vitro, as well as in vivo, and observation of the living microcirculation using intravital microscopy (Fig. 20.13), have delineated the coordinated sequence of events responsible for the tissue accumulation of circulating leukocytes. In the absence of inflammation, circulating leukocytes rarely adhere to the blood vessel wall which does not constitutively express adhesion molecules. However, following inhalation of allergen, cytokines (e.g. IL-1, IL-4, IL-13, and TNF-α) and mediators (e.g. histamine) released in the local tissue, upregulate local endothelial cell adhesion molecule expression. The local upregulation of adhesion molecule expression by endothelium at the site of allergen challenge localizes circulating leukocytes to that site. Circulating leukocytes are tethered to adhesion molecules expressed by endothelium via a transient adhesive interaction that results in leukocytes rolling along the endothelium of postcapillary venules (Figs 20.13 and 20.14). The selectins expressed by endothelium and their glycoprotein ligands expressed by leukocytes largely mediate this process, although the very late antigen-4 (VLA-4) integrin is also able to subserve this tethering function in eosinophils and lymphocytes. Subsequent activation of leukocyte integrins by chemoattractants (e.g. chemokines, anaphylatoxins, formylated peptides, and lipid mediators) causes the rolling leukocyte to arrest, firmly adhere, and flatten (reducing exposure to shear forces and increasing surface area in contact with endothelium) (Fig. 20.14). Integrins and Ig superfamily members mediate these steps of leukocyte firm adhesion to endothelium. Finally, the leukocytes migrate between endothelial cells (diapedesis) into the interstitium and move towards the source of the stimulus (chemotaxis). The importance of leukocyte adhesion molecules to leukocyte tissue recruitment is suggested from genetic disorders which result in defective leukocyte integrin adhesion molecules [leukocyte adhesion deficiency I (LAD I)], or defective leukocyte sialyl Lewis X (sLe^x) expression (LAD II). Patients with either of these leukocyte adhesion deficiencies have neutrophil adhesion defects, tissues which lack neutrophils, associated blood neutrophilia, and recurrent infections as neutrophils cannot bind to endothelial cells and emigrate into infected tissues to mediate host defense against infection.

Selectins and leukocyte adhesion to endothelium

The three members of the selectin family (E-, L-, P- selectin) (Fig. 20.15) are expressed on endothelium (E- and P-selectin), platelets (P-selectin), and leukocytes (L-selectin). The selectin family members share a common modular structure consisting of an N-terminal lectin ligand binding domain, an epidermal growth factor (EGF) domain, and complement binding domains or consensus repeats (CR), a transmembrane segment, and a short cytoplasmic domain at the C terminus. Although the EGF and CR domains contribute to full adhesive function of the selectins, it is the carbohydrate-recognizing N-terminal lectin domain that is directly responsible for ligand binding.

L-selectin

L-selectin is expressed constitutively on the surface microvilli of all leukocyte classes. The exposure of neutrophils to inflammatory mediators causes L-selectin to be rapidly shed from the cell surface via the action of a protease (Table 20.8). Leukocyte (including eosinophil) rolling and trafficking is diminished in L-selectin-deficient mice and in wild-type mice treated with anti-L-selectin antibodies.

P-selectin

P-selectin is synthesized and stored in Weibel-Palade bodies in endothelial cells. Stimulation of endothelial cells with inflammatory mediators such as histamine, thrombin, and C5a, rapidly induces preformed P-selectin stored in Weibel-Palade bodies to be expressed at the endothelial cell surface (Table 20.8). P-selectin is also upregulated transcriptionally by numerous inflammatory cytokines, including TNF-α and the Th2 cytokine IL-4 which are expressed during episodes of allergic inflammation. The importance of P-selectin to eosinophil adhesion to endothelium is suggested from studies in P-selectin-deficient mice which have significantly diminished eosinophil rolling and cell trafficking to sites of inflammation. The reduced eosinophil accumulation in the lung in allergen-challenged P-selectin knock-out mice is associated with reduced AHR.

E-selectin

E-selectin is expressed exclusively on endothelial cells where its expression is transcriptionally regulated by cytokines (e.g. IL-1, TNF-α) and LPS (Table 20.8). Expression of E-selectin peaks around 4 hours after exposure to cytokines and persists for 12 hours. An E-selectin monoclonal antibody (mAb) blocks

Table 20.7 Adhesion molecules in leukocyte–endothelial cell adhesion

Adhesion Proteins Mediating Leukocyte Cell Adhesion Interactions

Adhesion family	Adhesion molecule	Alternative designation	Gene	Localization	Ligand	Function
Selectin	L-selectin	CD62L	1q21-24	All leukocytes	CD34, MAdCAM	Rolling
	P-selectin	CD62P	1q21-24	Endothelial cells, platelets	PSGL-1	Rolling
	E-selectin	CD62E	1q21-24	Endothelial cells	PSGL-1, ESL-1	Rolling
Integrin	$\alpha_L\beta_2$	CD11a/CD18, LFA-1	$16(\alpha_1)\ 21(\beta_2)$	All leukocytes	ICAM-1, ICAM-2, ICAM-3	Adhesion
	$\alpha_M\beta_2$	CD11b/CD18, Mac-1	$16(\alpha_M)\ 21(\beta_2)$	Granulocytes, monocytes	ICAM-1, C3bi, fibrinogen	Adhesion
	$\alpha_x\beta_2$	CD11c/CD18, P150.95	$16(\alpha_x)\ 21(\beta_2)$	Granulocytes, monocytes	C3bi, fibronectin	Adhesion
	$\alpha_4\beta_1$	CD49d/CD29, VLA-4	$2(\alpha_4)\ 10(\beta_1)$	Lymphocytes, monocytes, eosinophils, basophils	VCAM-1, CS-1 Domain of fibronectin	Adhesion or rolling
	$\alpha_4\beta_7$	CD49d/β_7	$2(\alpha_4)\ 12(\beta_7)$	Lymphocytes, eosinophils	MAdCAM-1, VCAM-1, fibronectin CS-1 domain	Adhesion
Immunoglobulin	ICAM-1	CD54	19p13.2	Endothelium, monocytes	LFA-1, Mac-1	Adhesion
	ICAM-2	CD102	17q23-25	Endothelium	LFA-1	Adhesion
	VCAM-1	CD106	1p31-32	Endothelium	VLA-4	Adhesion or rolling
	PECAM-1	CD31	17q23	Endothelium, leukocytes, platelets	PECAM-1 (homophilic) $\alpha_v\beta_3$ (heterophilic)	Emigration
	MAdCAM-1	–	19p13.3	Endothelium	$\alpha_4\beta_7$, L-selectin	Adhesion or rolling

ESL, E-selectin ligand; ICAM, intercellular adhesion molecule; LFA, lymphocyte-function-associated antigen; MAdCAM, mucosal vascular addressin cell adhesion molecule; PECAM, platelet/endothelial cell adhesion molecule; PSGL P-selectin glycoprotein ligand; VCAM, vascular cell adhesion molecule; VLA, very late antigen.

neutrophil migration in the late-phase response to allergen challenge in monkeys, but does not block eosinophil accumulation or AHR. Furthermore, in vitro flow chamber and in vivo intravital microscopy studies suggest that E-selectin is more important to neutrophil tethering to endothelium than to eosinophil tethering to endothelium under conditions of blood flow.

Selectin ligands

As selectins bind to many different putative ligands in vitro with a range of affinities, identifying which are the physiologic ligands in vivo still requires further study. However, significant insights into potential selectin ligands have been derived from in vivo studies of leukocyte adhesion in mutant mice lacking individual selectin ligands.

Physiologic selectin ligands (Fig. 20.16) are a diverse group of glycosylated proteins and glycolipids that recognize one or more of the selectins. However, the minimal carbohydrate epitope recognized by all three selectins is the sialylated, fucosylated sLe^x comprised of four sugars, and its stereoisomer sLe^a. The enzymes involved in the synthesis of sLe^x and its stereoisomer sLe^a in leukocytes have been identified as α2, 3-sialyl-transferases and α1, 3-fucosyl-transferases. Mice

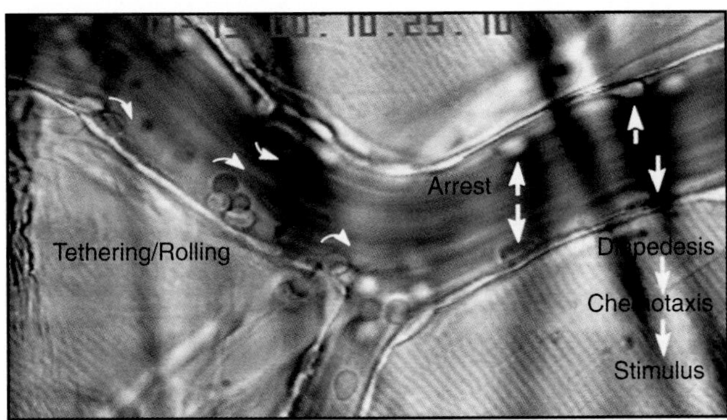

Fig. 20.13 Postcapillary leukocyte recruitment. The photograph shows the stages of leukocyte recruitment in a postcapillary venule of a mouse cremaster muscle. The picture was taken 10 minutes after initiating surgery. (Courtesy of Dr Keith Norman, University of Sheffield.)

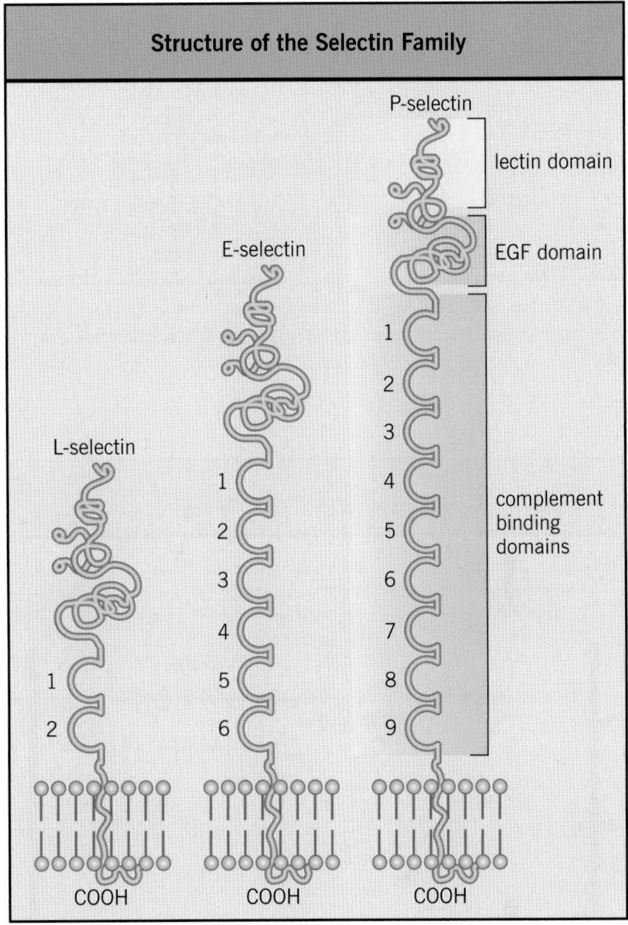

Fig. 20.15 Molecular structure of the selectin family. Each selectin contains a lectin ligand binding domain, an epidermal growth factor (EGF)-like domain, and different numbers of complement binding domains or consensus repeats (numbered 1–9).

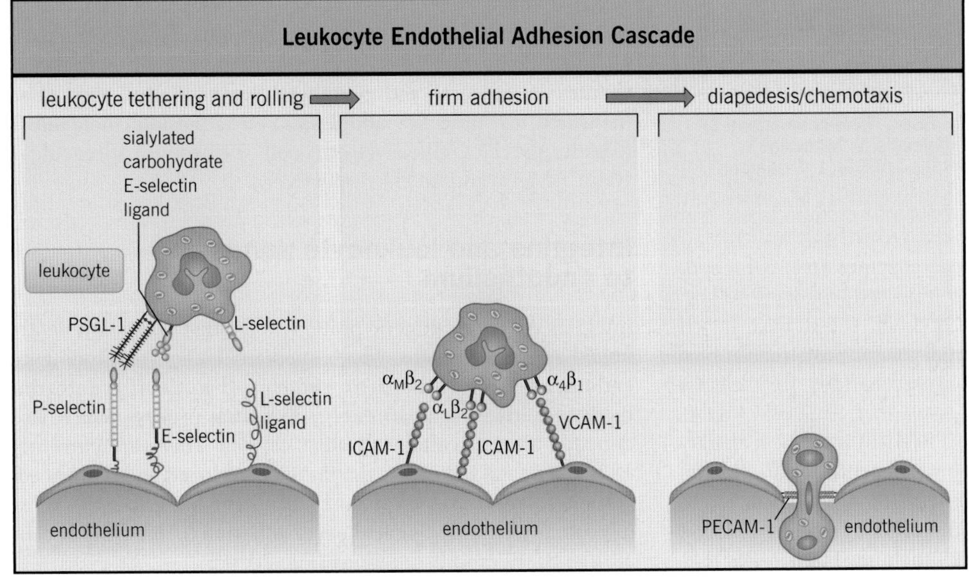

Fig. 20.14 The leukocyte endothelial cell adhesion cascade. Circulating leukocytes initially tether via selectins to endothelium, firmly adhere to endothelium via β1 and β2 integrins, and subsequently diapedese between endothelial cells. ICAM-1, intercellular adhesion molecule-1; PECAM-1, platelet endothelial cell adhesion molecule-1; PSGL-1, P-selectin glycoprotein ligand 1; VCAM-1, vascular cell adhesion molecule-1.

Table 20.8 Modulation of selectin expression

Modulation of Selectin Expression			
Selectin	**Constitutive**	**Inducible**	**Stimulus**
L-selectin	Yes	No	Downregulated by chemoattractants including chemokines
P-selectin	No	Yes	C5a, histamine, leukotriene C_4, thrombin, TNFα, LPS, IL-4
E-selectin	No	Yes	IL-1, TNFα, LPS

IL, Interleukin; LPS, lipopolysaccharide; TNF, tumor necrosis factor.

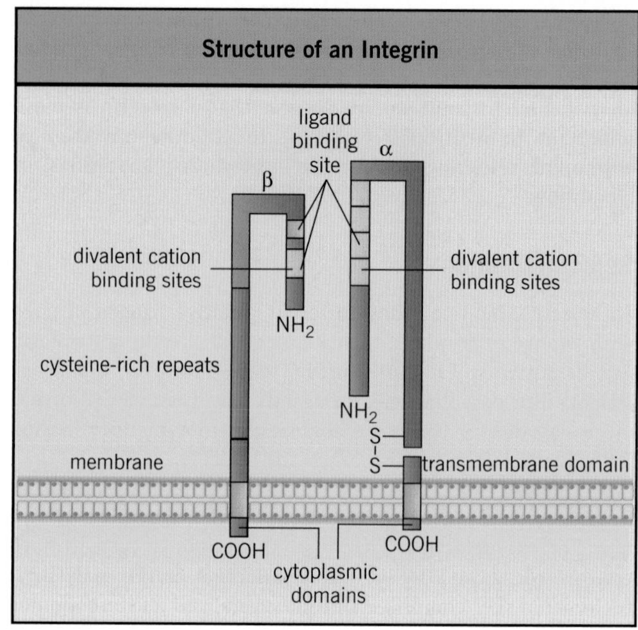

Fig. 20.17 The structure of an integrin heterodimer with its α and β subunits. Examples of integrin heterodimers include: β1 integrins (α4β1 or VLA-4), β2 integrins (α_L β_2 or LFA-1), and B7 integrins (α4β7).

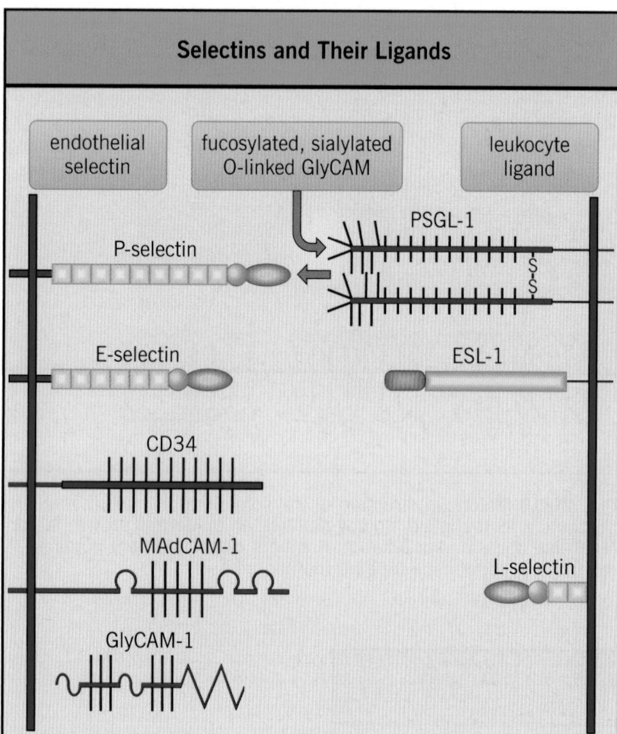

Fig. 20.16 Selectins and their ligands. ESL-1, E-selectin ligand-1; GlyCAM-1, glycosylated cell adhesion molecule 1; MAdCAM-1, mucosal addressin cell adhesion molecule-1; PSGL-1, P-selectin glycoprotein ligand 1.

genetically deficient in one of these enzymes (α1, 3-fucosyltransferase VII, or Fuc T VII) show impaired leukocyte rolling. As leukocyte expression of PSGL-1 in these Fuc T VII deficient mice is normal, the essential role of post-translational glycosylation with fucosylated oligosaccharides for selectin adhesion is evident.

P-selectin glycoprotein ligand 1 (PSGL-1) is the best characterized selectin ligand, whose counter-receptor is P-selectin. PSGL-1, a homodimer of two 120 kDa subunits, is localized to microvilli on all leukocytes and is therefore in a prime position to bind P-selectin expressed by endothelium. Human PSGL-1 is sulfated on tyrosine residues and the removal of sulfate eliminates binding to P-selectin. Skin homing T cells express a glycoform of PSGL-1, the adhesion molecule cutaneous lymphocyte antigen (CLA). CLA mediates T-cell binding to the counter-receptor E-selectin in skin blood vessels.

Although selectins bind to many different glycoconjugates with a range of affinities, experiments with blocking monoclonal antibodies and targeted genetic deletion in mice demonstrate that PSGL-1 is the principal ligand on leukocytes that is recognized by P-selectin and L-selectin. PSGL-1 is also a ligand for E-selectin, as indicated by impaired tethering of PSGL-1-deficient leukocytes, although a second, as yet unidentified E-selectin ligand appears to contribute to rolling. Thus in mice, PSGL-1 is a physiologically relevant ligand for P-selectin, and also may play a role in L- and E-selectin mediated adhesion.

While the ligand for L-selectin on postcapillary venules is not yet confirmed, L-selectin ligands on high endothelial venules in mucosal and peripheral lymph nodes have been identified as mucosal addressin cell adhesion molecule-1 (MAdCAM-1), glycosylated cell adhesion molecule-1 (GlyCAM-1), and CD34 respectively.

Integrins and leukocyte adhesion to endothelium

Integrins are heterodimeric proteins consisting of non-covalently linked α and β chains which mediate leukocyte binding to endothelial cells and matrix proteins (Fig. 20.17). Integrin-mediated adhesion is an energy requiring process which also depends on extracellular divalent cations. There are currently 15 α chains and 8 β chains that have been cloned and sequenced. Although leukocytes express 13 different integrins, the most important for mediating leukocyte adhesion to endothelial cells are the β_1, β_2, and β_7 integrins (Fig. 20.18).

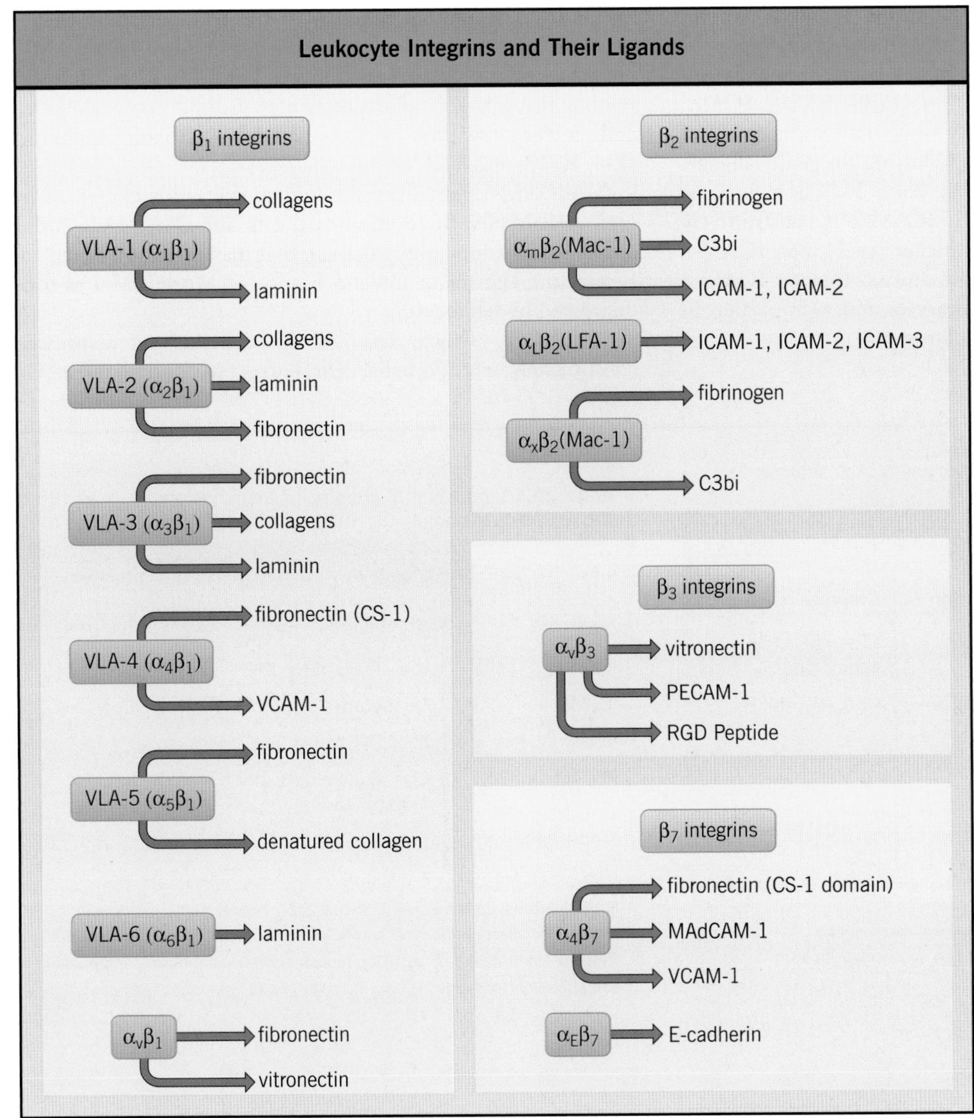

Fig. 20.18 Leukocyte integrins and their ligands. Leukocyte bind through β1, β2, β3, and β7 integrins to counter-receptors expressed on endothelial cells (VCAM-1, ICAM-1), as well as to extracellular matrix components (e.g. laminin, collagen, fibronectin). ICAM-1, intercellular adhesion molecule-1; MAdCAM-1, mucosal addressin cell adhesion molecule-1; PECAM-1, platelet/endothelial cell adhesion molecule-1; VCAM-1, vascular cell adhesion molecule-1.

The β_1 integrin VLA-4 ($\alpha_4\beta_1$) is expressed on circulating leukocytes important to allergic inflammation (including eosinophils, T cells, basophils, mononuclear cells), but not significantly on neutrophils. VLA-4 binds to counter-receptors expressed by endothelial cells (i.e. VCAM-1), as well as to receptors in the extracellular matrix (the CS-1 region of fibronectin). The α_4 integrins support firm adhesion of leukocytes to VCAM-1, and can also support leukocyte rolling on endothelium in vivo.

The β_2 integrin subfamily is highly expressed on all circulating leukocytes and consists of a common β subunit (β_2/CD18) linked to one of four α subunits: CD11a [lymphocyte function-associated antigen (LFA-1) or $\alpha_L\beta_2$], CD11b (Mac-1 or $\alpha_M\beta_2$), CD11c ($\alpha_X\beta_2$), or CD11d ($\alpha_D\beta_2$). The leukocyte β_2 integrins mediate firm adhesion of leukocytes to ICAM-1 expressed by endothelial cells. Thus firm adhesion of leukocytes to endothelium can either be mediated by leukocyte β_1 integrin binding to endothelial-expressed VCAM-1, or by leukocyte β_2 integrin binding to endothelial-expressed ICAM-1. Lymphocytes express primarily CD11a/CD18 (LFA-1 or $\alpha_L\beta_2$) while neutrophils, eosinophils, and monocytes express all four β_2 integrins. On neutrophils, surface expression of CD11b (Mac-1 or $\alpha_M\beta_2$) is rapidly increased after exposure to chemoattractants (Table 20.9) due to mobilization from intracellular granule stores. In contrast, CD11a (LFA-1) is constitutively expressed and a change in the conformation of this integrin regulates its affinity for its counter-receptor ICAM-1.

β_7 integrins ($\alpha_4\beta_7$) are expressed on eosinophils and a subset of gut-homing lymphocytes. On eosinophils, $\alpha_4\beta_7$ mediates binding to two different ligands on endothelial cells (VCAM-1, and MAdCAM-1). As MAdCAM is not significantly expressed in the lung compared to the GI tract, MAdCAM plays an important role in homing of cells expressing $\alpha_4\beta_7$ to the gut, but less of a role in mediating eosinophil recruitment to the lung via $\alpha_4\beta_7$ integrins.

The immunoglobulin superfamily

The immunoglobulin (Ig) superfamily includes ICAM-1, ICAM-2, ICAM-3, VCAM-1, and platelet endothelial cell adhesion molecule-1 (PECAM-1) (Fig. 20.19). ICAM-1 comprises a single transmembrane polypeptide having five Ig domains. Binding sites for CD11a are in ICAM-1 domains 1 and 2 and for CD11b in ICAM-1 domain 3. ICAM-1 is constitutively expressed at low levels on endothelial cells but is transcriptionally upregulated by various cytokines and LPS (Table 20.10). ICAM-1 deficient mice show substantially impaired lymphocyte and eosinophil trafficking into airways following antigen challenge. ICAM-2 has two Ig domains that have 34% homology to the first two domains of ICAM-1. ICAM-2 is constitutively expressed on endothelial cells at higher levels than ICAM-1 and it is not upregulated by inflammatory cytokines. ICAM-3 is expressed at high levels on leukocytes and is important in mediating interactions between leukocytes.

VCAM-1 is another member of the Ig superfamily that is expressed on endothelial cells. The major form of VCAM-1 consists of seven Ig domains. Domains 1 and 4 mediate VCAM-1 binding to VLA-4. Basal expression of VCAM-1 on endothelial cells is very low, and is upregulated by cytokines including IL-4, IL-13, and TNF.

MAdCAM-1 contains three Ig domains and is expressed by endothelial cells. In addition to the Ig domains, MAdCAM-1 also contains a mucin-like domain that may serve as a ligand for L-selectin. The major integrin ligand for MAdCAM-1 is $\alpha_4\beta_7$ expressed by leukocytes.

PECAM-1, which has six Ig domains, is expressed constitutively on endothelial cells, leukocytes, and platelets. On

Table 20.9 Modulation of leukocyte integrin expression and function

Modulation of Integrin Expression and Function

Molecule	Expression/function	Stimulus
$\alpha_L\beta_2$ integrin	Increased function	C5a, PAF, LTB4, chemokines
$\alpha_M\beta_2$ integrin	Increased expression and function	C5a, PAF, fMLP
$\alpha_x\beta_2$ integrin	Increased expression and function	IL-8
$\alpha_4\beta_1$ integrin	Increased function	Eotaxin, GM-CSF
$\alpha_4\beta_7$ integrin	Increased function	PAF

fMLP, formyl-Met-Leu-Phe; GM-CSF, granulocyte–macrophage colony-stimulating factor; IL, interleukin; LTB, leukotriene B; PAF, platelet-activating factor.

Table 20.10 Induction of endothelial immunoglobulin superfamily expression

Induction of Endothelial Ig Superfamily Member Expression

Molecule	Stimulus
ICAM-1	IL-1, TNFα, IFNγ, LPS
ICAM-2	Constitutive
VCAM-1	IL-1, TNFα, IL-4, IL-13, LPS
PECAM-1	Constitutive: IL-1 and IFNγ induce redistribution
MAdCAM-1	Constitutive

ICAM, intercellular adhesion molecule; IFN, interferon; IL, Interleukin; LPS, lipopolysaccharide; TNF, tumor necrosis factor; MAdCAM, mucosal vascular addressin cell adhesion molecule; PECAM, platelet/endothelial cell adhesion molecule; VCAM, vascular cell adhesion molecule.

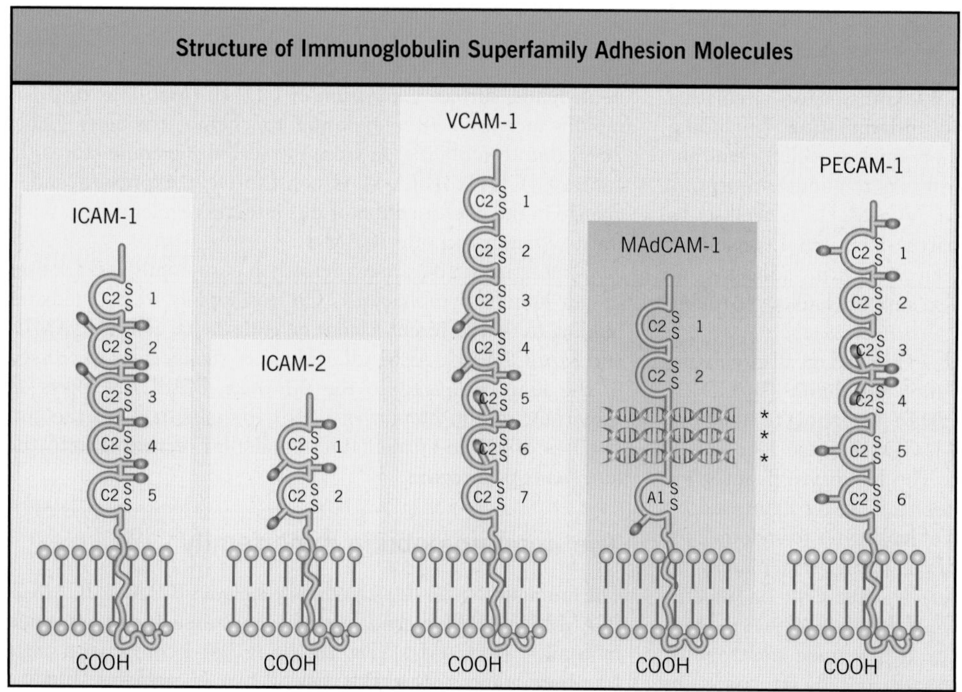

Fig. 20.19 Molecular structure of immunoglobulin superfamily adhesion molecules. Immunoglobulin superfamily adhesion molecules express variable numbers of extracellular constant Ig domains (C2). MAdCAM-1 also contains an extracellular IgA domain (A1) and a mucin domain (*). ICAM-1, intercellular adhesion molecule-1; MAdCAM-1, mucosal addressin cell adhesion molecule-1; PECAM-1, platelet/endothelial cell adhesion molecule-1; PSGL-1, P-selectin glycoprotein ligand 1; VCAM-1, vascular cell adhesion molecule-1.

endothelial cells, stimulation with the same inflammatory cytokines that induce the upregulation of ICAM-1 results in a redistribution of PECAM-1 to the endothelial cell periphery without affecting the total amount expressed by each cell. This redistribution of PECAM may facilitate leukocyte migration between adjacent endothelial cells. Studies using intravital microscopy in PECAM-deficient mice demonstrate that neutrophils are able to adhere to endothelium but are not able to diapedese between endothelial cells, suggesting an important role for PECAM in neutrophil diapedesis between endothelial cells. In contrast, studies with eosinophils suggest that PECAM is not important to eosinophil tissue recruitment. PECAM-1 undergoes homotypic as well as heterotypic adhesion, the latter being to $\alpha_v\beta_3$, which is expressed on several cell types including leukocytes and endothelial cells.

Soluble forms of adhesion molecules

Soluble forms of most of the endothelial adhesion molecules (Table 20.11) can be detected in plasma, suggesting that they are released from the cell surface or secreted. A metalloproteinase, 'L-selectin sheddase', which is distinct from other known matrix metalloproteinases, mediates this cleavage. Understanding the regulation of L-selectin sheddase may be important for controlling leukocyte migration from the blood. For P-selectin, an alternatively spliced mRNA variant from which the exon encoding the transmembrane domain is removed, has been identified. Thus, plasma levels of this selectin could be due to release of this form, or the loss of P-selectin from the cell surface, or both. The presence of other adhesion molecules in plasma could arise by similar mechanisms. These secreted adhesion molecules may be involved in regulation of the inflammatory responses by acting as endogenous inhibitors of adhesion.

Adhesion molecule signaling by integrins

In general, integrins are not constitutively active and require activation to bind to a ligand. In classical 'outside-in signaling' integrin cell surface receptors bind ligand and transduce signals from the extracellular integrin domain to the cytoplasm. 'Outside-in' signaling is the result of a cell surface integrin receptor transmitting a signal to the cell cytoplasm, leading to functions such as chemotaxis, the secretion of specific cytokines, the killing of invasive pathogens, gene expression, and apoptosis (Fig. 20.20). For example, ligation of the eosinophil β_2 integrin subunit triggers cell activation and degranulation. Cell surface integrin engagement stimulates the activity of numerous signaling molecules, including the Rho family of GTPases, tyrosine phosphatases, cyclic adenosine monophosphate (cAMP)-dependent protein-kinase, and protein kinase C. Integrins promote actin assembly via the recruitment of molecules that directly activate the actin polymerization machinery or physically link it to sites of cell adhesion.

Integrins also possess the unique ability to dynamically regulate their adhesiveness, through a process termed 'inside-out signaling' (Fig. 20.20). In 'inside-out signaling', stimuli are initially received by non-integrin cell-surface receptors (e.g. C5a, eotaxin, or IL-8 receptors) which subsequently initiate intracellular signals that impinge on integrin cytoplasmic domains and alter their adhesiveness for integrin extracellular ligands. Within minutes of a leukocyte binding an inflammatory mediator (e.g. C5a, eotaxin, or IL-8) to its respective leukocyte

Table 20.11 Soluble adhesion molecules and their mechanism of production

Soluble Adhesion Molecules	
Adhesion molecule	**Mechanism of production**
L-selectin	Shedding via L-selectin 'sheddase'
P-selectin	Shedding; alternatively spliced mRNA
E-selectin	Shedding via proteolytic cleavage
ICAM-1	Shedding; alternatively spliced mRNA
ICAM-2	?
ICAM-3	Shedding
VCAM-1	Shedding; alternatively spliced mRNA
PECAM-1	Shedding; alternatively spliced mRNA

ICAM, intercellular adhesion molecule; PECAM, platelet/endothelial cell adhesion molecule; VCAM, vascular cell adhesion molecule.

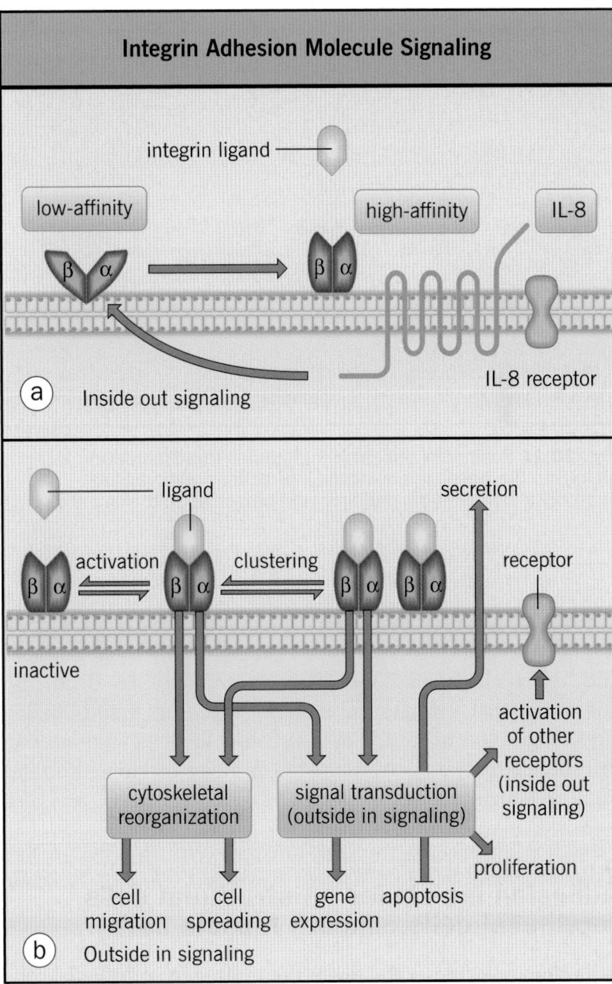

Fig. 20.20 Signaling events triggered by integrin–ligand binding. (a) Integrin receptor clustering induces classic 'outside in signaling' from the cell surface integrin receptor. (b) Activation of a chemokine receptor (e.g. IL-8 receptor) can activate the cytoplasmic domain of the integrin receptor to change its conformation from a 'low affinity' to a 'high affinity' state through 'inside out' integrin signaling.

Table 20.12 Adhesion molecule expression in asthma. The table compares the expression of adhesion molecules on lung microvascular endothelial and bronchial epithelial cells

Expression of Cell Adhesion Molecules on Human Long Endothelial and Epithelial Cells

Adhesion molecule	Bronchial epithelial cells		Lung microvascular endothelial cells	
	Basal	Stimulated	Basal	Stimulated
ICAM-1	−/+	+++	+	+++
ICAM-2	−	−	++	++
ICAM-3	−	−	−	−
E-selectin	−	−	−	+++
P-selectin	−	−	−	++
VCAM-1	−	−	−	+++

ICAM, intercellular adhesion molecule; VCAM, vascular cell adhesion molecule.

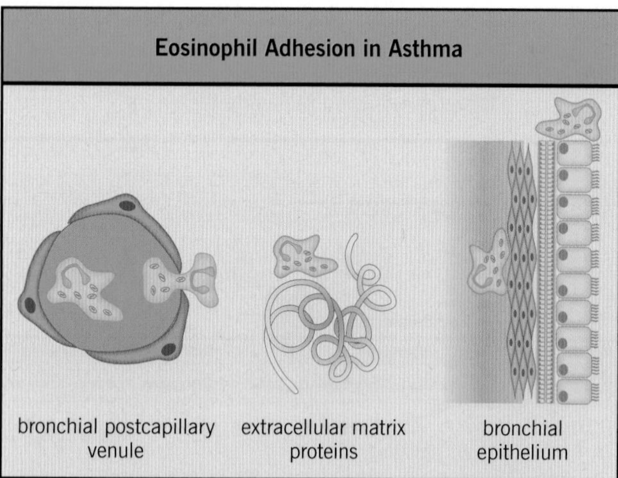

Fig. 20.21 Eosinophil adhesion in asthma. The illustration highlights the possible eosinophil interactions with vascular endothelial cells, matrix proteins, and bronchial epithelial cells.

Table 20.13 Adhesion molecule expression and function on intrapulmonary cells

Expression and Function of Cell Adhesion Molecules on Intrapulmonary Cells

Cell	Function
Bronchial epithelial cells	Eosinophil-mediated damage; β_6-integrin-mediated repair
Mast cells	Integrin-dependent degranulation
Macrophages	Activation via integrins/PSGL-1
Nerve cells	VLA-4-mediated damage by eosinophils
Dendritic cells	Activation via integrins/PSGL-1
T cells	Antigen presentation; activation

PSGL, P-selectin glycoprotein ligand; VLA, very late antigen.

cell surface receptor, integrin receptors on the same cell surface acquire the ability to adhere to ligands on other cell surfaces and extracellular regions. This is thought to occur by conformational changes in integrin receptor ligand-binding sites. This type of 'inside-out' signaling involves non-integrin cell surface receptor activation of G-proteins including Rho and Rac, although kinases including PI-3K and PKC are also involved.

Adhesion molecules on structural cells (epithelial cells, smooth muscle cells)

Adhesion molecule expression is not limited to endothelial cells and leukocytes, but is also present on structural cells (e.g. epithelial cells, smooth muscle cells, nerves, fibroblasts). Bronchial epithelial cells express ICAM-1 although, unlike lung microvascular endothelial cells, they do not express VCAM-1, PECAM-1, or selectins (Table 20.12). Another difference is that IFNγ is the most effective stimulus of epithelial ICAM-1 expression while TNF-α shows weak activity. Epithelial cell ICAM-1 mediates the adhesion of eosinophils to epithelium and this may be an important mechanism by which these two cells are brought into close proximity, leading to epithelial cell injury (Fig. 20.21). Other adhesion-molecule-expressing cells in the lung include mast cells (Table 20.13), which express β_1 integrins that bind to matrix proteins. Effective mast cell degranulation requires α_4-mediated adhesion to fibronectin. Airway nerves express ligands for VLA-4, which mediates eosinophil adhesion and potential nerve damage, in a manner analogous to eosinophil-mediated epithelial cell damage.

Modulators of adhesion molecules as therapeutics

Targeting adhesion molecules in allergic inflammation may be beneficial by reducing leukocyte trafficking as well as by

Table 20.14 Therapeutic modulation of adhesion molecule expression and function

Modulators of Adhesion Molecule Expression and Function as Therapeutics	
Suppress cell surface expression:	**Inhibit function:**
• Cytokines and cytokine-receptor antagonists	• Monoclonal antibodies
• Antisense oligonucleotides	• Soluble adhesion molecule constructs
• Fucosyl transferase inhibitors	• Small-molecule antagonists
	• Oligosaccharides
	• Glycomimetics
	• Integrin activation inhibitors

inhibiting cellular activation. A number of approaches to modulate adhesion molecule expression and function are possible (Table 20.14). Blocking the cytokines that induce adhesion molecule expression (e.g. TNF-α, IL-1, IL-4, IL-13) is one way, although it will be a rather non-specific effect as many effects other than adhesion will be influenced. Blocking adhesion molecule function with mAbs has been extensively tested in vitro and in vivo. For example, anti-ICAM-1 mAb reduces eosinophil trafficking and airway hyperresponsiveness in a monkey model. However, results with an anti-ICAM-1 mAb have thus far not been reported in humans with asthma. As blocking ICAM-1 would also block neutrophil recruitment, safety studies will need to demonstrate that asthmatics treated with an anti-ICAM-1 Ab do not have a significant increased incidence of infections. As VCAM-1 interacts with VLA-4 expressed by eosinophils, T cells, and basophils, neutralizing the VCAM-1/VLA-4 pathway has also been considered an important therapeutic approach to selectively blocking cells participating in the LPR while not inhibiting recruitment of cells important to host defense such as neutrophils (which do not express VLA-4). However, thus far results of human studies with VLA-4 antagonists in asthma have been disappointing, probably because adhesion pathways independent of VCAM/VLA-4 (e.g. P-, E-selectin, ICAM-1) can be used if the VCAM/VLA-4 pathway is blocked.

CONCLUSION

Cytokines, chemokines, and adhesion molecules play a key role in regulating the immune and inflammatory response in allergic inflammation. An improved understanding of the complex molecular mechanisms of allergic diseases will help to identify potential novel targets for therapeutic intervention. Clinical trials with agents such as cytokine antagonists, chemokine inhibitors, adhesion molecule antagonists, or compounds that interfere with the transcription of genes which regulate expression of chemokines, cytokines, and adhesion molecules, will improve our understanding of the function of these individual molecules in allergic inflammation. The use of any of these antagonists in clinical practice will be dependent on their relative potency in inhibiting allergic inflammation (e.g. therapeutic efficacy), as well as evidence that they do not significantly impair host defense to infection or immune surveillance (e.g. side-effect profile).

Acknowledgement

The author acknowledges the contributions of James Lordan and Paul Hellewell to this chapter in the 2nd edition of Allergy. The chapter has been substantially revised for the 3rd edition.

FURTHER READING

Barnes PJ. Cytokine-directed therapies for the treatment of chronic airway diseases. Cytokine Growth Factor Rev 2003; 14:511–522.

Davenpeck KL, Bochner BS. Leukocyte-blood vessel interactions. Clin Allergy Immunol 2002; 16:125–141.

Escoubet-Lozach L, Glass CK, Wasserman SI. The role of transcription factors in allergic inflammation. J Allergy Clin Immunol 2002; 110:553–564.

Holgate ST, Broide D. New targets for allergic rhinitis – a disease of civilization. Nat Rev Drug Discov 2003; 2:902–914.

Karin M, Yamamoto Y, Wang QM. The IKK NF-kappa B system: a treasure trove for drug development. Nat Rev Drug Discov 2004; 3:17–26.

Kay AB. Immunomodulation in asthma: mechanisms and possible pitfalls. Curr Opin Pharmacol 2003; 3:220–226.

Luster A. Anti-chemokine immunotherapy for allergic diseases. Curr Opin Allergy Clin Immunol 2001; 1:561–567.

Robinson DS, Kay AB, Wardlaw A. Eosinophils. Clin Allergy Immunol 2002; 16:43–75.

Romagnani S. 2004 Immunologic influences on allergy and the TH1/TH2 balance. J Allergy Clin Immunol 2004; 113:395–400.

Zimmerman N, Hershey GK, Foster PS, et al. Chemokines in asthma: cooperative interaction between chemokines and IL-13. J Allergy Clin Immunol 2003; 111:227–242.

Chapter 21

Definition:

The allergic response is initiated by mast cell activation. In addition to stimulating the symptoms of the early phase response, mast cell cytokines activate Th2 lymphocytes to secrete further cytokines which result in the influx of eosinophils, neutrophils and basophils to cause allergic inflammation.

Effector Cells of Allergy

Catherine M Hawrylowicz, Donald W MacGlashan, Hirohisa Saito, Hans-Uwe Simon, and Andrew J Wardlaw

PROGENITORS, AND CELL DIFFERENTIATION AND MATURATION

Whereas most structural cells within tissues divide and mature within the tissues, the effector cells of allergy – namely mast cells, basophils, eosinophils, neutrophils, and monocytes – are produced in the bone marrow. Some of these cells – specifically basophils, eosinophils, and neutrophils – also undergo maturation within the bone marrow and are released into the blood as mature leukocytes. In contrast, mast cells are released into the blood as precursor cells and only mature into recognizable mast cells in the tissues. Cells of the monocyte–macrophage lineage are somewhat of a 'halfway house', being released into the blood as functional monocytes and then undergoing a second phase of tissue specific maturation to form heterogeneous macrophage populations e.g. Kupffer cells in the liver, alveolar macrophages in the lung.

The current model of cell development in the bone marrow is based on the concept that all cells originate from a common totipotent stem cell that gives rise to pluripotent stem cells, which in turn differentiate into a series of more committed precursors with restricted capacity for change of lineage (Fig. 21.1). In general, the production of stem cells is stimulated by interleukin-3 (IL-3), which is lineage non-specific, and by growth factors from stromal cells, including endothelial cells, epithelial cells, and fibroblasts. Growth factor production by stromal cells is enhanced by cytokines such as tumor necrosis factor α (TNFα) and IL-1, both of which are increased in inflammation.

Mast cells

Mast cells cannot be readily identified until they mature in the tissues and express their characteristic granules and high-affinity receptor for IgE (FcεRI). It is considered that they enter the circulation from the bone marrow as immature precursors expressing CD34, a cluster determinant normally associated with precursor cells within the bone marrow, and c-kit receptors for stem cell factor (SCF), the primary growth factor for human mast cells. From the blood, the precursors migrate into the tissues where, under the influence of local microenvironmental factors, they undergo their final phases of differentiation and maturation into recognizable mast cells. Several helper T cells type 2 (Th2) cytokines such as IL-4 and IL-6 can slightly enhance human mast cell proliferation and maturation in vitro only in the place where considerable levels of SCF are present. Increased production of mast cells is often observed in the tissues where fibroblasts expressing membrane-bound SCF are abundant. The number of mast cells is also increased in inflammatory tissues in

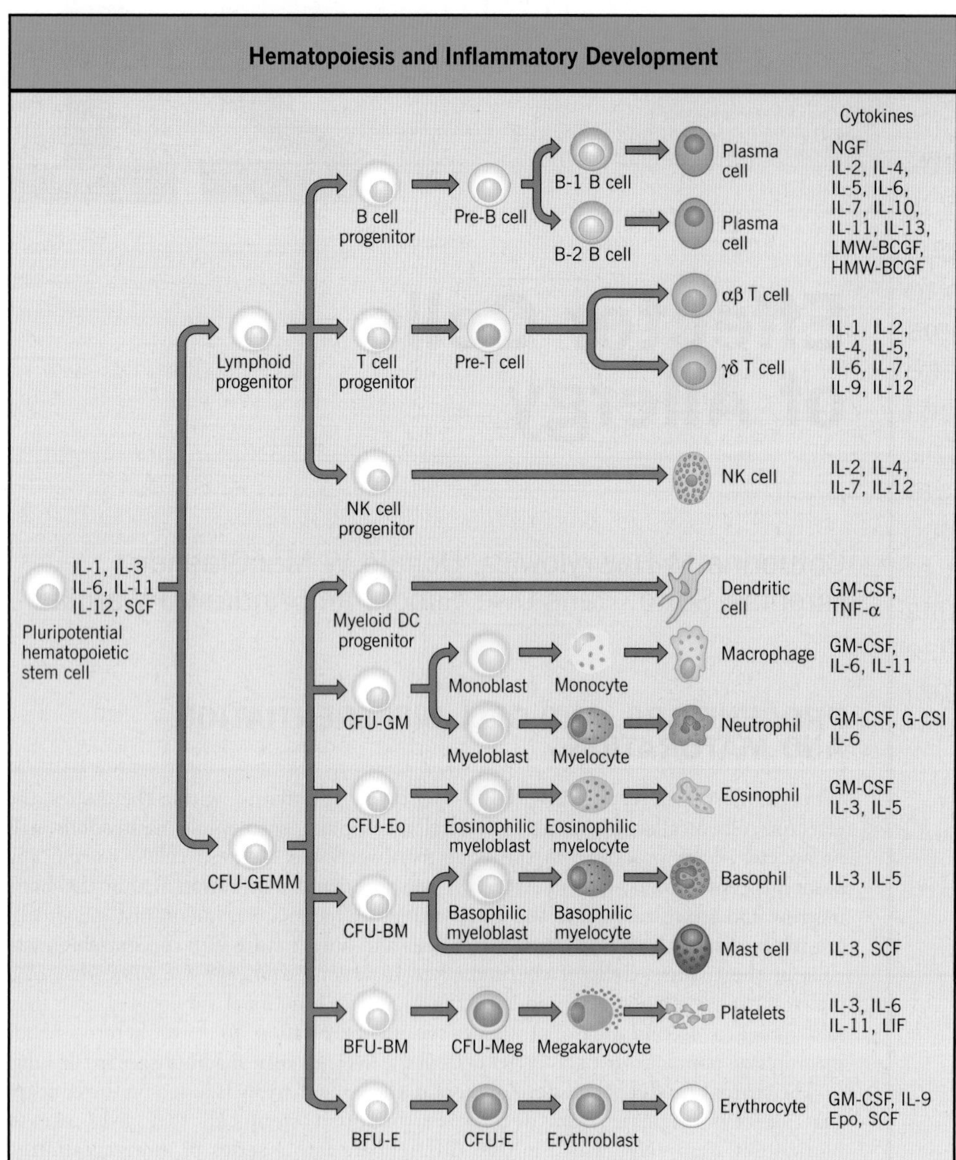

Fig. 21.1 Hematopoiesis and inflammatory cell development. (BFU, blast forming unit; DC, dendritic cell; E, erythrocyte; Eo, eosinophil; Epo, erythropoietin; GM, granulocyte–monocyte; GM-CSF, granulocyte–macrophage colony-stimulating factor; IL, interleukin; L (H) MW-BCGF, low (high) molecular weight B cell-derived growth factor; LIF lymphocyte inhibition factor; Meg, megakaryocyte; NGF, nerve growth factor; NK, natural killer; SCF, stem cell factor; TNF, tumor necrosis factor. (Modified with permission from Middleton E Jr, Reed CE, Ellis EF, et al, eds. Allergy, principles and practice, 5th edn. St Louis: Mosby; 1998.)

allergic diseases. However, it is still controversial whether the number of mast cell precursors is increased in circulating blood or only localized mast cells grow in the tissue.

Maturation of mast cells in the tissues is described in more detail later in this chapter. It should be pointed out at this stage that, although basophils were originally thought to be circulating mast cells, they are related more closely to eosinophils, developing in the bone marrow from granulocyte precursors and entering the circulation only when fully mature.

Eosinophils and basophils

Eosinophils and basophils are thought to arise from a common mononuclear stem cell, which is stimulated to divide by the cytokines IL-3 and granulocyte–macrophage colony-stimulating factor (GM-CSF) acting in concert with stromal factors.

The production of these cells, both of which enter the circulation as mature leukocytes, is limited in normal conditions. However, in allergy, increased levels of GM-CSF and IL-5 result in increased eosinophil production, demonstrable by eosinophilia in the blood and tissues. Little is known of the factors that increase basophil production. Both eosinophils and basophils are primarily tissue cells with a very limited life-span in the blood. For eosinophils, the life-span in the blood is about 24 hours and the tissue-to-blood ratio is about 100:1.

Neutrophils

Neutrophils are produced constitutively by the bone marrow in large numbers. Because of the large number produced and the relatively short life-span (less than 24 hours), more than half of the work done by the bone marrow is dedicated to the production of neutrophils. In inflammation, increased levels of inflammatory cytokines stimulate enhanced neutrophil production. IL-3, IL-6, GM-CSF, and TNFα are the cytokines that are most likely to be involved.

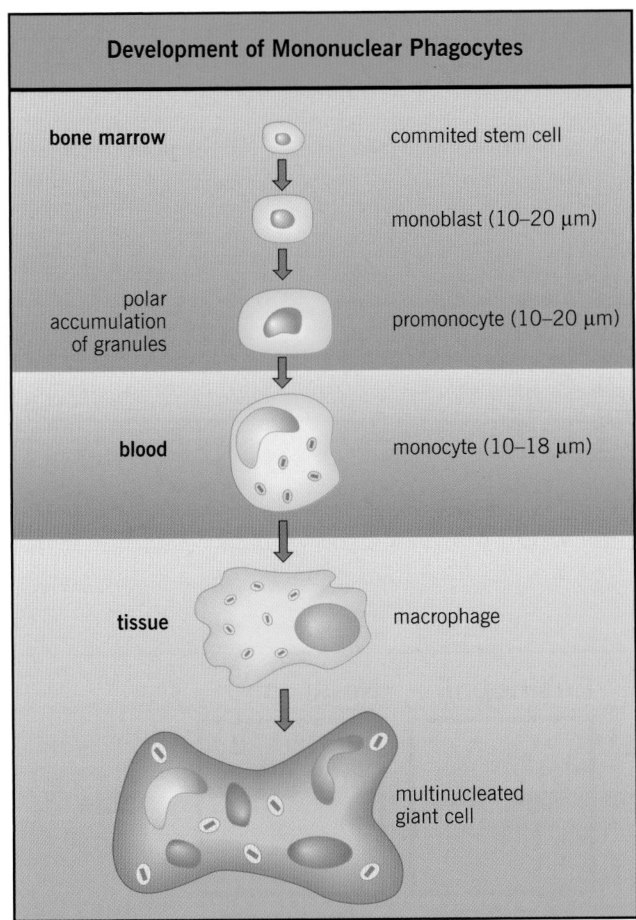

Fig. 21.2 Development of cells of the monocyte–macrophage lineage from bone marrow precursor cells.

Table 21.1 Cells of the mononuclear phagocyte system in normal and inflamed tissue

Cells of the Mononuclear Phagocyte System in Normal and Inflamed Issue

Cells	Localization
Committed stem cells	Bone marrow
Monoblasts	Bone marrow
Promonocytes	Bone marrow
Monocytes	Bone marrow (1 day) Blood (3 days)
Macrophages	Tissues
Free, normal state	
Histiocytes	Connective tissues
Alveolar macrophages	Lung
Pleural/peritoneal	Serous cavities
Fixed normal state	
Kupffer cells	Liver
Osteoclasts	Bone
Microglial cells	Central nervous system
Synovial A cells	Joints
Mesangial cells	Kidney
Fixed-tissue macrophages	Spleen, lymph nodes, bone marrow
Inflammation	
Exudative macrophages	Any inflamed tissue
Activated macrophages	Any inflamed tissue
Multinucleated giant cells	Chronic infection

Monocytes and macrophages

Mononuclear phagocytes originate in the bone marrow from pluripotent stem cells that differentiate into a common committed progenitor cell for the granulocyte and monocyte–macrophage lineage (Fig. 21.2). Colony-stimulating factors (CSFs) and glycoproteins such as IL-3, GM-CSF, and macrophage CSF (M-CSF) regulate the development of monocytes into committed cells of the mononuclear granulocyte lineage and then into monoblasts. Monoblasts have a half-life of approximately 12 hours and undergo one round of cell division to become promonocytes and then monocytes, which remain in the bone marrow for up to 24 hours before entering the bloodstream. In healthy people, monocytes constitute 1–6% of the total white blood cell count and have a half-life of approximately 3 days. Monocytes circulate around the body via the blood and migrate into extravascular tissues and spaces after adhesion to and passage between endothelial cells. Monocytes differentiate into macrophages in the tissues, where they can exist for several months. Monocyte differentiation is influenced by local factors, leading to considerable heterogeneity between cells from different tissues (Table 21.1). Furthermore, recent studies confirm a common bone-marrow precursor of both macrophages and dendritic cells and show that monocytes can also differentiate into immature dendritic cells.

Macrophages are found in body cavities and interstitial tissue. They can be resident or newly elicited as a result of local inflammatory events, or they can be activated as a result of inflammatory insult. In the lung, for example, several distinct populations are observed, including interstitial tissue macrophages and alveolar macrophages, newly recruited monocytes, and dendritic cells. Under extreme conditions of activation, as in granuloma formation during infection, macrophages fuse to form multinucleated giant cells. Continual destruction and replenishment of macrophages occurs, and feedback from sites of local inflammation leads to increased production of bone-marrow progenitor cells. Signals for the recruitment of macrophages into inflammatory sites include chemokines such as monocyte chemotactic protein 1, bacterial peptides such as fMLP (formyl-Met-Leu-Phe), and the complement component C5a. In the absence of inflammation, migration of monocytes into tissues occurs in an apparently random fashion. The basal production rate of monocytes is estimated to be around 7 million cells/hour/kg which is increased approximately three or four times during inflammation. Changes in functional characteristics of mononuclear phagocytes with maturation are summarized in Table 21.2.

PRINCIPLES OF APOPTOSIS

Apoptosis, or programmed cell death, is the most common form of physiologic cell death and is essential for organ development during embryogenesis. After a multicellular organism has completed its development, it must renew many cell lineages. For example, red and white blood cells are generated constantly throughout life from hematopoietic

Table 21.2 Changes in the cellular characteristics of mononuclear phagocytes with maturation

Changes in Cellular Functional characteristics with Maturation of Mononuclear Phagocytes				
Property	**Promonocyte**	**Monocyte**	**Immature macrophage**	**Mature macrophage**
Proliferation	+ + + +	+ + +	+ +	0
Azurophilic granules	+ + +	+ +	±	0
Lysosomes	+	+ +	+ + + +	+ + + +
Glass adherence	+	+ +	+ + +	+ + +
Endocytosis	±	+	+ +	+ + + +
Fc receptors	+	+ +	+ + +	+ + +
Lymphocyte interactions	?	+ +	+ + + +	+ + + +
Non-specific esterase	+ + +	+ + +	+ + +	+ + +
Lysosomal secretion	?	+ +	+ +	+ +

progenitor cells and, therefore, a physiologic cell death is a necessary process to maintain correct cell numbers. Apoptotic cells are removed by neighboring phagocytic cells without loss of their potentially harmful cell contents. In contrast to apoptosis, necrosis is a pathologic form of cell death resulting from acute cellular injury; it is always associated with loss of intracellular mediators and enzymes into the extracellular environment and the consequential induction of an inflammatory response.

Mechanisms of apoptosis

The morphology of apoptosis is associated with characteristic changes within the dying cell. The most readily observed features involve the nucleus, where the chromatin becomes extremely condensed before complete collapse of the nucleus occurs. A reduction in cell volume is also clearly detectable. Figure 21.3 demonstrates these two morphologic changes of apoptosis in both eosinophils and neutrophils. Furthermore, when apoptotic cells are not immediately phagocytosed, cells undergoing apoptosis can break up into apoptotic bodies. In contrast, in necrosis there are no nuclear changes and the cell swells rapidly before undergoing lysis.

Biochemically, apoptosis is characterized by a controlled autodigestion of the cell. Intracellular proteases are essential players of the apoptotic death machinery. These proteases, called caspases, all belong to one protein family. Caspases are processed by cleavage at specific aspartate residues to form active heterodimeric enzymes. It appears that caspases work in a hierarchical system similar to other proteolytic cascades such as complement activation or blood coagulation. Recent data suggest that an initial activation of the caspases cascade is reversible; however, in overt intracellular proteolysis the cell has to die, owing to irreversible damage.

Caspase-mediated proteolysis results in cytoskeletal disruption, cell shrinkage, and membrane blebbing. Caspases also activate endonucleases, which degrade nuclear DNA and are responsible for nucleus condensation and the internucleosomal DNA fragmentation that is often observed in apoptotic cells. This specific type of DNA fragmentation, or DNA laddering, is often used to demonstrate an apoptotic death in many cellular systems. Thus, all of the above-mentioned morphologic changes can be explained by the proteolytic activity within apoptotic cells.

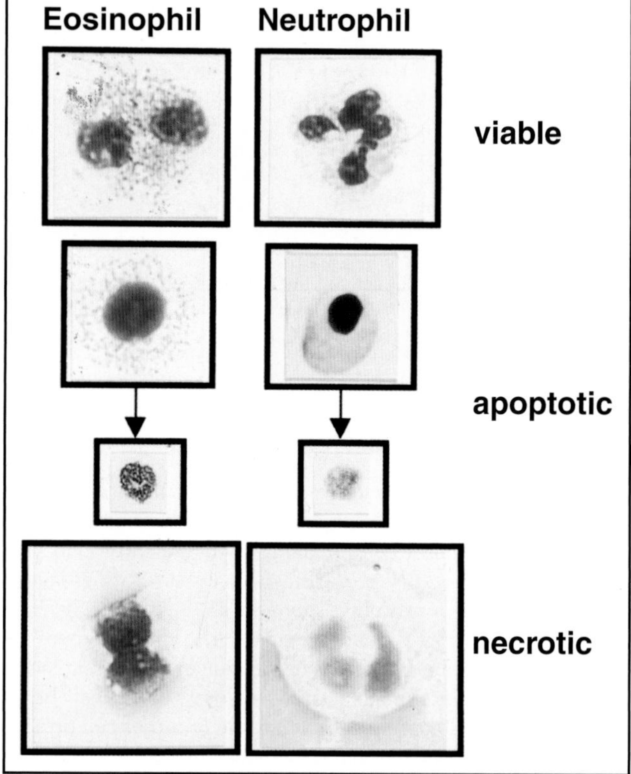

Fig. 21.3 Morphologic features of apoptotic and necrotic granulocytes. Apoptosis was induced by anti-Fas monoclonal antibody. Two stages of apoptosis are shown: first, pyknosis of the nucleus, and secondly, nuclear fragmentation and reduced cell volume. Note that, even at this late stage of apoptosis, these cells have an intact cell membrane. Necrosis was induced by treating the cells with water. In contrast to apoptosis, necrosis is a lytic process associated with inflammation. No changes in the morphology of the nucleus are observed in necrosis.

Table 21.3 Cytokines involved in apoptosis

Mediators and Cytokines That Induce or Inhibit Apoptosis		
	Eosinophils	**Neutrophils**
Antiapoptotic signals		
IL-3	+	+
IL-5	+	–
GM-CSF	+	+
G-CSF	–	+
IFNγ	+	+
Fibronectin	+	?
CD40 ligand	+	?
Glucocorticoids	–	+
Apoptotic signals		
Fas ligand	+	+
TNFα	–	(+)
Glucocorticoids*	+	–
TGFβ*	+	?
Survival factor withdrawal	+	+
CD69 ligand*	+	?

*These signals may not directly activate apoptotic pathways but they may block survival signals. G-CSF, granulocyte colony-stimulating factor; GM-CSF, granulocyte–macrophage colony-stimulating factor; IL, interleukin; IFN, interferon; TGF, transforming growth factor; TNF, tumor necrosis factor.

Regulation of apoptosis by cytokines and 'death factors'

It has been suggested that the apoptotic pathway in normal cells is a default program that must be actively blocked by autocrine and paracrine survival factors if a cell is to survive. Thus, cells from most organs will undergo apoptosis if cultured individually in vitro in the absence of exogenous survival factors. The survival of granulocytes also depends on the presence of survival signals, which are received in vivo from the local environment (e.g. IL-5, derived from T cells and mast cells, is a survival factor for eosinophils) (Table 21.3).

In addition to prolonging survival, local environmental factors acting at cell surface receptors may also actively induce apoptosis. Granulocytes express on their cell surface at least one member of the TNF nerve growth factor receptor family, a family that includes the Fas receptor and that is associated with 'death signaling'. Thus, ligands for this receptor family can induce apoptosis in many different cell types.

Contribution of dysregulated eosinophil apoptosis to allergic inflammation

Although apoptosis is a physiologic form of cell death, it can be dysregulated and may then contribute to a number of different pathogenic processes (e.g. defective regulation of apoptosis may play a part in the etiology of cancer, acquired immunodeficiency syndrome, autoimmune diseases, and neurodegenerative disorders). It also appears that dysregulated apoptosis plays a role in allergic inflammation since delayed eosinophil apoptosis represents a mechanism that leads to tissue eosinophilia.

One mechanism of delayed eosinophil apoptosis in allergic diseases is the overproduction of eosinophil survival factors such as IL-5 and GM-CSF. Evidence has been accumulated to suggest that allergic disorders are associated with increased T-cell activation and secretion of these cytokines. In addition, mast cells and eosinophils themselves contribute to the production of eosinophil survival factors.

The disruption of death signals may represent a second mechanism to inhibit eosinophil apoptosis. For example, it has recently been demonstrated that nitric oxide, the production of which is increased in inflammation, prevents Fas receptor-mediated apoptosis in eosinophils. Nitric oxide-mediated resistance to Fas receptor-mediated apoptosis appears to be of pathophysiologic relevance since eosinophils in allergic tissues do not usually undergo apoptosis after Fas receptor cross-linking. Therefore, nitric oxide concentrations within allergic inflammatory sites may be important in determining whether an eosinophil survives or undergoes apoptosis upon Fas ligand stimulation.

MAST CELLS

Morphology and heterogeneity of human mast cells

Human mast cells are a heterogeneous group of multifunctional, tissue-dwelling cells with roles in conditions as diverse as allergy, the response to parasite infestation, inflammation, angiogenesis, and tissue remodeling. The cells were initially named mastzellen (mastos is Greek for 'breast') in 1878 by Paul Ehrlich because he believed that the intracellular granules, which appeared purple in color when stained with aniline blue dyes (Fig. 21.4), contained phagocytosed materials or nutrients. This change in color, or metachromasia, we now know to represent the strong binding accompanied by polymerization of the basic dye molecules with the highly acidic (basophilic) heparin contained within mast cell granules.

Immunocytochemical studies have indicated the presence within the tissues of two mast cell phenotypes that are distinguishable by their neutral protease content (Fig. 21.5):

- the MC_T phenotype, which contains abundant levels of tryptase but scant of chymase; and
- the MC_{TC} phenotype, which contains abundant levels of both tryptase and chymase.

Initially, these respective subtypes were suggested to be the equivalents of the 'mucosal' and 'connective tissue' previously described in experimental animals. It is now being realized that variable amounts of MC_T and MC_{TC} are present within any given tissue, their relative abundance changing with disease (e.g. allergy or fibrosis). However, some rules may exist (Table 21.4). Thus, MC_T appear to be 'immune system-related' mast cells with a primary role in host defense, whereas MC_{TC} appear to be 'non-immune system-related' mast cells with functions in angiogenesis and tissue remodeling rather than immunologic protection. However, it should be remembered that both

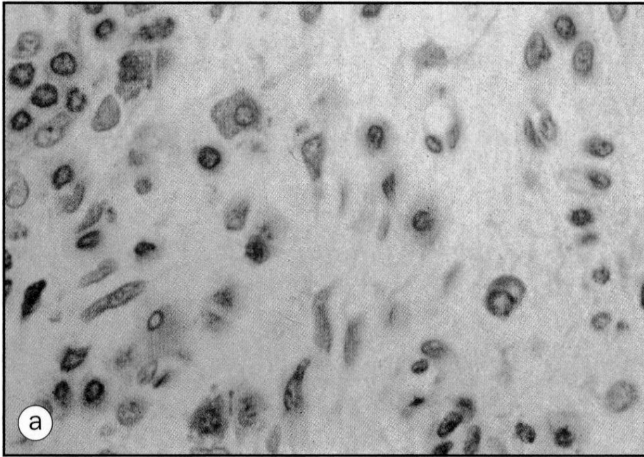

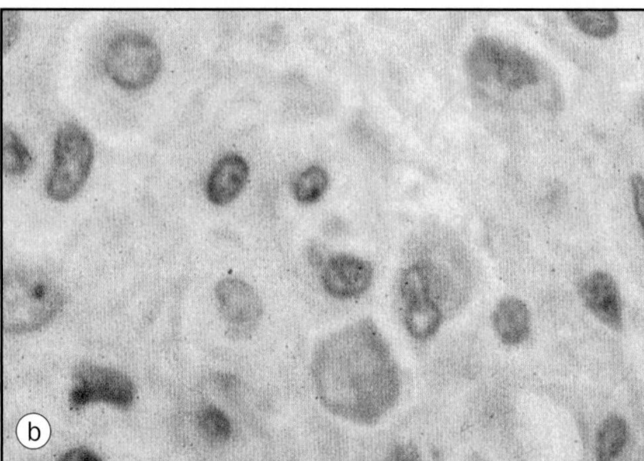

Fig. 21.4 Mast cells in a human biopsy. The cells are stained with (a) acid toluidine blue – note the reddish metachromasia of the mast cell granules – and (b) antimast cell tryptase (AA1 monoclonal antibody). (Courtesy of S Wilson and P Howarth.)

phenotypes express FcεRI and may, therefore, participate fully in IgE-dependent allergic or parasitic reactions.

It is now becoming obvious that the turning on of the genes that encode tryptase and chymase in mast cells are only two of many events that may occur as a consequence of their maturation in a particular local environment. Consequently, it is not surprising that there are forms of mast cell functional heterogeneity that are unrelated to immunocytochemical heterogeneity (Table 21.5). For example, human skin mast cells express CD88, the receptor for the anaphylatoxin C5a, allowing them to be activated in complement-mediated disease. In addition, skin mast cells alone respond to a variety of basic non-immunologic secretagogues, including neuropeptides and drugs such as morphine, codeine, and muscle relaxants. The mast cell heterogeneity between tissues is generally considered to be due to the local environmental factors. For example, priming with IL-4 upregulates the expression of FcεRI α chain, chymase, and the production of cytokines such as IL-13, while priming with IFNγ upregulates FcεRI expression and Toll-like receptor 4 and thereby increases the production of cytokines such as TNFα upon stimulation with their corresponding ligands. On the other hand, skin mast cells retain their unique characters such as substance P responsibility after long-term culture only with SCF.

Mast cell mediators

Preformed mediators

The secretory granule of the human mast cell contains a crystalline complex of preformed inflammatory mediators ionically bound to a matrix of proteoglycan. When mast cell activation occurs, the granules swell, lose their crystalline nature as the mediator complex becomes solubilized, and the individual mediators, including histamine, proteases, and proteoglycans, are expelled into the local extracellular environment by a process of compound exocytosis (Fig. 21.6).

The mediator most readily associated with the mast cell, the simple diamine histamine, is present in the granules at about 1–4 pg per cell. Histamine exerts many effects pertinent to the immediate phase of allergic responses, including vasodilatation, increased vasopermeability, contraction of bronchial and intestinal smooth muscle, and increased mucus production. However, these effects are normally of relatively short duration because histamine is rapidly metabolized, usually within 1–2 minutes – 30% of the histamine is metabolized by histamine-*N*-methyltransferase and 30% is metabolized by diamine oxidase (histaminase).

The dominant proteoglycan in human mast cells is heparin, which constitutes some 75% of the total, a mixture of chondroitin sulfates making up the remainder. Human heparin is composed of a single-chain, 17.6 kDa peptide core containing a region of alternating serine–glycine residues to which the glycosaminoglycan (GAG) side-chains are attached. Within the granule, proteoglycan may be viewed as a storage matrix because the acidic sulfate groups of the GAGs provide binding sites for the other pre-formed mediators. Once released, heparin stabilizes the active tetramer of β-tryptase. Other actions include anticoagulant, anticomplement, and antikallikrein effects, the ability to sequester eosinophil major basic protein, enhancement of collagen binding to fibronectin, and numerous growth factor-enhancing activities.

The major mast cell protease, present in all mast cells, regardless of subtype, is tryptase, a tetrameric serine protease with a molecular weight of approximately 130 kDa that is encoded on chromosome 16. It is stored in a fully active form in the granule. There appear to be at least two distinct forms of tryptase with 90% amino acid sequence homology, α-tryptase and β-tryptase. Interestingly, β-tryptase predominates in allergic reactions while both α -tryptase and β-tryptase are found in mastocytosis. β-Tryptase is recently identified as a potent growth factor for human airway smooth muscle cells, and thus it may contribute to airway remodeling of the asthmatics. Although there appear to be no endogenous inhibitors of tryptase, in the absence of heparin the biologically active tetrameric form of tryptase rapidly dissociates into inactive monomers.

Chymase is a 30 kDa monomeric protease encoded on chromosome 14. It is stored in the same secretory granules as tryptase. Chymase degrades the neuropeptide neurotensin, but not substance P or vasoactive intestinal peptide. It cleaves angiotensin I to angiotensin II more effectively than angiotensin-converting enzyme, an action which has led to much interest in chymase from cardiac mast cells in the control of the

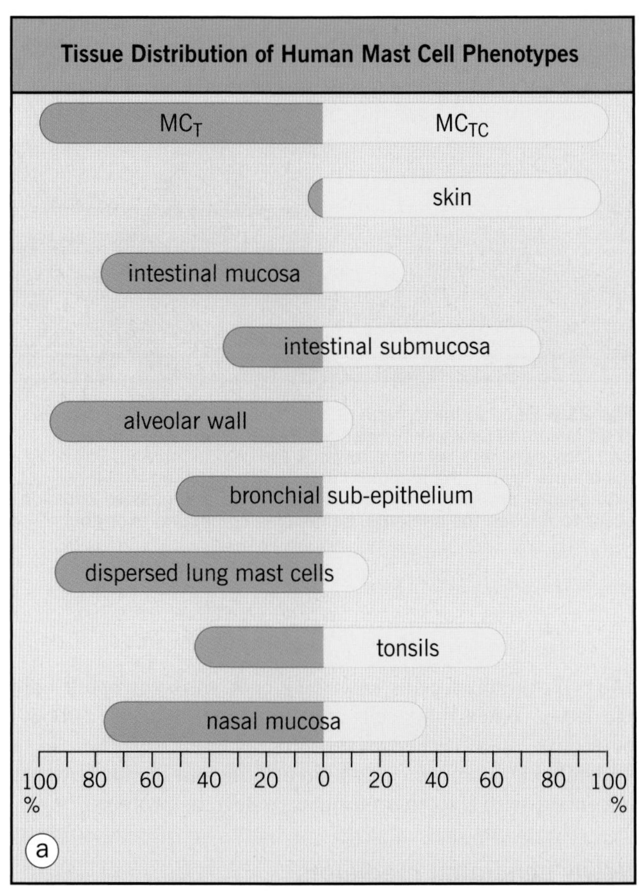

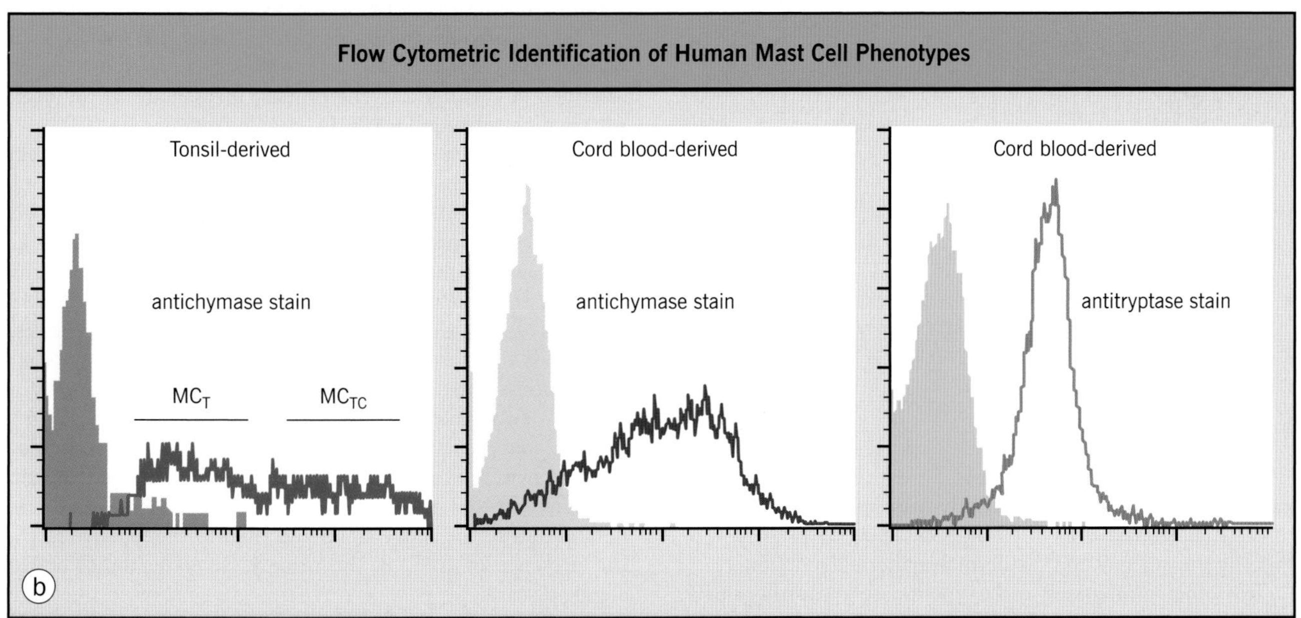

Fig. 21.5 Mast cell phenotypes. (a) Tissue distribution of human mast cell phenotypes. (b) Flow cytometric identification of human MC_T and MC_{TC}. Human mast cells can be immunohistochemically classified into chymase-positive (MC_{TC}) and -negative (MC_T). However, by intracytoplasmic flow cytometric analysis, they can be recognized as chymase-abundant and chymase-scant as shown in tonsil-derived mast cells. It should be noted that strength of chymase staining is widely distributed as compared to that of tryptase staining as shown in human cord blood-derived cultured mast cells (shaded areas indicate the results obtained with isotype-matched control antibody). [(a) – Courtesy of Dr A-M Irani and Dr LB Schwartz.]

Table 21.4 The characteristics of the two types of mast cells. MC_T appear to be immune system related mast cells, whilst MC_{TC} are non-immune system related

Characteristics of the Two Types of Mast Cells

MC_T	MC_{TC}
Immune system associated mast cell	Non-immune system associated mast cell
Proteases Tryptase	Proteases Tryptase Chymase Carboxypeptidase Cathepsin G
Characteristics Increased around sites of Th-cell activation Increased in allergic and parasitic diseases Decreased in AIDS and chronic immunodeficiency diseases	Characteristics Increased in fibrotic disease Unchanged in allergic and parasitic diseases Unchanged in AIDS and chronic immunodeficiency diseases

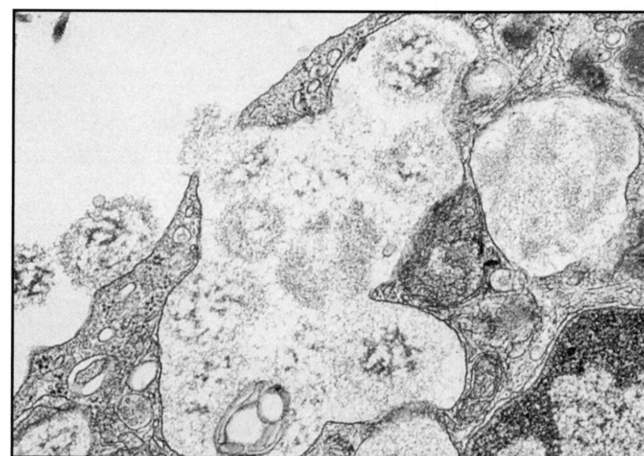

Fig. 21.6 Electron micrograph of compound exocytosis stimulated in an isolated human skin mast cell by IgE-dependent activation. Granules swell as they move towards the cell membrane. Following membrane fusion, the granular contents are exposed to the extracellular environment where ion exchange and passive diffusion occur to release the contents, so causing compound exocytosis.

Table 21.5 Mast cell heterogeneity

Heterogeneity of Human Mast Cells

	Lung	Intestinal (mucosae)	Skin	Uterus
Proteases				
Tryptase	+	+	++	++
Chymase	–	–	+	+
Stimuli				
IgE	+	+	+	+
C5a (CD88)	–	–	+	–
Substance P	–	–	+	–
Inhibitors				
β-stimulants	++	++	++	++
Cromolin sodium	±	++	–	?

The data in this table are generalized – all tissues contain a minority of mast cells whose properties are different from those specified here. Furthermore, populations of mast cells may be modified by disease.

vasculature in coronary disease. Chymase may also contribute to the role of mast cells in tissue remodeling by cleaving type IV collagen and splitting the dermal–epidermal junction.

Two other proteinases, carboxypeptidase and cathepsin G, have been associated mainly with the MC_{TC} type human mast cells. Carboxypeptidase is a unique, 34.5 kDa metalloproteinase that removes the carboxyl terminal residues from a range of peptides, including angiotensin, leu^5-enkephalin, kinetensin, neuromedin N, and neurotensin. Cathepsin G is a chymotryptic enzyme with a structure identical to that of neutrophil cathepsin G. Interestingly, the genes that encode mast cell chymase and cathepsin G are closely linked on chromosome 14q11.2, the mast cell transcribing both and neutrophils only the latter. When mast cells are activated, chymase, carboxypeptidase, and cathepsin G are released together in a 400–500 kDa complex with proteoglycan and are likely to act in concert with the other enzymes to degrade proteins.

Newly generated mediators

Immunologic activation of mast cells induces the liberation of membrane-derived arachidonic acid, a fatty acid that is then oxidized to eicosanoids. The detailed synthesis of eicosanoids is described in Chapter 24. The primary eicosanoids of the mast cell are prostaglandin D_2 (PGD_2) and leukotriene C_4 (LTC_4).

PGD_2 has the two different receptors, namely, D prostanoid receptor (DP) and chemoattractant receptor-homologous molecule expressed on Th2 cells (CRTH2). CRTH2 is coupled with Gi-type G protein and DP is coupled with Gs-type G protein. Ovalbumin-induced airway hypersensitivity of asthma model systems is suppressed in DP-deficient mice. CRTH2 mediates PGD_2-dependent cell migration of Th2 cells, eosinophils, and basophils. PGD_2 is rapidly degraded to another bronchoconstrictor agent, $9\alpha,11\beta$-PGF_2. LTC_4 is made by a variety of inflammatory cells in the lung. The mast cells are its primary source in the early-phase allergic response; predominance switches to the basophil in the late phase and allergic inflammation. In the extracellular environment, LTC_4 is metabolized to the active LTD_4 and then to the inactive LTE_4. The presence of LTE_4 in the urine is an indicator of active allergic disease.

The effects of the leukotrienes include potent contraction of bronchial and vascular smooth muscle, enhanced permeability of postcapillary venules, increased bronchial mucus secretion, and eosinophil chemoattraction, most of which are mediated by LTD_4. Because of their potent effects on the airways and their possible upregulation in allergic patients, leukotrienes are regarded as important molecules in the pathogenesis of asthma in particular.

Mast cell cytokines

Cytokines generated by both resident and freshly recruited cells are responsible for the initiation and coordination of many local processes, including allergic inflammation and tissue remodeling. In IgE-dependent allergic inflammation, it would be logical to expect that the mast cell would generate a spectrum of cytokines directed at initiating and maintaining allergic inflammation. Human mast cells generate:

- IL-4 (only immunohistochemically detected) and IL-13, which are involved in switching the B lymphocyte to IgE production;
- IL-5 and GM-CSF, which attract and prime eosinophils and prolong their life; and
- TNFα, a key cytokine in allergic inflammation that is involved in mRNA induction of various adhesion molecules and chemokines via nuclear factor κB (NF-κB) upregulation, priming leukocytes for mediator secretion, and increasing bronchial responsiveness.

The synthesis and secretion of all of these cytokines is upregulated following FcεRI activation. In addition, mast cells generate IL-3 and IL-6, both of which are proinflammatory cytokines, I-309, IL-8, RANTES, and IL-5, which are involved in granulocyte chemotaxis and activation. The ability of every sensitized mast cell to respond to stimulation with any individual allergen, as opposed to T cells, where only the small percentage of cells specific to that allergen respond, makes mast cells potentially important cytokine-generating cells in allergy. Furthermore, the presence within mast cells of preformed cytokines, which is not the case with T cells, suggests that they are available for rapid secretion.

Mast cell activation

All mast cells have as their cell surface high affinity receptors for IgE (FcεRI). The cross-linkage of two or more adjacent IgE molecules by allergen causes their associated receptors to be brought into juxtaposition. This event activates the biochemical processes that result in secretion of preformed mediators and the de novo synthesis of newly generated mediators including eicosanoids and cytokines. The biochemistry of mast-cell activation is described in more detail in Chapter 18.

Primary functions in allergy

In allergy, the release of mast-cell mediators by allergen has long been acknowledged to be the initiating step of the early-phase response. This finding is supported by the many studies that show increased levels of histamine and tryptase in blood or tissue samples in allergic asthma, rhinitis, conjunctivitis, and systemic anaphylaxis. More recently, the number of mast cells is increased in airway smooth muscle layers derived from asthmatic patients (Fig. 21.7). Since LTD_4 and tryptase stimulate the proliferation of the muscle cells, mast cells seem to play an important role in airway remodeling. In addition, mast cells, particularly through their generation of other proteases, leukotrienes, and cytokines, are critical in the initiation and control of allergic inflammation.

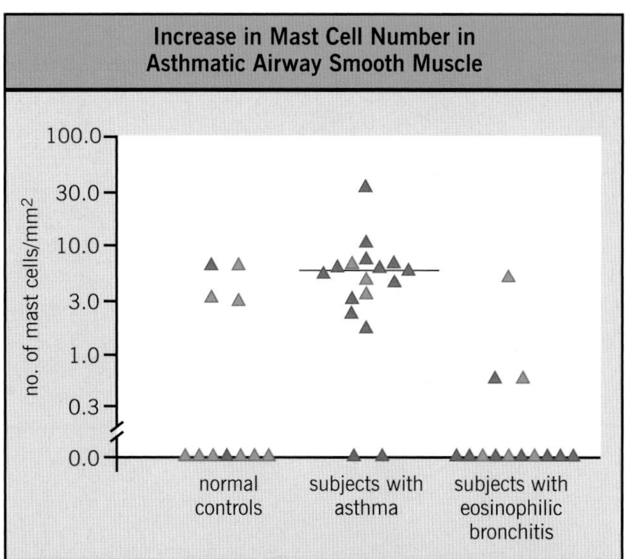

Fig. 21.7 Numbers of tryptase-positive mast cells in airway smooth muscle in normal controls, subjects with asthma, and subjects with eosinophilic bronchitis (red triangles represent atopic subjects, green triangles non-atopic subjects, and the horizontal lines represent the median values).(Adapted from Brightling CE, Bradding P, Symon FA, et al. Mast-cell infiltration of airway smooth muscle in asthma. N Engl J Med 2002; 346:1699–1705.)

BASOPHILS

Generation and morphology

Basophil granulocytes are generated in the bone marrow by precursor cells that are first shared with eosinophils and further back in lineage, with mast cells. After entering the circulation as mature cells, their passage is relatively rapid, with estimates of 0.5–2 days. Recently studies suggest that there is a period of about 6 days from the time that a precursor cell acquires the characteristics of a basophil until it is lost from circulation. The basophil has characteristics that resemble the tissue mast cell, expressing the tetrameric form of the high affinity IgE receptor and storing histamine in mature granules containing a variety of other proteases. While the precise lifetimes of mast cells and basophils are not well known in humans, a rough calculation suggests there may be 25 billion new mast cells generated every 3 months and 10–25 billion basophils generated. The basophil's characteristics suggest it can be readily recruited to tissue sites to generate mediators similar to mast cells. The basophil can be distinguished, with practice, from the mast cell under both the light and electron microscope; basophils have a bi-lobed nucleus and sparser granules than mast cells (Fig. 21.8). But there are now antibodies that can discriminate basophils from mast cells. The techniques for purifying basophils have been steadily refined over the last couple of decades and while they represent a relatively rare type of leukocyte, a wide variety of studies have provided a much clearer picture of their characteristics.

Cell surface receptors

Basophils share a variety of surface markers and receptors that are found on other leukocytes. For example, adhesion receptors

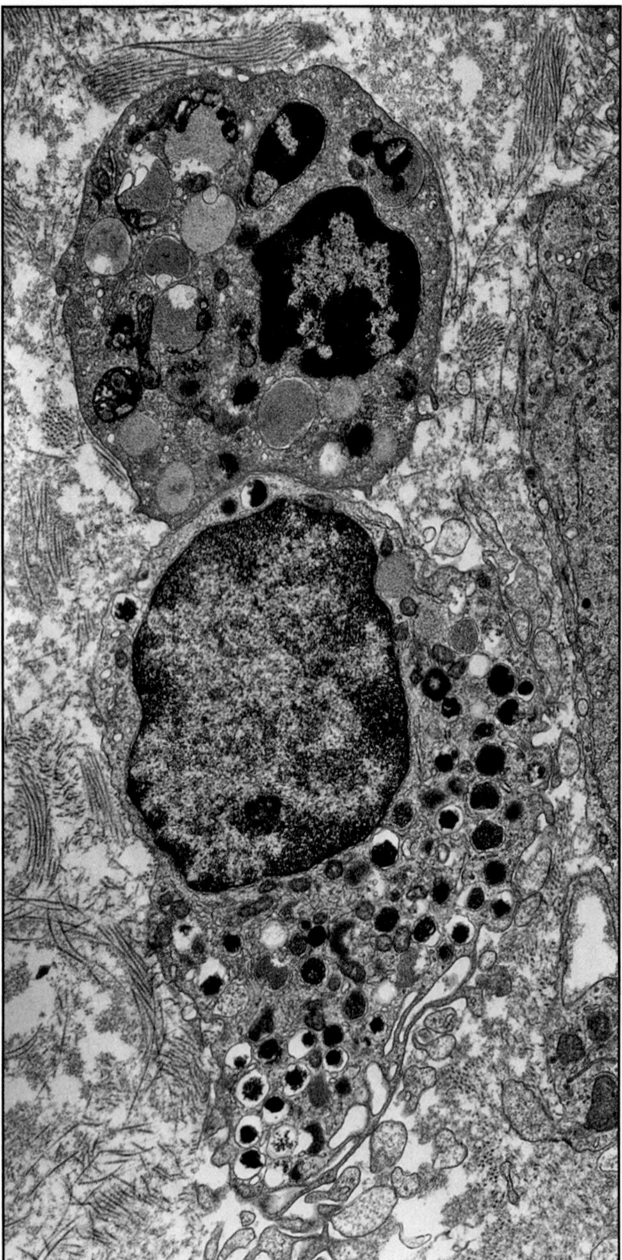

Fig. 21.8 Electron micrograph of a basophil and a mast cell together in a tissue section. (Reproduced with permission from Dvorak AM, Monahan RA, Osage JE, et al. Crohn's disease: transmission electron microscopic studies. Hum Pathol 1980; 11:606–619.)

and ligands on basophils are often found on eosinophils and, to some extent, on neutrophils. Likewise, there are a variety of peptide receptors, like fMLP and C5a, and chemokine receptors that are found on neutrophils and eosinophils. However, it is evident from studies of various inflammatory conditions that basophils can be selectively recruited and these observations suggest that there are several unique adhesion and chemokine receptors. Table 21.6 outlines some of the similarities and differences, compared with eosinophils.

There are several new classes of receptors being defined for granulocytes. For example, the leukocyte inhibitory receptors (LIRs) are known to have both activating and deactivating behaviors and recent evidence suggests that basophils and eosinophils share LIR-2 and LIR-7, with weak expression of LIR-2. A number of new members of the histamine and leukotriene families have been identified. The H_2 receptor was identified several decades ago but the newer H_3 and H_4 receptors may also be expressed. Likewise, there is evidence that cysteinyl leukotriene 1 ($CysLT_1$) and $CysLT_2$ receptors are expressed and modulate survival. Cytokines determine the maturation and survival of basophils and the basophil expresses IL-3, Il-5 and GM-CSF receptors. However, the IL-3 receptor is expressed at remarkably high densities. There is only one other cell type in circulation that expresses such high levels of IL-3 receptor, one of the recently identified precursors of dendritic cells. Indeed, it is possible to select basophils from the circulation on the basis of their coincident high expression of both the IL-3 receptors and FcεRI. It is no longer the case that basophils are the only circulating cells that express FcεRI. There is good evidence that monocytes and precursors to dendritic cells (pDC2) also express this receptor. However, basophils do express 10–1000 fold higher levels of FcεRI. There is some evidence to suggest that it is the expression of the FcεRI β subunit that provides for the higher level of expression in basophils (and mast cells).

Mediators

Basophils secrete mediators that have been grouped into three classes (Table 21.7). Granule-associated mediators, like histamine, are preformed and secreted rapidly (5–20 minutes at optimal stimulation). There are two newly generated mediator classes, lipids like leukotriene C_4 that are secreted rapidly (5–20 minutes) and newly synthesized cytokines/proteins that require hours. Although it is often reported that eosinophils secrete leukotriene C_4, the literature suggests that basophils may secrete 10–100-fold more LTC_4. Likewise, basophils appear to secrete considerably more IL-4 than eosinophil. Indeed, recent studies indicate that basophils may be a primary source of IL-4, with a majority of the IL-4 found in an inflammatory reaction coming from basophils (if they are a participant in the reaction), greater than antigen-specific T lymphocytes. It is possible that basophils represent the source of early IL-4 secretion from mast cells but it is not found in supernatants of cultured human mast cells following stimulation. Basophils also secrete IL-13 and this cytokine only needs IL-3 as a stimulus for its generation. There is no evidence that eosinophils secrete IL-13. These later two cytokines should have some role in cell recruitment and inducing the IgE switch in lymphocytes.

Activation

The very high levels of FcεRI expression in basophils lead to a condition of great sensitivity to allergen challenge. In atopic subjects, basophils express 200 000–700 000 FcεRI per cell. However, the basophil only needs 1000–5000 antigen-specific IgE molecules to respond maximally to antigen. The cells continue to secrete, albeit at lower levels, with one-tenth this density. For some subjects, allergen-specific IgE represents 50% of total IgE although it is more commonly the case that 1% of the total IgE has specificity for a given antigenic protein. It is the mix of antigens in an environmental allergen that cumulatively

Table 21.6 Receptor expression on human basophils and eosinophils

	Basophils	Eosinophils
Adhesion:	VLA-4, LFA-1 Mac-1, P150-95 $\alpha_d\beta_2$ $\alpha_4\beta_7$ VLA-6	VLA-4, LFA-1 Mac-1, P150-95 $\alpha_d\beta_2$ $\alpha_4\beta_7$ VLA-5
Histamine receptors:	H_2, (H_3, H_4)*	H_2, H_3, H_4
Leukotriene receptors:	cysLT1, cysLT2	
Chemokine receptors:	CCR1, CCR3 CXCR2, CXCR4 CCR2, CCR4, CCR7 CXCR1	CCR1, CCR3 CXCR2, CXCR4 CCR6
Active chemokines (weak):	MCP-2, -3,- 4 Eotaxin-1, -2, -3 RANTES, TECK, SDF-1α MCP-1, MIP-3, HCC-4 MIP-3β, SLC, 1-309, GCP-2	MCP-2, -3, -4 Eotaxin-1, -2, -3 RANTES, SDF-1α MIP-1α, MDC IL-8
Other chemotactic receptors:	C5a, C3a, PAF, LTB_4 PGD_2 fMLP, antigen	C5a, C3a, PAF, LTB_4 PGD_2
LIR:	LIR-2, -3, -7	LIR-2, -3,-7
Siglec:	Siglec-8	Siglec-8
Cytokine receptors:	IL-3, IL-5, GM-CSF NGF IL-1	IL-5, IL-3, GM-CSF NGF IL-1

* mRNA present. fMLP, formyl-Met-Leu-Phe; GM-CSF, GM-CSF, granulocyte–macrophage colony-stimulating factor; HCC, human CC; IL, interleukin; LFA, lymphocyte function-associated antigen; LIR, leukocyte inhibitory receptor; MCP, monocyte chemotactic peptide; MIP, macrophage inflammatory protein; NGF, nerve growth factor; PGD, prostaglandin.

Table 21.7 Secretagogues and the mediators they release from human basophils and eosinophils

	Basophils	Eosinophils
Secretagogues:	C5a, C3a, fMLP PAF (weak) MBP, polyamines MCP-1, SDF-1α, MIP-1α antigen	C5a, C3a, PAF fMLP (weak) chemokines
Mediators:	Histamine, 1 μg/10^6 LTC_4, 60 pmol/10^6 IL-4, 1000 pg/10^6 IL-13, 200 pg/10^6 Tryptase (weak)	None LTC_4, 2 pmol/10^6 IL-4, 20 pg/10^6 (intracellular) none

fMLP, formyl-Met-Leu-Phe; IL, interleukin; LTC_4, leukotriene C_4; MCP, monocyte chemotactic peptide; MBP, major basic protein; MIP, macrophage inflammatory protein; PAF, platelet-activating factor; SDF, stromal cell derived factor.

leads to high specific to total ratios. These considerations are a factor in understanding both the mast cell and basophil response to therapies that reduce IgE levels in the circulation. Considerable reduction is required to have an impact on allergen-driven secretion, a reduction of 2000–10 000 fold if receptor regulation is not considered. However, FcεRI expression is also under the control of IgE. Evidence to date indicates that IgE stabilizes the presence of FcεRI on the cell surface. Synthesis of the receptor is constitutive – not influenced, at least, by IgE – but its normal loss from the cell surface is inhibited by IgE binding. Even with the downregulation of FcεRI that occurs following reduction of free circulating IgE, significant loss of allergen-driven secretion requires 100-fold reductions in IgE in atopic patients. This IgE-dependent expression of FcεRI also appears to apply to other cells that express this receptor. Antigen-induced activation requires aggregation of FcεRI. Aggregation leads to recruitment of non-receptor tyrosine kinases (e.g. syk kinase) to the inner leaflet of the plasma membrane and this enzymatic activity initiates signal transduction cascades. Similar kinases are now known to be employed by a variety of immunoreceptors.

There are a variety of other agents that induce secretion from basophils. Many leukocytes express receptors for the bacterial tripeptide, fMLP and basophils are extremely responsive to activation of this receptor. Anaphylatoxins such as C5a and C3a are also secretagogues and under some circumstances platelet-activating factor (PAF) induces secretion. Finally, several chemokines [e.g. stromal cell derived factor-1α (SDF-1α), monocyte chemotactic peptide-1 (MCP-1)] also induce secretion (see Table 21.7). However, each of the non-IgE -dependent secretagogues operates by signal transduction pathways that depend on seven transmembrane receptors and heterotrimeric GTP binding proteins. These receptors are often associated with the functions of innate immunity. Because the signal transduction pathways are different, secretion and functional consequences are different. Notably, these secretagogues do not usually induce secretion of cytokines. However, an important way of modulating basophil secretion is to also expose the cell to cytokines like IL-3. Under these conditions, there are indications that even receptors such as C5a can induce modest secretion of IL-4.

Primary functions

Because basophils express FcεRI, it is reasonable to assume they participate in allergic reactions. There is considerable evidence to support this view although a formal demonstration of their role is not yet at hand. Recent studies have identified their presence in lung tissue following deaths due to asthma. Their presence can be elicited in tissues and airways fluids by experimental antigen challenge. Finally, there is a very strong inverse correlation between the sensitivity of basophils to allergen challenge and seasonal symptom scores. There are also indications that basophils selectively migrate into skin with exoparasitic infections, such as ticks.

EOSINOPHILS

Morphology

The association between eosinophils and allergic disease has long been established, although until the 1980s it was thought they may be antiinflammatory. This view changed with the realization that eosinophil granule proteins are highly toxic for both helminthic parasites and mammalian cells, including airway epithelial cells. Eosinophils are currently considered to be proinflammatory cells that mediate many of the features of asthma and related allergic diseases.

Eosinophils are non-dividing bone marrow-derived cells. They are approximately 8 μm in diameter and have a bi-lobed nucleus. The cytoplasm of each cell contains about 20 membrane-bound, core-containing, specific granules, which contain the

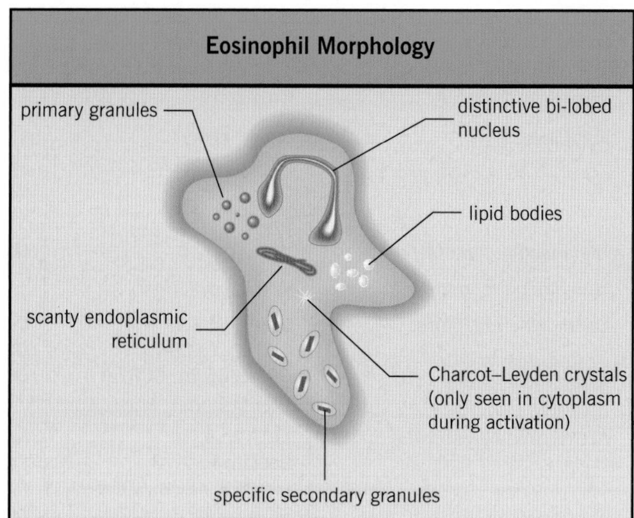

Fig. 21.9 Key morphologic features of the eosinophil.

basic proteins. These granules avidly take up acidic dyes such as eosin to give the eosinophils their characteristic microscopic appearance. In addition, the cells contain a number of primary granules, which lack a core and are of variable size. These granules contain Charcot–Leyden crystal protein (CLC protein), a characteristic feature of asthmatic sputum. Normal eosinophils contain about five, non-membrane-bound lipid bodies, which are the principal store of arachidonic acid. They also contain the enzymes cyclooxygenase and 5-lipoxygenase, which are required to synthesize prostaglandins and leukotrienes. Other granules contain acid phosphatase and aryl sulfatase (Fig 21.9).

Activated eosinophils have increased numbers of lipid bodies, primary granules, and vesicotubular structures. CLC protein is found diffusely in the cytoplasm. Specific granules may be partially emptied of their contents having undergone 'piecemeal' degranulation. At sites of inflammation eosinophils can appear necrotic although in culture they undergo apoptosis.

Cell surface receptors and antigens

Adhesion, chemoattractant, and cytokine receptors

A primary necessity of eosinophils is to be able to migrate from the blood into tissues. Tissue accumulation of eosinophils in allergic disease is likely to be due to a combination of factors, including:

- selective adhesion pathways;
- selective chemoattraction; and
- prolonged survival under the influence of locally generated cytokines, particularly IL-5 and GM-CSF.

Eosinophils express a number of adhesion receptors (Table 21.8). As well as migration from blood into tissue, adhesion receptor interactions influence: hematopoiesis, egress from the bone marrow, survival in tissues through matrix protein interactions, interactions with resident cells such as epithelium, and removal of apoptotic cells by macrophages. Migration into tissue requires a number of steps, including initial tethering to the endothelium, activation, engagement of integrins, and transmigration under the influence of chemotactic factors (see

Table 21.8 Eosinophil adhesion receptors. Note that GlyCAM-1 is secreted

Eosinophil Adhesion Receptors		
Eosinophil receptor	**Endothelial receptor**	**Matrix protein**
Integrin		
VLA-4 ($\alpha_4\beta_1$)	VCAM-1	Fibronectin
VLA-6 ($\alpha_4\beta_1$)	MAdCAM-1/VCAM-1	Laminin
(α_4/β_7)	ICAM-1, ICAM-2	Fibronectin
LFA-1	ICAM-1	Fibrinogen/heparin
Mac-1	?	
p150,95	?	
CD11d		
Immunoglobulin like		
PECAM	PECAM ($\alpha_v\beta_3$)	Glycosaminoglycans
ICAM-3 (binds LFA-1)		
Selectins		
L-selectin	GlyCAM-1, CD34, MAdCAM-1	
Carbohydrate		
PSGL-1	P-selectin/E-selectin	
?	E-selectin	
Others		
CD44		Hyaluronate

GlyCAM-1, glycosylated cell adhesion molecule-1; ICAM-1, intercellular cell adhesion molecule-1; LFA-1, lymphocyte function-associated receptor; MAdCAM-1, mucosal addressin cell adhesion molecule-1; PECAM, platelet/endothelial cell adhesion molecule; PSGL-1, P-selectin glycoprotein ligand-1; VCAM-1, vascular cell adhesion molecule-1.

Chapter 20). For eosinophils, selectins and α_4 integrins are likely to be important in the capture step; CD18 integrins and α_4 integrins mediate arrest; and C–C chemokines such as eotaxin, as well as PAF, are likely to be involved in mediating transmigration, although this also requires matrix metalloprotease-9 (MMP-9) and platelet/endothelial cell adhesion molecule (PECAM) to penetrate the basement membrane (Fig. 21.10). The exact nature of the activation signal is currently uncertain. In terms of specificity, eosinophils bind better to P-selectin than neutrophils do; the reverse appears to be true for E-selectin.

Once in the tissue, eosinophils can generate their own survival-inducing cytokines, in particular GM-CSF, that through outside-in signaling interact between very late antigen-4 (VLA-4) and VLA-6 and between tissue fibronectin and laminin. Of the eosinophil cytokines, IL-5 is the most characteristic. As well as being central to eosinophilopoiesis, IL-5 enhances mature eosinophil function – priming the cell for chemotactic and degranulatory responses and adhesion and cytotoxicity – and prolongs survival. Eosinophils can respond to a number of C–C chemokines, mainly through the CCR3 receptor (Table 21.9). Eosinophils also express low levels of CCR1. CCR3 has generated considerable excitement as a promising target for selective inhibition of eosinophil migration.

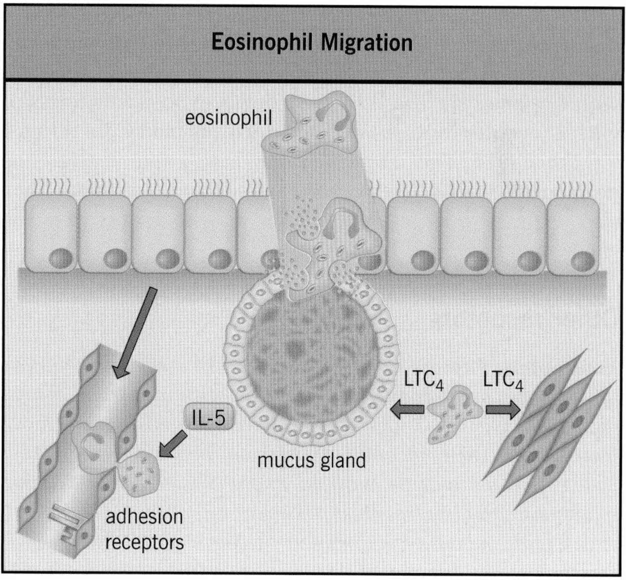

Fig. 21.10 The molecular events leading to eosinophil migration. IL, interleukin; LTC_4, leukotriene C_4.

Immunoglobulin and complement receptors

Eosinophils express Fc receptors for IgG, IgA, and IgE. The principal IgG receptor is CD32 (FcεRII), although expression of CD64 (FcεRI) and CD16 (FcγRIII) is induced by IFNγ. The FcαR on eosinophils has a higher molecular weight than the FcαR on neutrophils and monocytes as a result of differential glycosylation.

Despite intensive research there is still a degree of uncertainty about the nature and functional importance of IgE receptors on eosinophils. A subset of highly activated eosinophils expresses CD23. Eosinophils also express the IgE-binding

Table 21.9 Eosinophil receptors. Adhesion receptors are not shown

Eosinophil Receptors (other than adhesion)
Chemokines CCR3 CCR1 CXCR1 (only on primed cells) CXCR2 (only on primed cells)
Mediators Il-5, GM-CSF, IL-3 C5a, C3a, PAF, LTB_4
Immunoglobulin CD32, FcαR, FcεR, Galectin 3
Newly expressed CD69, CD25, CD4, ICAM-1, CD16
Other receptors CD40, CD9, CD45

GM-CSF, granulocyte–macrophage colony-stimulating factor; IL, interleukin; LTB_4, leukotriene B_4; PAF, platelet-activating factor.

Table 21.10 Eosinophil-derived mediators

Eosinophil-derived Mediators
Granule-associated mediators
Basic proteins: MBP, ECP, EDN, EPO Enzymes: lysophospholipase (CLC protein), catalase, acid phosphatase Cytokines: IL-1, IL-2, IL-3, IL-4, IL-5, IL-6, IL-8, GM-CSF, IL-16, TGFα, TGFβ Chemokines: RANTES, MIP-1α
Membrane-derived mediators
LTC_4; PAF; 15-HETE; PGE_1; PGE_2; TXB_2

CLC, Charcot–Leyden crystal; ECP, eosinophil cationic protein, EDN, eosinophil-derived neurotoxin; EPO, eosinophil peroxidase; GM-CSF, granulocyte–macrophage colony-stimulating factor; 15-HETE, 15-hydroxyeicosatetraenoic acid; IL, interleukin; MBP, major basic protein; MIP, macrophage inflammatory protein; LTB_4, leukotriene B_4; PAF, platelet-activating factor; PGE_1, PGE_2, prostaglandin E_1, E_2; TGF, transforming growth factor; TXB_2, thromboxane B_2.

protein, galectin 3 (Mac-2). However, neutrophils also express this receptor but are unable to interact functionally with IgE. Peripheral blood eosinophils express low levels of the high-affinity IgE receptor (FcεRI). Whether this receptor has a functional role in mediating eosinophil degranulation in allergic disease remains to be determined. Sepharose beads coated with immunoglobulin are effective at causing eosinophil degranulation with IgA (particularly secretory IgA), which is more effective than with IgG, which in turn is more effective than with IgE. Degranulation is considerably enhanced by priming the cells with cytokines such as IL-5. Eosinophils express low levels of CR1, a receptor for C3b, and can effectively bind C3bi through CD11b–CD18. This interaction may have a role in triggering degranulation in the presence of complement activation. They also express low levels of CR1 and receptors for the chemotaxins C3a and C5a.

Other receptors

Eosinophils express a large number of receptors whose importance in eosinophil function is still uncertain. These include CD9, CD40, CD4, and HLA-DR. As eosinophils move into tissue, their receptor expression becomes modulated. These changes include induced expression of the activation markers CD69, intercellular adhesion molecule-1 (ICAM-1), and CD25, increased expression of Mac-1, and shedding of L-selectin. The functional significance of these changes is also still unclear, but nonetheless it is important to appreciate that the phenotype and functional capacity of tissue eosinophils may be quite different from those of blood eosinophils.

Mediators

Basic proteins

The principal mediators produced by eosinophils include presynthesized granule-derived proteins, newly synthesized lipid mediators, and cytokines (Table 21.10).

The major granule proteins include major basic protein, eosinophil cationic protein, eosinophil peroxidase, and eosinophil-derived neurotoxin. They are all stored in the specific granules and they are all highly basic proteins with molecular weights in the region of 15–20 kDa. A brief description of the function of these proteins is shown in Table 21.11. However, a key feature of the basic proteins is that they are toxic for parasite larvae as well as for some mammalian cells and are either totally or largely exclusive to eosinophils. More than any other feature they set the eosinophil apart from other leukocytes. Cytokines as well as a number of enzymes of uncertain significance are stored in eosinophil granules.

Lipid mediators

Eosinophils are one of the major producers of leukotrienes in allergic inflammation. Maximum stimulation of eosinophils by calcium ionophore results in the production of about 50 ng of LTC_4 per 10^6 cells, while amounts in the region of 5 ng per 10^6 cells are produced on stimulation through Fc receptors. Eosinophils can also generate physiologically significant amounts of PAF.

Cytokines

Eosinophils have been shown by a combination of polymerase chain reaction, immunocytochemistry, and enzyme-linked immunosorbent assay to store and synthesize a large number of cytokines (Table 21.12). This action potentially greatly expands the functional role of eosinophils. For example, synthesis of TNFα may be important in wound healing. Several cytokines may be important in modulating eosinophil function in tissue; for example, the survival enhancing properties of GM-CSF and the apoptosis-inducing effects of transforming growth factor β (TGFβ). Generally, the amount of cytokines produced by eosinophils is very low compared to that produced by other cell types, which limits their likely functional effects.

Table 21.11 Functions of eosinophil granule proteins

Functions of Eosinophil Granule Proteins	
Protein	**Function**
MBP	Toxicity towards helminthic parasites such as schistosomulae of *S. mansoni* Cytotoxicity towards guinea pig and human airway epithelium at 10 mg/mL Bronchoconstriction and increased BHR on inhalation in rats and monkeys Non-cytotoxic release of histamine from basophils Strong platelet agonist Activates complement through alternate pathway
ECP	Ribonuclease activity (100 times less potent than EDN) Toxic for helminthic parasites and mammalian epithelial cells Causes Gordon phenomenon
EPO	Toxic for mammalian cells through ability to oxidize halides in presence of H_2O_2 to reactive hypohalous acids. Thiocyanate which forms the weak oxidant hypothiocyanous acid may be preferred halide in vivo
EDN	Only weakly toxic for parasites or mammalian cell Induces Gordon phenomenon

BHR, bronchial hyperresponsiveness; ECP, eosinophil cationic protein, EDN, eosinophil-derived neurotoxin; EPO, eosinophil peroxidase; MBP, major basic protein.

Table 21.12 Cytokine generation by eosinophils

Cytokine Generation by Eosinophils	
Cytokine	**Comments**
IL-1α	Syntheses triggered by LPS and phorbol esters
TGFα	mRNA +ve and immunoreactive eosinophils detected in association with healing wounds, HES, and squamous carcinoma
TGFβ	Detected in eosinophils in nasal polyps and Hodgkin's lymphoma
GM-CSF	Secreted in response to IFNγ and calcium ionophore stimulation
IL-2	IL-2 immunoreactivity detected in 10% of peripheral blood eosinophils
IL-3	IL-3 production inhibited by FK506, rapamycin and ciclosporin
IL-4	75 pg/10^6 cells detected within eosinophils. mRNA detected by RT-PCR
IL-5	mRNA expression detected in eosinophils by in situ hybridization and immunoreactivity in a number of conditions including HES, celiac disease, and BAL cells in asthma. Small amounts released following Fc receptor stimulation
IL-6	IL-6 stored in unstimulated eosinophil granules
IL-8	Stored in eosinophil granules, released by calcium ionophore
TNFα	Found in various eosinophilic conditions in association with granules
TNFα/RANTES	Expression of mRNA in nasal polyp eosinophils, skin eosinophils after allergen challenge, and HES eosinophils shown by in situ hybridization

BAL, bronchoalveolar lavage; GM-CSF, granulocyte–macrophage colony-stimulating factor; HES, hypereosinophilic syndrome; IFN, interferon; IL, interleukin; LPS, lipopolysaccharides; RT-PCR, reverse transcriptase polymerase chain reaction; TNF, tumor necrosis factor.

Activation

In peripheral blood and uninflamed tissue, eosinophils are in a resting state to prevent unwanted tissue damage from eosinophil-derived mediators. To mount an effective inflammatory response, eosinophils must first become primed – a process whereby effector functions such as migration, adhesion, and phagocytosis are enhanced – and then be triggered to release their mediators. Priming, which is mediated by both chemoattractants and growth factors, is required before effective triggering can occur. Activation involves both priming and triggering. Although many of the external signals that regulate this process in eosinophils are known, the signaling events are still being unraveled (Table 21.13). The most effective priming agents are the cytokines IL-5, GM-CSF, and IL-3, although PAF and LTB_4 are also active. One of the major uncertainties in eosinophil biology is the mechanism by which the often florid eosinophil degranulation that is seen in allergic disease occurs.

Eosinophils are designed to secrete their mediators on to the surface of a large, opsonized parasite in a process described as frustrated phagocytosis. In this case the opsonins are either immunoglobulin or derived from complement with triggering of secretion via Fc or complement receptors. However, in allergic disease there is neither an obvious target nor an opsonin, which suggests that different triggering mechanisms are involved. Chemokines, although effective chemoattractants, appear unable to cause mediator release. Interaction with matrix proteins such as fibronectin and laminin can result in sufficient GM-CSF synthesis to support autocrine survival and may have a modest priming effect as a result. IL-5 in eosinophils signals through the STAT-1, Jak2 tyrosine kinase pathway resulting in activation of mitogen activated protein (MAP) kinases. Following activation, eosinophils may undergo necrosis, which results in the indiscriminate and tissue-damaging release of granule proteins, or they may be disposed of by apoptosis, a pathway that is also triggered by removal of growth factors. Consistent with their status as end-stage cells, eosinophils express little or no Bcl-2. They do, however, express the survival promoting Bcl-xL. The major antisurvival member of the Bcl-2 family in eosinophils is Bax.

Table 21.13 Eosinophil chemoattractants and priming agents

Eosinophil Chemoattractants and Priming Agents	
Lipids	PAF LTB_4 LTC_4 18s, 15s, diHETE
Small MW peptides	C5a C3a fMLP
Chemokines	CC family RANTES MIP-1α MCP-3 MCP-4 Eotaxin-1 Eotaxin-2 newly expressed
CXC family	IL-8
Growth factors/cytokines	IL-5 IL-3 GM-CSF IFNγ TNFα

diHETE, di-hydroxyeicosatetraenoic acid; fMLP, formyl-Met-Leu-Phe; GM-CSF, granulocyte–macrophage colony-stimulating factor; IL, interleukin; IFN, interferon; MCP, monocyte chemotactic peptide; MIP, macrophage inflammatory protein; LTC_4, B_4, leukotriene C_4, B_4; PAF, platelet-activating factor; TNF, tumor necrosis factor.

Primary functions in allergy

Blood and tissue eosinophilia is a hallmark of all allergic diseases, including atopic asthma, allergic rhinitis and conjunctivitis, atopic dermatitis, and urticaria. An eosinophilia is also found in diseases such as intrinsic asthma, nasal polyposis, non-atopic rhinitis with eosinophilia, and episodic angioedema, which, although not obviously IgE dependent, are thought to have a broadly similar immunologic mechanism. Even if intact eosinophils are not seen in tissues from these patients, there is often extensive deposition of granule proteins.

There is currently a consensus that regards eosinophils and their mediators as important proinflammatory agents causing the pathologic abnormalities that are characteristic of allergic disease. This consensus rests on three types of evidence:

- Eosinophils are a consistent feature of inflammation associated with allergic diseases.
- Eosinophil-derived mediators have properties that can lead to many of the features of these diseases.
- Removal of eosinophils is associated with amelioration of the disease process.

The evidence to support this consensus is both extensive and largely consistent. For example, numerous carefully controlled studies, both in experimentally-induced allergic responses by allergen challenge and in clinical disease, have shown increased numbers of eosinophils and eosinophil granule proteins in tissue, with a broad correlation between numbers of eosinophils and markers of severity. Basic proteins have been shown to be toxic to airway epithelium, and LTC_4 is of undoubted relevance to the asthma process (Fig. 21.11). Countless animal studies in

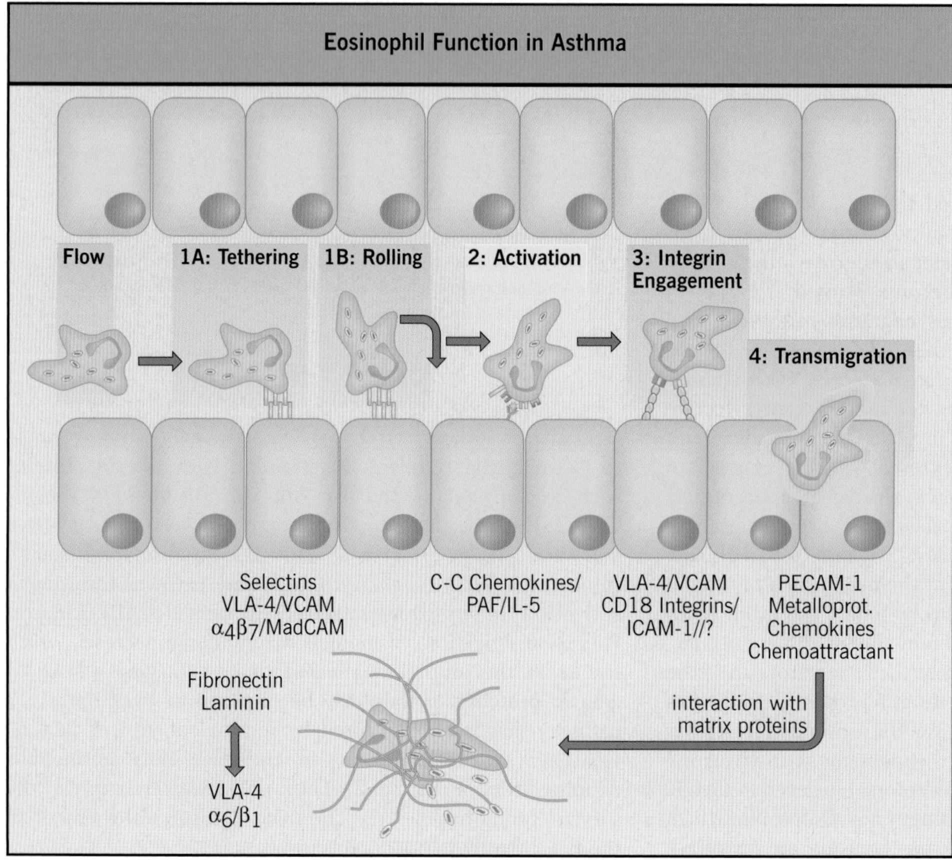

Fig. 21.11 Eosinophil function in asthma. Eosinophils are directed into tissues under the influence of adhesion receptors, epithelial-derived CC chemokines, and Th2 cell-derived IL-5. They are then triggered to release their mediators, including granule proteins that are toxic for epithelial cells and sulfidopeptide leukotrienes, which cause bronchoconstriction and mucus hypersecretion. ICAM, intercellular adhesion molecule; IL, interleukin; MAdCAM, mucosal addressin cell adhesion molecule; PAF, platelet-activating factor; PECAM, platelet/endothelial cell adhesion molecule; VCAM, vascular cell adhesion molecule; VLA, very late antigen.

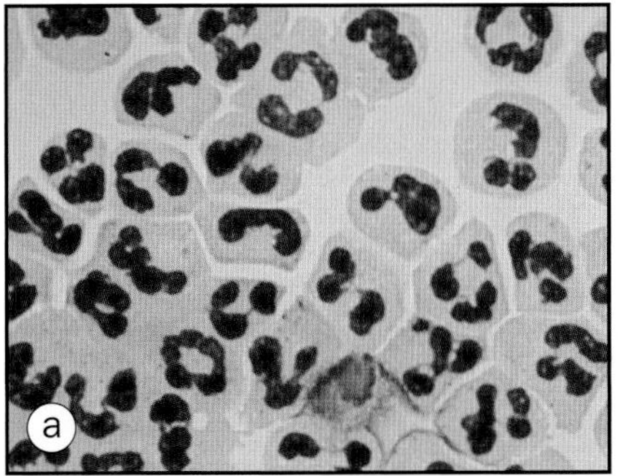

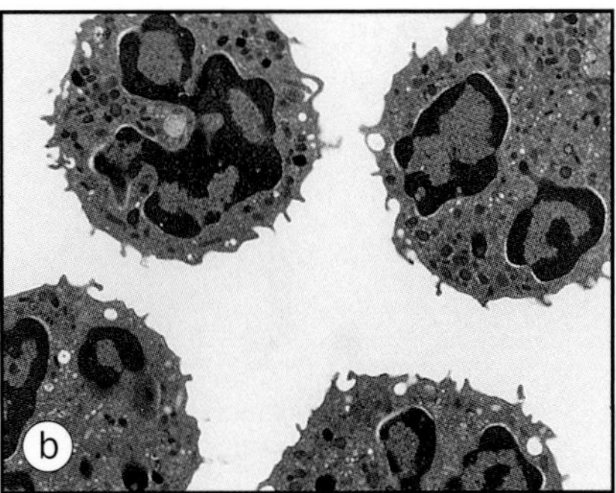

Fig. 21.12 Morphology of neutrophils. (a) Light microscopy of a cytospin preparation of purified human neutrophils, stained with Wright's modified Giemsa. Note the slightly pink cytoplasm and lobulated nucleus with loosely granular chromatin (oil immersion × 1000). (b) Electron micrograph of human neutrophils. Note the large numbers of cytoplasmic granules (× 12 000). (Courtesy of Jan Henson.)

several species have been undertaken in which an airway eosinophilia has been induced by antigen challenge and the eosinophilia has then been inhibited by antagonists of a variety of mediators. Prevention of the airway eosinophilia has usually been accompanied by reduction in tissue damage and airway hyperresponsiveness.

Lastly, one of the most marked effects of corticosteroids in asthma is a reduction in airway and blood eosinophils. As a result, there is a considerable effort by the pharmaceutical industry to develop strategies that will prevent the access of eosinophils to the tissue, in particular antagonists of adhesion receptors, chemokines, and IL-5.

However, a degree of caution is required. The evidence, although convincing, remains circumstantial. The increase in eosinophils in allergic disease is often modest and is remarkable largely because eosinophils are virtually absent from the normal airway and skin. In addition, it is not specific because increased numbers of eosinophils are seen in exacerbations of smoking-related airflow obstruction although not during stable periods. Many patients have a florid airway eosinophilia with mild asthma whereas some patients with severe asthma have few eosinophils in their airways. The evidence for toxicity of eosinophil granule proteins is largely from animal models and, furthermore, high concentrations of these proteins are required. Matrix metalloproteinases derived from a range of inflammatory cells may be more potent at detaching airway epithelial cells. Not all animal studies have shown a correlation between inhibition of airway eosinophilia and amelioration of pathology and, in any case, animal studies are limited as models of allergic disease.

Thus, while the evidence justifies the efforts of drug companies, inevitably the final proof that eosinophils are as important as they appear to be in causing allergic disease awaits the development of a selective antagonist.

NEUTROPHILS

Morphology

Neutrophils, or neutrophilic polymorphonuclear leukocytes, are about 7 μm in diameter and are easily recognized in conventional cytologic preparations by their pinkish cytoplasm and distinctive polymorphic nuclei (Fig. 21.12). When neutrophils are viewed under the electron microscope, a number of heterogeneous granules are obvious. The larger of these, the so-called primary or azurophilic granules, are peroxidase-positive whereas the smaller ones, the so-called secondary or specific granules, are peroxidase-negative. Other subcellular structures, such as Golgi apparatuses, are scarce.

Cell surface antigens and receptors

Neutrophils are the primary defense cells against infection and tissue injury. Consequently, it is necessary for them to express adhesion proteins on their cell surface so that they can infiltrate inflamed tissues rapidly and in large numbers.

Several adhesion proteins have been identified on the neutrophil (Table 21.14). Of these, the integrin, Mac-1, which is the ligand for ICAM-1, appears to be particularly important. This is evidenced by the ability of blocking antibodies to Mac-1 to inhibit the accumulation of neutrophils at sites of inflammation in experimental models.

The requirement for neutrophils to move rapidly to an inflammatory site once in the extravascular space, no matter what the cause, means that they must also express high levels of receptors for a wide range of chemotactic agents (Fig. 21.13). Of these, IL-8 and LTB_4 have received most attention, particularly since activated neutrophils generate large quantities of these two agents, thereby enhancing the stimulus for further neutrophil accumulation.

Mediators

Neutrophil mediators may be divided functionally into two groups (Table 21.15). The first group is commensurate with their primary function to phagocytose and digest bacteria and other foreign particles, including enzymes and oxygen radicals. The second group comprises mediators that attract and activate more neutrophils. These mediators include lipid mediators and cytokines.

Enzymes

Neutrophil lysosomal granules contain more than 20 enzymes, including proteinases, elastase, gelatinase, and collagenase, lysozyme, cathepsin G, and defensins. Intracellularly, these enzymes digest ingested bacteria but many are also liberated into the extracellular environment during inflammation. However, their potential to cause tissue damage is limited by the presence of antiproteinases, such as α_2-antiproteinase and α_2-macroglobulin, which penetrate the tissues from the plasma during inflammation. Therefore, the importance of the neutrophil in causing overt tissue damage in the presence of normal levels of antiproteinases is unclear. In antiproteinase deficiency, however, as has been suggested in emphysema, the potential for neutrophil-induced tissue damage is enhanced.

Table 21.14 Neutrophil adhesion proteins

Cell type	Workshop cluster designation	Common nomenclature	Ligand(s)
Adhesion Molecules and Ligands Relevant to Neutrophil/Endothelial Interactions			
Integrins			
Neutrophil	CD11a/CD18	LFA-1	ICAM-1, ICAM-2, ICAM-3 (immunoglobulin superfamily)
Neutrophil	CD11b/CD18	CR3 (Mac-1)	C3bi ICAM-1 Fibrinogen
Neutrophil	CD11c/CD18	p150,95	C3bi? Endothelial ligand Fibrinogen
Selectins			
Neutrophil	W/D	L-selectin (mel 14 mouse)	Endothelial CHO
Endothelial	–	GMP-140 PADGEM	Sialylated Lewis X antigen (CD15 on neutrophil)
Endothelial	–	ELAM-1	Sialylated Lewis X antigen (CD15 on neutrophil)
Others Neutrophil	CD44	HCAM?	Hyaluronate receptor

ELAM, endothelial leukocyte adhesion molecule; ICAM-1, intercellular cell adhesion molecule-1; LFA-1, lymphocyte function-associated receptor-1; PADGEM, platelet activation dependent granule-external membrane protein.

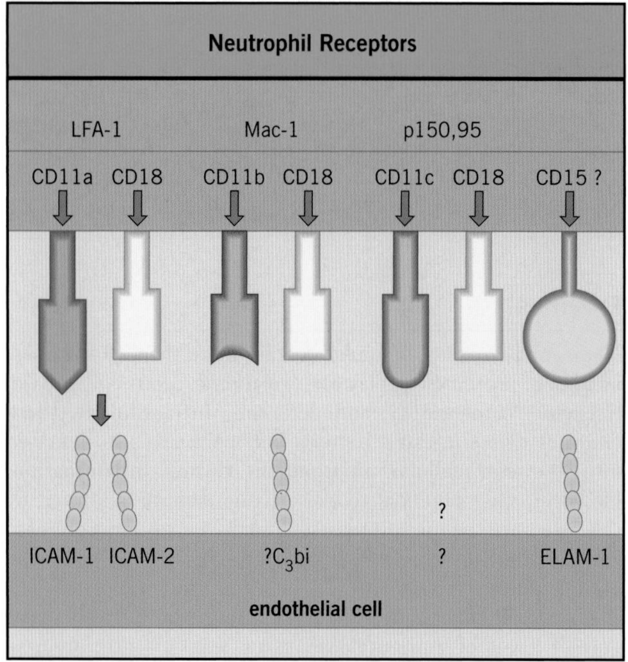

Fig. 21.13 Neutrophil receptors. ELAM, endothelial leukocyte adhesion molecule; ICAM, intercellular adhesion molecule; LFA, lymphocyte function-associated antigen.

Oxygen radicals

A characteristic of neutrophil activation is the stimulation within seconds of a respiratory burst. This leads to the generation of the oxygen radicals, hydrogen peroxide (H_2O_2) and superoxide (O_2^-). These are converted into the even more toxic hypohalous acid (HOCl) by the actions of neutrophil myeloperoxidase, and into hydroxyl ions (OH^-) by reduction of ferrous to ferric ions. While these radicals are clearly bactericidal, their role in allergic disease is not so clear.

Lipid mediators

Neutrophils are a major source of the chemotactic LTB_4. In the neutrophil, an epoxide hydrolase converts the arachidonate-derived lipid intermediate, LTA_4, into LTB_4. This is in contrast to eosinophils, in which a specific glutathione-S-transferase links glutathione to LTA_4 to produce LTC_4. Neutrophils can also generate physiologically significant amounts of PAF.

Cytokines

Because the neutrophil is essentially an end-stage cell with a short life-span, its ability to synthesize proteins de novo is limited. However, it has been demonstrated that neutrophils generate IL-1, TNFα, and IL-8, which serve to recruit and

Table 21.15 Neutrophil mediators

Constituents of Human Neutrophil Granules		
	Azurophil granules	**Specific granules**
Microbicidal enzymes	Lysozyme Myeloperoxidase	Lysozyme
Neutral proteinases	Elastase Collagenases Cathepsin G	Collagenase
Acid hydrolases	Phosphatases Lipases Sulfatases Histonase Cathepsin D β Glycerophosphatase esterase Neuraminidase 5′ nucleotidase	Phosphatases
Others	Bactericidal/permeability-inducing protein Defensins Cationic proteins Glycosaminoglycans Chondroitin sulfate Heparan sulfate	Lactoferrin V IT B_{12} binding protein C3bi Receptor Cytochrome B Flavoproteins

activate further neutrophils, and IL-6, IL-12, macrophage colony-stimulating factor (M-CSF), and GM-CSF, which stimulate hematopoiesis, a process that is necessary for the production of more neutrophils.

Activation

In order to mount a maximal secretory response and respiratory burst, neutrophils, like eosinophils, need to be exposed to the effects of both priming and activating stimuli. Priming agents, which upregulate the baseline activity of the cell but do not themselves initiate secretory events, include lipopolysaccharide, TNFα, and PAF. Activating stimuli, such as IL-8, C5a, and fMLP then activate the complex biochemical pathway that leads to enzyme secretion, upregulate the NADPH (reduced form of nicotinamide adenine dinucleotide phosphate) oxidase system to form oxygen radicals, and initiate phospholipid metabolism, which leads to the generation of LTB_4. Furthermore, a variety of inflammatory mediators, including GM-CSF, are able to extend the active life-span of neutrophils by delaying apoptosis.

Primary functions in allergy

Tissue neutrophilia is the hallmark of all inflammation. In allergic inflammation in humans, neutrophil accumulation in allergen-challenged sites precedes that of eosinophils. Moreover, the peak time of neutrophil accumulation is approximately 8 hours, which coincides with the peak of the late-phase response. However, no causal relationship between the neutrophil and the symptoms of allergic disease or asthma has been established. Even so, it would be surprising if local tissue damage caused by activated neutrophils did not contribute to the long-term pathogenicity of allergic inflammation, particularly at mucosal surfaces.

MONOCYTES AND MACROPHAGES

Morphology and heterogeneity of monocytes and macrophages

Macrophages represent the major mature cell of the mononuclear phagocyte system and are found in essentially every human tissue and body cavity. They originate from precursors in the bone marrow, which are released into the blood as monocytes and then marginate into tissues by following a defined pathway of maturation, trafficking, and differentiation. Blood monocytes have a kidney-bean shaped nucleus, and a granular cytoplasm containing lysosomes and phagocytic vacuoles. Once established in tissues, macrophages may assume many different forms (Table 21.1). Mononuclear phagocytes function in both the natural and acquired arms of the immune system and participate in a wide range of physiologic and pathologic processes (Table 21.16). An important role in the disease process seen in allergy is played by both:

- mononuclear phagocyte activation leading to the release of numerous soluble mediators that regulate inflammatory and immune processes; and
- the presentation of antigen to T lymphocytes and the regulation of T-lymphocyte activation.

Cell surface antigens and receptors

The capacity of mononuclear phagocytes to respond to changes in their environment is mediated by a large array of plasma membrane receptors. The use of monoclonal antibodies to

Table 21.16 General properties of mononuclear phagocytes

General Properties of Mononuclear Phagocytes
Ingestion and killing of invading microbes and tumor cells
Release of numerous soluble mediators involved in host defense and inflammation
Removal of tissue debris and wound repair
Regulation of hemopoiesis
Processing and presentation of antigen to and activation of T lymphocytes

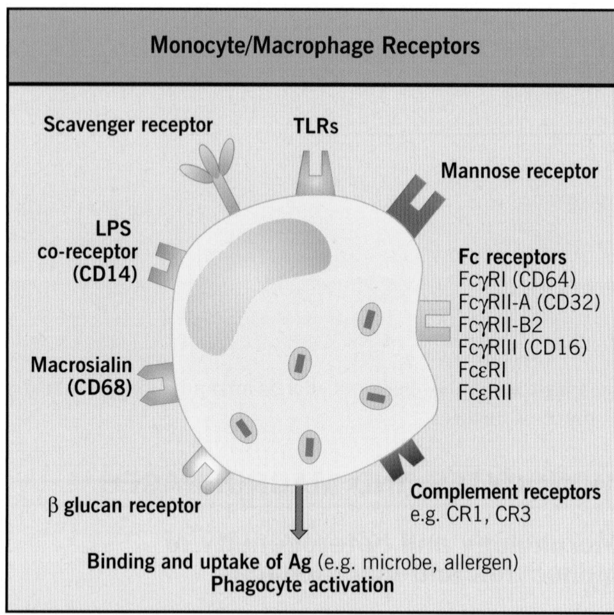

Fig. 21.14 Monocyte–macrophage receptors. LPS, lipopolysaccharide.

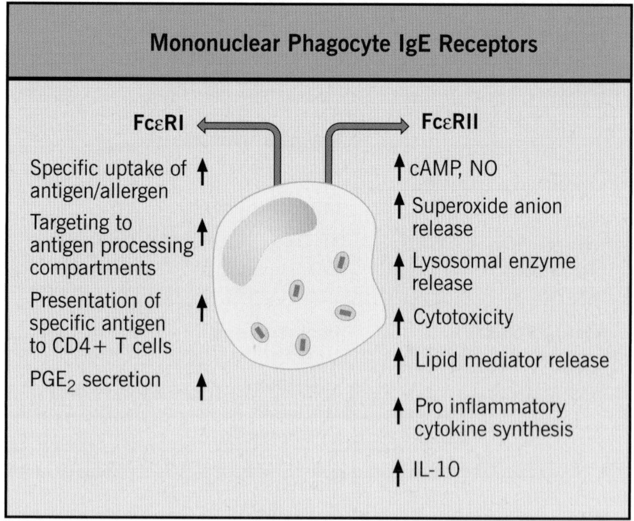

Fig. 21.15 Monocyte phagocyte IgE receptors. Expression by mononuclear phagocytes of low (FcεRII) and high (FcεRI) affinity receptors for IgE and the functional consequences of IgE receptor cross-linking. cAMP, cyclic adenosine monophosphate; IL, interleukin; PGE_2, prostaglandin E_2.

detect these and additional antigens expressed is an important aspect of cellular identification, although none of these antigens is completely lineage specific (Fig. 21.14). In humans, important markers are:

- CD14, a glycosyl phosphatidylinositol-anchored cell surface glycoprotein with a molecular weight of 55 kDa, which is also found in a soluble form; it functions as a co-receptor for Gram-negative bacterial endotoxins;
- CD64, a receptor for the constant portion of immunoglobulin, FcεR1; and
- CD68, a highly glycosylated protein that is found mainly intracellularly and is a homolog of the murine macrosialin protein.

Expression of major histocompatibility class II antigens, which are essential for presentation of antigen to CD4+ T lymphocytes, together with the lack of expression of defined T-, B- and natural killer (NK)-cell markers, are also useful for identification of this lineage.

Mononuclear phagocytes carry a number of receptors for the recognition of foreign antigens such as microbes and allergens. These facilitate binding and internalization of particulate and soluble ligands with great efficiency and selectivity, and lead to distinct patterns of intracellular signaling and cellular activation. Several families of receptors that recognize conserved molecular patterns permit recognition of microbial ligands, but also some host molecules, by cells of the innate immune system including monocytes, macrophages and dendritic cells. These include the Toll-like receptor family (TLR 1-10), scavenger receptors, c-type lectin-like receptors and the mannose receptor. These receptors recognize lipoproteins, glycoproteins, and carbohydrates. Fc receptors, which bind the Fc or constant portion of immunoglobulin, and receptors for complement components allow the recognition and endocytosis of opsonized antigen. Monocytes and macrophages express receptors for the complement components C3b, C3bi, and C3d, which are increased in allergic disease. In addition, receptors for IgG monomers, IgG complexes, and IgE immune complexes are also expressed by these cells. Increased expression of both the high-affinity receptor for IgE, FcεRI , and the low-affinity receptor for IgE, FcεRII (CD23), is observed on monocytes, macrophages, and dendritic cells in allergy. Major receptors are illustrated in Figure 21.15.

Mediators

The capacity of monocytes and macrophages to regulate T-lymphocyte activation, control microbial invasion, and regulate inflammatory events is mediated in large part by the synthesis and secretion of soluble mediators (Fig. 21.16). These biologically active molecules vary in molecular weight and range from simple chemical species such as nitric oxide to complex glycoproteins such as cytokines.

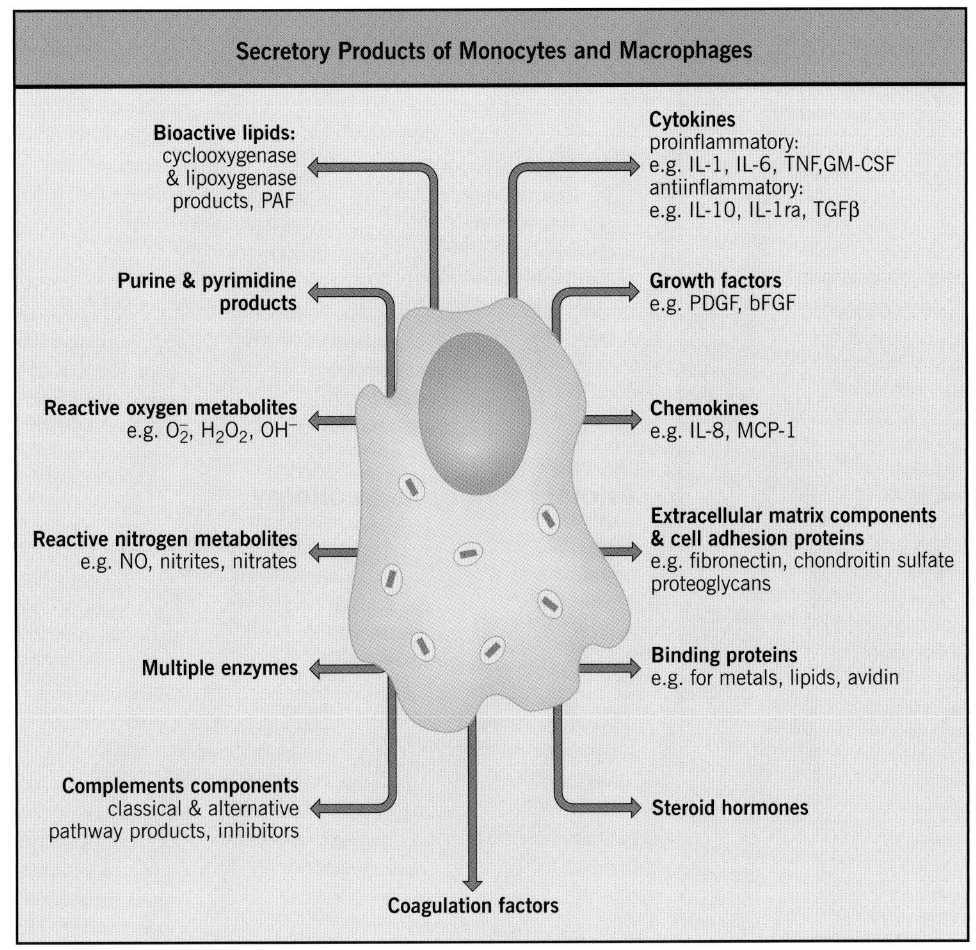

Fig. 21.16 Secretory products of monocytes and macrophages. bFGF, basic fibroblast growth factor; GM-CSF, granulocyte–macrophage colony-stimulating factor; IL, interleukin; MCP, monocyte chemotactic peptide; PAF, platelet-activating factor; PGDF, platelet-derived growth factor; TGF, transforming growth factor; TNF, tumor necrosis factor.

Production of reactive oxygen metabolites and reactive nitrogen intermediates

Cytokines, endocytosis of opsonized particles, and IgE-immune complexes all activate monocytes and macrophages for increased oxygen consumption and oxidation of glucose by the hexose-monophosphate shunt, termed the 'respiratory burst'. This leads to the generation of superoxide anions (O_2^-), hydrogen peroxide (H_2O_2) and hydroxyl radicals ($OH^•$). O_2^- has been implicated in the induction of inflammation, bronchoconstriction, and airway hyperreactivity in animal models. Human alveolar macrophages from patients with allergic asthma spontaneously release increased amounts of O_2^- compared to the alveolar macrophages of normal subjects, and this release is increased further by segmental allergen bronchoprovocation in atopic patients.

Nitric oxide is the final product of the oxidation of guanidino-nitrogen of L-arginine by nitric oxide synthase. This reactive nitrogen intermediate is increased in asthmatic patients, as is expression of inducible nitric oxide synthase. Important sources in asthmatic airways are likely to be epithelial cells and macrophages. Human monocytes and macrophages are stimulated for increased production by cross-linking of the low-affinity receptor for IgE, FcεRII, and by certain proinflammatory cytokines. It has been proposed that nitric oxide has a role in atopic disease, through its actions in promoting the production of proinflammatory mediators and its potential to cause tissue damage and through inhibition of the generation of Th1 cells and the likely increase in Th2 cells.

Lipid mediators

Monocytes and macrophages are triggered to synthesize and release several lipid mediators, including leukotrienes, hydroxyeicosatetraenoic acid, thromboxanes, prostaglandins, and PAF, which exhibit diverse proinflammatory effects. An important trigger for the production of these mediators in allergy includes FcεRII-dependent pathways mediated by IgE immune complexes. The functions of these mediators are reviewed in Chapters 22 and 23. The production of a number of these mediators is increased in monocytes and alveolar macrophages that are derived from atopic asthmatic patients.

Cytokines

Monocytes and macrophages have the capacity to synthesize numerous cytokines that exhibit both proinflammatory and antiinflammatory functions. Selective upregulation of several proinflammatory cytokines, including IL-1, IL-6, IL-8, TNFα, and GM-CSF, by peripheral blood monocytes or alveolar macrophages, or both, is observed in allergy and asthma (see Chapter 20). These cytokines are likely to promote the allergic process by enhancing recruitment and adhesion of granulocytes and lymphocytes to the allergic inflammatory site, by regulating

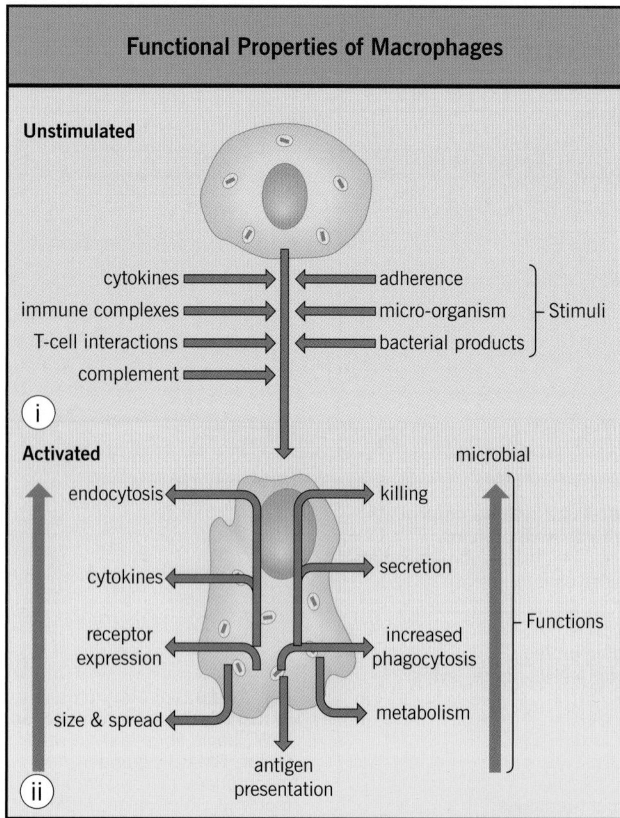

Fig. 21.17 Functional properties of macrophages. (i) Pathways of mononuclear phagocyte activation. (ii) Changes in the functional properties of mononuclear phagocytes following activation. (Modified from Gordon S, Clarke S, Greaves D, et al. Molecular immunobiology of macrophages: recent progress. Curr Opin Immunol 1995; 7:24–33 and de Waal Malefyt R, Figdor CG, Huijbens R, et al. Effects of IL-13 on phenotype, cytokine production and cytotoxic function of human monocytes: comparison with IL-4 and modulation by IFN or IL-10. J Immunol 1993; 151:6370–6381.)

the functions of mononuclear phagocytes and lymphocytes and, in the case of GM-CSF, by promoting the survival and activation of eosinophils, as well as enhancing both the recruitment and an antigen-presenting cell phenotype in monocytes, macrophages and dendritic cells. In contrast, the antiinflammatory cytokine IL-10 is reduced in both blood monocytes and alveolar macrophages from allergic patients with asthma.

Pathways of macrophage activation

Bacteria or their products, particulate antigens, cytokines, complement components, antibodies, immune complexes, cognate interactions with T lymphocytes, and adherence can all activate mononuclear phagocytes (Fig. 21.17). Activation results in increases in cell size, spreading and adherence, endocytic capacity, cytotoxic and other antimicrobial activity, and release of cytokines and soluble mediators. However, the nature of the activating stimulus greatly influences the response that is observed, leading, for example, to distinct patterns of cytokine synthesis. In many well-studied infectious models, Toll-like receptors and Th1-derived cytokines such as IFNγ are critical for increasing macrophage phagocytic and antimicrobial activities.

Signals for macrophage activation of likely importance in allergy include IL-4 and IL-13. These Th2 cell-derived cytokines induce an alternative pathway of mononuclear phagocyte activation leading to enhanced antigen presentation and migration, as also described for GM-CSF. Cross-linking of FcεRII by IgE immune complexes induces the release of proinflammatory cytokines and other soluble mediators. Triggering through FcεR1 enhances specific uptake of antigen and leads to highly increased presentation of specific antigen for the activation of CD4+ T lymphocytes. Activation of mononuclear phagocytes through cross-linking of FcRs by IgE-bound allergen therefore has the potential to greatly exacerbate the allergic inflammatory process (see Fig. 21.15). Conversely, IL-10 inhibits proinflammatory cytokine production and antigen presentation by mononuclear phagocytes.

Primary functions in allergy

Two basic functions of mononuclear phagocytes are likely to regulate and exacerbate the allergic inflammatory condition. One parameter is their capacity to secrete soluble proinflammatory mediators, including biologically active lipids, reactive oxygen and nitrogen metabolites, cytokines, and chemokines. Although the capacity to synthesize these mediators is not unique to monocytes and macrophages, it is their capacity to synthesize many different products in large quantities that is likely to contribute to and exacerbate the allergic inflammatory state. Activation leading to proinflammatory mediator secretion probably occurs partly through mediators secreted by other local cells such as mast cells and epithelial cells. However, allergen-specific activation is also likely to be important following the increased production of allergen-specific IgE and enhanced expression of low- and high-affinity receptors for IgE by mononuclear phagocytes in allergic and asthmatic patients (see Fig. 21.15).

The second function of mononuclear phagocytes is their capacity to present antigen to T lymphocytes and to activate T lymphocytes. The biology of processing and presentation of antigen and the activational requirements of CD4+ T cells are described in detail in Chapter 19. However, clear differences in the capacity of monocytes and macrophages to regulate CD4+ T-lymphocyte activation have been described in atopic and asthmatic patients. Recent data show that targeting antigen to the high-affinity receptor for IgE, which is increased on the surface of human monocytes of atopic patients, results in a 100-fold or greater increased efficiency in activating antigen-specific T cells. This process is also likely to enhance antigen uptake and presentation by dendritic cells and potentially also by macrophages in allergy. In addition, antigen presentation and activation of T lymphocytes in the lung appears very different in normal and atopic asthmatic donors. The lung is a very delicate organ which is both continually exposed to foreign and particulate antigens, including allergens, and perfused by large numbers of recirculating memory T lymphocytes. This combination of foreign antigen and antigen-primed T cells would be predicted to result in T-lymphocyte activation and consequent lung inflammation. This event is largely prevented in normal healthy subjects by a unique population of alveolar macrophages. These alveolar macrophages not only present antigen poorly for T-lymphocyte activation but also appear to suppress antigen-presenting function of local dendritic cells and T cells. These cells maintain strong phagocytic and antimicrobial activity, which enables them to function in the innate immune response and promote the local clearance of pathogens. In allergic inflammation, changes occur in the alveolar macrophage population, which results in an enhanced capacity to present antigen and a loss of their immunosuppressive phenotype. This is attributed to changes in the local environment with evidence for an important role of GM-CSF. In addition, an increase in newly recruited monocytes that demonstrate increased antigen-presenting function is likely to contribute to enhanced antigen presentation in the asthmatic lung. The likely importance of mononuclear phagocytes in the pathogenesis of allergic inflammation is highlighted by the sensitivity of these cells to the immunosuppressive effects of antiinflammatory agents that provide considerable benefit to the vast majority of atopic people.

FURTHER READING

Bieber T. FcRI on antigen presenting cells. Curr Opin Immunol 1996; 8:773–777.

Bochner BS, Schleimer RP. Mast cells, basophils, and eosinophils: distinct but overlapping pathways for recruitment. Immunol Rev 2001; 179:5–15.

Brightling CE, Bradding P, Symon FA, et al. Mast-cell infiltration of airway smooth muscle in asthma. N Engl J Med 2002; 346:1699–1705.

de Waal Malefyt R, Figdor CG, Huijbens R, et al. Effects of IL-13 on phenotype, cytokine production and cytotoxic function of human monocytes: comparison with IL-4 and modulation by IFN or IL-10. J Immunol 1993; 151:6370–6381.

Dugas B, Mossalayi MD, Damais C, et al. Nitric oxide production by human monocytes: evidence for a role of CD23. Immunol Today 1995; 16:574–580.

Dvorak AM. Cell biology of the basophil. Int Rev Cytol 1998; 180:87–236.

Gordon S, Clarke S, Greaves D, et al. Molecular immunobiology of macrophages: recent progress. Curr Opin Immunol 1995; 7:24–33.

Gordon S. Alternative activation of macrophages. Nature Rev Immunol 2003; 3:23–35.

Hirai H, Tanaka K, Yoshie O, et al. Prostaglandin D2 selectively induces chemotaxis in T helper type 2 cells, eosinophils, and basophils via seven-transmembrane receptor CRTH2. J Exp Med 2001; 193:255–261.

Johnson RB. Monocytes and macrophages: current concepts. N Engl J Med 1988; 318:747–752.

Lee TH. Eicosanoids in asthma. In: Robinson C, ed. Lipid mediators in allergic diseases of the respiratory tract. Florida: CRC Press, 1994:121–145.

Liu YJ. Dendritic cell subsets and lineages, and their functions in innate and adaptive immunity. Cell 2001; 106:259–262.

MacGlashan D Jr, Gauvreau G, Schroeder JT. Basophil in airway disease. Curr Allergy Asthma Rep 2002; 2(2):126–132.

Macrophages and related cells. In: Horton MA, ed. Blood cell biochemistry, vol. 5. New York: Plenum Press; 1993.

Matsuoka T, Hirata M, Tanaka H, et al. Prostaglandin D2 as a mediator of allergic asthma. Science. 2000; 287:2013–2017.

Nathan CF. Secretory products of macrophages. J Clin Invest 1987; 79:319–326.

Okumura S, Kashiwakura J, Tomita H, et al. Identification of specific gene expression profiles in human mast cells mediated by Toll-like receptor 4 and FcεRI. Blood 2003; 102:2547–2554.

Peters JH, Gieseler R, Thiele B, et al. Dendritic cells: from ontogenetic orphans to myelomonocytic descendants. Immunol Today 1996; 17:273–277.

Saini SS, MacGlashan D. How IgE upregulates the allergic response. Curr Opin Immunol 2002; 14(6):694–697.

Takeda K, Kaisho T, Akira S. Toll-like receptors. Annu Rev Immunol 2003; 21:335–376.

van Furth R. Origin and turnover of monocytes and macrophages. Curr Topic Pathol 1989; 79:125–150.

Chapter 22

Definition:

The early-phase allergic response is that which occurs within 30 minutes of allergen challenge. It is initiated largely by mast cell activation with histamine and cysteinyl leukotrienes being the dominant mediators. The clinical manifestations are organ specific and include:

- in the upper airways: sneezing, itching, rhinorrhea, and nasal congestion;
- in the lower airways: bronchoconstriction, dyspnea, wheezing, and cough;
- in the skin: wheal, flare, and itching

Cellular and Mediator Mechanisms of the Early-Phase Response

Burton Zweiman, Paul M O'Byrne, Carl GA Persson, and Martin K Church

INTRODUCTION

The early-phase allergic response is initiated by the release of mast cell mediators following allergen challenge of a sensitized individual. Although the spectrum of mediators is essentially the same in all tissues, the symptoms provoked are different due to differences in the anatomy of their target tissues, e.g. bronchoconstriction in the lower airways, rhinorrhea and blockage in the nose, a wheal-and-flare response in the skin, and cardiovascular collapse in systemic anaphylaxis.

CHARACTERISTICS OF EARLY-PHASE ALLERGIC RESPONSES

The inhalation of allergen by sensitized individuals results in airway narrowing which develops within 10–15 minutes, reaches a maximum within 30 minutes, and generally resolves within 1–3 hours – this is the early asthmatic response (Fig. 22.1). In some of these subjects, the airway narrowing either does not return to baseline values or recurs after 3–4 hours and reaches a maximum at 6–12 hours – this is the late asthmatic response (see Fig. 22.1). The late asthmatic response need not necessarily be preceded by a clinically evident early response. Thus, in a subset of sensitized subjects, allergen inhalation induces an isolated late response at 3–8 hours in the absence of a clinically demonstrable early response.

In the nose, topical allergen challenge of sensitized individuals causes immediate nasal reactions involving itching, sneezing, obstruction, and watery discharges. The early response usually abates within 1–3 hours. In contrast to the dual allergic response in the lower airways, distinct late-phase responses are not common in the nose although low-grade nasal inflammation and symptoms may continue well beyond the first 3 hours after challenge with large amounts of allergen. Furthermore, nasal allergen challenge has a 'priming' effect, the nasal mucosa exhibiting an increased responsiveness to histamine or to a second allergen challenge on the day after the initial challenge.

In the skin, intradermal injection of allergen induces a characteristic 'triple response' first described by Thomas Lewis in 1927. The first symptom to be observed, which occurs almost immediately, is an initial reddening at the site of allergen injection. This is followed by the development within 5–10 minutes of an area of edema, or wheal, whose size is dose dependent and may be up to 20 mm in diameter (Fig. 22.2a). During this time, an area of erythema, or flare, develops around the wheal. The size

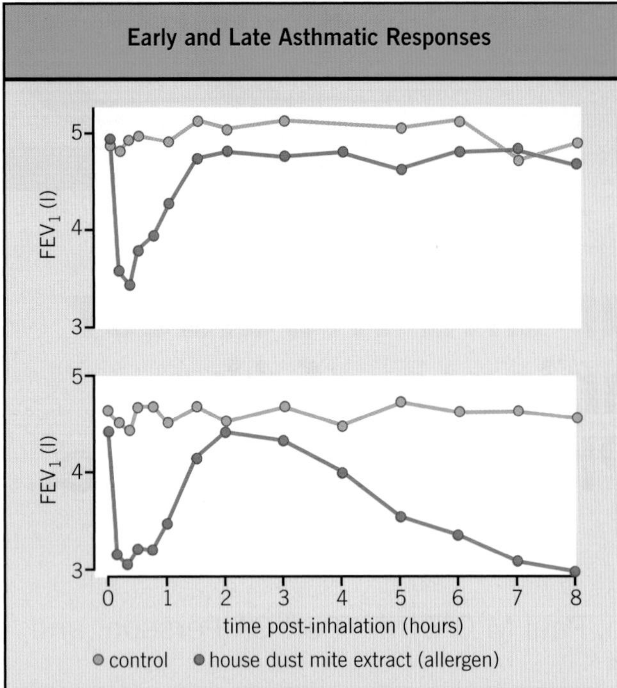

Fig. 22.1 Early and late asthmatic responses. (top) An isolated early asthmatic response following the inhalation of house dust mite (*Dermatophagoides pteronyssinus*) extract. Airway narrowing has developed 10–15 minutes after exposure to the allergen and has resolved within about 2 hours. (bottom) An early followed by a late asthmatic response following the inhalation of house dust mite extract. Airway narrowing recurs after about 3 hours, gradually worsens, and reaches a maximum at about 8 hours. The control measurements are made after inhalation of the diluent alone. FEV_1, forced expiratory volume in 1 second.

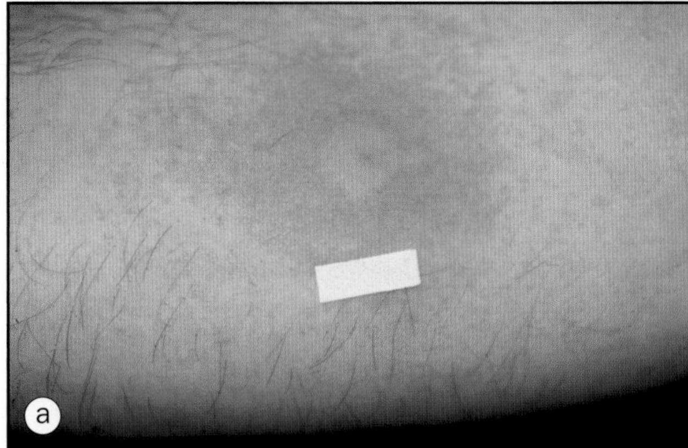

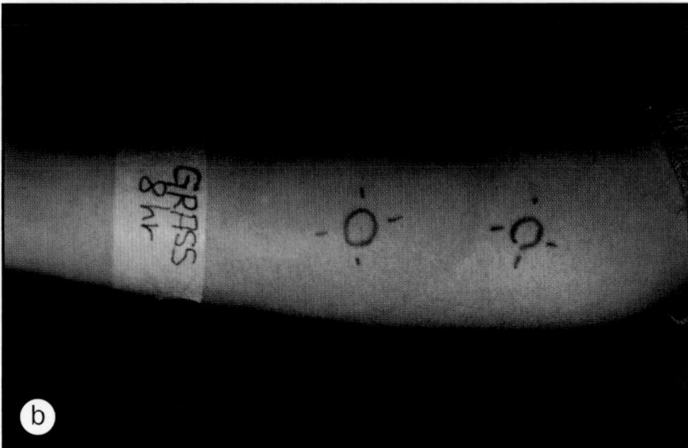

Fig. 22.2 The cutaneous response to allergen. (a) A wheal-and-flare response 10 minutes after the intradermal injection of allergen into a sensitized individual; (b) a late cutaneous response 8 hours after the intradermal injection of allergen into a sensitized individual.

of the flare is again dose dependent and may measure several centimeters across (see Fig. 22.2a). The wheal-and-flare generally resolves within about 30 minutes. However, in up to 50% of very sensitive subjects challenged with large doses of allergen the immediate wheal evolves gradually into an indurated erythematous inflammatory reaction. The latter reaches a peak at about 6 –8 hours and often persists for 24 hours (Fig 22.2b). It is very unusual to see a late-phase reaction without a preceding early-phase response.

CELLS AND THE EARLY-PHASE RESPONSE

It is now established that allergens initiate early-phase allergic responses through IgE-dependent mechanisms. The pivotal role of IgE has recently been demonstrated conclusively by the treatment of allergic subjects with a recombinant humanized monoclonal anti-IgE antibody omalizumab, a recombinant humanized monoclonal anti-IgE antibody which decreases the level of free IgE in the serum by forming biologically inactive immune complexes with free IgE. Such binding prevents binding of the IgE to the high-affinity IgE receptor (FcεRI). As a consequence, there is decreased expression of FcεRI on mast cells and basophils and a significantly reduced severity of the consequential early-phase response following challenge.

The current accumulated evidence, as listed below, indicates that the cell which initiates the early-phase allergic response is the mast cell.

- Mast cells are present as resident cells in all tissues capable of mounting allergic responses.
- Mast cells bind IgE with high affinity to FcεRI on their cell surface membranes.
- Cross-linking of IgE bound to the high-affinity IgE receptor (FcεRI) results in degranulation of local mast cells to release their preformed mediators. Studies in the skin have shown that this mast cell degranulation starts within 10 seconds after intradermal allergen challenge in sensitive subjects. Mast cells in such sites are also stimulated to synthesize and liberate its spectrum of newly generated mediators, including prostaglandin (PG) D_2 (PGD_2) and leukotriene (LT) C_4 (LTC_4).
- Following allergen challenge in vivo, increased levels of histamine and tryptase are demonstrable in bronchoalveolar lavage (BAL) fluid in allergic asthma, in nasal washings in rhinitis, in tears in conjunctivitis, and in sites of early-phase whealing reactions in the skin. Also, increased levels of the stable leukotriene end-product LTE_4 are demonstrable in the urine.
- Drugs, such as cromolin sodium, whose putative mechanism of action is the inhibition of mast cell mediator release, prevent allergen-induced early-phase responses.

- In contrast, there is evidence that any histamine liberated during late phase reactions in the nose, eye, and skin comes predominantly from basophils accumulating in the reaction site.

MEDIATORS AND THE EARLY-PHASE RESPONSE

To show that a specific mediator is involved in the pathogenesis of an allergic response it is necessary to demonstrate that the mediator or its metabolites are measurable in biological fluids during induced allergic responses, that exogenous administration of the mediator mimics aspects of the allergic response, and that inhibition of the synthesis or action of the mediator prevents or attenuates the response.

Histamine

Histamine has long been recognized to be a mediator of acute allergic reactions in humans and was one of the first chemical substances to be associated with mast cells. β-Imidazolyl-ethylamine was first synthesized in 1907 and was later named 'histamine' (from the Greek histos, for 'tissue') because of its ubiquitous presence in animal tissues. In classic pharmacologic studies, Henry Dale demonstrated the potent bronchospastic and vasodilator activity of histamine when it was injected intravenously into animals. Thirteen years later, in the same laboratory, it was noted that many of the symptoms of injection of antigen into a sensitized animal could be reproduced by histamine, and it was therefore considered to be a humoral mediator of the acute allergic response. With the description of the wheal-and-flare response in human skin, Lewis further expanded upon the vascular actions of histamine, which suggested that this mediator could be released from cellular stores within the skin on appropriate stimulation.

An increase in urinary histamine metabolites has been demonstrated during the allergen-induced early asthmatic response and following allergen instillation into the upper airways. Also, the use of a sensitive radioimmunoassay has shown rises in plasma histamine allergen provocation of the airways and induction by allergen of a wheal-and-flare response.

Histamine has wide-ranging biological activities mediated through the activation of specific cell surface receptors. The discovery of chemical entities that specifically antagonize the pharmacologic effects of histamine has led to the definition of four receptor subtypes, termed H_1, H_2, H_3 and H_4 receptors. The occupation of H_1 receptors by histamine results in the contraction of airway and gastrointestinal smooth muscle. In humans the bronchospastic response to inhaled histamine has been used as a test for defining the degree of airway non-specific reactivity, which has been found useful in the diagnosis of asthma. When injected intradermally histamine causes a wheal-and-flare response and, when instilled into the nose, it causes many of the symptoms of rhinitis.

The importance of histamine as a vasoactive mediator in human allergic disease is testified by the efficacy of H_1 receptor antagonists in modifying diseases associated with IgE-dependent reactions. H_1 receptors are constitutively expressed in active and inactive forms which interact with each other. Histamine binding stabilizes the active form of the receptor leading to the events described above. In contrast, the H_1 antihistamines bind to the inactive conformation and thus counteract actions of histamine. H_1 antihistamines have found a particular use in the treatment of allergic rhinoconjunctivitis, local and systemic anaphylactic reactions, and urticaria. At therapeutic doses antihistamines can inhibit about 75% of the skin wheal-and-flare response induced by intradermal allergen, suggesting an important role for histamine in this mast-cell-mediated event. The therapeutic success of antihistamines in the treatment of rhinitis and urticaria suggests that histamine plays a major, though not the sole, role in the pathogenesis of these diseases.

In the lower airways, histamine, in combination with leukotrienes, is largely responsible for allergen-induced bronchoconstriction in asthma, as demonstrated by the ability of pretreatment with a combination of an antileukotriene and antihistamine to almost completely abolish the early asthmatic response. The residual bronchoconstriction not attenuated by antileukotrienes is likely to be histamine mediated. Also, antihistamines effectively reduce symptoms such as sneezing, itching, and plasma exudation with rhinorrhea after nasal allergen challenge. However, antihistamines are much less effective in reducing nasal congestion.

Cysteinyl leukotrienes

The cysteinyl leukotrienes (CysLTs) LTC_4 and LTD_4 are derived from arachidonic acid following its oxidation by 5-lipoxygenase (5-LO). The synthesis of leukotrienes is initiated by the action of the enzyme phospholipase A_2, which selectively cleaves arachidonic acid from phospholipid. Arachidonic acid is converted sequentially to 5-hydroperoxyeicosatetraenoic acid (5-HPETE) and then to LTA_4 by a catalytic complex consisting of 5-LO and the 5-LO-activating protein (FLAP). This interaction occurs at the perinuclear membrane, where FLAP is localized. Subsequently, in the presence of LTC_4 synthase, glutathione is added to LTA_4 to yield LTC_4, which is exported extracellularly, where the glutamic acid moiety is cleaved by γ-glutamyltranspeptidase to form LTD_4. Cleavage of the glycine moiety from LTD_4 by a variety of dipeptidases results in the formation of LTE_4. As they each contain cysteine, these molecules are known as the cysteinyl leukotrienes (CysLTs) and constitute the material formerly known as slow-reacting substance of anaphylaxis (SRS-A).

All three CysLTs have the same range of biological effects although LTE_4 is much less potent than its precursor molecules, and is the excretory metabolite. Mast cells, eosinophils, and alveolar macrophages are the cells in the lung that possess the enzymatic activities to produce the CysLTs.

The CysLTs are released from human lungs after allergen challenge in vitro; increases in urinary LTE_4 have been observed after allergen challenge in vivo, the magnitude of which correlates with the magnitude of the early asthmatic responses, demonstrating the production and release of leukotrienes in association with early-phase responses. Evidence from immuno-cytochemical studies has indicated that the source of CysLTs in the early-phase response is the mast cell. This contrasts with the late phase where eosinophils take over as their major source. In the skin, there is no release of CysLT during the first hour of allergen challenge. Some, but not all, have found CysLT release later, during developing late-phase response.

The CysLTs were initially demonstrated to be very potent constrictors of human airway smooth muscle in vitro. Inhaled LTC_4 and LTD_4 have been demonstrated to be potent broncho-constrictors in both normal and asthmatic subjects (Fig. 22.3),

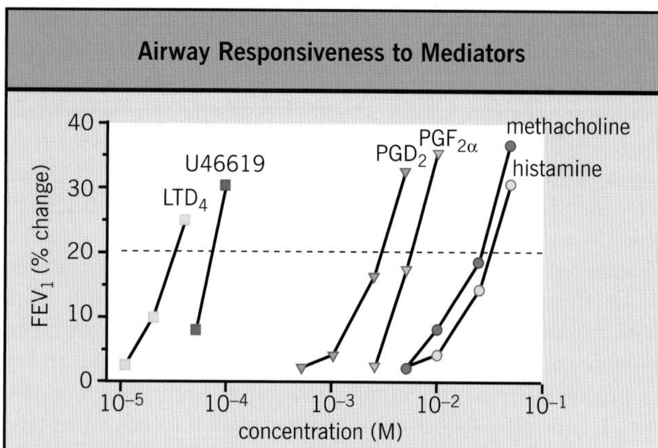

Fig. 22.3 Airway responses to inhaled bronchoconstrictor mediators in asthma. The relative potency of the mediators differs, with the cysteinyl leukotrienes and the thromboxane mimetic U46619 being the most potent studied to date in human subjects. FEV_1, forced expiratory volume; LTD_4, leukotriene D_4; PGD_2, $PGF_{2\alpha}$, prostaglandin D_2, prostaglandin $F_{2\alpha}$.

being up to 10 000 times more potent than methacholine in some normal subjects. The CysLTs have also been shown to have a longer duration of action than inhaled histamine. The bronchoconstrictor effects of inhaled LTD_4 are generally resolved within 1 or 2 hours but are not followed by the development of a late-phase bronchoconstrictor response. CysLTs also increase microvascular permeability, and stimulate the secretion of mucus, both of which may be involved in the pathophysiology of early-phase responses.

Pretreatment of patients with specific $CysLT_1$-receptor antagonists and LT-biosynthesis inhibitors markedly attenuates allergen-induced early asthmatic responses, as well as partially attenuating late asthmatic responses, providing further evidence for a role of CysLTs in the development of allergen-induced responses. No studies with antileukotrienes have demonstrated complete protection against early allergen asthmatic responses. Also, leukotriene receptor antagonist treatment does significantly inhibit early-phase reactions to allergen in the skin.

Prostaglandins and thromboxane

The oxidative metabolism of arachidonic acid by the enzyme cyclooxygenase produces the cyclic endoperoxides, PGG_2 and PGH_2. The subsequent action of prostaglandin isomerases produces either PGD_2 or PGE_2, reductive cleavage produces $PGF_{2\alpha}$, while the action of one of two terminal synthetases on the endoperoxide produces PGI_2 and thromboxane (TX) A_2 (TXA_2). Cyclooxygenase appears to be present in most cells although the cyclooxygenase metabolite(s) released from a particular cell are quite specific, e.g. PGD_2 is generated by the mast cell, TXA_2 by the platelet, and PGI_2 by the endothelial cell. This suggests that terminal synthetases are cell specific. All of the cyclooxygenase products of arachidonic acid metabolism have been synthesized and, with the exception of TXA_2, are readily available for study. TXA_2 has an exceedingly short half-life, about 30 seconds, limiting its use to a few, very limited, experimental preparations, none of which is in the upper or lower airways. Also, while a wide variety of cyclooxygenase inhibitors exist and have been extensively studied, again with the exception of TXA_2, no selective synthetase inhibitors or receptor antagonists are available for the other prostaglandins. The prostaglandins are most easily considered in two classes to evaluate their possible role in asthma. These are stimulatory prostaglandins, such as PGD_2 and $PGF_{2\alpha}$, which are potent bronchoconstrictors, and inhibitory prostaglandins, such as PGE_2, which can reduce allergen-induced bronchoconstrictor responses and can attenuate the release of acetylcholine from airway nerves.

PGD_2 is known to be released from stimulated dispersed human lung cells in vitro. In vivo, the release of PGD_2 into nasal washings, BAL fluid, skin chamber/dialysis fluids, and venous blood has been observed following allergen provocation of the upper airways, the lower airways, and the skin, respectively, of allergic human subjects following allergen provocation.

PGD_2 is a bronchoconstrictor of human airways and is more potent when inhaled by human subjects than $PGF_{2\alpha}$. PGD_2 causes bronchoconstriction directly through the stimulation of a specific contractile receptor, which appears to be a single contractile receptor for all bronchoconstrictor prostaglandins and thromboxane and is called the TP_1 receptor, as well as indirectly through presynaptically stimulating acetylcholine release from airway cholinergic nerves. Thus PGD_2 released in human airways after allergen inhalation has the potential to cause both acute bronchoconstriction and increase airway hyperresponsiveness to other constrictor mediators. However, specific receptor antagonists for PGD_2 or inhibitors of its production are not available to allow a precise evaluation of the importance of this cyclooxygenase metabolite in causing asthmatic responses. PGE_2 is released after the first hour of allergen challenge in the skin. Although PGE_2 has proinflammatory effects in the skin, pretreatment with a potent cyclooxygenase-1 (COX-1) inhibitor did not alter early phase or late phase skin test responses to allergen.

TXA_2 is a potent constrictor of smooth muscle. Several studies have demonstrated increased levels of TXB_2 in plasma following allergen challenge. However, plasma TXB_2 measurements must be viewed with caution because of the possibility of local platelet generation of TXB_2 and measurements should be confirmed by assaying the 2,3-dinor metabolite of TXB_2, which cannot come from platelet activation alone. However, studies (which have examined either a thromboxane synthetase inhibitor or a TP-receptor antagonist on airway responses after allergen challenge) have demonstrated a slight but significant inhibition in the magnitude of the early asthmatic response. These studies taken together suggest that TXA_2 is released following allergen challenge and is partly responsible for the early asthmatic response. There are no published studies demonstrating a beneficial effect of thromboxane synthesis inhibitors or receptor antagonists in the allergic responses in the upper airways.

When considered together these studies have demonstrated that allergen inhalation into the upper and lower airways in sensitized subjects causes histamine, CysLTs, PGD_2 and, at least in the lower airways, TXA_2 release, which together result in the early-phase response. In the upper airways, histamine appears mainly to mediate allergen-induced sneezing and itching, while the CysLTs mediate nasal congestion. In the lower airways, the CysLTs are mainly responsible for allergen-induced bronchoconstriction. In the skin, histamine appears to be the major mediator in early-phase wheal response while the flare is due to vasodilatation caused by an antidromal neural reflex.

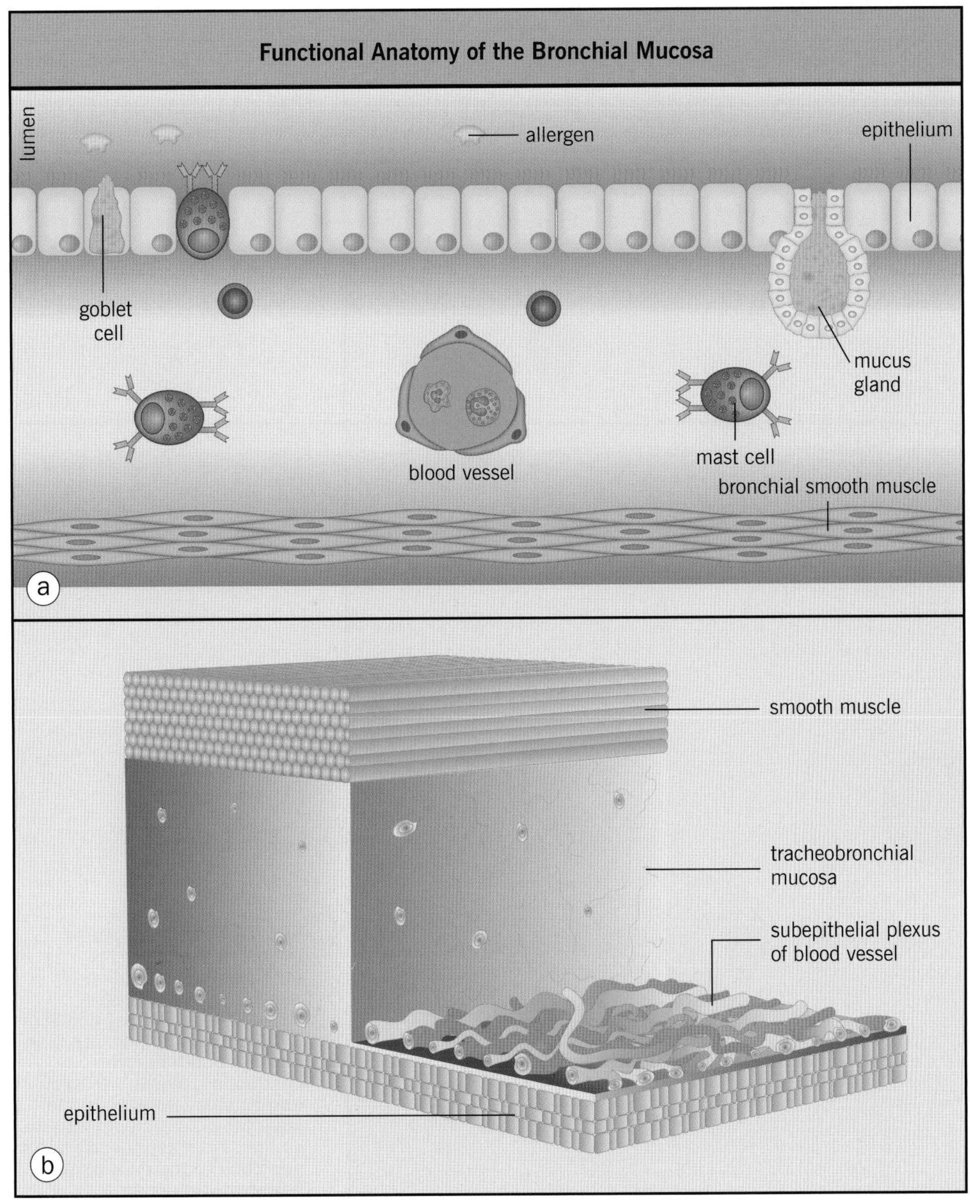

Fig. 22.4 Functional anatomy of the bronchial mucosa. (a) Gross structural anatomy of the bronchial mucosa; (b) the dense vascular plexus just beneath the epithelial lining of the bronchial mucosa.

PATHOPHYSIOLOGY OF EARLY-PHASE RESPONSES

As stated above, the symptoms accompanying early-phase responses depend on the anatomy of the target organs and the responsiveness of their constituent tissues to inflammatory mediators.

In the lower airways, the primary targets for mast-cell mediators are the mucous lining (and its secretory glands), the blood vessels, and the bronchial smooth muscle (Fig. 22.4). Bronchoconstriction is the main clinical manifestation of the early-phase response. This is manifested by dyspnea, chest tightness, wheezing, and cough. The mechanism of bronchoconstriction is complex and results from a combination of bronchial smooth muscle contraction, increased vascular permeability leading to edema, and increased airway mucus production (Fig. 22.5). Histamine, PGD_2, and CysLTs all have the ability to contract human bronchial smooth muscle. However, the exquisite sensitivity of this muscle to CysLTs suggests that these are potentially important bronchoconstrictor mediators (Fig. 22.6). Furthermore, the time course of recovery of the bronchoconstriction during the early asthmatic response is consistent with the recovery from bronchoconstriction induced by inhaled LTC_4 and LTD_4. In addition to causing bronchoconstriction, histamine and the CysLTs can increase vascular permeability and stimulate mucus production. It should be noted that only about half of asthmatics find benefit with leukotriene receptor antagonists, suggesting that leukotrienes are only important in a genetically predisposed subpopulation.

In the nose, the mucosa is underpinned by cartilage which confers a relatively rigid structure. However, the nasal mucosa is rich in mucous glands, nerves, blood vessels, and venous sinuses, all of which are potential targets for mast cell mediators (Fig. 22.7). Thus, the symptoms of the early-phase allergic response in the upper airways are a watery nasal discharge

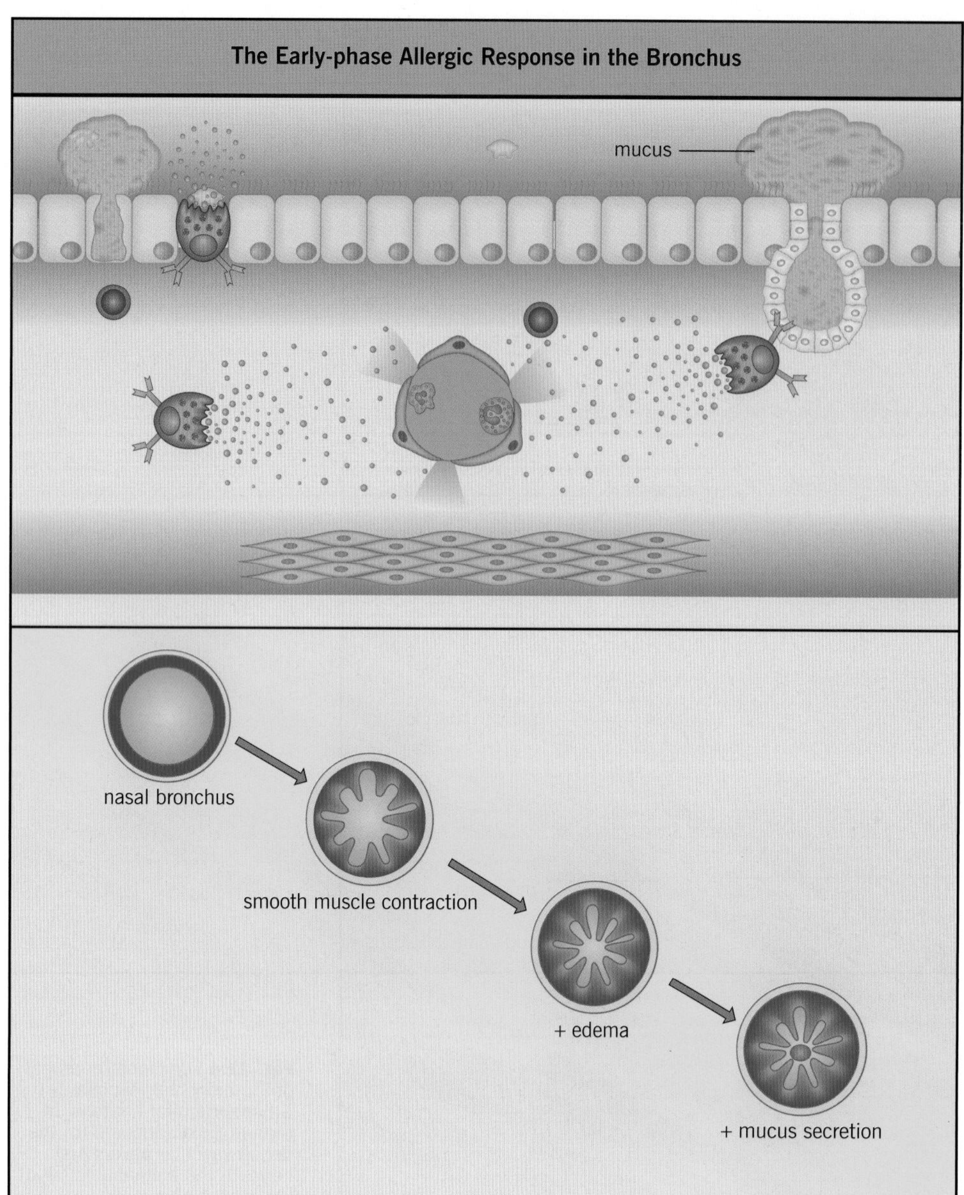

Fig. 22.5 The early-phase allergic response in the bronchus. (a) Inhalation of allergen into the airways causes mast cell degranulation – the liberated mediators then cause smooth muscle contraction, mucus secretion and plasma leakage; (b) the contribution of smooth muscle contraction, edema and mucus secretion to the early-phase asthmatic response.

(rhinorrhea), itching and sneezing, and nasal blockage (Fig. 22.8). Rhinorrhea, caused by a combination of local vasodilatation and mucous gland stimulation, is largely histamine mediated, thus explaining the effectiveness of antihistamines in treating these symptoms (see Fig. 22.6). As most of the early-phase obstruction to airflow in the upper airways is reversed by α-adrenoceptor vasoconstrictor drugs, it appears that acute filling of venous sinuses rather than tissue edema is responsible for nasal blockage. This symptom is poorly inhibited by antihistamines and is possibly mediated by nerves or local bradykinin production.

In the skin, most mast cells are concentrated in the superficial dermis, an area particularly rich in blood vessels and nerves, both potential targets for mast-cell mediators (Fig. 22.9). As described above, intradermal allergen injection causes a characteristic triple response resulting in a wheal-and-flare (Fig. 22.10). The initial local erythema is caused largely by a mixed histamine H_1- and H_2-receptor-mediated arteriolar vasodilatation. The wheal is a local edematous response resulting from a direct histamine effect leading to the contraction of endothelial cells of postcapillary venules with the consequential exudation of plasma fluid. The more widespread flare response is initiated by the stimulation of receptors on afferent non-myelinated nerves, which results in the release of calcitonin-gene-related peptide (through antidromic neural conduction) and possibly other neuropeptides and vasodilatation over a relatively large area. Nerve stimulation also results in itch. Most of the wheal-and-flare reaction is largely a histamine H_1-receptor response. However, the failure of histamine H_1 antagonists to clear the response completely indicates that other mediators, and possibly the stimulation of H_2 receptors, are also involved in its mediation. Another possibility is that the early entry of leukocytes into the dermis may play a pathogenic role. Such a leukocyte accumulation starts within 1 hour in the site of whealing responses to allergen, but not to histamine, injection.

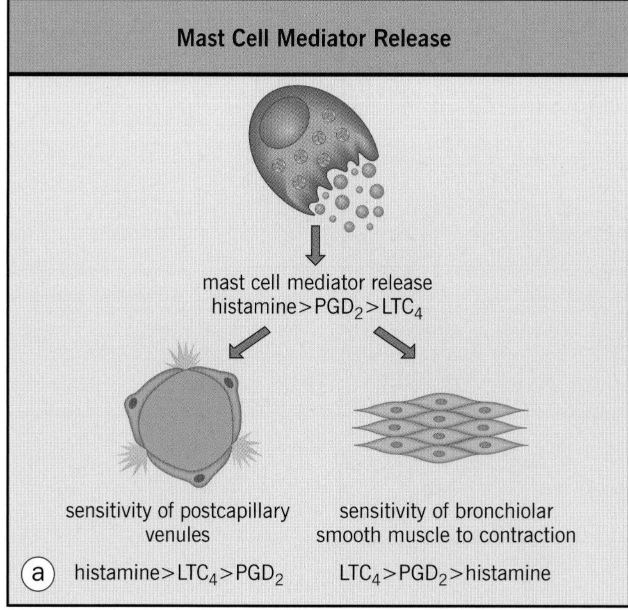

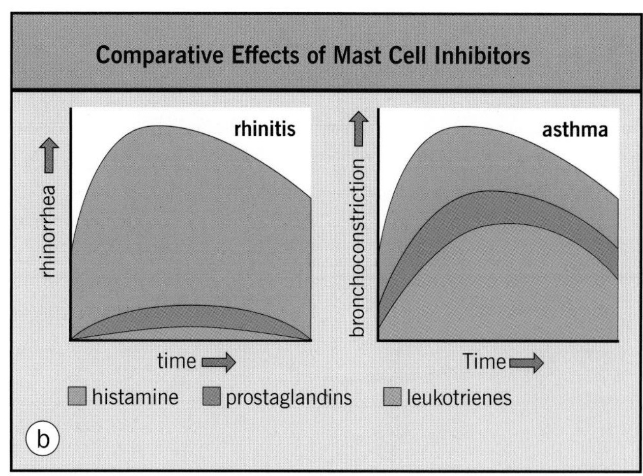

Fig. 22.6 The comparative effects of mast cell mediators showing the comparative effects of mast cell mediators in the bronchi and nose. (a) The differential effects of mediators on vascular endothelial cells and bronchial smooth muscle; (b) their relative contribution to rhinorrhea and bronchoconstriction. LTC_4, leukotriene C_4; PGD_2, prostaglandin D_2.

Mechanism of plasma exudation

In both the upper and lower airways, the early-phase response includes secretory and exudative components, mucinous secretions from mucosal glands and goblet cells, mixed with serous exudate following edema, accounting for the major part of the acute airway exudation.

Although the plasma exudation response may involve only small volumes, it effectively distributes plasma-derived proteins and peptides into the extracellular matrix of the mucosal tissue. The microvessels that participate in the exudative process belong to a profuse microcirculation positioned just beneath the airway epithelial lining (Fig. 22.11a and b). Immediately after the topical challenge of the mucosa, vasopermeability mediators such as histamine and CysLTs act directly on the wall of post-capillary venules producing tiny gaps between the venular endothelial cells (Fig. 22.11c). So long as these gaps are kept open, which is for about 1 hour during the early-phase response, non-sieved plasma is moved into the lamina propria, the epithelium and, in the airways, into the lumen.

A valve-like function of the apical junctions between epithelial lining cells readily permits luminal entry of an almost non-sieved plasma exudate without compromising the tightness of the epithelium as an absorption barrier. An exception may occur during inhalational exposure to certain allergens such as those of house dust mites which exert enzymatic effects that enhance protein absorption through the epithelial barrier. The epithelial crossing of a macromolecular exudate occurs within the first few minutes after allergen challenge. While a swift luminal entry may prevent formation of mucosal edema, it allows the convenient monitoring of vascular permeability increases in the airways. The appearance of large plasma proteins such as α_2-macroglobulin in mucosal surface samples, e.g. lavage fluids and sputum, may thus reflect the intensity and the duration of early- and late-phase responses as a biphasic increase in airway microvascular permeability. Also, preformed cytokines and eosinophilic proteins are avidly bound by α_2-macroglobulin and may acutely be brought into the airway lumen by the plasma exudation response. This latter mechanism may explain the appearance of cytokines in luminal samples during the early phase, although the de novo release of these mediators in the airway mucosa does not occur until several hours after an acute allergen challenge.

The plasma exudation process may not directly cause airway symptoms, except in already compromised lower airways, where a viscous exudate and mucosal edema may contribute to an acute episode. The general importance of the plasma exudation process may lie in the dynamic and biologically active molecular milieu (Fig. 22.12) that it creates in the allergic airway mucosa in vivo.

Initiation of allergic inflammation

Although often considered purely as an isolated acute event, the early-phase allergic response also lays the foundations for the development of allergic inflammation. An intravascular accumulation of inflammatory cells is seen within minutes of allergen challenge in the guinea pig (Fig. 22.13) and biopsies taken at 1 hour have indicated an increased expression of adhesion proteins, particularly E-selectin and intercellular adhesion molecule-1, on the vascular epithelium. Sequential skin biopsies in sites of allergen challenge in sensitive subjects have shown increased accumulation of neutrophils and eosinophils starting within 20 minutes, and increased vascular expression of E-selectin within 1 hour. Current research has also suggested that, during the first few hours after allergen challenge, there may be early signs of complex and severe airway inflammation, including eosinophil cytolysis, and epithelial injury and repair events, which traditionally have not been considered components of the early-phase response.

Functional Anatomy of the Nasal Mucosa

mast cell
epithelial cell
nerve
mucous gland
venous sinusoid
capillary
arteriole
periosteum and bone
(a)
venous sinusoids
nasal mucosa
(b)

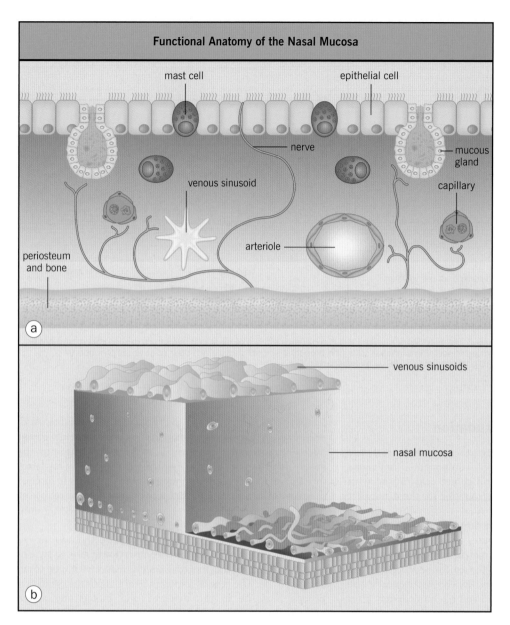

Fig. 22.7 The functional anatomy of the nasal mucosa. (a) The gross structural anatomy of the nasal mucosa; (b) the dense plexus of capillary–venular microvessels just beneath the epithelial lining of the nasal mucosa. The major obstructive mechanisms in rhinitis are congestion and blood-filling of the venous sinusoids in the nasal passages.

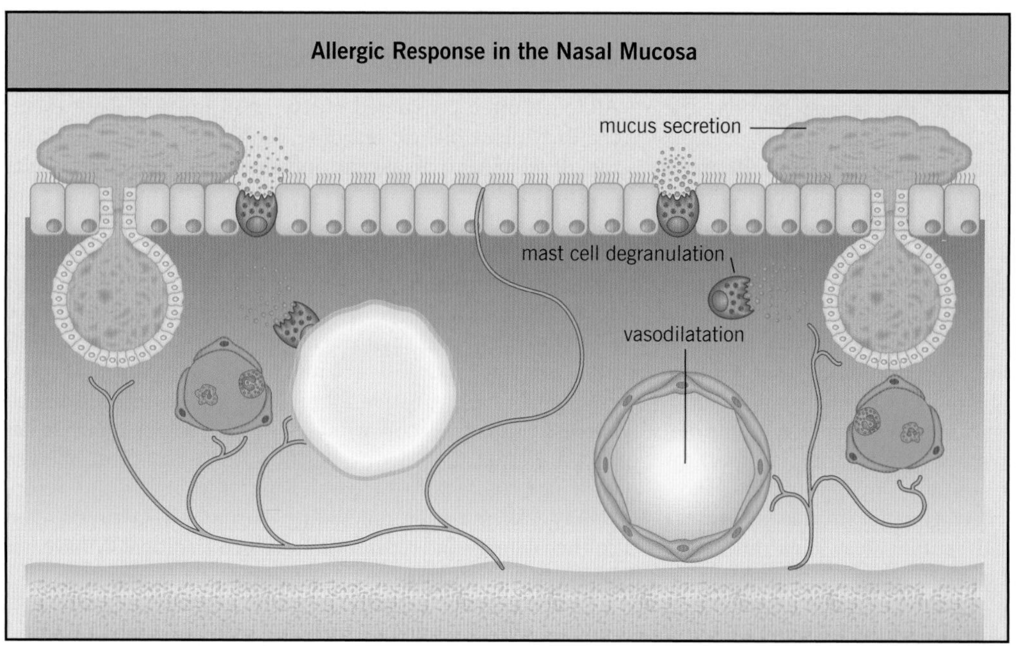

Fig. 22.8 The early-phase allergic response in the nasal mucosa. Instillation of allergen into the nose causes mast cell degranulation. The liberated mediators then cause mucus secretion, vasodilatation, plasma leakage, and congestion of the venous sinusoids.

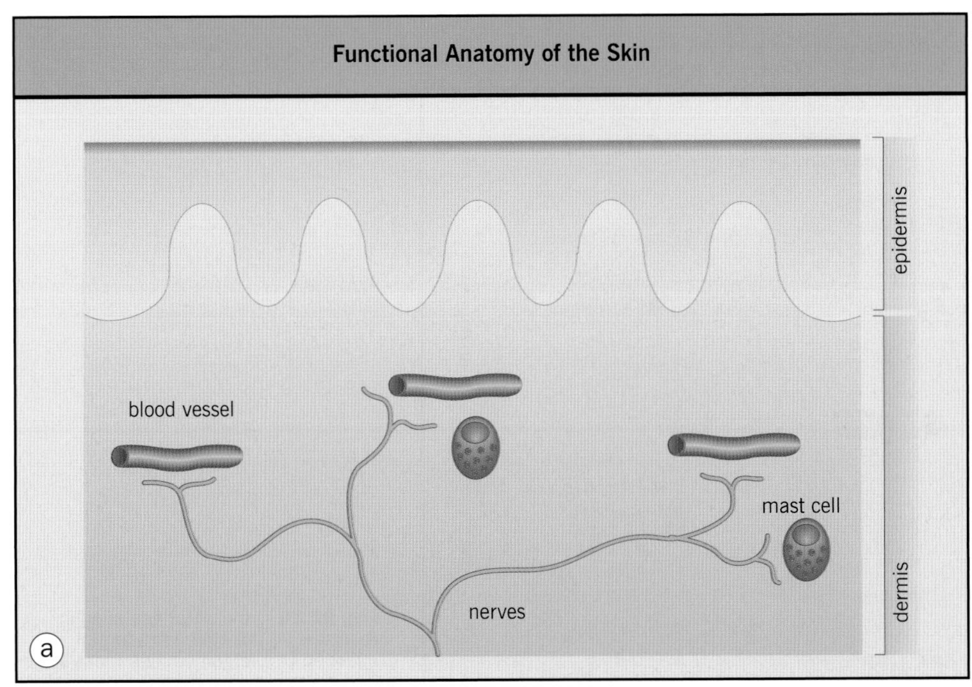

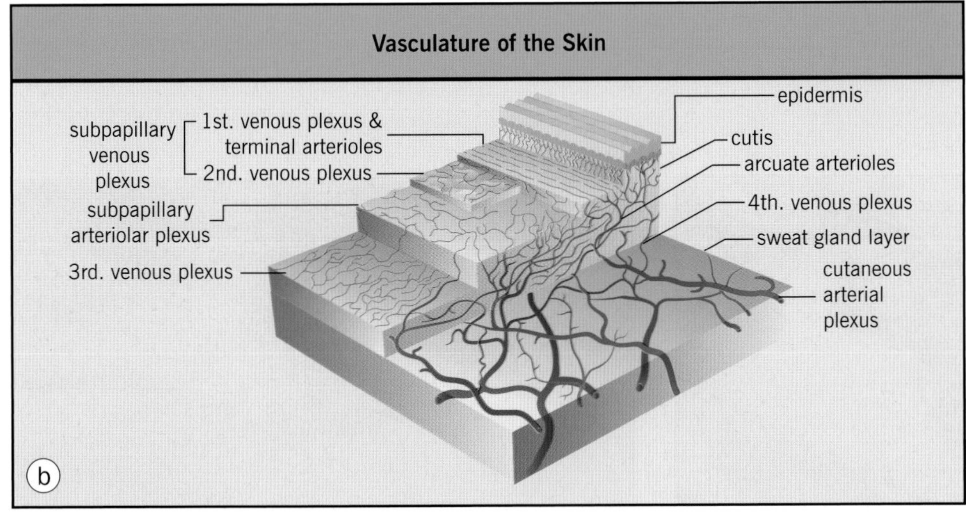

Fig. 22.9 The functional anatomy of the skin. (a) The gross structural anatomy of the skin; (b) the complex vascular plexus of the dermis.

METHODS FOR EVALUATING THE EARLY-PHASE RESPONSE

Relationship of the early-phase to the late-phase reaction

As noted earlier, only some allergic individuals will manifest a late phase reaction following an early-phase response to allergen challenge. Studies in the skin have shown similar patterns of mediator release and inflammatory cell responses during the first hour of allergen challenge whether or not a gross late reaction follows the early-phase reaction. Is there a particular type of mast cell activation during the early-phase reaction that leads to late-phase reactions? A clue may come from injection of opiates in the skin which induces a prominent wheal-and-flare with marked mast cell degranulation but no subsequent late-phase reaction or local inflammatory cell responses. Since opiates generally stimulate release of preformed but not newly synthesized mast cell mediators, the latter activity may be required for development of late-phase response.

Upper airways

The human nose is a gratifying locale for safe, versatile, and well-controlled investigations into the inflammatory response of the airways. Since several early-phase effects, including mast cell release and plasma exudation, are well developed within 10 minutes after allergen exposure, cumulative dose-response evaluations involving a wide range of allergen doses can be carried out in the nose (Fig. 22.14). A common procedure (completed in 30–40 minutes) involves the topical application of three cumulative doses, from a threshold effective dose up

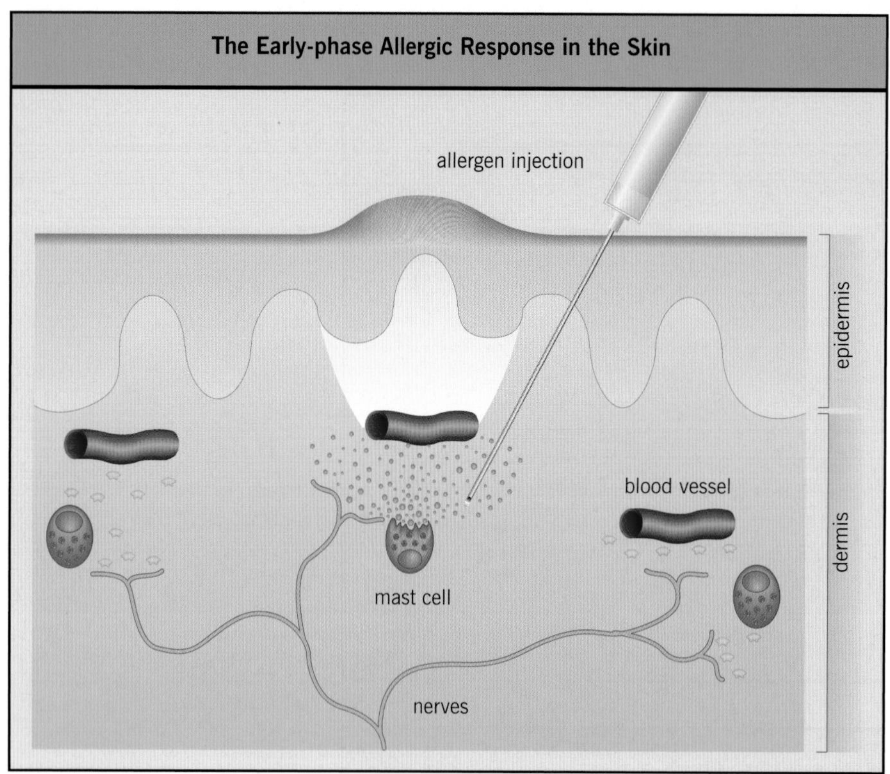

Fig. 22.10 The early-phase allergic response in the skin. Intradermal injection of allergen causes mast cell degranulation. The liberated mediators then cause local vasodilatation and vascular leakage (the wheal) and stimulate nerve axon reflexes to cause a more widespread erythema (the flare).

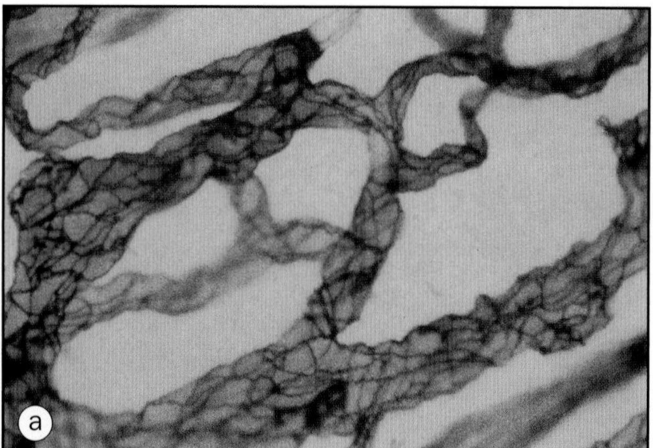

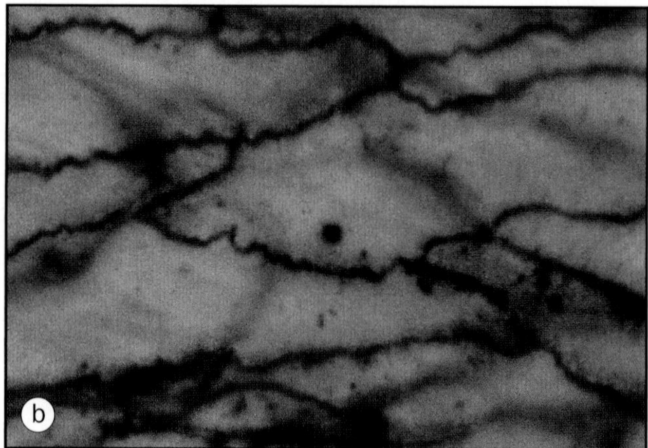

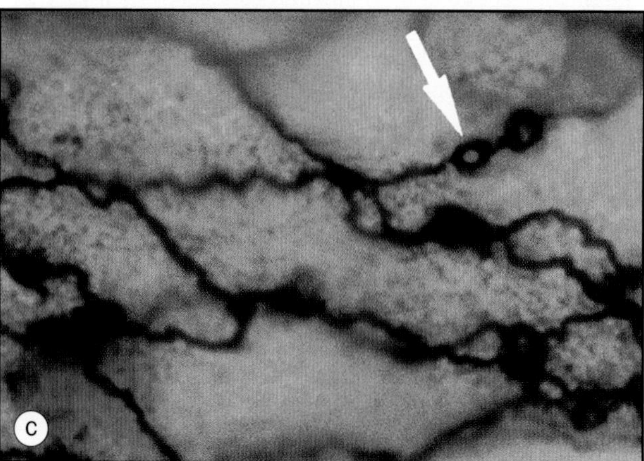

Fig. 22.11 Subepithelial venules in the airway mucosa. Light micrographs demonstrating subepithelial venules in airway mucosal whole-mount preparations. The venular endothelial cell borders are outlined as silver-stained black lines. They are intact in baseline conditions (a, b). In airways challenged with allergen (sensitized airways) or with a great variety of inflammatory mediators or chemicals, the endothelial cells respond by producing round gaps occupying tiny stretches of the cell border (c, arrow). Bulk plasma exits through these gaps. In the late-phase response leukocytes will also traverse the venular wall between endothelial cells but not through the plasma exudation gaps. (Reproduced with permission from Persson CGA, Erjefält J, Greiff L, et al. Plasma-derived proteins in airway defense, disease and epithelid injury-repair. Eur Resp J 1998; 11:1–13. These micrographs were kindly provided by Dr Jonas Erjefält, University of Lund.)

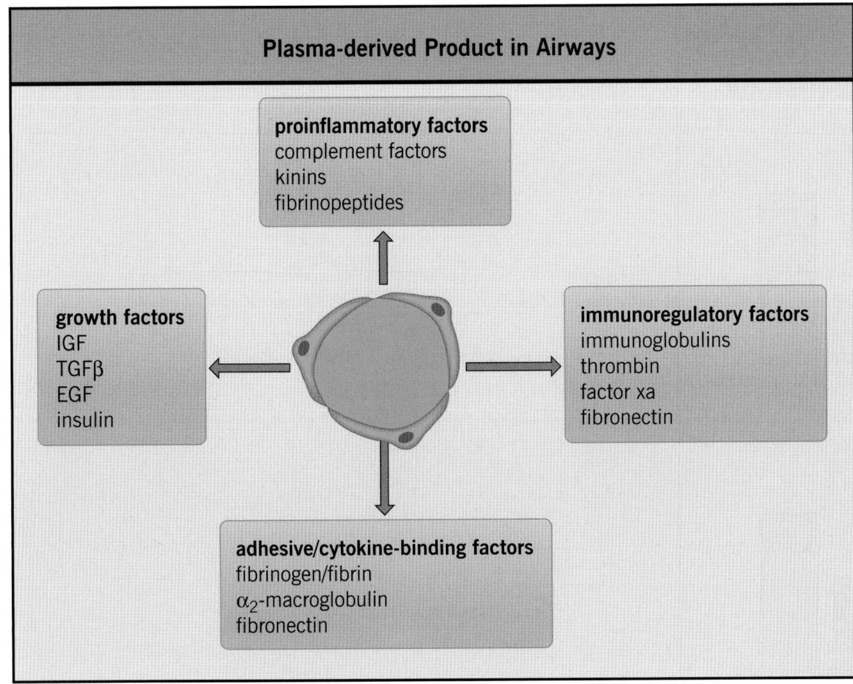

Fig. 22.12 Plasma-derived products in airways. These are only a fraction of the biologically active plasma-derived molecules that will 'flood' the lamina propria, move across the epithelial basement membrane, pass up between airway epithelial cells and, due to the plasticity of the apical epithelial junctions, gently seep into the airway lumen at sites of allergen exposure. EGF, epidermal growth factor; IGF, insulin-like growth factor; TGF, transforming growth factor.

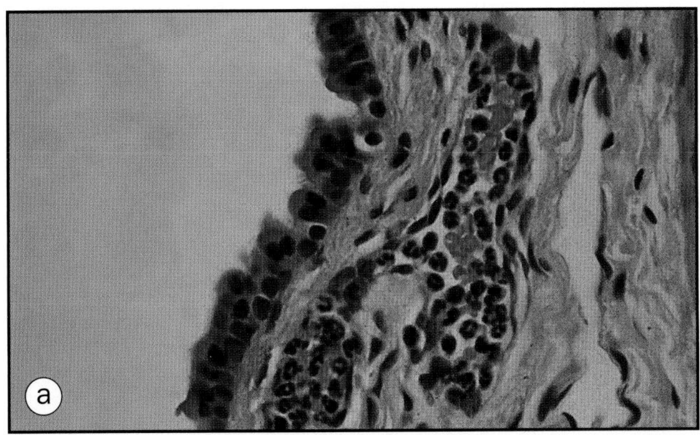

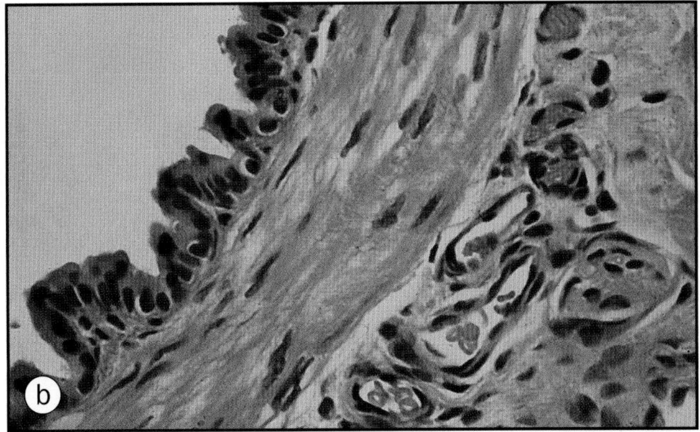

Fig. 22.13 Inflammatory cell accumulation during the early-phase allergic response. A light micrograph of the bronchial mucosa of a sensitized guinea pig 8 minutes after the inhalation of (a) allergen and (b) saline. Note the accumulation of inflammatory cells, both neutrophils and eosinophils, in the blood vessels.

to a 100-times-greater dose (100, 1000, and 10 000 protein nitrogen standard quantity units) of the appropriate allergen extract (birch, grass, or ragweed pollen extract). A handheld nasal spray pump delivering 50 μL per actuation effectively delivers the allergen to the entire surface of the ipsilateral nasal cavity. Symptoms of the subject are recorded and, when feasible, the extent of nasal congestion is estimated by rhinomanometry or acoustic rhinometry.

Prior to and in between each allergen challenge, nasal lavage may be performed. Using a compressible pool device, a large and well-defined mucosal surface area can be efficiently lavaged. The nasal pool method is also used to keep the nasal mucosa exposed to known concentrations of mediators, drugs, and tracers. After the exposure time has passed, the instilled pool fluid is quantitatively recovered into the pool device. Thus, mucosal surface indices are sampled exclusively from the area of interest. As a lavage procedure the nasal pool method can be repeated at will, apparently without causing any disturbances of the nasal mucosa.

The mucosal application of paper disks soaked with allergen challenges and samples from only a small surface area; the paper itself may cause tissue responses. However, the high concentrations of solutes sucked into the disks from the mucosal tissue and surface are advantageous for the quantitative assessment of cytokines in the airway mucosa. This paper disk method has the further advantage that lavage is not required. Lavage results in dilution of mucosal exudates and may not be completed satisfactorily without prior treatment with a vasoconstrictor nasal spray. Use of the latter interferes with the quantitation of nasal congestion.

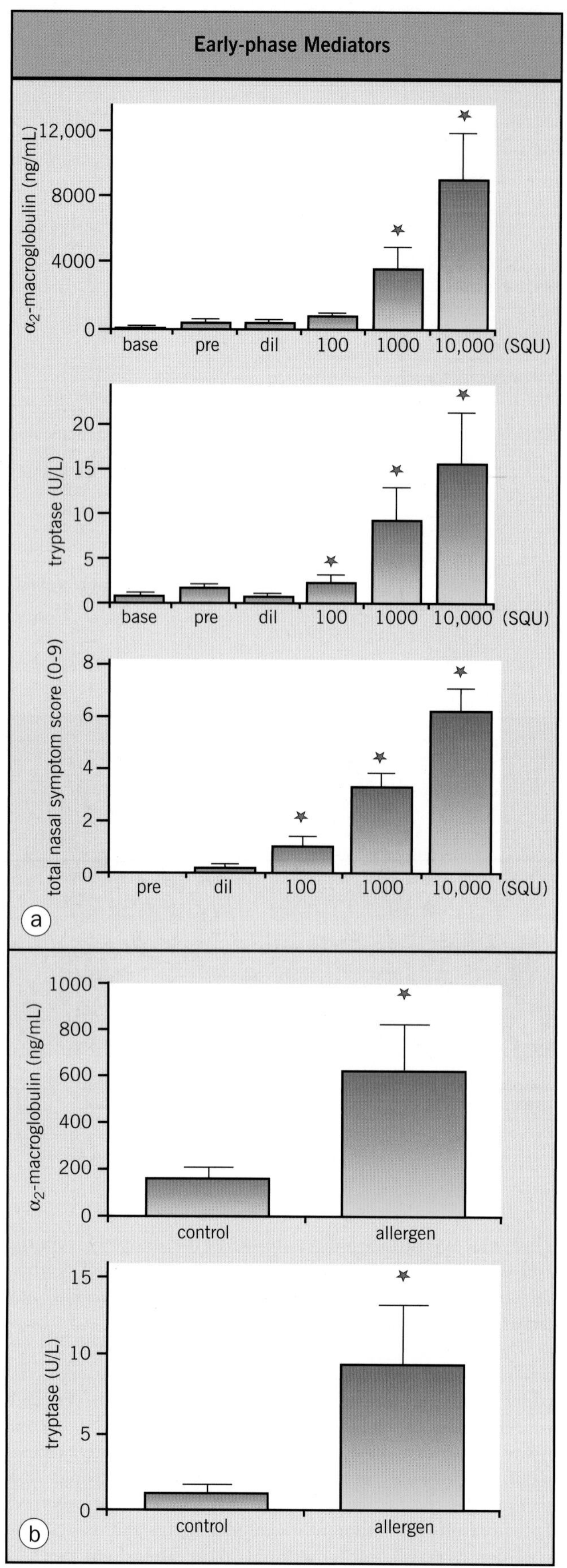

Fig. 22.14 Immediate mucosal responses to allergen challenge. (a) Nasal lavage fluid levels of α2-macroglobulin and tryptase, and total nasal symptoms score (mean ± standard error of the mean) after consecutive nasal challenges with increasing doses of allergen. The total nasal symptoms score (0–9) was calculated from the sum of nasal blockage score (0–3), secretion score (0–3), and number of sneezes transformed into scores (0–3) (*$p < 0.05$). Diluent challenge versus 100, 1000 and 10 000 standardized quantity units (SQU) of allergen, respectively; (b) bronchoalveolar lavage fluid levels of α2-macroglobulin and tryptase after endobronchial challenge with saline (control) and allergen (*$p < 0.05$). Base, baseline; Pre, prechallenge; Dil, diluent challenge. (Reproduced with permission from Greiff L, Pipkorn U, Alkner U, et al. The 'nasal pool' device applies controlled concentrations of solutes on human nasal airway mucosa and samples its surface exudations/secretions. Clin Exp Allergy 1990; 20:253–259, Blackwell Science Ltd.)

Lower airways

Most studies examining the allergen-induced asthmatic responses have been carried out in the laboratory using allergen inhalation tests. However, methods of allergen inhalation have not been uniform. In one widely used method, doubled concentrations of allergen are inhaled for 2 minutes from a Wright nebulizer. The starting allergen concentration is chosen from the results of skin prick tests of increasing concentrations of the allergen extract in use. Generally, the lowest allergen concentration causing a 2 mm wheal skin response is the initial concentration inhaled; however, Cockcroft et al have described a formula which includes information from the skin test titration and the degree of airway responsiveness, to more accurately predict the concentration of inhaled allergen which will give a 20% fall in the forced expired volume in 1 second (FEV_1).

Baseline measurements of airway caliber, most commonly FEV_1, are made before inhalation of the allergen. Then the measurements are repeated 10 minutes after each allergen inhalation. If the FEV_1 has fallen less than 10%, the next allergen concentration is inhaled. If the FEV_1 has fallen 10–20%, the measurement is repeated every 10 minutes until the maximal fall in FEV_1 has occurred. If this fall has not exceeded 20% some care must be taken in choosing the next allergen dose. Specifically, if the next doubling concentration is inhaled for 2 minutes, a severe early response may result. For this reason, the next doubling concentration should be inhaled for 75 or 90 seconds rather than 2 minutes to give a fall in FEV_1 of 20–30%. Once this has been achieved, the inhalations are discontinued and the FEV_1 is measured every 10 minutes up to 30 minutes, then every 15 minutes up to 90 minutes, then again at 120 minutes to establish the magnitude of the early asthmatic response, and every hour for 8–12 hours if a late asthmatic response is being evaluated.

Skin

Several approaches have been used to evaluate early- and late-phase allergic reactions in the skin.

- The visual examination of the mean diameter or area of wheal-and-flare responses has traditionally been used to estimate the intensity of the reaction, particularly when the reactions to injections of serial dilutions of the allergen are compared. However, scanning laser–Doppler imaging techniques can assess more quantitatively the increased skin blood flow which occurs in the areas of flare during the early phase response.
- Dermal microdialysis techniques using microcatheters placed under the dermis in sites then challenged with allergen can assess the profile of inflammatory mediators and cytokines released in such sites.

The temporal patterns of release of mediators and cytokines have also been established using skin chamber approaches. Skin blisters with the base at the dermal–epidermal junction are induced by combined heat and suction. These are unroofed and collection chambers with ports for introducing and removing contents are appended to the blister base. It is also feasible to biopsy the blister base to compare patterns of mediator release with inflammatory cell profiles in the underlying dermis.

FURTHER READING

Cockcroft DW, Murdock KY, Kirby J, et al. Prediction of airway responsiveness to allergen from skin sensitivity to allergen and airway responsiveness to histamine. Am Rev Respir Dis 1987; 135:264–267.

Dahlen SE, Hedqvist P, Hammarstrom S, et al. Leukotrienes are potent constrictors of human bronchi. Nature 1980; 288:484–486.

Greiff L, Pipkorn U, Alkner U, et al. The 'nasal pool' device applies controlled concentrations of solutes on human nasal airway mucosa and samples its surface exudations/secretions. Clin Exp Allergy 1990; 20:253–259.

Manning PJ, Stevens WH, Cockcroft DW, et al. The role of thromboxane in allergen-induced asthmatic responses. Eur Respir J 1991; 4:667–672.

Persson CGA, Erjefält J, Greiff L, et al. Plasma-derived proteins in airway defence, disease and epithelial injury-repair. Eur Respir J 1998; 11:1–13.

Persson CGA, Erjefält J. 'Chronic' airway inflammation following allergen exposure - Eosinophil cytolysis and epithelial injury-repair in a plasma exudation-derived molecular milieu. Allergy Clin Immunol Int 1998; 10:45–55.

Roquet A, Dahlen B, Kumlin M, et al. Combined antagonist of leukotrienes and histamine produces predominant inhibition of allergen-induced early and late phase airway obstruction in asthmatics. Am J Respir Crit Care Med 1997; 155:1856–1863.

Samuelsson B. Leukotrienes: mediators of immediate hypersensitivity reactions and inflammation. Science 1983; 220:568–575.

Togias AG, Naclerio RM, Proud D, et al. Mediator release during nasal provocation. A model to investigate the pathophysiology of rhinitis. Am J Med 1985; 79:26–33.

Chapter 23

Definition:

Allergic inflammation is characterized in its early phases by mediator release and in its later phases by influx and activation of inflammatory leukocytes particularly T cells and eosinophils.

Cellular and Mediator Mechanisms of Allergic Inflammation

Jay J Prochnau, William W Busse, and Stephen T Holgate

INTRODUCTION

The scope of the allergic inflammatory reaction can no longer be described in simple terms because many components of the normal immune defense system are involved. This amplified biological response typically involves mast cell degranulation and eosinophil recruitment. It has become apparent that allergic inflammation of the airway wall involves activation of normal epithelial cells and of extracellular matrix, and both seem to make an important contribution to the inflammatory process. The challenge involved in understanding allergic inflammation lies in the recognition of the key cellular interactions that drive the process forward and in understanding those factors that are responsible for the initiation, persistence, and resolution phases of inflammation.

EPITHELIAL BARRIER AND TRANSPORT FUNCTIONS

Epithelial cells maintain the integrity of underlying tissues by regulating exposure to potential antigens (Fig. 23.1). Although the skin has a relatively impervious keratinized squamous epithelium, the respiratory tract is relatively vulnerable and relies on both epithelial structure and function. The airways are lined from the nose to terminal bronchioles by columnar epithelium. In the larger airways, this epithelium is stratified and includes ciliated, secretory, neuroendocrine, brush, and basal cells. In the bronchioles, pseudostratification gives way to simple, non-ciliated columnar epithelium.

The epithelial surface is protected by a discontinuous mucous bilayer generated by submucosal glands and secretory goblet cells. The outer *gel layer* is formed by viscous mucin glycoproteins, which trap inhaled particles. Underneath lies a thin liquid *sol layer*, which permits free movement of the cilia and lifts mucus towards the oropharynx. In non-ciliated bronchioles, mucus is cleared by airway macrophages and by coughing.

The epithelial barrier is maintained by tight junctions and the *zonula adherens* which, together with complex desmosomal adhesion structures, attach the adjacent cells. The adhesion molecule E-cadherin is concentrated in the zonula adherens. Transport through cytoplasm by the transcellular path is a selective and highly regulated process that allows the cell to maintain normal electrochemical gradients. The paracellular path between cells forms a charge- and size-selective passive barrier to ions and macromolecules. Most environmental antigens are unable to cross these epithelial pathways and so remain on the airway surface, vulnerable to phagocytosis by macrophages and neutrophils.

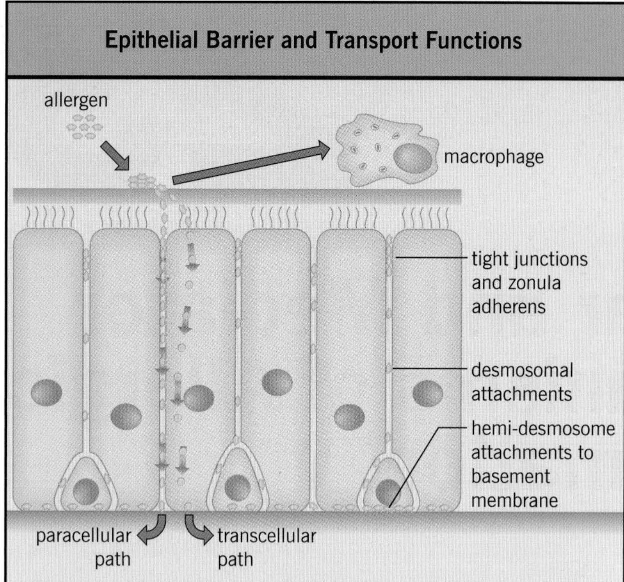

Fig. 23.1 Epithelial barrier and transport functions. Aeroallergen on the mucous lining of the airway may be phagocytosed by airway macrophages or cleared by the mucociliary escalator. To make contact with the underlying immune system the aeroallergen must traverse the epithelial barrier via the paracellular or transcellular pathways.

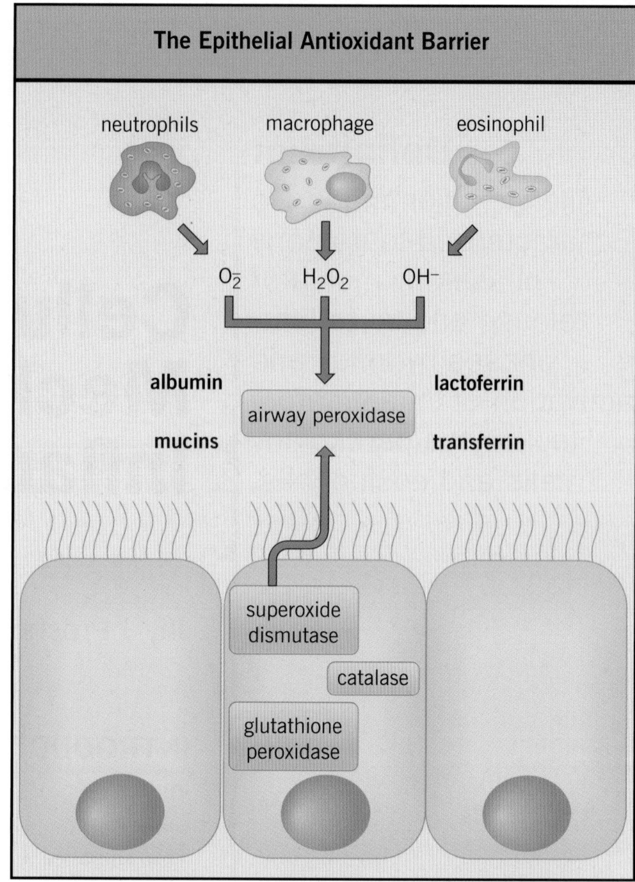

Fig. 23.2 The epithelial antioxidant barrier. Epithelium- and serum-derived antioxidant substances protect epithelial cells from damage by oxidant radicals. Oxidant radicals are generated by inflammatory cells recruited to the airway. Superoxide anion (O_2^-), hydrogen peroxide (H_2O_2), and hydroxyl ions (OH^-) are oxidant radicals generated by inflammatory cells recruited to the airway. Epithelium- and serum-derived antioxidants protect the epithelium from oxidant-mediated damage.

The means by which allergens cross the epithelium are not clear; however, it may be that their physical properties, such as high molecular weight, stability, and solubility, defeat mucosal barriers. In addition, the recently described proteolytic function of some allergens (e.g. Der p 1, Asp f 13, and Pen ch 18) confers additional properties that facilitate their penetration through the cleavage of intercellular adhesion molecules.

Antioxidant systems

Epithelial cells contribute to the maintenance of an appropriate antioxidant environment in the airway wall. This is important because oxidizing agents, such as ozone, nitrogen oxide, and agents produced by inflammatory cells, are potent mediators of cell injury. Neutrophils, macrophages, and eosinophils generate superoxide anions (O_2^-), hydrogen peroxide (H_2O_2), and hydroxyl ions (OH^-), which are released into the local environment around the migrating cells (Fig. 23.2). These oxidizing substances are able to damage cell membranes by lipid peroxidation and protein degradation. The inhaled oxidant gases – ozone and nitrogen dioxide – have been observed to increase non-specific airway hyperresponsiveness; however, it is probably the reactive oxidant products of inflammatory cells that are of greater significance in the allergic inflammatory process.

The region around epithelial cells is rich in productive antioxidant substances derived from a number of sources, including neutrophils, macrophages, and eosinophils. In particular, uric acid, ascorbic acid, mucous glycoproteins, and albumin are able to neutralize oxidant radicals, while lactoferrin and transferrin from serum avidly bind ferric ion, which is essential for the formation of hydroxyl radicals (see Fig. 23.2). In common with other lung cells, airway epithelial cells express three major intracellular antioxidant systems: glutathione, superoxide dismutase, and catalase. These antioxidants can also be generated and released by the epithelium and contribute to the antioxidant activity of epithelial lining fluids. Superoxide dismutase converts the superoxide radical to hydrogen peroxide, which is in turn reduced to water by catalase.

Proteases

Activated inflammatory cells release large amounts of proteases in the extracellular environment. These enzymes are capable of degrading cell and matrix proteins and are responsible in part for the tissue destructive effects of the inflammatory process. Four classes of proteases have been described: serine proteases, cysteine proteases, metalloproteases, and aspartate proteases. In normal circumstances, the airway epithelium and lung tissue are protected from proteases by an excess of antiprotease activity derived from serum and from structural lung cells (Fig. 23.3). α_2-Macroglobulin, which is derived from serum and released by macrophages, is active against all four protease classes, while the α_1-protease inhibitor (α_1-antitrypsin) and α_1-antichymotrypsin inactivate serine proteases. Epithelial cells generate class-specific antiproteases – secretory leukoprotease

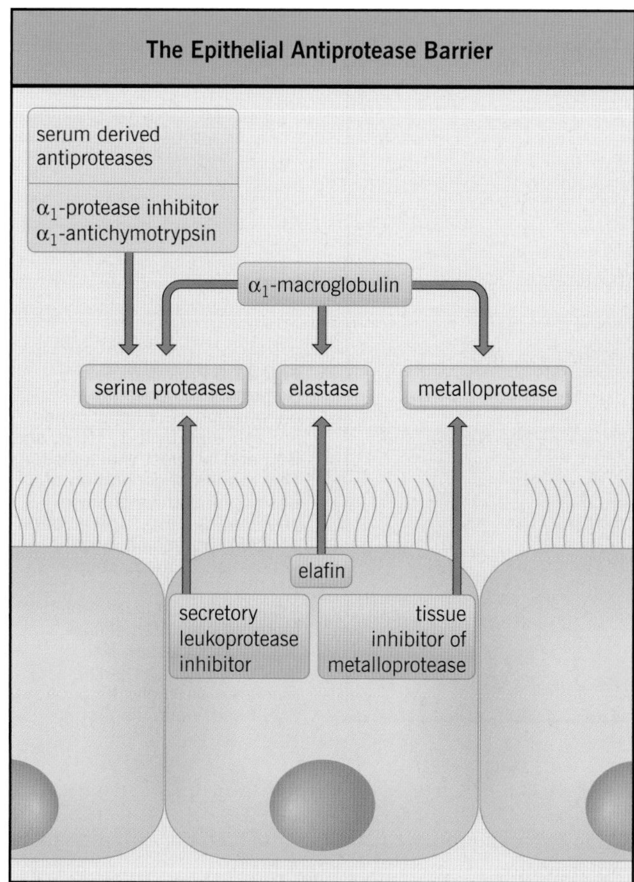

Fig. 23.3 Epithelial antiprotease barrier. Proteases generated by inflammatory cells tend to degrade cellular and extracellular matrix proteins. Protective antiproteases are derived from epithelial cells and serum.

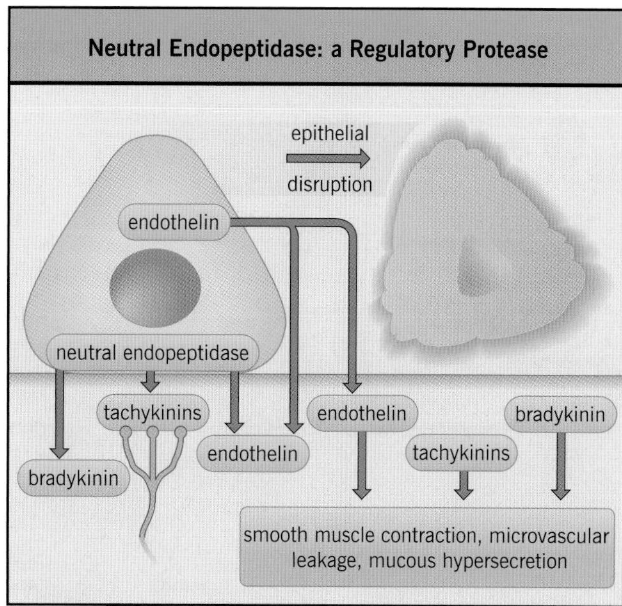

Fig. 23.4 Neutral endopeptidase – a regulatory protease. Neutral endopeptidase is a protease generated by basal epithelial cells. It has significant antiinflammatory activity because it degrades the proinflammatory mediators bradykinin, endothelin-1, and the tachykinins.

inhibitor, elafin, and tissue inhibitor of metalloproteases (TIMPs). These antiproteases contribute to the ability of epithelial cells to maintain the structural integrity of epithelium and extracellular matrix during infiltration by inflammatory cells. An abundance of proteases, released by inflammatory cells migrating towards a chemotactic stimulus, allows matrix degradation to occur, facilitates cell movement, and provides a basis for tissue remodeling.

Epithelium and promotion of the allergic response

Neutral endopeptidase is a membrane-bound protease with important antiinflammatory activity. It is located on basal epithelial cells adjacent to sensory C fiber nerve terminals and is able to degrade bradykinin, endothelins, and the tachykinins – neurokinin A and substance P – which are released by sensory nerve fibers as well as by activated macrophages and dendritic cells (Fig. 23.4). Epithelial cells are also able to metabolize histamine through the action of histamine *N*-methyl transferase.

Despite these important homeostatic functions, the airway epithelium is able to recognize the initiation of allergic inflammation and to play an active role in its propagation. Epithelial cells are activated by the early-response cytokines, interleukin (IL)-1β and tumor necrosis factor TNFα, by the lymphocyte cytokine interferon γ (IFNγ), and by direct viral infection. In response to these factors, epithelial cells generate chemokines, cytokines, and autacoid mediators, which promote the allergic response (Fig. 23.5). In particular, epithelial products have powerful chemoattractant activity for eosinophils, lymphocytes, macrophages, and neutrophils. It is becoming clear that the epithelium is able to create a directional chemotactic gradient by the preferential secretion of IL-8 and RANTES onto the apical surfaces rather than basal cell surfaces. The epithelium is a major source of chemoattractant CCR3 receptor ligands, RANTES, monocyte chemotactic peptide-4 (MCP-4), and eotaxin, which are highly effective eosinophil chemoattractants. Chemoattractants for memory (CD45RO+) CD4+ T lymphocytes generated by the epithelium include RANTES, MCP-1, and IL-16.

Epithelium in asthma

In the asthmatic airway, epithelial cells upregulate the expression of intercellular adhesion molecule (ICAM)-1 when they are stimulated by IL-1β, TNFα, and IFNγ. This allows the epithelium to maintain contact with any recruited leukocyte expressing the CD11/CD18 complex.

Recently, the epithelium has also been shown to express vascular cell adhesion molecule (VCAM)-1, whose counter-ligand is very late antigen-4 (VLA-4) expressed on eosinophils, basophils, and helper T cells type 2 (Th2) lymphocytes. In turn, this interaction promotes leukocyte activation and maturation. In common with other inflammatory cells, the epithelium generates mediators that influence smooth muscle tone. In particular, prostaglandin $F_{2\alpha}$ ($PGF_{2\alpha}$) and endothelin-1 promote bronchoconstriction, while PGE_2, nitric oxide (NO), neutral endopeptidase, and histamine *N*-methyltransferase favor bronchodilatation. Active transforming growth factor β (TGFβ),

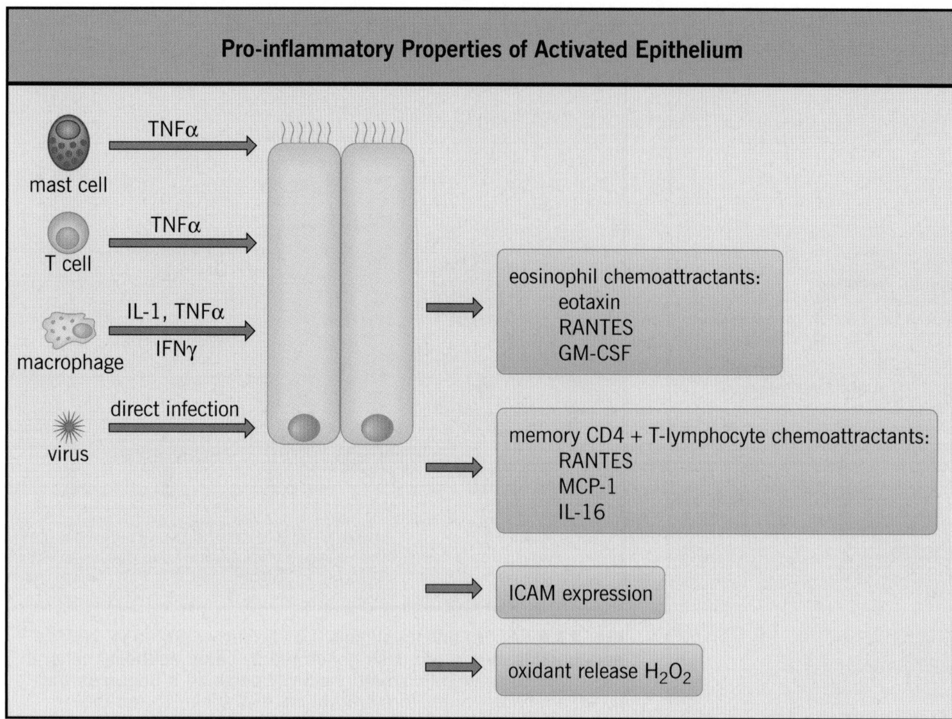

Fig. 23.5 Proinflammatory properties of activated endothelium. Epithelial cells are activated by IL-1, TNFα, and IFNγ and by direct viral infection. This results in generation of eosinophil and lymphocyte chemoattractants, upregulation of ICAM expression, and generation of the oxidant H_2O_2. GM-CSF, granulocyte–macrophage colony-stimulating factor; ICAM, intercellular adhesion molecule; IFN, interferon; IL, interleukin; MCP, monocyte chemotactic peptide; TNF, tumor necrosis factor.

basic fibroblast growth factor (b-FGF), insulin-like growth factor-1 (IGF-1), platelet-derived growth factor (PDGF), and fibronectin fragments released by epithelial cells are probably responsible for myofibroblast recruitment, proliferation, and activation for metalloprotease, collagen, and mediator release. In the region adjacent to the epithelium, major histocompatibility complexes (MHC) can be induced on epithelial cells, implying a role in antigen presentation, although an in vivo role has yet to be established.

NO is produced by a variety of cells, including epithelial cells, by inducible nitric oxide synthase (iNOS), in response to proinflammatory cytokines. Although the role of NO in the pathogenesis of asthma is not completely understood, its biologic properties include bronchodilation and increased airway mucus secretion. It has been proposed that the fractional concentration of exhaled NO (FE_{NO}) may provide a useful surrogate marker of inflammation, as levels of FE_{NO} are typically elevated in acute exacerbations of asthma, and levels typically decrease with corticosteroid therapy.

THE ROLE OF FIBROBLASTS IN ALLERGIC INFLAMMATION

Fibroblasts are widely distributed throughout the airway wall below the basement membrane. It is becoming clear that these structural cells play an important role in altering the composition of the airway wall after the initiation of an allergic response. Fibroblasts proliferate in response to several cytokines and mediators generated by inflammatory cells (Fig. 23.6). Recognized fibroblast mitogens include histamine, heparin, and tryptase derived from mast cells, and major basic protein (MBP) and eosinophil cationic protein (ECP) from eosinophils. The cytokines IL-1β, PDGF, TGFβ, b-FGF, IGF-1, and endothelin released from epithelial cells and macrophages in the airway wall promote fibroblast proliferation, differentiation, and activation.

Epithelial cells and fibroblasts have a mutually dependent relationship, which regulates the growth and function of both cell types (Fig. 23.7). Fibroblasts release extracellular matrix and cytokines such as keratinocyte growth factor, which regulates epithelial repair and function. Upon injury, the epithelium also secretes epidermal-like growth factors, including epidermal growth factor (EGF), TGFα, and heparin-binding (HB) EGF. Through autocrine mechanisms involving EGF receptors, which subsequently drive epithelial proliferation, these epidermal growth factors may be largely responsible for triggering the release of epithelial cytokines, chemokines, and mediators.

In common with epithelial cells, fibroblasts are activated by the early-response cytokines (e.g. IL-1β) to initiate synthesis and secretion of a range of proinflammatory mediators, enzymes, chemokines, and cytokines that amplify the allergic response and tissue restructuring. Fibroblasts can also generate the chemoattractants IL-8, macrophage inflammatory protein (MIP-1), MCP-1, and RANTES, which promote the recruitment of macrophages, lymphocytes, eosinophils, and neutrophils. IL-1, IL-6, IL-11, and oncostatin-M enhance lymphocyte development and are profibrogenic, while granulocyte–macrophage colony-stimulating factor (GM-CSF) rescues fibroblasts and eosinophils from apoptosis. Fibroblasts and myofibroblasts can upregulate the production of proinflammatory cytokines in an autocrine manner. In this way, contact of the fibroblasts with IL-1, TGFβ, and PDGF increases production of the specific cytokines.

Extracellular matrix is synthesized and released from fibroblasts in response to IGF-1, b-FGF, TGFβ, IL-6, IL-11, and oncostatin-M. TGFβ is produced by macrophages, epithelial cells, eosinophils, and fibroblasts. It enhances production of a range of extracellular matrix components, but it decreases

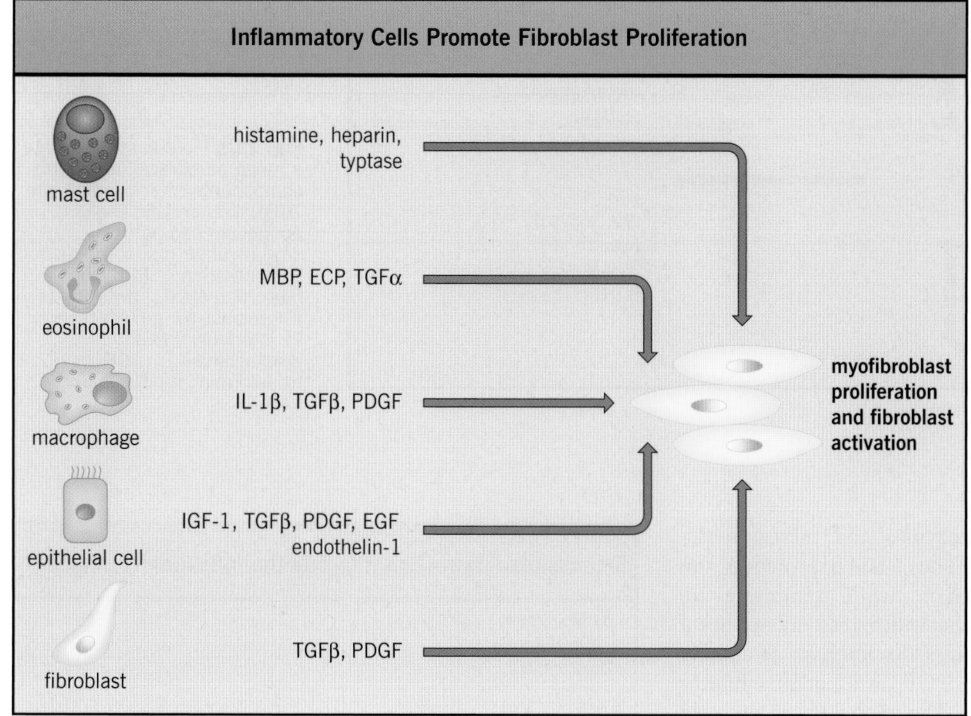

Fig. 23.6 Fibroblast proliferation in response to cytokines and mediators generated by inflammatory cells. Several substances produced by inflammatory cells and structural airway cells are fibroblast mitogens. ECP, eosinophil cationic protein; EGF, epidermal growth factor; IGF, insulin-like growth factor; IL, interleukin; MBP, major basic protein; PDGF, platelet-derived growth factor; TGF, transforming growth factor.

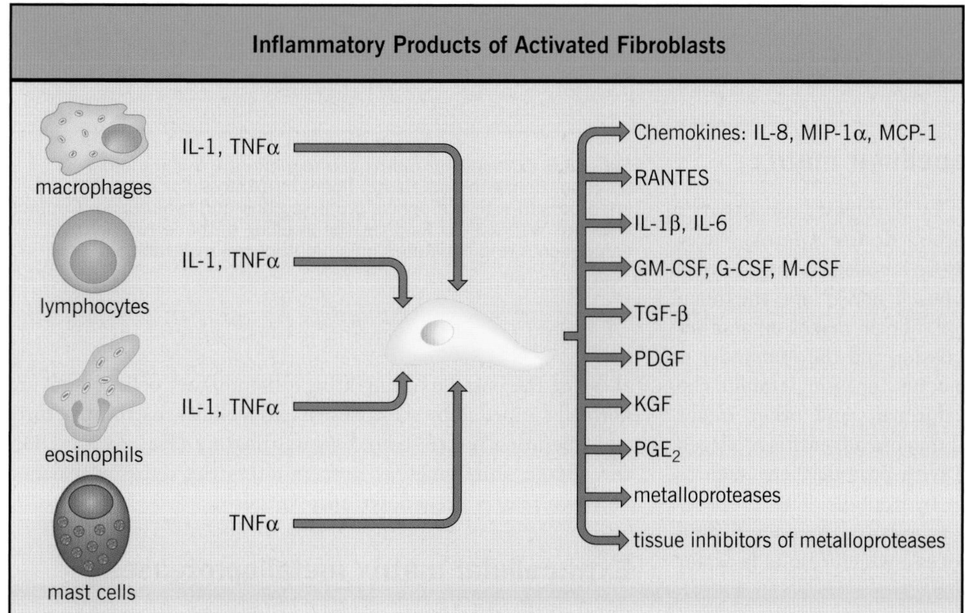

Fig. 23.7 Activation of fibroblasts by IL-1 or TNFα or by direct viral infection results in the generation of a range of proinflammatory substances. G-CSF, granulocyte colony-stimulating factor; GM-CSF, granulocyte–macrophage colony-stimulating factor; IL, interleukin; KGF, keratinocyte growth factor; MCP, monocyte chemotactic peptide; MIP, macrophage inflammatory protein; M-CSF, macrophage colony-stimulating factor; PDGF, platelet-derived growth factor; TNF, tumor necrosis factor.

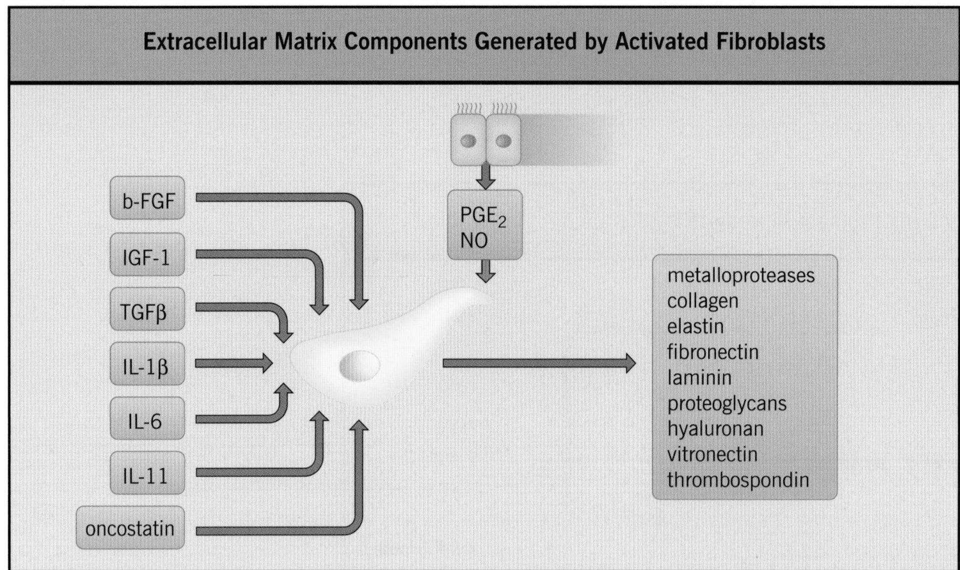

Fig. 23.8 Fibroblasts generate a range of extracellular matrix components after contact with TGFβ, IL-1, or IL-6. The epithelium can act to downregulate matrix production by generation of PGE_2. b-FGF, basic fibroblast growth factor; IGF, insulin-like growth factor; IL, interleukin; PGE_2, prostaglandin E_2; TGF transforming growth factor.

synthesis of matrix-degrading enzymes and increases the synthesis of protease inhibitors. Thus, TGFβ promotes the deposition of extracellular matrix while inhibiting its degradation, and contributes to the widespread subepithelial extracellular matrix deposition that is characteristic of chronic allergic inflammation. Conversely, TGFβ is a potent inhibitor of EGF-mediated epithelial repair. The epithelium is also able to downregulate extracellular matrix production by fibroblasts by producing large amounts of PGE_2 and NO. Both these substances have been shown to suppress fibroblast production of glycoproteins (Fig. 23.8).

PROPERTIES OF EXTRACELLULAR MATRIX

Composition of the extracellular matrix

The extracellular matrix produced by fibroblasts consists of a variety of proteins and complex carbohydrates. Approximately one-third of the dry mass of lung tissue is collagen, largely types 1, 3, and 5, whereas collagen types 4 and 7 are the main components of basement membrane. Elastin makes up another one-third of the dry mass of lung tissue, and the remainder is composed of glycoproteins – fibronectin, tenascin, laminin, the proteoglycan heparan sulfate, hyaluronan, and other minor matrix components. Within the submucosa adventitia, collagen and elastin fibers are interspersed with proteoglycans such as versican and hyaluronan, which are hydrophilic. This property becomes important when matrix is exposed to edema fluid generated by the inflammatory process, which results in water retention by proteoglycans.

The composition of matrix elements is also altered by several products of the allergic inflammatory response. Matrix-degrading proteases, especially the matrix metalloproteases (MMPs), endoglycosidases and exoglycosidases, and reactive oxidant radicals, are capable of degrading high-molecular-weight proteins and proteoglycans to low-molecular-weight species. This changes their hydration state and molecular form, thereby allowing the passage of migrating inflammatory cells, which are normally impeded by the cohesive extracellular matrix structure, and liberating matrix-bound growth factors (Fig. 23.9). Thus, the allergic inflammatory process alters the dynamic balance between matrix breakdown and synthesis.

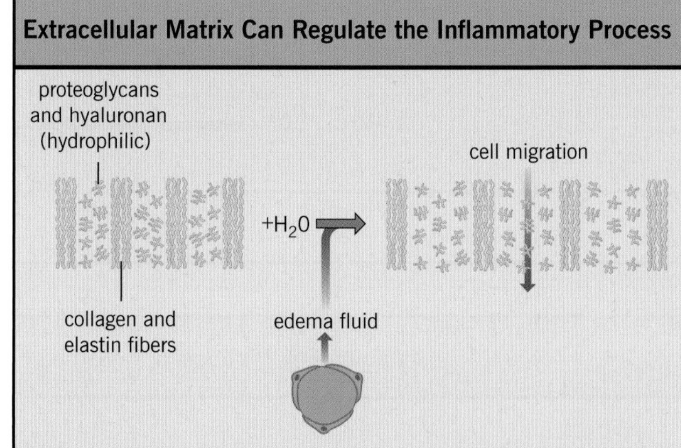

Fig. 23.9 Extracellular matrix can regulate the inflammatory process. Collagen and elastin fibers in extracellular matrix are interspersed with hydrophilic proteoglycans and hyaluronan. Contact of matrix with edema fluid causes swelling of these two matrix components and facilitates inflammatory cell migration.

Extracellular matrix metalloproteases

Matrix metalloproteases are zinc-dependent endopeptidases that have specific and selective activity against many components of the extracellular matrix. They are generated by inflammatory cells in response to IL-1β, TNFα, PDGF, TGFβ, and b-FGF, and are secreted as inactive high-molecular-weight zymogens. The metalloproteases MMP-2 (gelatinase A) and especially MMP-9 (gelatinase B) are present in increased concentrations

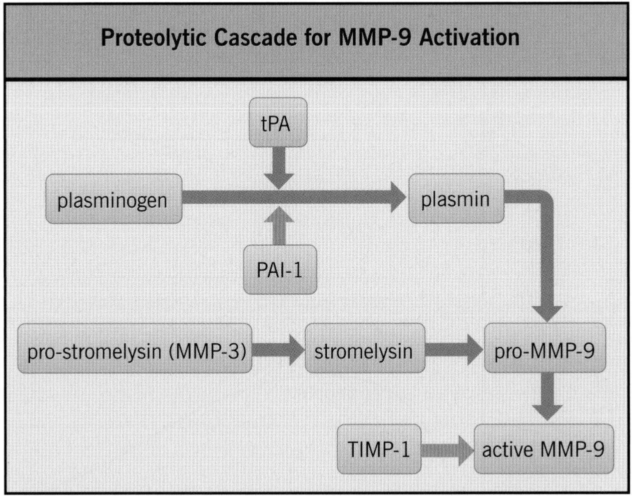

Fig. 23.10 Proteolytic cascade for MMP-9 activation. tPA, tissue plasminogen activator; PAI-1, plasminogen activator-1; TIMP-1, tissue inhibitor of metalloprotease-1; MMP-3 (stromelysin) expressed in the asthmatic epithelium and in submucosal mast cells; MMP, matrix metalloprotease.

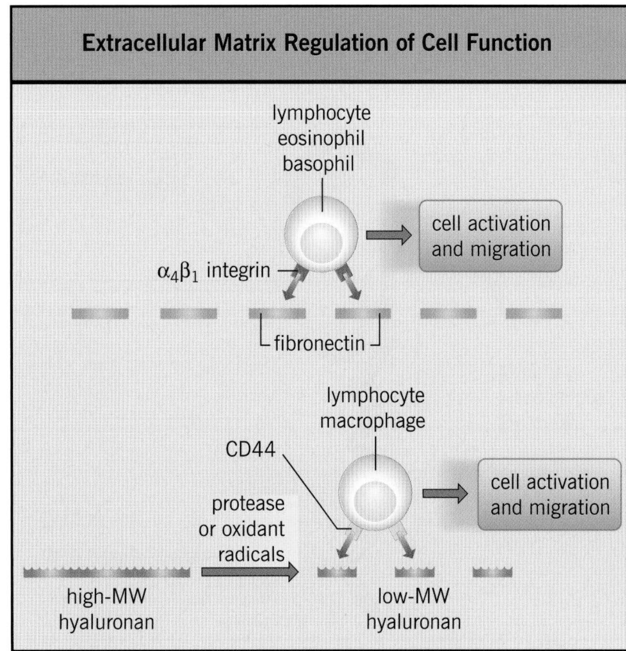

Fig. 23.11 Regulation of cell function by the extracellular matrix. Lymphocytes, eosinophils, and basophils expressing the $\alpha_4\beta_1$ surface receptor are able to interact with the CS-1 domain of fibronectin. This interaction results in cell activation and promotes cell migration. CD44 on lymphocytes and macrophages can interact with the low-molecular-weight (MW) form of hyaluronan but not the high-molecular-weight form. These interactions suggest the extracellular matrix can significantly influence the function of migrating inflammatory cells.

in bronchoalveolar lavage fluid from patients with asthma, with further increases after allergen challenge. All MMPs are inhibited by related compounds called tissue inhibitors of metalloproteases (TIMPs). TIMP-1 binds to both pro-MMP-9 and active MMP-9, while TIMP-2 inhibits MMP-2. A major source of MMP-9 is the eosinophil, which releases the enzyme in its inactive 92 kDa form. Cleavage of this to the active 66 kDa component occurs in the endothelium, submucosa, and epithelium through the actions of plasmin and stromelysin-1 (MMP-3). Tissue plasminogen activator (tPA) released from endothelial and epithelial cells with stromelysin-1 is located in mast cells (Fig. 23.10). In addition to overexpression of these pro-MMP-9 activating enzymes, there is also impaired TIMP-1 production by endothelial cells in asthma, which leads to the unregulated activation of eosinophil-derived MMP-9.

The functions of many of the matrix metalloproteases have recently been discovered. Several MMPs, such as MMP-2 and MMP-3, can directly modulate the activity of growth factors and chemokines. Matrix protein fragments released by MMP proteolysis can also serve as chemoattractants for inflammatory cells. Metalloproteases may also play a role in the development of bronchial hyperresponsiveness and airway remodeling. The recent discovery of increased expression of the ADAM33 gene in fibroblasts and bronchial smooth muscle in asthmatics seems to support a role of metalloproteases in the pathogenesis of asthma. The altered ADAM (a disintegrin and metalloproteinase) 33 gene product may promote myogenic fusion between airway smooth muscle cells, and may participate in the release of proliferative factors that affect airway remodeling in the asthmatic lung (Chapter 14).

Binding of extracellular matrix and inflammatory cells

In addition to providing a medium through which inflammatory cells can migrate, the extracellular matrix can also actively regulate cell function (Fig. 23.11). Many leukocytes express surface receptors that are able to bind to elements of the extracellular matrix. The most important receptor class is the integrins, which bind to matrix proteins containing an arginine–glycine–aspartate sequence. In this way, matrix proteins can signal to migrating inflammatory cells by 'outside-in' signaling.

The $a_4\beta_1$ integrin (VLA-4) is present on eosinophils, lymphocytes, and basophils. It binds to the CS-1 domain of fibronectin as well as to the adhesion molecule VCAM-1. This interaction promotes cell migration through the matrix, but it also regulates aspects of the cell function through priming and activation. By rescuing eosinophils from programmed cell death (apoptosis), interaction between VLA-4 and fibronectin enhances local retention of eosinophils. Another function of this integrin receptor is to provide (along with CD28 and B7) a co-stimulus to lymphocytes undergoing T-cell receptor-MHC (TCR-MHC) class II-mediated antigen presentation. Elements of the extracellular matrix may also enhance the efficiency of antigen presentation by 'non-professional' antigen-presenting cells, which themselves lack adequate surface molecules to provide the needed co-stimulus.

The condition of the matrix can also determine the effectiveness of the interaction between the matrix and the cell receptors. CD44 is a surface receptor found on epithelial cells, lymphocytes, and macrophages. Isoforms of CD44 can be generated by the insertion of alternative exons in the extracellular domain of the glycoprotein, and are labeled V1–V11. Some isoforms of CD44, such as V3, are able to bind low-molecular-weight hyaluronan and a variety of growth factors,

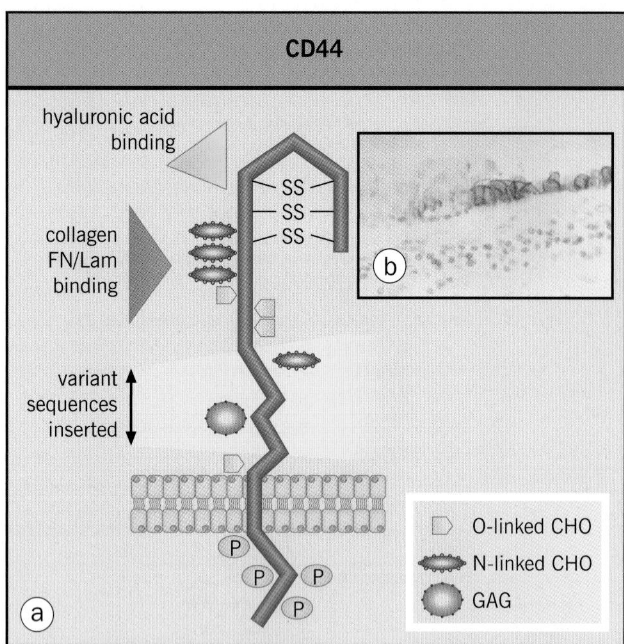

Fig. 23.12 CD44 is a cell adhesion molecule involved in epithelial repair. (a) Structure of CD44 showing the binding sites for cytokines and growth factors. (b) Immunoreactive CD44 expression on damaged epithelium in asthmatic bronchial mucosa.

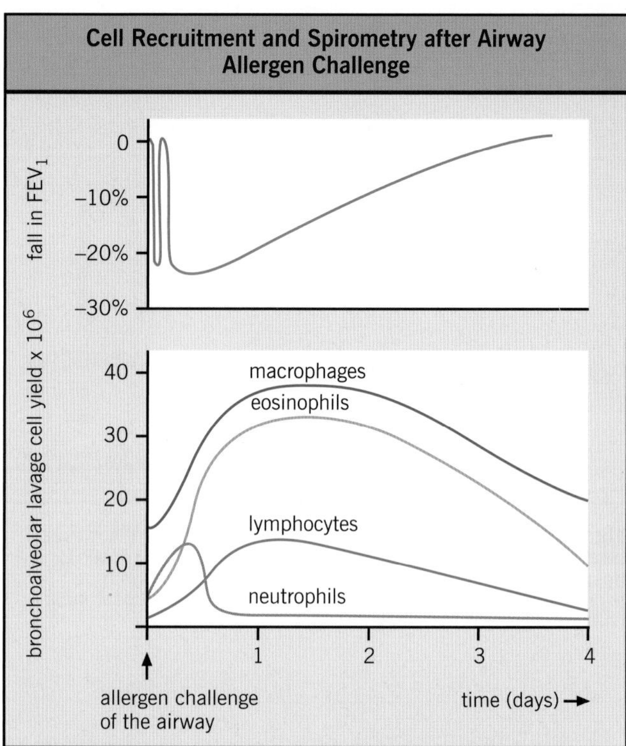

Fig. 23.13 Effects of experimental allergen challenge on the airway. Experimental allergen challenge of the airway can result in early- and late-phase falls in forced expiratory volume in 1 second (FEV_1). The late-phase response is associated with an initial transient influx of neutrophils followed by rises in lymphocyte, eosinophil, and macrophage numbers over several days.

including HB-EGF. The epithelial V3 isoform of CD44 is overexpressed in the injured asthmatic epithelium, thereby facilitating local interactions of HB-EGF with its c-erb B receptors and enabling an interaction between EGF receptors and CD44 through eserine, moiesin, and actin filaments, which are involved in cell motility and epithelial repair (Fig. 23.12). Intact matrix contains the high-molecular-weight (> 10^3 kDa) form of hyaluronan, which is broken down by proteases or oxidant radicals into low-molecular-weight (< 5 x 10^2 kDa) fragments. The specificity of the CD44 receptor for this low-molecular-weight form implies that the cell-hyaluronan interaction will only occur in matrix that has been partially degraded and in the presence of oxidant radicals generated by other inflammatory cells. The CD44–hyaluronan interaction provides a co-stimulus for activating macrophages. In addition, CD44 may be shed from the cell surface, possibly through the involvement of the ADAM family of enzymes. This soluble CD44 may play a role in the organization of the extracellular matrix.

Extracellular matrix may act as a tissue reservoir for cytokines. Negatively charged proteoglycans, such as heparan sulfate, decorin, and CD44V3, are able to bind b-FGF, TGFβ, and HB-EGF, respectively. Heparin and histamine released from mast cells are able to displace some of these cytokines from their proteoglycan binding sites, while others (e.g. TGFβ) are released through proteolytic and glycosidic cleavage of the matrix molecules themselves. MMPs, heparinase, arylsulfatase, and plasmins are all active in this regard.

PATTERNS OF INFLAMMATORY CELL INFLUX

Experimental models show that the recruitment of inflammatory cells during the allergic response is a highly variable process and depends on characteristics of the subject and the circumstances surrounding allergen exposure. Large differences in cell number and the pattern of cell influx are seen between subjects responding to standardized administration of allergen to the skin, nasal mucosa, conjunctivae, or the lower airways. Following the mast cell-mediated early response, which is largely the result of the release of cysteinyl leukotrienes, PGD_2, and histamine, neutrophils are first seen adjacent to engorged blood vessels 10 minutes after allergen exposure. After 30 minutes this cellular infiltrate becomes enriched with eosinophils and by 6–8 hours there are neutrophils, eosinophils, basophils, and mononuclear cells (lymphocytes and macrophages) with a preferential accumulation of CD4+ T lymphocytes expressing Th2 cytokines (Fig. 23.13).

Similarly, allergen challenge of the asthmatic airway results in a variable, but often dramatic, increase in cell concentration and in the total yield of cells obtained by bronchoalveolar lavage. Total cell counts obtained may rise as much as 20-fold. A transient influx of neutrophils is followed by eosinophils, basophils, lymphocytes, and macrophages, which then revert to baseline values over several days. A notable feature of these allergen challenge models is that the allergic inflammatory response does not persist. The mechanisms responsible for the persistence of inflammatory disease in clinical settings are unknown, although, as discussed above, an important interaction occurs between inflammatory cells and the altered tissue matrix. Autopsy studies of patients who have died from asthma show intense infiltration of the airway wall by eosinophils, neutrophils, lymphocytes, and macrophages. Increased numbers

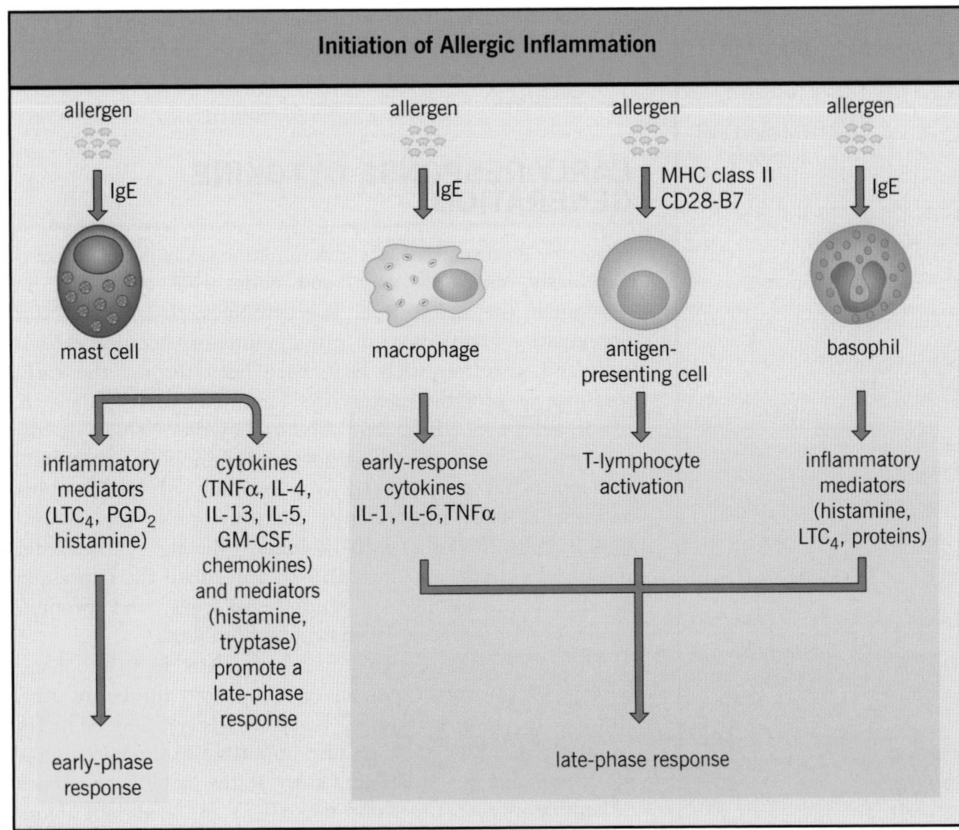

Fig. 23.14 The initiation of allergic inflammation. Mast cell degranulation is responsible for the early-phase response and tends to promote a late-phase response. Macrophages, antigen-presenting cells, and basophils are able to recognize allergens and contribute to initiation of a late-phase response.

of mast cells and dendritic cells have also been reported in the epithelium and submucosa.

THE INITIATION OF ALLERGIC INFLAMMATION

Fundamental questions concerning the ability of allergens to initiate the allergic response remain unanswered. Although several common allergens contain peptide sequences similar to serine proteases, there appears to be no common amino acid structure that confers the ability of a protein to initiate allergic disease. Occupational allergens also share no common structural features and are represented by a wide variety of low- and high-molecular weight compounds, including metal anhydrides, amines, wood dusts, metals, organic chemicals, animal and plant proteins, and biological enzymes. Platinum salts and low-molecular-weight acid anhydrides can interact with mast cells by acting as haptens and are recognized by IgE only after conjugation with a protein.

The best-described mechanism involves binding of an allergen to allergen-specific IgE on the mast cell surface, resulting in degranulation and an early-phase response (Fig. 23.14). It is important to recognize that although mast cell degranulation often precedes a late-phase response, it may be neither sufficient nor necessary for the development of this late reaction. Experimental allergen challenge models in the skin and airway consistently show the presence of isolated early-phase responses, or isolated late-phase responses. This implies that allergens are in part able to provoke late-phase allergic inflammation by mechanisms that are independent of the mast cells. Mechanisms involved in the initiation of a late-phase cellular response are not well defined and probably involve the coordinated action of several cells, each of which is able to respond directly to the presence of allergenic protein. In particular, macrophages express large numbers of surface receptors that are able to recognize a variety of substances including foreign antigens, immunoglobulins, cytokines, hormones, proteins, and lipids. Allergen-specific IgE is able to bind to macrophages via FcεRII (CD23), the low-affinity IgE receptor, allowing the macrophage to respond directly to the presence of specific allergen in a manner similar to that of the mast cell. A notable consequence of macrophage activation is the synthesis and release of early-response cytokines, such as IL-8, IL-6, and TNFα.

A key event in initiating allergen sensitization and for elaborating a specific T-cell response is the uptake, processing, and presentation of allergen by dendritic cells that are dedicated to this purpose. After contact with an antigen, these cells take up antigen both non-specifically (via clathrin-coated pits) and specifically (via FcεRII and FcεRI). Dendritic cells process the antigens into peptides, and in the presence of GM-CSF and TNFα migrate to regional lymph nodes where the peptide fragments are presented to the T-cell receptor of naïve T lymphocytes via MHC class II. Dendritic cells initiate the polarization of Th subsets with the aid of co-stimulatory molecules, such as B7-1 (CD80), B7-2 (CD86), and CD40. T lymphocyte polarization and activation profoundly influence the nature of the subsequent inflammatory reaction through the generation of cytokine profiles, either of the Th2 or Th1 types.

In the presence of a large allergen load, basophils recruited from the bloodstream can contribute to late-phase inflammation by IgE-mediated late-phase degranulation.

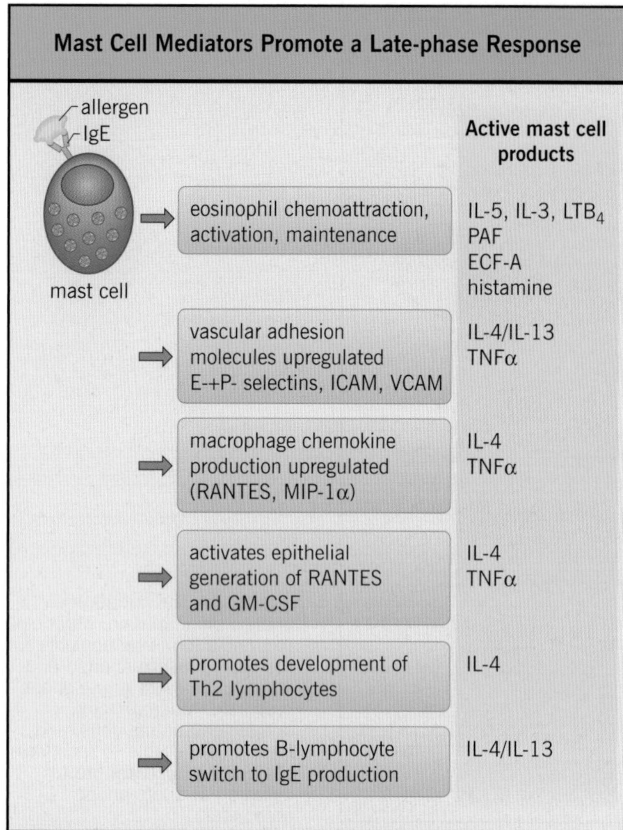

Fig. 23.15 Several products of mast cell degranulation promote generation of the late-phase inflammatory response. ECF-A, eosinophil chemotactic factor A; ICAM, intercellular adhesion molecule; IL, interleukin; LTB_4, leukotriene B_4; MIP, macrophage inflammatory protein; PAF, platelet-activating factor; TNF, tumor necrosis factor; VCAM, vascular cell adhesion molecule.

MAST CELL MEDIATORS PROMOTE A LATE-PHASE RESPONSE

Although mast-cell-derived mediators are chiefly responsible for the appearance of an early-phase response and may not be necessary for a late phase, mast cell products do contribute to the development of the late-phase reaction (Fig. 23.15). Reported effects of mast cell products include eosinophil recruitment, activation and maintenance – notably by TNFα, IL-4, IL-5, IL-13, and GM-CSF. The vascular adhesion molecules E- and P-selectins, ICAM-1, and VCAM-1 are upregulated by TNFα, as well as IL-4 or IL-13. These cytokines also stimulate macrophages and epithelial cells to generate important lymphocyte and eosinophil chemoattractants, including RANTES, MIP-1α, and GM-CSF. Interleukin-4 (but not its homolog, IL-13) promotes development of Th2 lymphocytes rather than Th1 lymphocytes and is necessary for B-lymphocyte switching to IgE production. The consequences of mast cell degranulation also encourage the influx of inflammatory cells in an indirect manner. This influx is accomplished by promotion of vascular leak and tissue edema with release of large amounts of mast cell-derived leukotriene C_4 (LTC_4), histamine, and matrix-degrading proteases, including stromelysin (MMP-3), tryptase, and chymotryptase. The recent finding that treatment with omalizumab, an anti-IgE monoclonal antibody, allowed asthmatic patients to reduce their oral and inhaled corticosteroid use by 50%, and produced improvement in pulmonary function, symptoms, and β_2-agonist use, further supports a role for IgE and the mast cell in clinical asthma.

EARLY-RESPONSE CYTOKINE GENERATION

A notable feature of allergic inflammation is the involvement of fibroblasts, epithelial cells, and endothelial cells that are resident in the airway wall. Two cytokines, IL-1β and TNFα, upregulate a broad range of proinflammatory activity in these cells and, together with IL-6, have been termed the early-response or proinflammatory cytokines. Macrophages are the major source of IL-1β and TNFα; however, TNFα is also released by mast cells, lymphocytes, eosinophils, fibroblasts, and epithelial cells. IL-1β is a product of lymphocytes, endothelial cells, neutrophils, dendritic cells, and smooth muscle cells. TNFα and IL-1β initiate further synthesis and release of cytokines and mediators, upregulate the expression of adhesion molecules on endothelial cells, and promote production of extracellular matrix by fibroblasts.

The early-response mediators are generated by macrophages in response to contact with allergens and by a number of other stimuli, including endotoxin, IL-1β and IFNγ, and NO. The early-response mediators are also important in the initiation of other non-allergic, proinflammatory states, notably the septic inflammatory response syndrome (SIRS), and so are not unique to allergic inflammation. However, alone or together, they are probably responsible for some of the non-specific features of the allergic response, such as bronchial hyperresponsiveness and increased mucus secretion.

IL-6 belongs to a family of acute response cytokines that also includes IL-11 and oncostatin, and is produced by macrophages, epithelial cells, and fibroblasts. Fungal and dust mite proteases, viral infections, and histamine increase IL-6 production by epithelial cells. IL-6 promotes the activation, growth, and differentiation of T lymphocytes, and promotes IgE synthesis by B lymphocytes (in conjunction with IL-4 or IL-13). The antiinflammatory properties of IL-6 include suppression of the production of TNFα and IL-1 by macrophages. IL-11 has recently been shown to be a powerful stimulus for hyperplasia of airway smooth muscle and the synthesis of collagen by fibroblasts; it can also activate B cells via a T-lymphocyte-dependent mechanism.

MACROPHAGE ACTIVATION

Macrophage activation is an event of profound importance in the generation of a cellular allergic inflammatory response (Fig. 23.16). In addition to IgE-mediated activation, macrophage activity is upregulated by several other products of the allergic response – IL-4 and IL-13, TNFα, and IFNγ. As a result, macrophages generate not only the early-response mediators but also products that promote eosinophil chemoattraction. Leukotrienes released by activated macrophages consist mainly of the dihydroxyarachidonic acid metabolite LTB_4, rather than the cysteinyl leukotriene LTC_4, although for alveolar macrophages that express FcεRII receptors this may not be true. LTB_4 has important neutrophil chemotactic activity and activates the oxidative respiratory burst, resulting in release of reactive oxygen species. Although neutrophil recruitment and activation

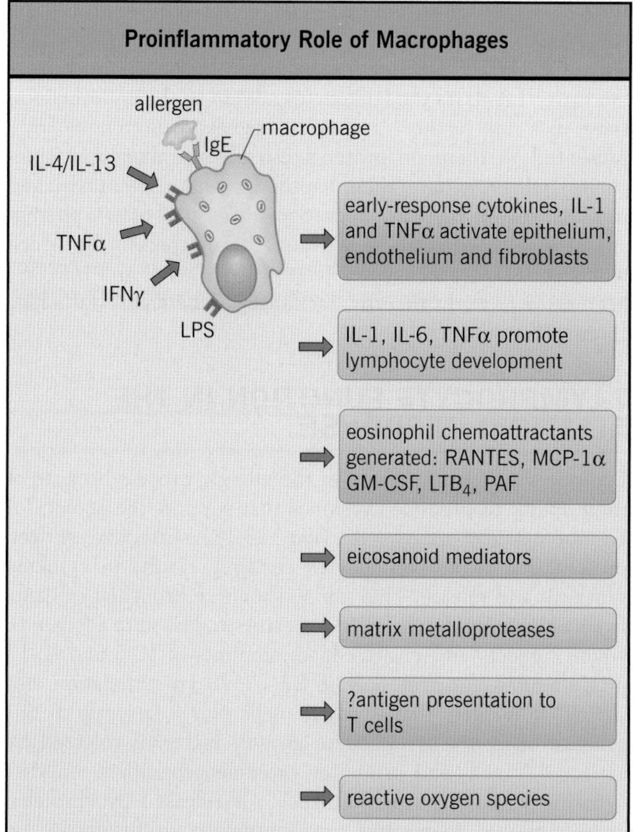

Fig. 23.16 The proinflammatory role of macrophages. Macrophage activation may occur directly by IgE-mediated allergen recognition or by contact with cytokines such as IL-4, TNFα, and IFNγ. A range of proinflammatory mediators is generated by activated macrophages, including the early-response cytokines, IL-1 and TNFα. IFN, interferon; GM-CSF, granulocyte–macrophage colony-stimulating factor; IL, interleukin; LPS, lipopolysaccharide; LTB_4, leukotriene B_4; MCP, monocyte chemotactic peptide; PAF, platelet-activating factor; TNF, tumor necrosis factor.

is important in other inflammatory states, its role in allergic inflammation is probably restricted to the initial component of the late-phase response. Neutrophils may be especially important in severe asthma and in asthma provoked by respiratory viruses.

Macrophages are also able to regulate T-lymphocyte function vis-à-vis antigen presentation. The effective activation of T cells by tissue macrophages is critically dependent on the activation state of both cells and on the tissue microenvironment in which the antigen presentation takes place. The timing and location of antigen presentation by macrophages to T lymphocytes in inflamed tissues is not well established; however, several lines of evidence suggest that these cells are able to present antigen effectively to recently activated memory (CD45RO+) T cells and effector CD4+ T cells in inflamed tissues. Alveolar macrophages usually have limited expression of the co-stimulatory molecules B7-1 (CD80) and B7-2 (CD86); these molecules engage CD28 on the T cell for effective antigen presentation. Thus, luminal macrophages may produce T-cell anergy and T-cell apoptosis as a result of antigen presentation in the absence of co-stimulation, or when B7 engages cytotoxic T-lymphocyte antigen (CTLA-4). These downregulatory mechanisms may become ineffective in the microenvironment of the inflamed airway wall either because of the reduced co-stimulatory requirements of highly activated effector T cells, or because of the provision of alternative co-stimulatory signals. Interstitial macrophages in the airway wall are clearly different from luminal macrophages and, along with B cells and dendritic cells, are able to more effectively present antigen to T cells.

Macrophage and T-lymphocyte responses to antigens can also be regulated by factors intrinsic to the antigen itself. Receptors that recognize pathogen-associated molecular patterns (PAMPs) are present on macrophages, and are an important part of innate immunity. Chief among these receptors are the Toll-like receptors (TLRs). The Toll receptor, first described in the *Drosophila* fruit fly, is important in activating antifungal defense mechanisms. Functionally homologous receptors in the human have been termed TLRs, and at present nine different TLRs have been described. TLR4, in the presence of the lipopolysaccharide (LPS) receptor CD14, plays an important role in the recognition of bacterial LPS, with subsequent upregulation of IL-12 and IL-18, and eventual Th1-polarized immune responses. TLR9, which recognizes unmethylated cytosine–guanine (CpG) motifs found in bacterial DNA, also plays an important role in innate immunity and the upregulation of Th1 immune responses. The clinical importance of TLRs is evident in that polymorphisms in the promoter for the CD14 gene, which result in increased levels of soluble CD14 and increased signaling via TLR4, has been shown to lead to decreases in the total level of serum IgE. The immunomodulatory potential of TLR9 has also been exploited by conjugating allergens with CpG motifs in an effort to modify the allergic response by upregulating the Th1 response, and by cross-inhibition, decreasing the Th2 response, to the allergen.

Several macrophage products actively inhibit inflammation. One such product is IL-10, which downregulates cytokine production by macrophages and Th2 lymphocytes. Recent studies point to reduced production of IL-10 in asthmatic and rhinitic airways; this reduction in IL-10 may lead to decreased control over Th2 responses. Another product of macrophages is the IL-1 receptor antagonist, which competes with IL-1β for binding to a common receptor site and prevents induction of a range of gene products in target cells. TGFβ is generated by macrophages and other cells and is recognized as having both proinflammatory and antiinflammatory effects.

ENDOTHELIAL CELLS IN THE ALLERGIC RESPONSE

Vascular endothelium serves as a gateway for cells that leave the bloodstream and enter interstitial tissue (Fig. 23.17). In the systemic circulation this is thought to occur in postcapillary venules by a process that involves the migrating cells rolling over the endothelial cells, firmly adhering to the endothelial cells, and finally migrating between the endothelial cells. Expression of adhesion molecules on the vascular endothelium is central to this process, as is the presence of appropriate and activated counter-receptors on the cells. In allergic diseases, P-selectin, E-selectin, ICAM-1, and VCAM-1 are all upregulated in the microvessels of the skin, nose, conjunctivae, and airways. After allergen challenge, this occurs in a time-dependent manner and is a major factor in the regional recruitment of inflammatory cells. P-selectin, which is expressed following exposure to histamine and leukotrienes, and E-selectin, which is expressed following exposure to endotoxin, IL-1β and TNFα, initiate leukocyte rolling by interacting with lectin ligands such as sialyl Lewis[x]. Recently, a truncated form of P-selectin has been shown to be selective for eosinophils by interacting with a unique carbohydrate moiety expressed on these cells. For effective recruitment of eosinophils, basophils, and T cells, further interaction is required between integrins expressed on these leukocytes and ICAM-1 and VCAM-1. ICAM-1 interacts with CD11/CD18 integrins whereas VCAM-1 selectively binds to VLA-4. As the leukocytes adhere to the endothelium, they pick up further 'activation' signals from chemokines presented to them on proteoglycan glycosaminoglycan side-chains, which initiate their haptotaxis and chemotaxis, and prime them for mediator secretion. Release of active plasmin and stromelysin (MMP-3) provides the mechanism by which leukocyte MMP-proenzymes (especially MMP-2 and MMP-9) become activated, thereby facilitating leukocyte trafficking through the matrix.

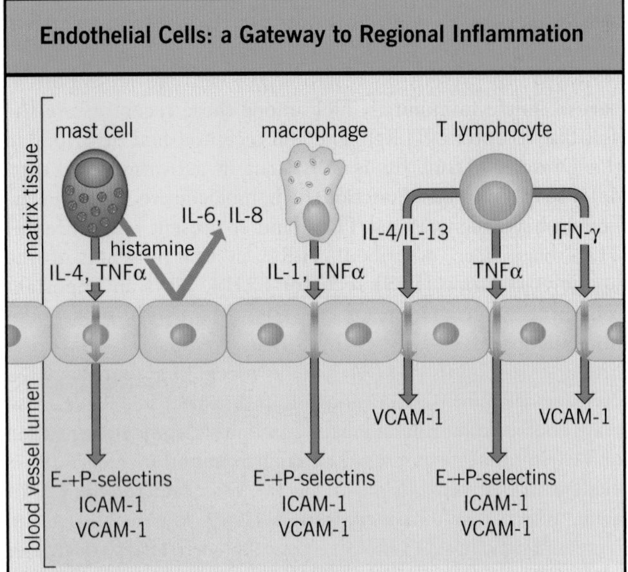

Fig. 23.17 Mast cell, macrophage, and T-lymphocyte cytokines upregulate expression of adhesion molecules on endothelial cells. This upregulation promotes recruitment of inflammatory cells from the bloodstream. ICAM, intercellular adhesion molecule; IFN, interferon; IL, interleukin; VCAM, vascular cell adhesion molecule.

T-LYMPHOCYTE FUNCTION IN THE ALLERGIC RESPONSE

Lymphocytes are important in the allergic process because of their ability to produce cytokines that support the activity of eosinophils and mast cells (Fig. 23.18). Effective antigen presentation to T lymphocytes certainly results in cytokine synthesis and release. This can be shown in bronchial explants from asthmatic airways, as on exposure to dust mite allergen to which subjects are sensitive large amounts of IL-5 and IL-13 production result, but only if B7–CD28 co-stimulation also occurs. It is likely that dendritic cells play a key role in this process. IL-2, the lymphocyte growth factor, is released by activated T cells and promotes cytokine generation. Another cytokine-generating stimulus, IL-15, is released by epithelial cells, activated monocytes, and fibroblasts; it results in the production of IL-5 by T lymphocytes through mechanisms that

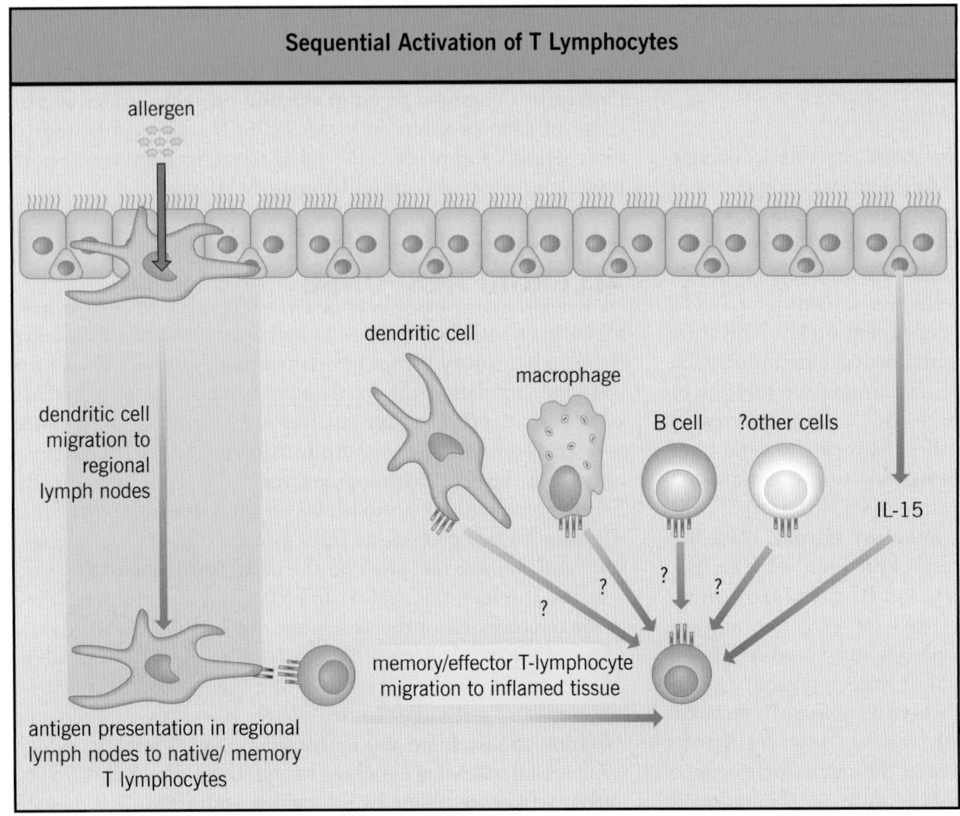

Fig. 23.18 Contact with allergen causes dendritic cells to migrate to regional lymph nodes, where antigen presentation to lymphocytes takes place. Activated lymphocytes then migrate to inflamed tissue. Mechanisms then responsible for cytokine generation by these lymphocytes are not well defined. IL, interleukin.

are independent of IL-2 or the T-cell receptor–CD3 complex. IL-15 may be important because it represents a means by which inflammatory cells can promote cytokine generation from a heterogeneous population of T and B lymphocytes, independent of the stringent allergen-specific requirements of antigen presentation.

$CD4^+$ lymphocytes in the asthmatic airway express a range of surface activation markers – CD25 (IL-2Rα), CD69, CD71, and HLA-DR – and represent a mixed population of Th0 (naïve), Th1, and Th2 cells. However, it is the Th2 cytokines that are considered responsible for the eosinophil response. Th2 cells express CCR4 receptors, and are activated by monocyte-derived chemokine (MDC) and thymus- and activation-regulated cytokine (TARC). Epithelial cells from asthmatic patients are known to express TARC, and increased concentrations of TARC are found in the bronchoalveolar lavage (BAL) of patients with asthma. TARC is likely an important chemokine in the recruitment of CD4+ Th2 cells into the airway. CD4+ lymphocyte populations isolated from the airway after allergen challenge actually generate a number of different cytokines – IL-4, IL-5, IFNγ, and IL-10 – and it may be the relative proportions of these cytokines that influence the nature of the inflammatory response. The magnitude of the CD4+ T-cell response to an allergen depends on the number of cells that recognize the antigen, the cell activation state, the efficiency of antigen presentation with adequate co-stimuli, and possibly the presence of IL-15. CD4+ T cells initiate a B-cell switch to IgE production through the generation of IL-4 and by direct interaction via CD40 ligand (CD154), which is the B-cell CD40 receptor.

It has become apparent that the Th1–Th2 dichotomy may represent an oversimplification of the T-lymphocyte response to antigen. The immune responses of both Th1 and Th2 subsets may be downregulated by CD4+ T-regulatory cells. Although it is unclear exactly how T regulatory lymphocytes exert their immunosuppressive effects, it appears that IL-10 is important for this process. Currently, three subsets of T regulatory cells have been defined. The CD4+CD25+ (Treg) subset constitutively expresses the IL-2Rα subunit (CD25), and may be important in the prevention of autoimmunity. Depletion of CD4+CD25+ cells leads to the development of the *immune dysregulation, polyendocrinopathy enteropathy X-linked* (IPEX) syndrome. The Tr1 subset also produces IL-10 and may play a role in the suppression of chronic inflammation. The Th3 subset produces TGFβ in addition to IL-10, and likely plays a role in oral tolerance. Although the relationship between the different types of regulatory T-lymphocytes is not clear at present, it does appear that the environment from which they develop is important. The Tr1 subset may be important in the regulation of immune responses in the lung, where dendritic cells produce IL-10, and the Th3 subset may be more important in the gastrointestinal system, where dendritic cells produce both IL-10 and TGFβ.

Although CD4+ T-cell numbers in the blood and airway correspond to the severity and activity of the disease and to eosinophil survival, it is now recognized that a population of CD8+ T cells, the so-called Tc2 subset (for *c*ytotoxic *T* cell) are also capable of producing Th2-type cytokines. A role for CD8+ T lymphocytes in allergic inflammation has not been well established. Viral-specific CD8+ T cells, when grown in the presence of IL-4, may be induced to switch their cytokine profile to type 2 cytokines, i.e. IL-5. Tc2 lymphocytes therefore may play a putative role in the association between respiratory infections and asthma exacerbations. CD8+T cells may also be important in occupational allergy, where they are present in increased numbers in the airway. It has been suggested that the small chemicals implicated in occupational asthma may be processed via the MHC I pathway, with subsequent presentation to CD8+ T lymphocytes.

PROINFLAMMATORY PROPERTIES OF EOSINOPHILS

Eosinophils contribute to allergic inflammation by producing mediators that directly damage tissue (Fig. 23.19). Eosinophils are found in large numbers in all tissues undergoing a late-phase or chronic allergic response. Circumstantial evidence supporting their pathogenic role in allergic inflammation is strong. In asthma, increased numbers of activated eosinophils are found in the blood, sputum, BAL fluid, bronchial biopsy specimens, and autopsy specimens of involved airways. Their presence correlates with airway hyperresponsiveness and disease severity. The half-life of eosinophils in the blood is less than 24 hours and they quickly enter tissue by interaction with the selectins, ICAM-1, and VCAM-1, in a process that takes 1–2 hours. Once in the extracellular matrix, eosinophil survival is enhanced by GM-CSF and IL-5 and by interaction between VLA-4 and the fibronectin components of extracellular matrix. Normal eosinophil life-span in tissue is about 2–5 days but, under the influence of these factors, survival may be extended to 14 days or more by rescue from apoptosis; this prolongation of the life-span contributes to the increased eosinophil numbers observed at sites of allergic inflammation.

Mature eosinophils have cytoplasmic granules that contain several proteins that are toxic to parasites and to a variety of airway cells. Major basic protein (MBP) is stored as an inactive preprotein, which becomes highly basic on account of its high content of arginine residues when released. ECP and eosinophil-derived neurotoxin (EDN) contribute to the cytotoxic activity of eosinophils. The highly basic nature of these proteins is considered to be the factor that makes them toxic to the respiratory epithelium. Eosinophil peroxidase (EPO) can also damage epithelium through the production of hypophalous acids, which are synthesized in the presence of hydrogen peroxide and halide.

In established allergic disease, activated eosinophils are the major source of cysteinyl leukotrienes, which cause smooth muscle contraction, mucus hypersecretion, microvascular leakage, eosinophil chemotaxis, and airway hyperresponsiveness. Thromboxane A_2 and platelet-activating factor are also generated. The precise mechanism responsible for eosinophil activation in asthma is not known, although mast cell tryptase, IgA, and the secretory component of IgA are all capable of stimulating eosinophil mediator release. Hypodense eosinophils at sites of allergic inflammation have released granule products, and they stain with the monoclonal antibody EG-2, which is directed at an epitope expressed on granule eosinophil cationic protein. The major eosinophil chemoattractants currently identified are eotaxin-1, eotaxin-2, RANTES, and MCP-4, all of which interact with CCR3 receptors; various other cytokines and mediators also have chemoattractant activity. Increased expression of eotaxin-1, eotaxin-2, MCP-3, and MCP-4 occurs in the asthmatic airway and correlates well with airway

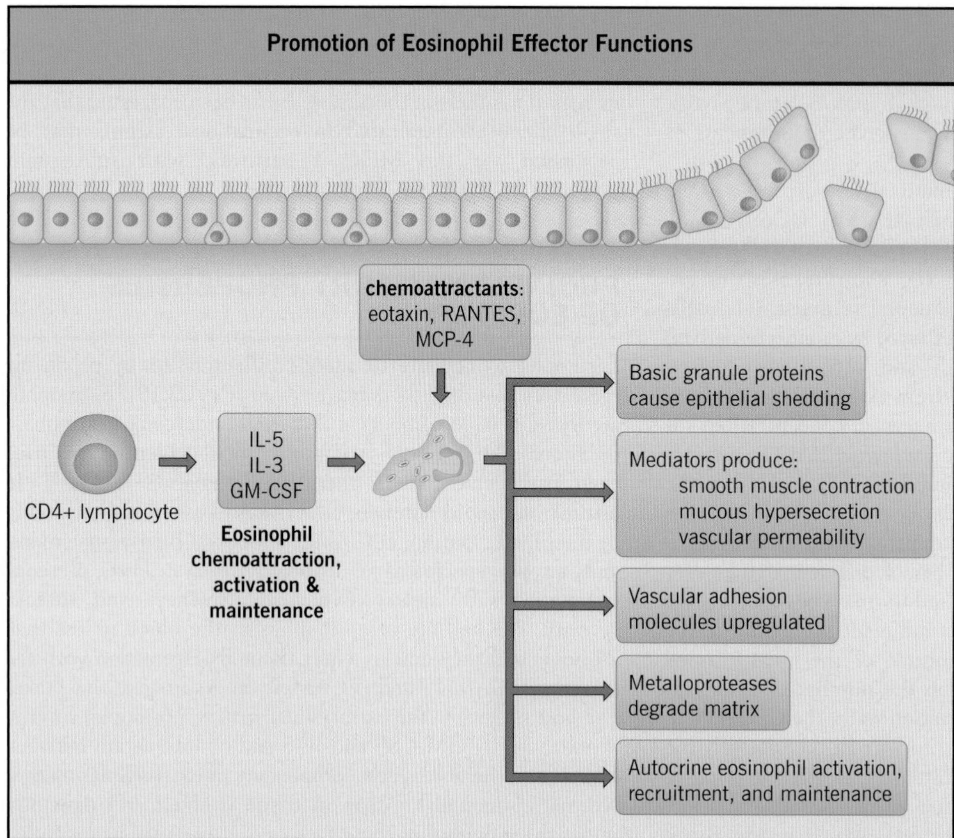

Fig. 23.19 Eosinophils migrate towards inflamed tissue under the influence of chemoattractants: eotaxin, RANTES, and MCP-4. Activation and maintenance of eosinophils is promoted by CD4+ T-lymphocyte cytokines – IL-3, IL-5, and GM-CSF. Eosinophils generate a variety of proinflammatory mediators. GM-CSF, granulocyte–macrophage colony-stimulating factor; IL, interleukin; MCP, monocyte chemotactic peptide.

hyperresponsiveness. Eosinophil development from precursors is mediated by IL-3, IL-5, and the CCR3 ligands.

THE ROLE OF BASOPHILS

In contrast to mast cells, which are resident in tissue, basophils circulate freely. They are recruited to sites of late-phase inflammation by interaction with the adhesion molecules E-selectin, ICAM-1, and VCAM-1. Basophil chemotactic factors include IL-3, IL-5, IL-8, GM-CSF, C5a, and platelet-activating factor. Basophil degranulation occurs after cross-linking of surface-bound IgE, or after contact with a number of cytokines, including MCP-1 and the eosinophil granule protein MBP. Important basophil mediators include histamine, cysteinyl leukotrienes, prostanoids, kallikreins, and Th2 cytokines, especially IL-4 and IL-13. Basophils act to support the role of eosinophils by generating these mediators in late-phase and chronic allergic inflammation of the skin, nose, and airways, especially in the presence of high antigen exposure.

CHOLINERGIC MECHANISMS OF AIRWAY INFLAMMATION

Stimulated cholinergic nerves in the airway wall can rapidly induce smooth muscle contraction, cause vasodilatation, and mucus hypersecretion. There is experimental evidence that cholinergic overactivity, characteristic of asthmatic airways, results from several mechanisms (Fig. 23.20). Cholinergic tone is increased by an excess of central vagal output, resulting from the activity of local reflexes involving sensory nerves. Non-specific chemical and physical irritants, bradykinin, histamine, leukotrienes, and prostaglandins can trigger this reflex arc, particularly after the loss of overlying epithelium. Mast cell products (especially histamine and PGD_2) and eosinophil mediators upregulate the activity of the cholinergic ganglia. Impaired inhibition of acetylcholine release from postganglionic fibers is a consequence of dysfunction of the prejunctional inhibitory muscarinic M_2 receptors. M_2 receptor (M_2R) dysfunction may be mediated in part by CD8+ T lymphocytes, type I interferons, and IFNγ. Additionally, MBP released from eosinophils can act as an M_2R antagonist. A relative reduction of acetylcholinesterase activity in airways undergoing allergic inflammation has also been reported.

TACHYKININS – INFLAMMATORY NEUROPEPTIDES

Tachykinins are immunoactive peptides released from sensory non-myelinated (C) nerve fibers and macrophages in the airway and are co-localized. They have a number of effects that contribute to airway inflammation. Neurokinin (NK)-A, which acts via NK-2 receptors, causes smooth muscle contraction, particularly in peripheral airways. Substance P, acting preferentially via NK-1 receptors, augments mucus secretion from airway submucosal glands and induces microvascular leak from postcapillary venules. This peptide also promotes degranulation of chymase-containing mast cells (MC_{TC}) in connective tissue, chemotaxis and degranulation of eosinophils, and proliferation of blood vessels. A third tachykinin, the calcitonin gene-related peptide (CGRP), acts directly on

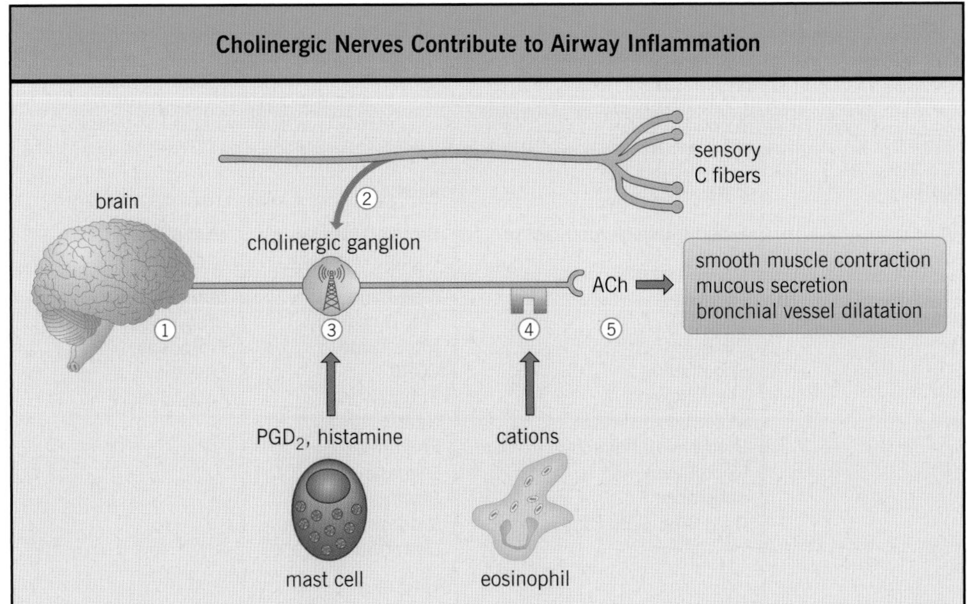

Fig. 23.20 Cholinergic overactivity may result from (1) increased vagal nerve output, (2) activation of a local reflex sensory arc based on the regional cholinergic ganglion, (3) the cholinergic activity of mast cell products acting on the cholinergic ganglia, (4) damage to the prejunctional M_2 receptor, or (5) increased levels of junctional acetylcholine (Ach). PGD_2, prostaglandin D_2.

vascular smooth muscle receptors to cause arteriolar dilatation, which further potentiates postcapillary leakage. Tachykinins also activate macrophages and T cells and induce the generation of IL-6. Substance P and NK-A cause proliferation and chemotaxis of fibroblasts via NK-1 and NK-2 receptors. Tachykinins are inactivated by epithelial-derived neutral endopeptidase; deficiency of this endopeptidase accompanies epithelial damage in asthma, thereby increasing the local bioavailability of these mediators.

CONSEQUENCES OF ALLERGIC AIRWAY INFLAMMATION

Allergic inflammation alters the structure of the airway wall because of the action of multiple mediators and proinflammatory cytokines (Table 23.1). The onset of inflammation is characterized by smooth muscle contraction, owing to the action of cholinergic and sensory nerves. Mast cell degranulation soon follows, causing mucus hypersecretion, vasodilatation, microvascular leak, and sustained smooth muscle contraction. Histamine, cysteinyl leukotrienes, and PGD_2 are the predominant mast cell products associated with the early reaction, being supplemented by tryptase, bradykinin, and endothelin-1. In established allergic inflammation, eosinophils are the dominant source of cysteinyl leukotrienes and also secrete platelet-activating factor and a range of prostanoids. Structural alterations to the components of the airway wall evolve as epithelium is damaged and replaced, smooth muscle and fibroblasts respond to mitogens, and extracellular matrix is broken down and replaced. The inflammatory process resolves as proinflammatory cells are lost into the airway or undergo apoptosis, and are not replaced by newly recruited cells. Although many mediators are involved in the inflammatory process, the relative contribution of each mediator to the inflammatory process and its subsequent resolution is unclear.

PATHOLOGIC FEATURES OF ALLERGIC INFLAMMATION

The normal airway wall has an intact epithelial layer, a thin lattice collagen basement membrane, and a sparse distribution of mast cells, lymphocytes, and macrophages. In small airways, bronchial vessels lie deep to the smooth muscle. In larger airways, vessels lie above and below the muscle layer.

The early allergic response in the airway shows the effects of mast cell degranulation (i.e. vascular dilatation, edema of extracellular matrix, and mucus hypersecretion). Late-phase inflammation is characterized by an initial and transient infiltration by neutrophils followed by a more sustained recruitment of eosinophils, macrophages, and lymphocytes, which become distributed through the full thickness of the airway wall.

Asthma is predominantly a disease of the airways and not of the alveoli. However, recent evidence does suggest that eosinophils can accumulate in the alveolar interstitium in association with nocturnal exacerbations of asthma and in fatal asthma exacerbations. Damage to the epithelium is a common feature of airway wall inflammation. Columnar cells detach from their basal cells through cleavage of desmosomes and tight junctions, leaving basal cells attached. In addition, subjects with asthma of even a mild degree show an apparent thickening of the basement membrane. This is due to deposition of types III and V 'repair' collagens in the lamina reticularis underneath the types IV and VII 'reticular' collagens, which largely make up the basement membrane. The altered sub-basement membrane region also contains fibronectin, tenascin, and lamin-C, which are indicative of the induction of morphogenic genes. Myofibroblasts that lie just below the basement membrane and whose numbers are increased in asthma are the source of these matrix products that are recruited after allergen or other environmental exposure; these myofibroblasts receive growth factor activation signals from the overlying but phenotypically altered repairing epithelium. The asthmatic airway also

Table 23.1 Consequences of allergic airway inflammation. Allergic inflammation can be considered as a process with immediate, early, late, and repair phases. The mediators and cells that have activity corresponding to the pathologic features of these phases of allergic inflammation are listed

Consequences of Allergic Airway Inflammation

	Immediate	**Early →**	**Late**	
Effect	Smooth muscle contraction	Smooth muscle contraction	Bronchial vessel dilatation or leak	Mucus hyper secretion
Causes	Cholinergic nerves Neurokinin A	Histamine LTC_4, LTD_4 PGD_2, $PGF_{2\alpha}$ Endothelins-1, -2, -3, Thromboxane A_2 Major basic protein Bradykinin (indirectly) Neurokinins and substance P C5a, C4a, C3a, C2a	Histamine PAF, Bradykinin Nitric oxide CGRP Substance P Neurokinin A, Endothelin-1, Tryptase Chymase, Cathepsin-D, C5a, D4a, C3a, C2a	Substance P Bradykinin Proteases Endothelin-1 Acetylcholine
			Late →	
Inflammatory cell influx	Epithelial damage	Smooth muscle hypertrophy hyperplasia	Fibroblast proliferation	Extracellular-remodeling
Eosinophils Lymphocytes Macrophages Mast cells	Eosinophil basic granule proteins Reactive oxygen species PAF Proteases	LTD_4 Thromboxane A_2 Endothelin-1 Histamine IL-1 Growth factors: EGF ILGF PDGF FGF Colony-stimulating factor	IL-1 Growth factors Fibroblast, Platelet-derived Histamine Heparin Tryptase Eosinophil basic granule proteins Fibronectin Endothelin-1	Proteases: Tryptases Chymases Elastases MMPs
		Repair →		
Effect	Epithelial regrowth	Matrix depositon	Inflammatory cell attrition	
Due to	Fibronectin Epidermal growth factor TGFβ Retinoic acid	TGFβ IL-1 IL-4	Chemoattraction Adhesion molecules Apoptosis Loss of cells into the airway	

CGRP, calcitonin gene-related peptide; EGF, epidermal growth factor; FGF, fibroblast growth factor; IL, interleukin; ILGF, insulin-like growth factor; LTC_4, D_4, leukotriene T_4, D_4; MMP, matrix metalloprotease; PAF, platelet-activating factor; PDGF, platelet-derived growth factor; PGD_2, $F_{2\alpha}$, prostaglandin D_2, $F_{2\alpha}$; TGF, transforming growth factor.

demonstrates smooth muscle hypertrophy and hyperplasia, fibroblast proliferation, and extracellular matrix deposition, which is responsible for overall thickening of the airway wall. Bronchial vessels, which are also present in greater numbers in asthma, are dilated and leak edema fluid.

Whether an excess of new vessels is formed by angiogenesis is controversial. Submucosal glands are enlarged while goblet cells within the epithelium are metaplastic. It is notable that the pathologic features of chronic allergic airway disease are identical to those seen in all types of chronic asthma (i.e. extrinsic, intrinsic, and occupational asthma), and no clear distinction between the structural changes induced by these different forms of asthma has yet been identified.

Resolution of allergic inflammation in non-asthmatic but allergic individuals follows attrition of the inflammatory cells that have invaded the airway wall. Damage to epithelium is followed by a vigorous restoration process – adjacent ciliated cells lose their cilia, goblet cells discharge granules into the edge of the wound, and a plasma-derived gel that contains fibronectin, fibrin, and growth factors forms over the basement membrane. Remaining epithelial cells flatten and proliferate to form an undifferentiated epithelial layer within about 8 hours of an acute injury. Full differentiation of the newly formed epithelium may take 5 days unless repeated injury occurs. Thus, in the presence of severe inflammation, epithelial resuscitation is delayed with the epithelium switching to secrete a range of new mediators, including IL-8, GM-CSF, eotaxin, NO, prostanoids, and a series of mediators such as fibrogenic and smooth muscle growth factors (TGFβ, IGF-1, b-FGF, PDGF, endothelin-1). Chronic inflammation is also associated with more substantial extracellular matrix deposition, fibroblast proliferation, smooth muscle hyperplasia, and hypertrophy.

AIRWAY OBSTRUCTION BY MUCOUS PLUGS

The allergic process has profound consequences for the functional integrity of the airway. Mucous impaction, smooth muscle spasm, thickening of the swollen airway wall, and possibly mechanical dissociation from adventitia and cartilage all promote airway narrowing and airflow obstruction. The mucous plugs that form adjacent to the inflamed airway are composed of mucus derived from submucosal glands and epithelial goblet cells. Plasma proteins also leak through extracellular matrix and into the airway lumen. The epithelium is shed, probably as a result of action of toxic basic proteins, proteolytic enzymes, and reactive oxygen species derived from inflammatory cells, including eosinophils. Migrating inflammatory cells lost into the lumen contribute to the burden of cellular debris. Lysis of these cells is associated with release of sticky DNA, which tends to bind components of the mucous plug.

An understanding of the pathophysiologic processes leading to airway function is providing a rational basis for treatment. Most guidelines now place inhaled corticosteroids as the principal 'controller' drug through their effects in suppressing the Th2- and epithelium-mediated inflammatory cascade. The advent of new therapies that selectively inhibit cytokine effects, remove IgE, or selectively block eosinophil recruitment are based on an understanding of the pathogenesis of airway inflammation. Clearer understanding of what initiates asthma and results in its chronic and relapsing features is likely to reveal important and novel targets against which to develop new drugs.

FURTHER READING

Bates CA, Silkoff PE. Exhaled nitric oxide in asthma: from bench to bedside. J Allergy Clin Immunol 2003; 111:256–262.

Boushey HA. New and exploratory therapies for asthma. Chest 2003; 123:439S–445S.

Carroll N, Cooke C, James A. The distribution of eosinophils and lymphocytes in the large and small airways of asthmatics. Eur Respir J 1997; 10:292–300.

Jordana M, Sarnstrand B, Sime PJ, et al. Immune-inflammatory functions of fibroblasts. Eur Respir J 1994; 7:2212–2222.

Kalish RS, Askenase PW. Molecular mechanisms of CD8+ T cell-mediated delayed hypersensitivity: Implications for allergies, asthma, and autoimmunity. J Allergy Clin Immunol 1999; 103:192–199.

Mori A, Suko M, Kaminuma O, et al. IL-15 promotes cytokine production of human T helper cells. J Immunol 1996; 156:2400–2405.

Sabroe I, Parker LC, Wilson AG, et al. Toll-like receptors: their role in allergy and non-allergic inflammatory disease. Clin Exp Allergy 2002; 32:984–989.

Thompson AB, Robbins RA, Romberger DJ, et al. Immunological functions of the pulmonary epithelium. Eur Respir J 1995; 8:127–149.

Umetsu DT, Akbari O, DekRuyff RH. Regulatory T cells control the development of allergic disease and asthma. J Allergy Clin Immunol 2003; 112:480–487.

VanEedewegh P, Little RD, Dupuis J, et al. Association of the ADAM33 gene with asthma and bronchial hyperresponsiveness. Nature 2002; 418:426–430.

Chapter 24

Definition:
The principles of drug treatment are to relieve symptoms and treat underlying inflammation.

Drugs for the Treatment of Allergic Disease

Martin K Church and Sohei Makino

INTRODUCTION

Allergy comprises a wide spectrum of conditions affecting many organs, each of which requires treatment with different drugs. The principles, however, are the same. In its early stages, allergy may present as isolated episodes of asthma, rhinitis, or urticaria. However, as the condition progresses, an underlying pathology of allergic inflammation develops leading to chronic disease in which the episodic exacerbations, or attacks, are more severe. The drugs used to treat allergy may, therefore, be classified into two groups: those aimed primarily at the relief of the symptoms of the acute exacerbations and those primarily for treatment of the underlying inflammation. These categories, however, are not completely watertight as some drugs aimed principally at providing relief from immediate symptoms may also influence the underlying inflammation.

EPINEPHRINE AND β-ADRENOCEPTOR STIMULANTS

The use of epinephrine (adrenaline) in the relief of asthma symptoms and as a life-saving drug in systemic anaphylaxis has been established for almost 100 years. In the latter use, the ability of epinephrine to stimulate both α- and β-receptors, as illustrated in Fig. 24.1, contributes to its beneficial effects. Of particular note are its bronchodilator properties, its capacity to inhibit mast-cell-mediator secretion, and its restoration of a satisfactory circulation by its action on the heart, blood vessels, and renin–angiotensin system. However, in the treatment of bronchial asthma, many of these effects are not desired, with the cardiovascular effects, particularly stimulation of cardiac arrhythmias, being of particular concern. Many of those problems have now been overcome by chemical modifications of the epinephrine molecule and by developing preparations with a satisfactory pharmacokinetic profile when administered to the lung by inhalation.

The first clue that chemical modification of epinephrine may modify its receptor selectivity came in 1941 when the terminal methyl group on the side-chain was replaced by an isopropyl group (Fig. 24.2). This increase in the bulk of the side-chain produced isoproterenol, a drug which acts almost exclusively at β-receptors. Further increases in the bulk of this substituent produced drugs which, although having decreased absolute potency, have an increased degree of selectivity for β_2-receptors over β_1-receptors. Examples of such drugs are shown in Figure 24.2. It should be emphasized, however, that such chemical maneuvers do not confer an absolute specificity for β_2-receptors but only selectivity. Thus, with high systemic concentrations, β_1-receptor-mediated effects on the heart may become apparent.

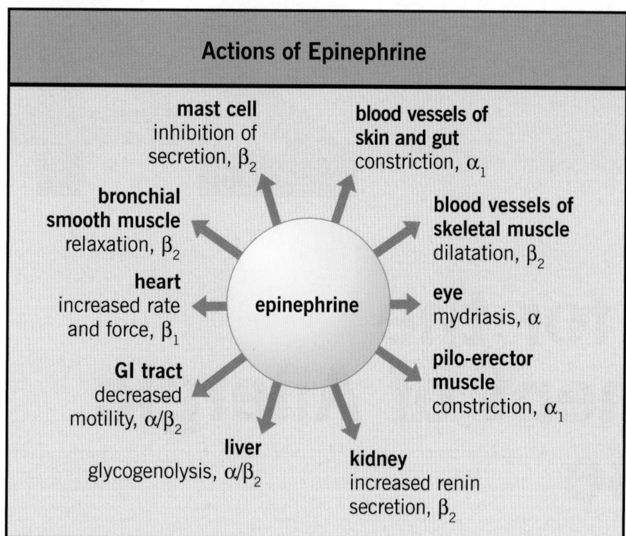

Fig. 24.1 Actions of epinephrine.

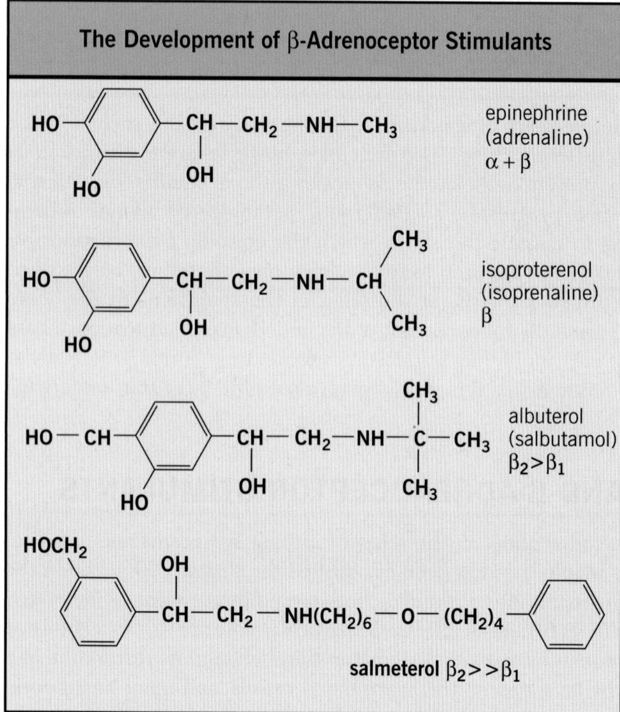

Fig. 24.2 Chemical development of β-adrenoceptor agonists.

The second objective of chemical manipulation was to increase the duration of action of sympathomimetic bronchodilators. Epinephrine is rapidly inactivated by two enzymatic processes:

- monoamine oxidase (MAO) in neuronal tissue;
- catechol-O-methyltransferase (COMT) in extraneuronal tissues.

Besides conferring β-receptor selectivity, increasing the bulk of the side-chain precludes neuronal uptake of the drug, thus preventing its access to MAO. To prevent metabolism by COMT, drugs have been synthesized in which the native catechol group has been substituted or removed (see Fig. 24.2). Metabolism of these drugs occurs in the liver. The duration of action of β_2-selective stimulants is shown in Table 24.1.

Table 24.1 Duration of action of β-stimulants

Duration of Action of β-Stimulants	
β-Stimulant	**Hours**
Albuterol	4–5
Terbutaline	4–5
Formoterol	10–12
Salmeterol	> 12

Mechanism of action

More is probably known about the biochemical mechanism of action of β-adrenoceptor stimulants than any other of the drugs used in the treatment of allergic diseases. The actions of β-adrenoceptor stimulants are summarized in Figure 24.3. Briefly, interaction of a β-stimulant with its receptor unit initiates the binding of guanosine triphosphate (GTP) to the α subunit of the regulatory G protein leading to its dissociation from the G protein complex. This subunit then complexes with adenylate cyclase (AC), the catalytic unit of the complex, activating it to generate cyclic adenosine monophosphate (AMP) from adenosine triphosphate (ATP). Cyclic AMP (cAMP) then acts as a second or intracellular messenger to activate a series of cAMP-dependent protein kinases (cAMP-dPK) which phosphorylate a number of proteins crucial to many intracellular biochemical events.

By these mechanisms, β-stimulants cause potent relaxation of bronchial smooth muscle, from which the term bronchodilator is derived. As this is a direct action, β-agonists are able to relax bronchial smooth muscle regardless of the contractile stimulus, thus giving rise to the term functional antagonists. Similarly, β-adrenoceptor stimulants prevent the activation of mast cells, but not basophils, to release their mediators. In this respect, β-stimulants are considerably more effective than the archetypal mast cell stabilizer, cromolin sodium. As the highest concentration of β-receptors in the lung is found on the luminal aspect of bronchial epithelial cells, it is postulated that β-agonists stimulate these cells to release their bronchorelaxant factors.

All of these events contribute to the effectiveness of β-stimulants as inhibitors of the early asthmatic response, indicative of their ability to provide symptomatic relief in asthma. As such, they are the first-line treatment used on an 'as required' basis for the reversal of acute asthmatic attacks. Recently much debate has raged about the suitability of β-stimulants to suppress the long-term bronchial inflammation associated with asthma. The consensus of opinion, at present, is that they are not suitable. Indeed, two recent studies, in which β-stimulants were given on a regular basis, have shown a small deterioration rather than an improvement in objective parameters of airway function over a prolonged period. For this reason, it is advisable to treat the inflammatory aspects of the

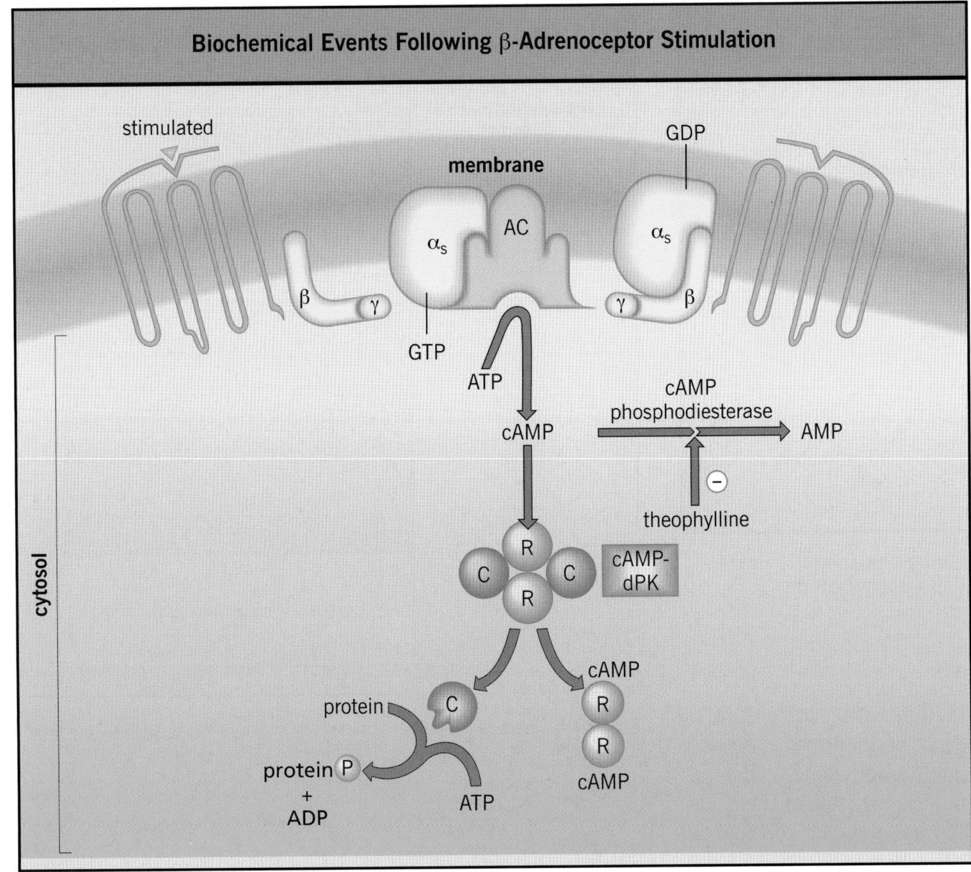

Fig. 24.3 Activation of adenylate cyclase and protein kinases. The diagram shows two β -adrenoceptor molecules, each of which is composed of three transmembrane loops. Stimulation of the receptor (left) causes its activation, in which the α_s unit of the heterotrimeric G_s protein binds GTP and dissociates from the complex to the adenylate cyclase catalytic unit (AC). Activated AC catalyzes the formation of cyclic adenosine monophosphate (cAMP), which binds to the regulatory units (R) of cAMP-dependent protein kinases (cAMP-dPK), thus freeing the catalytic units (C) to phosphorylate specific proteins. The activated state exists only transiently, ATP hydrolysis to ADP leading to reassociation of the $\alpha_s\beta\gamma$ complex of G_s, inactivation of AC, receptor regeneration, and the breakdown of AMP by phosphodiesterases.

disease with an antiinflammatory agent, such as an inhaled corticosteroid, while providing β-stimulants for their bronchodilator actions on an 'as required' basis during periods of enhanced bronchoconstriction.

Long-acting β_2-agonists, such as salmeterol and formoterol, have duration of bronchodilatation lasting 10–12 hours, and can be beneficial to patients when added to inhaled corticosteroids, particularly in the control of night-time symptoms.

Uses and administration

Epinephrine is the drug of choice for acute anaphylactic shock. Patients at risk should carry with them – at all times – a preloaded syringe, such as an 'Epipen'. Epinephrine should be administered subcutaneously or intramuscularly (not intravenously) as soon as the early symptoms of anaphylactic shock manifest themselves. The patient should then seek immediate specialized medical attention (see Ch. 11).

In asthma, the choice of the most appropriate route of administration of β-stimulants is of paramount importance. In all but the most severe asthmatics, inhalation of an aerosol provides an effective topical treatment by delivering the drug directly to the luminal surface of the bronchus where it can act on superficial mast cells and gain ready access to the bronchial smooth muscle. Onset of action is rapid, within 5–15 minutes, a vital factor when trying to reverse a developing or established bronchoconstriction. With the older bronchodilators, the duration of action of 4–5 hours is not long enough to allow the nocturnal asthmatic a full night's sleep. However, the prolonged duration of the second-generation drugs, which are given once or twice daily, has overcome this problem (see Table 24.1). The major drawbacks to inhalation therapy are problems of poor administration techniques by the patients, particularly young children and geriatric patients, and poor drug penetration into the airways of patients with severe obstruction. Systemic side-effects of β-adrenoceptor therapy are usually minimal with inhaled drugs, but may become a problem with over usage, a point which must be stressed to the patient. These side-effects include:

- skeletal muscle tremor to which tolerance develops;
- hyperglycemia in diabetes;
- cardiovascular effects, cardiac arrhythmias acutely, and a possibility of myocardial ischemia in the long term; and
- hypokalemia.

β-Adrenoceptor stimulants may also be given orally, although the use of this route is declining with the introduction of long-acting inhaled agents. Oral administration may be advantageous when patients cannot use an inhaler effectively or when prolonged duration of action is required. The obvious disadvantages are the unwanted systemic effects. Parenteral administration is usually reserved for acute severe asthma (status asthmaticus) where it may have life-saving potential when used in conjunction with other appropriate supportive therapy.

METHYLXANTHINES

Methylxanthines, in the form of coffee and extracts from the tea plant, have been used for the treatment of bronchial asthma for almost 700 years. Today the predominant methylxanthine

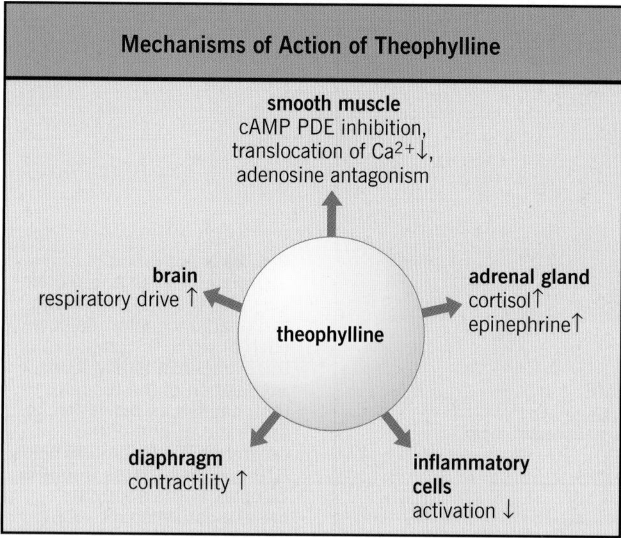

Fig. 24.4 Proposed mechanisms of action of theophylline. cAMP, cyclic adenosine monophosphate; PDE, phosphodiesterase.

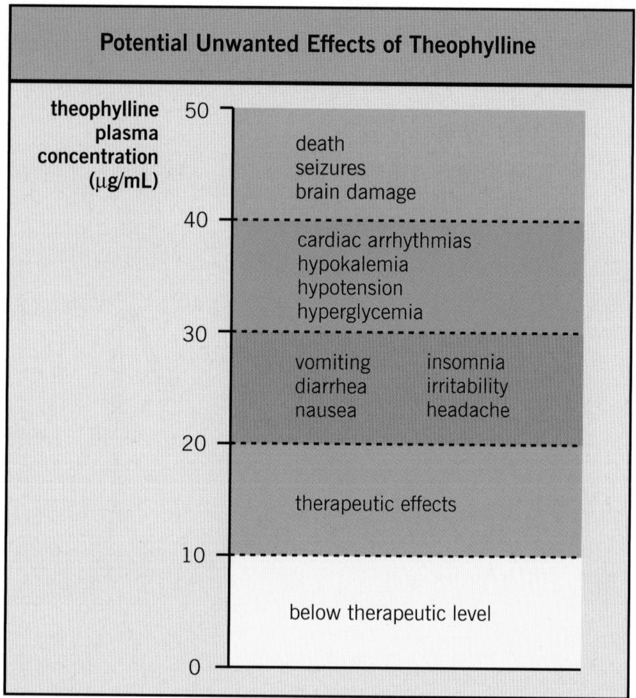

Fig. 24.5 Dose-related therapeutic and toxic effects of theophylline.

in clinical use is theophylline, given either as the native drug, as its water-soluble ethylene diamine salt, aminophylline, or as a long-acting conjugate, such as choline theophyllinate. The use of these drugs is somewhat enigmatic: they are one of the drugs of choice in North America and some parts of continental Europe but are rarely used in the UK and Australasia.

Theophylline

Mechanism of action

The precise mechanism by which theophylline acts as an antiasthma drug is still somewhat obscure. Clearly it has the potential to inhibit cAMP phosphodiesterase (PDE), thus causing the elevation of intracellular levels of cAMP by preventing its breakdown (see Fig. 24.3). The theory for this mechanism of action in asthma has been based on biochemical and in vitro studies that use theophylline at concentrations which would be toxic in vivo. Consequently, a variety of alternative mechanisms have been proposed, which are summarized in Figure 24.4. However, the PDE inhibition theory has recently gained more credence from two lines of evidence. First is the observation that, at therapeutic doses, there is evidence in leukocytes in vivo of increased levels of cAMP, suggesting that even a small and subtle action on PDE at these concentrations may be sufficient to confer clinical activity. Second is the identification of seven families of PDE isozymes, many of which contain multiple subtypes that are encoded by distinct genes, and the synthesis of specific inhibitors for them. Of particular note is that bronchial smooth muscle and inflammatory cells, including mast cells, have type 4 PDE (PDE4). Initial studies with inhibitors of this isoenzyme indicate that they carry the beneficial actions of theophylline while being devoid of many of the side-effects. Drugs of this class are undergoing intense clinical trial at present and are described later.

The major disadvantage with theophylline is its narrow therapeutic window (Fig. 24.5). The beneficial effects of the drug in long-term management are observed only with plasma levels in the range of 5–15 mg/mL. Below 10 mg/mL, the drug is comparatively ineffective and, above 20 mg/mL, toxic effects are observed which increase in number and in severity with increasing plasma concentrations. Because of this relationship, the prudent physician will regularly monitor serum theophylline levels and adjust the dose so that possible life-threatening toxicity is avoided.

Uses and administration

Theophylline is only weakly active and of transient duration when given by inhalation and is, therefore, given routinely by oral administration. Rectal preparations of aminophylline are available and may be well suited for young children. Theophylline and aminophylline are rapidly and completely absorbed from the intestinal tract. Theophylline is metabolized in the liver with a half-life of approximately 6 hours in normal individuals. Because of this relatively short duration of action, many slow-release preparations have been formulated to extend its duration to 8–12 hours. However, care must be taken with such preparations, as large fluctuations in plasma concentrations may occur, bringing with them either lack of efficacy or potential toxicity. These problems may arise in two ways. First, the presence of food in the gastrointestinal tract may lead to erratic absorption with changes in gastric emptying, so causing 'dumping' of enteric-coated preparations into the intestine. Second, other disease processes or the use of other drugs may markedly alter the rate of metabolism of theophylline, the half-life being around 20 hours in hepatitis and 4 hours in heavy cigarette smokers. As a consequence, a conservative approach to therapy should be adopted, and the dose titrated to suit individual patients. In acute severe asthma, intravenous theophylline may be used by infusion, rather than by bolus

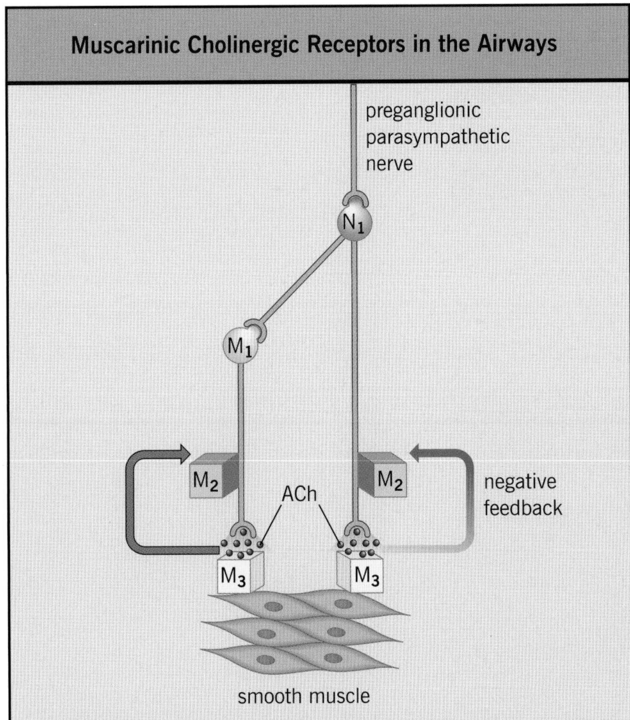

Fig. 24.6 Muscarinic cholinergic receptors in the airways. Postganglionic fibers are excited by the action of ACh at N_1-receptors. These fibers go directly to smooth muscle where the ACh released interacts with M_3-receptors to cause contraction. ACh also feeds back to stimulate M_2- receptors on the nerves and to reduce ACh release. The site of M_1-receptors is speculative but they are thought to be present as secondary stimulant nerves which augment parasympathetic stimulation in the airways. ACh, acetylcholine.

injection, with a view to obtaining plasma levels within but not above the therapeutic range.

ANTICHOLINERGIC AGENTS

Antimuscarinic agents, particularly from the smoking of leaves of stramonium, belladonna, and hyoscyamus, have been used for the treatment of asthma for centuries. Today, chemically modified derivatives of atropine are used as bronchodilator drugs.

Mechanism of action

Stimulation by acetylcholine of muscarinic M_3-receptors on bronchial smooth muscle initiates its contraction by a cyclic guanosine monophosphate (cGMP)-mediated pathway. Atropine and related drugs are competitive and reversible antagonists of this effect of acetylcholine, thereby producing a dose-related inhibition of smooth muscle contraction (Fig. 24.6).

Uses and administration

Atropine is well absorbed, even following inhalation, and produces systemic inhibition of parasympathetic nervous system activity. This severely limits its use as a bronchodilator. However, ipratropium bromide and oxitropium bromide, both potent topical anticholinergics and bronchodilators with poor systemic absorption and hence few systemic side-effects, are widely available. In adults, topical anticholinergics are used primarily for the treatment of chronic obstructive pulmonary disease. These agents have found little place in the treatment of asthma in adults in competition with β_2-adrenoceptor stimulant bronchodilators although they do have a role as adjuncts to β_2-stimulant therapy, particularly in acute severe asthma. However, in infants in whom the bronchial tree is not fully developed, topical anticholinergics are used with good effect in cases of wheeze where β_2-stimulant bronchodilators are ineffective.

H_1 ANTIHISTAMINES

Histamine, released from mast cells and basophils, plays a major role in the pathophysiology of all allergic diseases, including rhinitis, urticaria, asthma, and systemic anaphylaxis. Therefore, prevention of its ability to stimulate its target organs has presented an obvious goal in drug development. Over the last two decades it has become apparent that the actions of histamine are initiated following its interaction with one of four distinct receptors (Table 24.2). In allergic disease, it is the H_1 antihistamines which are of primary benefit, although H_2 antihistamines may have some therapeutic benefit.

H_1 antihistamines are usually classified into the older, or first-generation antihistamines, and the newer, or second-generation, antihistamines. The commonly used members of these drug classes are listed in Table 24.3 and the chemical structures of some of them shown in Figure 24.7. The main differences between the two generations of drugs are their propensity to cause central nervous system (CNS) sedation and their side-effects. The highly lipophilic nature of the first-generation antihistamines allows them to penetrate well into the CNS where they induce sedation. Although this sedative effect may have some clinical benefit in the treatment of night-time exacerbations of allergy responses, especially in children, it severely compromises such drug use in ambulatory patients in whom doses capable of causing only a 3–5-fold shift of the histamine dose-response curve may be given. The potential to enhance the central effects of alcohol and other CNS sedatives further limits such use. In addition, many of these drugs also have actions which reflect their poor receptor selectivity, including an atropine-like effect and blockade of both α-adrenergic and 5-hydroxytryptamine receptors.

The second-generation H_1 antihistamines cause much-reduced CNS sedation and are essentially free of this effect at doses recommended for the treatment of rhinitis or urticaria. Consequently, the shift of the histamine dose-response curve that can be achieved with these drugs is much greater. Also, these drugs have little or no atropine-like activity or effects at other receptors. Some second-generation drugs have been suggested to have antiallergic and antiinflammatory effects which may contribute to their therapeutic benefit. An example of this is a recent trial, the so-called ETAC study, in which children of 1–2 years of age with atopic dermatitis were treated with cetirizine for 18 months. The results showed a significant reduction in the development of asthma during this period in those who were sensitive to pollen or house dust mite. There was also a concomitant reduction in other allergic symptoms, including urticaria and allergic reactions to foods.

Table 24.2 Receptor-mediated effects of histamine

Target tissue	Effect	Receptor
Airways		
Bronchial smooth muscle Bronchial epithelium Secretory glands	Contraction Increased permeability Increased glycoprotein secretion Secretion Stimulation Cough receptors	H_1 H_1 H_1, H_2 H_1
Blood vessels		
Postcapillary venules	Dilatation Increased permeability	H_1
Nerves		
Sensory nerves Central nervous system	Stimulation Neuroregulation	H_1 H_3
Nose	Rhinorrhea Edema	H_1 H_1
Leukocytes	Increased proliferation; chemotaxis and activation	H_2, H_4

Table 24.3 Common H_1-receptor antagonists

First generation	Second generation
Hydroxyzine	Acrivastine
Diphenhydramine	Cetirizine
Chlorphenamine	Desloratadine
	Fexofenadine
	Levocetirizine
	Loratadine
	Mequitazine

Mechanism of action

H_1 antihistamines are not receptor antagonists as previously thought, but are inverse agonists. When neither histamine nor antihistamine is present, the active and inactive states of the H_1 receptor are in equilibrium or a balanced state. Histamine combines preferentially with the active form of the receptor to stabilize it and shift the balance towards the activated state and stimulate the cell (Fig. 24.8). In contrast, H_1 antihistamines stabilize the inactive form and shift the equilibrium in the opposite direction. Thus, the amount of histamine-induced stimulation of a cell or tissue depends on the balance between histamine and H_1 antihistamine.

Histamine effects stimulated through the H_1 receptor include: pruritus, pain, vasodilatation, vascular permeability, hypotension, flushing, headache, tachycardia, bronchoconstriction, and stimulation of airway vagal afferent nerves and cough receptors; and decreased atrioventricular-node conduction. Although most of the effects of histamine in allergic diseases are mediated by H_1 receptor stimulation, hypotension, tachycardia, flushing, and headache, cutaneous itching and nasal congestion have been suggested to have a minor component mediated through both H_1 and H_2 receptors.

Through H_1 receptors histamine has proinflammatory activity and is involved in the development of several aspects of antigen-specific immune response, including the maturation of dendritic cells and modulation of the balance of helper T cell type 1 (Th1) and Th2 towards Th1. Histamine also induces the release of proinflammatory cytokines. Because histamine has such effects on allergic inflammation and the immune system, treatment with H_1 antihistamines reduces the expression of proinflammatory cell adhesion molecules and the accumulation of inflammatory cells, such as eosinophils and neutrophils. Major clinical effects of H_1 antihistamines are seen in suppression of the early response to allergen challenge in conjunctiva, nose, lower airway and skin.

In the CNS, the effects histamine exerts through H_1 receptors include cycle of sleep and waking, food intake, thermal regulation, emotion and aggressive behavior, locomotion memory and learning. First-generation H_1-antihistamines, such as chlorphenamine, diphenhydramine, hydroxyzine and promethazine, penetrate readily into the brain, in which they occupy 50–90% of the H_1 receptors, as shown by positron-emission tomography (PET). The result is CNS sedation. On the other hand, second-generation H_1 antihistamines penetrate the CNS poorly, as they are actively pumped out by P-glycoprotein, an organic anion transporting protein that is expressed on the luminal surfaces of vascular endothelial cells

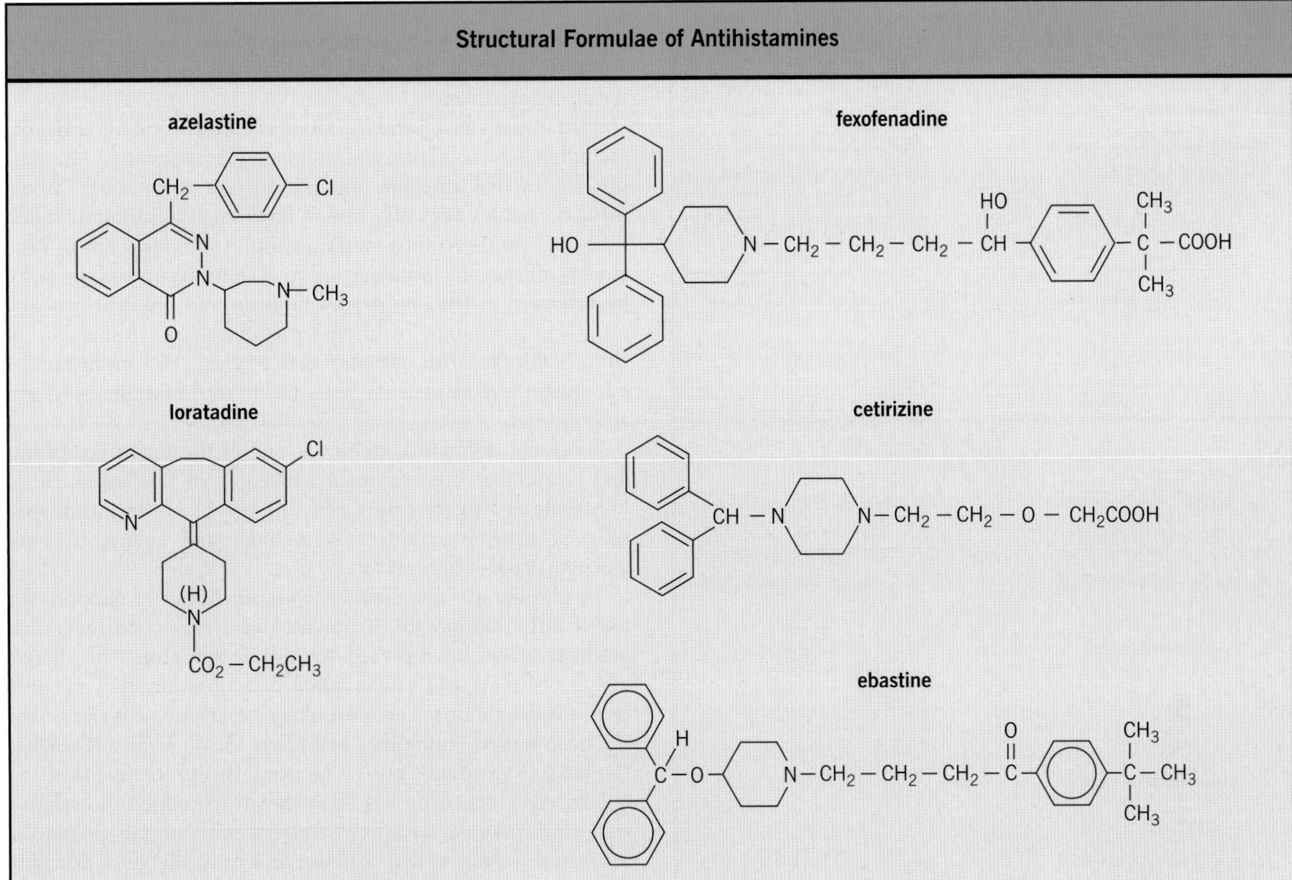

Fig. 24.7 Structural formulae of some antihistamines.

in the blood vessels that constitute the blood–brain barrier. Their propensity to occupy H_1 receptors in the CNS varies from 0% for fexofenadine to 30% for cetirizine. Thus, second-generation H_1 antihistamines are relatively free of sedating effects and impairment of driving performance. Currently, desloratadine, fexofenadine, and loratadine are the H_1 antihistamines for which pilots can receive a waiver for use from the Federal Aviation Administration.

Cardiac toxic effects induced by H_1 antihistamines occur rarely and independently of the H_1 receptor. Two early second-generation H_1 antihistamines, astemizole and terfenadine, which are no longer marketed, potentially prolong the QT interval and have been shown to cause torsades de pointes. No such effects occur with new second-generation H_1 antihistamines.

Uses and administration

All H_1-receptor antagonists are well absorbed from the gastrointestinal tract after oral dosage. With most oral H_1 antihistamines, symptomatic relief is observed within 1–3 hours. Their duration of action varies from several hours to 24 hours, that of the second-generation drugs being generally around 24 hours. No tolerance to the suppressive effects on skin test reactivity to histamine is observed for at least 3 months. Residual suppression of skin test reactivity to allergens may last for up to 7 days after the discontinuation of an H_1 antihistamine.

Although topical intranasal and ophthalmic H_1 antihistamines differ in their pharmacokinetics, most of the topical preparations need to be administered twice daily because of the washout from the nasal mucosa or conjunctiva.

All of the first-generation H_1 antagonists and some of the second-generation antihistamines are oxidatively metabolized by the hepatic cytochrome P450 system, the main exceptions being levocetirizine, cetirizine, and fexofenadine. Levocetirizine and cetirizine are excreted largely unchanged in urine and fexofenadine is excreted largely in the feces. Hepatic metabolism has several implications: prolongation of the serum half-life in patients with hepatic dysfunction and those receiving concomitant cytochrome P450 inhibitors, such as ketoconazole and erythromycin. Also, longer duration of action is found in elderly patients who have reduced liver function. In these patients there is a possibility of precipitating serious unwanted cardiac or CNS effects. Such adverse effects are more likely to occur when first-generation antihistamines rather than second-generation antihistamines are used.

In patients with allergic rhinitis both first- and second-generation H_1 antihistamines have been proven to be useful in ameliorating sneezes, itching, and nasal discharge but are less effective in relieving nasal blockage. H_1 antihistamines provide relief of allergic rhinitis comparable to that provided by intranasal cromolin sodium 4%, but are generally found to be less potent than intranasal corticosteroids in the management of severe allergic rhinitis symptoms, particularly in ameliorating nasal blockage. Leukotriene receptor antagonists have been

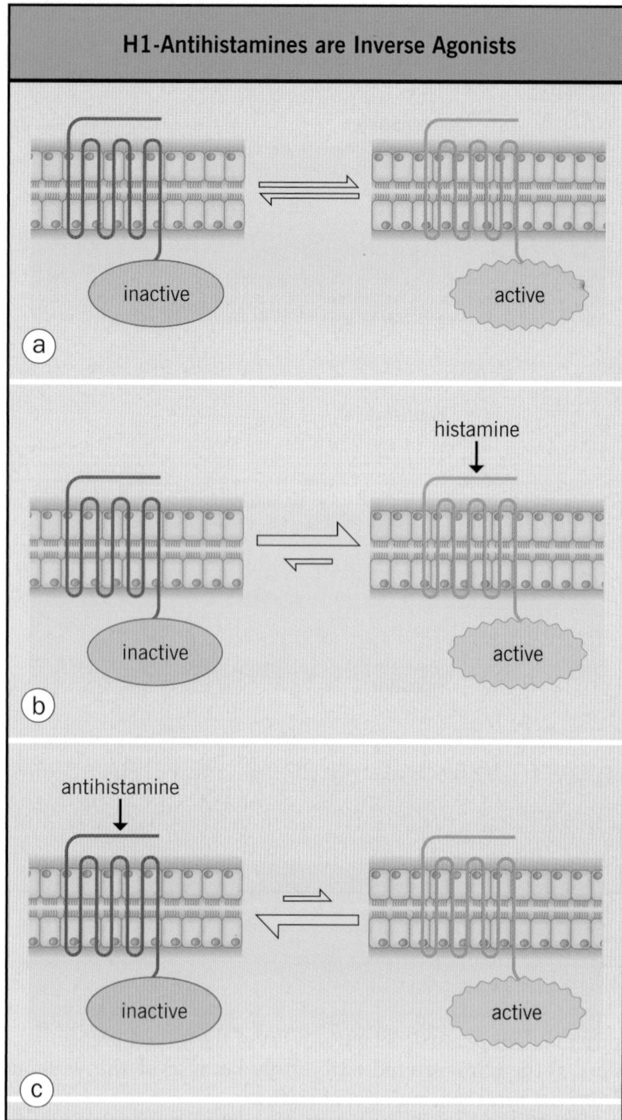

Fig. 24.8 This diagram shows the two compartment model of the histamine receptor. The transmembrane histamine H_1 receptors are shown in their inactive (left) and active (right) forms. Panel (a) shows that the inactive and active conformations of the H_1 receptor are in equilibrium in the absence of either histamine or an H_1 antihistamine. In reality, the equilibrium would be very much in favor of the much more stable inactive form. Panel (b) shows the effect of histamine, which has a preferential affinity for the active conformation of the receptor. Histamine combines with the active form of the receptor to stabilize it and thus cause the equilibrium to shift in favor of the activated form. Panel (c) shows the effect of an antihistamine, which has a preferential affinity for the inactive conformation of the receptor. Consequentially, the antihistamine combines with the inactive form of the receptor to stabilize it and thus cause the equilibrium to shift in the opposite direction. (Adapted from Leurs R, Church MK, Taglialatela M. H_1 antihistamines: inverse agonism, anti-inflammatory actions and cardiac effects. Clin Exp Allergy 2002; 32:489–498.)

proven to be effective to allergic rhinitis. Combination of a leukotriene receptor antagonist with an antihistamine has been shown to reduce nasal symptoms more than monotherapy with each of the agents.

In allergic conjunctivitis, the ocular symptoms induced by allergen, such as itching, tearing, and reddening are reduced by administration of H_1 antihistamines either systemically or locally as eye drops.

Histamine can reproduce all of the symptoms of urticaria, including wheal, flare, and itching. Consequently, H_1 antihistamines are first-line medications in acute and chronic urticaria and are very effective in providing symptomatic relief. Both first- and second-generation antihistamines seem to have similar efficacy in chronic urticaria. H_1 antihistamines appear to be effective in treating dermographism and physical urticaria including cholinergic, cold, and pressure-induced urticaria. In some patients with chronic urticaria an H_2 antihistamine administered concurrently with an H_1 antihistamine may give added relief.

In atopic dermatitis, itching is one of the major symptoms and scratching often causes a worsening of the lesion. Since histamine is a major pruritogen, the use of H_1 antihistamines relieves pruritus, reduces scratching, and seems to have glucocorticoid-sparing effects.

In chronic asthma, current evidence does not support the use of antihistamines for treatment. However, second-generation antihistamines are reported to reduce symptoms of allergic asthma patients and exacerbation of asthma in adult patients with allergic rhinitis. The most likely explanation for this is that the nose warms, humidifies and filters the air before it reaches the lung. If a patient's nose is blocked, this protective function is lost. Also, cetirizine has been shown to reduce the relative risk of developing asthma in infants with atopic dermatitis sensitized to grass pollen or house dust mite allergens, probably due to its antiinflammatory effects.

Although most of the symptoms of anaphylaxis can be reproduced by histamine, the treatment of choice for this condition is injection of epinephrine. H_1-receptor antagonists can be useful for adjunctive relief of pruritus, urticaria, rhinorrhea, and other symptoms.

Adverse effects

The most obvious adverse effects of first-generation H_1 antihistamines are those on the CNS, including drowsiness, impaired driving performance, fatigue, lassitude, and dizziness. In addition, dry mouth, urinary retention, gastrointestinal upset, and appetite stimulation may occur. Clinical tolerance to the sedating effects of first-generation antihistamines has been suggested but has not been found consistently in objective tests. If taken by mothers, first-generation drugs may cause irritability, drowsiness, or respiration suppression in nursing infants. The incidence of CNS sedation from second-generation H_1 antihistamines, when used at the manufacturers' recommended doses, is greatly reduced or absent.

Some of the first-generation H_1 antihistamines may cause sinus tachycardia, reflex tachycardia and supraventricular arrhythmia, and prolongation of the QT interval in a dose-dependent manner. The potential unwanted serious cardiac effects of astemizole and terfenadine, which are not marketed now, have been described previously.

Some of the oral H_1 antihistamines including cetirizine, loratadine, and emedastine, are considered relatively safe for use during pregnancy (FDA category B: no adverse effect in animals, but no data in humans, or adverse effects in animals but no adverse effects in humans).

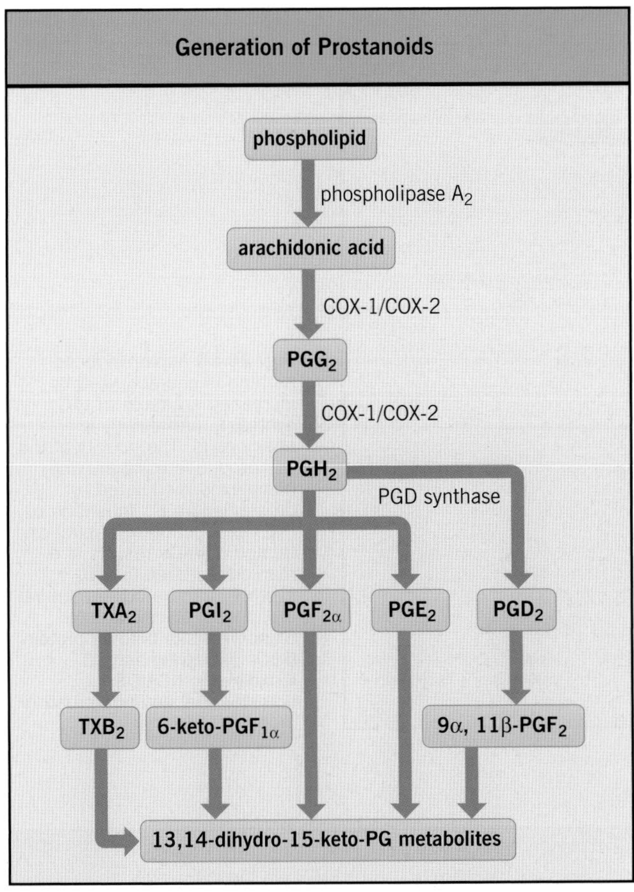

Fig. 24.9 Generation of prostanoids. COX, cyclooxygenase; PG, prostaglandin; TX, thromboxane.

PROSTANOID SYNTHESIS INHIBITORS AND RECEPTOR ANTAGONISTS

Prostanoids are ubiquitous intracellular and intercellular messengers. They are synthesized de novo when required, by the action of cyclooxygenases (COX) on the 20-carboxy fatty acid, arachidonic acid (Fig. 24.9). Recent studies have shown that there are two distinct cyclooxygenases:

- COX-1, which is constitutive and present in the majority of tissues; and
- COX-2, whose presence in inflammatory cells is induced over a period of hours following an inflammatory stimulus.

While COX-1 and COX-2 activity both eventually result in prostaglandin H_2 (PGH_2), further processing into individual prostaglandins depends on the presence of the requisite enzymes within particular cells. Five principal bioactive prostaglandins are generated in vivo including thromboxane A_2 (TXA_2), PGD_2, PGE_2, PGI_2, and $PGF_{2\alpha}$ (Fig.24.9) Of particular relevance to allergy are the production of PGD_2 and TXA_2 by mast cells and other inflammatory cells, both of which contribute to bronchoconstriction in asthma following their interaction with the TXA_2 receptor (TP) and/or PGD_2 receptor (DP) (Table 24.4). Thus, either inhibition of the formation of these prostanoids or prevention of their effects provides a therapeutic target in asthma and rhinitis.

Mechanism of action

Non-steroidal antiinflammatory drugs

Cyclooxygenase inhibition is the primary mechanism of action of all non-steroidal antiinflammatory drugs (NSAIDs), such as aspirin, indomethacin, ibuprofen, or flurbiprofen. Consequently, they have the ability to cause a dose-related inhibition of the

Table 24.4 Prostanoids and their receptors

Prostanoids	Receptors	Effects	Antagonist
TXA_2	TP	Smooth muscle constriction	Seratrodast Ramatroban
PGD_2	DP	Smooth muscle relaxation, vasodilation	
	CRTh2	Eosinophil chemotaxis and activation	Ramatroban
PGE_2	EP1 EP2 EP3 EP4	Bronchoconstriction Relaxation, antiinflammatory? Bronchoconstriction Antiinflammatory and/or proinflammatory	
PGI_2	IP	A regulator of airway inflammation	
$PGF_{2\alpha}$	FP	Bronchoconstriction	

CRTh2, chemoattractant receptor-homologous molecule expressed on Th2 cells ; DP, PGD_2 receptor; TP, TXA_2 receptor; PGD_2, E_2, I_2, $F_{2\alpha}$, prostaglandin D_2, E_2, I_2, $F_{2\alpha}$; TXA_2, thromboxane A_2. (Data based on Hata AN, Breyer RM. Pharmacology and signaling of prostaglandin receptors: Multiple roles in inflammation and immune modulation. Pharmacol Ther 2004; 103(2):147–166.)

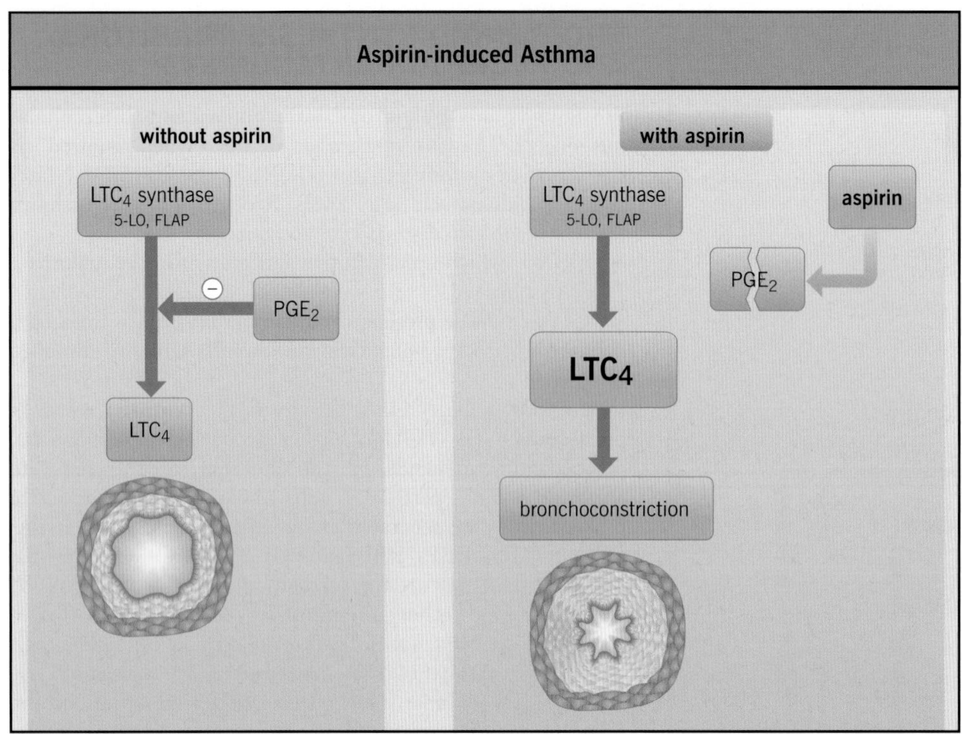

Fig. 24.10 Aspirin-induced asthma is characterized by increased amounts of LTC_4 synthase, particularly in eosinophils. The activity of the leukotriene-forming enzyme complex is modulated by prostaglandin E_2. Inhibition of PGE_2 production by aspirin and related NSAIDs results in a marked increase in LTC_4 synthesis and a consequential bronchoconstriction. FLAP, 5-lipoxygenase binding protein; 5-LO, 5-lipoxygenase; LT, leukotriene; NSAIDS, non-steroidal antiinflammatory drugs; PG, prostaglandin.

formation of all prostaglandins, whether potentially harmful or beneficial. In asthma, non-specific inhibition of the production of prostanoids, including the bronchoconstrictors PGD_2 and TXA_2, has some beneficial effects in acute allergen provocation but appears to have little benefit in clinical asthma. PGE_2 has been suggested to shift the balance of T cells in favor of a Th2 response in part by PGE_4-mediated mechanisms. On the other hand, NSAIDs may precipitate aspirin-induced asthma (AIA) in 4–28% of adult patients, a property which precludes their indiscriminate use in asthma. AIA is characterized by increased production of cysteinyl leukotrienes, although the exact mechanism by which aspirin acts on cylooxygenases to trigger bronchoconstriction remains unknown (Fig. 24.10).

Thromboxane A_2 modifiers (Figs 24.11 and 24.12)

TXA_2-induced bronchoconstriction has been largely overcome by the development of TXA_2 synthase inhibitors, such as ozagrel, which suppresses antigen-induced early and late airway responses in both sensitized guinea pigs and humans and decreases the airway responsiveness to inhaled acetylcholine in asthmatic patients. Ozagrel has been marketed in Japan for the treatment of asthma.

The development of prostanoid antagonists has concentrated on agents that prevent the interaction of TXA_2 and PGD_2 with the thromboxane TP receptor and/or the PGD_2 DP receptor. In guinea pigs, TxA_2 receptor antagonists suppress antigen-induced early and late asthmatic responses and suppress eosinophil infiltration 6 hours after antigen. Seratrodast also inhibits the bronchoconstriction induced by the TXA_2 analog U46619 but not histamine. So far only seratrodast has been marketed for the treatment of asthma.

Ramatroban is another potent TP receptor antagonist with significant efficacy against allergic rhinitis in many animal models and patients with allergic rhinitis. Ramatroban can also block the newly identified PGD_2 receptor, a chemoattractant receptor-homologous molecule expressed on Th2 cells (CRTh2). PGD_2 induces migration and degranulation of eosinophils through CRTh2 and contributes to late-phase inflammation and cell damage.

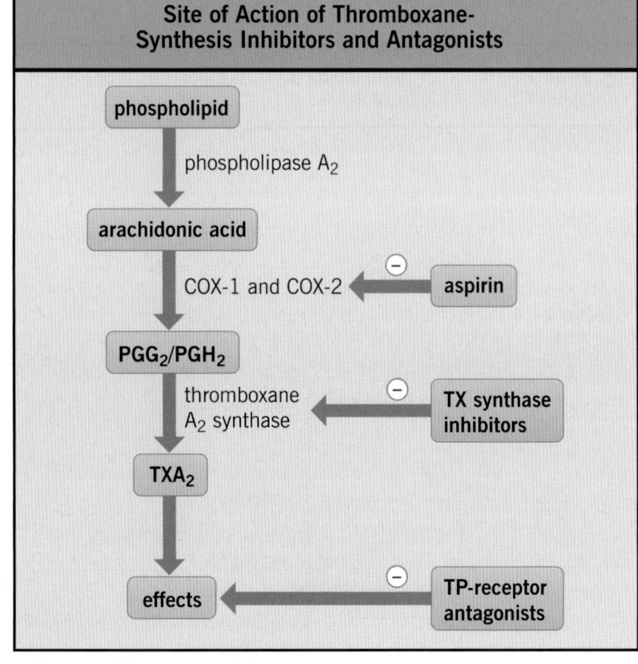

Fig. 24.11 Site of action of thromboxane synthesis inhibitors and antagonists. COX, cyclooxygenase; PG, prostaglandin; TP, TXA_2 receptor; TX, thromboxane.

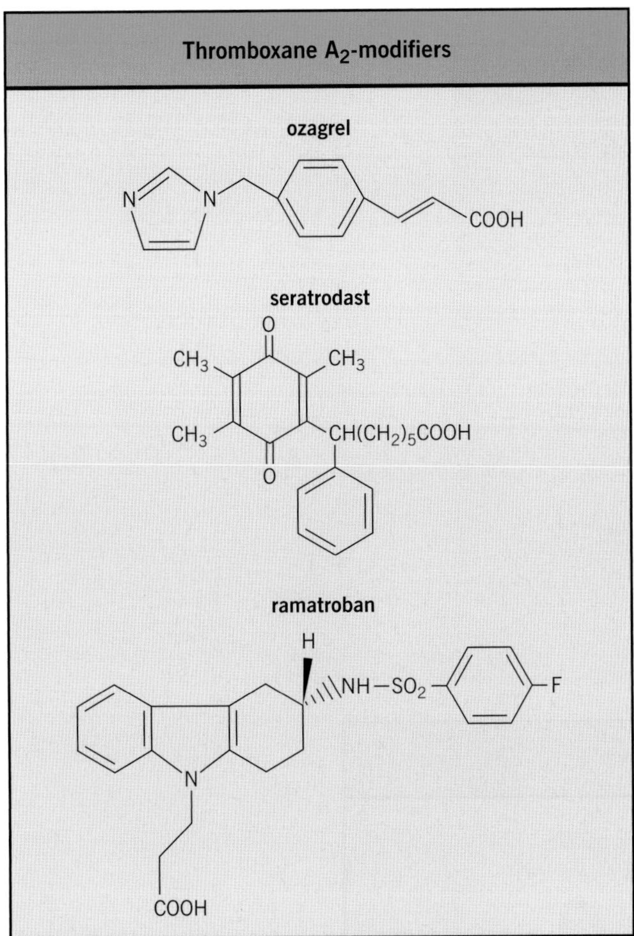

Fig. 24.12 Chemical structures of ozagrel, seratrodast and ramatroban.

Uses and administration

As stated above, the use of cylooxygenase inhibitors in asthma is not usually recommended and is contraindicated to adult patients with AIA. However, they may be of some use in conjunction with antihistamines in the control of the cutaneous symptoms of systemic mastocytosis where they inhibit the synthesis of mast cell-derived PGD_2.

Ozagrel (200 mg twice daily) is indicated for the treatment of asthma. Inhibitors of TXA_2 synthase are relatively new in clinical practice. In a multicenter double-blind clinical trial of ozagrel in adults with mild-to-moderate asthma, the global improvement rating was assessed to be moderately or markedly effective in 48% of subjects taking ozagrel compared with 16% of subjects taking placebo. No significant adverse effects were reported in this trial. The decrease of symptom score and medications was greater in the ozagrel group.

Seratrodast (80 mg once daily) is indicated for the treatment of asthma. A multicenter double-blind clinical trial has also been performed with the TXA_2 receptor antagonist, seratrodast, in adults with mild-to-moderate asthma. The global improvement rating of 48% of the patients taking 80 mg seratrodast daily was assessed to be moderately or markedly effective compared with 41% of patients taking 40 mg daily and 19% of patients taking a placebo. Rare, but severe, liver dysfunction restricts conventional use of this agent in the treatment of asthma.

Ramatroban (75 mg twice a day) is indicated in the treatment of allergic rhinitis in adults in Japan. Efficacy of ramatroban was compared with terfenadine in a randomized double-blind trial in patients with perennial allergic rhinitis. A moderate to marked improvement in symptoms was reported in 67.4% of patients on ramatroban and 43% of patients on terfenadine ($p = 0.002$). Ramatroban was well tolerated without significant adverse effects.

These findings indicate that the TXA_2 synthase inhibitor, ozagrel, and the TXA_2-receptor antagonist, seratrodast, can be considered for the treatment of mild-to-moderate asthma. Another TXA_2 receptor antagonist, ramatroban, is indicated in the treatment of allergic rhinitis. The results of further trials with these drugs are awaited.

LEUKOTRIENE SYNTHESIS INHIBITORS AND RECEPTOR ANTAGONISTS

Leukotrienes (LTs) are important inflammatory lipid mediators derived from arachidonic acid following its oxidation by 5-lipoxygenase (5-LO) on the nuclear envelope. There are two types of LTs, the dihydroxy acid LTB_4 and the cysteinyl LTs (CysLT: LTC_4, LTD_4, LTE_4). 5-LO mediates the conversion of arachidonic acid into the unstable epoxide LTA_4, which is converted by LTA_4 hydrolase into LTB_4 or by LTC_4 synthase into LTC_4, depending on cell type: eosinophils predominantly produce CysLTs, whereas neutrophils mainly produce LTB_4. Once LTC_4 is released from inflammatory cells, it is converted into LTD_4 by γ-glutamyl transpeptidase and subsequently into stable LTE_4 by a dipeptidase. LTB_4 has a specific LTB receptor and acts mainly as a neutrophil chemoattractant.

CysLTs show activities through two different receptors, $CysLT_1$ and $CysLT_2$ receptors (Table 24.5). The $CysLT_1$ receptor seems to be very important for the induction of asthmatic reaction as it induces constriction of airway smooth muscle, increases microvasculature leakage and secretion of bronchial mucosa, and induces the inflammation of the airways, including eosinophil infiltration, and finally hypertrophy of bronchial smooth muscle. Hypertrophy of smooth muscle is a component of airway remodeling seen in asthma (Fig. 24.13). In addition, the $CysLT_1$ receptor has important roles in allergic reactions, such as allergic rhinitis, atopic dermatitis, and chronic urticaria.

CysLTs are produced in response to allergic or other stimuli. Allergen-induced provocation of asthma is associated with the increased leukotriene levels in bronchoalveolar lavage fluids. Furthermore, increased urinary levels of the stable leukotriene metabolite, LTE_4, are found in both allergen- and aspirin-induced asthma.

Importantly, CysLTs have been found in bronchoalveolar lavage fluids despite treatment with low to high doses of corticosteroids although corticosteroids are the most potent antiinflammatory agents used in the treatment of asthma, supporting the theory that corticosteroids do not directly reduce the production of CysLTs. Consequently, drugs which interfere with either the synthesis of leukotrienes or their receptor actions are likely to be beneficial in asthma. Both of these have been successful, leading to the development of new drugs for the treatment of asthma.

The LT receptor antagonists (LTRAs), montelukast, zafirlukast, and pranlukast were approved in 1998, 1996 in the

Table 24.5 Summary of the properties of human CysLT receptors

	Receptor	
	Human CysLT$_1$	**Human CysLT$_2$**
Amino acid	337	346
Chromosome	Xq13-q21	13q14.2
Binding affinity	LTD_4 >> LTC_4 > LTE_4	LTD_4 = LTC_4 > LTE_4
Antagonist	Montelukast Zafirlukast Pranlukast	
Expression	Lung smooth muscle PBL including eosinophils Spleen	Heart, adrenal medulla Pulmonary vein, PBL

LTC_4, D_4, E_4, leukotriene C_4, D_4, E_4; PBL, peripheral blood lymphocyte.
(From Evans JF. Cysteinyl leukotriene receptors. Prostaglandins Other Lipid Mediators 2002; 68–69:587–597.)

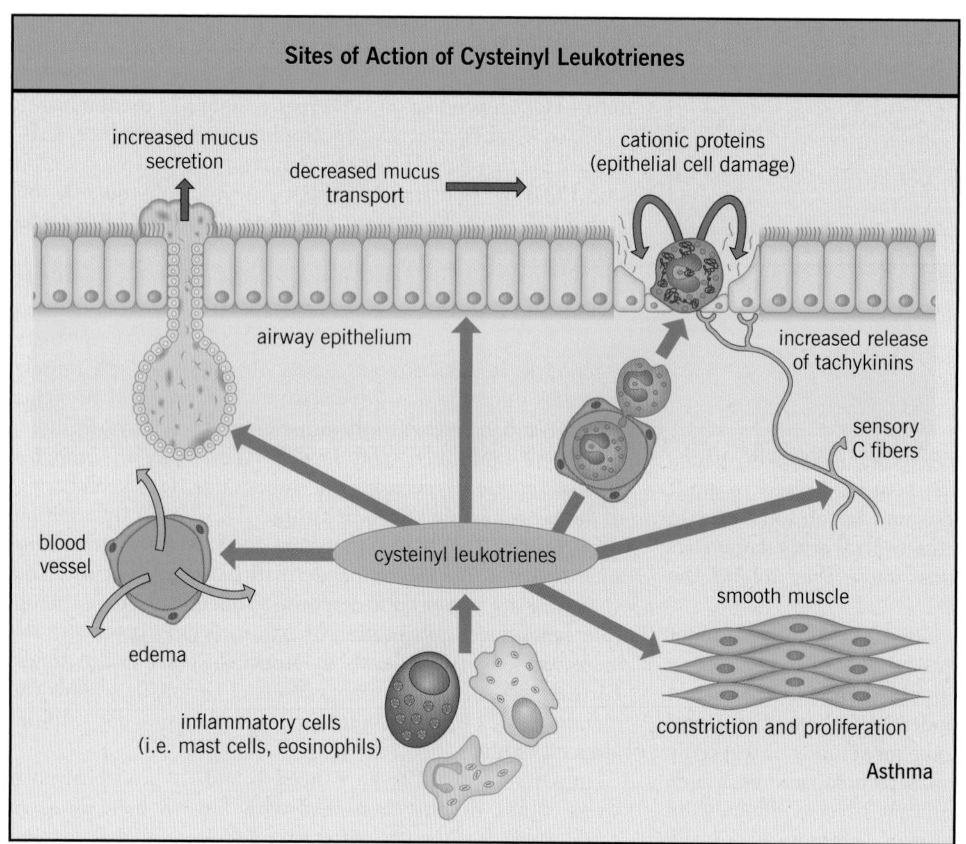

Fig. 24.13 The actions of cysteinyl leukotrienes in asthma.

USA, and 1995 in Japan, respectively. Both montelukast and pranlukast are approved for the treatment of allergic rhinitis in adults. In 1996 the leukotriene synthesis inhibitor, zileuton, was approved for use in the USA. However, it is not currently marketed.

Mechanism of action

The development of drugs to inhibit the synthesis of leukotrienes has been aimed at two targets, 5-LO and 5-LO-activating protein (FLAP). Zileuton is an antioxidant inhibitor of 5-LO.

However, it is not entirely specific as it inhibits some other oxidizing enzymes, such as hepatic microsomal cytochrome enzyme, CYP3A4, involved in the metabolism of terfenadine, theophylline, and warfarin. Following allergen challenge of atopic asthmatic subjects, zileuton produces inhibition of the early, but not the late asthmatic response. The degree of inhibition of bronchospasm is correlated with the reduction of urinary LTE_4. Zileuton also suppresses AIA, in which a reduction of the urinary excretion of LTE_4 is also observed.

Although FLAP inhibitors have shown activity in experimental models and have been used to suppress early and late asthmatic response in humans, none has yet been marketed, largely because of their lack of potency.

LTRAs have been developed to prevent the interaction of LTC_4 and LTD_4 at the $CysLT_1$ receptor, responsible for many of the effects of asthma as described. The human $CysLT_1$ receptors are expressed in peripheral blood leukocytes (eosinophils, subsets of monocytes, macrophages, basophils and pregranulocytic CD34+ cells), lung smooth muscle cells and interstitial macrophages, and spleen, and less strongly in the small intestine, pancreas and placenta. Human $CysLT_2$ receptors are expressed in heart (myocytes, fibroblasts, and vascular smooth muscle cells), adrenal medulla, peripheral blood leukocytes, spleen, lymph nodes, CNS, interstitial macrophages and smooth muscle cells in the lung. Because LTRAs have relatively high receptor selectivity and do not block the $CysLT_2$ receptor, they usually have fewer unwanted effects than leukotriene synthesis inhibitors. LTRAs suppress airway inflammation including eosinophil infiltration. In sensitized experimental animals, LTRAs suppress antigen-induced early and late responses and eosinophil infiltration in bronchoalveolar lavage fluid. In asthma patients, prolonged administration of LTRAs suppresses eosinophils in sputum and the airway wall. They also suppress allergen-induced early and late asthmatic responses.

In antigen-sensitized/challenged animal models montelukast has been reported to have anti-remodeling activities, such as reduction of smooth muscle hypertrophy and subepithelial fibrosis and pranlukast abolished LTD_4 epithelium growth factor-induced human airway smooth muscle proliferation in vitro (Table 24.6).

As enhanced leukotriene production is a primary feature in AIA, it is hardly surprising that $CysLT_1$-receptor antagonists inhibit this response.

Table 24.6 Effects of leukotriene antagonists in the airways in asthma

Effects of $CysLT_1$-receptor Antagonists in the Airway in Asthma
Suppression of: • Constriction of bronchial smooth muscle • Increased vascular permeability • Increased mucus production • Increased airway hyperresponsiveness • Airway inflammation including eosinophil migration and activation • Airway remodeling including airway smooth muscle hyperplasia

In chronic asthma, zafirlukast and intravenous/oral montelukast show a rapid increase of the forced expired volume in 1 second (FEV_1), suggesting that leukotrienes are continuously released in chronic asthma, thereby causing bronchoconstriction and enhancing non-specific airway hyperresponsiveness.

Uses and administration

LTRAs (montelukast 10 mg once daily, zafirlukast 20 mg twice daily, and pranlukast 225 mg twice daily in adults) have shown improvement of pulmonary function and symptoms in patients with mild-to-severe asthma. In children, montelukast (1 year of age or older), zafirlukast (5 years of age or older) and pranlukast (1 year of age or older) are indicated for asthma. In both adults and children, LTRAs provide significant protection against exercise- and antigen-induced bronchoconstriction as well as AIA. In addition to beneficial effects on pulmonary functions, LTRAs decreased markers of airway inflammation. Recently, LTRAs were approved for treatment of allergic rhinitis. Moreover, LTRAs are generally safe and well tolerated.

Randomized, double-blind, placebo-controlled clinical trials have demonstrated the efficacies of LTRAs (montelukast 10 mg once daily, zafirlukast 20 mg twice daily, and pranlukast 225 mg twice daily) in improving pulmonary function, symptoms, and quality of life and decreasing risk of asthma exacerbation in patients with mild-to-moderate asthma as compared with placebo.

LTRAs can be an alternative therapy to low-dose inhaled corticosteroids in mild persistent asthma, although LTRAs are less effective. In a double-blind extension trial in adults and children 6 years of age and older, the efficacy of an LTRA (montelukast 10 mg once daily) and beclomethasone 200 μg twice daily was similar. In addition to the significant efficacy of monotherapy, LTRAs have additive effects with inhaled corticosteroids.

There is evidence that LTRAs used as add-on therapy reduce the dose of inhaled corticosteroids required by patients with moderate-to-severe asthma or improve asthma control in patients whose asthma is not controlled with low to high doses of inhaled corticosteroids. In patients inadequately controlled by low–medium dose inhaled corticosteroids, inhaled corticosteroids plus LTRAs or a double dose of inhaled corticosteroids showed similar progressive improvement in several measures of asthma control compared with baseline. Moreover LTRAs plus inhaled corticosteroids showed faster onset of action than a double dose of inhaled corticosteroids. Adding montelukast 10 mg once daily to the treatment of patients whose symptoms remain uncontrolled with inhaled corticosteroids could provide equivalent clinical control compared with adding long acting inhaled β-stimulants.

LTRAs decrease the number of eosinophils in sputum and peripheral blood suggesting that part of the effect of LTRAs is antiinflammatory. LTRAs prevent exercised-induced asthma. No tolerance to the bronchoprotective effects has been observed with LTRAs.

In patients with seasonal rhinitis, with or without concomitant asthma, LTRAs improved nasal, eye, and throat symptoms as well as quality of life. Concomitant montelukast, together with the antihistamine, loratadine, provided effective improvement of daytime nasal symptoms as compared to placebo and each agent alone.

In AIA, 4–28% of adult patients have asthma exacerbation by taking aspirin or other NSAIDs with anti-cyclooxygenase activity. These patients show increased production of cysteinyl leukotrienes. Inhaled corticosteroids continue to be the mainstay of therapy and LTRAs can be useful for additional control of underlying diseases.

An advantage of LTRAs is their administration as a tablet rather than an inhaler, since compliance is an especially critical element in controlling asthma.

LTRAs are generally safe and well tolerated. The incidence of adverse effects of LTRAs in asthma patients was similar to those seen in placebo in double-blind, placebo-controlled trials. To date, no specific adverse effects have been reported with these drugs but, as with all new drugs, there is a possibility of rare hypersensitivity or idiosyncratic reactions that were not detected in premarketing trials. Churg–Strauss syndrome (CSS) is an eosinophilic vasculitis which has been reported with all three LTRAs. An incidence of approximately 60 cases per million patients treated with LTRAs per year is similar to those in the general population. It is speculated that they unmask an underlying vasculitic syndrome that was suppressed by previous corticosteroid therapy.

The 5-LO inhibitor, zileuton, is effective in chronic asthma. A 4-week study in 46 patients with a mean FEV_1 at 60% of predicted values showed that a dose of 4.6 g a day significantly increased FEV_1, decreased β-agonist use and decreased symptoms. Zileuton is indicated for long-term control and prevention of symptoms in mild persistent asthma for patients over 12 years of age. As stated earlier, its primary potential adverse effects are elevation of liver enzymes and inhibition of the metabolism of terfenadine, warfarin, and theophylline.

In a multicenter double-blind trial in 157 adult patients with mild-to-moderate asthma, the global improvement rating with 225 mg twice a day of the $CysLT_1$-receptor antagonist, pranlukast hydrate, was moderate or marked in 57% of cases compared with 11.5% of cases for the placebo. The decrease of both clinical symptoms and escape medication was greater in the pranlukast group but the incidence of the adverse effects was not significantly different.

Clinical trials with two $CysLT_1$-receptor antagonists, zafirlukast, used at a dose of 40 mg twice daily, and montelukast, at a dose of 10 mg once daily, showed them to be superior to the placebo in observations, including reducing the number of night-time awakenings and mornings with asthma, and daytime symptom scores, increasing morning and evening peak expiratory flow (PEF), reducing the use of β_2-agonists and improving quality of life. Efficacy was maintained during the trial periods.

Zafirlukast, montelukast, and pranlukast have now been marketed for the long-term control and prevention of symptoms in mild-to-moderate adult asthma and asthma induced by NSAIDs. Administration of zafirlukast with meals decreases its bioavailability, so it should be taken at least 1 or 2 hours after a meal.

In summary, findings from these studies support the hypothesis that LTRAs improve pulmonary functions and symptoms in patients with mild to moderate asthma, mediate antiinflammatory effects, and complement the antiinflammatory properties of corticosteroids. In patients with moderate-to-severe asthma, LTRAs permit corticosteroid tapering. Observations that inhaled medication cannot penetrate into small airways, nor inhaled or systemic corticosteroids suppress leukotriene production thus provide a rational argument for the use of LTRAs as complementary therapy to inhaled corticosteroids in more severe asthma. LTRAs increase the therapeutic options for patients with asthma, and based on recent data, it is expected that future guidelines will include expanded uses for these agents.

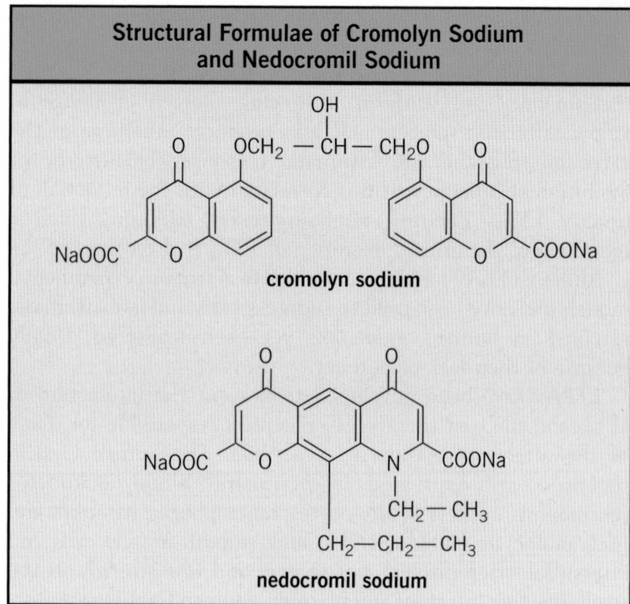

Fig. 24.14 Structures of cromolin sodium and nedocromil sodium.

CROMOLYN SODIUM AND NEDOCROMIL SODIUM

Cromolyn sodium and nedocromil sodium (Fig. 24.14) are often termed 'antiallergic drugs', which are defined here as drugs capable of inhibiting both the early-phase response to challenge and chronic allergic inflammation. Cromolyn sodium was originally introduced as a mast cell stabilizer for the treatment of asthma while nedocromil sodium was marketed as a drug to reduce allergic inflammation. The similarity in the mechanisms of action of the two drugs indicates that they both have the two effects, the effect on the mast cell being responsible for their ability to prevent and treat immediate hypersensitivity responses and the effect on allergic inflammation, especially the influx and activation of eosinophils, contributing to their ability to reduce the severity of chronic allergic disease.

While cromolin sodium and nedocromil sodium were both originally introduced for the treatment of asthma, they are now used widely as topical therapies for allergic rhinitis and conjunctivitis.

Mechanism of action

The possible sites of action of antiallergic drugs are shown in Figure 24.15. The mechanism by which cromolin sodium and nedocromil sodium act at the biochemical level is still unclear. Phosphorylation of a 78 kDa protein, a substrate for protein kinase C, has been proposed, but inhibition of a unique chloride channel is now thought to be the primary target. While an action on mast cells may explain the action of the drugs on bronchoconstriction induced by allergen, exercise, and cold air,

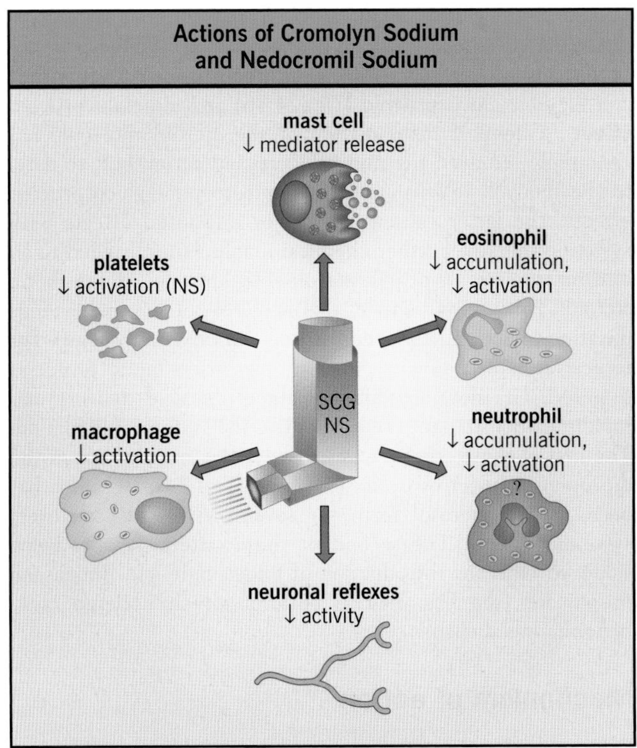

Fig. 24.15 Target sites for cromolin sodium (SCG) and nedocromil sodium (NS).

the effect on that induced by irritant agents, such as sulfur dioxide, is unlikely to be mast cell mediated. An effect on neuronal reflexes, possibly involving C-fiber sensory neurons, has been postulated. The ability of nedocromil sodium to inhibit bronchoconstriction induced by bradykinin and capsaicin would support this theory. Thus, there are probably two complementary mechanisms by which cromolin sodium and nedocromil sodium may exert their beneficial effects against the early phase of acute asthma attacks.

Besides inhibiting the early-phase response, cromolin sodium and nedocromil sodium also protect against allergen-induced late-phase responses which, in asthma, are associated with the acquisition of bronchial hyperresponsiveness. As these events are associated with the accumulation and activation of inflammatory cells, particularly eosinophils, an inhibitory effect on these aspects of allergic disease must be considered. In vitro, activation of eosinophils, neutrophils, and macrophages is reduced by cromolin sodium and nedocromil sodium, the latter again being approximately 10 times more potent. In vivo studies have shown that cromolin sodium inhibits eosinophil migration into the lung both following allergen challenge and in clinical asthma. Furthermore, nedocromil sodium, but not cromolin sodium, inhibits platelet activation in aspirin-sensitive patients.

Uses and administration

Both cromolin sodium and nedocromil sodium (see Fig. 24.14) are acidic drugs with pKa values of 1.0–2.5 and, consequently, exist almost exclusively in the ionized form at physiologic pH (~7.4). These physicochemical characteristics mean that the drugs have negligible absorption from the gastrointestinal tract and must be given topically. Aerosols are available for asthma, both drops and sprays for rhinitis, and drops for conjunctivitis. In addition, oral solutions have been suggested for the topical treatment of gastrointestinal allergy. A major advantage of the drugs existing almost exclusively in the ionized form is that any drug absorbed systemically remains in the extracellular compartment, thus giving negligible toxicity.

Both cromolin sodium and nedocromil sodium have achieved a well-established place in the control of mildly to moderately severe asthma but are less effective in severe asthma. Their ability to treat both immediate and late-phase bronchoconstrictor events and to prevent the acquisition of bronchial hyperresponsiveness provides a uniquely wide spectrum of activity. However, their major drawback is their relatively weak action and the fact that they are ineffective in approximately 30% of patients.

When used for the prevention of an early-phase allergic response, a single prophylactic inhaled dose has been shown repeatedly to be effective. However, to have an effect against bronchial hyperresponsiveness, courses of at least 1–2 months are necessary. The unwillingness of patients and physicians to wait this length of time before experiencing the beneficial effects of the drugs is one of the major reasons why antiallergic drugs are often considered to be ineffective. However, skilled management of patients with cromolin sodium or nedocromil sodium may provide a single asthma therapy which is free from the potential hazards associated with β-stimulants, corticosteroids, or theophylline.

The most common unwanted effects following inhalation are transient cough and mild wheezing.

Although not as effective as topical corticosteroids, cromolin sodium and nedocromil sodium drops and nasal sprays have found a place in the treatment of allergic rhinitis and are often the drugs of first choice in children. For maximal effect, treatment should begin 2–3 weeks before the hayfever season and continue throughout its duration. The only unwanted effect is local irritation of the nasal mucosa, very rarely associated with transient bronchospasm.

Cromolyn sodium and nedocromil sodium drops are also effective in the treatment of allergic conjunctivitis. Again, their freedom from unwanted effects may make them preferable to topical corticosteroids and systemic antihistamines.

Cromolyn sodium and nedocromil sodium may, therefore, be particularly useful drugs for the treatment of allergic disease in patients, especially young children, where the unwanted effects of drugs of other classes may be a problem.

CORTICOSTEROIDS

Corticosteroids, or steroids as they are often loosely termed, have been the drug of choice for the treatment of chronic severe asthma since their introduction in 1950. More recently it has been recognized that the treatment of milder asthma with steroids may also help to reduce bronchial inflammation and control the progression of the disease. In addition, their ability to reduce allergic inflammation has led to the widespread use of steroids in all allergic diseases, including those of the nose, eye, skin, and gastrointestinal tract. However, it must be stressed that steroids have potentially debilitating, unwanted effects when used incorrectly or inappropriately.

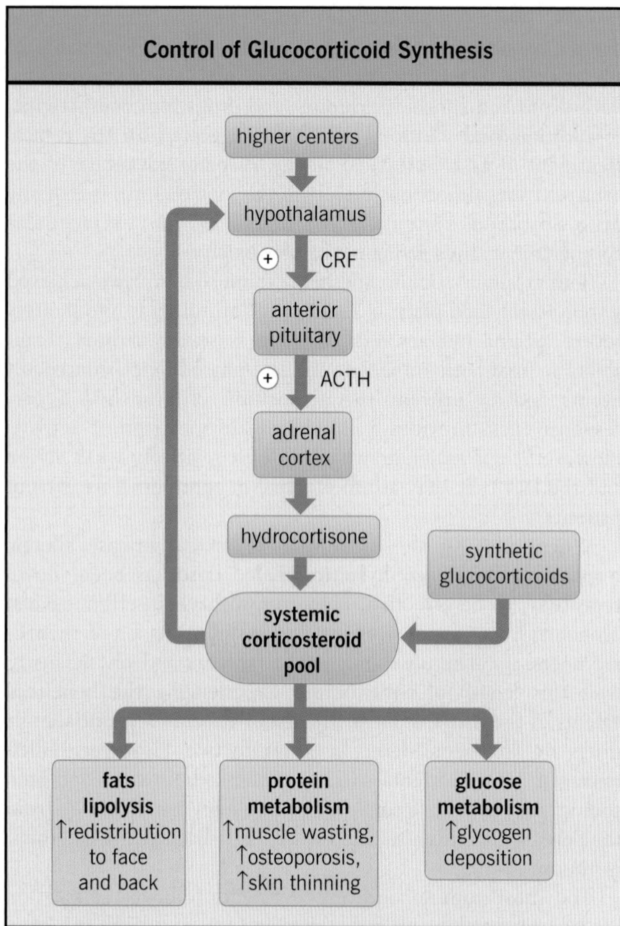

Fig. 24.16 Control of secretion and metabolic effects of glucocorticosteroids. In normal individuals, the positive signals of corticotrophin-releasing factor (CRF) and adrenocorticotrophic hormone (ACTH) from the hypothalamus and pituitary gland, respectively, induce the secretion of hydrocortisone from the adrenal cortex. Both hydrocortisone and exogenous glucocorticoids exert a negative effect on the hypothalamus to reduce natural hydrocortisone secretion.

The natural glucocorticoid released from the zona fascicularis of the human adrenal cortex is hydrocortisone. While possessing potent antiinflammatory effects, hydrocortisone carries with it considerable glucocorticoid (Fig. 24.16) and mineralocorticoid effects. Chemical manipulation of the steroid molecule has essentially removed the mineralocorticoid action but, to date, has been unable to separate antiinflammatory and glucocorticoid effects, the latter causing the major unwanted effects with systemic therapy. Further chemical manipulation has led to an optimization of the pharmacokinetic profile of synthetic steroids. For systemic activity, this increases potency and extends duration of action (e.g. prednisolone and dexamethasone). For topical administration, a different pharmacokinetic profile is required, viz. slow absorption from the site of delivery and rapid metabolism once the drug enters the systemic circulation. The first of these criteria was met with the introduction of the dipropionate ester of beclomethasone (Fig. 24.17), which has been used in aerosol form for several years without overt systemic effects. The second of these criteria is now being achieved with the introduction of budesonide and fluticasone propionate (see Fig. 24.17), both of which undergo rapid systemic metabolism.

Mechanism of action

Both natural and synthetic steroids are highly lipophilic and largely bound to either of two plasma proteins: transcortin, a specific corticosteroid-binding globulin which binds glucocorticoids with high affinity, and albumin, which binds all steroids with low affinity. Free steroid molecules diffuse across the cell membrane where they interact with glucocorticoid receptors (GR) in the cytoplasm (Fig. 24.18). In the absence of glucocorticoids, inactive glucocorticoid receptors (GRi) are maintained in their resting state by being bound to a 90 kDa heat-shock protein. Interaction with a glucocorticoid molecule leads to shedding of the heat-shock protein to expose the active

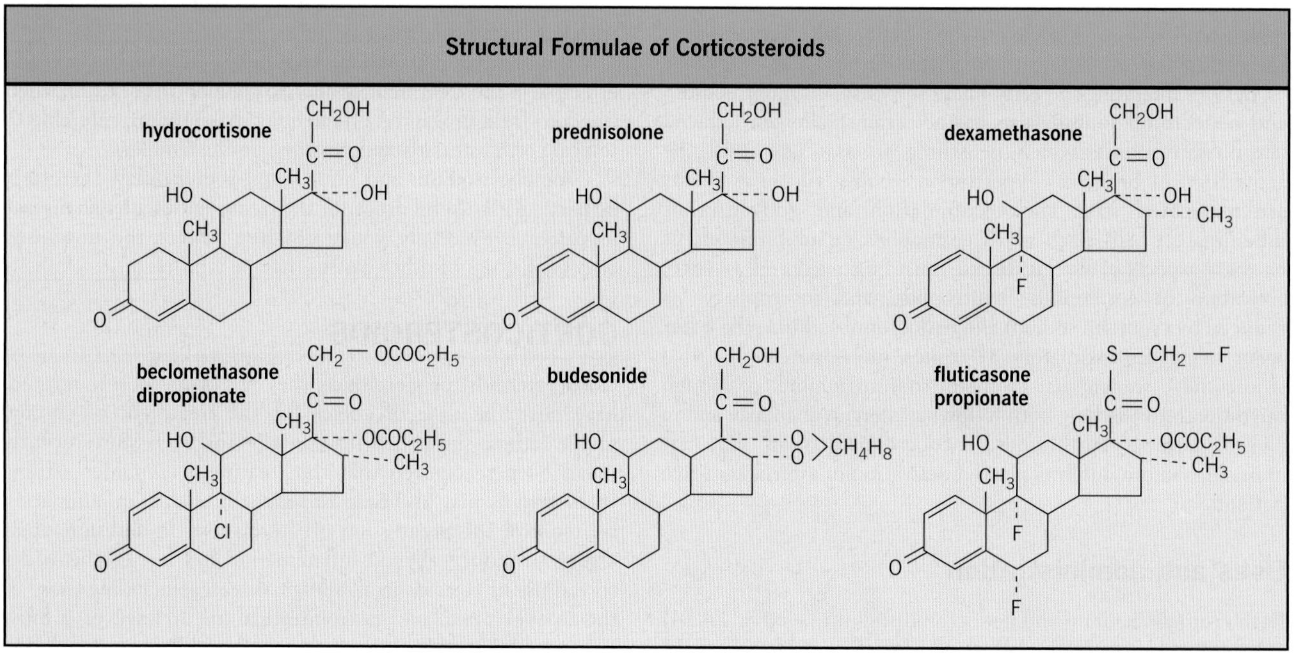

Structural Formulae of Corticosteroids

hydrocortisone · prednisolone · dexamethasone · beclomethasone dipropionate · budesonide · fluticasone propionate

Fig. 24.17 Structural formulae of common corticosteroids.

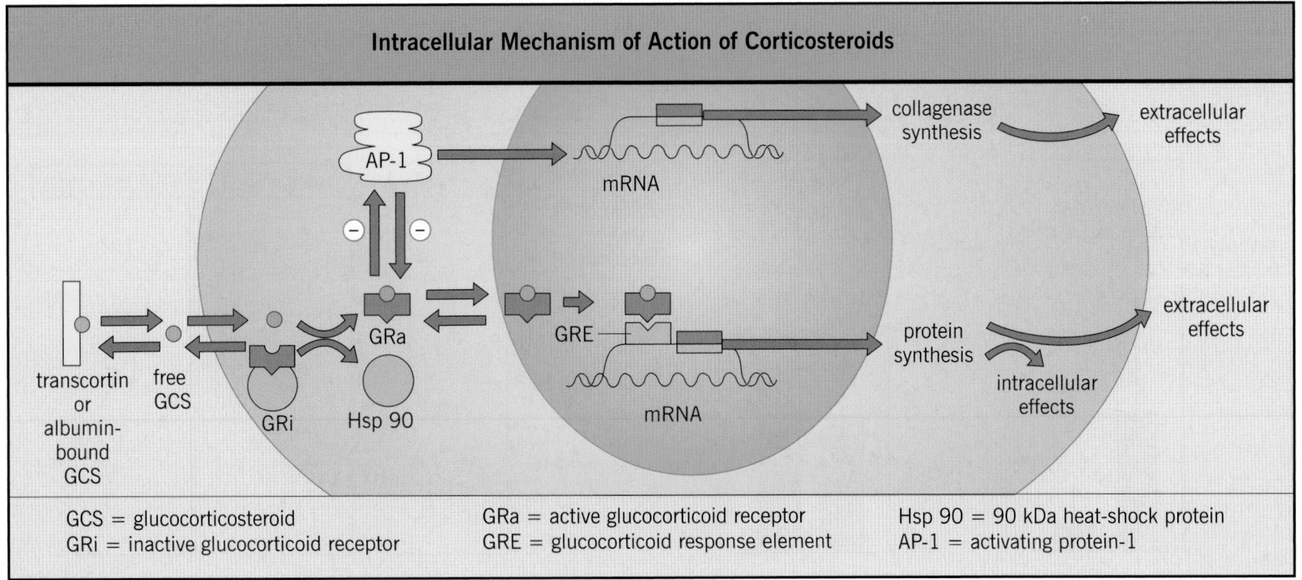

Fig. 24.18 Intracellular mechanisms of action of corticosteroids (see text).

site. The resultant activated receptor (GRa) then diffuses into the nucleus where it interacts with a specific glucocorticoid response element (GRE) on the chromatin of the DNA to influence transcription and, consequently, de novo synthesis of steroid-susceptible proteins. Two examples of proteins whose synthesis are upregulated are lipomodulin, which exerts an antiinflammatory activity by inhibiting the activity of phospholipase A_2 and inhibitory factor κB (IκB), the inhibitory factor of nuclear factor κB (NF-κB) which is the transcription factor responsible for the synthesis of many proinflammatory cytokines and adhesion proteins. Glucocorticoids may also downregulate transcription. An example of this is the inhibition of transcription of activating protein-1 (AP-1), a factor responsible for the synthesis of many proinflammatory cytokines and growth factors. In addition, corticosteroids may reduce the stability of messenger RNA for cytokines, such as IL-4. The complexities of these processes account for the considerable time delay of 6–12 hours, even after intravenous administration, before the beneficial effects of corticosteroids begin to be observed.

At the cellular level, glucocorticoids suppress both acute and chronic inflammation, irrespective of cause, by inhibiting many steps in the inflammatory process. Some cellular actions pertinent to allergy are shown in Figure 24.19. Of these, corticosteroid reduction of proinflammatory cytokine production from many cells, including Th2 lymphocytes, mast cells, and eosinophils, reduction of eosinophil and mast cell influx and maturation, and promotion of apoptosis in inflammatory cells are likely to be the mechanisms by which corticosteroids achieve their long-term antiinflammatory effects in chronic allergic disease (Fig. 24.20). Their life-saving effects, which are apparent within 8–12 hours of intravenous injection in acute severe asthma, are more likely to be due to the ability of the drugs to reduce edema, reduce the local generation of eicosanoids following lipomodulin generation, reduce inflammatory cell influx and activation, and reverse adrenoceptor downregulation.

The intracellular events which are responsible for the anti-inflammatory effects of glucocorticoids cannot be separated from their effects on glucose, protein, and lipid metabolism and their suppressive effects on the hypothalamo–pituitary–adrenal (HPA) axis. These effects are summarized in Figure 24.16. It should be noted that all glucocorticoids, whether natural or synthetic, will exert these effects when present in the systemic circulation. Furthermore, the magnitude of the side-effects is dependent on:

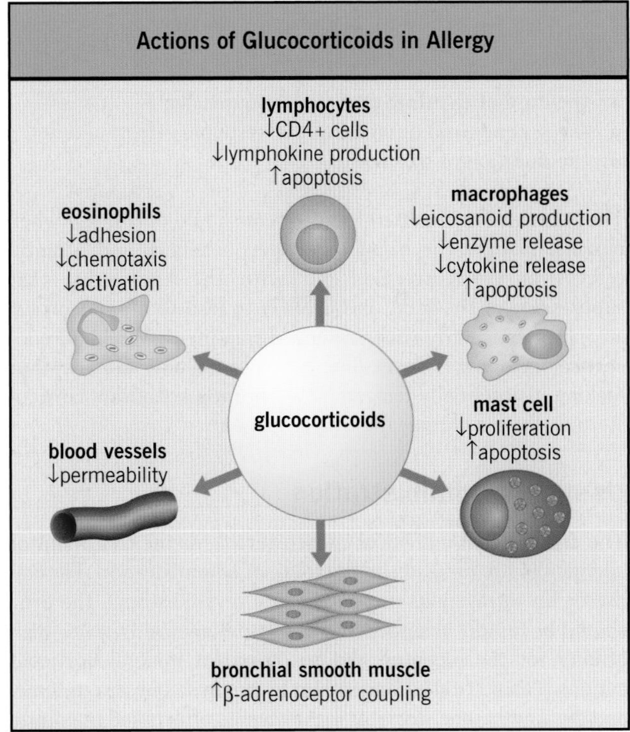

Fig. 24.19 Possible mechanisms by which corticosteroids reduce allergic diseases.

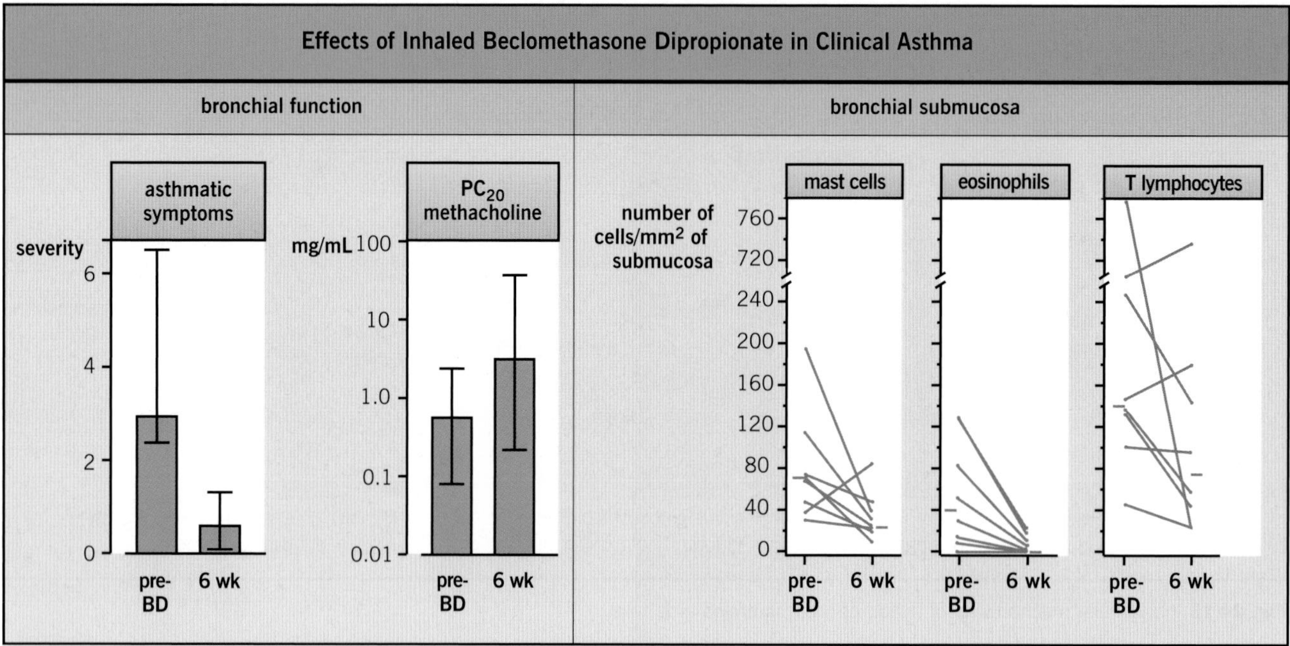

Fig. 24.20 The effect of beclomethasone dipropionate in asthma. Patients were examined before and after treatment with beclomethasone dipropionate (BD), 1000 µg a day by inhalation. Improvements were observed in subjective symptoms and bronchial hyperresponsiveness to methacholine. These were paralleled by significant falls in submucosal mast cell and eosinophil numbers as assessed in bronchial biopsies.

- the dose of the drug absorbed systemically;
- the potency and duration of the systemic effect; and
- the duration of treatment.

Thus, instigation of systemic treatment should only begin when bearing in mind the balance between beneficial and harmful effects of corticosteroids and with the knowledge that suppression of the HPA axis is likely to lead to adrenocortical atrophy, particularly with prolonged treatment. While adrenocortical atrophy is reversible, this occurs only slowly, thus making it potentially dangerous to abruptly withdraw corticosteroids from a chronically treated patient.

Uses and administration

The choice of an individual corticosteroid for the treatment of allergic disease depends on the route of administration. For oral use or for intravenous use, as in acute severe asthma, the drug should be rapidly absorbed and slowly metabolized, have a high affinity for the receptor, and be devoid of mineralocorticoid actions. These criteria are best met by prednisolone, prednisone, and dexamethasone. To minimize unwanted effects and maximize effectiveness, large initial doses should be used followed by systematic reduction to the lowest possible maintenance dose. Alternatively, intermittent high-dose therapy may be used, thus allowing the body periods of recovery between administrations.

In less severe conditions, a corticosteroid should be administered topically whenever possible. The ideal pharmacokinetic properties of such a drug are slow absorption from the site of deposition and rapid metabolism once absorbed systemically. These criteria are met most closely by beclomethasone dipropionate, budesonide, and fluticasone. Experience with inhaled steroids, since the early 1970s, has shown that original fears about long-term adverse effects appear not to have been borne out, with only occasional reports of candidiasis and reversible dysphonia and rare reports of systemic effects. Only with inhaled doses of around 1000–2000 mg a day have mild systemic effects and some degree of HPA suppression been reported. In rhinitis and conjunctivitis, the total dose of steroid is small enough to make it essentially free from systemic effects. Treatment of inflammatory diseases of the skin, however, may still result in systemic effects, particularly when it is necessary to apply steroids to large areas of the body. Thus, the increasing tendency to use topical corticosteroids as antiinflammatory agents in allergic disease appears to be a logical and relatively safe therapeutic development. However, it should still be a maxim of the practicing physician to use as low a dose as possible, particularly in children.

Guidelines for the use of steroids in asthma have now been formulated in many countries. Briefly, they suggest the introduction of inhaled preparations even in relatively mild asthma, increased inhaled doses as asthma becomes more severe, and the use of oral therapy only when the disease cannot be controlled satisfactorily by inhaled therapy.

In rhinitis, steroid nasal sprays, such as beclomethasone dipropionate and fluticasone propionate, are used to reduce the influx of mast cells and other inflammatory cells into the nasal mucosa. As they do not inhibit mast cell degranulation, they do not provide immediate relief. For maximal benefit in seasonal rhinitis, topical steroid therapy should be instituted 2–3 weeks before the hayfever season. Unwanted effects are negligible with conventional doses. Systemic therapy should only be used in extremely debilitating conditions.

Steroid eye drops are very effective in the treatment of many forms of conjunctivitis, including allergic conjunctivitis. In extreme conditions, the drug may also be given systemically. However, in eye disease, steroids should only be used under expert medical supervision because of their local unwanted effects. The most potentially dangerous of these are as follows.

- Aggravation of 'red eye', a condition of dendritic ulceration caused by the herpes simplex virus may occur. The local immunosuppressive effects of steroids worsen this condition and may lead to loss of sight or even of the eye.
- In persons predisposed to chronic simple glaucoma, steroid eye drops may induce 'steroid glaucoma' after a few weeks' use. Again, this may be sight threatening.
- Use of high doses of steroids for conjunctival inflammation, particularly when given systemically, is associated with the development of 'steroid cataract'. This problem is both dose and duration related. For example, daily oral dosage with 15 mg of prednisolone (or equivalent with other steroids) for prolonged periods carries a risk of 'steroid cataract' of around 75%.

In the skin, steroid creams and ointments are used for a wide variety of inflammatory conditions, including eczema and atopic dermatitis. They act to suppress symptoms and are in no sense curative, rebound exacerbations often occurring on cessation of treatment. They are of limited value in urticaria and are contraindicated in rosacea and ulcerative conditions, which they worsen. Because of their local unwanted effects (Table 24.7) and their ability to be absorbed through the skin and cause systemic effects, steroids should not be the drugs of first choice but reserved for the more problematic conditions. Even then, the lowest strength of the least potent steroids should be used. Also, short courses are recommended wherever possible. The use of topical steroids in the skin of children is discouraged because of the systemic effects.

In conclusion, steroids afford effective therapy in allergic disease when the appropriate formulations are given and the physician observes with diligence the basic rules to avoid unwanted effects.

HUMANIZED MONOCLONAL ANTI-IMMUNOGLOBULIN ANTIBODY

Immune responses mediated by IgE are important in the pathogenesis of allergic asthma. Recently, a recombinant humanized monoclonal antibody directed against IgE (anti-IgE, omalizumab, rhuMAb-E25) has been introduced in the USA for the treatment of patients with moderate-to-severe asthma, with seasonal and perennial allergic rhinitis and with concomitant allergic asthma and rhinitis. In particular, clinical trials have shown that injection of anti-IgE improves asthma control in allergic asthma in patients who remained symptomatic despite regular use of inhaled corticosteroids.

Table 24.7 Possible detrimental effects of steroids in the skin

Possible Detrimental Effects of Steroids in the Skin
Spread and worsening of untreated infection
Thinning of the skin, which may be only partially reversible
Irreversible striae atrophicae
Increased hair growth
Perioral dermatitis
Acne at the site of application
Mild depigmentation of the skin

Mechanisms of action

Anti-IgE is humanized monoclonal antibody to the domain of human IgE which binds to the FcεRI on mast cells and basophils (Fig. 24.21). Consequently, when anti-IgE forms a complex with IgE, the IgE can no longer bind to the FcεRI and, thus, cannot sensitize mast cells and basophils. This has been shown in vivo in a study where anti-IgE infusion decreased serum IgE levels, the density basophil surface IgE and FcεRIα, and antigen-induced basophil histamine release. As the FcεRI-binding domain is hidden once IgE is bound to FcεRI, anti-IgE cannot activate mast cells or basophils and cause anaphylaxis. Furthermore, dendritic cells, which are crucially involved in allergen presentation in allergic individuals, also have cell surface FcεRI. Thus, anti-IgE would be expected to lead to a reduction in allergen presentation, Th2 cell activation, and proliferation. This has been demonstrated in humans where anti-IgE reduced submucosal T-cell and B-cell numbers. In seasonal allergic rhinitis anti-IgE inhibited the allergen-induced seasonal increases in circulating and tissue eosinophils.

The effects of anti-IgE antibody are dependent on its presence in the serum. After the final infusion with anti-IgE, subjects slowly regain levels of IgE, reaching 18% of preinfusion levels at 8 weeks in one study. Basophil IgE and FcεRIα surface density and antigen-induced basophil histamine release responses rose in parallel with free IgE.

Uses and administration

The efficacy of anti-IgE has been demonstrated in patients with moderate-to-severe asthma, in patients with seasonal allergic rhinitis and perennial allergic rhinitis, and in subjects with concomitant allergic asthma and rhinitis. Several large-scale, randomized, double-blind, placebo-controlled clinical trials of anti-IgE, mostly given every 2–4 weeks depending on serum IgE level, have demonstrated the benefits of this agent in adult patients with moderate-to-severe allergic asthma who remain symptomatic despite treatment with systemic or inhaled corticosteroids. The trials have shown consistently that administration of anti-IgE is associated with fewer asthma exacerbations per patient despite significant reductions in corticosteroid dose, stable symptom control despite concomitant reductions in rescue medication use, improvement of lung function and improvement in quality of life compared with the placebo. Regression analysis of pooled data from the two studies in adults with moderate-to-severe asthma showed the most marked benefit of anti-IgE therapy was observed in patients with a history of frequent emergency asthma treatment and in patients receiving high inhaled corticosteroids doses. In moderate-to-severe childhood asthma, like adult asthma, administration of anti-IgE has been shown to be associated with fewer exacerbations, and less use of rescue medication in both the stable steroid period and steroid reduction phases.

Anti-IgE has been shown to be safe and well tolerated, there being no significant differences in the incidence of adverse effects when compared to placebo in many clinical trials. Mild-to-moderate urticaria has been reported occasionally after the

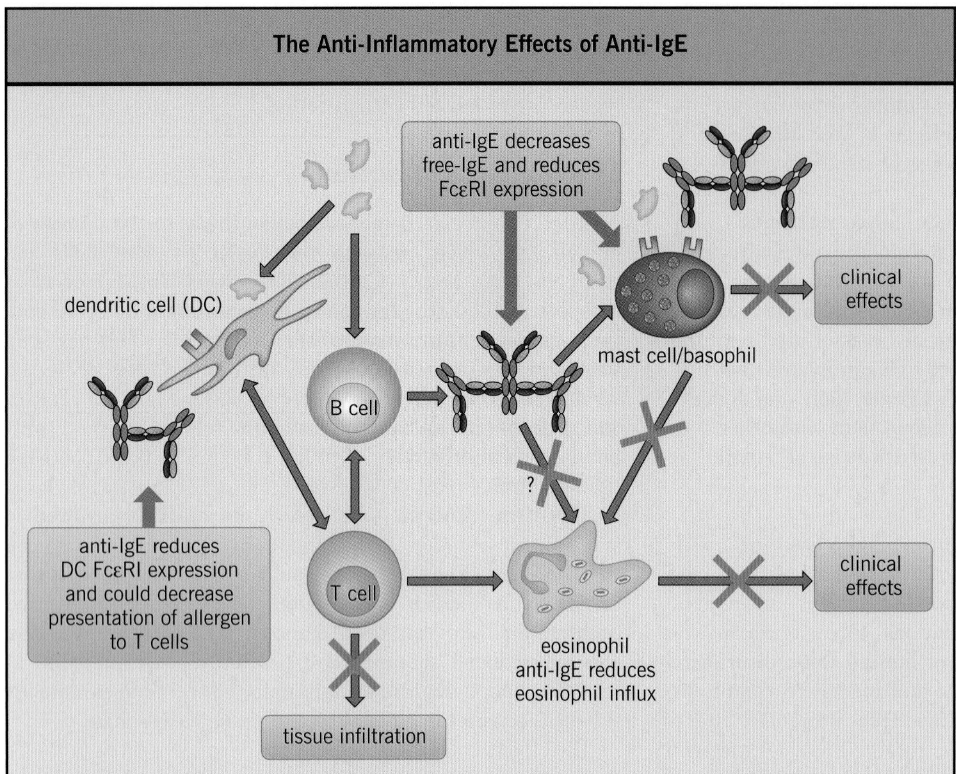

Fig. 24.21 Proposed mechanisms of action of recombinant humanized monoclonal antibody to IgE (omalizumab). (Adapted from Holgate S, Casale T, Wenzel S, et al. The anti-inflammatory effects of omalizumab confirm the central role of IgE in allergic inflammation. J Allergy Clin Immunol 2005; 115:459–465.)

anti-IgE infusion. Other reported events are headache and bruising at the injection site. It has been shown that even after 20 weeks of treatment, no antibodies against anti-IgE were detectable. The absence of immunogenicity of anti-IgE may be attributed to the humanization of the antibody and to protein engineering that resulted in a non-complement-fixing molecule with a human IgGκ framework.

DRUGS IN DEVELOPMENT

The prevalence of allergic diseases is rising, particularly in the developed world. Current drug therapy is not reaching its objectives either in reversing this increase or in satisfactorily treating the allergic symptoms. Of particular concern is that the prevalence of asthma and the incidence of asthma deaths are still rising. Thus, the quest for newer and more effective drugs must continue. As drugs in development are described here only in general terms, the reader is referred to more specialized texts for details. Approaches toward achieving bronchodilatation and symptomatic relief in asthma are now discussed.

Calcium antagonists

Calcium antagonists reduce the stimulus-induced entry of calcium into bronchial smooth muscle and thus decrease its contractility. Due to their lack of specificity, effects on the cardiovascular system are of major concern.

Potassium-channel-opening drugs

Potassium-channel-opening drugs lead to hyperpolarization and, consequently, a reduction in contractile sensitivity of bronchial smooth muscle. One of these agents, cromakalim has been shown to reduce 'morning dipping' in human nocturnal asthma, and to inhibit histamine-induced bronchoconstriction. Although it has shown some efficacy, cromakalim is associated with significant adverse vascular effects including orthostatic hypotension, headache, and flush. The possibility of delivering such drugs to the airways by aerosol inhalation may present a useful means of therapy.

Tachykinin-receptor antagonists

Tachykinins, particularly substance P and neurokinin A (NKA), are widely distributed in the endings of some primary afferent neurons in the airways of many species, including humans. Stimulation of NK-1 and NK-2 receptors by these tachykinins has many effects relevant to asthma, including bronchoconstriction, vasodilatation, plasma extravasation, and inflammatory effects, such as eosinophil accumulation in the airway and upregulation of the expression of adhesion molecules on vascular endothelial cells. Stimulation of NK-2 receptors may induce cough responses. There are few studies on the effects of NK-1 and NK-2 tachykinin-receptor antagonists in humans. A mixed NK-1 and NK-2 antagonist inhibits bradykinin-induced bronchoconstriction in patients with asthma. Further development of more potent and bioavailable antagonists and clinical trials is needed to decide the usefulness of tachykinin-receptor antagonists.

Phosphodiesterase type 4 inhibitors

Inhibition of PDE4 acts by increasing intracellular concentration of cAMP, which has a broad range of antiinflammatory

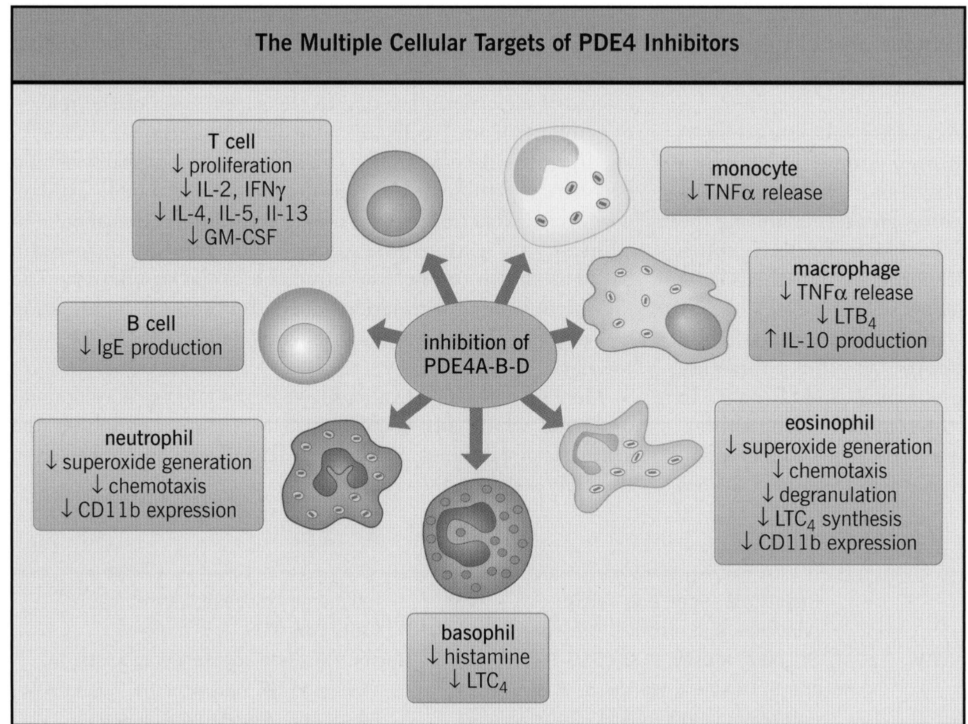

Fig. 24.22 Potential antiinflammatory and immunomodulatory effects of phosphodiesterase 4 (PDE4) inhibitors. (Quoted from Banner K, Trevethick MA. PDE4 inhibition: a novel approaches from the treatment of inflammatory bowel disease. Trends Pharmacol Sci 2004; 25:430–436.)

effects on various key effector cells involved in airway inflammation in asthma and chronic obstructive pulmonary disease (COPD) (Fig. 24.22). Orally active, selective PDE4 inhibitors including roflumilast and cilomilast have antiinflammatory effects and have been shown to be effective for the treatment of asthma and COPD.

PDE4 belong to an important family of proteins that regulate the intracellular levels of cyclic nucleotide second messengers. Targeting PDE4 with selective inhibitors may offer novel therapeutic strategies in the treatment of airway inflammatory diseases including asthma and COPD. The rationale for such an approach stems, in part, from the clinical efficacy of theophylline, an orally active drug that is purportedly a nonselective PDE inhibitor with significant antiinflammatory effect at low doses.

PDE4 is present in various inflammatory cells, including eosinophils, basophils, neutrophils, macrophages, monocytes, T cells, B cells, and epithelial cells. Intracellular cAMP levels regulate the function of many of these cells thought to contribute to the pathogenesis of respiratory diseases such as asthma and COPD. At present two PDE4 inhibitors, cilomilast and roflumilast, are undergoing clinical trials.

In vitro and in vivo experiments have shown multipathway antiinflammatory properties of these PDE4 inhibitors that may translate into continuous and sustained improvements in the lung function of patients with asthma. In animal models of asthma, PDE4 inhibitors reduce tumor necrosis factor α (TNFα) release and airway hyperresponsiveness. The PDE4 inhibitor roflumilast has been reported to suppress activation of neutrophils, eosinophils, macrophages/dendritic cells, CD4+T cells [release of interleukn-2 (IL-2), -4, -5 and interferon γ (INFγ)]. In addition to antiinflammatory effects, roflumilast has been reported to relax smooth muscle and modulate the activity of pulmonary nerves.

The therapeutic ratio for PDE4 inhibitors is thought to be determined by selectivity on receptor subtypes for relative effects on PDE4B (antiinflammatory) and PDE4D (emesis). Higher selectivity to PDE4B will give a superior therapeutic ratio.

Randomized, double-blind, multicenter studies on roflumilast, 500 μg per day, have been carried out on stable asthma patients whose baseline FEV_1 was 73% of predicted and baseline PEF was 77% of predicted. Roflumilast improved lung function; the mean increase of peak inspiratory flow rate being 24.21 ± 2.58 L/min compared a baseline of 360 L/min at the end of the 12 week trial. Roflumilast showed a rapid onset of bronchodilatation and reached clinically relevant levels of the improvement. Roflumilast has activity in asthma as assessed by its attenuation of allergen and exercise challenges. It shows clinical efficacy equivalent to that of beclomethasone dipropionate 400 μg daily.

Roflumilast is thought to be indicated to stabilize asthma of moderate severity and provide weak but rapid onset of efficacy and steady, continuous improvement of lung function. In COPD cilomilast, 15 mg twice daily, and roflumilast, 500 μg once daily, have shown variable but significant effects on exacerbations and quality of life, with small improvement in measures of pulmonary function.

One of the major issues to be resolved is the tolerability profile associated with this drug class (i.e. emesis and headache). Cilomilast and roflumilast have low emetic potential.

Ciclosporin, FK506, and rapamycin

The network of immune processes involved in allergic inflammation provides numerous opportunities for therapeutic intervention in allergic diseases, including bronchial asthma, allergic rhinitis, conjunctivitis, and atopic dermatitis. Obvious therapies undergoing intensive preclinical investigation include use of stimulants of eosinophil apoptosis, modulators of IgE production and function, and peptide fragments of common allergens.

Ciclosporin, FK506, and rapamycin have inhibitory effects on several inflammatory cells, the most important of which appears to be inhibition of T-cell activation. Cyclosporine acts at an early stage in the T-cell activation process, inhibiting the transcriptional activity of NF-AT to block T-cell receptor-mediated signal transduction. Cyclosporine inhibits the release of IL-5 from isolated human mononuclear cells, thereby reducing recruitment of eosinophils in allergic inflammation. In sensitized animals, ciclosporin suppresses the pulmonary accumulation and activation of eosinophils and T cells. In patients with chronic severe corticosteroid-dependent asthma, ciclosporin has been reported to decrease disease exacerbation and improve lung function. A significant reduction of activated T cells in peripheral blood and reduced expression of activation markers on peripheral blood CD4+ cells parallel clinical improvement, strongly suggesting that the antiasthmatic effects of ciclosporin are due to the suppression of the release of cytokines from T cells. Because of its potential renal toxicity and hypertensive effects, the use of ciclosporin probably should be restricted to corticosteroid-dependent intractable asthma, with renal function being monitored during treatment. In addition to asthma, systemic and topical ciclosporin has been shown to improve intractable atopy significantly. The microemulsion formulation used for topical application was reported to have good bioavailability and to be well tolerated.

More recently, investigations have begun into the development of agents which either antagonize the actions or inhibit the synthesis of cytokines, particularly IL-5. These are, however, in the early stages.

FURTHER READING

Barnes PJ. Theophylline and phosphodiesterase inhibitors. In: Adkinson NF, Yunginger JW, Busse WW, et al, eds. Allergy: principles and practice. 6th edn. St Louis: Mosby; 2003:823–833.

Busse W, Corren J, Lanier BQ, et al. Omalizumab, anti-IgE recombinant humanized monoclonal antibody, for the treatment of severe allergic asthma, J Allergy Clin Immunol 2001;108:184–190.

Dogne JM, De Leval X, Benoit P, et al. Thromboxane A_2 inhibition: therapeutic potential in bronchial asthma. Am J Respir Med 2002; 1:11–17.

Edwards AM, Holgate ST. The chromones: cromolin sodium and nedocromil sodium. In: Adkinson NF, Yunginger JW, Busse WW, et al, eds. Allergy: principles and practice. 6th edn. St Louis: Mosby; 2003:915–927.

Holgate S, Casale T, Wenzel S, et al. The anti-inflammatory effects of omalizumab confirm the central role of IgE in allergic inflammation. J Allergy Clin Immunol 2005; 115:459–465.

Kemp JP. Recent advances in the management of asthma using leukotriene modifiers. Am J Respir Med 2003; 2:139–156.

Leurs R, Church MK, Taglialatela M. H_1-antihistamines: inverse agonism, anti-inflammatory actions and cardiac effects. Clin Exp Allergy 2002; 32:489–498.

Lipworth BJ. Phosphodiesterase-4 inhibitors for asthma and chronic obstructive pulmonary disease, Lancet 2005; 365:167–175.

Nelson HS. Beta-adrenergic agonists. In: Adkinson NF, Yunginger JW, Busse WW, et al, eds. Allergy: principles and practice. 6th edn. St Louis: Mosby; 2003:803–821.

Schleimer RP, Spahn JD, Covar R, et al. Glucocorticoids. In: Adkinson NF, Yunginger JW, Busse WW, et al, eds. Allergy: principles and practice. 6th edn. St Louis: Mosby; 2003:870–913.

Simons FER, Advances in H_1-antihistamines, New Engl J Med 2004; 351:203–217.

Glossary

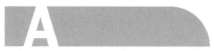

Acute phase proteins: Serum proteins whose levels increase during infection or inflammatory reactions.
Adhesion: The sticking of migratory leukocytes to endothelial or structural cells by the interaction of complementary adhesion proteins.
Adhesion proteins: Complementary cell surface molecules expressed on leukocytes, endothelial and structural cells that allow leukocyte adherence.
Adjuvant: A substance that non-specifically enhances the immune response to an antigen.
Agretope: The portion of an antigen or antigen fragment which interacts with a MHC molecule.
A-kinase (cAMP dPK): Cyclic AMP dependent protein kinase; a family of enzymes activated by cyclic AMP which catalyze intracellular phosphorylation reactions.
Allergen: A foreign protein or hapten which induces the formation of anaphylactic antibodies and which may precipitate an allergic response.
Allergenic: Behaving like an allergen.
Allergy: Initially embraced immunology, but now focused on the host tissue-damaging or irritation effects of immunologic responses.
Anaphylactoid reaction: An allergic-like reaction but produced by non-immunologic mechanisms.
Anaphylatoxins: Complement peptides C3a and C5a which cause smooth muscle contraction, increased microvascular permeability, leukocyte migration and activation, and degranulation of some types of mast cells.
Anaphylaxis: The consequences of an allergic reaction in an isolated organ or systemically.
Antibody: A molecule produced by the immune system in response to antigen that has the property of combining specifically with the antigen which induced its formation.
Antidromic reflex: *See* axon reflex.
Antigen: A molecule that induces the formation of antibody.
Antigen presentation: The process by which certain cells in the body (antigen-presenting cells) express antigen on their cell surface in a form recognizable by lymphocytes.
Antigen processing: The conversion of an antigen into a form in which it can be recognized by lymphocytes.
Antiserum: Serum containing antibodies to a specific antigen.
APCs (antigen-presenting cells): A variety of mobile or tissue-fixed cells, usually of the monocyte/macrophage family, which present antigen to lymphocytes through MHC class II molecules.
Apoptosis: Programmed cell death in which one cell engulfs another, usually senescent, cell in order to prevent liberation of its potentially toxic constituents.
Arachidonic acid: A 20-carbon fatty acid liberated from membrane phospholipid that may be converted into prostaglandins of the 2 series and leukotrienes of the 4 series.
Atopy: The ability to produce IgE antibodies to common allergens; demonstrable by RAST or skin prick tests.
Axon reflex: Local propagation of a nerve reflex by retrograde or antidromic stimulation of nerve axons resulting in the release of neuropeptides.

B

Bradykinin: A vasoactive nonapeptide that is probably the most important mediator generated by the kinin system.

C

C1–C9: The components of the complement classical and lytic pathways that are responsible for mediating inflammatory reactions, opsonization of particles, and lysis of cell membranes.
C domains: The constant domains of antibodies and T-cell receptors. These domains do not contribute to the antigen-binding site and show relatively little variability between receptor molecules.
CD markers: Surface molecules of cells, usually leukocytes and platelets, which are identified with monoclonal antibodies and may be used to distinguish cell populations.
CD3+ cells: Lymphocytes with pan-T cell marker CD3 on their surface.
CD4+ cells: T lymphocytes with CD4 surface marker, usually equitable with helper T cells.
CD8+ cells: T lymphocytes with CD8 surface marker, usually equitable with suppressor T cells.
CD23: A cell membrane molecule associated with the low affinity receptor for IgE (FcεRII).
Cell line: A collection of cells that divide continuously in culture. May be either monoclonal or polyclonal and may have been transformed naturally or be an artificial hybridization.
Challenge: Administration of an implicated allergen to an allergic subject, in order to provoke an allergic response.
Charcot–Leyden crystal: Lysolecithin crystals found in sputum of asthmatic subjects.
Chemokinesis: Increased random migratory activity of cells in response to a chemical stimulus.
Chemotaxis: Increased directional migration of cells particularly in response to concentration gradients of certain chemotactic factors (chemotaxins).
Chymase: A neutral protease of the mast cell granule found only in the MC_{TC} subpopulation of human mast cells.
Ciclosporin: An immunosuppressive drug with an action primarily on CD4+ lymphocytes.
Class I/II/III MHC molecules: Three major classes of molecule within the MHC. Class I molecules have one MHC encoded peptide associated with β_2-microglobulin. Class II molecules have two MHC encoded peptides that are non-covalently associated, and class III molecules are other molecules including complement components.
Class switching: The process by which an individual B cell can link new immunoglobulin heavy chain C genes to its recombined V gene to produce a different class of antibody with the same specificity. This process is also reflected in the overall class switch seen during the maturation of an immune response.
Clone: A family of cells or organisms having a genetically identical constitution.
CMI (cell-mediated immunity): A term used to refer to immune reactions that are mediated by cells, usually lymphocytes, rather than by antibody or other humoral factors.

Complement: A group of serum proteins involved in the control of inflammation, the activation of phagocytes and the lytic attack on cell membranes. The system can be activated by interaction with the immune system.

Conjugate: A reagent that is formed by covalently coupling two molecules together such as fluorescein coupled to an immunoglobulin molecule.

Constant regions: The relatively invariant parts of immunoglobulin heavy and light chains, $\alpha\beta$ and $\gamma\delta$ chains of the T-cell receptor.

CR1, CR2, CR3: Receptors for activated C3 fragments.

CSFs (colony-stimulating factors): A group of cytokines that control the differentiation of hemopoietic stem cells.

Cytokines: A generic term for soluble molecules that mediate interactions between cells.

Cytophilic: Having a propensity to bind to cells.

Cytostatic: Having the ability to stop cell growth.

Cytotoxic: Having the ability to kill cells.

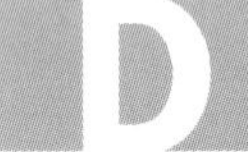

DAG (diacylglycerol): A potent protein kinase C activator usually generated from the action of phospholipases on membrane phospholipids.

Degranulation: Exocytosis of granular products from inflammatory cells, usually mast cells, basophils, eosinophils, and neutrophils.

Dendritic cells: A set of antigen-presenting cells present in epithelial structures and in lymph nodes, spleen, and at low levels in blood, which are particularly active in presenting antigen and stimulating T cells.

Desensitization: A protocol of repeated injections of allergen or modified allergen with the aim of reducing a patient's allergic responsiveness to that allergen.

Desetope: The part of an MHC molecule which links to antigen or processed antigen.

Diapedesis: The movement of a blood leukocyte through a blood vessel wall into the extravascular compartment.

Domain: A region of a peptide having a coherent tertiary structure. Both immunoglobulins and MHC class I and class II molecules have domains.

DTH (delayed type hypersensitivity): This term includes the delayed skin reactions associated with type IV hypersensitivity.

ECP: Eosinophil chemotactic protein released following eosinophil degranulation.

Edema: Tissue swelling due to extravasation of plasma proteins.

EDN: Eosinophil-derived neurotoxin released following eosinophil degranulation.

Eicosanoids: Group name of products derived from 20-carbon fatty acids which includes prostaglandins, leukotrienes, thromboxanes, and lipoxins.

ELAM-1 (E-selectin): Endothelial leukocyte adhesion molecule-1, expressed on vascular endothelial cells, and involved in neutrophil recruitment.

ELISA (enzyme-linked immunosorbent assay): Technique used to quantitate small amounts of material by use of specific monoclonal antibodies.

Endothelium: Cells lining the blood vessels that contract to allow extravasation of plasma proteins and which express endothelial adhesion proteins.

Epitope: A single antigenic determinant. Functionally it is the portion of an antigen that combines with the antibody paratope.

EPO: Eosinophil peroxidase, released following eosinophil degranulation.

Fab: The part of antibody molecule which contains the antigen combining site, consisting of a light chain and part of the heavy chain.

Fc: The portion of antibody that is responsible for binding to antibody receptors on cells and the C1q component of complement.

Flare: The red area of neurogenic origin, surrounding a skin wheal response to allergen, histamine, or like substance.

G-CSF (granulocyte colony-stimulating factor): A cytokine involved in the proliferation and maturation of granulocytes.

Genetic association: A term used to describe the condition where particular gene associations are found with particular diseases.

Genome: The total genetic material contained within the cell.

Genotype: The genetic material inherited from parents; not all of it is necessarily expressed in the individual.

Giant cells: Large multinucleated cells sometimes seen in granulomatous reactions and thought to result from the fusion of macrophages.

GM-CSF (granulocyte–macrophage colony-stimulating factor): A cytokine involved in the proliferation and maturation of granulocytes and macrophages.

G-protein: A guanosine triphosphate-dependent membrane-protein complex that transduces many receptor-dependent events.

Granulocytopoiesis: Production of granulocytes in the bone marrow.

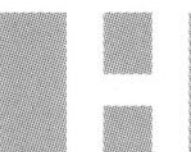

H_1, H_2 and H_3 receptors: Subtypes of the histamine receptor family that transduce the action of histamine.

Haplotype: A set of genetic determinants located on a single chromosome.

Hapten: A small molecule which is incapable of inducing an antibody response by itself but can, when bound to a protein carrier, act as an epitope, e.g. penicilloic acid.

Heavy chain: Larger molecules of the bi-heterodimer that comprises an immunoglobulin. Heavy chains are characteristic for each antibody class. Each heavy chain is composed of constant domains at the C-terminal (Fc end) and variable domains at the N-terminal (Fab end). *See also* light chain.

HETE: Hydroxyeicosatetraenoic acids, lipoxygenase products of arachidonic acid. Often preceded by a number, e.g. 5- or 15-, which identifies individual chemical structures.

Histamine: A major vasoactive amine released from mast cells and basophil granules.

Histocompatibility: The ability to accept grafts between individuals.

HLA: The human major histocompatibility complex.

Humoral: Pertaining to the extracellular fluids, including the serum and lymph.

Hybridoma: Cell line created in vitro by fusing two different cell types of which one is a tumor cell. Lymphocyte hybridomas are usually used for making monoclonal antibodies.

5-Hydroxytryptamine (5-HT, serotonin): A vasoactive amine present in platelets and some rodent, but not human, mast cells.

Hyperreactivity: A state of increased reactivity to a provoking stimulus, e.g. bronchial hyperreactivity in asthma. Specifically, a greater magnitude of response to a given concentration of stimulus.

Hyperresponsiveness: A state of increased responsiveness to a provoking stimulus, e.g. bronchial hyperresponsiveness in asthma. Specifically, the ability to respond, either in magnitude or sensitivity, to a lower concentration of stimulus.

Hypersensitivity: Synonymous with allergy (by usage).

ICAM-1: Intercellular adhesion molecule-1 expressed on endothelial and other cells that interacts with LFA-1 (CD11b/CD18) expressed on leukocytes.

Idiotype: A single antigenic determinant on an antibody V region.

IFNs (interferons): Members of the cytokine family originally associated with resistance to viral infections. IFN_ is now recognized as a pluripotent cytokine, particularly associated with cell-mediated immunity.

ILs (interleukins): Members of the cytokine family which were originally conceived as intercellular messengers between leukocytes but are now perceived as having wider immunologic and inflammatory effects.

Immune complex: An aggregate of antibody and antigen that may induce a hypersensitivity response, often by stimulating the complement cascade.

Immunoblotting: A technique of contact transference of proteins from SDS polyacrylamide gel to nitrocellulose so that they may be identified by monoclonal antibodies.

Immunocytochemistry: A technique used to identify cellular constituents by use of specific monoclonal antibodies.

Immunofluorescence: A technique used to identify particular antigens microscopically in tissues or on cells by the binding of a fluorescent antibody conjugate.

Integrin: A family of cell-adhesion molecules most frequently found on leukocytes, consisting of a common β chain, but different α chains, and involved in leukocyte recruitment.

IPs (inositol phosphates): Intracellular messengers (e.g. inositol 1,4,5-triphosphate) involved in elevation of intracellular calcium from intracellular or extracellular stores.

Isoelectric focusing: Separation of molecules on the basis of charge. Each molecule will migrate to the point in a pH gradient at which it has no net charge.

J chain: A monomorphic polypeptide present in, and required for the polymerization of polymeric IgA and IgM.

Kinins: A group of vasoactive peptides comprising bradykinin, kallidin (lysyl-bradykinin) and des-arg-bradykinin.

Langerhans'cells: Antigen-presenting cells of the skin which emigrate to local lymph nodes to become dendritic cells; they are active in presenting antigen to T cells.

LFAs (leukocyte function antigens): A group of leukocyte adhesion proteins composed of CD11/CD18 heterodimers.

Ligand: A linking or binding molecule usually used to define a specific antigenic determinant to which an antibody binds.

Light chains: Smaller molecules of the biheterodimer that comprises an immunoglobulin. They may be of κ or λ subtypes, regardless of immunoglobulin class. Present only in the Fab end of the immunoglobulin and composed of both variable and constant domains. *See also* heavy chain.

LPs (lipopolysaccharide): A product of some Gram-negative bacterial cell walls that can act as a B-cell mitogen.

LTs (leukotrienes): Members of the eicosanoid family, lipoxygenase products, usually of arachidonic acid, with potent myogenic, cardiovascular, and inflammatory effects.

Lymphokines: A generic term for molecules other than antibodies which are involved in signaling between cells of the immune system and are produced by lymphocytes (cf. interleukins).

MALT (mucosa-associated lymphoid tissue): Generic term for lymphoid tissue associated with the gastrointestinal tract, bronchial tree, and other mucosa.

MBP (major basic protein): A basic arginine-rich protein making up the electron-dense core of the eosinophil granule and which may be released during eosinophil degranulation.

M-CSF (macrophage colony-stimulating factor): A member of the cytokine family, involved in the proliferation and maturation of macrophages.

MC_T and MC_{TC}: Mast cell subtypes defined by their granular content of tryptase (MC_T) and tryptase and chymase (MC_{TC}).

Mediator: A chemical substance released by one cell that stimulates another, e.g. mast cell mediators.

MHC (major histocompatibility complex): A genetic region found in all mammals where products are primarily responsible for the rapid rejection of grafts between individuals, and function in signaling between lymphocytes and cells expressing antigen.

MHC class II: The histocompatibility antigens expressed on cells of the monocyte/macrophage family which present antigen to the T-cell receptor on T lymphocytes.

MIF (migration inhibition factor): A group of peptides produced by lymphocytes that are capable of inhibiting macrophage migration.

Mitogen: A substance that causes cells, particularly lymphocytes, to undergo cell division.

Monoclonal: Derived from a single clone, e.g. monoclonal antibodies, which are produced by a single clone and are homogenous.

Myeloma: A lymphoma produced from cells of the B-cell lineage.

Neuropeptide: Peptides released from nerves following stimulation. The many neuropeptides now recognized include substance P, vasoactive intestinal polypeptide (VIP), neurotensin, and bombesin.

NK (natural killer) cells: A group of lymphocytes that have the intrinsic ability to recognize and destroy some virally infected cells and some tumor cells.

Nude mouse: A genetically athymic mouse which also carries a closely linked gene producing a defect in hair production.

Opsonization: A process by which phagocytosis is facilitated by the deposition of opsonins (e.g. antibody and C2b) on the antigen.

PAF (platelet activating factor): A lipid-derived product generated by many inflammatory cells which activates platelets and induces bronchial hyperresponsiveness.

Paratope: The part of an antibody molecule which makes contact with the antigenic determinant (epitope).

Pathogen: An organism that causes disease.

PCA (passive cutaneous anaphylaxis): The technique used to detect antigen-specific IgE, in which the test animal is injected intravenously with the antigen and dye, the skin having previously been sensitized with antibody.

PGs (prostaglandins): Members of the eicosanoid family cyclooxygenase products usually of arachidonic acid, including PGA_2, PGD_2, PGE_2, and $PGF_{2\alpha}$.

Phagocytosis: The process by which cells engulf material and enclose it within a vacuole (phagosome) in the cytoplasm.

Phagolysosome: A phagosome containing proteolytic enzymes capable of degrading the ingested particles.

Phagosome: An intracellular vacuole containing material ingested by phagocytosis.

Phenotype: The morphologic characteristics of a cell or animal resulting from genetic expression.

Pinocytosis: The process by which liquids or very small particles are taken into the cell.

PK reaction (Prausnitz–Küstner reaction): The passive transfer of allergic responsiveness to an unresponsive recipient by intradermal injection of serum from an allergic donor.

Plasma cell: An antibody-producing B cell that has reached the end of its differentiation pathway.

Polyclonal: A term that describes the products of a number of different cell types (cf. monoclonal).

Primary lymphoid tissues: Lymphoid organs in which lymphocytes complete their initial maturation steps; they include the fetal liver, adult bone marrow and thymus, and the bursa fabricius in birds.

Primary response: The immune response (cellular or humoral) following an initial encounter with a particular antigen. Synonymous with sensitization.

Promyelocyte: A precursor cell of the myelocyte family.

RANTES: Regulated on activation, normal T-cell expressed and secreted.

RAST (radioallergosorbent test): A laboratory technique for the detection of circulating IgE with specific allergen determinants.

Receptor: A specific protein or group of proteins, usually on the cell surface, capable of recognizing and binding a specific ligand.

Respiratory burst: Increase in oxidative metabolism following stimulation of granulocytes, usually by phagocytosis.

RIA (radioimmunoassay): A technique for the laboratory assay of small amounts of materials by competition for antibody binding with known amounts of radioactive substance.

Rosetting: A technique for identifying or isolating cells by mixing them with particles or cells to which they bind (e.g. sheep erythrocytes to human T cells). The rosettes consist of a central cell surrounded by bound cells.

SCF (stem cell factor): A cytokine released by stromal cells that interacts with the *c-kit* receptor on mast cells to stimulate cell maturation and activation.

SDS-PAGE (sodium dodecyl sulfate polyacrylamide gel electrophoresis): A method of separating proteins by gel electrophoresis.

Secondary response: The immune response that follows a second or subsequent encounter with a particular antigen.

Sensitization: The stimulation of allergic antibody production usually by an initial encounter with a specific allergenic substance. Synonymous with primary response.

Serotonin: See 5-hydroxytryptamine.

Skin prick test: The detection of allergen to specific allergens through the production of a wheal-and-flare response by pricking the skin through droplets of allergen or injecting them intradermally.

SLE (systemic lupus erythematosus): An autoimmune disease of humans usually involving antinuclear antibodies.

Substance P: A common neuropeptide that is likely to be involved in the neurogenic spread of the skin flare response.

TCR (T-cell receptor): The T-cell antigen receptor consisting of either α/β dimer (TCR2) or a γ/δ dimer (TCR1) associated with the CD3 molecular complex.

T-dependent/T-independent antigens: T-dependent antigens require immune recognition by both T and B cells to produce an immune response. T-independent antigens can directly stimulate B cells to produce specific antibody.

TGFβ (transforming growth factor β): A cytokine involved in the stimulation of fibroblasts for collagen synthesis.

Th cells (helper T cells): A functional subclass of T cells that can help to generate cytotoxic T cells or cooperate with B cells in production of antibody response. Helper cells recognize antigen in association with class II MHC molecules.

Th1 cells: A subdivision of Th cells involved in cell-mediated immunity and characterized by their production of IFNγ, TNFα, and IL-2.

Th2 cells: A subdivision of Th cells involved in allergy by their influence on B cells to produce IgE and proinflammatory effects. Characterized by their production of IL-3, IL-4, and IL-5.

TNF (tumor necrosis factor): A multifunctional cytokine initially identified for its effects on tumor cells.

Tolerance: A state of specific immunologic unresponsiveness.

Tryptase: The major neutral protease of the mast cell granule found in all human mast cells.

TXA_2 (thromboxane A_2): A member of the cyclooxygenase product family of eicosanoids from arachidonic acid. Synthesized by platelets and other cells, its many actions include platelet aggregation, bronchoconstriction.

VCAM-1 (vascular cell adhesion molecule-1): An adhesion molecule expressed on vascular endothelial cells.

V domains: The variable N-terminal (Fab) domains of antibody heavy and light chains and the α, β, γ, and δ regions of the T-cell receptor that are responsible for antigen recognition.

VLA (very late antigen): A series of integrins expressed on the surface of leukocytes involved in cell recruitment, especially T cells and eosinophils.

Wheal: An area of edema produced at the site of intradermal introduction of allergen, histamine or similar provocant. Stimulation of axon reflexes in the wheal area gives rise to the larger flare response.

Index

NOTE: Page numbers in *italics* refer to figures. *vs* indicates differential diagnosis

A

D

E

F

G

H

I

J

K

L

M

N

O

P

R

S